Reversibility of Chronic Disease and Hypersensitivity, Volume 4
The Environmental Aspects of Chemical Sensitivity

Reversibility of Chronic Disease and Hypersensitivity, Volume 4

The Environmental Aspects of Chemical Sensitivity

William J. Rea, M.D.
Environmental Health Center
Dallas, Texas, USA

Kalpana D. Patel, M.D.
Allergy and Environmental Health Center
Buffalo, New York

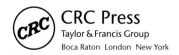

CRC Press
Taylor & Francis Group
Boca Raton London New York

CRC Press is an imprint of the
Taylor & Francis Group, an **informa** business

CRC Press
Taylor & Francis Group
6000 Broken Sound Parkway NW, Suite 300
Boca Raton, FL 33487-2742

First issued in paperback 2022

© 2018 by Taylor & Francis Group, LLC
CRC Press is an imprint of Taylor & Francis Group, an Informa business

No claim to original U.S. Government works

ISBN-13: 978-1-439-81350-8 (hbk)
ISBN-13: 978-1-03-233934-4 (pbk)
DOI: 10.1201/9781315374826

Publisher's Note

The publisher has gone to great lengths to ensure the quality of this reprint but points out that some imperfections in the original copies may be apparent.

Visit the Taylor & Francis Web site at
http://www.taylorandfrancis.com

and the CRC Press Web site at
http://www.crcpress.com

This volume is massive because the new information seals the mechanism of diagnosis and treatment of chemical sensitivity, which now should be classified as a real disease entity. Thus, this volume is dedicated to all the chemically sensitive patients who have suffered from poor determination for their diagnosis and treatment. It is also dedicated to all the physicians and scientists who were much maligned for treating these patients.

Contents

Preface

The clinical aspects of the diagnosis and treatment of chemical sensitivity and chronic degenerative disease presented in this volume are now complete. This volume is for people interested in the origin of the clinical aspects of chemical sensitivity and chronic degenerative disease. The clinical aspects of chemical sensitivity are growing in leaps and bounds and need to be known and considered in every case of chronic degenerative disease.

In treating chronic degenerative disease, healthcare providers must consider every aspect of chemical sensitivity. In this way, they will be able to help more patients obtain health and prevent advanced disease. Also, considering the aspects of chemical sensitivity will help each clinician to direct research for the prevention of advanced irreversible end-stage disease. Modern technology has contributed to the advancement of chemical sensitivity, and it should be brought to bear on the solution of the problem.

Acknowledgments

Thanks to the great environmental clinicians and scientists who based their clinical findings on not only sound observations but also basic scientific facts of anatomy, physiology, and biochemistry. These astute physicians and surgeons include Drs. Theron Randolph, Laurence Dickey, Carlton Lee, Herbert Rinkle, Joseph Miller, Dor Brown, James Willoughby, French Hansel, Ed Binkley, Al Lieberman, Harris Husen, Marshal Mandel, Jean Monro, Sherry Rogers, Jonathan Maberly, Jonathan Wright, Joe Morgan, Klaus Runow, Clive Pyman, Colin Little Richard Travino, John Boyles, Wallace Rubin, Daniel Martinez, Jonathan Brostoff, Phyllis Saifer, Gary Oberg, Satosi Ishikawa and his group, and countless others.

Thanks to Chris Bishop and Dr. Yaqin Pan, whose help in analyzing the data and preparing the manuscript and illustrations was invaluable; their efforts were herculean, and the book could not have been completed without them. Thanks also to Drs. Alfred Johnson, Gerald Ross, Ralph Smiley, Thomas Buckley, Nancy Didriksen, Joel Butler, Ervin Fenyves, John Laseter, and Jon Pangborn, who supplied cases, data, reports, and critiques of what should and should not be done. Additional thanks to Drs. Sherry Rogers, Allan Lieberman, Bertie Griffiths, and Kalpana D. Patel, who proofread and helped compile sections of the book; to the staff at the EHC-Dallas for all of their support; to the members of the American Academy of Environmental Medicine and the Pan American Allergy Society for their contribution to and support of the EHC-Dallas; to the American Environmental Health Foundation, who lent financial support to this effort; to Doris Rapp, Theron Randolph, Lawrence Dickey, John MaClennen, Dor Brown, Carlton Lee, James Willoughby Sr., George Kroker, Jean Monro, Jonathan Maberly, Klaus Runow, Colin Little, Marshall Mandell, Jozef Krop, Hongyu Zhang, Satoshi Ishikawa, Miko Miyata, Joseph Miller, and Ronald Finn for advice and for freely exchanging information.

We are especially indebted to Dr. Jonathan Pangborn, William B. Jakoby, Andrew L. Reeves, Thad Godish, Steve Levine, Alan Levin, Felix Gad Sulman, and Eduardo Gaitan, whose research, books, and papers provided an invaluable foundation for the preparation of this text.

William J. Rea, MD
Kalpana D. Patel, MD

Special Recognition

Special recognition goes to Yaqin Pan, MD, who constructed the tables in this volume, Alexis Plowden who did the majority of the references and editing, and Gladys Morris who did the multiple typings and organization of the book, as well as many of the references.

Authors

William J. Rea, MD, FACS, FAAEM, is a thoracic, cardiovascular, and general surgeon with an added interest in the environmental aspects of health and disease. Founder of the Environmental Health Center—Dallas (EHC-Dallas) in 1974, Dr. Rea is currently the director of this highly specialized Dallas-based medical facility.

Dr. Rea was awarded the Jonathan Forman Gold Medal Award in 1987 for outstanding research in environmental medicine, The Herbert J. Rinkle Award in 1993 for outstanding teaching, and the 1998 Service Award, all by the American Academy of Environmental Medicine. He was named Outstanding Alumnus by Otterbein College in 1991. Other awards include the Mountain Valley Water Hall of Fame in 1987 for research in water and health, the Special Achievement Award by Otterbein College in 1991, the Distinguished Pioneers in Alternative Medicine Award by the Foundation for the Advancement of Innovative Medicine Education Fund in 1994, the Gold Star Award by the International Biographical Center in 1997, Five Hundred Leaders of Influence Award in 1997, Who's Who in the South and Southwest in 1997, The Twentieth Century Award for Achievement in 1997, the Dor W. Brown, Jr., M.D. Lectureship Award by the Pan American Allergy Society, and the O. Spurgeon English Humanitarian Award by Temple University in 2002. He is the author of 10 medical textbooks, and Vol II The Effects of Environmental Pollutants on the Organ System *Chemical Sensitivity (V. 1–4)*, *Reversibility of Chronic Degenerative Disease and Hypersensitivity, V. 1: Regulating Mechanisms of Chemical Sensitivity*, and the coauthor of *Your Home, Your Health and Well-Being*. He also published the popular book on how to build less polluted homes, *Optimum Environments for Optimum Health and Creativity*. Dr. Rea has published more than 150 peer-reviewed research papers related to the topic of thoracic and cardiovascular surgery as well as that of environmental medicine.

Dr. Rea currently serves on the board and is the president of the American Environmental Health Foundation. He is vice president of the American Board of Environmental Medicine and previously served on the board of the American Academy of Environmental Medicine. He previously held the position of chief of surgery at Brookhaven Medical Center and chief of cardiovascular surgery at Dallas Veteran's Hospital, and he is a former president of the American Academy of Environmental Medicine and the Pan American Allergy Society. He has also served on the Science Advisory Board for the U.S. Environmental Protection Agency, on the Research Committee for the American Academy of Otolaryngic Allergy and on the Committee on Aspects of Cardiovascular, Endocrine and Autoimmune Diseases of the American College of Allergists, Committee on Immunotoxicology for the Office of Technology Assessment, and on the panel on Chemical Sensitivity of the National Academy of Sciences. He was previously adjunct professor with the University of Oklahoma Health Science Center, College of Public Health. Dr. Rea is a fellow of the American College of Surgeons, the American Academy of Environmental Medicine, the American College of Allergists, the American College of Preventive Medicine, the American College of Nutrition, and the Royal Society of Medicine.

Born in Jefferson, Ohio and raised in Woodville, Ohio, Dr. Rea graduated from Otterbein College in Westerville, Ohio, and Ohio State University College of Medicine in Columbus, Ohio. He then completed a rotating internship at Parkland Memorial Hospital in Dallas, Texas. He held a general surgery residency from 1963 to 1967 and a cardiovascular surgery fellowship and residency from 1967 to 1969 with The University of Texas Southwestern Medical School system, which includes Parkland Memorial Hospital, Baylor Medical Center, Veteran's Hospital and Children's Medical Center. He was also part of the team that treated Governor Connelly when President Kennedy was assassinated.

From 1969 to 1972, Dr. Rea was an assistant professor of cardiovascular surgery at the University of Texas S.W. Medical School; from 1984 to 1985, Dr. Rea held the position of adjunct professor of environmental sciences and mathematics at the University of Texas; while from 1972 to 1982, he acted as a clinical associate professor of thoracic surgery at The University of Texas Southwestern Medical School. Dr. Rea held the First World Professorial Chair of Environmental Medicine at the

University of Surrey, Guildford, England from 1988 to 1998. He also served as adjunct professor of psychology and guest lecturer at North Texas State University.

Kalpana D. Patel, MD, FAAP, FAAEM, is a pediatrician with an added interest in the environmental aspects of health and disease. Dr. Patel is a founder of the Environmental Health Center-Buffalo (EHC-Buffalo) in 1985, a specialized Buffalo-based medical facility. Dr. Patel was awarded the Jonathan Forman Gold Medal Award in 2006 for outstanding research in environmental medicine and the Herbert J. Rinkle Award in 2008 for outstanding teaching by the American Academy of Environmental Medicine. She was a recipient of the prestigious Hind Ratna award by the NRI organization in India. She is a coauthor of the medical textbooks *Reversibility of Chronic Degenerative Disease and Hypersensitivity, V. 1: Regulating Mechanisms of Chemical Sensitivity*. Dr. Patel has published many peer-reviewed research papers related to the topic of environmental medicine. Dr. Patel currently serves on the board and is the president of the Environmental Health Foundation of New York. She was a president of the American Board of Environmental Medicine and previously served on the board of the American Academy of Environmental Medicine. She previously held the position of Director of Child Health at Department of Health, Erie County and chief of Pediatrics at Deaconess Hospital Buffalo, New York. Dr. Patel is a fellow of the American Academy of Environmental Medicine.

Dr. Patel was born in Pune, India and was raised in Ahmedabad, India. She graduated from St Xavier's College with honors in the state of Gujarat, India, and also with honors from B. J. Medical College, Gujarat University in Ahmedabad, India. She then completed a rotating internship at Bexar County Hospital in San Antonio, Texas. She held a pediatric residency from 1969 to 1972. Dr. Patel is an assistant professor of pediatrics at the State University of New York at Buffalo since 1973.

Martha Stark, MD, a graduate of Harvard Medical School and the Boston Psychoanalytic Institute, is a holistic (adult, adolescent, and child) psychiatrist/psychoanalyst and integrative medicine specialist in private practice in Boston, Massachusetts.

Martha serves as faculty at Harvard Medical School, codirector/faculty at the Center for Psychoanalytic Studies, faculty at Psychiatry Redefined, faculty/scientific advisory board of The Academy of Comprehensive Integrative Medicine, and adjunct faculty at William James College and Smith College School for Social Work, and is former faculty at Boston Psychoanalytic Institute, Massachusetts Institute for Psychoanalysis, Massachusetts Association for Psychoanalytic Psychology, Boston Institute for Psychotherapy, Psychoanalytic Couple and Family Institute of New England, and Three Ripley Street.

Martha is the author of seven critically acclaimed books: *Integrative Psychiatry (Working with Resistance*; *A Primer on Working with Resistance*; *Modes of Therapeutic Action*; *The Transformative Power of Optimal Stress*; *Psychotherapeutic Moments*; *How Does Psychotherapy Work?*; and *Relentless Hope: The Refusal to Grieve)*—award-winning "mandatory reading" at psychoanalytic training institutes and in psychodynamic psychotherapy programs both in the United States and abroad.

Board Certified by the American Association of Integrative Medicine, Martha has contributed chapters to integrative medicine textbooks—including Rattan and Le Bourg's *Hormesis in Health and Disease* and Greenblatt and Brogan's *Integrative Therapies for Depression*—and also articles to peer-reviewed toxicology/environmental medicine journals—including *Critical Reviews in Toxicology*; *Dose-Response: Nonlinearity in Biology, Toxicology, and Medicine*; and *Journal of Nutritional and Environmental Medicine*.

Martha also serves on the editorial/advisory boards of various holistic health publications—including *Alternative Therapies in Health and Medicine*; *Integrative Medicine: A Clinician's Journal*; *Journal of the American Association of Integrative Medicine*; *Advances in Mind-Body Medicine*; *Gavin Journal of Psychiatry and Cognitive Behavior*; and *International Journal of Clinical Toxicology*.

1 Outdoor Emissions

INTRODUCTION

The environmental aspects of health and disease basically involve pollutants delivered to the body through air, foods, and water and how the body deals with it. The evaluation and measurement of these pollutants have become quite complex and the tracing of the metabolites of the detoxification systems is very complex as well. The pollutants enter the body through a rhinocerebral-hypothalamic route, the pulmonary route, skin, Genitourinary (GU), and the Gastrointestinal (GI) tracts. The clinician must know the tools to analyze the pollutants that are measurable and how to apply knowledge to help diagnose and treat each specific patient.

We know that the environment, epigenetics, and specific genetic makeup are the causes of health and diseases. Unfortunately, most of the research into the millions to billions of dollars has been on genetics, which may result in helping about 1% of the health problems. However, at present, more research should be and is being directed to the environment and epigenetics. The single and multiple environmental incitants are the specific triggers of most of the diseases. The incitants can be microbes, biologics, toxic chemicals, Electromagnetic frequency (EMF), and radioactivity. They can overload metabolism and the genetics, causing malfunction and disease.

Clearly, at present, there are over 80,000 chemicals, 500,000 molds, and mycotoxins, pollens, multiple bacteria, viruses, parasites and thousands of particulate matter (PM), and dirty electricity and EMF waves, which make up the total environmental pollutant load. These substances, when entering into the body, combine with the body's nutrition for detoxification, immune system, and genetics, which make up the total body pollutant load. This total body pollutant load usually determines how the body responds. Some specific pollutants such as an organophosphate insecticide, a natural gas stove, lead or mercury, or a mycotoxin or an adverse EMF wave may affect the human body. Other parts of the total environmental pollutant load may be much heavyweight, causing disturbances in the immune system. Both *innate* and the *adaptive* immune systems are involved; T or B lymphocytes, complements, gamma globulin or subsets, autoantibodies, and many other mechanisms can be triggered by the nonspecific or total body pollutant load like enzyme detoxification systems, neurotransmitters, cytokines, membrane changes, etc.

This volume tries to combine and categorize the pollutants entering with the triggering of these systems and many more body mechanisms, which try to maintain normal homeostatic body function in spite of the total environmental pollutant load. At times there is an acute immediate reaction with a hypersensitivity response, and chemical sensitivity develops. At other times, there is a gradual deterioration of the enzyme detoxification systems, nutrients, and immune system, which results in years of oxidative stress (OS) and inflammation, resulting later in not only chemical sensitivity but eventually arteriosclerosis, cancer, or neurovascular degenerative disease. The environmental aspects of each phase of this ill health will be described.

This volume deals with the effects of the individual and complete total load of environmental stressors, which can act as the triggering agents of ill health and disease if the body cannot handle the pollutant load, especially if this combination of pollutants is found in the case of chemical sensitivity. This load includes pollutants in outdoor air, indoor air, food, and water. For most of the individuals, the most contaminated part of their environment is indoor air. However, in some of the great cities of this world like Mexico City (MC), Mexico, and Los Angeles, California, United States, and many more in Asia, the Middle East, and Europe, the outdoor environment is also extremely polluted, triggering much ill health and disease. That is the thrust of this volume.

Outdoor pollutants entering the body must be utilized, catabolized, or parked. Depending on the toxicity and sensitivity, the pollutants can trigger any symptoms and pathology ranging from a slight irritation to acute and chronic responses to death. The modern informed physician will want to stifle pollutant entry and injury to prevent end-stage diseases such as cardiovascular and pulmonary failure, arteriosclerosis, cancer, and neurodegenerative disease.

Manipulation and decrease in pollutant entry, injury, and increase in nutrition with immune manipulation will help the patient live a vigorous life and prevent chemical sensitivity and chronic degenerative disease (CDD).

The big mechanism that is most frequently overlooked is that when a pollutant triggers the body's detoxification mechanisms is that of 1–3 protein kinase which when phosphorylated can trigger a hypersensitivity of up to 1000 times. Often this occurs through the nerves, creating a lot of pain, motor deregulation, and often neurological dysfunction. Some of the therapies are based on treating the hypersensitivity phase. When this is missed, the patient will not get well. The clinician must learn about the newer methods of desensitization.

OUTDOOR POLLUTANTS: POLLENS, DUST, MOLD, HEAT CHANGES, CARBON DIOXIDE

POLLENS

Pollens, dust, and molds are considered to be part of the total environmental pollutant load and will eventually influence the total body load. Pollens are seasonal and depend on where the patient is on Earth and the seasons. These depend upon the season and appear to be common knowledge and will be discussed in Chapter 1 of Vol. 5.

Higher levels of CO_2 and a warming climate are likely to worsen the global burden of allergic disease, which has increased in prevalence in the industrialized world for more than 50 years.[1] Worldwide, between 10% and 30% of the people suffer periodically from allergic rhinitis, and up to 40% are sensitized (by the presence of IgE antibodies and nonimmune triggering to environmental proteins).[1] Warmer temperatures lengthen the pollen season in temperate climates because plants bloom early in the spring. In Texas, in 2014, we have had the worst mountain cedar season ever in January, February, and March. The regular pollen season starts in April giving no break between a severe mountain cedar season and spring pollen season of oak, hackberry, ash, etc. Between 1995 and 2009, the pollen season lengthened 13–27 days above 44° north in the United States.[2] Higher levels of CO_2 in the atmosphere have been found to increase pollen productivity and the allergic potency (relative allergen protein content) of pollen.[3,4] Extreme weather events involving high winds, heavy precipitation, and thunderstorms, which may increase the incidence over midlatitudes due to climate change[5] may also contribute to large and sudden bursts of allergen release.[6,7]

Higher pollen concentrations have been associated with increased prevalence of allergic sensitization[8] and increased healthcare use for allergic disease, measured in terms of over-the-counter allergy medication use,[9] and emergency department (ED) and physician office visits for allergic disease.[10,11] In the future, more potent allergy seasons are likely to be especially detrimental to people with asthma. Experimental studies have found reduced lung function and increased pulmonary inflammation in subjects with asthma, exposed to pollen.[12,13]

Numerous studies in temperate climates have found increases in asthma and wheeze-related ED visits in association with high pollen concentrations.[14–17] Some studies have linked asthma outbreaks to thunderstorms with peaks in allergen release.[6,7,18] There may be adverse synergistic effects of increases in both air pollution and pollen for people with allergy and/or allergic asthma. Higher levels of PM and ozone lower the bronchoconstrictive threshold to environmental allergens such as pollen and increase the subsequent production of IgE and nonallergic hypersensitivity and cytokines, which may promote hypersensitive respiratory disease.[19–22]

Increases in allergen exposure may also result in health effects beyond allergic disease. At least one study identified an increase in cardiovascular and respiratory mortality in association with higher pollen levels, a concerning finding that deserves further scientific investigation.[23] We also see a host of microvascular leisons (see vascular chapter) due to hypersensitivity.

According to Rice et al.,[24] climate change is likely to increase the frequency and intensity of a number of "extreme" weather events, including heat waves, hurricanes and tropical storms, and droughts. These changes have already been reported in recent decades.[5] The 2013 Intergovernmental Panel on Climate Change (IPCC) report projects with 90%–100% certainty that in the heat waves over most of the land areas, there is an increase in the intensity and frequency of heavy precipitation over midlatitudes and wet tropical areas, and an increase in the frequency and/or magnitude of extremely high sea levels (which may result in floods). The confidence levels for an increase in drought on a regional to global scale (66%–100%) and increased tropical cyclone activity (>50%–100%) in the late-twenty-first century are lower.[5]

Heat waves have well-documented adverse health effects. It is therefore highly concerning that climate models project almost 50% increase in the frequency of the hottest (i.e., the top fifth percentile based on historical records) days by midcentury.[25,26] Extreme heat increases all-cause mortality. The heat wave that hit Western Europe in August 2003 resulted in an excess of 15,000 deaths in France alone.[27] Studies have found that the elderly and those with chronic respiratory or cardiovascular disease are particularly susceptible to heat-related death.[28,29] Some of these deaths are due to a "harvesting effect," or short-term mortality displacement, wherein people who would have died within 1–2 months die a few weeks earlier. However, only 30%–40% of the estimated deaths from recent heat waves in the United States have been attributed to a harvesting effect, and the remainder constitutes actual life-years lost.[30] A study of the 2003 heat wave mortality in France found no evidence of harvesting.[27] As average temperatures increase, populations will adjust to a higher temperature range, but they will continue to be vulnerable at temperature extremes.[31]

Extreme heat events are associated with exacerbations of respiratory and cardiovascular disease. Hot, humid days trigger asthma symptoms and have shown to increase airway resistance, most likely by stimulating airway C-fiber nerves.[32,33] Studies in the United States have associated acute increases in temperature and humidity with increased ED visits and hospitalizations for asthma in children[34] and adults.[35] A case-crossover study in England and Wales examining hourly temperature and incidence of myocardial infarction found that higher ambient temperatures above a threshold of 20°C were associated with an increased risk of myocardial infarction 1–6 hours after exposure.[36] There is also evidence that extreme heat may trigger exacerbations of congestive heart failure.[37]

Warming temperatures cause an intensification of the water cycle that increases the frequency of both droughts and floods and promotes storm formation. Hot temperatures increase the rate of evaporation of moisture in the soil, resulting in droughts. Warmer air also holds more moisture, leading to heavier precipitation and floods. Additionally, high sea surface temperatures increase wind velocities, which promotes storms. Tropical storms will only form in the presence of warm ocean waters of at least 26.5°C to a minimum depth of 50 m.[38] The melting of sea ice and a rising sea level also increase the vulnerability of coastal areas to storm surges. The IPCC projects a rise in the sea level of 0.3–0.8 m by 2100 compared with 1986 to 2005 levels and a rise in sea surface temperatures by up to 2°C.[5]

Although extreme weather events such as droughts, floods, and storms are low-probability events, the human health costs of any one event can be catastrophic. In 2011, in the United States, there were 14 weather-related disasters costing more than $1 billion in damages, which was a national record.[39] Hurricane Katrina killed more than 1300 people and displaced approximately 30,000 persons.[40] Though the United States ranks first among the world's nations in terms of the frequency of coastal hurricanes, there are many regions of the world that are much less equipped to manage these natural disasters and suffer greater loss of life.[38] In 1999, for example, 30,000 people died as a result of storms followed by floods and landslides in Venezuela.[41] South Asia and Latin America have been identified as the most vulnerable areas to floods and tropical cyclones in terms of the human death toll and number of people affected.[42] Studies of recent storms have identified drowning and severe injuries as the most common cause of death.[42] The decreased sanitation and crowding after storms and floods promote the spread of infectious respiratory disease, and damage to the health-care infrastructure, including disruption of electricity to clinics, hospitals, and intensive care units, impairs virtually every dimension of public health.[38]

Desertification and droughts are a major public health concerns for arid climates. Malnutrition is one of the top global health challenges, and climate change further threatens the ability of low-resource areas to maintain adequate food production. The World Health Organization (WHO) ranked malnutrition as the largest global health problem associated with climate change.[43] The risk of drought-related health effects depends on the severity of the drought and resources to mitigate impacts of the drought.[44] Sub-Saharan Africa and South Asia, where food supplies are already limited are anticipated to have the largest reductions in food supply as a result of climate change.[45] A large proportion of global deaths from pneumonia in children under the age of 5 years is attributed to malnutrition,[46] and pediatric pneumonia deaths in low-resource arid climates may rise as a result of an increasing frequency of droughts.

Molds and terpenes are also large problems in outdoor air pollution. They are so large that separate chapters are dedicated to them (see Chapter 1, Vol. 5 on molds and Chapter 8, Vol. 4 on terpenes.

Carbon Dioxide

According to Rice et al.,[24] as early as in 1896, it was found that carbon dioxide in the Earth's atmosphere causes an imbalance between infrared light-transmitting and absorbing properties and an increased black carbon-radiation effect in the atmosphere that elevates the temperature at the surface and in the lower atmosphere or surface.[47] Human activities that burn fossil fuels release additional CO_2 into the atmospheres. CO_2 levels have risen dramatically since industrialization and continue to rise at alarming rates. The 2013 IPCC report concluded that CO_2 concentrations have risen by 40% since preindustrial times, primarily due to fossil fuel emissions, and periodically have reached levels "unprecedented in the onset of the last 800,000."[5] Other human activities release other greenhouse gases with similar effects, including methane, nitrous oxide, and sulfur dioxide, in addition to naturally occurring ozone and water vapor.

Particulate *black carbon* is released from fossil fuel, biomass, and forest burning and directly absorbs solar radiation, which warms surface temperatures, and also deposits on snow and ice, which reduces the reflectivity and further contributes to global warming. Over 200 tons of Hg is released each year with melting of the polar ice caps.[48]

There is no dispute among climate scientists that the Earth's climate system is warming. Figure 1.1 shows globally averaged surface and ocean temperatures since 1850 (relative to 1961–1990 levels) and illustrates the global warming trend since the 1950s. The 2013 IPCC report concluded that

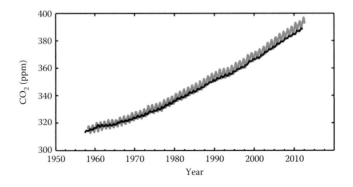

FIGURE 1.1   Atmospheric CO_2 from Mauna Loa, Hawaii (light) and South Pole (black) since 1958.

global warming is "unequivocal" and that with 95%–100% certainty, the observed warming since the 1950s is primarily due to human activity.[5] Global temperatures rose 0.6–0.7°C from 1951 to 2010, of which 0.5–1.3°C is attributed to greenhouse gases, −0.6°C to 0.1°C from other human emissions including the cooling effect of aerosols, −0.1°C to 0.1°C from natural forcings, and −0.1°C to 0.1°C from internal variability.[5]

According to Rice et al.,[24] disruption of the global climate promotes extreme weather patterns (as shown in Chapter 2) that effect human health. These include heat waves, droughts, thunderstorms and heavier precipitation, and hurricanes and tropical cyclones. Secondary consequences of these changes include worsening air quality (due to high temperatures, forest fires, and dust storms), floods, and desertification.

Black Carbon PM

The primary outdoor air pollutants associated with environmental changes that are of particular relevance to health are black carbon, ozone, carbon monoxide, sulfur dioxide, nitrogen dioxide, pesticides, herbicides, and PM.

Black carbon is released from fossil fuel combustion (including diesel, coal, and gas fuel), cooking with biomass fuels (which is widespread in the developing world), and the burning of forest and crop residue for agricultural purposes. Black carbon has been identified as an important climate-forcing emission along with CO_2[48] and has climate-forcing effects that last for decades (compared with centuries for CO_2). In addition to its effects on climate, black carbon is an air pollutant (a constituent of fine PM) with well-described respiratory and cardiovascular health effects at increased concentrations, including worsening of preexisting cardiovascular disease with neurological dysfunction,[49] worsening lung and brain function[50] and increases in chronic obstructive pulmonary disease (COPD) hospitalization and mortality[51] and cardiovascular neurological mortality.[52] Household air pollution, consisting of black carbon smoke from indoor cooking particularly in the developing world, has been ranked as the third largest contributor to the global burden of disease, largely because of its associations with childhood respiratory infections, COPD in women, and cardiovascular disease in men.[53] Natural gas stoves are the number one offender along with pesticides in the home (Randolph, T. G. 1985, personal communication) of the chemically sensitive. Mold and mycotoxins are also a growing problem, while pesticides, herbicides, and fumigants are other major problems. EMF waves are now the absconding pollutant that wreaks havoc on the individual.

The following section will briefly review the major outdoor air pollutants which are detailed throughout the book. Many human and natural activities produce more than one class of pollutants. The final part of this section will briefly discuss standards for common outdoor air pollutants as well as pollutant sources for other major problems.

Microbial Organisms

There is an ongoing debate about the potential role of the airway microbiome for the development of asthma and also other respiratory and cardiovascular diseases. A number of studies have shown that the bronchoalveolar lavage fluid and induced sputum of patients with asthma is primarily colonized with γ-proteobacteria, that is, *Haemophilus influenzae, Moraxella catarrhalis*, and *Streptococcus pneumoniae*.[54–56] These cross-sectional studies do not allow, however, outcoming of the primary cause. The question is does asthma result in distant airway colonization in the presence and the absence of inhaled steroids, or is a certain airway microbiome causally related to disease onset? Only prospective studies can address these questions, by assessing the airway microbiota before the development of asthma occurs. The Copenhagen Prospective Studies on Asthma in Childhood (COPSAC) birth cohort has collected all necessary data, and the investigators have shown that colonization of the hypopharynx with *H. influenzae, M. catarrhalis*, and *S. pneumoniae* at age of 4 weeks preceded the onset of childhood asthma, thereby suggesting a causal role.[57] However, pollutant entry was not assessed and probably may well be the initial cause that lets these bacteria colonize.

Vissing and colleagues[58] from the COPSAC cohort report that colonization with *H. influenzae*, *M. catarrhalis*, and *S. pneumoniae* is a risk for the subsequent occurrence of severe pulmonary infections (pneumonia and bronchiolitis) up to age of 3 years.[56] One might argue that this finding is expected, as pneumonia and bronchiolitis may precede asthma development. However, the association between colonization with these bacteria and severe pulmonary infections was only seen among children not developing asthma; therefore, there may be a protective effect of this bacterial invasion.

This inverse interaction implies that the association of bacterial colonization with asthma is more pronounced in children without pulmonary infections. In other words, this bacterial colonization associates with either asthma or pulmonary infections, which is partially in conflict with the earlier unstratified analysis.[57] Furthermore, the interaction implies that the presence or the absence of colonization with *H. influenzae*, *M. catarrhalis*, and *S. pneumoniae* determines the strength of the association between asthma and pulmonary infections. The resulting complex pattern of interactions brings into question the specificity and thereby predictive power of such colonization.

The idea of unspecific colonization is furthermore supported by another finding from the COPSAC cohort: The incriminated bacteria were detected not just in an asymptomatic state at 4 weeks of age but also during manifest episodes of wheezing and clinical pneumonia, respectively.[59] Interestingly, there was again, no difference between the detection rate of these and other bacteria (and also viruses) between episodes of wheezing and pneumonia. This lack of specificity may be attributable to difficulties in clinically distinguishing episodes of asthma and pneumonia in young children, although the COPSAC team made every effort to carefully differentiate between various combinations of symptoms. Hypersensitivity to these and other (air pollutants) bacteria, virus, foods, and chemicals was not considered. Therefore, if the underlying etiology may have been missed for any of these, it can cause immune deregulation and at times immune suppression.

As a result of recent advances in high-throughput sequencing and the formation of microbiome consortia, the previous dichotomy of pathogens and commensals currently yields a more coevolutionary perspective of host–microbiome interactions. Within the Lung HIV Microbiome Project[60] and other investigations,[56,61] a pulmonary core microbiome of healthy individuals has been proposed. This contains, among others, the genera *Streptococcus*, *Haemophilus*, and *Pseudomonas*, the latter belongs to the same order as *M. catarrhalis*. In this light, the detection of *S. pneumoniae*, *H. influenzae*, and *M. catarrhalis* might reveal not causal pathogens for asthma or severe pulmonary infections, but merely the local airway microbiome that introduces or stabilizes immunity. These complex relations may not be understood unless one or more underlying environmental (NO_2, pesticides, traffic) or genetic factor(s) are identified. A candidate genetic factor might be found in the chromosome 17 loci, as it has recently been reported to interact with asthma and rhinovirus-triggered wheezy illness in the COPSAC cohort.[62] If the chromosome 17 loci were additionally associated with pneumonia, then the true underlying association with this gene locus might be the pattern of microbial colonization. The environmental factors may be legion but the odds are that the pollutants that the patient is surrounded by are usually the underlying culprits like SO_2, NO_2, ozone, CO, particulate, mycotoxins, pesticides, natural gas, EMF, etc.

The authors have furthermore shown in the COPSAC 2010 cohort that *M. catarrhalis* and *H. influenzae*, but not *S. pneumoniae*, colonization was associated with an inflammatory immune response of the nasal mucosal lining fluid at age of 4 weeks.[63] Whether colonization results in inflammation or inflammation leads to particular colonization remains unanswerable in such a cross-sectional analysis. It is, however, conceivable and now known that any type of pollutant exposure can lower local and general resistance, thus allowing a trigger for the inflammation.

VIRUS

These are covered well in the modern medicine and will not be discussed but as part of the total body pollutant load and must be considered daily.

ENDOTOXIN

According to Matsui et al.,[64] the effect of endotoxin on asthma morbidity in urban populations is unclear. Their objectives were to determine if indoor pollutant exposure modifies the relationships between indoor airborne endotoxin and asthma health and morbidity.

According to Matsui et al.,[64] 146 children and adolescents with persistent asthma underwent repeated clinical assessments at 0, 3, 6, 9, and 12 months. Home visits were conducted at the same time points for assessment of airborne nicotine, endotoxin, and nitrogen dioxide (NO_2) concentrations. The effect of concomitant pollutant exposure on relationships between endotoxin and asthma outcomes was examined in stratified analyses and statistical models with interaction terms.

Both air nicotine and NO_2 concentrations modified the relationships between airborne endotoxin and asthma outcomes. Among children living in homes with no detectable air nicotine, higher endotoxin was inversely associated with acute visits and oral corticosteroid bursts, whereas among those in homes with detectable air nicotine, endotoxin was positively associated with these outcomes (interaction p-value = 0.004 and 0.07, respectively). Among children living in homes with lower NO_2 concentrations (<20 ppb), higher endotoxin was positively associated with acute visits, whereas among those living in homes with higher NO_2 concentrations, endotoxin was negatively associated with acute visit (interaction p-value = 0.05). NO_2 also modified the effect of endotoxin on asthma symptom outcomes in a similar manner, showing that pollutant exposure and total body pollutant load must be considered in evaluation of this and other problems.

In conclusion, the effects of household airborne endotoxin exposure on asthma are modified by coexposure to air nicotine and NO_2, and these pollutants have opposite effects on the relationships between endotoxin and asthma-related outcomes.

Each of the sources of contamination in Table 1.1 will be briefly discussed.

TABLE 1.1

Major Sources of Chemical Air Pollution[a] Affecting the Individual with Chemical Sensitivity

1. Transportation—autos, buses—i.e., Mexico City, Sao Paulo, Los Angeles, Beijing, Delhi, Jakarta
2. Fuel combustion and emanation in stationary sources, refineries, factories, power plants, oil, and fracking of gas fields.
3. Industrial processes (zinc, nickel, electronics)
4. Forest fires and grass fires
5. Solid waste disposal
6. Chemical dumps—United States—60,000
7. Aerial spraying of farms—United States, Mexico, Canada
8. Volcanoes—United States
9. Oil spills—Gulf of Mexico, Alaska, etc.
10. Dust storm (Africa and Gobi dusts)
11. Nuclear explosions—Fukashima, Chernobyl
12. The Gulf War sensitized many troops and civilians
13. Lyme diseases has infected many individuals around the United States and contributed to immune deregulation
14. The greatest environment conformation has come from the electromagnetic generators of electricity, radio, TV, computers, Wi-Fi, smart meters, mobile phones, and towers

Source: Environmental Health Center-Dallas. Modified from Chemical Sensitivity, Volume II, page 641, table 3. With permission.

[a] Listed from highest to lowest emission, 1–14.

MAJOR TYPES AND SOURCES OF OUTDOOR
AIR POLLUTION: TRANSPORTATION

The greatest exposure to air toxic pollution that increases the total body pollutant load occurs in large urban areas where there is excess traffic such as Los Angeles, California, United States[65]; MC, Mexico[65]; Sao Paulo, Brazil[65]; Beijing and Shanghai, China[65]; Delhi and Bombay, India; Karachi, Pakistan; Cairo, Egypt; Jakarta, Indonesia[65]; Denver, Colorado, United States[65]; and areas where there is year-round aerial spraying of insecticides in the surrounding countryside, such as in the Rio Grande Valley in Texas, the Fresno Valley in California,[66] and the Bitter Root Valley in Idaho. Electromagnetic pollution sources include radio, TV, power line, Wi-Fi, and smart meters, which are being prolifically placed at a rapid rate around the world.

It is evident that traffic-related air pollution affects human health. These effects comprise negative health outcomes in many aspects, including reduced lung function in children,[67] increased susceptibility to airway infections,[68] inducing OS and airway inflammation, with olfactory, neurological, brain dysfunction, as well as important cardiovascular endpoints, such as increased risk for myocardial infarction and cardiovascular disease mortality.[69–72,923,924] These adverse effects can have a considerable variety of manifestations depending on the type of exposure, including airway inflammation,[73,74] arrhythmias,[75] and reduced lung function.[76]

Based on extensive epidemiological evidence, the association between air pollution, primarily of traffic-related origin, and cardiorespiratory morbidity and mortality is well established. There are likely multiple complex and interdependent mechanistic pathways that link air pollution to cardiorespiratory disease. Presently, there is growing evidence that pulmonary and systemic OS and inflammation play important roles. However, within the concept of epidemiological studies, it is not possible to address causality (i.e., what individual parts of the complex air pollution mixture that impact disease). Neither are epidemiological studies able to disentangle the individual effects of specific pollutants within the multifaceted ambient air pollution mix, with a good environmental control unit to sift out individual and a mixture of air pollutants. Here, randomized experimental human exposure studies have certain advantages; however, there are also shortcomings. As suggested by Van Hee and Pope,[77] studies using an experimental design may be ideal for understanding mechanisms of air pollution-induced cardiac and pulmonary disease in humans. Such studies are nevertheless of limited importance when it comes to who can be exposed as well as the duration and intensity of exposure, given several practical and ethical concerns. Studies in the environmental control unit are most important for defining specific environmental incitants and the use of their symptoms and signs. Experimental studies are favored, as they can use exposure to a single air pollutant at the time, yet, as stated above, they are not suitable to address long-term effects of air pollution in humans.

Ozone

The ozone molecule contains three oxygen atoms (O_3) instead of the usual two oxygen atoms (O_2). In the stratosphere, ozone plays a vital role in blocking out harmful ultraviolet light from the sun, but at the ground level, ozone is toxic to humans. Ozone can be produced by a number of processes such as lightning,[78] electronic devices like photocopiers,[79] and by atmospheric reactions of transportation involving volatile organic chemicals, nitrogen oxides, and sunlight; this indirect ozone production is most efficient during warm weather.[79]

According to Rice et al.,[24] ozone formation increases on sunny, cloudless days and at higher temperatures.[80] The frequency and intensity of ozone episodes during summer months are projected to increase as a result of rising temperatures[81,82] and excess transportation vehicles. Some recent heat waves have been associated with ozone levels that exceeded air quality standards.[83]

Short-term elevations in ozone have been associated with increases in all-cause mortality in relatively polluted Latin American cities[84] and in less-polluted cities in Western Europe and North

America.[85] The deadly heat wave of 2003 in Europe was associated with high levels of ozone that are believed to have contributed to excess mortality in addition to the mortality caused by the heat itself.[83,925] Ozone has also been found to exacerbate preexisting respiratory diseases in both children and adults. Because ozone is a respiratory irritant that causes bronchial inflammation and hyper-responsiveness,[19,86] people with preexisting obstructive lung disease are particularly susceptible to some adverse respiratory effects of ozone. A substantial body of evidence has shown that modest short-term increase in ground-level ozone increases risk of acute care visits and hospitalization for asthma[87–90] and COPD.[91,92] Ozone exposure has been associated with deterioration in asthma control in studies in the United States and Europe, resulting in increased medication use and missed school and work days.[93–95] There is emerging evidence that obesity may increase susceptibility to respiratory effects of ozone exposure, which is concerning given the increasing prevalence of obesity in many parts of the world.[96,97]

Like particulates, ozone can travel for thousands of kilometers. The atmospheric half-life of ozone is 1–2 weeks in summer and 1–2 months in winter.[98]

Table 1.2 shows the people at risk in the 25 most ozone polluted cities in the United States. It shows that traffic-generated ozone causes problems and those where wind currents are minimal or air inversions are frequent.

Table 1.3 shows the 25 top ozone counties in the United States. Most are heavily populated areas or areas where the wind currents are not available enough to sweep ozone out.

Table 1.4 shows the cleanest outdoor air counties. These counties though shill have moderate population centers have winds that will sweep ozone out.

Table 1.5 shows the cleanest cities for air outdoor as air pollution. These have both less population and winds that will help clear ozone.

Ozone: Inhalation of Reactive Oxygen Species

As stated earlier, ozone is a major component of photochemical smog and is derived from multiple sources, including automobile exhaust. While ozone is not a radical, it is a reactive oxygen species and powerful inhaled oxidizing agent. Once in the lung or olfactory area, ozone interacts with proteins and lipids to create modified proteins/lipids, carbon/oxygen-centered radicals, and toxic compounds.[99] For example, breakdown products from the interaction of ozone with lipids produce ozonides and cytotoxic aldehyde by-products, which have been implicated in the extrapulmonary like the brain and cardiovascular systems effects of ozone.[99,100] As a consequence, ozone is well known to activate pulmonary macrophages recruit neutrophils to the lung, and is linked to OS, airway inflammation, and dysfunction of innate immunity in the lung.[101]

However, ozone is also associated with CNS effects. Recent studies with animal models have shown that OS induced by acute or chronic ozone exposure can lead to brain lipid peroxidation,[102,103] dopaminergic neuron death in the substantia nigra,[104] neuronal morphological damage,[104] motor deficits,[103,105] and memory deficits.[106] Further, prenatal exposure to ozone has been shown to alter neurotransmitter expression in adult rats,[107] suggesting there may be a developmental impact on CNS development. In addition, some ozone effects are associated with the cerebral vasculature. For example, ozone exposure in adult rats was shown to cause cytokine production in the brain, where it enhances IL-6 and TNF-α expression which was localized to astrocytes close to capillary walls.[108] In addition, ozone exposure upregulated the expression of vascular endothelial growth factor in rat brains, which was believed to be a compensatory and beneficial response.[108] Thus, there is increasing experimental evidence that ozone causes neuroinflammation, lipid peroxidation in the brain, neuron damage, memory deficits, and motor deficits. We see this inflammatory phenomena in the ozone exposed chemically sensitive patient. Elimination often leads to the subsiding of the chemical sensitivity and reexposure yields an exacerbation of the chemical sensitivity. These fluctuations of chemical sensitivity not only occurs with alterations of ozone but many of the other outdoor pollutants like sulfur dioxide (SO_2), carbon monoxide (CO), nitrous oxide (NO_2) pesticides, and volatile organic chemicals as well.

TABLE 1.2

People at Risk in 25 Most Ozone-Polluted Cities

2013 Rank[a]	Metropolitan Statistical Areas	Total Population[b]	Under 18[c]	65 and Over[c]	Pediatric Asthma[d,e]	Adult Asthma[e,f]	COPD[g]	CV Disease[h]	Poverty[i]
1	Los Angeles–Long Beach–Riverside, CA	18,081,569	4,542,151	2,021,451	325,187	1,139,030	587,808	3,983,369	3,038,607
2	Visalia–Porterville, CA	449,253	145,232	431,010	10,398	25,559	13,074	86,663	113,766
3	Bakersfield–Delano, CA	851,710	254,658	77,793	18,232	50,187	25,296	167,656	200,571
4	Fresno–Madera, CA	1,095,829	321,487	114,718	23,016	65,120	33,800	224,505	272,942
5	Hanford–Corcoran, CA	153,765	42,382	12,366	3034	9354	4504	29,646	27,949
6	Sacramento–Arden–Arcade–Yuba City, CA-NV	2,489,230	606,325	319,042	43,295	158,254	88,544	586,151	386,342
7	Houston–Baytown–Huntsville, TX	6,191,434	1,708,164	552,120	137,217	33,104	237,213	1,462,793	1,056,710
8	Dallas–Fort Worth, TX	6,853,425	1,881,791	648,640	151,163	369,858	286,821	1,640,113	1,052,759
9	Washington–Baltimore–Northern Virginia, DC-MD-VA-WV	8,670,607	2,025,927	964,445	191,397	577,502	385,948	2,191,845	808,337
10	El Centro, CA	177,057	50,986	18,749	3650	10,603	5513	36,633	43,259
11	Merced, CA	259,898	80,991	25,034	5798	15,039	7658	50,722	68,371
11	San Diego-Carlsbad-San Marcos, CA	3,140,069	726,602	362,928	52,020	203,011	106,254	707,051	462,997
13	Modesto, CA	518,522	146,498	56,563	10,488	31,303	16,547	110,394	119,325
14	Birmingham-Hoover-Cullman, AL	1,212,800	287,870	162,832	30,184	73,803	89,406	393,595	200,725
14	Cincinnati–Middletown–Wilmington, OH-KY-IN	2,179,965	537,575	270,708	52,080	163,904	132,373	590,680	307,286
16	Las Vegas–Paradise–Pahrump, NV	2,013,326	497,829	241,449	29,400	122,240	109,798	497,456	333,690
17	Louisville, Jefferson County-Elizabethtown–Scottsburg KY-IN	1,440,607	343,686	185,720	29,991	113,046	105,848	438,810	215,950

(*Continued*)

TABLE 1.2 (*Continued*)
People at Risk in 25 Most Ozone-Polluted Cities

2013 Rank[a]	Metropolitan Statistical Areas	Total Population[b]	Under 18[c]	65 and Over[c]	Pediatric Asthma[d,e]	Adult Asthma[e,f]	COPD[g]	CV Disease[h]	Poverty[i]
17	New York–Newark–Bridgeport, NY-NJ-CT-PA	22,214,083	5,027,088	2,963,886	472,117	1,634,531	973,420	5,601,883	3,056,701
19	Charlotte–Gastonia–Salisbury, NC-SC	2,442,564	614,338	280,468	52,534	160,312	124,668	630,498	388,999
20	Beaumont–Port Arthur, TX	390,535	95,311	51,293	7656	22,226	17,372	105,287	67,523
20	Oklahoma City–Shawnee, OK	1,348,333	335,791	162,124	31,610	97,487	84,284	374,335	216,926
20	Philadelphia–Camden–Vineland, PA-NJ-DE-MD	6,562,287	1,513,270	886,837	145,153	461,724	305,296	1,699,047	867,174
23	Phoenix–Mesa–Glendale, AZ	4,263,236	1,107,303	540,544	93,175	302,805	166,853	963,671	727,056
24	Pittsburgh–New Castle, PSA	2,450,281	487,427	424,058	48,891	175,676	134,681	705,328	304,860
25	St. Louis, St. Charles-Farmington, MO-IL	2,907,732	682,579	395,222	52,616	198,808	171,525	814,289	394,418
25	Tulsa–Bartlesville, OK	998,438	251,983	133,087	23,720	71,733	64,452	286,681	147,999

Source: American Lung Association, 2009.

a Cities are ranked using the highest weighted average for any county within that combined or metropolitan statistical area.

b Total population represents the at-risk populations for all counties within the respective combined or metropolitan statistical area.

c Those under 18 and 65 years and over are vulnerable to $PM_{2.5}$ and are therefore included. They should not be used as population denominators for disease estimates.

d Pediatric asthma estimates are for those under 18 years of age and represent the estimated number of people who had asthma in 2011 based on state rates (BRFSS) applied to population estimates (U.S. Census).

e Adding across rows does not produce valid estimates, for example, summing pediatric and adult asthma.

f Adult asthma estimates are for those 18 years and older and represent the estimated number of people who had asthma in 2011 based on state rates (BRFSS) applied to population estimates (U.S. Census).

g COPD estimates are for adults 18 years and over who have been diagnosed within their lifetime, based on state rates (BRFSS) applied to population estimates (U.S. Census).

h CVD disease is cardiovascular disease and estimates are for adults 18 years and over who have been diagnosed within their lifetime based on state rates (BRFSS) applied to population estimates (U.S. Census).

i Poverty estimates come from the U.S. Census Bureau and are for all ages.

Because ozone is reactive with a short half-life, it is unlikely to physically reach the brain but molecules derived from ozone and lung tissue interactions can. These have been proposed to mediate nonpulmonary ozone effects.[109,110] However, the specific signals from the lung to the brain responsible for CNS pathology are unknown. While one hypothesis is that radical species generated in the lung enter the blood and transfer to the brain,[109] this seems unlikely due to the reactivity and again,

TABLE 1.3

People at Risk in 25 Most Ozone-Polluted Counties

2013 Rank[a]	County	ST	Total Population[b]	Under 18[c]	65 and Over[c]	Pediatric Asthma[d,e]	Adult Asthma[d,e]	COPD[f]	CV Disease[g]	Poverty[h]	Weighted Average[i]	Grade[i]
											High Ozone Days in Unhealthy Ranges 2009–2011	
								At Risk Groups				
1	San Bernardino	CA	2,065,377	593,206	188,958	42,470	123,780	62,735	416,898	391,911	121.5	F
2	Riverside	CA	2,239,620	623,094	268,723	44,609	136,046	73,244	488,747	371,930	102.2	F
3	Tulare	CA	449,253	145,232	43,101	10,398	25,559	13,075	86,663	113,766	87.5	F
4	Los Angeles	CA	9,889,056	2,378,370	1,099,904	170,275	631,724	328,847	2,187,906	1,788,681	81.8	F
5	Kern	CA	851,710	254,658	77,793	18,232	50,187	25,926	167,656	200,571	78.3	F
6	Fresno	CA	942,904	278,349	96,955	19,928	55,881	28,859	191,544	238,977	58.3	F
7	Kings	CA	153,765	42,382	12,366	3034	9354	4504	29,656	27,949	36.2	F
8	Sacramento	CA	1,436,105	362,155	164,643	25,928	90,380	48,063	321,109	250,842	35.3	F
9	Unitah	UT	33,163	11,005	3021	743	1950	905	5755	3845	27.8	F
10	Harris	TX	4,180,894	1,165,484	350,212	93,623	222,920	155,592	959,756	803,895	27.3	F
11	Tarrant	TX	1,849,815	515,160	160,223	41,383	99,250	71,169	438,244	307,362	23.7	F
12	El Dorado	CA	180,938	40,081	27,785	2870	11,395	7173	49,004	18,496	21.0	F
13	Harford	MD	246,489	59,086	31,665	5444	15,763	11,356	65,860	20,309	20.3	F
14	Placer	CA	357,138	85,6332	56,457	6131	22,901	13,526	91,482	29,985	19.7	F
15	Madera	CA	152,925	43,138	17,763	3088	9239	4941	32,961	33,965	18.0	F
16	Denton	TX	686,406	187,155	50,520	15,034	36,863	25,093	156,026	62,240	17.3	F
17	Imperial	CA	177,057	50,986	18,749	3650	10,603	5513	36,633	43,259	16.3	F
18	San Diego	CA	3,140,069	726,602	362,928	52,020	203,011	106,254	707,051	462,997	16.2	F
18	Merced	CA	259,898	80,991	25,034	5798	15,039	7658	50,722	68,371	16.2	F
20	Ventura	CA	831,771	210,361	100,114	15,060	52,329	28,516	191,413	94,625	15.3	F
20	Stanislaus	CA	518,522	146,498	56,563	10,488	31,303	16,547	110,394	119,325	15.3	F
20	Brazoria	TX	319,973	88,132	31,569	7080	17,332	12,720	78,226	37,492	15.3	F
23	Dallas	TX	2,416,014	666,960	215,670	53,577	129,337	91,285	56,864	475,446	13.3	F
24	Jefferson	AL	658,931	154,664	87,341	16,217	40,237	48,459	213,021	120,760	12.8	F
24	Hamilton	OH	800,362	187,735	106,776	18,778	60,469	46,5646	214,359	144,388	12.8	F

Source: American Lung Association, 2009.

a   Counties are ranked by weighted average.

b   Total population represents the at-risk populations in counties with PM₂₅ monitors.

c   Those under 18 and 65 years and over are vulnerable to PM2.5 and are therefore included. They should not be used as population denominators for disease estimates.

d   Pediatric asthma estimates are for those under 18 years of age and represent the estimated number of people who had asthma in 2011 based on state rates (BRFSS) applied to population estimates (U.S. Census).

e   Adding across rows does not produce valid estimates, for example, summing pediatric and adult asthma.

f   Adult asthma estimates are for those 18 years and older and represent the estimated number of people who had asthma in 2011 based on state rates (BRFSS) applied to population estimates (U.S. Census).

f   COPD estimates are for adults 18 years and over who have been diagnosed within their lifetime, based on state rates (BRFSS) applied to population estimates (U.S. Census).

g   CVD disease is cardiovascular disease and estimates are for adults 18 years and over who have been diagnosed within their lifetime based on state rates (BRFSS) applied to population estimates (U.S. Census).

h   Poverty estimates come from the U.S. Census Bureau and are for all ages.

TABLE 1.4
Cleanest Counties for Ozone Air Pollution

County	State	Metropolitan Statistical Area	County	State	Metropolitan Statistical Area	County	State	Metropolitan Statistical Area
Yukon–Koyukuk Census Area	AK		Lee	FL	Cape Coral-Fort Myers, FL	Winnebago	IL	Rockford-Freeport-Rochelle, IL
Colbert	AL	Florence–Muscle Shoals, AL	Leon	FL	Tallahassee, FL	Delaware	IN	Muncie, IN
Elmore	AL	Montgomery–Alexander City, AL	Pasco	FL	Tampa-St. Petersburg–Clearwater, FL	Huntington	IN	Fort Wayne–Huntington–Auburn, IN
Etowah	AL	Gadsden, AL	St. Lucie	FL	Port St. Lucie-Sebastian-Vero Beach, FL	Madison	IN	Indianapolis-Anderson-Columbus, IN
Houston	AL	Dothan–Enterprise–Ozark, AL	Volusia	FL	Orlando–Deltona–Daytona Beach, FL	Wyandotte	KSA	Kansas City–Overland Park–Kansas City, MO-KS
Morgan	AL	Huntsville–Decatur, AL	Chatham	GA	Savannah–Hinesville–Fort Stewart, GA	Bell	KY	
Tuscaloosa	AL	Tuscaloosa, AL	Chattooga	GA		Carter	KY	
Neston	AR		Coweta	GA	Atlanta Sandy Springs-Gainesville, GA-AL	Hardin	KY	Louisville–Jefferson County–Elizabethtown–Scottsburg, KY-IN
Navajo	AZ		Glynn	GA	Brunswick, GA	Perry	KY	
Glenn	CA		Sumter	GA		Pike	KY	
Humboldt	CA		Honolulu	HI	Honolulu, HI	Pulaski	KY	
Lake	CA		Bremer	IA	Waterloo-Cedar Falls, IA	Warren	KY	Bowling Green, KY
Marin	CA	San Jose–San Francisco–Oakland, CA	Clinton	IA		Ouachita Parish	LA	Monroe–Bastrop, LA
Mendocino	CA		Linn	IA	Cedar Rapids, IA	Androscoggin	ME	Portland–Lewiston–South Portland, ME

(Continued)

TABLE 1.4 (*Continued*)
Cleanest Counties for Ozone Air Pollution

County	State	Metropolitan Statistical Area	County	State	Metropolitan Statistical Area	County	State	Metropolitan Statistical Area
San Francisco	CA	San Jose–San Francisco–Oakland, CA						
Santa Cruz	CA	San Jose–San Francisco–Oakland, CA	Montgomery	IA		Aroostook	ME	
Siskiyou	CA		Palo Alto	IA		Oxford	ME	
Sonoma	CA	San Jose–San Francisco–Oakland, CA	Polk	IA	Des Moines–Newton–Pella, IA	Sagadahoc	ME	Portland–Lewiston–South Portland, ME
Garfield	CO		Scott	IA	Davenport–Moline–Rock Island, IA-IL	Becker	MN	
Mesa	CO	Grand Junction, CO	Story	IA	Ames-Boone-IA	Carlton	MN	Duluth, MN-WI
Alachua	FL	Gainesville, FL	Van Buren	IA		Goodhue	MN	Minneapolis–St. Paul–St. Cloud, MN-WI
Baker	FL	Jacksonville, FL	Warren	IA	Des Moines-Newton-Pella, IA	Lake	MN	
			Butte	ID		Lyon	MN	
Brevard	FL	Palm Bay-Melbourne-Titusville, FL	Kootenal	ID	Coeur d'Alene, ID	Mille Lacs	MN	
Broward	FL	Miami–Fort Lauderdale–Pompano Beach, FL	Clark	IL		Olmsted	MN	Rochester, MN
Collier	FL	Naples–Marco Island, FL	Effingham	IL		Scott	MN	Minneapolis–St. Paul–St. Cloud, MN-WI
Columbia	FL		Randolph	IL		St. Louis	MN	Duluth, MN-WI
Highlands	FL		Rock Island	IL	Davenport-Moline-Rock Island, IA-IL			
Holmes	FL							

Note: This list represents countries with no monitored ozone air pollution in unhealthful ranges using the Air Quality Index based on 2008 NAAGS.

TABLE 1.5

Cleanest U.S. Cities for Ozone Air Pollution

Metropolitan Statistical Area	Population	Metropolitan Statistical Area	Population
Ames–Boone, IA	115,918	La Crosse, WI-MN	134,488
Bellingham, WA	203,663	Laredo, TX	256,496
Bend–Prineville, OR	181,177	Lincoln, NE	306,503
Bismarck, ND	110,879	Logan, UT-ID	127,549
Brownsville–Harlingen–Raymondville, TX	436,218	Madison–Baraboo, WI	638,757
Brunswick, GA	112,923	McAllen–Edinburg-Pharr, TX	797,810
Burlington–South Burlington, VT	212,535	Medford, OR	204,822
Cape Coral–Fort Myers, FL	631,330	Monroe–Bastrop, LA	205,259
Cedar Rapids, IA	260,575	Muncie, IN	117,660
Charleston–North Charleston–Summerville, SC	682,121	Naples–Marco Island, FL	328,134
Palm Bay–Melbourne–Claremont–Lebanon, NH-VT	218,057	Titusville, FL	543,566
Coeur d'Alene, ID	141,132	Port St. Lucie–Sebastian–	
Columbia, MO	175,831	Vero Beach, FL	566,768
Davenport–Moline–Rock Island, IA-IL	381,342	Rapid City, SD	128,361
Des Moines–Newton–Pella, IA	650,137	Rochester, MN	187,162
Dothan–Enterprise–Ozark, AL	247,132	Rochester-Batavia-Seneca Falls, NY	1,150,469
Duluth, MN-WI	279,815	Rockford–Freeport–Rochelle, IL	449,038
Eugene–Springfield, OR	353,416	Santa Fe-Espanola, NM	186,094
Fargo–Wahpeton, ND-MN	235,008	Savannah–Hinesville–Fort Stewart, GA	436,163
Florence–Muscle Shoals, AL	147,293	Sioux City–Vermillion, IA-NE-SD	158,113
Gadsden, AL	104,303	Sioux Falls, SD	232,433
Gainesville, FL	266,369	Spokane, WA	473,761
Grand Junction, CO	147,083	Tuscaloosa, AL	221,553
Honolulu, HI	963,607	Utica Rome, NY	298,447
Janesville, WI	160,092	Waterloo–Cedar Falls, IA	168,289
		Wausau–Merrill, WI	163,002

Source: American Lung Association, 2009.

Note: This list represents cities with no monitored ozone air pollution in unhealthful ranges using the Air Quality Index based on the 2008 ozone NAAGS.

the consequent short half-life of the radicals. Alternatively, aldehyde ozone–lipid by-products,[109] ozone-modified soluble proteins,[109] activated circulating monocytes, or cytokines from the proinflammatory lung response (systemic inflammation) could exert harmful CNS effects. Interestingly, systemic TNF-α administration[111] causes lipid peroxidation in the brain and TNF-α is elevated in brains of animals exposed to ozone,[108] supporting that a cytokine could link a peripheral response to brain lipid peroxidation, a noted effect of ozone administration in animals. However, animal studies have shown that low levels of ozone exposure have failed to result in a systemic inflammatory response.[112] Further, ozone administration has been used as a treatment to attenuate pain in humans[113] and animals[114] with varying results, suggesting that the concentration and duration of ozone exposure may determine the nature of the effects. Another avenue would be up the sensitized olfactory nerve going to the hypothalamus. (See hypothalamic-rhino inflammation and prefrontal cortex—Chapter 4, Vol. 5.)

CARBON MONOXIDE

Carbon monoxide (CO) is a product of incomplete combustion. Its main sources are combustion processes from vehicles, heating, coal-fired power generation, and biomass burning.[78] Carbon monoxide is produced in larger amounts if combustion is not efficient (i.e., a poorly tuned engine), in colder weather or at high altitudes.[79] Carbon monoxide has an atmospheric half-life of 1–2 months and can also travel for thousands of kilometers away from its source[98] just as ozone can.

Carbon monoxide (CO) is a colorless, nonirritating, odorless, and tasteless gas ubiquitous in the atmosphere. It is a primary pollutant mainly from the incomplete combustion of fossil fuels and biomass. Toxic effects of CO are mainly caused by its ability to bind to heme and alter the function and metabolism of heme proteins. The formation of carboxyhemoglobin decreases the O_2 from hemoglobin for its use in tissues.

In the outdoor environment, the major sources of carbon monoxide are petroleum and coal combustion from transportation and industry. Carbon monoxide may accumulate to dangerous levels when certain weather conditions are present in specific locations on Earth (see Chapter 4). Due to its location adjacent to the eastern side of the Rocky Mountains and due to cold winter weather conditions with inversion, both of which combine to inhibit dispersion of pollutants, Denver, for example, is known for its high incidence of air pollution due to carbon monoxide. The major indoor sources of carbon monoxide are unvented kerosene heaters, gas stoves, gas appliances, and cigarette smoking.

The well-known, acute effects of CO include cardiac effects (angina, ventricular arrhythmia), pulmonary effects (edema), visual effects (decreased light sensitivity, dark adaptation, tunnel vision), auditory effects (central hearing loss), neuropsychiatric effects (seizures, agitation, coma, thermoregulation), dermatologic effects (bullae, alopecia, sweat gland necrosis), and metabolic effects (lactic acidosis, myonecrosis, hyperglycemia, proteinuria). Chronic effects involve the heart (decreased voltage, premature ventricular contractions, conduction block, lower defibrillatory threshold), neuropsychiatric functions (decreased cognitive ability, psychosis, parkinsonism, incontinence), and hematologic function (increased HB and HCT, increased erythroprotein, increased reticulocyte count, and disseminated intravascular coagulation). Such diffuse effects of carbon monoxide on the general population are inevitably intensified in the chemically sensitive, making this population particularly vulnerable to carbon monoxide at any concentration. These effects are due to the adverse responses seen in the enzyme detoxification systems that are already malfunctioning in the chemically sensitive.

CO inhibits the cytochrome oxidase system (e.g., cytochrome A_3, cytochrome P-450) by binding to hemoproteins. It also inhibits most of the oxidation, degradation, and conjugation reactions. Therefore, its intake into the body, even in low levels, may adversely affect detoxification systems and allow for the accumulation of toxic substances that are usually eliminated by these systems. For the already vulnerable chemically sensitive, this physiological response to exposure to carbon monoxide results in exacerbation of signs and symptoms of their illness.[115] The current exposure threshold limit value for healthy people is 9 ppm for 8 hours and 35 ppm for 1 hour. No safe exposure threshold has been established for 7 days/week, 24 hours/day for people who are already damaged by disease or other toxic exposures. For the chemically sensitive, none of these levels apply since these appear to be little safe levels.

However, recent studies suggested that exogenous CO at lower concentrations may have beneficial anti-inflammatory effects under certain circumstances.[116–118] This does not seem true in the chemically sensitive patient. Current toxicologic and epidemiologic research has focused on examining health effects of low-level CO exposures (50 ppm and less) that did not result in overt CO poisoning.[119,120] Findings of earlier epidemiologic studies were mixed.[119,121]

Only a few recent population-based investigations have been conducted to specifically examine the health effects of environmentally relevant CO exposure,[122,123] and there was significant heterogeneity in the effect estimates among cities. Heterogeneity in mortality effects of exposure to CO were reported for four Chinese cities of different development levels; CO was associated with an increased risk of mortality in the megacity of Guangzhou, whereas in a smaller city of Zhongshan, a 0.5-ppm increase of CO was associated with a 3.5% and 2.4% decrease in cardiovascular and total mortality, respectively.[123] Protective effect of CO on daily mortality was also indicated in a study of 10 U.S. cities: 1-ppm increase of CO was associated with a 0.7% decrease in daily mortality.[124]

Currently, Hong Kong outdoor CO levels are low and well below the WHO guideline of 10 mg/m^3 (8.7 ppm) since it is a windswept island. In 2010, the highest 8-hour average concentration of CO was 3.0 ppm in Hong Kong. CO emission in Hong Kong arises mainly from gasoline-powered automobiles, although this source has declined significantly over the past several decades because of the use of catalytic converters and other emission control devices on modern passenger vehicles.[125]

Despite the measured low concentrations of CO, the intake fraction, which is the fraction of total emissions that is inhaled by a receptor population, can be high because of the city's high population density and traffic density. The intake fraction of CO in Hong Kong was estimated to be 270 ppm per emission, much higher than that previously reported for vehicle emissions in U.S. urban areas, Helsinki, and Beijing.[126] Hong Kong is one of the world's most densely populated cities. It has a small land area of 1100 km^2, of which 21% has been developed as an urban area. The land population density was 6620 per km^2 in 2012, whereas the district with the highest population density is Kwantung, with 56,200 per km^2.[127] Hong Kong's road density is also among the highest in the world at 254 vehicles per kilometer of road.[128]

The antimicrobial effects of CO have been extensively reviewed in the literature[129–133] but there are no population-based data on the effects of CO on infectious diseases. They conducted a time series study to estimate the association between short-term exposure to outdoor CO and risk of respiratory tract infection (RTI) hospitalizations in Hong Kong.

Table 1.6 provides descriptive statistics on pollution, weather, and hospitalization data. CO concentrations were low during the study period with a daily average of 0.6 pmp in background stations and 1.0 pmp in roadside stations, compared with the WHO 8-hour air quality guideline for

TABLE 1.6

Summary Statistics of Pollution, Weather, and Health Data for Hong Kong during 2001–2007

Variables	Days	Mean	SD	Min	25%	50%	75%	Max
Background Pollution								
CO, ppm	2.554	0.6	0.2	0.1	0.5	0.6	0.8	1.9
PM$_{10}$, µg/m^3	2545	52.1	27.3	13.2	29.1	46.7	70.4	144.2
NO$_2$, µg/m^3	2549	42.5	17.1	5.0	30.2	41.1	52.5	129.2
Roadside Pollution								
CO, ppm	2553	1.0	0.3	0.4	0.8	1.0	1.2	1.9
PM$_{10}$, µg/m^3	2553	74.4	24.7	24.1	54.5	70.5	91.4	144.7
NO$_2$, µg/m^3	2535	95.3	26.5	30.7	72.4	96.2	114.9	159.5
Weather								
Temperature, °C	2556	23.6	4.9	8.2	19.6	24.9	27.7	31.8
Humidity, %	2556	78.3	9.9	31.3	73.5	79.3	84.9	98.1
RTI Admissions								
Children, <15	2556	43	17	4	32	42	53	122
Adults, 15–64	2556	16	6	2	12	16	20	50
Elderly, >65	2556	52	28	8	26	52	70	154
All	2556	111	39	24	86	112	132	250

Source: Tian, L. et al. 2013. Ambient carbon monoxide associated with reduced risk of hospital admissions for respiratory tract infections. *American Journal of Respiratory and Critical Care Medicine.* 188(10): November 15, 2013.

Definition of abbreviations: CO = carbon monoxide, NO$_2$ = nitrogen dioxide; PM$_{10}$ = particulate matter with aerodynamic diameter <10 µm; RTI = respiratory tract infection.

CO: 8.7 pmp. From January 1, 2001 to December 31, 2007, a total of 284,622 hospital admissions through accident and emergency were recorded from RTI, which had daily admissions of 111 on average.

Table 1.7 shows the percentage change in total emergency hospital admissions for RTI per unit increase in the concentrations of CO, NO_2, and PM_{10} at lag 0, 1, 2, and 02 days in single-pollutant and two-pollutant models. Both NO_2 and PM_{10} were associated with increased risks of RTI hospitalizations. The effect estimates for CO, however, were negative for all three single-day lags, and the lag 1 day CO was associated with the largest RTI risk reduction, respectively. Similar results were generated by using roadside CO monitoring data. Sensitivity analysis found that the effect estimates of CO were largely robust to the degree of adjustment for seasonality and trend, model specifications for weather variables, the lag of CO exposure, CO monitoring station coverage, and the usage of other CO measurement (1-hour maximum). The results from these *a priori* models were also comparable with those from case-crossover analyses and those GAM models chosen by minimizing the partial autocorrelation function of residuals.

This was the first population-based study to demonstrate the negative correlation between ambient CO and hospital admissions for RTI. After adjustment for NO_2 and PM_{10}, the negative associations of CO with RTI became stronger. Stronger effect estimates were observed for the adults than for the children and the elderly.

Because the primary CO source in cities is traffic, they considered confounding by other traffic-related pollutants: NO_2 and PM_{10}. After adjustment for NO_2 and PM_{10}, the negative associations of CO with RTI became stronger. Many of the earlier epidemiologic studies showing the adverse effects of CO did not adjust for the confounding effect of copollutants. In the studies that did evaluate multipollutant models, positive associations between CO concentrations and respiratory outcomes did not persist when adjusted for NO_2 and PM_{10}.[134–136] As reviewed in a recent U.S. Environmental Protection Agency (EPA) report, although there is clear evidence of ambient CO being associated with ischemic heart diseases and other cardiovascular outcomes, few studies found associations

TABLE 1.7

Percentage Change (Excess Risk % with 95% Confidence Interval) in Total Emergency Hospital Admissions for Respiratory Tract Infection per Unit Increase in the Concentrations of CO, NO_2, and PM_{10} at Lag 0, 1, 2, and 02 days in Single-Pollutant and Two-Pollutant Models[a]

CO Monitor	Days of Lag	CO Only	NO_2 Only	PM_{10} Only	CO Adjusted for NO_2	CO Adjusted for PM_{10}
Background	0	−3.2 (−6 to −0.4)	0.9 (0.5–1.3)	0.6 (0.4–09)	−7.7 (−10.7 to −4.7)	−7.6 (−10.6 to −4.6)
	1	−3.8 (−6.6 to 0.9)	0.9 (0.5–1.3)	0.7 (0.5–1.0)	−8.3 (−11.2 to −5.2)	−8.9 (−11.8 to −5.9)
	2	−3 (−5.8 to −0.1)	0.9 (0.5–1.2)	0.7 (0.5–1.0)	−6.7 (−9.6 to 3.6)	−7.9 (−10.7 to −4.9)
	02	−5.7 (−9.2 to −2.1)	1.6 (1–2.1)	1.0 (0.7–1.4)	−12 (15.5 to −8.3)	−11.7 (−15.3 to −8.1)
Roadside	0	−2.2 (−4.9 to 0.6)	0.9 (0.6–1.2)	0.7 (0.4–0.9)	−7.9 (−10.8 to −4.9)	−6.5 (−9.4 to −3.5)
	1	−3.5 (−6.2–0.8)	0.9 (9.6–1.2)	0.7 (0.4–0.9)	−9.6 (−12.4 to −6.8)	−8.2 (−11 to −5.3)
	2	−1.7 (04.4–1.1)	0.8 (0.6–1.1)	9.6 (0.4–0.9)	−6.7 (−9.6 to −3.8)	−6.1 (−8.9 to −3.2)
	02	−5.1 (−8.5 to −1.6)	1.3 (0.9–1.6)	1.0 (0.6–1.3)	−12.8 (16.3 to −9.2)	−11.4 (−15 to 7.7)

Source: Tian, L. et al. 2013. Ambient carbon monoxide associated with reduced risk of hospital admissions for respiratory tract infections. *American Journal of Respiratory and Critical Care Medicine.* 188(10): November 15, 2013.

[a] Effects of CO were estimated for a parts per million increase of CO concentrations; effects of NO_2 and PM_{10} were estimated for 10 µg/m³ increase of NO_2 or PM_{10} concentrations.

Definition of abbreviations: CO = carbon monoxide; NO_2 = nitrogen dioxide; PM_{10} = particulate matter with aerodynamic diameter <10 µm.

between CO and respiratory outcomes that persisted after accounting for other air pollutants.[119] Even with the cardiovascular outcomes, the positive association of CO with hospital admissions was attenuated with the adjustment of traffic-related pollutants, particularly NO_2,[137] the estimated increase in cardiovascular mortality associated with CO was reduced by 47% (using 8 df per year approach) after adjustment for NO_2.[122]

The negative association between CO and RTI hospitalizations seemed to be stronger in the adults than in the children and the elderly. As the largest subpopulation, adults experience about 60% of the overall intake fraction for motor vehicle emissions in Hong Kong.[124]

The short-term protective effects of ambient CO against RTI are biologically plausible. The antimicrobial effects have been extensively reviewed in the literature.[129–133] Exogenous administration of CO, by coreleasing molecules, were able to kill bacteria.[129] Inhaled CO resulted in preservation of organ function and improved survival of rodents previously treated with endotoxin.[116,138] CO enhances the phagocytosis of *Escherichia coli* p38-mediated expression of toll-like receptor (TLR) 4 on the surface RAW 264.7 murine macrophages.[139] Heme oxygenase-derived CO improved microbial sepsis because heme oxygenase-1-deficient mice were more vulnerable to polymicrobial infections; exogenous CO prevented the sepsis-induced death of the heme oxygenase-1-deficient mice.[140] Water-soluble CO releaser (CO-releasing molecules-3) decreased bacterial counts in the spleen and increased survival in immunocompetent and immunosuppressed mice after *Pseudomonas aeruginosa* bacteremia.[141] It was proposed that increased CO levels can augment and heighten the inflammatory response in common infections, initially to clear the microbe followed by a rapid resolution of the inflammatory response.[131] The anti-inflammatory activity of CO may have a further protective effect against viral infections, such as hepatitis, influenza, and possibly HIV.[130]

Moreover, the effect of prolonged CO exposure on RTI is unknown. In the current time series study, they examined only the effects of ambient CO on emergency admissions of RTI, but did not analyze the effects on scheduled outpatient clinic visits. The current study design only allows us to infer about the acute effects but not the long-term effects, which needs to be examined by experimental studies or epidemiologic designs such as cohort or case–control studies. Indeed, contrast has been observed for the acute and chronic effects of CO on the cardiac system. Although acute exposure to low CO levels is considered beneficial and cardioprotective, prolonged exposure seems deleterious for cardiovascular health.[120]

Further research is needed to evaluate the overall health effects of exposure to low environmental CO levels.

In conclusion, they found low environmental CO to be associated with reduced risk of daily RTI hospitalizations.

Carbon monoxide (CO) exposure at high concentrations is recognized in both the lay and medical communities as the cause of a toxic syndrome manifested by neurologic and cardiac side effects that can lead to death. Exposure to carbon monoxide in controlled settings at low concentrations, however, is increasingly identified as a possible mediator of the inflammatory response to injury, with potentially beneficial effects. In preclinical models, carbon monoxide has been shown to inhibit cell death,[142,143] as well as to exhibit anti-inflammatory properties,[138] among other protective effects. Low-dose inhaled carbon monoxide in animal models has been associated with prolonged survival and protection from ventilator-associated lung injury in rodents.[144] In addition, anti-inflammatory properties have been observed after administration of inhaled CO to humans with COPD.[145]

Defining the safe and effective dose and duration of CO exposure in humans presents one of the challenges to development of CO as a novel therapy at this early stage. Moreover, parsing the benefits of CO exposure at low concentrations from the potential toxicities at higher concentrations is an area of interest not only in the context of clinical trials but also in the setting of environmental health.

This effect may relate to CO's anti-inflammatory properties; for example, CO has been shown in animal models to decrease inflammation in the setting of LPS administration[146] and to attenuate early neutrophil recruitment in the setting of acid aspiration.[147] Interestingly, the authors report that environmental CO concentrations in their study were low, with daily averages ranging from 0.6

to 1.0 ppm. Despite this low exposure, the authors saw a statistically significant decrease in RTI rates with each incremental increase of 1 ppm in CO concentration. As the authors point out, these exposure levels are much lower than those administered in preclinical studies and human clinical trials, but occurred continuously. In addition, individuals' exposures may actually have been higher depending upon their proximity to tall buildings or the concentration of motor vehicles in the vicinity.

In addition, the authors report that the observed decrease in RTI rates was more marked in adults, as compared with children and the elderly. This could be explained, as outlined in the manuscript, with the higher intake fraction of adults in this community.

Alternatively, children and the elderly may be more susceptible to toxicities at these exposure rates, which could account for a higher RTI prevalence in these groups. Thus, measured CO concentration must be put in context of potential modifying factors, such as duration of exposure susceptibility of the host, and the environmental conditions in which exposure occurs, when assessing the potential beneficial effects of such exposure, particularly in an environmental setting.

The authors acknowledge the challenges that they experienced in establishing the true definition of exposure in this context. Because the monitoring stations in Hong Kong were clustered, and potentially not fully representative of all of the factors contributing to the levels of contact with CO in different areas, they may not have been representative of the varying exposures across the general population. This is particularly important as personal CO exposure is mostly influenced by microenvironmental levels, and the association with outdoor monitors is weak, with a correlation ranging from a median of 0.19–0.30.[148,149]

SULFURS

Sulfur dioxide emissions have lessened in the United States since antipollution devices have been placed on cars; the emissions that continue are a result of a massive increase in motor vehicles on the roadways coupled with excessive emissions from sulfur-containing sour (sulfur) gas fields and refineries, and coal-burning areas, and these emissions create problems (Figure 1.2).

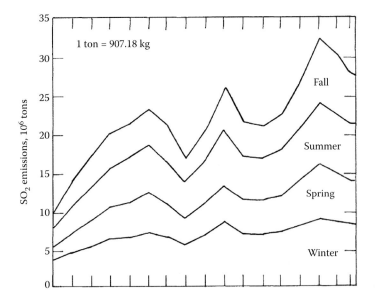

FIGURE 1.2   Overall trend in SO_2 emissions from 1900 to 1980 for the United States and by fuel type for each study year. (From Gschwandtner, G. et al. 1986. Historic emissions of sulfur and nitrogen oxides in the U.S. from 1900 to 1980. *J.A.P.C.A.* 36(2):139–149. With permission.)

TABLE 1.8
SO_2 Emissions around the World

Rank	Country	Rank	Country
#1	Belgium	#8	Germany
#2	Korea, South	#9	Slovakia
#3	Jamaica	#10	Bulgaria
#4	Czech Republic	#11	Chile
#5	Korea, North	#12	Netherlands
#6	Kuwait	#13	Egypt
#7	United Kingdom		

Source: Nation Master, Environment > SO2 emissions per populated area: http://www.nationmaster.com/country-info/stats/Environment/ SO2-emissions-per-populated-area, Ian Graham.

Acid rain, for instance, can be caused by sulfur dioxide emissions. Approximately, 15% of outdoor air pollutants are made up of sulfur dioxide. Background sulfur dioxide is 1 ppb. Maximum hourly concentrations in cities are from 1.5 to 2.3 ppm.

Hydrogen sulfide has a background of 0.05 ppb. It has a "rotten egg" odor. Natural sources are decaying organic matter, natural hot springs, and volcanoes, all of which account globally for 100×10^2 tons. Man-made sources are oil and gas extraction, petroleum refining, paper mills, rayon manufacturing, and coke ovens, which taken together account for 3×10^6 tons.[150] Carbon disulfides also emanate from the latter sources and cause adverse health effects. Most chemically sensitive people react adversely to any kind of sulfur exposure because their sulfur detoxification systems are easily overloaded. For more information, see Chapter 4 on inorganics (Table 1.8).

Nitrogen Compounds

Many nitrogen compounds are known to harm the chemically sensitive. A few of the most common that can easily contribute to the total body pollutant load and thus increase chemical sensitivity are discussed in the following pages. Some of these compounds have been seen to induce chemical sensitivity. Most are detoxified by similar detoxification mechanisms; thus, their effects on the chemically sensitive may be cumulative.

The nitrous oxides, nitrogen dioxide, and nitric oxide are discussed together since they may occur together and may be converted to each other. All can adversely affect the chemically sensitive.

The major sources of nitrogen dioxide (NO_2) in outdoor air are coal and oil combustion, gas-fired transportation, and nitrogen fertilizers. For indoor air, these pollutants are generated in kerosene heaters, gas stoves, gas heaters, and arc welding. Nitric oxide (NO) and nitrous oxide (N_2O) are quickly converted to nitrogen dioxide at concentrations below 50 ppm. Therefore, high concentrations of NO may occur with low levels of NO_2, and as their levels drop, nitrogen dioxide appears. The main health effect of NO is that it forms methemoglobin and subsequently acts on the nervous system. Also in humans, it can be generated naturally and can create a toxic substance peroxynitrite. Animal experimentation indicates that NO is about one-fifth as toxic as NO_2 (assuming minimal contamination with NO_x and no synergistic action, which may be quite unrealistic). Again, it should be emphasized that the data are limited, and levels may need to be much less due to synergisms and increased total load. (For more data, see Chapter 2.)

Emissions of nitrous oxides occur when there is heavy traffic in the city or that occur in farm country as a result of extensive fertilization with nitrogen fertilizers pose air pollution problems. Nitrous oxides are also a product of anaerobic bacteria. These oxides can evaporate, form clouds, and yield acid rain. When oxides are exposed to sunlight, they become one of the prime sources of ozone generation. (For more information, see Chapter 4.) Chemically sensitive patients do poorly in areas of high nitrous oxide pollution, as their detoxification systems become overloaded by pollutant exposure (Tables 1.9 through 1.11).

TABLE 1.9
NO_2 Emissions by Country

Rank	Country	Rank	Country
#1	Libya	#8	Germany
#2	United Arab Emirates	#9	Iceland
#3	Belgium	#10	Netherlands
#4	United Kingdom	#11	Japan
#5	Botswana	#12	Cambodia
#6	Egypt	#13	United States
#7	Namibia		

Source: Data from List of countries by greenhouse gas emissions, https://en.wikipedia.org/wiki/List_of_countries_by_greenhouse_gas_emissions.

TABLE 1.10
Urban NO_2 Concentrations around the World

Rank	Country	Rank	Country
#1	Mexico	#12	Egypt
#2	Italy	#13	Poland
#3	Bulgaria	#14	Israel
#4	United Arab Emirates	#15	Libya
#5	Benin	#16	Denmark
#6	Paraguay	#17	Austria
#7	Saudi Arabia	#18	Canada
#8	Chile	#19	Jordan
#9	Ghana	#21	China
#10	Turkmenistan	#22	Hungary
#11	Zambia	#37	United States

Source: Data from Scientists relate urban population to air pollution, https://www.sciencedaily.com/releases/2013/08/130819185352.htm, *Science Daily*.

TABLE 1.11
CO Emissions by Countries

Rank	Country	Rank	Country
#1	United States	#6	Germany
#2	China	#7	United Kingdom
#3	Russia	#8	Canada
#4	Japan	#9	Italy
#5	India	#10	Mexico

Source: Data from Boden, T., B. Andres, G. Marland. National CO_2 emissions from fossil-fuel burning, *Cement Manufacture, and Gas Flaring*: 1751–2011.

Studies Supporting Outdoor Pollutant Damage

As a compromise, the use of "quasi-experimental" studies has been developed (i.e., that mechanistic inferences are allowed during long-term exposure under "real-world" conditions). Given the considerable decrease in ambient air pollution concentrations during the 2008 Beijing Olympics, this gave unique possibilities to use this study concept.

A study by Rich and colleagues[70] also used a quasi-experimental approach to study young healthy adults. They aimed to investigate whether markers related to pathophysiological pathways of cardiovascular disease were sensitive to changes in air pollution and focused on biomarkers for systemic inflammation and thrombosis along with measuring heart rate and blood pressure (BP). Similar to the study of Huang and coworkers,[69] they reported substantial decrease in concentrations of particulate and gaseous pollutants by −13% to −60% between the pre- and during-Olympics periods, whereas ozone concentrations increased by 24%. The findings of the present study include statistically significant decreases in sCD62P and von Willebrand factor, implying the importance of thrombosis–endothelial dysfunction mechanism, along with statistically non-significant decreases in sCD40L, heart rate, and BP between pre- and during-Olympics periods. Although the reductions in von Willebrand factor and sCD62P were detected in healthy young subjects, where the findings are of uncertain clinical significance, these data may be particularly important when considering the increased air pollution-related cardiovascular health risks in an elderly population.

In another study investigating acute respiratory inflammation in relation to the 2008 Beijing Olympics, Lin and coauthors[71] recruited healthy schoolchildren and schoolchildren with asthma. They conducted a 2-year panel study covering the periods before and during the Olympics, using eNO as a biomarker for acute respiratory inflammation, along with on-site monitoring of hourly mean ambient air concentrations of black smoke (bc), $PM_{2.5}$, CO, SO_2, and NO_2. They observed a wide range of pollutant exposures, especially for bc and $PM_{2.5}$, although with 0–24-hour concentrations 4 versus 70% lower during the Olympic period. eNO concentrations varied considerably from 1.3 to 71.5 ppb, but the concentration of eNO decreased by about 27% during the Olympics compared with the other time periods. It was found that bc averaged over 0–48 hours had the strongest association with eNO. Taken together, the findings from this study suggest that the decrease in air pollution during the Olympics was rapidly followed by a decrease in respiratory inflammation in children, measured as eNO. In addition, the authors showed a robust association between ambient bc and acute airway inflammation based on an almost linear exposure–response relationship on a wide range of measured bc concentration. This was the fact, even though bc accounted for only 3% of the total $PM_{2.5}$ mass, suggesting that traffic-related air pollution is of importance in this case, and also that other combustion constituents may play a role.

Finally, in a study with a similar quasi-experimental design but without direction relation to the Olympics, Langrish and colleagues[151] investigated the benefits of reducing personal exposure to urban air pollution in almost 100 patients with coronary heart disease. These patients walked along a predefined route in Central Beijing, either with or without a highly efficient face mask. Personal air pollution exposure was determined using monitoring equipment, and symptoms and cardiovascular endpoints were observed throughout a 24-hour study period. It was shown that the urban air pollution was dominated by traffic-derived fine and ultrafine PM (UFPM), contained OC and polycyclic aromatic hydrocarbons (PAHs), and was highly oxidizing. The face mask reduced the personal PM exposure from 89 $\mu g/m^3$ to ~2 $\mu g/m^3$ and was associated with a decrease in self-reported symptoms and a reduction of maximal ST segment depression. Furthermore, mean arterial pressure was lower, and heart rate variability (HRV) increased. In summary, this study shows that reducing personal exposure to air pollution by means of a highly efficient face mask appeared to reduce symptoms and improve a range of cardiovascular health outcomes in patients with coronary heart disease. This suggests the potential to reduce the incidence of cardiovascular events in highly susceptible populations.

Based on more than 1900 children in the Swedish birth cohort BAMSE, Schultz and coworkers[67] addressed the role of timing of long-term air pollution exposure in relation to lung function decrements in children. The children were followed with repeated questionnaires, dynamic spirometry, and IgE measurements until 8 years of age. The authors related time-weighted average air pollution exposure during different time windows and spirometry at 8 years by linear regression. An association was found between traffic-related average $PM < 10 \mu m$ (PM_{10}) exposure during infancy and decreased lung function (FEV[1]) in children up to 8 years of age, with stronger effects suggested in children sensitized to common allergens. Of importance, air pollution exposure after the first year of life seemed to have less impact on lung function at 8 years of age. Challenge studies under environmentally controlled conditions at the EHC-Dallas and the EHC-Buffalo have confirmed fuel oil sensitivity in the chemically sensitive patients.

In an editorial, Grigg[152] put forward that more than one-half of the world's population now live in urban areas and that African megacities rank among the most polluted in the world. This information indicates that the long-term effects of traffic-derived air pollution on children's respiratory health are of major significance globally, and there is now sufficient evidence to reduce children's exposure to traffic pollution to protect their long-term respiratory health.

Inflammation, Increased Susceptibility to Infection, and Sensory Nerve Damage

Previous data indicate that exposure to diesel exhaust enhances allergic inflammation and that exposure to air pollution is associated with increased susceptibility to viral respiratory infections. In a recent study, Noah and coauthors[153] addressed the issue of whether acute exposure to diesel exhaust would modify inflammatory responses to influenza virus in normal and allergic individuals. After exposure to diesel exhaust at a particular concentration of ~100 $\mu g/m^3$ or air for 2 hours, virus was administered, followed by serial nasal lavages with markers of inflammation and viral quantity as endpoints. Diesel exposure was shown to be associated with an increase in IFN-γ. Furthermore, linked to allergy, increases in cotaxin-1, eosinophil cationic protein, and influenza RNA sequences in nasal cells was found after exposure to diesel exhaust. Taken together, these data denote that prior exposure to diesel exhaust exacerbates influenza virus-induced nasal inflammation, in particular by promoting eosinophilic activation in subjects with allergic rhinitis, along with signs of reduced virus clearance. Studies at the EHC-Dallas and the EHC-Buffalo on the influenza virus show that the neutralization dose of the virus under environmentally controlled conditions can run from 1:5 dilutions to more the 1:3000. These dilutions will stop the influenza for people with air pollution exposure as well as that of the patients living in a clear nonpolluted environment when administered every 4 hours at the onset of symptoms.

As shown at the beginning of this volume, sensory nerves are necessary for monitoring the input of pollutants. Some literature is now showing that the sensory input tracts can be injured.[154] These especially include the olfactory apparatus, the trigeminal ganglion, the bronchial-pulmonary area, the dermal, the genitourinary and the gastrointestinal tract. Both hypersensitivity and hyposensitivity (from the masking phenomenon) occur to odors. A study in MC by Calderon-Garciduenas et al.[155] confirmed how badly outdoor pollutants can damage dogs as well as humans. Calderon observed air pollution-induced cognitive defects and brain abnormalities. The injuries occurred in four places, mainly the olfactory areas and the neurovascular system of the brain were involved, as was the bronchopulmonary tree and the dermal areas.[155]

MC residents are exposed to severe air pollution, especially car exhausts, and exhibit olfactory bulb (OB) inflammation.[156]

Urban air pollution influences on olfactory function and pathology in exposed children and young adults compared the olfactory function of individuals living under conditions of extreme air pollution to that of controls from a relatively clean environment. They explored associations between olfaction scores, apolipoprotein E (APOE) status, and pollution exposure. The OBs of 35 MC residences and 9 controls aged 20.8 ± 8.5 years were assessed by light and electron microscopy. The University of Pennsylvania Smell Identification Test (UPSIT) was administered to 62

MC/25 controls 21.2 ± 2.7 years. MC subjects had significantly lower UPSIT scores: 34.24 ± 0.42 versus controls 35.76 ± 0.40, $p = 0.03$. Olfaction deficits were present in 35.5% MC and 12% of the controls. MC APOE ε 4 carriers failed 2.4 ± 0.54 items in the 10-item smell identification scale from the UPSIT related to Alzheimer's disease, while APOE 2/3 and 3/3 subjects failed 1.36 ± 0.16 items, $p = 0.01$. MC residents exhibited OB endothelial hyperplasia, neuronal accumulation of particles (2/35), and immunoreactivity to β-amyloid $βA_{42}$ (29/35) and/or α-synuclein (4/35) in neurons, glial cells, and/or blood vessels. Ultrafine particles were present in OBs, endothelial cytoplasm, and basement membranes. Control OBs were unremarkable. Air pollution exposure is associated with olfactory dysfunction and OB pathology, APOE 4 may confer greater susceptibility to such abnormalities, and ultrafine particles could play a key role in the OB pathology. This study contributes to our understanding of the influences of air pollution on olfaction and its potential contribution to neurodegeneration.[156]

Air pollution is a complex mixture of PM, gases, organic and inorganic compounds present in outdoor and indoor air. Children living in MC exhibit evidence of chronic inflammation of the upper and lower respiratory tracts, accumulation of particulates in nasal respiratory epithelium, breakdown of the nasal respiratory epithelial barrier, systemic inflammation, brain inflammation, cognitive deficits, and MRI brain abnormalities.[155,157–162] UFPM < 100 nm is found in the OBs of children and young adults exposed to the highly polluted atmosphere of MC.[159,162] Healthy dogs living in MC also exhibit disruption of nasal and olfactory barriers, increased apurinic and apyrimidinic DNA sites in OB and hippocampus tissues, and white matter hyperintense prefrontal lesions by MRI similar to those present in children.[155,163,164]

The observation that MC teenagers with an APOE ε 4 allele accumulate Aβ42 in OB neurons concomitantly with markers of OS, mitochondrial abnormalities, and dysfunction of the proteasomal system[165,166] is very important. The APOE ε 4 allele is a major genetic risk factor for the development of Alzheimer's disease and older adult ε 4 carriers perform poorly on odor identification tests.[167–172] Also relevant to this study, Kozauer et al.[173] have shown an association between cognitive decline and APOE ε 4 in young individuals. Specifically, ε 4 carriers first seen at an average age of 29.3 years and followed up for 22 years scored lower in the Mini-Mental State Examination (MMSE) and three tests of verbal learning: immediate recall, delayed recall, and word recognition.[173] Kozauers' study suggests that the association between APOE ε 4 and cognitive decline is likely an early one, emphasizing the need to explore olfactory deficits in younger individuals carrying the ε 4 allele.[173]

MC represents an extreme of urban growth and environmental pollution[172,173] being much of the problem. The MC Metropolitan Area (19° 25′N latitude and 99° 100′W longitude) lies in an elevated basin at an altitude of 2240 m above mean sea level and its urbanized area covers around 2000 km².

The northwest sector of MC—the residency area of the exposed cohort—corresponds to a mixed medium-income residential and industrial area with heavy traffic. Although PM_{10} (PM with aerodynamic diameters of <10 μm) and $PM_{2.5}$ (PM with aerodynamic diameters of <2.5 μm) concentrations over this sector are not the highest in the metropolitan area, their levels represent a health concern to its residents.[174]

Air quality MC data clearly indicate that during the period of the study, residents in NWMC were exposed to significant concentrations of PM_{10} and $PM_{2.5}$. The annual $PM_{2.5}$ average concentrations from 2004 to June 2008 registered by the local official monitoring network (Partisol $PM_{2.5}$ samplers) in MC, ranged from 23.6 to 24.3 μg/m³.[175] The interpolated annual $PM_{2.5}$ average concentration for the study area (parabolic interpolation method as suggested in EPA, 1977) for any 12-month period combination between December 2005 and June 2008 was 21.03 μg/m³ (9.2 μg/m³ SD). For comparison, the annual mean air quality standard for $PM_{2.5}$ stands at 15.0 μg/m³. In terms of short-exposure 24-hour levels, the exploratory statistical analysis for the NWMC December 2005–June 2008 data period indicated that in 8% of this period (~77 days) $PM_{2.5}$ 24-hour concentrations were above 35 μg/m³, while the median was 19.9 μg/m³ and the maximum was 57.35 μg/m³. In general, $PM_{2.5}$

composition or its spatial distribution in MC has not changed significantly in the last 10 years.[174,175] Organic carbon (OC) has been shown to be the major component, accounting for ~48%.[176] Secondary inorganic aerosols are the second major component of $PM_{2.5}$, accounting for 26%, and elemental carbon (soot) resulting from incomplete combustion accounts for ~17%.

Environmental risk factors have been implicated in the development of neurodegenerative diseases such as Alzheimer's and Parkinson's disease (PD), and a disturbed sense of smell is seen early in the course of these two major neurodegenerative diseases.[169,177–182] Occupational exposures to airborne particulates and aerosolized metals (i.e., welding) have been associated with smell loss and some forms of central nervous system (CNS) degeneration.[183,184] The present study suggests that a relationship exists between olfactory deficits in young healthy individuals and their sustained exposures to a complex mixture of air pollutants. Thus, more than one-third of the MC young healthy adults had odor identification deficits independent of APOE status.

Calderón-Garcidueñas et al.[156] did not know nor did they state how many exhibited hypersensitivity to odors but other studies suggest at least one-third or more exhibited hypersensitivity to odors. Therefore, at least 60% of the population may have altered olfactory responses to air pollution in the city. Moreover, carriers of an APOE ε 4 allele with less residency time in MC failed significantly more UPSIT items known to be sensitive to Alzheimer's disease than their APOE 2/3 and 3/3 MC and control counterparts, implying that a combination of environmental factors and genetics plays a role in influencing olfactory function.

The pathology findings in MC children and young adults indicate that PM accumulates in the respiratory nasal epithelium, olfactory epithelium, and Bowman glands, as well as in OB neurons.[157,162] The presence of UFPM in the endothelium and basement membranes of OB arterioles was associated with endothelial inflammation, as shown by neutrophils attaching to the vessel walls, and endothelial hyperplasia with significant reduction of vessel lumen.[162,185] MC subjects exhibited OB/nerve immunoreactivity of βA_{42} in 83% and α-synuclein in 11% of the cases, indicating that the abnormal protein accumulation is a very common response in highly exposed subjects.

At least five critical OB-related issues could be pertinent to subjects exposed to air pollution: (1) the olfactory transport into the brain of toxic materials, including PM[183,186,187,930]; (2) the role of ultrafine particulates (UFPM) in the enhancement rate of protein fibrillation potentially affecting amyloid, β_{42}, and α-synuclein[188–192]; (3) the OB accumulation of β-amyloid$_{1-42}$ and α-synuclein[180,193,194]; (4) the OB neuroinflammation observed in individuals exposed to air pollutants.[162,195]; (5) and the impact of the OB pathology upon the neuronal populations, including the migrating progenitor cells from the subventricular zone (SVZ).[196–200]

The olfactory nerve/OB pathway is a well-known route of access of toxins and PM to the brain for experimental animals and occupational exposures.[183,186,201] Both the olfactory and the trigeminal (responsible for the nasal perception of cold, pungent, or burning sensations) pathways are likely portals of entry in urban residents.[162] There has been a growing interest in the identification of fine PM and UFPM in urban air, and their health effects.[202–204] Ultrafine particles have a very large surface-to-volume ratio, and are not membrane bound, which allows for direct access to intracellular proteins, organelles, and DNA, enhancing their toxic potential.[205,206] The release of nanoparticles in the environment as aerosols from traffic, waste, and industry processes strongly suggests that inhalation is an important access route in humans and dogs.[207] Transport of nanoparticles across an epithelium is dependent on concentration, temperature, and size. Chen et al. and Des Rieux et al.[187,208] have recently published papers showing the effects of aluminum oxide nanoparticles in brain endothelial cell cultures and intact rats. Nano-alumina produced significant endothelial OS and disrupted the expression of tight junction proteins.[187]

These experimental observations are very relevant to MC subjects, since Calderón-Garcidueñas et al.[162] have described alterations of zonula occludens (ZO-1) immunoreactivity with a breakdown of the BBB in the frontal cortex of exposed children.[162] Factors such as age, gender, weight, race, nostril shape, exercise level, minute ventilation, and outdoor time all contribute to the particle deposition, and to lesser or higher risk from inhalation of pollutant PM in ambient air.[209] Approximately

5%–20% of the nasal air flow passes through the olfactory region,[210] and in a recent human nasal computational fluid dynamic model using particles ranging in size from 5 to 50 μm and volumetric flow rates of 7.5, 15, and 30 L/minute, the olfactory region had a PM deposition efficiency maximum value of 3%.[211] These data are critical for children given that their respiratory frequency is higher than adults and thus their PM olfactory deposition could be higher.

The novel observation that nanoparticles can significantly enhance the rate of protein fibrillation[188–192,206] and the ability of synthetic polymers to interact and alter polypeptide conformations[212] adds a new important facet to the issue of environmental (natural and man-made) nanoparticles playing a role in neurodegeneration.

The fact that pollutants can damage proteins and enzymes like protein kinases A and C, which are combined with Ca^{2+} and then phosphorylated causing an increase in cell especially nerve sensitivity at least 1000 times is highly significant in the chemically sensitive patient. Also, as Pall has shown, the NO can trigger the OS and hydrogen peroxide pathway, causing more damage to the blood–brain barrier.[211]

ER protein kinase activates phosphorylation cascades increasing the expression, which acts as molecular chaperons to establish ER folding or promote ER deregulation or destruction of misfolded proteins to adjust to the changing environment. Failure of adaptation gives ER stress-yielding expression of genes and will eventually lead to chronic body malfunction and programmed death.

The clinician is obligated to the patient to enforce the process of decreasing the total body pollutant load in the chemically sensitive and episodic CDD patient using massive avoidance of the pollutants in air, food, and water; intradermal neutralization when possible; and nutrient supplementation to keep the detoxification full.

The mammalian OB receives new neurons throughout the life, progenitors migrate from the SVZ located in the walls of the lateral ventricles facing the striatum, the septum, and the corpus callosum.[197,199,213,214] Within the OB, young neurons mature into various types of local inhibitory interneurons.[199] Different interneuron subtypes are produced at different ages and play a crucial role in olfactory processing; thus, neuronal accumulation of ultrafine particles and/or abnormal proteins could likely alter the plasticity of postnatal olfactory circuits and impair olfactory circuits with functional consequences such as change in memory, balance, and confusion. Furthermore, the endothelial and basement membrane changes Calderón-Garcidueñas describe in OB vessels likely also alter the delicate balance between the neuro-glial-vascular components of the olfactory glomeruli.[200,215] Specifically, in these structures, there is a close interaction between axon terminals, presynaptic and postsynaptic dendrites, glial cells, and the capillary/arteriolar network. Thus, gliosis, alterations in the Virchow–Robin spaces, breakdown of the BBB, endothelial hyperplasia, reduction of the arteriolar lumen, and thickening of arteriolar walls could alter the blood perfusion in relation to neuronal activity in an anatomical and functional unit onto which all olfactory sensory axons that express the same odor receptors converge.[200,216] This anatomical variation could cause pathophysiological changes, thus altering brain and bodily functions (Table 1.12) (Figure 1.3).

Particulates

Particulates comprise a wide range of materials, which are solid or liquid in the air and are a concentration of <10 μm in diameter (PM_{10}). These particulates are capable of penetrating deep into the respiratory tract and the nasal–hypothalamic–limbic area of the brain. The nanoparticles <200 μg/m can cause disease in any organ as they can cross the nasal and pulmonary vascular barrier. The sources of particulates are many and include dust from soil and roads, diesel exhaust emissions from combustion and industrial processes, construction and demolition, powdered pesticides, bioaerosols, and volcanic ash.[79,217] Such particulates may travel thousands of kilometers in the air across oceans and deposit themselves onto other continents,[218,219] that is, African dust travels to United States in mid-May to mid-September, then goes to the Amazon in South America the other

TABLE 1.12
Monthly Periodicity (ppb) Pollutant Counts

Month	CO	O_3	SO_2	$PM_{2.5}$
January	819 ± 60	33.65 ± 0.83	2.90 ± 0.40	7.45 ± 0.44
February	688 ± 50	37.13 ± 1.12	6.02 ± 0.68	7.79 ± 0.40
March	566 ± 36	43.60 ± 1.20	4.53 ± 0.55	8.87 ± 0.57
April	543 ± 47	49.18 ± 1.47	7.46 ± 1.15	10.99 ± 0.53
May	470 ± 24	57.27 ± 2.01	9.45 ± 1.43	10.48 ± 0.53
June	378 ± 19	56.93 ± 2.80	4.50 ± 0.65	10.62 ± 0.62
July	408 ± 17	73.69 ± 2.76	4.11 ± 0.70	13.10 ± 0.54
August	474 ± 22	82.58 ± 2.19	4.50 ± 0.54	11.54 ± 0.54
September	607 ± 37	64.05 ± 2.56	4.08 ± 0.70	10.71 ± 0.62
October	579 ± 48	49.40 ± 1.47	6.44 ± 1.00	9.84 ± 0.69
November	754 ± 74	36.92 ± 1.37	3.21 ± 0.41	9.20 ± 0.69
December	740 ± 71	30.15 ± 0.86	3.78 ± 0.60	6.45 ± 0.40

Source: Environmental Health Center-Dallas 2012.

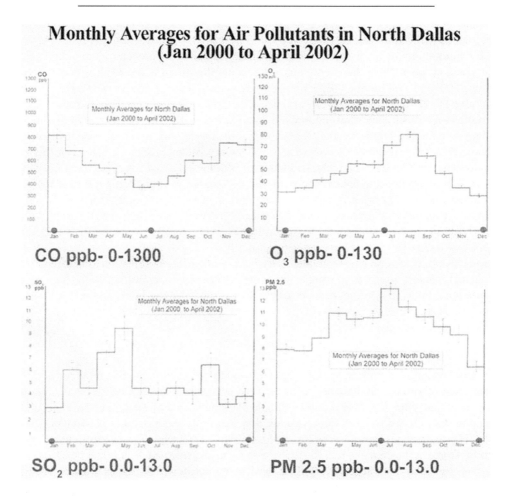

FIGURE 1.3   People at risk in 25 most ozone-polluted counties. (From American Lung Association, 2009.)

months; Gobi dust goes to Western United States. We have developed antigens for African dust and have multiple patients who get relief from the injection of the neutralization dose every 4 days.

Biomass burning of wood, leaves, crops, and forests is the largest source of particulates in many parts of the world. A study of 15 U.S. cities found that woodburning produced 36%–95% of wintertime airborne $PM_{2.5}$ from all sources.[220] Smoke from large forest fires in Indonesia and Quebec has been found to greatly increase airborne particulates in areas many hundreds of kilometers away.[221,222]

According to Rice et al.,[24] climate change is expected to contribute to dangerous elevations in PM by fostering conditions favorable to forest fires and, in some arid parts of the world, promoting sand storms. Climate models indicate that with 1°C of warming, wildland fire risk may increase two- to sixfold over the 1950–2003 baseline in most of the continental United States, west of the Mississippi.[223]

Although forest fires may ignite in certain regions only, their smoke plumes may extend over great distances. During the Russian heat wave of 2010, for instance, smoke from more than 500 wildfires stretched across more than 1800 miles, roughly the distance from San Francisco to Chicago.[224] Studies in the United States, Europe, and Australia have associated exposure to wildland fire smoke with asthma and COPD exacerbations and hospitalizations,[225,226] congestive heart failure events,[227] and overall mortality.[228]

Rising temperatures and increasing frequency of droughts are projected to increased desertification in areas with dry climates.[228] Desertification and droughts promote dust storms,[229] which are public health hazards, particularly for people with pulmonary disease. Desert dust particles contain quartz, which has been found to cause airway inflammation in animal studies.[230,231] Exposure to airborne dust particles transported from regional deserts (in some cases more than 4000 km away) has been associated with increases in cardiovascular and respiratory mortality,[232] cardiopulmonary emergency room visits,[233] stroke,[234] and admissions for asthma[235] and pneumonia[236] in studies from Spain, Taiwan, and California.

PM emissions tend to increase during heat waves in regions where electricity is supplied by coal-fired power plants, as a consequence of increased electrical energy use for cooling. There is evidence that high temperatures and PM interact to cause greater mortality that would be expected from the same level of PM at cooler temperatures, even in developed countries where particulate levels are relatively low.[237–239] PM concentrations have declined substantially in the developed world in recent decades as a result of air quality regulations and tightening emissions standards. Even if average PM concentrations continue to decrease in the future, the relative toxicity of PM may rise during higher temperature periods because of this interaction.

According to Block et al.,[240] ultrafine (nano-size particles) and fine particles are the most notorious of air pollution components, penetrating olfactory apparatus and lung tissue compartments to reach the capillaries and circulating cells, or constituents (e.g., erythrocytes),[241] giving OS and inflammation. Vasculitis in the chemically sensitive occurs with OS and tissue inflammation. Experimentally, inhalation or nasal instillation of ultrafine particles in rodents results in the translocation of the particles to the systemic circulation[242] and to the brain.[243] The nasal olfactory pathway is believed to be a key portal of entry, where inhaled nanoparticles have been shown to reach trigeminal nerves, brainstem, and hippocampus,[244,245] which are involved in chemical sensitivity. Very recently, nano-sized PM was identified in the human brain.[246] Specifically, PM has been observed in human OB and periglomerular neurons, and particles smaller than 100 nm were observed in intraluminal erythrocytes from frontal lobe and trigeminal ganglia capillaries.[246] These observations in highly exposed subjects confirm that air pollution components reach the brain,[204] even penetrating deep into the parenchyma and yielding OS and inflammation and eventually chemical sensitivity.

However, once the particles reach the CNS, there is considerable debate on what the mechanisms of toxicity are. Most hypotheses are derived from traits conferred by the physical and chemical constitution of the PM. For example, ultrafine particles have a large surface-to-volume ratio[247] and easily penetrate cellular membranes.[205] This provides insight into why UFPM is able to traverse traditional barriers in the lung and the BBB, including why PM is found in neurons and carried in erythrocytes causing OS and inflammation.

Another hypothesis builds on the premise that the particles themselves may stimulate innate immunity in the brain. Pattern recognition receptors are present in the brain's resident innate immune cells, microglia, and identify large pathogen-associated molecular patterns, such as charge and protein aggregates.[248] Studies examining the toxic effects of nanometer-sized carbon (carbon black, a model of PM missing adsorbed compounds) confirm that inhalation of carbon black alone is known to cause inflammation,[249] suggesting that something inherent in the particle may be culpable. Indeed, UFPM exposure in mice induces the production of pro-inflammatory cytokines (ILa-β, TNF-α, and INF-γ) in the OBs of exposed animals.[248] Work by Veronesi et al.[250] reports that the inflammatory response to PM in both respiratory epithelial cells[110,250] and microglia[251] (brain macrophages) relates to physiochemical features of the particles, such as surface charge. Thus, PM itself may indeed be a proinflammatory stimulus once it reaches the brain.

Interestingly, nanoparticles are proposed as an ideal vehicle to enhance drug entry to the CNS.[252] Thus, it has been suggested that the particle components of air pollution may also represent an effective delivery system for diverse environmental toxicants to reach the brain. We do see this in the chemically sensitive individuals who are exposed to nanoparticles like manganese, lead, mercury, arsenic, volatile organics, pesticides, mycotoxins, molds, foods, etc. Additionally, some adsorbed compounds are soluble and may become a toxic stimulus independent of the particle itself.[204] Indeed, the toxicity and immune-stimulating characteristics of PM, such as diesel exhaust particles (DEPs) in the lung, have been linked to both the adsorbed chemicals on the outside of the carbon particle (e.g., transition metals and lipopolysaccharides)[253,254] and the physical characteristics of the particle itself.[255] These nanoparticles would then trigger chemical sensitivity.

Many of the adsorbed compounds present on PM are neurotoxic. For example, manganese is a component of urban air pollution, where concentrations in the air vary based on location, season, and source.[109] Acute manganese exposure typically occurs as an occupational exposure in humans and is likened to dopaminergic neurotoxicity and PD symptoms.[256] One source of manganese content in the air is industrial derived, arising due to emissions from ferroalloy production, iron and steel foundries, and coke ovens. In addition, manganese is also dispersed as air pollution due to gasoline engine combustion, when the gasoline contains methylcyclopentadienyl manganese tricarbonyl as an antiknock agent.[255] Recently, both traffic and environmentally derived manganese in air pollution was linked to increased risk for PD diagnosis.[109,255] We do see a subset of chemically sensitive patients who have increased manganese levels in the hair and urine analysis. This could trigger cerebral toxicity leading to chemical sensitivity. Also, we see a significant number of chemically sensitive patients who have metal or synthetic implants who develop cerebral triggering from their implant. They have to either have them removed or we intradermal neutralize them to counteract their incitant capacity.

Laboratory studies suggest that exposure to fine PM ($\leq\mu$m in diameter) ($PM_{2.5}$) can trigger a combination of pathophysiological responses that may induce the development of hypertension. However, epidemiological evidence relating $PM_{2.5}$ and hypertension is sparse, though we have produced it by intradermal challenge. Chen et al.[257] conducted a population-based cohort study to determine whether exposures to ambient $PM_{2.5}$ are associated with incident hypertension. They assembled a cohort of 35,303 nonhypersensitive adults from Ontario, Canada, who responded to one of four population-based health surveys between 1996 and 2005 and were followed up until December 31, 2010. Incident diagnoses of hypertension were ascertained from the Ontario Hypertension Database, a validated registry of persons diagnosed with hypertension in Ontario (sensitivity = 72%, specificity = 95%). Estimates of long-term exposure to $PM_{2.5}$ at participants' postal code residences were derived from satellite observations. Chen et al.[257] used Cox proportional hazards models, adjusting for various individual and contextual risk factors, including body mass index (BMI), smoking, physical activity, and neighborhood-level unemployment rates. Between 1996 and 2010, they identified 8649 incident cases of hypertension and 2296 deaths. For every 10-μg/m^3 increase of $PM_{2.5}$, the adjusted hazard ratio of incident hypertension was 1.13 (95% CI: 1.05–1.22). Estimated associations were comparable among all sensitivity analyses.

This study supports an association between $PM_{2.5}$ and increase incidence of hypertension (Tables 1.13 through 1.16).

Texas has had problems with particulates especially in Houston–Beaumont–Port Arthur coastal area where the petrochemical complexes are as well as part of El Paso where there is dust and pollution coming across the Rio Grande from the Mexican city of Jaurez, Mexico. One can see that Texas lowered its primary annual for particulates 2.5 from 15 to 12 $\mu g/m^3$. Table 1.17 shows the annual design for particulate 2.5 in various cities.

INCREASED MONITORING AT CHAMIZAL

Prior to 2011, El Paso Chamizal had data only from the FRM monitor, which samples every sixth day. In 2011, an FEM monitor was also installed at Chamizal, resulting in an increase in sampling days. The increased monitoring captured more high PM days, causing an increase in the annual average $PM_{2.5}$. Some of those high days are exceptional events (typically dust events).

TABLE 1.13
Recent Standard for Outdoor Air Concentration of Common Criteria Outdoor Air Pollutants

Country	Particulates in $\mu g/m^3$	Ozone in $\mu g/m^3$	Carbon Monoxide in mg/m^3	Sulfur Dioxide in mg/m^3	Nitrogen Dioxide in mg/m^3	Lead in $\mu g/m^3$
U.S. EPA	PM_{10} Annual 50 Daily 150 2009 = 18 2010 = 18	1 hour—240	1 hour 40 8 h 10	0.365 Annual 0.08 1680 m/tons	Annual 0.1	3 months mean 1.5–52
Japan	PM_{10} Annual 200 Daily 100 2009 = 30 2010 = 30	1 hour—120	8 h 22.8	Daily 0.26 Annual 0.11 970,000 m/tons	Daily 0.04–0.06	*
Germany	PM_{10} Annual 100 Daily 200 2009 = 16 2010 = 16	*	1 hour—30	Daily 0.40 annual 0.14 5100 m/tons	Daily 0.3 Annual 0.1	*
India	PM_{10} 2009 = 103 2010 = 96		1,007,980	1150	29.68	
Mali	18–121					
WHO	Total soluble particulates TSP annual 60–90 daily 150–230	1 hour—200	1 hour—30 8 hour 10	Daily 0.20 Annual 0.09	1 hour 0.190–0.320	*1

Source: U.S. EPA (1982, 1987, 1997, 2000, 2009, and 2010) Environmental Management Center (2006 World Bank 1995–2009–2010). Adverse Health Effect of Outdoor Air Pollutants. *Literature Review* 2009. DOI: 10.1016/j.envint.2006.03.012. https://www.ncbi.nlm.nih.gov/pubmed/16730796

* Pollutant levels without an ambient standard yet.

TABLE 1.14

PM > 2.5 µg/m³—2009–2012 by State

State	$PM_{2.5}$ Annual Value	
	2010–2012	2009–2011
Alabama	9.5–13.0	9.8–12.2
Alaska	4.5–11.5	4.7–12.0
Arizona	4.0–10.3	4.3–11.0
Arkansas	10.8–12.2	10.2–12.1
California	3.5–1.9	3.3–18.2
Colorado	5.9	6.3
Connecticut	5.7–9.4	5.7–9.6
Delaware	8.1–10.4	8.4–10.7
District of Columbia	10.1–10.4	10.3–10.6
Florida	5.9–9.5	5.9–9.9
Georgia	10.0–13.1	10.1–13.4
Hawaii	4.9–15.5	5.2–15.5
Idaho	6.6–14.7	5.2–12.0
Illinois	9.3–13.5	9.6–13.0
Indiana	10.4–13.2	10.2–13.5
Iowa	8.8–11.8	9.0–12.1
Kansas	7.7–10.2	8.1–10.4
Kentucky	8.9–12.1	9.1–12.8
Louisiana	8.4–11.8	8.6–11.1
Maine	4.6–8.4	4.5–8.2
Maryland	8.8–11.3	9.1–11.1
Massachusetts	7.2–8.8	7.8–10.2
Michigan	6.0–11.5	6.0–10.9
Minnesota	5.3–9.8	5.4–10.0
Mississippi	9.4–011.6	9.4
Missouri	9.5–11.9	9.5–12.0
Montana	6.9–11.5	6.0–11.4
Nebraska	7.3–11.5	7.1–11.0
Nevada	4.0–7.9	3.7–7.7
New Hampshire	6.0–9.1	5.8–9.6
New Jersey	7.6–11.2	7.6–11.4
New Mexico	4.6–13.5	4.2–11.9
New York	4.3–11.8	4.4–11.7
North Carolina	7.7–11.1	8.7–11.1
North Dakota	4.4–8.0	4.3–8.1
Ohio	8.9–13.0	9.0–13.8
Oklahoma	9.3–10.5	9.3–10.8
Oregon	5.6–10.5	6.1–10.7
Pennsylvania	7.2–14.8	9.0–15.0
Rhode Island	6.3–8.0	8.2
South Carolina	8.9–10.7	9.2–11.3
South Dakota	3.8–9.3	5.9–9.0
Tennessee	9.1–12.2	8.6–12.3
Texas	8.1–12.1	8.5–11.6
Utah	5.1–8.8	4.2–9.7
Vermont	5.1–9.6	5.2–7.3

(Continued)

TABLE 1.14 (*Continued*)
PM > 2.5 µg/m³—2009–2012 by State

| State | PM$_{2.5}$ Annual Value | |
	2010–2012	2009–2011
Virginia	8.5–10.2	8.7–10.4
Washington	5.9–8.7	6.3–8.9
West Virginia	9.3–12.8	9.6–13.0
Wisconsin	5.3–11.3	5.5–11.7
Wyoming	4.7–8.3	4.4–8.5

Source: Data from U.S. EPA (2012).

TABLE 1.15
Cleanest U.S. Cities for Year-Round Particle Pollution (Annual PM$_{2.5}$)[a]

Rank[b]	Design Value[c]	Metropolitan Statistical Area	Population
1	4.1	Cheyenne, WY	92,680
2	4.2	Santa Fe-Espanola, NM	186,094
2	4.2	St. George, UT	141,666
4	4.3	Prescott, AZ	211,888
5	4.5	Farmington, NM	128,200
6	5.2	Pocatello, ID	91,457
7	5.3	Redding, CA	177,774
8	5.4	Tucson, AZ	989,569
9	5.9	Albuquerque, NM	898,642
9	5.9	Colorado Springs, CO	660,319
9	5.9	Flagstaff, AZ	134,511
9	5.9	Rapid City, SD	128,361
13	6.1	Salinas, CA	421,898
14	6.2	Anchorage, AK	387,516
15	6.3	Fort Collins–Loveland, CO	305,525
16	6.6	Duluth, MN-WI	279.815
16	6.6	Palm Bay–Melbourne–Titusville, FL	543,566
18	6.8	Reno–Sparks–Fenley, NV	481,477
18	6.8	Sarasota–Bradenton–Punta Gorda, FL	869,866
20	6.9	Bismarck, ND	110,879
20	6.9	Cape Coral–Fort Myers, FL	631,330
22	7.3	Bangor, ME	153,786
22	7.3	Burlington–South Burlington, VT	212,535
24	7.4	Boise City–Nampa, ID	627,664
25	7.5	Lakeland–Winter Haven, FL	609,492
25	7.5	Miami–Fort Lauderdale–Pompano Beach, FL	5,670,125
25	7.5	Orlando–Deltona–Daytona Beach, FL	2,861,296

[a] This list represents cities with the lowest levels of annual PM$_{2.5}$ air pollution.

[b] Cities are ranked by using the highest design value for any within that metropolitan area.

[c] The design value is the calculated concentration of a pollutant based on the form of the National Ambient Air Quality Standard and is used by the EPA to determine whether the air quality in a county meets the standard.

TABLE 1.16

Top 25 Cleanest Counties for Year-Round Particle Pollution (Annual PM$_{2.5}$)[a]

2013 Rank[b]	County	State	Design Value[c]
1	Lake	CA	3.3
2	Jackson	SD	3.8
3	Laramie	WY	4.1
4	Washington	UT	4.2
4	Santa Fe	NM	4.2
6	Billings	ND	4.3
6	Yavapai	AZ	4.3
8	Park	WY	4.4
10	Teton	WY	4.5
10	San Juan	NM	4.5
10	Hancock	ME	4.5
10	Custer	SD	4.5
14	Maui	HI	4.9
15	Siskiyou	CA	5.1
16	Bannock	ID	5.2
17	Shasta	CA	5.3
18	Pima	AZ	5.4
19	Ashland	WI	5.5
20	San Benito	CA	5.6
20	Sweetwater	WY	5.6
22	Litchfield	CT	5.7
22	Douglas	CO	5.8
24	Be Lma	NH	5.8
25	Coconino	AZ	5.9
25	El Paso	CO	5.9
25	Pennington	SD	5.9
25	Bernalillo	NM	5.9

[a] This list represents counties with the lowest levels of monitored long-term PM$_{2.5}$ air pollution.

[b] Counties are ranked by design value.

[c] The design value is the calculated concentration of a pollutant based on the form of the National Ambient Air Quality Standard and is used by the EPA to determine whether the air quality in a county meets the standard.

One can see the graft Figure 1.4, which shows a decrease in particulates from 2006 to 2012. In 2013, there were only 5 exceptional days when the PM$_{2.5}$ exceeded the limits.

Cross-Border Air Quality Planning Instituted around 2010

The Paso Del Norte Air Basin comprised El Paso, parts of Dona Ana County in New Mexico, and Ciudad Juarez in the Mexican state of Chihuahua were involved. This area is located between the Franklin Mountains and Sierras de Juarez. It has a unique topography, meteorology, population, and economy. There are jurisdictional obstacles in controlling cross-border emissions. The Regional Air Quality Planning was formal cross-border cooperation through which the Joint Advisory Committee for the Improvement of Air Quality in the Paso Del Norte was instituted.

TABLE 1.17

2012 PM$_{2.5}$ Design Values (DV) Particulate Matter

CBSA FRM[a]	Number of 2012 Monitors	Annual Design Value µg/m³ (Standard: 12.0 µg/m³)	24-Hour Design Value µg/m³ (Standard: 35 µg/m³)	Monitors with Annual Design Value above 12.0 µg/m³
Austin-Round Rock	2	10.2	21	0
Corpus Christi	2	10.4	30	0
Dallas–Fort Worth–Arlington	2	10.8	22	0
El Paso	2	10.8	30	0
Houston-The Woodlands–Sugar Land	3	12.1[b]	24	1[b]
McAllen–Edinburg–Mission	1	10.3	23	0
San Antonio–New Braunfels	2	9.0	23	0
Texarkana	1	11.1	21	0
Marshall	1	10.9	22	0

[a] FRM: Federal Reference Method.

[b] Includes exceptional events such as Saharan dust events and smoke from Central American agricultural burning.

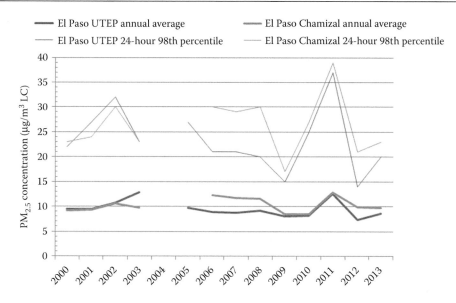

FIGURE 1.4 Trends of annual averages and 98th percentiles of 24-hour averages for long-term particulate matter of 2.5 µm or less in diameter (PM$_{2.5}$) monitoring sites in the El Paso area including exceptional event days.

Control measures included woodburning regulations, alley paving, and street sweeping.

From 1991 through 2010, the percentage of unpaved alleys decreased from 66% to 16% of the total alleys in the El Paso area. The city of El Paso discontinued garbage collection in alleys in 1997 dramatically, reducing traffic in alleys. The reclaimed asphalt pavement (RAP) has been used to cover some unpaved alleys and has proven to be as effective as paving.

The toxicity of particulates depends greatly on their size, with particulates <10 µm (PM$_{10}$) or 2.5 µm (PM$_{2.5}$) being considered especially dangerous since they can easily penetrate the nasal sinus cavity and lungs, then through the alveoli go to the vascular system and brain. Currently, there are some questions as to whether the PM_{10}, $PM_{2.5}$ particulates are more important to human health.[258] Toxicity of particulates also varies depending upon their chemical compositions with nanoparticles <200 μm being the worst because they can enter the body and especially the brain so easily. Particulates of special concern include toxic metals like lead and mercury, PAHs, persistent organic toxicants such as dioxins,[217,259] and pesticides. The main outdoor sources of PAHs are motor vehicles, coal/oil-fired power plants, and biomass burning.[260] (See Chapter 2 for more information.)

PATHWAYS OF AIR POLLUTION INTO THE BRAIN AND INTERBRAIN DYSFUNCTION AS WELL AS THE REST OF THE BODY

The direct route of translocation of inhaled nanoparticles is the olfactory nerve in the nose leading to the OB of the brain.[79] Nanoparticles with a size about 35 nm were detected in the brain OB after inhalation exposure. The route of brain entry was suggested to be by migration along the olfactory nerve into the OB of the brain after deposition on the olfactory mucosa in the nasal region.[243]

It has been reported that the inhaled nanoparticles not only subsequently reach the brain, the lungs, and the blood but may also reach other target sites such as the liver, heart, or blood cells.[261–263]

With decreasing size, there is a major increase in alveolar and nasal deposition. Studies specifically dealing with the toxicity of nanoparticles have only appeared recently and, although now emerging in the literature, are still rare.[264]

Data on the behavior of the particles are also available from pharmaceutical studies in which formulations involving nanoscale components are used to solve problems dealing with insolubility of drug formulations and for drug delivery. However, these small pollutants can further damage brain tissues.

Compounds of the nanoparticles size induced nasal, cerebral, lung OS, inflammation as well as epithelial damage in rats at greater extent than their larger counterparts. In addition, chemicals absorbed on the surface may affect the reactivity of nanoparticles.

Fractions isolated from particulate air pollutants (DEPs) were demonstrated to exert toxic effects on cells *in vitro*.[265] Nanoparticles in ambient air can have a very complex composition, and these components, such as organics and metals, can interact. Metallic iron was able to potentiate the effect of carbon black nanoparticles, resulting in enhanced reactivity, including OS.[266]

One has to be aware that particles in ambient air as part of pollution of combustion origin are coated with all kinds of reactive chemicals (solvents, pesticides, metal, mycotoxins), including biological compounds such as endotoxin.[267–269]

STATIONARY INDUSTRY-POWER PLANTS, FUEL COMBUSTION, AND REFINERIES: STATIONARY, OIL, AND GAS FIELDS

Additional city pollution is generated by heavy industry that uses nuclear power, coal, oil, and gas. Also contributing to city pollution are factories, including electricity-generating plants; facilities that make steel, iron, aluminum, and other metals; plastic factories of many types; refineries or pesticide processing plants; etc.; and the so-called clean industries of manufacturing of microchips, computers, radios, watches, etc. Electrical generation is also prominent. Tables 1.13 and 1.14 show the daily average criteria for pollutants in Dallas and the United States, while Figures 1.2 and 1.3 and Tables 1.13 through 1.15 show a years' monthly average for outdoor pollutants. Other pollutants are shown for local areas in the Dallas–Fort Worth area. These include power plants, cement factories, industrial pollution (Figure 1.5), air traffic, while Figure 1.6 shows the toxic release for the United States.

Power plants are another source of air pollution and can cause local as well as distal pollution.[269] An example of this type pollution would be the emanation of fumes from power plants in the Midwestern United States where their fumes are dumped on the upper northeast coast of the United

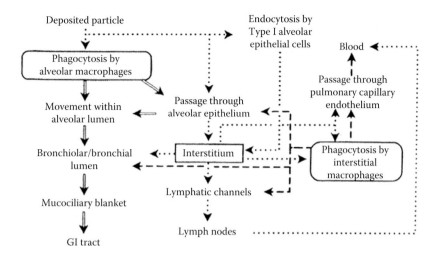

FIGURE 1.5 Nanoparticles enter the body. (From Europa DG Health and Consumer Protection. Public Health. Scenihr.)

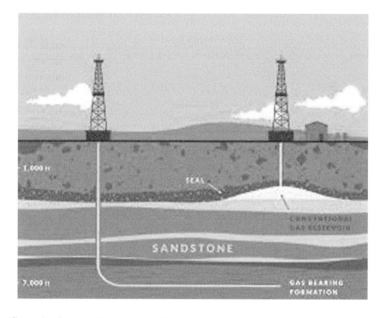

FIGURE 1.6 (**See color insert.**) Horizontal drilling—fracking.

States and lower southeast areas of Canada.[269] Toxic chemicals have been and are dumped around most military bases.[269]

Military bases and their surrounding areas are usually extremely toxic. Other man-made air pollution comes from *fluorocarbons*, which are emitted from air-conditioning and industry, gas and oil fields. Fracking for natural gas is another pollutant generative that can cause disease in those exposed.

A summary of data regarding chemical contamination in the Texas City and La Marque areas in Texas is shown (Tables 1.18 through 1.21). The section is an example of what is the output of refineries.

SWAPE has attained data from various air monitoring stations. Graphical summaries of the monitoring data demonstrate elevated levels of volatile organic compounds (VOCs), ozone, sulfur dioxide, and nitrogen oxides in this area and those towns.

TABLE 1.18
Early Devastating Fires in the Northern Hemisphere

Year	Size	Name	Area	Note
1825	3,000,000 acres (1,200,000 ha)	Miramichi Fire	New Brunswick	Killed 160 people
1846	450,000 acres (180,000 ha)	Yachina Fire	Oregon	
1853	320,000 acres (130,000 ha)	Nestucca Fire	Oregon	
1868	1,000,000 acres (400,000 ha)	Silverton Fire	Oregon	Worst recorded fire in state's history
1868	300,000 acres (120,000 ha)	Coos Fire	Oregon	
1870	964,000 acres (390,000 ha)	Saguenay Fire	Quebec	
1871	1,200,000 acres (490,000 ha)	Peshtigo Fire	Wisconsin	Killed over 1700 people and has the distinction of the conflagration that caused the most deaths by fire in U.S. history. It was overshadowed by the Great Chicago Fire that occurred on the same day
1871	2,500,000 acres (1,000,000 ha)	The Great Michigan Fire	Michigan	It was overshadowed by the Great Chicago Fire that occurred on the same day
1876	500,000 acres (200,000 ha)	Bighorn Fire	Wyoming	
1881	1,000,000 acres (400,000 ha)	Thumb Fire	Michigan	Killed 200+ people
1889	300,000 acres (120,000 ha)	Santiago Canyon Fire of 1889	California	
1894	160,000 acres (65,000 ha)	Hinckley Fire	Minnesota	Killed 418 people and destroyed 12 towns
1903	464,000 acres (188,000 ha)	Adirondack Fire	New York	
1910	3,000,000 acres (1,200,000 ha)	Great Fire of 1910	Idaho-Montana-Washington	Killed 86 people, including 78 firefighters

Source: Data from Wikipedia. https://en.wikipedia.org/wiki/List_of_wildfires#Canada_and_the_United_States.

They found two peer-reviewed health studies showing that sulfur dioxide concentrations were high enough (above 50 μg/m^3) to cause a sensitive child to have an asthma attack.

The Texas City 34th Street air monitor showed ~10% of the year, an individual should wear a respirator while being active due to ozone. BP's immense VOC releases are the primary source for ozone in the area.

The maps show the pollutant generators of the toxics and their locations. The toxics such as H_2S, SO_2, NO_x, and other volatiles such as benzene, toluene, hexane, pentane, CO, and ozone are shown in close proximity to their refineries.

The objective of this sampling assessment was to measure concentrations of "PAHs" in samples of dust at residential properties and churches surrounding the BP facility. This report presents the laboratory analytical results for these results for these samples and a discussion of the preliminary findings of this assessment.

TABLE 1.19
Who Is Polluting the Community?

Rank	Facility	City	Pounds
1	Lyondell Chemical Co.	Channelview	4,394,822
2	DuPont La Porte Plant	La Porte	2,492,552
3	Deer Park Refining L.P.	Deer Park	2,102,403
4	Merisol, U.S.A. LLC	Houston	2,077,666
5	TM Deer Park Services LLC	Deer Park	2,049,733
6	ExxonMobil Refining and Supply Baytown Refy.	Baytown	1,968,828
7	ExxonMobil Baytown Chemical Plant	Baytown	1,558,218
8	Equistar Chemicals LP	Channelview	1,350,052
9	Rohm and Haas	Deer Park	1,205,960

Source: Pollution Locator Scorecard Community Center, Harris County, Texas. Reported Environmental Releases from TRI Sources in 2002.

TABLE 1.20
What Are the Major Pollutants?

Rank	Chemical Name	Pounds
Reported Environmental Releases from TRI Sources in 2002		
1	Methanol	5,864,510
2	Ethylene	3,074,225
3	Nitrate compounds	2,972,526
4	Propylene	2,870,318
5	Sulfuric acid	1,272,878
6	Ethylbenzene	1,055,090
7	*n*-Hexane	953,652
8	Toluene	953,407
9	Styrene	878,948
10	Ammonia	854,647
11	Benzene	850,679
12	Vinyl acetate	835,348
13	Phenol	721,984
14	Xylene (mixed isomers)	694,522
15	Acetophenone	678,227
16	Methyl ethyl ketone	660,220
17	Hydrochloric acid	614,395
18	Methyl *tert*-butyl ether	518,151
19	1,3-Butadiene	494,102

Source: Pollution Locator Scorecard Community Center, Harris County.

Dust samples were collected in Texas City and La Marque, Texas from October 6 through 8, 2010. The sampling locations included 14 single-family residences, 5 churches, and 1 Shell Service Station building. Three types of dust (media) samples were collected as part of this preliminary assessment: (1) air filter samples, (2) air duct samples, and (3) settled attic dust samples. Air filter and duct samples were collected from residential and commercial heating, ventilating, and

TABLE 1.21
Occupational Hazards Associated with Waste Handling

Infections:
- Skin and blood infections resulting from direct contact with waste and from infected wounds.
- Eye and respiratory infections resulting from exposure to infected dust, especially during landfill operations.
- Different diseases that result from the bites of animals feeding on the waste.
- Intestinal infections that are transmitted by flies feeding on the waste.

Chronic diseases:
- Incineration operators are at risk of chronic respiratory diseases, including cancers resulting from exposure to dust and hazardous compounds. Also, exacerbation of chemically sensitive will occur.

Accidents:
- Bone and muscle disorders resulting from the handling of heavy containers.
- Infecting wounds resulting from contact with sharp objects.
- Poisoning and chemical burns resulting from contact with small amounts of hazardous chemical waste mixed with general waste.
- Burns and other injuries resulting from occupational accidents at waste disposal.

air-conditioning (HVAC) systems. Attic dust samples were collected from attic spaces inside residences and church buildings. Fourteen air filter media samples and nine duct media samples were analyzed by TestAmerican Laboratory, Inc. (TestAmerica) in West Sacramento, California. The nine attic dust samples were placed on hold and were not analyzed.

All 14 filter media samples were found to contain detections of phenanthrene. Fluoranthene and pyrene were also frequently detected in the samples. The BP facility is a "major" source of air pollutants and has reported emissions of PAHs, including phenanthrene, to federal and state regulatory agencies, including the U.S. EPA and Texas Commission on Environmental Quality (TCEQ).

Publicly available data on BP's emissions demonstrate that the BP facility has emitted large quantities of phenanthrene into the local atmosphere. For example, in 2000, BP reported emitting over 12,000 pounds of phenanthrene into the atmosphere from the BP Texas City refinery facility. The BP facility and BP's nearby dockyard property in Texas City are the only facilities that reported phenanthrene releases to the TRI in the zip code 77590. Based on BP's reporting to the TRI, these BP facilities released more than 23,000 pounds of phenanthrene to the atmosphere between 1995 and 2009. For the period from 1995 and 2009, the BP facility and dockyard property were responsible for ~98% of all phenanthrene releases to the atmosphere reported to TRI for Galveston County. Phenanthrene was detected in 100% of the air filter samples collected for this assessment.

Two filter media samples (Lab I.D.s #9 and #16) were found to contain certain other PAHs (benzo[*a*]anthracene, benzo[*a*]pyrene, benzo[*a*]fluoranthene, benzo[*hi*]perylene, benzo[*k*]fluoranthene, and indeno[1,2,3-*cd*] pyrene) that distinguish them from the other samples (Table 1.3). These samples (Lab I.D.s #9 and #16) were collected from a church property situated adjacent to the Emmett F. Lowry Expressway and from a Shell Service Station property at 901 6th Street N in Texas City, respectively. Both these locations would be expected to have high traffic density compared to other sampling locations in this study; therefore, the results demonstrate patterns of PAHs resulting from vehicular sources. The PAHs benzo[*hi*]perylene and indeno[1,2,3-*cd*] pyrene have been associated with vehicular exhaust in numerous scientific studies in the literature.

Two samples (Lab I.D.s #1 and #31) were reported with low detections of phenanthrene, fluoranthene, and pyrene. PAHs were not detected above the laboratory reporting limits in the seven other duct samples collected and analyzed for this assessment. The low levels of detectable PAHs found in the duct media samples suggest that atmospheric PAHs are largely deposited as particulates onto air filter media.

Air filter media samples collected and analyzed for this preliminary assessment demonstrate that PAHs are present in ambient air at locations of residences and other building such as churches in the

Texas City area. Phenanthrene, fluoranthene, and pyrene were the most commonly detected PAHs in the air filter media samples. Phenanthrene and other PAHs are associated with petroleum refining operations and have been reported as emissions by BP at the Texas City facility.

HEALTH CONDITIONS

A study from Cape Town South Africa by White et al.[270] shows us how meteorology enters into the significance as well as those missing and location.[270]

A meteorologically derived exposure metric was calculated with the refinery as the putative point source. The study aimed to determine whether (1) asthma symptom prevalences were elevated compared to comparable areas in Cape Town and (2) whether there was an association between asthma symptom prevalences and the derived exposure metric.

The results support the hypothesis of an increased prevalence of asthma symptoms among children in the area as a result of refinery emissions and provide a substantive basis for community concern. Asthma symptoms, lung function, and markers of OS and inflammation in children exposed to oil refinery pollution are legion.

According to Rusconi et al.,[271] little is known about the effects of exposure to petroleum refinery emissions on respiratory health in children. They evaluated lung function and markers of inflammation and OS in children and adolescents with and without asthma or wheezing symptoms living in a petrochemical polluted area (Sarroch, Sardina) versus a reference area (Burcei).

Parents of 275/300 six-to-fourteen-year-old children living in Sarroch and parent of 214/323 children living in Burcei answered a questionnaire on respiratory symptoms and risk factors. Measurements of forced expiratory volume after 1 second (FEV[1]) and of forced expiratory flow rates at 25%–75% of vital capacity (FEF[25–75]) were available in 27 and 23 asthma/wheezing-positive subjects and in 7 and 54 asthma/wheezing-negative subjects in Sarroch and in Burcei, respectively; for fractional exhaled nitric oxide (FE(NO)) corresponding figures were 27 and 24 and 8 and 55 in Sarroch and in Burcei, respectively. Malondialdehyde-deoxyguanosine (MDA-dG) adduct levels in nasal mucosa were measured in 12–14-year-old adolescents (8 and 1 asthma/wheezing-positive and 20 and 28 asthma/wheezing-negative subjects in Sarroch and in Burcei, respectively). Air pollutants were assessed during 3 weeks, starting 1 week before lung function, FE(NO), and MDA-dG measurements. Generalized linear models were used to estimate the effect of the area of residence adjusting for confounders.

Weekly average concentrations of sulfur dioxide were 6.9–61.6 $\mu g/m^3$ versus 1.7–5.3 $\mu g/m^3$; and of benzene, 1.8–9.0 $\mu g/m^3$ versus 1.3–1.5 $\mu g/m^3$, respectively. Children living in Sarroch versus children living in the reference area showed an increase in wheezing symptoms (adjusted prevalence ratio = 1.70 [90% CI = 1.01; 2.86]); a decrease in lung function (variation in FEV[1] = −10.3% [90% CI = −15.0; −6.0%] and in FEF [25–75] = 123.9% (90% CI = 20.7; −4.3%)]; an increase in bronchial inflammation [variation in FE(NO) = +35% (90% CI = 11.7; 80.1%]; and an increase in MDA-dG adducts of +83% (90% CI = 22.9; 174.1%).

Data from this small study are consistent with the role of environmental pollutants on lung function and inflammation.

Meteorologically estimated exposure but not distance predicts asthma symptoms in schoolchildren in the environs of a petrochemical refinery: a cross-sectional study.

According to White et al.,[270] community concern about asthma prompted an epidemiological study of children living near a petrochemical refinery in Cape Town, South Africa.

Potential confounding factors that were controlled in the analysis included passive smoking and family atopy (reported family history of asthma or hay fever), both of which were common in this population. Distance from a major road was included as a proxy for traffic exposure.

Other potential environmental exposures could vary by area and account for higher respiratory symptoms aeroallergens. Annual monitoring of pollen counts over a period which included the study dates in both this area and a comparison suburb 10 miles away showed some differences.[271] A very strong grass pollen peak was recorded in spring, that is, after the study period, in the study area compared with the control area. The counts of certain other pollens derived from trees, weeds, and fungal spores were higher in the control area. As pollen data were not available for most of the areas covered by the 2002 ISAAC study, no inference about the role of pollen as a potential confounding factor could be drawn.

It was not possible in this study to identify which component of refinery admissions might be responsible for symptom aggravation, or alternatively whether a mixture was responsible.

Environmental monitoring of indicator pollutants has been carried out at sites near the refinery for a number of years by the local authority.[272] At the instigation of a local air monitoring task group, monthly reports were produced at the time of the study for three sites, one to the northwest of the petrochemical refinery, one to the southeast and (Bothasig), and a third moveable monitor close to the refinery (Killarney). In addition to SO_2, particles with an aerodynamic diameter <10 μm (PM_{10}), oxides of nitrogen, and hydrogen sulfide are continuously monitored.

SO_2 has long been the focus in the ongoing concern about the air pollution impact of refinery operations. The Department of Health of the City of Cape Town has been using the U.K. standards for SO_2 to report air quality since 2000,[273] particularly in the form of guideline exceedances. For example, a short-term guideline level for SO_2 of 266 μg/m³ (100 ppb) as a 15-minute mean was adopted. Mean data were available only as monthly means.

In the year of the study, SO_2 monthly means in the area averaged below 10 μg/m³ (3.75 ppb), well below the guideline annual mean SO_2 of 20 μg/m³ (8 ppb).[274] However, short-term exceedances are of greater interest. The refinery in question produced up to 18 tons per day during the year of the study. The air monitoring data for 2002, the year of the study, show 38 exceedances of the 15-minute guideline at the Killarney monitoring site closest to the refinery.[272] The highest level recorded was 605 μg/m³ (227 ppb). From the experience of year on air monitoring from 2002 onward, it has been observed that a number of these exceedances occur during operational maintenance at the refinery. Maintenance shutdowns at the petrochemical refinery have also been recorded to result in significant lowering of monthly mean SO_2 concentrations.[274]

It is thus possible that SO_2 peaks against a background of relatively low-average SO_2 concentrations might underlie the asthma symptom excess and geographic pattern noted in this study. In a recent study of asthma hospitalizations and emergency room visits among children living near two petroleum refineries in Montreal, Smargiassi et al.[275] found same-day SO_2 peaks to be a better predictor of such asthma episodes than daily SO_2 means. However, even in studies where SO_2 effects have been observed, these may be difficult to distinguish from the effects of copollutants such as particulates.[276,277] During the study year, mean monthly PM_{10} concentrations in the area averaged around 3 μg/m³ again below the guideline annual mean of 40 μg/m³.[278] Particles with an aerodynamic diameter <2.5 μm ($PM_{2.5}$ levels to be no higher in the study area than in other parts of the city).[279]

According to Smargiassi et al.,[275] this study is an extension of an ecologic study that found an increased rate of hospitalizations for respiratory conditions among children living near petroleum refineries in Montreal (Canada).

Smargiassi et al.[275] used a time-stratified case-crossover design to assess the risk of asthma episodes in relation to short-term variations in sulfur dioxide levels among children 2–4 years of age living within 0.5–7.5 km of the refinery stacks. Health data used to measure asthma episodes included ED visits and hospital admissions from 1996 to 2004. They estimated daily levels of SO_2 at the residence of children using (1) two fixed-site SO_2 monitors located near the refineries and (2) the American Meteorological Society/Environmental Protection Agency Regulatory Model (AERMOD) atmospheric dispersion model.

The risks of asthma ED visits and hospitalizations were more pronounced for same-day (lag 0) SO_2 peak levels than for mean levels on the same day, or for other lags, respectively.

Short-term episodes of increased SO_2 exposures from refinery stack emissions were associated with a higher number of asthma episodes in nearby children.

Smargiassi et al.[275] initiated this study to clarify whether higher hospital admission rates for respiratory problems for children in the east end of Montreal were related to short-term variations in refinery emissions. Their results suggest that same-day SO_2 peak levels, rather than daily mean levels, were associated with asthmatic episodes in young children who lived in close proximity to the refineries.

The first finding was that children residing in the areas around the petrochemical refinery reported a higher prevalence of asthma symptoms than children of the same age and socioeconomic status in other areas of the city. These findings are similar to those found in the La Marque and Texas City areas in the United States.

An individual's exposure to a putative point source emission is dependent on how far away they live from the source, how often the wind blows toward them from the source, and how hard the wind blows with stronger winds, resulting in greater dilution of emissions.

On theoretical grounds, this metric would be expected to perform better than simple distance from the refinery. This expectation was strongly confirmed in the study, as distance from the refinery alone was not predictive of any symptom, whereas MEE was. A similar principle of "wind adjusted distance," although a different model, was used in a case–control study of asthma attacks in children in Puerto Rico living in proximity to a number of industrial plants.[280] In that study, simple proximity to a number of the plants was predictive of asthma attacks, with wind adjustment making a difference only in the case of one plant. Nevertheless, the current study has shown that wind adjustment may make an appreciable difference to inferences about associations of symptoms with point sources.

A number of studies of children living in the vicinity of industrial and petrochemical plants have shown associations between specific pollutants or proximity to the plants and aggravation of asthma or worse respiratory health,[275,280–283] and to a lesser extent with doctor-diagnosed asthma.[281,283] Whether asthma can be caused *de novo* by typically occurring levels of ambient air pollutants is less clear.[284] If such an effect exists, it may involve interactions with airborne sensitizers.[285,286] In this study, while there was no association between MEE and reported asthma or hay fever, strong associations were found with having to take an asthma inhaler to school, frequent waking at night with wheezing, and recent sneezing at rest. The findings are thus compatible with the hypothesis that the effect of refinery emissions is to aggravate asthma.

ACTIVE AND UNCONTROLLED ASTHMA AMONG CHILDREN EXPOSED TO AIR STACK EMISSIONS OF SULFUR DIOXIDE FROM PETROLEUM REFINERIES IN MONTREAL, QUEBEC

The results of the study by Deger et al.[287] suggest that the prevalence of active asthma and poor asthma control among children living nearby in the east end of Montreal.

Results of the study by Deger et al.[287] suggest a relationship between exposure to refinery stack emissions of SO_2 and the prevalence of active and poor asthma control in children living in east-end Montreal who live and attend school in proximity to refineries.

Their results concur with those of Charpin et al.,[288] Dales et al.,[289] and Yang et al.[281] who reported an increased prevalence of respiratory symptoms in industry-polluted communities with higher levels of SO_2 compared with low-pollution areas. These results are also in agreement with studies reporting an increased prevalence of asthma[270,290,291] or asthma-related symptoms[79,270,292] among children living in proximity to industrial areas, including refineries and petrochemical plants, where SO_2 emissions occur.

The prevalence of parental atopy was quite high in this study with >60% in children with active asthma and poor control of their disease, and 33% in children without asthma.

In fact, the prevalence of declared parental atopy among immigrants was approximately one-half of that among the domestic population (North American origin).[293]

Furthermore, other studies did not find an association between proximity to areas with SO_2-emitting industrial facilities and asthma-related outcomes.[294,295] These inconsistencies may be due to the fact that most studies failed to properly classify exposure. Exposure may be better estimated with the use of dispersion modeling than by proximity to industrial facilities.

Given the multifactorial etiology of asthma, it is also possible that pollutants derived from indoor sources contribute to the aggravation of the disease. Yet, they controlled for ETS exposure in the home—the most probably confounder or effect modifier among environmental and lifestyle risk factors for asthma. Analyses controlling for the presence of reported mold or humidity in the house, as well as road traffic density on the street of the residence were also performed, with no confounders to the associations with SO_2 levels observed (data not shown).

Results of the present study suggest an association between exposure to SO_2 from refinery stack emissions and the prevalence of active and poor asthma control.

NATURAL GAS FRACKING

The recent discovery of natural gas in the United States has many people concerned about the air contamination as well as if their drinking water wells will be protected from contamination. As gas wells are drilled, eager developers propose to pump tens of thousands of gallons of chemicals into the ground to fracture the rock and stimulate the flow of gas to their wells.

These companies want to use a process hydraulic fracturing or "fracking." Fracking is an engineering technique that injects liquid (gel + sand + water + chemicals) into a well at high pressure to create cracks in deep rock. These cracks allow natural gas to flow more freely into the well.

The trouble with this type of chemical drilling is that it is exempt from many federal laws that protect public health and the environment and, for many years, the liquid contents injected into the wells have been treated as trade secrets by the industry.

Hydraulic fracturing, or fracking, wrenches open rock deep beneath the Earth's surface, freeing the natural gas that is trapped inside. Gas recovery is a game changer, a bridge to the future. The gas, primarily methane, is cheap and relatively clean.

But along with these promises have come alarming local incidents and national reports of blowouts, contamination, and earthquakes. Fracking opponents contend that the process poisons air and drinking water and may make people sick. What is more, they argue, fracking leaks methane, a potent greenhouse gas that can cause explosion in homes.

Research suggests methane leaks do happen. The millions of gallons of chemical-laden water used to fracture shale deep in the ground have spoiled land and waterways. There is also evidence linking natural gas recovery to earthquakes, but this problem seems to stem primarily from wastewater disposal rather than the fracturing process itself.

Hydraulic fracturing has been cranking up output from gas and other wells for more than 50 years. But not until fracking joined up with another existing technology, horizontal drilling, was the approach used to unlock vast stores of previously inaccessible natural gas. The real fracking boom has kicked off in just the last decade.

Conventionally drilled wells tap easy-to-get-at pockets of natural gas. Such gas heats homes and offices, fuels vehicles, and generates electricity. But as easily accessible reserves have been used up, countries seeking a steady supply of domestic energy have turned to natural gas buried in difficult-to-reach places, such as deep layers of shale.

Gas does not flow easily through shale or other impermeable rock. Drilling a conventional well into such formations would gather gas only from a small area right around the well. For shale in particular, many formations in the United States extend hundreds of kilometers across but are <100 m thick, hardly worth sending a vertical well into it.

Combining hydraulic fracturing with horizontal drilling offers a way to wrest gas from these untapped reserves. By drilling sideways into a rock formation and then sending cracks sprawling through the rock, methane can bubble into a well from a much larger area.

Today, hydraulic fracturing is used in about 9 out of 10 onshore oil and gas wells in the United States, with an estimated 11,400 new wells fractured each year. In 2010, about 23% of the natural gas consumed in the United States came from shale beds.

While the immediate output is gas, the uptick in this type of extraction has also fueled fears over fracking's potential dangers such as drinking water contamination.

One of the most explosive issues, literally, is whether fracking introduces methane into drinking water wells at levels that can make tap water flammable or can build up in confined spaces and cause home explosions.

Studies are few, but a recent analysis suggests a link. Scientists who sampled groundwater from 60 private water wells in Northeastern Pennsylvania and upstate New York found that average methane concentrations in wells near active fracturing operations were 17 times as high as in wells in inactive areas. Methane naturally exist in groundwater—in fact, the study found methane in 51 of the 60 water wells but the high levels near extracting sites were prominent.[294]

To get at where the methane was coming from, the researchers looked at the gas's carbon, which has different forms depending on where it has been. The carbon's isotopic signature, and the ratio of ethane to other hydrocarbons, suggested that methane in water wells near drilling sites did not originate from surface waters but came from deeper down. But how far down and how the methane traveled is not clear.[1118]

He proposed four possibilities. The first most contentious—the least likely—is that the extraction process opens up fissures that allow methane and other chemicals to migrate to the surface. A second possibility is that the steel tubing lining the gas well, the well casing, weakens in some way. Both scenarios would also allow briny water from the shale and fracking fluid to migrate upward. The well water analysis found no evidence of either.

Third, newly fracked gas wells could also be intersecting with old, abandoned gas or oil wells, allowing methane from those sites to migrate. Many old wells have not been shut down properly. In some places in Pennsylvania, West Virginia and elsewhere (especially those with existing coal beds), methane turned up in well water long before hydraulic fracturing became widespread.

A fourth possibility is that the cement between the well casing and the surrounding rock is not forming a proper seal. Cracking or too little cement could create a passageway, allowing methane from an intermediate layer of rock to drift into water sources near the surface. Such cases have been documented. In 2007, for example, the faulty cement seal of a fracked well in Bainbridge, Ohio, allowed gas from a shale layer above the target layer to travel into an underground drinking water source. The methane built up enough to cause an explosion in a homeowner's basement.

Accompanying these concerns are worries that methane leaking into the air will have consequences for the climate and human health. Burning methane creates fewer greenhouse gas emissions and smog ingredients than other fossil fuels; therefore, natural gas is considered relatively clean. However, evidence suggests that methane frequently escapes into the air during drilling and shipping, where it acts as a greenhouse gas and traps heat. Such leaching undermines the gas's "clean" status.

A case report occurred near Arlington, Texas where there was fracking recently. Air analyses showed high levels of methane (1800 ppb) and other hydrocarbons in both the outdoor (8000 ppb) and indoor (1000 ppb) air. In the family, all became ill with chemical sensitivity. Breath analyses showed high levels of methane and other related chemicals (900 ppb). The patients moved out of the fracking area and gradually improved until they lost their chemical sensitivity and became functional again.

Methane leaking into the air can also cause ozone to build up locally, leading to worries about headaches, inflammation, and other ills among people who live nearby.

A typical fracked well uses between 2 million and 8 million gallons of water. At the high end, it is enough to fill 12 Olympic swimming pools. Companies have their own specific mixes, but generally, water makes up about 90% of the fracking fluid. About 9% are "proppants." Stuff, that is, sand or glass beads that prop open the fissures. Other 1% consists of additives, which include chemical compounds and other materials (such as walnut hulls) that prevent bacterial growth, slow corrosion, and act as lubricants to make it easier for proponents to get into cracks.

As the gas comes out of a fracked well, a lot of this fluid comes back as waste. Until recently, many companies would not reveal the exact chemical recipes of their fluids, citing trade secrets. A report released in April 2011 by the House Energy and Commerce Committee did provide some chemical data: From 2005 to 2009, 14 major gas and oil companies used 750 different chemicals in their fracking fluids. Twenty-five of these chemicals are listed as hazardous pollutants under the Clean Air Act, 9 are regulated under the Safe Drinking Water Act, and 14 are known or possible human carcinogens, including naphthalene and benzene.

In addition to the fracking fluid, the flowback contains water from the bowels of the Earth. This "produced" water typically has a lot of salt, along with naturally occurring radioactive material, mercury, arsenic, and other heavy metals.

It is not just what you put into the well. The shale itself has chemicals, some of which are quite nasty. A report analyzing the risks associated with fracking was released by the Energy Institute.

Wastewater is dealt with different ways. Sometimes, it is stored on-site in lined pits until it is trucked off. When these pits are open to the air, they can release fumes or overflow, with possibly hazardous consequences.

The Energy Institute report cites one case in West Virginia in which about 300,000 gallons of flowback water was intentionally released into a mixed hardwood forest. Trees prematurely shed their leaves, many died over a 2-year study period, and ground vegetation suffered. In 2009, leaky joints in a pipeline carrying wastewater to a disposal site allowed more than 4000 gallons to spill into Pennsylvania's Cross Creek, killing fish and invertebrates.

For obvious ethical reasons, controlled studies exposing people to fracking fluid do not exist. And long-term population studies comparing pre- and postfracking health have not yet been done. However, these incidents and the known dangers of some of the chemicals used raise alarms about the possible consequences of human exposure.

Local geology in some areas may also allow fracking chemicals and produced water to seep up from deep below into water sources. A study published in July in the *Proceedings of the National Academy of Sciences* found a geochemical fingerprint of briny shale water in some aquifers and wells in Pennsylvania.[296] Local geology probably also played a role in fracking fluid getting into drinking water in Pavillion, Wyoming, a site that has been at the heart of the fracking controversy.

Still, several reviews of where fracking chemicals and wastewater have done harm find that the primary exposure risks relate to activities at the surface, including accidents, poor management, and illicit dumping.

An accepted disposal route is injecting the water into designated wastewater wells. However, that strategy can cause an additional problem: earthquakes. Hydraulic fracturing operations have been linked to some small earthquakes, including a magnitude 2.3 quake near Blackpool, England, last year. However, some agree such earthquakes are extremely rare, occurring when a well hits a seismic sweet spot, and are avoidable with monitoring. There were multiple quakes in a fracking area in Oklahoma in 2013.

Of greater concern is earthquakes associated with the disposal of fracking fluid into wastewater wells. Injected fluid essentially greases the fault, a long-known effect. In the 1960s, a series of Denver earthquakes was linked to wastewater disposal at the Rocky Mountain arsenal, an Army site nearby. Wastewater disposal was also blamed for a magnitude 4.0 quake in Youngstown, Ohio, 2013.

A study headed by Ellsworth[297] of the U.S. Geological Survey in Menlo Park, California, documents a dramatic increase in earthquakes in the Midwest coinciding with the start of the fracking boom.[296] From 1970 to 2000, the region experienced about 20 quakes per year measuring at or above magnitude 3.0. Between 2001 and 2008, there were 29 such quakes per year. Then, there were 50 in 2009, 87 in 2010, and 134 in 2011.[296]

However, the earthquakes were not happening near active drilling; they seemed to be clustered around wastewater wells.

It is hard to look back without prequake data and figure out what triggers a single earthquake, notes Ellsworth. There are several pieces of the geology equation that, if toggled, can tip a fault from stable to unstable.

A recent study examining seismic activity at wastewater injection wells in Texas linked earthquakes with injections of more than 150,000 barrels of water per month. However, not every case fit the pattern, suggesting the orientation of deep faults is important.

Ellsworth advises that injection at active faults be avoided. Drill sites should be considered for their geological stability, and seismic information should be collected. Only about 3% of the 75,000 odd hydraulic fracturing setups in the United States in 2009 were seismically monitored.[296]

Ultimately, unless people are willing to cut way back on their energy use, the risks associated with natural gas recovery have to be weighed against the risks that come with coal, nuclear power, and other energy sources.

FRACKING FOOTPRINT: POTENTIAL HAZARDS

1. *Blowout*: When blowout prevention equipment is absent or fails, pressurized fluid and gas can explode out of the wellhead, injuring people and spewing pollutants.
2. *Gas leak*: Methane, the primary gas in natural gas, may be present in layers of rock above the target layer. Cracks in the cement that seal the well to the surrounding rock can provide a path for this methane to travel into the water table.
3. *Air pollution*: Flare pipes that burn methane so that it does not build up, diesel truck exhaust, and emissions from wastewater evaporation can dirty the air near a drill site. When methane is released without being burned, it acts as a potent greenhouse gas, trapping 20 times as much heat as carbon dioxide.
4. *Wastewater overflow*: Fracking fluid, about 1% of which is made up of chemicals (sometimes including carcinogens), is increasingly recycled for use in other wells. However, sometimes it is stored in open pits that emit noxious fumes and can overflow with rain.
5. *Other leaks*: There are some worries that local geology in particular areas would allow fracking-produced fluid and methane to travel upward. However, most evidence of exposure stems from surface problems such as spills or illicit dumping.
6. *Home explosions*: If methane does get into the water table because of cracked cement, local geology, or the effects of old wells, it can build up in homes and lead to explosions.

GEOLOGY: DISTANT EARTHQUAKES CAN LOOSEN FAULTS NEAR GAS EXTRACTION SITES

Earthquakes near hydraulic fracturing and waste fluid injection wells in the Central United States may be being triggered by massive earthquakes thousands of miles away, according to a new study.[298]

The study notes the recent rise in the United States of small to midsized earthquakes. It points to a relationship between that rise and the increased deep underground injection of large amounts of water and wastewater for hydraulic fracturing, or fracking, for natural gas and oil.

The researchers looked at past earthquake recordings near three U.S. hydraulic fracturing injection sites. They found that pressure in faults at these sites was already approaching critical levels when major earthquakes occurred far away. The distant earthquakes triggered a rise in frequency and intensity of local tremors.[299]

The injected fluids are driving the faults to their tipping point.[298] The remote triggering by big earthquakes is an indication that the area is critically stressed and this can give future problems.

The study points to a magnitude 8.8 quakes in Chile in 2010 that sent surface waves ripping across the planet. Sixteen hours later, the powerful quake triggered a magnitude 4.1 earthquake near Prague, Oklahoma, site of several injection wells. Over the years, swarms of quakes have affected Prague as well as injection well sites in Colorado and Texas.[298]

Probably the largest quake associated with wastewater injection—a magnitude 5.7 tremor—occurred in Prague, Oklahoma in 2011. That quake destroyed 14 homes and injured 2 people.

Ellsworth states that although there is rapid growth in the worldwide use of fracturing technologies and an increase in earthquake activity, the exact relationship between the two remains unclear.[297]

The research has practical consequences. Building codes near fracturing and injection sites might need to be modified.

According to McFarland,[300] making most of our fuels and chemicals from fossil hydrocarbons is unsustainable. Proven reserves of natural gas have doubled in the last decade,[301] mainly from increase in "unconventional" gas found with shale (shale gas), coal (coal bed methane), and in low-permeability "tight" sandstones (tight gas) (Figure 1.7).

Today, as it is not easy to convert methane into heavier molecules, natural gas (composed largely of methane) is mostly burned for heating and electrical power generation, a tiny fraction is used in vehicles. Natural gas and pesticides are the number one trigger of chemical sensitivity. Cost-effective conversion of natural gas into higher-value chemical intermediates and liquid products could reduce our need for oil and help lower its shipping costs, which are higher than those of petroleum or coal on an energy-delivered basis. In addition, such processes might recover the large quantities of gas now flared or vented from fossil reservoirs.

The challenge in converting natural gas into liquids, olefins, alcohols, ethers, and other high-value products is to exploit reactions that only partially oxidize alkanes and stop short of complete combustion to CO_2. Process chemistry—including free-radical routes or catalytic partial oxidation—already allows a fraction of the heavier alkanes in natural gas (ethane, propane, and butane) to be converted into more valuable chemical products.

A single commercial plant in the Middle East uses a molybdenum-based oxide catalyst to convert very low-cost ethane to acetic acid; substantial improvements in ODH catalysts are still needed for widespread adoption.

Butadiene is the number one pollutant found in the breath analyses in many chemically sensitive patients. We do not know whether this is a natural isoprene or a synthetic one. Acetic acid is often

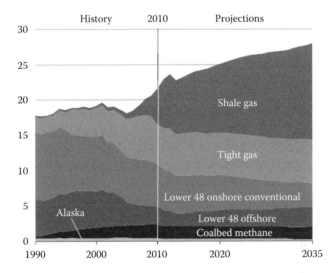

FIGURE 1.7 **(See color insert.)** Changing production sources. Worldwide, about half of the known natural gas is in "conventional," highly permeable geologic formations, often together with liquid petroleum. The other half is the "unconventional gas" found in more diffuse, low-permeability geologic formations. In the United States, convention gas production peaked in the 1990s and today represents less than half of the annual U.S. gas production. (From E.I.A, Annual Energy Outlook 2012. Report Number DOE/EIA-0383, U.S. Energy Information Administration: Washington, DC.)

the number two chemical found in a chemically sensitive patient's breath analysis. It too could be synthetic coming from ethane generation (EHC-Dallas).

Natural gas can create chemical sensitivity and humans should be cautious in their exposure and not be breathing it 24 hours a day.

OTHER INDUSTRIAL PROCESSES

Zinc, nickel, manganese, and electronics are some of the so-called clean industries' contaminates of outside air. Also computers, electronics, and electrical industries come in this category. Many put out nanoparticles of ultrafine particles which over time can bother the normal population and especially the chemically sensitive and high manganese levels are often found in the chemically sensitive patient at the EHC-Dallas, which usually triggers their chemical sensitivity but at times may cause it.

Occupational lung diseases are caused by repeated, long-term exposures or a single, severe exposure to harmful particles, especially nanoparticles <200 μm chemicals, vapors, or gases. This wide spectrum of diseases incorporates a variety of interstitial lung diseases as well as inflammatory airway diseases. Neurovascular degenerative disease also occurs frequently. We often see small vessel vasculitis in these chemically sensitive patients.

The committee of The American Thoracic Society reported that there is strong evidence for occupational exposures as a nonsmoking cause of COPD.[302] A recent review puts the population attributable risk percent linked to occupational exposure-associated COPD at ~15%.[302] Furthermore, several other work-related airway disorders have been identified, such as occupational asthma, chronic bronchitis, and "asthma-like disorders"[302] as well as neurovascular problems.

Numerous inorganic/organic dusts, gases, and pollutants have been shown to contribute to the development of these airway and neurovascular ailments. In addition, close to 3 billion people (one-half the world's population) still rely on biomass fuels for cooking and heating in poorly ventilated houses, with known health consequences, such as acute respiratory infections, asthma, COPD, and lung cancer.[302] Biomass-induced histopathological lung changes, in terms of inflammatory cell recruitment and septum thickening, have also been seen in young children at autopsy.[302]

High-tech industry of electronics is also a problem because of its use of plaster, glue, and especially electromagnetic pollutant generators. These can cause not only nasal sinus and respiratory dysfunction but also neurovascular dysfunction. Neurodegenerative disease like PD, Alzheimer's, ALS, and multiple sclerosis are some of the most prominent problems. Zinc is prominent but not so harmful, whereas nickel is a highly sensitizing agent. Nickel accounts for one-third of the sensitivities in the titanium alloys found in metal implants at the EHC-Dallas. Electronics is famous for their general fatigue and short-term memory degeneration.

MANGANESE

Manganese causes impaired dopaminergic, glutameteric, GABAergic transmission.

Manganese is a trace mineral that is present in tiny amounts in the body. It is found mostly in bones, liver, kidneys, and pancreas. Manganese helps the body form connective tissue, bones, blood-clotting factors, and sex hormones. It also plays a role in fat and carbohydrate metabolism, calcium absorption, and blood sugar regulation. Manganese is also necessary for normal brain and nerve function and can be an outlier in chemical sensitivity.

Manganese is a component of the antioxidant enzyme superoxide dismutase (SOD), which helps fight free radicals. Free radicals occur naturally in the body but can damage cell membranes and DNA. They may play a role in aging, as well as the development of a number of health conditions, including heart disease and cancer. Antioxidants, such as SOD, can help neutralize free radicals and reduce or even help prevent some of the damage they cause.

Low levels of manganese in the body can contribute to infertility, bone malformation, weakness, and seizures. It is fairly easy to get enough manganese in the diet as this nutrient is found in whole grains, nuts, and seeds but some experts estimate that as many as 37% of the Americans do not get the recommended dietary intake (RDI) of manganese in their diet.

The American diet tends to contain more refined grains than whole grains, and refined grains only provide half the amount of manganese as whole grains.

However, too much manganese in the diet could lead to high levels of manganese in the body tissues. Abnormal concentrations of manganese in the brain, especially in the basal ganglia, are associated with neurological disorders similar to, including chemical sensitivity, PD. Early-life manganese exposure at high levels, or low levels, may impact neurodevelopment. Elevated manganese is also associated with poor cognitive performance in schoolchildren.

METAL EMISSIONS AND URBAN INCIDENT PD: A COMMUNITY HEALTH STUDY OF MEDICARE BENEFICIARIES BY USING GEOGRAPHIC INFORMATION SYSTEMS

PD associated with farming and exposure to agricultural chemicals has been reported in numerous studies; little is known about PD risk factors for those living in urban areas. The authors investigated the relation between copper, lead, or manganese emissions and PD incidence in the urban United States, studying 29 million Medicare beneficiaries in 2003. PD incidence was determined by using beneficiaries who had not changed residence since 1995. Over 35,000 nonmobile incident PD cases, diagnosed by a neurologist, were identified for analysis. Age-, race-, and sex-standardized PD incidence was compared between counties with high cumulative industrial release of copper, manganese, or lead (as reported to the EPA) and counties with no/low reported release of all three metals. PD incidence in counties with no/low copper/lead/manganese release was 274.0 (95% CI: 226.8, 353.5). Incidence was greater in counties with high manganese release: 489.4 (95% CI: 368.3, 689.5) (relative risk [RR] = 1.78%, 95% CI: 1.54, 2.07) and counties with high copper release 304.2 (95% CI: 276.0, 336.8) (RR = 1.1%, 95% CI: 0.94, 1.31). Urban PD incidence is greater in counties with high-reported industrial release of copper or manganese. Environmental exposure to metals may be a risk factor for PD in urban areas. Certainly, PD has an environmentally triggered etiology.

Although essential, Mn is toxic at high concentrations. Mn neurotoxicity has been attributed to impaired dopaminergic (DAergic), glutamatergic, and GABAergic transmission, mitochondrial dysfunction (MD), OS, and neuroinflammation. As a result of preferential accumulation of Mn in the DAergic cells of the basal ganglia, particularly the globus pallidus, Mn toxicity causes extrapyramidal motor dysfunction. First, described as "manganism" in miners during the nineteenth century, this movement disorder resembles PD characterized by hypokinesia and postural instability. To date, a variety of acquired causes of brain Mn accumulation can be distinguished from an autosomal recessively inherited disorder of Mn metabolism caused by mutations in the SLC30A10 gene. Both, acquired and inherited hypermanganesemia, lead to Mn deposition in the basal ganglia associated with pathognomonic magnetic resonance imaging appearances of hyperintense basal ganglia on T1-weighted images. Current treatment strategies for Mn toxicity combine chelation therapy to reduce the body Mn load and iron (Fe) supplementation to reduce Mn binding to proteins that interact with both Mn and Fe.

Dystonia with brain manganese accumulation resulting from SLC30A10 mutations, a new treatable disorder, occurs according to Stamelou et al.[303]

Stamelou et al.[303] wishes to highlight this rare disorder, which, together with Wilson's disease, is the only potentially treatable inherited metal storage disorder to date, that otherwise can be fatal as a result of complications of cirrhosis.[304]

Mutations in SLC30A10 cause parkinsonism and dystonia with hypermanganesemia, polycythemia, and chronic liver disease according to Quadri et al.[304]

Chelation therapy can normalize the manganesemia, leading to marked clinical improvements. In conclusion, they show that SLC30A10 mutations cause a treatable recessive disease with pleomorphic phenotype, and provide compelling evidence that SLC30A10 plays a pivotal role in manganese transport. This work has broad implications for understanding of the manganese biology and pathophysiology in multiple human organs.

Syndrome of hepatic cirrhosis, dystonia, polycythemia, and hypermanganesemia caused by mutations in SlC30A10, a manganese transporter in man according to Tuschi et al.[305]

TOLL-LIKE RECEPTORS: ZINC AND NICKEL

Crucial role of TLRs in the zinc/nickel-induced inflammatory response occur in vascular endothelial cells. There is a zinc-induced inflammatory response in both vascular endothelial cells and promonocytes. Following screening of 15 metals, zinc and nickel were identified with a marked proinflammatory effect, as determined by ICAM-1 and IL-8 induction, on human umbilical vein endothelial cells (HUVECs).

Accumulation of zinc, nickel, lead, and cadmium occurs in some organs of rabbits after dietary nickel and zinc inclusion according to Kalafova et al.[306]

This study reports the effect of dietary nickel (Ni) and a combination of Ni and zinc (Zn) on the accumulation of lead (Pb), cadmium (Cd), Ni and Zn in muscles, liver, and kidneys of rabbits. Zn addition of 30 g to the diet caused an increase of Cd level in the kidney as well as in the liver. Ni and Zn treatment caused a significant decrease of Pb accumulation in the M. longissimus dorsi of rabbits. This study indicates that dietary inclusion of Ni and Zn caused specific interactions among the observed metals.

The content of cadmium, cobalt, and nickel in laryngeal carcinoma according to Janusz et al.[307] was found. The study was conducted on 43 patients with laryngeal carcinoma.

The imbalance in the level of nickel, cadmium, and cobalt in laryngeal cancer may be due to a changed cellular metabolism in the cancer process. However, the results of this study reveal the significant differences in the concentration of these metals between patients from urban and rural areas, which suggest that this fact may be related to environmental or occupational factors and therefore it requires further study.

On the other hand, cobalt (Co) is an essential trace element as a constituent of vitamin B_{12} (cyanocobalamin) and its deficiency results in anemia. However, different compounds of Co are also described as highly toxic and/or radiotoxic for individuals or the environment. The underlying mechanism of cobalt toxicity is not clearly established. According to Gault et al., the toxicity of Co(II) and or irradiation arises from production of reactive oxygen species.[308]

ROUTES OF NICKEL EXPOSURE

Air

Mean ambient air concentrations of nickel typically range between 6 and 20 ng/m³ and can be as high as 150 ng/m³ near anthropogenic sources of airborne nickel.[309] Schroeder et al.[310] reported nickel concentrations in PM in the U.S. atmosphere of 0.01–60, 0.6–78, and 1–328 ng/m³ in remote, rural, and urban areas, respectively. Nickel concentrations in PM ($PM_{2.5–8}$), collected in Spokane, Washington, from January 1995 to March 1999, averaged 1.2 ± 0.0 (1 SD) ng/m³.[311] The five states with the highest average concentrations of nickel in ambient air were (ng/m³): West Virginia (6.60), Utah (4.42), Delaware (4.10), New York (3.80), and Pennsylvania (3.69); the five states with the lowest concentrations were: Wyoming (0.127), South Dakota (0.157), North Dakota (0.211), Montana (0.311), and Vermont (0.311).

The results for Washington, DC, are in basic agreement with the results obtained from Kowalczyk et al.[312] In this study, 24-hour samples collected at 10 locations yielded average nickel concentrations ranging from 5.7 to 35 ng/m³, with a mean concentration of 17 ng/m³. The two major contributing sources are believed to be oil and coal combustion.

Nickel resulting from oil combustion is primarily nickel sulfate with lesser amounts of complex metal oxides and nickel oxide. Approximately 90% of nickel in fly ash from coal combustion consists of complex (primarily iron) oxides. Nickel silicate and iron–nickel oxides would be expected from the mining and smelting of lateritic nickel ore, whereas nickel matte refining would produce nickel subsulfide and metallic nickel. The primary nickel species from secondary nickel smelting and steel and nickel alloys production is iron–nickel oxide.

Dusts from power plants had a silicate characteristic with quartz and mullite predominant. Approximately 90% of the nickel from these facilities was in the residual fraction. Only 40%–60% of the nickel from metallurgical, chemical, and cement plants was in the residual fraction. Essentially none of the nickel from any of the industries was in an organic/sulfidic fraction. Dusts from metallurgical, chemical, and cement plants contained between 0% and 10% (typically 5%) of the nickel in the relatively mobile, cation-exchangeable fraction. Thirty percent of the nickel in dust from a slag processing facility was in this form.

See Chapter 5 on inorganics for detection.

FOREST AND GRASS FIRES AND OTHER NATURAL POLLUTANTS

WOOD FIRES

Often, forest and grass fires occur throughout the Southwest and Western United States and other parts of the world as just occurred in Washington State and Idaho and other western states in 2013 and 2014.[313] When they occur topographically, these can be devastating to the chemically sensitive patient who often has to move out of the area. Forest fires have three stages that bother the chemically sensitive. The first is the fire heat, the second is the solidified organic residue, and the third is the actual PM from smoke that occurs initially. Then when the fire is out, the remaining particulates, from the charred wood, grass, and carbon particulates, can cause nasal sinus, and respiratory dysfunction secondarily causes dysfunction of the cardiovascular and neurovascular systems. Some particles can damage the peripheral and central nervous systems. A litany of severe fires has occurred around the world.

In Asia, many fires have occurred. For example, in China, 1987—The Black Dragon fire burned a total of 72,884 km^2 (28,141 mi^2) of forest along the Amur River, and 3 million acres (4687.5 mi^2) were destroyed on the Chinese side.[314]

Indonesia

Forest fires in Indonesia occur annually. When there is a weather pattern disturbance because of strong El Nino, the number and the distribution of forest fires in Indonesia increased significantly. When there is a weather pattern disturbance because of strong La Nina, the number and the distribution of forest fire in Indonesia decreased. An El Nino is usually followed by La Nina on the following year. The strength of disturbance is determined by Southern Oscillation Index.

From 1982 and 1983, in massive forest fires in Kalimantan and East Sumatra, 36,000 km^2 (14,000 mi^2) of forest burned down. There were other forest fires in Java and Sulawesi in the same year. In 1987, 1991, and 1994, there were large-scale forest fires in Kalimantan and East Sumatra, Java, and Sulawesi in Indonesia. More than 3300 km^2 (1300 mi^2) of forest were destroyed by forest fire. From 1997 and 1998, in unprecedented forest fires in Kalimantan and East Sumatra, 97,000 km^2 (37,000 mi^2) of forest were destroyed, and >2.6 gigatonnes of CO$_2$ was released to the atmosphere. The underground smoldering fire on the *peat bogs* continues to burn and ignite new forest fires each year during dry season. There are other forest fires in Java and Sulawesi in the same year. From 1999 to 2005, there were annual forest fires in Boc Choi, Samatra, Java, and Sulawesi. Every year, the forest is burned by farmers and plantation owners and there is a continuous underground fire (since 1997). About 1345 km^2 (519 mi^2) of forest was destroyed by forest fire.

Japan

On April 27, 1971, 340 ha (840 acres) was lost in a forest fire at Kire, Western Honshu, Japan. Construction workers were using fire in order to wither weeds when a strong wind moved through the area, fueling the fire; 18 firefighters were killed. The fire lasted for one day.

Israel

The Mount Carmel forest fire in Israel, started on December 2, 2010 and burned 41 km² of forest, killing as many as 44 people, most of them Israel Prison Service officer cadets, who were on a bus evacuation and were trapped in flames.

South Korea

Gangwon-do Gangneung—2000 Gangwon Wildfire, 2013—Gyeongsangbukdo Pohang Wildfire.

Australia

Black Thursday bushfires of 1851 (Victoria), Black Friday bushfires of 1939 (Victoria), Black Sunday bushfires of 1955 (South Australia), 1961 Western Australian bushfires, 1967 Tasmanian fires, Ash Wednesday fires of 1980 and 1983 (Victoria and South Australia), 1994 Eastern seaboard fires, Black Christmas (bushfires) 2001–2002, Canberra bushfires of 2003, Black Tuesday bushfires of 2005 (Eyre Peninsula South Australia, Mount Lubra bushfire of 2006, Black Saturday bushfires of 2009—the deadliest bushfire event ever recorded in Australian history.

Europe

Germany: In the fire of the Luneburg Heath in Lower Saxony in August 1973, 74.18 km² (28.64 mi²) of heathland burned, killing firefighters.

Greece: Penteli Fire in the Penteli mountains which was in June and July, 1995 lasted for almost the entire weekend starting on Friday. In 1998, forest fires in Greece, a series of forest fires affected the Athens area, Avlona, Taygetus, and Olympus mountains and other places. The fire began in the beginning of the summer season. In 2000, forest fires in Greece, a series of forest fires affected Greece including Agioi Theodoroi and Eastern Corinthia at the beginning of July 2000. In 2005, East Attica Fire in Greece—Forest fires ravaged East Attica on July 28, 2005 from Agia Triada Rafinas to west of Rafina. The first began at around 11:00 (EET/UTC +3) consuming 70 km² of forests, properties, and farmlands. The fire spread quickly after a few hours with winds of up to 55–70 km/hour and spread near the suburban housings of Athens near Rafina area mostly on the hillside areas. Pine trees were devastated. On July 29, 2005, a day after the enormous Attica fire, another series of fires occurred throughout Greece entirely in Preveza, including Morrolithi, consuming properties and a campground, Ioannina and Xiromeni of Aerolia–Acamania. 2007 Greek forest fires, 2012 Chios forest fire.

Italy and France: 200 fires in Southern Europe in July 2000 consumed forests and buildings in Southern France, parts of Iberia, Corsica, and most of Italy, including the southern part during the heat wave that dominated Southern Europe with 40–43°C temperatures and caused the fire phenomena.

Poland: The Kuznia Raciborska fire in Poland burned 90.62 km² of forest and killed two firefighters on August 26, 1992. A third casualty is also mentioned but she did not die in the fire; she was involved in a collision with a fire engine that skidded.

Portugal: August 2003—Wildfires in August 2003.

Russia and Soviet Union: 1921 Mari wildfires, August 1935—Kursha-2 settlement was burned with 1200 victims. June–August 2010—drought and the hottest summer since records at drought began in 1890 cause that many devastating forest fires in European Russia.

Spain: July 17, 2005—Guadalajara province, Spain, a 130-km² forest fire and 11 dead firefighters. The fire brigade unit is not out of post because of this deadly toil. A barbecue sparked deadly blazes.

North America

There have been many fires in Canada and the United States. Table 1.18 shows a list of early devastating fires in our hemisphere.

OTHER NATURAL POLLUTANTS

Methane gas emanating from marshes and the earth make up 70% of the natural nonfire pollution and terpenes, which molecularly mimic toxic chemicals, emanate from pine, cedar, juniper, mesquite, other conifers, and many bushes and grasses and make up 29% of the natural air pollution.

Curiously, while this mound is basically adjacent to the onshore Los Angeles Basin, which is one of the best-known Cenozoic basins along the California coast for its prolific oil production, the methane emanating from the mound crest mound appears to be microbial in origin, based on the conventional interpretation of the C_1/C_2 (34,000) and δ^{13} values. Methane is the number one trigger of chemical sensitivity in our series, usually from indoor gas heat but also can be from outdoor amenities.

Numerous workers have been injured by inhalation of various fumes such as nitric acid fumes causing bronchiolitis obliterans[315] and also from house fires[316] with hydrogen cyanide gas causing toxicity from the burning of furniture and building material, with the use of polymers and antimony in combination with halogens used as flame retardents.[317] Acute inhalation also occurs.[317]

Bronchiolitis Obliterans Organizing Pneumonia Following Nitric Acid Fumes after a Fire Exposure

Lee et al.[318] describe a patient with clinical, radiological, and pathological features of bronchiolitis obliterans and organizing peneumonia.[318]

Erythema Nodosum after Smoke Inhalation-Induced Bronchiolitis Obliterans Organizing Pneumonia

Srivastava et al.[315] report the case of a lady who developed bronchiolitis obliterans organizing pneumonia and erythema nodosum simultaneously, several weeks after smoke inhalation in a house fire.[315]

Toxic Smoke Inhalation: Cyanide Poisoning in Fire Victims

According to Jones et al.,[319] the most common cause of death in fires is the inhalation of noxious gases rather than thermal injury.[319] During the first 4 months of 1986, toxic amounts of cyanide were found in four of six fatalities from house fires in Akron, Ohio.[320] These cases illustrate the increasing frequency of cyanide poisoning in household fires. Sources of cyanide toxicity include the increased use of synthetic polymers in building materials and furnishings. Survivors can be prone to chemical sensitivity and chronic degenerative disorder.

Antimony Toxicity in Firefighters: Florida, 2009

Antimony oxides, in combination with halogens, have been used as flame retardants in textiles since the 1960s. Uniforms made from fabric containing antimony are common among the estimated 1.1 million firefighters in the United States. In 2008, an outbreak of antimony toxicity among 30 firefighters who had elevated antimony levels was detected in hair samples. In February 2009, CDC administered questionnaires and collected urine samples from two groups of firefighters: 20 firefighters from the fire department showed elevated levels of antimony.

According to Stafanidou and Athanaselis,[321] most fatalities from fires are not due to burns, but are a result of inhalation of toxic gases produced during combustion.[321] Fire produces a complex toxic environment, involving flame, heat, oxygen depletion, smoke, and toxic gases. As a wide variety of synthetic materials is used in building (insulation, furniture, carpeting, electric wiring covering, decorative items), the potential for poisoning from inhalation of products of combustion is continuously increasing. The incidence of chemically sensitivity and chronic degenerative disorder increases.

Inhalation of Products of Combustion

According to Cohen and Guzzardi,[317] the atmosphere of fire is deadly to breathe. Firefighters or building occupants may be victims of the heat, irritating smoke, depleted oxygen, carbon monoxide, and such other toxic gases as cyanide, hydrogen chloride, and acrolein. Increasing numbers of homes and public building are being built and furnished with highly flammable synthetic materials that give off copious smoke and toxic gases when burned. Whether or not there are cutaneous burns, the possibility of inhalation injury must be considered in any fire victim. All victims of a fire environment should be presumed to have CO intoxication and should be treated with 100% oxygen until the HbCO level is within normal limits. In an extreme situation, cyanide intoxication should be suspected and administration of sodium thiosulfate may be lifesaving. Upper airway occlusion may result from thermal damage or edema secondary to burns from soluble toxic gases. Chemical injury to the lower airway and alveoli may result from inhalation of insoluble irritant gases and toxic gases adsorbed on carbon particles. Upper respiratory tract obstruction may be suggested by the clinical presentation (e.g., pharyngeal burns, stridor, hoarseness, dysphagia), but only by means of fiber-optic bronchoscopy can it be recognized or excluded with certainty. Intubation may be necessary. Lower respiratory tract injury may be manifested clinically by dyspneas, wheezing, and chest tightness, as well as by hypoxemia and reduced FEV(1) and FVC. Treatment is symptomatic, but close observation for progressive respiratory insufficiency is necessary.

According to Megahed et al.,[316] inhalation injury greatly increases the incidence of respiratory failure and the acute respiratory distress syndrome.[316] This study included 130 burn patients with inhalation injury admitted to Menoufiya University Hospital Burn Center, Egypt, from January 2004 to April 2008 (61 males and 69 females). They found that the presence of inhalation injury, increasing burn size, and advancing age were all associated with increased mortality ($p < 0.01$). The incidence of inhalation injury in their study was 4.3% (130 patients were identified as having inhalation injury out of 281). The overall mortality for patients with inhalation injury was 41.5% (54 patients out of 130) compared with 7.2% (11 patients out of 151) for patients without inhalation injury. These statistical data make it clear that inhalation injury is an important factor for the prediction of mortality in burn patients. Approximately 80% of the fire-related deaths are not due to the burn injury to the airway but due to the inhalation of toxic products, especially carbon monoxide and hydrogen cyanide gases. Inhalation injury is generally caused by thermal burns, mostly confined to the upper airways. Major airway, pulmonary, and systemic complications may occur in cases of inhalation injury and thus increase the incidence of burn patient mortality.

According to Heimbach and Waeckerie,[322] inhalation injuries occur in approximately one-third of all major burns and account for a significant number of deaths in those burn patients each year.[322] Victims die as a result of carbon monoxide poisoning, hypoxia, and smoke inhalation. These deaths can occur without thermal wounds as well as with burn injuries. However, many survive who have residual problems like chemical sensitivity and chronic degenerative disorder.

Thermal burns occurring in the upper airway are usually manifested within 48 hours of injury. Diagnosis is made by direct visualization of the upper airway, looking for signs of thermal injury. Admission for observation with humidified oxygen, attentive pulmonary toilet, bronchodilators as needed, and prophylactic endotracheal intubation as indicated are the mainstays of treatment. Resolution of the injury usually occurs within days. Carbon monoxide poisoning, the most common cause of death in inhalation injury is a result of combustion. Symptoms and signs correlate with blood levels, but arterial blood gases are used to determine the degree of carbon monoxide intoxication. Treatment is based on the principle that carbon monoxide dissociation occurs much faster if the patient is placed on 100% oxygen. The use of oxygen therapy 4.8 L/minute is often necessary for those who develop chemical sensitivity. Occasionally, the patient's symptoms may persist or get worse despite adequate treatment. Smoke inhalation significantly damages normal respiratory physiology, resulting in injury progressing from acute pulmonary insufficiency to pulmonary edema to bronchopneumonia, depending on the severity of exposure. Diagnosis is based on history, but clinical finds, arterial blood gases, and fiber-optic bronchoscopy are helpful; especially, PvO_2 is useful to define the state of oxygen extraction. Treatment is supportive with careful attention paid to fluid resuscitation in the patient with burns.

Toxic Leukoencephalopathy with Atypical MRI Features Following a Lacquer Thinner Fire

Toxic leukoencephalopathy is a structural alteration of the white matter following exposure to various toxic agents. Kao et al.[323] report a 49-year-old man exposed to an explosion of lacquer thinner with brain MRI features atypical from those of chronic toxic solvent intoxication.[323]

People have lived for tens of thousands of years in the presence of smoke from fires. That long period of adaptation tends to allow healthy younger adults in today's environments to be generally resistant to serious adverse health effects from smoke from sources such as wildfires, prescribed forest burns, agricultural field burns, and peat bog fires. This is not true for the chemically sensitive or CDD patients.

But a high percentage of people are not young, healthy adults. In the United States, nearly half of the population suffers from at least one chronic illness,[324] potentially placing them at risk for adverse effects from exposure to fire smoke. Children and older adults also are considered more vulnerable to smoke's effects.[325] The limited health research that is been carried out on smoke from large-scale fires has provided some refinements to these general categories of vulnerable people, and new information occasionally emerges. There also has been a trickle of information identifying the toxic substances that characterize smoke from various kinds of fires, and pinning down the specific body systems that are vulnerable and the pathways through which damage occurs.

The annual acreage burned is expected to increase to about 10–12 million acres within just a few years.[326] Among the areas expected to face the greatest increase in fire threats are the Southeast, Southwest, and West, although the Midwest and East also are expected to experience some increases.

Historically, people have caused most wildfires. Of the 63,591–96,386 fires that occurred each year from 2001 to 2010%, 89%–90% were human caused in any given year.[327] For acreage burned, lightning often plays a much bigger role; when lightning fires strike at country areas, they are more often allowed to burn. However, people still were the ignition source for 12%–65% of the acreage burned in any of those years.[327] Among the human causes of fires are arson, accidents, carelessness, and intentionally prescribed fires designed to reduce acute threats or remove vegetation for planning, wildlife management, or other purposes.

Buildings and other structures usually contain plastic materials and various stored chemicals, pesticides, insecticides, paint, solvents, cleaning solutions, etc. that release extremely toxic substances when burned. This can represent a significant source of toxic air pollutants in certain areas.

Globally, forest wildfire statistics are very scarce. In 2010, hard data were available for less than half the world's countries and only about three-fourths of the world's forests.[328] In a word, consistent methods and reporting make it impossible to determine realistic total numbers of fires and acreage burned for any given year, or to detect trends. However, it is clear from global satellite images that significant fires in all types of vegetation occur multiple times every year in all continents except Antarctica.[329] The percentage of these fires that are caused by humans is considered to be roughly 90%–95%.[330]

Although hard global data are not available, researchers have used models and satellite images to calculate that fires in grasslands and savannas account for 44% of the fire-derived carbon emissions, with 20% from tropical deforestation and degradation fires, 16% from tropical woodland fires, 15% from fires in forests outside the tropics, 3% from agricultural field burning, and 2% from peat fires.[331]

A global picture is also emerging for what are being termed "megafires."[331] The authors said that the megafire label applies when a burn cannot be controlled by people without the help of natural forces such as rain, and it causes significant long-lasting effects on an area's environment and social and economic structure. Prime examples covered in some detail in the report include fires in Australia (2009), Botswana (2008), Brazil (1998), Greece (2007), Indonesia (1997/198), Israel (2010), Russia (2010), and the United States (2003).

Other megafires have occurred in other years in some of these countries as well as in countries such as Canada, China, South Africa, Portugal, Spain, and Turkey. All were fueled in part by over-zealous fire suppression or land practices that substantially altered the more fire-resistant natural vegetation mosaic and allowed fuels to accumulate.[330] Drought and "extreme fire weather" (i.e., low humidity and high temperature combined with high winds) increased the hazard, and people almost always were the final straw, acting as the match in one way or another. Should these preventable fires increase as projected,[328] their size and inability to be controlled will escalate the number of people exposed to toxic smoke and the length of time they are at risk.

Smoke changes as it travels, and the PM might pose greater risk when it is closer to the source. Anytime that smoke results in elevated PM, it has health effects.[330] The chemically sensitive are much more prone to smoke injury.

Smoke can contain thousands of individual compounds, in categories such as PM, hydrocarbons and other organic chemicals, nitrogen oxides, trace minerals, carbon monoxide, carbon dioxide, and water vapor.[330] As just one example of the elements in a complex mix, a 2009 fire in a mixed-evergreen forest in Central Portugal generated emissions that included degradation products from biopolymers (such as levoglucosan from cellulose and methoxyphenols from lignin), n-alkanes, n-alkenes, n-alkanoic acids, n-alkanols, monosaccharide derivatives from cellulose, steroid, and terpenoid biomarkers, PAHs (with retene being the most abundant), and even-carbon-number homologs of monoglycerides (which the authors said were identified for the first time as biomarkers in biomass burning aerosols).[333] Many of these substances can trigger the chemical sensitivity. Often, they become sensitive to the terpenoid and aromatic hydrocarbons (Chapters 6 and 9).

Woodsmoke exposure may depress the respiratory immune defenses[334] and has been linked with ED visits for upper and lower respiratory effects.[335] The evidence regarding cardiovascular effects has been mixed, but recent research is reinforcing these health issues as a possible area of concern, though sometimes only for certain categories of people in any given study.[226,336–340] We see many of the chemicals emanating from fires that triggers chemically sensitivity and chronic degenerative disorder.

Other populations that might be vulnerable and deserve greater study include diabetics, fetuses, people with cystic fibrosis and primary pulmonary hypertension, and those carrying certain genetic polymorphisms.

Refinements to this information are surfacing as studies trickle out. For instance, a study of bushfires in the Darwin, Australia area in 2000, 2004, and 2005 found that indigenous people were significantly more vulnerable to a range of respiratory disorders, and had a statistically significant increase in hospital emissions for ischemic heart disease 3 days after initial exposure to smoke in relation to each 10-μg/m^3 increase in PM$_{10}$.[339] The patients may have been at greater risk than others in the area because of greater underlying cardiorespiratory problems.

According to Johnston et al.,[339] a severe smoke pollution event were to affect an indigenous community, the health outcomes are likely to be more serious, and public health officials would need to consider this when planning their responses.[339]

In an investigation of wildfires in Central and Northern California in 2008, it was found the PM collected in the city of Tracy over 2 days at the peak of the fires was about 10 times more damaging to alveolar macrophages than ambient PM collected in the area under normal conditions, on an equal-dose basis.[341] In California's Central Valley, another team of researchers investigated differences between air in an urban area, Fresno, and near a wildfire about 100 miles to the northwest near Escalon.[327] PM from each area induced very different inflammatory, OS, and xenobiotic responses in human bronchial epithelial cells, providing further evidence that it is probably inappropriate to simply extrapolate findings on urban pollution to wildfire pollution. However, it has been observed that fire smoke can trigger chemical sensitivity symptoms and signs and at times induce the chemical sensitivity.

However, urban air and wildfire smoke can have one thing in common, isocyanic acid, which was recently identified for the first time in outdoor air in each of these settings.[340] The limited information available indicates the acid could plausibly contribute to cardiovascular problems and inflammation, although effects at the concentrations present in wildfire smoke have yet to be observed.

Much more is generally known about the health risks posed by ground-level ozone, and a recent study indicates wildfires in Western United States can help spark the formation of the toxic substance, increasing ambient ozone by up to 50 ppb for a short period of time and potentially traveling long distances.[342] Such bursts of ozone could cause affected areas to exceed the current federal 8-hour ozone standard of 75 ppb[335]

In addition to polluting the air, wildfires can affect soil and water quality. In a study following fires in 2005 and 2006 in three watersheds in Southern California, researchers found that organic or particulate-bound mercury in surface soils can be more readily deposited in waterways after a fire.[335] Awareness of that tendency could lead to actions such as better testing of fish in affected waterways or improved sampling for water quality if the waterways are a drinking water source. However, it appears that this phenomenon may depend on local soils, vegetation, waterways, and weather because an analysis of 146 sites in Minnesota that had burned sometime between 1759 and 2004 found intense fires had reduced soil mercury concentrations for tens, even hundreds, of years.[343] In contrast, such reductions lasted only a year or so in the California settings.[344]

The U.S. Federal, state, and other agencies have conducted prescribed burns on about 2.2 million acres per year in the past decade.[345] Prescribed fires are also widely used globally, though hard data are scant.

Research on the health effects of prescribed burns is very limited. In a study of South Carolina prescribed fires, it was found that plots in which the vegetation had been mechanically chipped in advance of burning emitted significantly less PM and carbon monoxide than nonchipped plots.[346] The authors said this has implications for both firefighters and nearby communities. In Georgia, another team found emissions of most VOCs were much higher during the smoldering phase of prescribed fires in pine forests compared with the flaming phase.[347] They also found emissions of several pinene compounds from prescribed fires were much higher than those from fireplace wood-burning. The α- and β-pinenes have been found to trigger chemical sensitivity when challenged at the EHC-Dallas in hundreds of patients.

A study of prescribed burns in Arizona ponderosa pine forests found the emissions, which included PM, PAHs OC, elemental carbon, potassium, chlorine, sulfur, and silicon, were characteristic of smoldering, low-intensity burns.[348] On the basis of the information in this and other studies, Robinson[347] would argue that the biggest health effects associated with prescribed burns are short term and involve susceptible individuals like the chemically sensitive living in neighboring communities.[347]

Problems could be significant in some settings, though. Another study of the Darwin, Australia area found that when PM_{10} from fires (many of which were prescribed burns) exceeded 40 $\mu g/m^3$, ED admissions for asthma increased sharply.[348] That concentration is far below the current 24-hour standard of 150 $\mu g/m^3$ established by the U.S. EPA[349] and even the level of 65–75 $\mu g/m^3$ recommended in September 2010 by the agency's Clean Air Scientific Advisory Committee.[350] Other researchers report that smoke from prescribed fires in Australian bushlands contained acrolein, formaldehyde, and carbon monoxide at levels of concern.[351] Formaldehyde has been found to be the number three trigger of chemical sensitivity after pesticides and methane gas.

A large June 2008 peat bog fire in North Carolina that burned about 6 weeks generated smoke affecting significant portions of the state. The fire, smoldering in peat 3–15 ft deep, had a poor oxygen supply and generated extensive smoke due to incomplete combustion. There were periods of $PM_{2.5}$ concentration greater that 200 $\mu g/m^3$ at ground-based monitors 200 km from the fire.[226] The composition of peat fire emissions is known to differ substantially from forest fires, but the relative toxicity of these emissions is unknown. However, Mueller[342] points out that low-temperature or smoldering combustion such as that associated with peat fires (and fireplaces) is notorious for emitting high amounts of carbon monoxide.[342]

Whatever the specific toxic substances were, researchers studying cardiopulmonary-related ED visits associated with the 2008 peat bog fire found a 37% relative increase in heart failure (traits of the population studied, such as low income and high prevalence of health problems such as hypertension, diabetes, ischemic heart disease, and heart failure, may have contributed to susceptibility).[226] They also reported increases in ED visits for COPD (73% increase), asthma (65% increase), and pneumonia and acute bronchitis (59% increase).[226] Major peat fires were burning once again in North Carolina throughout late spring and summer of 2011.[352–354]

In agricultural fields, burning residue is a worldwide practice. It is done to kill pests, improve fertilization (by increasing nitrogen availability), and making planting easier, often at a lower cost than some other options such as mechanical tilling. Regions with the highest activity included the Russian Federation, Eastern Europe, and Central Asia.

In the United States, field burning averaged 43% of the equivalent area burned by wildfires from 2003 to 2007 and peaked at 79% of the equivalent area in 2003.[355] Field burning is a source of pollutants such as fine and coarse PM, nitrogen dioxide, sulfur dioxide, carbon monoxide, and methane.[356] The states with the highest emissions (largely from sugarcane, wheat, rice, and bluegrass fields) are Arkansas, California, Florida, Idaho, Texas, and Washington. In those six states alone, about 15.5 million people live in "source" counties (i.e., counties with crop-burning areas), although it is uncertain how many had significant smoke exposures.[357] The percentage of a state's population that lives in source counties can be quite high, such as 47% in Idaho and 25% in Arkansas.[356]

Field burning can occur for extended periods of time in any given area, leading to chronic exposures to the emissions.[356] Smoke can readily waft beyond the source counties, although as with forest fires, the distance at which toxic effects occur remains largely unknown.

The limited research on health effects of field burning has found some significant respiratory and cardiopulmonary problems. The threat is highly variable, based on (local farming) laws, air quality laws, crop type, and cultural practices of burning.

All together, there have been several dozens of studies of health effects related to wildfires, prescribed forest burns, peat bog fires, and agricultural field burning. That is a relatively small number given the huge variation in source material that can burn, the various underlying conditions of people who can be affected, and other variables (by comparison, more than 1700 health studies have been conducted for ground-level ozone). One reason for that dearth is the research is hard to be carried out.

WASTE DUMPS—LIQUID COLLECTIONS

Industrial pollution and waste pose potential threats to human and ecological health if not properly managed. The concerns range from toxic effects on fetuses and children to the health implications of low-level exposures to multiple pollutants and the degradation of habitats and ecosystems. Certainly, this composite will trigger chemical sensitivity. These concerns do not stop at the borders because some pollutant can travel long distances and waste is shipped to recycling and disposal sites across political boundaries.

Solid and liquid waste disposals (dumps) and chemical dumps will trigger air pollution, which bothers those who live near, on, or within a few miles in proximity to these areas. Frequently, mercury has been released from these dumps[358]; although 200 tons is dumped in the air from melting of the polar ice caps each year, the amount emanating from the dumps can be significant. Love Canal near Buffalo, New York, was the first of numerous chemical waste dumps investigated by the U.S. EPA because so many people were made ill by its emanations. Multitudes of people were made ill and many developed chemical sensitivity and CDDs.

The effects of certain toxic chemicals on the health and development of children and other vulnerable groups are a special concern. Researchers describe "windows of vulnerability" during fetal and child development in which toxic exposures can have particularly devastating effects. Although the traditional focus has been on overt health effects such as cancer, scientists are increasingly worried about the more subtle effects of low-level toxic exposures, such as impairments in endocrine, neurological functions, vascular disease, and hypersensitivity.

Industrial pollution and waste are important in the North American context because pollutants travel through the air and water to cross national borders and because waste is also shipped across borders for recycling, treatment, and disposal. The deposition of persistent contaminants in the distant north, in locations far from industrial sources, attests to the ability of pollutants to travel far from their points of origin, resulting in local and variant hypersensitivity and CDD.

Decisions on how to manage waste have environmental implications. Municipal waste incineration, medical waste incineration, burning of hazardous waste in cement kilns, and backyard waste burning were among the top sources of dioxins, according to the U.S. and Canadian inventories. Dioxins, like some other PBTYs can be dispersed long distances by air currents and other environmental pathways and tend to settle in colder regions, resulting in disease or OS and inflammation.

Whatever the differences, it is true that North American companies ship hundreds of thousands of tons of hazardous waste each year between Canada, Mexico, and the United States. When waste is sent to other jurisdictions for recycling, treatment, or disposal, the waste shipments must be transported along roads and railways and through populated areas before reaching their final destinations, often contaminating those people along the way.

Apart from its potential effects on humans and the environment, waste represents inefficiency in industrial production. Waste imposes costs on facilities; they must pay for waste management, regulatory compliance, and underutilized material inputs. From a societal perspective, the economic costs include paying for cleaning up contaminated sites, regulating waste-generating industries, and ensuring medical treatment for the adverse effects of environmental exposures. Usually, the medical costs are not even recognized or paid for. The nonmonetary costs include the depletion of nonrenewable resources, consumptive land use, and degradation of ecosystems (Figure 1.8).

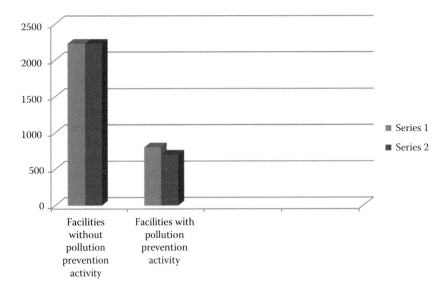

FIGURE 1.8   (**See color insert.**) Series 1 is year 2002, Series 2 is year 2004. Amounts represent millions of 1 kg.

According to Godri et al.,[359] waste transfer stations (WTSs) represent a hybrid of traffic and industrial microenvironments. These sites experience high volumes of heavy-duty diesel trucks and are often situated in densely populated urban centers.[360] They frequently are not recognized for the health hazard they are creating, which causes chemical sensitivity and chronic degenerative disability. These facilities serve as the link in the waste management system between the waste collection program and final disposal. Street waste collection vehicles discharge loads, avoiding uneconomic travel to distant landfill sites. Although this approach effectively decreases the overall air quality burden the waste management system poses on an urban center, communities in proximity to WTSs suffer from enhanced traffic flow and increased PM levels arising from vehicular tailpipe/nontailpipe emissions and dust releases from laden trucks.[361,362] Studies conducted in New York City[362–364] have reported that the highest PM concentrations in these urban centers occur at sampling sites influenced by WTS-related emissions.

Land use planning and climate change are just two of the other important environmental issues linked to industrial pollution and waste.

In the United States, as of 2008, 1581 sites (final and deleted) were on the Superfund program's National Priorities List and 3746 facilities are expected to need cleanup under the Federal Resource Conservation and Recovery Act. Numerous other sites are under local or state jurisdiction, and so the full extent of contaminated land is unknown. In Canada, about one-quarter of the 17,866 contaminated sites under federal responsibility are on native reserves, placing an additional burden on populations already vulnerable to environmental threats because of socioeconomic factors or geography. In Mexico, the federal government has identified 300 contaminated sites covering 200,000 ha. The location of polluting industries, landfills, and other waste management sites also raises questions of environmental justice.

Recycling and energy recovery of industrial waste enable the waste from one process to become the material inputs or energy source for another. More than a million tons of materials, mostly metals, were sent for recycling by PRTR-reporting facilities in 2004, and nearly 300,000 tons was sent for energy recovery. However, recycling and energy recovery can have their drawbacks. Recycling activities themselves can be sources of environmental contamination, and the air releases and residuals from energy recovery are a concern.

Industrial pollution and waste contribute to climate change as well. The anaerobic decomposition of waste in landfills produces methane, a potent greenhouse gas, and the number one cause of chemical sensitivity and waste incineration releases carbon dioxide. The transportation of waste to recycling, treatment, and disposal sites produces transportation-related carbon emissions. Finally, the materials disposed of as waste must be replaced by more raw materials, which imply further consumption of fossil fuels and additional carbon releases.

Industrial production contributes goods, services, and jobs, and is also a major source of pollution and waste. This pollution and waste can be classified into six categories: toxic chemicals, criteria air contaminants, greenhouse gases, hazardous waste, nonhazardous waste, and radioactive waste. Exposure to any of these for long term can trigger chemical sensitivity.

These substances are hazardous to human health and the environment causing chemical sensitivity and CDD. In 2004, North American industrial facilities generated over 5 million tons of toxic chemicals as production-related pollutants and waste. Despite this large amount, data for comparable industries and chemicals in Canada and the United States reveal encouraging trends. Over the period 1998–2004, total releases of carcinogens and developmental/reproductive toxicants declined by 26% in the United States and Canada (see graph in Figure 1.9), compared with a 15% reduction in all tracked chemicals. Mexican data are not available for this time period. Although releases to most media for these chemicals have declined over time, releases to underground injection have increased. This disposal method, in which fluids are released into subsurface wells, has increased by over 40% since 1998 for carcinogens and developmental/reproductive toxicants. Furthermore, even though facilities with the largest reported amounts have made progress in reducing toxic releases and transfers, the numerous facilities reporting smaller pollution amounts is tending to more in the opposite direction (Figure 1.9).

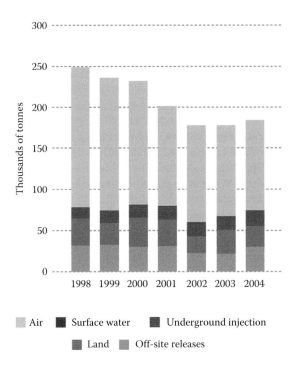

FIGURE 1.9   **(See color insert.)** Releases of carcinogens and developmental/reproductive toxicants. (From Canadian and U.S. data.)

CRITERIA AIR CONTAMINANTS

Greenhouse Gases

These gases, which include carbon dioxide (CO_2), methane, and nitrous oxide, are linked not only to global climate change but also to chemical sensitivity and CDD. Industrial energy use is a major source of CO_2 emissions in North America, roughly on par with the CO_2 emissions arising from energy use in the agricultural, commercial, and residential sectors combined. Although CO_2 emissions from industrial energy use dropped by >30% from 1980 to 2005, emissions from transportation increased by about 50%, and those from electricity generation and refineries by nearly 60% during the same time period. Total emissions of greenhouse gases in North American amounted to >8.5 billion tons of CO_2 equivalent in 2005.

Hazardous Waste

The amounts of hazardous waste being generated are significant. In the United States, nearly 34.8 million tons of hazardous waste was generated in 2005, mostly in the form of liquid waste. Government estimates put Canada's annual generation at about 6 million tons. In Mexico, data from over 35,000 facilities put the annual total at 6.17 million tons in 2004. Mexico's total generation of hazardous waste is not known, but 8 million tons a year is frequently cited.

Nonhazardous Waste

Nonhazardous industrial waste includes coal ash, foundry sands, cement kiln dust, mining- and mineral-processing waste, oil and gas production waste, and other waste that lacks the characteristics of hazardous waste. Although these waste streams are not classified as hazardous, their management is not without risk and generally legal requirements are in place for their proper treatment and disposal. In Canada, disposal of waste from nonresidential sources (industrial, commercial, and institutional) increased from 14.6 to 15.5 million tons between 2002 and 2004. In the United States and Mexico, overall estimates of nonhazardous industrial waste are not readily available, although estimates for various individual sources may exist.

Electronic waste, e-waste, e-scrap, or waste electrical and electronic equipment (WEEE) describes discarded electrical or electronic devices.

All electronic scrap components, such as cathode ray tubes (CRTs) may contain contaminants such as lead, cadmium, beryllium, or brominated flame retardants. Even in developed countries, recycling and disposal of e-waste may involve significant risk to workers and communities and great care must be taken to avoid unsafe exposure in recycling operations and leaking of materials such as heavy metals from landfills and incinerator ashes. Scrap industry and the U.S. EPA officials agree that materials should be managed with caution.[365]

"Electronic waste" may be defined as discarded computers, office electronic equipment, entertainment device electronics, mobile phones, television sets, and refrigerators. This definition includes used electronics which are destined for reuse, resale, salvage, recycling, or disposal. Others define the reusables (working and repairable electronics) and secondary scrap (copper, steel, plastic, etc.) to be "commodities," and reserve the term "waste" for residue or material which is dumped by the buyer rather than recycled, including residue from reuse and recycling operations. Because loads of surplus electronics are frequently commingled (good, recyclable, and nonrecyclable), several public policy advocates apply the term "e-waste" broadly to all surplus electronics. CRTs are considered one of the hardest types to recycle.[366]

CRTs have relatively high concentration of lead and phosphors (not to be confused with phosphorus), both of which are necessary for the display. The U.S. EPA includes discarded CRT monitors in the category of "hazardous household waste"[358] but considers CRTs that have been set aside for testing to be commodities if they are not discarded, speculatively accumulated, or left unprotected from weather and other damage.

The relationship between extended air pollutant exposure and increased prevalence of asthma symptoms has been well documented.[367–370] In New York City, asthma hospitalization rates were stratified by the geographic location within each of the city's boroughs. Children living in the Bronx, specifically the South Bronx, suffered from hospitalization rates for asthma 70% and 700% greater than the average for New York City and New York State, respectively (New York City Department of Health 1999). Sources contributing to adverse air quality in South Bronx include industrial facilities and vehicular traffic.[320,371] Nineteen WTSs housed in this low-income and densely inhabited community are also contributed significantly to increased PM exposures, with children experiencing elevated exposures due to the proximity of these facilities to schools, playgrounds, and residential buildings.[363] To date, it is not clear whether such health effects are simply due to residents experiencing elevated PM concentrations or whether the toxicity of PM derived from WTS-related activities is elevated above that of urban PM.

Recent literature has suggested that transition metals,[372] organic species (PAHs and quinines),[373] and endotoxin are associated with increased PM toxicity. The capacity of PM to induce toxicity (in particular, to elicit a respiratory and/or systemic inflammatory response) has been proposed to be a function of its oxidative potential,[374,375] that is, the ability of PM to generate reactive oxygen species directly or indirectly to engender oxidative injury to the lung[359,376,377] therefore evaluated PM oxidative potential to provide a simple aggregate measure of the particulate oxidative burden in the ambient airshed influenced by WTS emissions.

The objective of this study was to examine the pattern of elevated PM concentrations at a WTS located adjacent to a densely populated community in London. They used PM source apportionment techniques and microscale meteorological information to identify pollutant episodes attributed to specific local sources, and quantified PM oxidative potential derived from WTS activity emissions.

Elevated PM concentrations have been reported in proximity to WTS[362–364] but no study has yet examined whether there is a basis for believing odors from these industrial emissions may have enhanced toxicity, based on their chemical composition. They examined both the composition and oxidative properties of PM generated by WTS activity. Incorporation of PM oxidative potential into a receptor model source apportionment analysis is a novel aspect of this study.

A weekly pattern of local PM_{10} concentrations was observed at the sampling site: Elevated concentrations were found on weekdays and Saturdays, with much lower concentrations on Sundays. The PM_{10} mass concentration difference between weekday and Sunday samples was expected because the WTS was closed on Sundays. This general trend also extended to oxidative potential measurements. Intercomparison of weekday oxidative potential levels revealed variation regardless of the continual WTS operation during these days. The extent that industrial emissions influenced sampled PM_{10} concentration, as predicted by WD, was used to explain this weekday variation. Moreover, elevated PM oxidative potential was established when WTS emissions predominately contributed to PM sampled at this site.

Additionally, the measured PM oxidative potential was likely attributable to the compositional profile of the local PM_{10} fractions, given its high sensitivity to WD.

The oxidative potential of PM derived from WTS was compared with the PM total metal and bioavailable Fe content. Correlations between total transition metals and antioxidant depletion produced significant associations between metal species and GSH (Al, Pb) and AA (Fe, Pb) depletion. Moreover, the concentration of Pb was strongly associated with both Fe and Al, suggesting a common source(s). Total Fe and Pb exhibited a significant difference between weekday Saturday and Sunday concentrations following the pattern of locally produced PM_{10} at the sampling site.

Cu was not identified as a predicator of PM oxidative potential.[378,379] Differences in the traffic profile are likely accountable for this discrepancy: Cu is a marker of light-duty vehicle brake wear, whereas barium and antimony are characteristics of brake wear from heavy-duty vehicles.[380] The vehicle fleet servicing the WTS comprised predominantly the latter type, unlike the traffic profiles of the previously mentioned studies.

Bioavailable Fe content was considered for a subset of exposed samples. Weekday (Monday and Wednesday) samples were found to have the highest ferric ion content. This trend of elevated weekday Fe(III) concentrations also corresponded with the highest PM oxidative potential measurements reflective of WTS contributions to the sampling site rather than residential emissions. As the contribution of WTS emissions to sampling site declined, so too did the PM_{10} bioavailable iron pool.

Organic PM content, including PAHs, quinines, and endotoxin, were not measured in the present study, although they can also trigger the generation of reactive oxygen species, once inhaled, through metabolism and the induction of inflammation.[381] Of these components, only particulate quinone content would have influenced the measured PM oxidative potential in the acellular RTLF model because of its capacity to redox cycle[373] (Table 1.2). No significant antioxidant depletion was measured with PM_{10} samples were incubated with DTPA. This demonstrates that PM catalytic metal content explained much of the intrinsic capacity of these samples to catalyze damaging oxidation reactions.

PM_{10} exceedances at the sampling site were the result of WTS emissions linked to site activity. Detailed PM chemical characterization indicated that these high PM_{10} mass concentrations contained elevated transition metal levels. Concentrations of total Fe, Al, and Pb were especially high; WTS-soluble Fe emissions existed predominantly in the form of Fe (III). Assessment of the WTS PM oxidative potential revealed that it was associated with increased transition metal concentrations. Thus, PM_{10} generated by WTSs may be a potential health risk to neighboring communities. The resident population is exposed to a high PM mass concentration on a recurrent basis, and particulate emitted by these industrial emissions may have a greater capacity to drive damaging oxidation reactions in the lung compared to other PM sources in urban environments. Certainly, the fumes from this type of environmental disturbances affect the chemically sensitive and those with CDD.

CHEMICAL DUMPS INCLUDING THE USE OF SYNTHETIC TURF

Synthetic Turf

The health of thousands of children may be at risk due to long-term exposure to toxic chemicals from artificial turf that has become a popular replacement for grass on sporting ovals and school playgrounds around the country.

Australian scientists have raised the alarm over the potential dangers of the fake grass, and called for a moratorium on its use until its safety can be established.[382]

An investigation was carried out for the widespread concerns about the turf. These investigations are centered on a range of factors, from the cheap imported products that are not tested for toxic chemicals and made from unknown materials to what makes up the turf favored for soccer fields—crumb rubber that comes from recycled tires.

Warnings have also been issued around the world about cases of turf heating up to such temperatures that it can cause burns and heat stress.

Residents in some Sydney suburbs have successfully fought the introduction of synthetic grass, including at Arlington Recreation Reserve in Dulwich Hill, where they forced Marrickville Council to reverse its decision.

A series of studies in the United States, Denmark, and Italy has again raised concerns about long-term intensive exposure to artificial turf. Numerous studies around the world have had differing results, however, with some arguing no increased health risks.

A study released in 2010 by the Connecticut Department of Environmental Protection revealed the presence of chemical carcinogens in the air over an artificial field, but the findings were reportedly "softened" for public release.

Artificial turf has gained popularity in Australia in the past decade as a way of extending playing hours and cutting maintenance time and costs. Schools, councils, and sport groups have opted to use it to replace grass.

Yet, across the United States, schools have been digging up the turf and reinstating grass, concerned about toxic chemicals and heavy metals, including lead, which was used in some of earlier generations of turf.

Edwards said an overlooked issue was the heating of the turf to temperatures that could cause injury. He quoted a study by Brigham Young University in Utah that showed it reaching temperatures much higher than grass and in some cases almost three times the air temperature, recording 93.3°.[382]

The same study said one coach developed blisters on his feet, despite wearing tennis shoes, as a result of the extreme temperatures and that the New York State Department of Health had issued warnings.

Some of the famous chemical dumps include: (1) Love Canal, (2) Elba, Island Italy, (3) Queensland Australia, and (4) San Jacinto Waste Pits.

Love Canal

Love Canal is a neighborhood within Niagara Falls, New York located in the laSalle section of the city. It officially covers 36 square blocks in the far southeastern corner of the city, along 99th Street and Read Avenue. Two bodies of water define the northern and southern boundaries of the neighborhood: Bergholtz Creek to the north and the Niagara River one-quarter mile 9400 m) to the south. In the mid-1970s, Love Canal became the subject of national and international attention after it was revealed in the press that the site had formerly been used to bury 21,000 tons of toxic waste by Hooker Chemical (now Occidental Petroleum Corporation).

Hooker Chemical sold the site to the Niagara Falls School board in 1953 for $1 with a deed explicit detailing the presence of the waste and including a liability limitation clause about the contamination.[383] The construction efforts of housing development, combined with particularly heavy rainstorms, released the chemical waste, leading to a public health emergency and an urban planning scandal. Hooker Chemical was found to be negligent in their disposal of waste, though not reckless in the sale of the land, in what became a test case for liability clauses from 1976 through the evacuation in 1978. Potential health problems were first raised in July 1978.

The Love Canal incident was especially significant as a situation where the inhabitants "overflowed into the waste instead of the other way around."[384]

The Canal became a dumpsite for the City of Niagara Falls, with the city regularly unloading its municipal refuse into the pit. In the 1940s, the U.S. Army began using the site to dump waste from the war effort during World War II, including some nuclear waste from the Manhattan Project, the rest of which was dumped in nearby Lewiston, New York, at the Niagara Falls Storage Site.

Hooker was granted permission by the Niagara Power and Development Company in 1942 to dump waste in the canal. The canal was drained and lined with thick clay. Into this site, Hooker began placing 55-U.S. gallon (210 L) metal or fiber barrels. In 1947, Hooker bought the canal and the 70-ft wide (21 m) banks on either side of the canal.[385] The City of Niagara Falls and the army continued the dumping of refuse.

This dumpsite was in operation until 1953. During this time, 21,000 tons of chemicals such as "caustics, alkalines, fatty acids, and chlorinated hydrocarbons from the manufacturing of dyes, perfumes, solvents for rubber and synthetic resins" were added.[386] These chemicals were buried at a depth of 20–25 ft.[387] After 1953, the canal was covered with soil, and vegetation began to grow atop the dumpsite.

The Niagara Falls City School District needed land to build new schools, and attempted to purchase the property from Hooker Chemical that had been used to bury toxic waste. The corporation initially refused to sell citing safety concerns; however, the board refused to capitulate,[383] eventually faced with parts of the property being condemned and/or expropriated.

Hooker stated that the area should be sealed off "so as to prevent the possibility of persons or animals coming in contact with the dumped materials."[388]

Despite the disclaimer, the board began construction of the 99th Street School in its originally intended location. The kindergarten playground also had to be relocated because a chemical dump lay directly beneath. Upon completion in 1955, 400 children attended the school and it opened along with several other schools that had been built to accommodate students. That same year, a 25-ft area crumbled exposing toxic chemical drums, which then filled with water during rainstorms. This created large puddles that children enjoyed playing in.[384]

In 1950, a second school, the 93rd Street School, had opened six blocks away.

In 1957, the City of Niagara Falls constructed sewers for a mixture of low-income and single-family residences be built on lands adjacent to the landfill site. The school district had sold off the remaining land, and homes were to be built by private developers, as well as the Niagara Falls Housing Authority, who planned to build the Griffon Manor housing project. While building the gravel sewer beds, construction crews broke through the clay seal, breaching the canal walls.[383] Specifically, the local government removed part of the protective clay cap to use as fill dirt for the nearby 93rd Street School, and punched holes in the solid clay walls to build water lines and the LaSalle Expressway. This allowed the toxic waste to escape when rainwater, no longer kept out by the partially removed clay cap, washed them through the gaps created in the walls.[389] Hence, the buried chemicals had a further opportunity to migrate and seep from the canal. The land where the homes were being built was not a part of the agreement between the school board and Hooker; thus, none of these residents knew the history of the canal.[390] There was no monitoring or evaluation of the chemical waste which were being stored under the ground. Additionally, the clay cover of the canal which was supposed to be impermeable began to crack.[390] The subsequent construction of the LaSalle Expressway restricted groundwater from flowing to the Niagara River. Following the exceptionally wet winter and spring of 1962, the elevated expressway turned the breached canal into an overflowing pool. People reported having pebbles of oil or colored liquid in yards or basements.[391]

In 1976, two reporters tested several sump pumps near Love Canal and found toxic chemicals in them. The matter went quiet for more than a year and was resurrected when investigated potential health effects by carrying forth an informal door-to-door survey in early 1978, finding birth defects and many anomalies such as enlarged feet, heads, hands, and legs. Local residents created a protest group, which was led by resident Karen Schroeder whose daughter had many (about a dozen) birth defects. The New York State Health Department followed suit and found an abnormal incidence of miscarriages. The dumpsite was declared an unprecedented state emergency on August 2, 1978. Mr. Brown who wrote more than a hundred articles on the dump, also further tested groundwater and later found that the dump was three times the size officials knew, with possible ramifications beyond the original evacuation zone. He also discovered that highly toxic dioxin was present.

The neighborhood sat on top of 21,000 tons of buried chemical waste.[392]

Basements were often covered with a thick, black substance, and vegetation was also dying. In many yards, the only vegetation that grew were shrubby grasses.[393]

According to the U.S. EPA in 1979, residents exhibited a "disturbingly high rate of miscarriages." Love Canal family had birth defects, one girl was born deaf with a cleft palate, an extra row of teeth, and slight retardation, and a boy was born with an eye defect.[394] A survey conducted by the Love Canal Homeowners Association found that 56% of the children born from 1974 to 1978 have had at least one birth defect.[394]

The 99th Street School, on the other hand, was located within the former boundary of the Hooker Chemical landfill site. The school was closed and demolished but both the school board and the chemical company refused to accept liability. The 93rd Street School was closed some 2 years later due to concerns about seeping toxic waste.

At first, scientific studies did not conclusively prove that the chemicals were responsible for the residents' illnesses, and scientists were divided on the issue even though 11 known or suspected carcinogens had been identified, one of the most prevalent being benzene. There was also dioxin (polychlorinated dibenzodioxins in the water, a very hazardous substance). Dioxin pollution is usually measured in parts per trillions at Love Canal; water samples showed dioxin levels at 53 ppb.[395] Geologists were recruited to determine whether underground swales were responsible for carrying the chemicals to the surrounding residential areas. Once there, chemicals could leach into basements and evaporate into household air.

In 1979, the EPA announced the result of blood tests that showed high white blood cell counts, a precursor to leukemia,[394] and chromosome damage in Love Canal residents. In fact, 33% of the residents had undergone chromosomal damage; in a typical population, chromosomal damage affects 1% of people.[395] Other studies were unable to find harm.[396–400] The U.S. National Research Council (NRC) surveyed Love Canal health studies in 1991. The NRC noted that the major exposure of concern was the groundwater rather than drinking water, the groundwater "seeped into basements" and then led to exposure through air and soil.[401] It was noted that several studies reported higher levels of low-birth-weight babies and birth defects among the exposed residents[402] with some evidence; the effect subsided after the exposure was eliminated.[403] The NRC also noted a study which found that exposed children were found to have an "excess of seizures, learning problems, hyperactivity, eye irritation, skin rashes, abdominal pain, and incontinence" and stunted growth.[401] Voles in the area were studied and found to have significantly increased mortality compared with controls (mean life expectancy in exposed animals: 23.6 and 29.2 days, respectively, compared to 48.8 days for control animals).[404] New York State also has an ongoing health study of Love Canal residents[405]; in that year, the Albert Elia Building Co., Inc. now Sevenson Environmental Services, Inc., was selected as the principal contractor to safely rebury the toxic waste at the Love Canal Site.

Eventually, the government relocated more than 800 families and reimbursed them for their homes, and the U.S. Congress passed the Comprehensive Environmental Response Compensation, and Liability Act (CERCLA), or the Superfund Act. Because the Superfund Act contained a "retroactive liability" provision, Occidental was held liable for cleanup of the waste even though it had followed all applicable U.S. laws when disposing of it in 1994. Federal District Judge John Curtin ruled that Hooker/Occidental had been negligent, but not reckless, in its handling of the waste and sale of the land to the Niagara Falls School Board.[406] Curtin's decision also contains a detailed history of events leading up to the Love Canal disaster. Occidental Petroleum was sued by the EPA and in 1995 agreed to pay $129 million in restitution.[407] Residents, lawsuits were also settled in the years following the Love Canal disaster.[408]

Currently, houses in the residential areas on the east and west sides of the canal have been demolished. All that remains on the west side are abandoned residential streets. Some older eastside residents, whose houses stand alone in the demolished neighborhood, chose to stay. It was estimated that less than 90 of the original 900 families opted to stay.[395] They were willing to stay as long as they were guaranteed that their homes were in a relatively safe area.[409] On June 4, 1980, the Love Canal Area Revitalization Agency (LCARA) was founded to restore the area. The area, north to Love Canal, became known as *Black Creek Village*. LCARA wanted to resell 300 homes that had been bought by New York when the residents were relocated.[409] These homes were farther away from where the chemicals had been dumped. The most toxic area (16 acres (65,000 m)) has been reburied with a thick plastic liner clay and dirt. A 2.4-m (7 ft 109 in) high-barbed wire fence was constructed around this area.[410] It has been calculated that 248 separate chemicals including 60 kg (130 lb) of dioxin have been unearthed from the canal.[411]

Besides double the rate of birth defects to children born while living in Love Canal, a follow-up study two decades after the incident "showed increased risks of low birth weight congenital malformation and other adverse reproductive events."[412]

Love Canal, along with Times Beach, Missouri, are important in the U.S. environmental history as the two sites that in large part led to the CERCLA. CERCLA is much more commonly referred to as "Superfund" because of the fund established by the act to help clean-up of toxic pollution in residential locations such as Love Canal. It has been stated that Love Canal has "become the symbol for what happens when hazardous industrial products are not confined to the workplace but 'hit people where they live' in inestimable amounts."[413]

CHARACTERIZATION OF SULFIDE-BEARING WASTE ROCK DUMPS USING ELECTRICAL RESISTIVITY IMAGING: THE CASE STUDY OF THE RIO MARINA MINING DISTRICT (ELBA ISLAND, ITALY)

According to Mele et al.,[357] sulfide-bearing mine dumps are potential sources of pollution when acid mine drainage (AMD) occurs. Because the generation of AMD depends on the volume and composition of waste materials, their characterization is crucial for the evaluation of geochemical hazards and for the design of remediation strategies to minimize their environmental impact. In this paper, a cost-effective strategy for the characterization of an inactive mine dump in the Rio Marina mining district (Elba Island, Italy) using Earth resistivity imaging (ERI) is presented. As no information regarding the nature of waste rocks is found in reports for the mine, five ERI profiles were acquired at the top of the waste pile. The results show that waste rocks are heterogeneous with a maximum thickness of 30 m. Due to the large amounts of dispersed sulfide minerals, the waste rocks are characterized by an electrically conductive geophysical signature in comparison to the surrounding resistive metamorphic bedrock. A geostatistical approach was adopted to estimate the elevation of the edges of the mine dump, and the net volume of the waste rocks was computed through a raster analysis of the elevations of the upper and lower boundaries of the mine dump. High-conductivity anomalies were detected within the core of the mine dump. The integration of the hydrogeological, geochemical, and geological framework of the Rio Marina mining district suggests that these anomalies could be a geophysical signature of subsurface regions where AMD is currently generated or stored, thus representing sources of environmental pollution.

CRITICAL REVIEW OF THE EFFECTS OF GOLD CYANIDE-BEARING TAILINGS SOLUTIONS ON WILDLIFE

According to Donato et al.,[414] wildlife deaths associated with cyanide-bearing mine *waste* solutions have plagued the gold mining industries for many years; yet, there are little published data showing the relationship between wildlife mortality and cyanide toxicity. The perceived extent of the issue varies, with one study finding the issue inadequately monitored and wildlife deaths grossly underestimated.[414] In Nevada, United States, during 1990 and 1991, 9512 carcasses were reported of over 100 species, although there was underestimation due to reporting being voluntary. Of these, birds comprised 80%–91% of vertebrate carcasses reported annually.

At Northparkes, Australia, in 1995, it was initially estimated that 100 bird carcasses were present by mine staff following a tailings incident; when a thorough count was conducted, 1583 bird carcasses were recorded. Eventually, 2700 bird deaths were documented over a 4-month period. It is identified that avian deaths are usually undetected and significantly underestimated, leading to a perception that a risk does not exist. Few guidelines and information are available to manage the risks of cyanide to wildlife, although detoxification, habitat modification, and denying wildlife access have been used effectively. This places the onus on mining operations to document that no risk to wildlife exists. Cyanide-bearing tailing storage facilities (TSFs) are environmental control structures to contain tailings, a standard practice in the mining industry. Cyanide concentrations below 50 mg/L weak acid dissociable (WAD) are deemed safe to wildlife but are considered an interim benchmark for discharge into TSFs. Cyanide is a fast-acting poison, and its toxicity is related to the types of cyanide complexes that are present. Cyanide in biota binds to iron, copper, and sulfur-containing enzymes and proteins required for oxygen transportation to cells. The accurate determination of cyanide concentrations in the field is difficult to achieve due to sampling techniques and analytical error associated with loss and interferences following collection. The main WAD cyanide complexes in gold mine tailings are stable in the TSF environment but can release cyanide ions under varying environmental conditions, including ingestion and absorption by wildlife. Therefore, distinction between free, WAD, and total cyanide forms in tailings water for regulatory purposes is justified. From an environmental perspective, there is a distinction between ore bodies on the basis of their copper content. For example, wildlife deaths are more likely to occur at mines possessing copper–gold ores due to the formation of copper–cyanide complexes which is toxic to birds and bats. The formation of copper–cyanide complex occurs preferentially to gold–cyanide complex, indicating the relative importance of economic versus environmental considerations in the tailings water. Management of cyanide to a perceived threshold has inherent risks since cyanide has a steep toxicity response curve, is difficult to accurately measure in the field, and is likely to vary due to variable copper content of ore bodies and ore blending. Consequently, wildlife interaction needs to be limited to further reduce the risks. A gap in knowledge exists to design or manage cyanide-bearing mine waste solutions to render such facilities unattractive to at-risk wildlife species. This gap may be overcome by understanding the wildlife behavior and habitat usage of cyanide-bearing solutions.

SAN JACINTO RIVER WASTE PITS

A set of waste ponds, known as impoundments ~14 acres in size, were built in the mid-1960s for disposal of paper mill wastes. In 1965 and 1966, pulp and paper mill wastes (both solid and liquid) were transported by barge from the Champion Paper, Inc. paper mill in Pasadena, Texas and unloaded at these impoundments north of I-10, west of the main river channel of the San Jacinto River, and east of the City of Houston between two unincorporated areas now known as Channelview and Highlands.[415]

The Champion Paper Mill used chlorine as a bleaching agent, and the wastes deposited in the impoundments were contaminated with polychlorinated dibenzo-*p*-dioxins, polychlorinated furans (dioxins and furans), and some metals. Physical changes at the site in the 1970s and 1980s resulted in partial submergence of the impoundments north of I-10 and exposure of the contents to surface water. Dioxins and furans are "hazardous substances" as defined by Section 101(14) of CERCLA, 42 U.S.C. §(14).

The EPA issued an Action Memorandum on April 2010 for *time-critical removal action (TCRA)* to stabilize the waste pits and prevent direct human and benithic contact with the waste materials until the site is fully characterized and a remedy is selected.

A Remedial Investigation/Feasibility Study (RI/FS) is also being carried out to address the nature and extent of activities beginning with the preliminary perimeter. While the two impoundments are currently located directly north of the I-10 Bridge with one partially submerged in the San Jacinto River, an additional impoundment is suspected to be located directly south of the I-10 Bridge. Watershed management strategies will address permitted disposal activities within the permit areas of concern.

The Texas Department of State Health Services (DSHS) and the Agency for Toxic Substances and Disease Registry has released the *San Jacinto River Waste Pits Public Health Assessment— Public Comment Draft.*

HEALTH IMPACTS OF SOLID WASTE

With increase in the global population and the rising demand for food and other essentials, there has been a rise in the amount of waste being generated daily by each household. This waste is ultimately thrown into municipal waste collection centers from where it is collected by the area municipalities to be further thrown into the landfills and dumps. However, either due to resource crunch or inefficient infrastructure, not all of this waste gets collected and transported to the final dumpsites. If at this stage the management and disposal of waste are improperly done, it can cause serious impacts on health and problems to the surrounding environment. We have seen this problem in the chemically sensitive who are exposed to the air around waste pits.

Waste that is not properly managed, especially excreta and other liquid and solid waste from households and the community, is a serious health hazard and leads to the spread of infectious diseases. Unattended waste lying around attracts flies, rats, and other creatures that in turn spread disease. Normally, it is the wet waste that decomposes and releases a bad odor. This then leads to unhygienic conditions and an increase in the health problems. The plague outbreak in Surat, India is a good example of a city suffering due to the callous attitude of the local body in maintaining cleanliness in the city. Plastic waste is another cause for ill health. Thus, taking certain preventive measures should control excessive solid waste that is generated.

The group at risk from the unscientific disposal of solid waste includes—the population in areas where there is no proper waste disposal method, especially the preschool children; waste workers; and workers in facilities producing toxic and infectious material. Other high-risk groups include population living close to a waste dump and those, whose water supply has become contaminated either due to waste dumping or leakage from landfill sites. Uncollected solid waste also increases risk of injury and infection, and those who are chemically sensitive.

In particular, organic domestic waste poses a serious threat, since they ferment, creating conditions favorable to the survival and growth of microbial pathogens. Direct handling of solid waste can also result in various types of infectious and chronic diseases of which the waste workers and the rag pickers being the most vulnerable.

Exposure to hazardous waste can affect human health, children being more vulnerable to these pollutants and the chemically sensitive. In fact, direct exposure can lead to diseases through chemical exposure as the release of chemical waste into the environment leads to chemical poisoning. Many studies have been carried out in various parts of the world to establish a connection between health and hazardous waste.

Waste from agriculture and industries can also cause serious health risks. Other than this, codisposal of industrial hazardous waste with municipal waste can expose people to chemical and radioactive hazards. Uncollected solid waste can also obstruct stormwater runoff, resulting in the formation of stagnant water bodies that become the breeding ground of disease. Waste dumped near a water source also causes contamination of the water body or the ground water source. Direct dumping of untreated waste in rivers, seas, and lakes result in the accumulation of toxic substances in the food chain through the plants and animals that feed on it.

Disposal of hospital and other medical waste requires special attention since this can create major health hazards. This waste generated from the hospitals, healthcare centers, medical laboratories, and research centers such as discarded syringe needles, bandages, swabs, plasters, and other types of infectious waste are often disposed with the regular noninfectious waste.

Waste treatment and disposal sites can also create health hazards for the neighborhood. Improperly operated incineration plants cause air pollution, and improperly managed and designed landfills attract all types of insects and rodents that spread disease. Ideally, these sites should be located at a safe distance from all human settlement. Landfill sites should be well-lined and walled to ensure that there is no leakage into the nearby ground water sources.

Recycling too carries health risks if proper precautions are not taken. Workers working with waste containing chemical and metals may experience toxic exposure. Disposal of healthcare wastes require special attention since it can create major health hazards, such as hepatitis B and C, through wounds caused by discarded syringes. Rag pickers and others, who are involved in scavenging in the waste dumps for items that can be recycled, may sustain injuries and come into direct contact with these infectious items.

DISEASES

Certain chemicals if released untreated, for example, cyanides, mercury, and polychlorinated biphenyls are highly toxic and its exposure can lead to disease or death. Some studies have detected excess of cancer in residents exposed to hazardous waste. Many studies have been carried out in various parts of the world to establish a connection between health and hazardous waste and chemical sensitivity occur.

ROLE OF PLASTICS

The unhygienic use and disposal of plastics and its effects on human health has become a matter of concern. Colored plastics are harmful as their pigment contains heavy metals that are highly toxic. Some of the harmful metals found in plastics are copper, lead, chromium, cobalt, selenium, and cadmium. In most industrialized countries, color plastics have been legally banned. In India, the Government of Himachal Pradesh has banned the use of plastics and so has Ladakh district. Other states should emulate their example.

AERIAL SPRAYING

Aerial spraying in the United States, Mexico, and other countries for insect control has been toxic for many individuals and especially children and the chemically sensitive. It is used frequently to control so-called insect epidemics like mosquitoes for the West Nile virus (WNV), and tics to stop Lyme disease, etc.[416] Sacramento, California, and Dallas, Texas seemed to be the areas most affected by WNV, and aerial spraying was carried out. No data has ever been recorded on how much damage was caused to the human population who received the brunt of the spray. We have many chemically sensitive patients who are made ill by aerial spray. Most have to leave the area when it is being actively performed. Pesticides and herbicides along with natural gas are the number one cause of chemical sensitivity.

In rural areas, the biggest sources of pollutants are insecticides, herbicides, artificial nitrogen fertilizers, and sweet and sour gas from oil field emissions.[416]

In some rural areas, especially in the Midwest, intensive factory farming severely contaminates the air (usually with ammonia, pesticides, and herbicides), food, and water and is very detrimental to the health of the people living and working in the areas (some of the highest cancer rates in the United States) as well as to the plant and wildlife. Also, factory hog and chicken raising farms are extremely toxic especially after solvents and often toxic chemicals are used.[416] Ranching areas are less polluted but can contain some areas of herbicides and pesticides that are used for "enhancing" pastures.

The big studies for Dallas, Texas, and Sacramento, California show no harmful effects due to aerial spraying. These studies are flawed and ignore the facts of patient illness. However, we have seen many patients made ill from it. Crop dusting has been the worst of aerial spraying making personnel and their offspring ill. We have known of and seen cases of renal failure and neurovascular disease as well as chemical sensitivity.

Correlation between aerial insecticide spraying to interrupt WNV transmission and ED visits in Sacramento County, California have been performed.

According to Geraghty et al.,[416] insecticides reduce vector-borne pathogen transmission but also pose health risks. In August 2005, Sacramento County, California, underwent emergency aerial ultralow-volume (ULV) application of pyrethrin insecticide to reduce the population of WNV-infected mosquitoes and thereby interrupt enzootic and tangential transmission. Geraghty et al.[416] assessed the association between aerially applied pyrethrin insecticide and patterns of ED visit diagnoses.

They used geographic information systems software to determine ZIP Code-level exposure to pyrethrin.

Exposure to aerially applied insecticide was not associated with number of respiratory, gastrointestinal, skin, eye, and neurologic complaints in adjusted models but was inversely associated with ICD-9-CM code 799 (other ill-defined morbidity and mortality), with adjusted odds ratios (AORs) ranging from 0.31 to 0.36 for 0–3 lag days (95% CI: 0.17, 0.68). Spraying was also directly associated with ICD-9-CM code 553 with ORs ranging from 2.34 to 2.96 for 2–3 lag days.

However, they did not contact any chemically sensitive patients. To say this spraying was entirely safe is open to questions.

West Nile Encephalitis Epidemic in Dallas, Texas

According to Chung et al.,[417] after progressive decline over recent years, in 2012, WNV epidemics resurged nationwide, with the greatest number of cases centered in Dallas County, Texas.

The objective was to analyze the epidemiologic, meteorologic, and geospatial features of the 2012 Dallas WNV epidemic to guide future prevention efforts.

Public health surveillance of Dallas County, an area of 2257 km^2 and with a population of 2.4 million was conducted. Surveillance data included number of residents diagnosed with WNV infection between May 30, 2012 and December 3, 2012; mosquito trap results; weather data; and syndromic surveillance from area EDs.

The investigation identified 173 cases of WNND, 225 of West Nile fever, 17 WNV-positive blood donors, and 19 deaths in 2012. The incidence rate for WNND was 7.30 per 100,000 residents in 2012, compared with 2.91 per 100,000 in 2006, the largest previous Dallas County outbreak. An unusually rapid and early escalation of large number of human cases closely followed increasing infection trends in mosquitoes. The *Culex quinquefasciatus* species-specific vector index predicted the onset of symptoms among WNND cases 1 to 2 weeks later (count regression $\beta = 2.97$ [95% CI, 2.34–3.60]; $p < .001$). Although initially widely distributed, WNND cases soon clustered in neighborhoods with high housing density in the north central area of the county, reflecting higher vector indices and following geospatial patterns of WNV in prior years. During the 11 years since WNV was first identified in Dallas, the log-transformed annual prevalence of WNND was inversely associated with the number of days with low temperatures below 28°F (−2.2°C) in December through

February ($\beta = 0.29$ [95% CI, -0.36 to -0.21]; $p < .001$). Aerial insecticide spraying was not associated with increases in ED visits for respiratory symptoms ($\beta = -4.03$ [95% Cl, -13.76 to 5.70]; $p = .42$) or skin rash ($\beta = -1.00$ [95% Cl, -6.92 to 4.92]; $p = .74$).

Impact of aerial spraying of pyrethrin insecticide on *Cx. pipiens* and *Cx. tarsalis* (Diptera: Culicidae) abundance and WNV infection rates in an urban/suburban area of Sacramento County, California was found.

According to Elnaiem et al.,[418] in response to an epidemic amplification of WNV (family Flaviviridae, genus *Flavivirus*, WNV), the Sacramento and Yolo Mosquito and Vector Control District (SYMVCD) sprayed ULV formulations of pyrethrin insecticide (EverGreen EC 60-6: 6% pyrethrin insecticide, 60% piperonyl butoxide; MGK, Minneapolis, Minnesota, applied as 0.003 kg/ha [0.0025 lb/acre]) pyrethroids were applied over 218 km² in north Sacramento and 243.5 km² in south Sacramento on three consecutive evenings in August 2005. They evaluated the impact of this intervention in north Sacramento on the abundance and WNV infection rates of *Cx. pipients* L. and *Cx. tarsalis* Coquillett. Mortality rates of aged *Cx. tarsalis* sentinels ranged from 0% under dense canopy to 100% in open fields. A comparison of weekly geometric mean mosquito abundance in CO_2-baited traps in sprayed and unsprayed areas before and after treatment indicated a 75.0% and 48.7% reduction in the abundance of *Cx. pipiens* and *Cx. tarsalis*, respectively. This reduction was statistically significant for *Cx. pipiens*, the primary vector of WNV, with highest abundance in this urban area, but not for *Cx. tarsalis*, which is more associated with rural areas. The infection rates of WNV in *Cx. pipiens* and *Cx. tarsalis* collected from the spray zone was 8.2 and 4.3 per 1000 female mosquitoes in the 2 week before and the 2 week after applications of insecticide, respectively. In comparison, WNV infection rates in *Cx. pipiens* and *Cx. tarsalis* collected at same time interval in the unsprayed zone were 2.0 and 8.7 per 1000, respectively. Based on the reduction in vector abundance and its effects on number of infective bites received by human population, they concluded that the aerial application of pyrethrin insecticide reduced the transmission intensity of WNV and decreased the risk of human infection. Again no questions were asked about exacerbation of the chemically sensitive.

Pyrethroid pesticides were applied via ground spraying to residential neighborhoods in New York City during July–September 2000 to control mosquito vectors of WNV. They conducted this analysis to determine whether widespread urban pyrethroid pesticide use was associated with increased rates of ED visits for asthma. They recorded the dates and locations of pyrethroid spraying during the 2000 WNV season in New York City and tabulated all ED visits for asthma to public hospitals from October 1999 through November 2000 by date and ZIP Code of patients' residences. There were 62,827 ED visits for asthma during the 14-month study period, across 162 ZIP codes. The number of asthma visits was similar in the 3-day period before and after spraying (510 vs. 501, $p = 0.78$). Secondary analyses among children and for COPD yielded similar null results. However, there were no data on brain or vascular dysfunction which usually bothers the chemically sensitive.

Rocky Mountain Spotted Fever

According to Demma et al.,[419] Rocky Mountain spotted fever is a life-threatening, tickborne disease caused by *Rickettsia rickettsii*.

A total of 16 patients with Rocky Mountain spotted fever infection (11 with confirmed and 5 with probable infection) were identified. Of these patients, 13 (81%) were children of 12 years of age or younger, 15 (94%) were hospitalized, and 2 (12%) died. Dense populations of *Rhipicephalus sanguineus* ticks were found on dogs and in the yards of patients' homesites. All patients with confirmed Rocky Mountain spotted fever had contact with tick-infested dogs, and four had a reported history of tick bite preceding the illness. *R. rickettsii* DNA was detected in nonengorged *R. sanguineus* ticks collected at one home, and *R. rickettsii* isolates were cultured from these ticks.

This investigation documents the presence of Rocky Mountain spotted fever in eastern Arizona, with common brown dog ticks (*R. sanguineus*) implicated as a vector of *R. rickettsii*. The broad distribution of this common tick raises concern about its potential to transmit *R. rickettsii* in other settings.

MALARIA

Estimation of Human Body Concentrations of DDT from Indoor Residual Spraying for Malaria Control

Inhabitants of dwellings treated with DDT for indoor residual spraying showed high DDT levels in blood and breast milk. This is of concern since mothers transfer lipid-soluble contaminants such as DDT via breastfeeding to their children. Focusing on DDT use in South Africa, we employ a pharmacokinetic model to estimate DDT levels in human lipid tissue over lifetime of an individual to determine the amount of DDT transferred to children during breastfeeding, and to identify the dominant DDT uptake routes. In particular, the effects of breastfeeding duration, parity, and mother's age on DDT concentrations of mother and infant are investigated. Model results show that primiparous mothers have greater DDT concentrations than multiparous mothers, which causes higher DDT exposure to firstborn children. DDT in the body mainly originates from diet but can be from spraying in old houses. Generally, the modeled DDT levels reproduce levels found in South African biomonitoring data within a factor of 3.

Hazards Associated with Aerial Spraying of Organophosphate Insecticides in Israel

Aerial application of organophosphates can result in exposure to drift and leaf residues for pilots, ground crews, field workers, and residents near sprayed fields. Exposure can be by either the airborne or dermal route, and can produce illness (headaches, fatigue, diarrhea, cramps, and respiratory problems) even with low-grade depressions in cholinesterase. Alkyl phosphate metabolites have been shown to be "gold standard" measures of such exposures. Experience in Israel indicates that reduction of health hazards from exposure to drift and leaf residues may be attained by the use of a comprehensive "mix" of preventive measures. These measures include, first and foremost, reduction in total amount of organophosphates used, followed by substitution of less or more toxic organophosphates, reduction in length of spray season, banning the use of flagger, and greater reliance on tractor spraying. Cotton yield per hectare cultivated has increased despite a reduction in use of pesticides of all kinds and organophosphates in particular. Enclosure and air-conditioning (to prevent heat stress) of cockpits, protective clothing, training, and licensing of pilots have been implemented. Education and communication of information, in keeping with the right-to-know principle on hazards and how they should be controlled and monitored, is a part of a comprehensive strategy. Ground spraying should produce no drift in adjacent residential communities but this depends upon the wind. The criterion for achieving this goal is the absence of urine alkyl phosphate metabolites above the threshold of detection.

Symptoms and Cholinesterase Activity among Rural Residents Living near Cotton Fields in Nicaragua

100 residents, each 10 years of age or older, were randomly selected from a Nicaraguan community surrounded by actively sprayed cotton fields (the exposed community) and from a socioeconomically similar community far from agricultural spraying (the control community). Subjects working with pesticides were excluded and the study was conducted at the end of the 1990 cotton spraying season (August–December). Demographic information, exposure questions, and prevalence of 11 acute symptoms and 17 chronic symptoms were gathered from a structured interview. Finger stick erythrocyte cholinesterase (AChE) inhibitors are classified into four ordinal categories (asymptomatic, nonspecific, possible, probable).

Residents from the exposed community were significantly more likely to report recently sighting a spray plane near their community, exposure to pesticide from drift, crossing recently sprayed fields, eating home-grown food, and feeling ill after drift exposure. The mean AChE value was significantly lower for residents of the exposed community (4.9 vs. 5.3 IU/dL). The proportion of subjects complaining of one or more chronic or acute symptoms was significantly higher for the exposed community (87%) than for the controls (53%). Odd ratios for residents in the exposed community, by symptom categories, were nonspecific 1.6 (95% CI: 0.8–3.2), possible 4.1 (95% CI: 1.7–10.2), and probable 9.93 (95% CI: 2.9–34.4).

These findings indicate a strong association between exposure to aerial pesticides and symptoms. This study should be replicated with more quantitative exposure measures, for if confirmed, the results have relevance for millions in rural communities worldwide.

VOLCANOES

Volcanoes (Mt. St. Helens in Washington State, Kilauea in Hawaii, Popocatepetl in Mexico, Chaparrastique in San Miguel, El Salvador) are a common source of natural air pollution, as are forest fires.[420]

The major active volcanoes are situated in Mexico and the United States, the latter of which are located in Hawaii, Alaska, and Washington State. These increase both local and global air pollution. In terms of human health effects, this uncontrollable source of air pollution is very significant, as is indicated by the increased incidence of respiratory infection in the Mt. St. Helens area.

According to Chow,[420] its objective was to determine the autonomic cardiovascular control among residents of Hawaii who are exposed to varying levels of volcanic air pollution (vog), which consists largely of sulfur dioxide (SO_2) and acid aerosols.

According to Chow,[420] in a cross-sectional study between April 2006 and June 2008, the authors measured cardiovagal autonomic function by HRV in 72 healthy individuals who lived in four exposure zones on Hawaii Island: vog (volcanic air, pollutant) − free ($n = 18$); episodic exposure to $SO_2 > 200$ ppb and acid aerosol ($n = 19$); chronic exposure to $SO_2 \geq 30$ ppb and acid aerosol ($n = 15$); and chronic exposure to acid aerosols ($n = 20$). Individuals with diabetes or heart disease, or who had smoked in the preceding month were excluded. HRV was measured in all subjects during rest, paced breathing, and active standing (Ewing maneuver). HRV was analyzed in time and frequency domains and compared between the four exposure zones.

There were no significant differences between exposure zones in HRV, in either time or frequency domains, even after adjustment for age, gender, ethnicity, and BMI. There was no significant HRV change in three individuals in whom HRV was measured before and during an exposure to combined SO_2 100–250 ppb and concentration of respirable particles of diameter ≥ 2.5 μm ($PM_{2.5}$) >500 μg/m^3. Age was significantly correlated with time-domain parameters during paced breathing and the Ewing maneuver.

This study of healthy individuals found no appreciable effects of vog (volcanic air, pollution) on the autonomic nervous system.

Epidemiological studies show an association between urban air pollution and increased mortality and morbidity attributable to cardiovascular causes.[420–423] Decreased HRV, an indication of disordered autonomic regulation of cardiac rhythm, can predict cardiovascular and all-cause mortality.[424–427] Air pollution may induce lung inflammation and OS, which can cause cardiovascular distress,[428–430] short-term perturbations in sympathetic activity, and sympathovagal imbalance.[431] Sulfur dioxide (SO_2) can reduce vagal tone in asthmatic adults.[432] Studies report associations between the concentration of respirable particles of diameter ≤ 2.5 μm ($PM_{2.5}$) and changes in autonomic nervous system control as assessed by HRV in elderly volunteers.[433] In addition, perturbations in sympathetic activity resulting in sympathovagal imbalance from short-term effects of air pollution are reported.[434–437]

The association between volcanic air pollution and changes in HRV are not well studied. Hawaii's Kilauea volcano has released 300–7000 tons of SO_2 gas daily for more than 25 years, far more than any other stationary source in the United States.[438] SO_2 reacts with water, vapor, oxygen, and sunlight to produce highly acidic, respirable particles. The blend of SO_2 and acid aerosols that comprise volcanic air pollution is referred to locally as "vog."

Hawaii Island's terrain and its prevailing wind patterns create zones of different exposures to volcanic air pollution. Kilauea volcano is located on the southeast portion of the island. Kohala, at the northernmost tip of the island, is usually fog free. It is protected from volcanic air pollution by the prevailing winds from the northeast and by Mauna Kea, the tallest mountain on the island. Volcano Village, located slightly north of Kilauea volcano's summit, is normally upwind of the source during prevailing trade winds. During wind reversals or low wind conditions, however, hourly concentrations of SO_2 in Volcano Village can exceed 500 ppb. Ka'u district, 50 miles southwest and downwind of Kilauea's degassing vents, is chronically exposed, with ambient concentrations of SO_2 of ~30 ppb and $PM_{2.5}$ of 10–15 µg/m³. Kona, west of Kilauea volcano, receives acid particulates that trade winds carry around the southern tip of the island. Diurnal onshore, offshore wind patterns in the lee of the island can cause vog to linger on the Kona coast.

The objective of this study is to determine the association between volcanic air pollution and HRV. They tested the hypothesis that chronic exposure to volcanic air pollution disturbs sympathovagal balance. They measured HRV of individuals who live in the four different exposure zones: vog-free (Kohala), episodic high vog (Volcano Village), chronic SO_2 ~30 ppb and acid aerosol (Ka'u), and chronic high acid aerosol (Kona).

The highest hourly SO_2 level detected by SO_2 analyzers in Volcano Village within 72 hours before HRV testing was 453 ppb; $PM_{2.5}$ was not continuously monitored in Volcano Village. Hourly SO_2 levels in Ka'u were usually at 30 ppb. Concentrations of SO_2 and $PM_{2.5}$ in Ka'u, Kona, and Kohala were estimated from 4-week integrated samples of SO_2 and 2-week integrated samples of $PM_{2.5}$[439,440] conducted between 2002 and 2005, when volcanic emissions were ~1600 tons/day, and weather patterns were similar to the current study period. Their estimations of SO_2 and $PM_{2.5}$ at each site were consistent with ongoing monitoring by the Hawaii State Department of Health started in 2007 (http://www.his02index.info/ and http://airnow.gov/).

Seventy-two subjects from the four exposure zones were studied between April 2006 and July 2008. Characteristics of subjects from each zone indicate significant differences between the groups in percentage of men and in the mean BMI. Apparent differences in mean age and percentage of different ethnic groups did not reach statistical significance.

None of the subjects was excluded because of ectopic beats greater than 5% of the total tachograms. There were minimal atrial and ventricular arrhythmias. Only four ECG tracings required modification due to ectopic beats. All time- and frequency-domain measures were normally distributed and did not require log transformation or use of nonparametric analysis. Age was significantly correlated with SDNN during paced breathing ($r = -0.20$, $p = 0.04$) and Ewing maneuver ($r = 0.22$, $p = 0.05$). This was supported by the significant correlation between age and PNN_{50} during paced breathing ($r = 0.31$, $p = 0.008$) and Ewing maneuver ($r = 0.26$, $p = 0.02$). No significant correlation was noted between age and RMSSD. No correlation was noted between age and frequency-domain measures, such as high-frequency power and low-/high-frequency power ratio. No significant differences were noted between men and women in time- and frequency-domain measures.

Time-domain measures did not differ between the sites. Given the strong effects of age, and the unequal proportions of gender, ethnicity, and BMI between sites, adjustment of these covariants was performed. There were no significant differences in time-domain measures between sites even after adjustment for these covariants. It displaces spectral analysis during: (1) rest, (2) deep breathing, and (3) Ewing maneuvers. Frequency peaks were clearly delineated at each maneuver. There were no significant differences between the sites in the frequency domain variables, even after adjusting for gender, ethnicity, and BMI. The low-frequency power, high-frequency power, and ratio of low- to high-frequency power were not significantly different between the four zones. Combining all the exposed zones into one (any exposure to volcanic pollution) group and comparing it with the vog-free zone did not reveal any significant differences in time and frequency domains.

The observations in the cross-sectional study were further supported by a natural experiment in which increased emissions from Kilauea and conducive weather conditions caused SO_2 to exceed 500 ppb and $PM_{2.5}$ to exceed 500 µg/m^3 in Ka'u on several occasions. They were able to repeat studies in three of the Ka'u subjects during such an episode. Despite these conditions, there was no change in intraindividual time- or frequency-domain measures before and after this high vog episode.

This is the first study to examine the effects of volcanic pollution on autonomic function as assessed by HRV. The study area provides an uncommon opportunity because there is relatively little fossil fuel-derived air pollution in any area. This allows us to examine the long-term effects of SO_2 and acid aerosols with little confounding by other pollutants through four volcanic air pollution exposure zones.[441,442] These zones are determined by the rate of volcanic emission, wind speed and direction, and distance from the source and terrain. SO_2 and acid (sulfate) aerosol concentration at the times of HRV measurements were inferred from the volcanic emissions measured by the National Park Service/U.S. Geological Survey and wind speed and direction, measured by the National Weather Service.[439,440]

This study suggests that exposure to volcanic pollution, at the concentrations and composition that prevailed in these four zones between April 2006 and July 2008, is not associated with autonomic imbalance in healthy adults. These findings differ from an earlier study of 21 active 53- to 87-year-old subjects in Boston, in which ambient $PM_{2.5}$ (as high as 49 µg/m^3 or ozone (as high as 77 ppb) were associated with significantly decreased SDNN and r-MSSD, with a combined effect of a 33% reduction in the mean r-MSSD.[443] Similarly, a study of healthy young adults in MC, each increase in $PM_{2.5}$ of 30 µg/m^3 in the 2 hours before HRV measurement was associated with a significant decrease in pNN_{50}.[444] Indeed, a growing body of evidence confirms an association between $PM_{2.5}$ or ozone and diminished HRV.[364,423,430] One major reason for the difference in results is the different source and composition of Hawaii's volcanic air pollution. It does not result from combustion of carbonaceous fuels, as is typical of the ambient pollution in studies in urban or industrial settings. Fine particles that result from volcanic emissions are mainly sulfates, with little or no organic or oxidant compounds. There is no secondary production of ozone, an inflammatory component of urban pollution.[445]

The finding that SO_2, even at concentrations that exceed 400 ppb, was not associated with decreased HRV differs from that of Tunnicliffe et al., who showed that SO_2 of 200 ppb decreased HRV in 12 nonasthmatic and 12 asthmatic subjects.[441] Routledge et al.[446] similarly demonstrated decreased vagal control after the subject breathed SO_2 200 ppb. These chamber studies allowed the investigators to detect the time-dependent and transient nature of the response, which may have been missed in field studies. They had also excluded current smokers. Several studies indicate that cigarette smoking not only directly decreases HRV but also can synergistically augment the effect of SO_2.[447,448] HRV associated with small changes in ambient SO_2 in Korea (4 hour mean 67 ppb) was significantly reduced in 267 smokers compared with 700 nonsmokers.[449]

Moreover, while the lack of significant findings could still be due to a lack of statistical power, there did not seem to be a consistent pattern of differences about the mean among each community, which supports our conclusion that the observed variability in the study parameters was due to random variation.

Their study found no appreciable influence of volcanic air pollution on the autonomic nervous system. The lack of significant differences between the groups exposed to different levels of air pollution may be due to excluding people who were more susceptible to autonomic dysfunction, exposure to predominantly SO_2 gas and acid aerosols (and not organic compounds or strong oxidants), small sample size, or a combination of all these factors. More studies are needed to increase our understanding of the effects of higher levels of volcanic air pollution, or its effects on susceptible individuals with comorbidities such as COPD, asthma, diabetes, and cardiovascular disease.[450]

According to Longo et al.,[439] they investigated cardiorespiratory health effects associated with chronic exposure to volcanogenic sulfur dioxide (SO_2) and fine sulfate particle (< or = 0.3 µm) air pollution emitted from Kilauea Volcano, Hawaii.

An air study was conducted to measure exposure levels in the downwind area, and to confirm nonexposure in a reference area. Cross-sectional health data were collected from 335 adults, > or = 20 years of age, who had resided for > or = 7 years in the study areas. Prevalence was estimated for cardiorespiratory signs, and self-reported symptoms and diseases. Logistic regression analysis estimated effect measures between exposed and unexposed groups considering potential confounding including age, gender, race, smoking, dust, and BMI. Student's t-tests compared mean differences in BP, pulse, and respiratory rates.

The results were statistically significant positive associations between chronic exposure and increased prevalence of cough, phlegm, rhinorrhea, sore/dry throat, sinus congestion, wheezing, eye irritation, and bronchitis. The magnitude of the associations differed according to SO_2 and fine sulfate particulate exposure. Group analyses found no differences in pulse rate or BP; however, significantly faster mean pulse rates were detected in exposed nonmedicated, nonsmoking participants with BMI < 25, and in participants aged > or = 65 years. Higher mean systolic BP was found in exposed participants with BMI < 25.

Long-term residency in active degassing volcanic areas may have an adverse effect on cardiorespiratory health in adults. Further, study at Kilauea is recommended and the authors encourage investigations in communities near active volcanoes worldwide.

According to Hansell and Oppenheimer,[451] millions of people are potentially exposed to volcanic gases worldwide and exposures may differ from those in anthropogenic air pollution. A systematic literature review found few primary studies relating to health hazards of volcanic gases. SO_2 and acid aerosols from eruptions and degassing events were associated with respiratory morbidity and mortality but not childhood asthma prevalence or lung function decrements. Accumulations of H_2S and exposure to H_2S in geothermal areas were associated with increases in nervous system and respiratory diseases. Some impacts were on a large scale, affecting several countries (e.g., Laki fissure eruption in Iceland in 1783–1784). No studies on health effects of volcanic releases of halogen gases or metal vapors were located. More high-quality collaborative studies involving volcanologists and epidemiologists are recommended.

According to Ishigami et al.,[452] following a volcanic eruption in 2000, high concentrations of ambient sulfur dioxide (SO_2) are still observed on Miyake-jima, Japan despite the reversal 2 years ago of the ban on residents living on the island. This study examines the association between current levels of volcanic SO_2 and the incidence of acute subjective symptoms in volunteers on Miyake-jima.

Hourly incidence of cough, scratchy throat, sore throat, and breathlessness showed clear exposure–response relationships with SO_x concentrations. There were statistically significant risks of those symptoms at relatively low SO_2 levels. Thus, rate ratios in the 0.6–2.0 ppm exposure band (vs. <0.01 ppm) were for cough, 3.4 (95% CI 1.8–6.6) in men and 9.8 (3.9–24.9) in women; for sore throat, 3.2 (1.7–6.2) in men and 5.8 (2.0–16.5) in women; and for breathlessness 10.5 (4.2–26.6) in men and 18.5 (4.6–74.3) in women. Little evidence of SO_2 effects on sputum and nasal discharge/congestion was observed in this study. Eye and skin irritations showed inconsistent results between hourly maximal and hourly mean SO_2 concentrations.

The authors observed strong evidence of an exposure–response relationship between volcanic SO_2 and subjective acute respiratory symptoms among a healthy population on Miyake-jima. The results are consistent with reports that females and nonsmokers are more sensitive to irritant gas than males and smokers, respectively.

Relationship between Ambient Sulfur Dioxide Levels and Neonatal Mortality near Mt. Sakurajima Volcano in Japan

Shinkura et al.[453] examined the association between neonatal mortality and ambient sulfur dioxide (SO_2) levels in the neighborhood of Mt. Sakurajima, Yamashita public health district of Kagoshima City, during the period between 1978 and 1988. The analysis using Poisson regression models showed that the monthly average level of SO_2 was positively associated with the neonatal mortality

($p = 0.002$). When the SO_2 levels were categorized into four groups to estimate the RR of neonatal mortality using the lowest exposure category as a reference, the RR increased with elevated exposure levels (p for trend <0.001) and was the highest in the group with the highest level of exposure (RR = 2.2%, 95% CI: 1.2–4.1). Other than SO_2, they also examined the number of eruptions, the amount of ashfall, and the average level of suspended PM. None of these factors were associated with neonatal mortality. Although the present study suggests that increase in SO_2 levels has had an adverse effect on neonatal mortality in the neighborhood of Mt. Sakurajima, it is difficult to determine the source of the SO_2. Further studies are necessary to elucidate the mechanisms of the excess neonatal mortality probably associated with the volcanic SO_2 levels.

According to Horwell,[454] respirable crystalline silica (RCS) continues to pose a risk to human health worldwide. Its variable toxicity depends on inherent characteristics and external factors which influence surface chemistry. Significant population exposure to RCS occurs during volcanic eruptions, where ashfall may cover hundreds of square kilometers and exposure may last for many years. Occupational exposure also occurs through mining of volcanic deposits. The primary source of RCS from volcanoes is through collapse and fragmentation of lava domes within which cristobalite is mass produced. After 30 years of research, it is still not clear if volcanic ash is a chronic respiratory health hazard. Toxicological assays have shown that cristobalite-rich ash is less toxic than expected. They investigated the reasons for this by determining the physicochemical/structural characteristics which may modify the pathogenicity of volcanic RCS. Four theories are considered: (1) The reactivity of particle surfaces is reduced due to cosubstitutions of Al and Na for Si in the cristobalite structure; (2) particles consist of aggregates of cristobalite and other phases, restricting the surface area of cristobalite available reactions in the lung; (3) the cristobalite surface is occluded by an annealed rim; and (4) dissolution of other volcanic particles affects the surfaces of RCS in the lung.

The composition of volcanic cristobalite crystals was quantified by electron microprobe and differences in composition assessed by Welch's two-sample t-test. Sections of dome-rock and ash particles were imaged by scanning and transmission electron microscopy, and elemental compositions of rims determined by energy dispersive x-ray spectroscopy.

Volcanic cristobalite contains up to 4 wt. % combined Al_2O_3 and Na_2O. Most cristobalite-bearing ash particles contain adhered materials such as feldspar and glass. No annealed rims were observed.

The composition of volcanic cristobalite particles gives insight into previously unconsidered inherent characteristics of *silica mineralogy* which may affect *toxicity*. The structural features identified may also influence the hazard of other environmentally and occupationally produced silica dusts. Current exposure regulations do not take into account the characteristics that might render the silica surface less harmful.

According to Wilson et al.,[455] in July 1995, the Soufriere Hills volcano on the island of Montserrat began to erupt. Preliminary reports showed that the ash contained a substantial respirable component and a large percentage of the toxic silica polymorph, cristobalite. In this study, the cytotoxicity of three respirable Montserrat volcanic ash (MVA) samples were investigated: M1 from a single explosive event, M2 accumulated ash predominantly derived from pyroclastic flows, and M3 from a single pyroclastic flow. These were compared with the relatively inert dust TiO_2 and the known toxic quartz dust, DQ12.

The surface of the particles was measured with the Brunauer, Emmet, and Teller (BET) adsorption method and cristobalite content of MVA was determined by x-ray diffraction (XRD). After exposure to particles, the metabolic competence of the epithelial cell line A549 was assessed to determine cytotoxic effects. The ability of the particles to induce sheep blood erythrocyte hemolysis was used to assess surface reactivity.

Treatment with either MVA, quartz, or titanium dioxide decreased A549 epithelial cell metabolic competence as measured by ability to reduce 3-(4,5-dimethylthiazol-2-yl)-2,5-diphenyltetrazolium bromide (MTT). On addition of mannitol, the cytotoxic effect was significantly less with M1, quartz, and TiO_2. All MVA samples induced a dose-dependent increase in hemolysis, which, although less than the hemolysis induced by quartz, was significantly greater than that induced by TiO_2. Addition of mannitol and SOD significantly reduced the hemolytic activity only of M1, but not of M2 or M3, the samples derived from predominantly pyroclastic flow events.

Neither the cristobalite content nor the surface area of the MVA samples correlated with observed *in vitro* reactivity. A role for reactive oxygen species could only be shown in the cytotoxicity of M1, which was the only sample derived from a purely explosive event. These results suggest that in general the bioreactivity of MVA samples *in vitro* is low compared with pure quartz, but that the bioreactivity and mechanisms of biological interaction may vary according to the ash source.

According to Housley et al.,[456] the Soufriere Hills, a stratovolcano on Montserrat started erupting in July 1995, producing volcanic ash, both from dome-collapse pyroclastic flows and phreatic explosions. The eruptions/ash resuspension result in high concentrations of suspended PM in the atmosphere, which includes cristobalite, a mineral implicated in respiratory disorders.

Housley et al.[456] conducted toxicological studies on characterized samples of ash, together with major components of the dust mixture (anorthite, cristobalite), and a bioreactive mineral control (DQ12 quartz).

Rats were challenged with a single mass (1 mg) dose of particles via intratracheal instillation and groups sacrificed at 1, 3, and 9 weeks. Acute bioreactivity of the particles was assessed by increases in lung permeability and inflammation, changes in epithelial cell markers, and increase in the size of bronchothoracic lymph nodes.

Data indicated that respirable ash derived from pyroclastic flow (20.1% cristobalite) or phreatic explosion (8.6% cristobalite) had minimal bioreactivity in the lung. Anorthite showed low bioreactivity, in contrast to pure cristobalite, which showed progressive increases in lung damage.

The results suggest that either the percentage mass of cristobalite particles present in Montserrat ash was not sufficient as a catalyst in the lung environment, or its surface reactivity was masked by the nonreactive volcanic glass components during the process of ash formation.

Higuchi et al.[457] studied Mt. Sakurajima in Japan as one of the most active volcanoes in the world. This work was conducted to examine the effect of volcanic ash on the chronic respiratory disease mortality in the vicinity of Mt. Sakurajima.

The present work examined the standardized mortality ratios (SMRs) of respiratory diseases during the period 1968–2002 in Sakurajima town and Tarumizu city, where ashfall from the volcano recorded more than 10.000 $g/m^2/year$ on average in the 1980s.

The SMR of lung cancer in the Sakurajima–Tarumizu area was 1.61 (95% CI = 1.44–1.78) for men and 1.67 (95% CI = 1.39–1.95) for women while it was nearly equal to one in Kanoya city, which neighbors Tarumizu city but located at the further position from Mt. Sakurajima, and therefore has much smaller amounts of ashfall. Sakurajima–Tarumizu area had elevated SMRs for COPDs and acute respiratory diseases while Kanoya did not.

Cristobalite is the most likely cause of the increased deaths from those chronic respiratory diseases since smoking is unlikely to explain the increased mortality of respiratory diseases among women since the proportion of smokers in Japanese women is less than 20%, and SPM levels in the Sakurajima–Tarumizu area were not high. Further studies seem warranted.

The Sidoarjo mud flow or Lapindo mud (informally abbreviated as Lusi, a contraction of Lumpur Sidoarjo wherein lumpur is the Indonesian word for mud) is the result of an erupting mud volcano[458] in the subdistrict of Porong, Sidoarjo in East Java, Indonesia that has been in eruption since May 2006. It is the biggest mud volcano in the world; responsibility for it was credited to the blowout of a natural gas well drilled by PT Lapindo Brantas, although some scientists[459] and company officials contend it was caused by a distant earthquake.

At its peak, Lusi spewed up to 180,000 m^3 of mud per day.[460] By mid-August 2011, mud was being discharged at a rate of 10,000 m^3 per day with 15 bubblers around its gushing point. This was a significant decline from the previous year when mud was being discharged at a rate of 100,000 cubic meters per day with 320 bubbles around its gushing point.[461] It is expected that the flow will continue for the next 25–30 years.[460,462] Although the Sidoarjo mud flow has been contained by levees since November 2008, resultant floodings regularly disrupt local highways and villages, and further breakouts of mud are still possible.[463]

People with chemical sensitivity do poorly in volcanic areas like Hawaii. Our patients already have neurovascular membrane damage. Therefore, the exposures to not only the SO_2 gas but also the ash particles further damage the cellular and vascular membranes which then develop leaks and cause the increase in intracellular calcium, which when combined with protein kinases A and C and phosphorylated, increases the hypersensitivity response 1000 times. We have seen this response repeatedly. The increase in intracellular Ca^{2+} also releases several enzymes like endonuclease, proteases, and nitric oxide synthase. This suddenly influences metabolism and other body responses as well as nitric oxide which trigger the proximate mechanism.

The west coast of Central America is lined with volcanoes. Some of them are quiescent, some active. One of them, San Miguel (also known as Chaparrastique) in El Salvador, has erupted in modern times, as recently as 2002.

On December 29, 2001, it underwent a decent-sized paroxysm, blasting a cloud of ash, steam, and gas that rapidly expanded to about 40 km in width, blowing east and north for more than a hundred kilometers.

This area is a subduction zone, where one continental plate is sliding under another. Stress builds up in the rocky plates, which can slip suddenly and cause earthquakes. Magma from deep inside the Earth can make its way to the surface as well, so subduction zones are frequently dotted with volcanoes.

OIL SPILLS

Most oil spills not only devastate the wildlife but also the human population. The oil spill in Alaska and the one in the Gulf of Mexico are illustrations of the effects on both the wildlife and the human population. The Alaskan oil spill changed the life of many people as did the Florida and Gulf of Mexico spills.

The Gulf of Mexico oil spill damaged many more due to the populous cost of Western Florida, Mississippi, Louisiana, and Alabama.

The oil spill in the Gulf of Mexico poses direct threat to human health from inhalation or dermal contact with the oil and dispersant chemicals, and indirect threats to seafood safety and mental health. Physicians should be familiar with health effects from oil spills to appropriately advise, diagnose, and treat patients who live and work along the Gulf Coast or wherever a major oil spill occurs.[464]

The main components of crude oil are aliphatic and aromatic hydrocarbons. Lower-molecular-weight aromatics, such as benzene, toluene, and xylene, are VOCs and evaporate within hours after the oil reaches the surface. VOCs can cause respiratory irritation and CNS depression. Benzene is known to cause leukemia in humans, and toluene is a recognized teratogen at high doses. Higher-molecular-weight chemicals such as naphthalene evaporate more slowly. Naphthalene is "reasonably anticipated to cause cancer in humans" based on olfactory neuroblastomas, nasal tumors, and lung cancers in animals. Oil can also release hydrogen sulfide gas and contains traces of heavy metals, as well as nonvolatile PAHs that can contaminate the food chain. Hydrogen sulfide gas is neurotoxic and has been linked to both acute and chronic CNS effects; PAHs include mutagens and probably carcinogens. Burning oil generates PM, which is associated with cardiac and respiratory symptoms and premature mortality. The Gulf oil spill is unique because of the large-scale use of dispersants to break up the oil slick. By late July, more than 1.8 million gallons of dispersant had been applied in the Gulf. Dispersants contain detergents, surfactants, and petroleum distillates, including respiratory irritants such as 2,1-butoxyethanol, propylene glycol, and sulfonic acid salts. In addition to oil and its products (Chapter 6), these dispersants cause havoc with the chemically sensitive, causing an exacerbation of their symptoms (Figures 1.10 and 1.11).

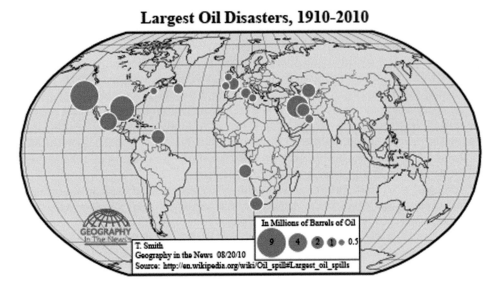

FIGURE 1.10   (**See color insert.**) Largest oil disasters, 1910–2010.

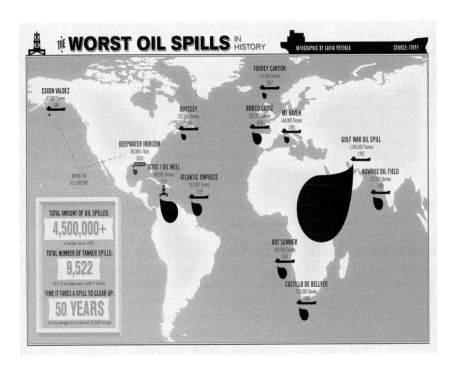

FIGURE 1.11   Worst oil spills in history. (Courtesy of Potenza, G. ITOPF (2011).)

Major Oil Spills

A brief summary of the top 20 major oil spills that have occurred since the Torrey Canyon in 1967 is given in Table 1.22 and the locations are shown in Figure 1.11; it is of note that 19 of the largest spills recorded occurred before the year 2000. A number of these incidents, despite their large size, caused little or no environmental damage as the oil was spilt some distance offshore and did not impact

TABLE 1.22

Major Oil Spills Since 1967 (Quantities Have Been Rounded to Nearest Thousand)

Position	ShipName	Year	Location	Spill Size (Tonnes)
1	Atlantic Empress	1979	Off Tobago, West Indies	287,000
2	ABT Summer	1991	700 nautical miles off Angola	260,000
3	Castillo de Bellver	1983	Off Saldanha Bay, South Africa	252,000
4	Amoco Cadiz	1978	Off Brittany, France	223,000
5	Haven	1991	Genoa, Italy	144,000
6	Odyssey	1988	700 nautical miles off Nova Scotia, Canada	132,000
7	Torrey Canyon	1967	Scilly Isles, United Kingdom	119,000
8	Sea Star	1972	Gulf of Oman	115,000
9	Irenes Serenade	1980	Navarino Bay, Greece	100,000
10	Urquiola	1976	La Coruna, Spain	100,000
11	Hawaiian Patriot	1977	300 nautical miles off Honolulu	95,000
12	Independenta	1979	Bosphorus, Turkey	95,000
13	Jakob Maersk	1975	Oporto, Portugal	88,000
14	Braer	1993	Shetland Islands, United Kingdom	85,000
15	Aegean Sea	1992	La Coruna, Spain	74,000
16	Sea Empress	1996	Milford Haven, United Kingdom	72,000
17	Khark 5	1989	120 nautical miles off Atlantic coast of Morocco	70,000
18	Nova	1985	Off Kharg Island, Gulf of Iran	70,000
19	Katina P	1992	Off Maputo, Mozambique	67,000
20	Prestige	2002	Off Galicia, Spain	63,000
35	Exxon Valdez	1989	Prince William Sound, Alaska, United States	37,000
131	Hebei Spirit	2007	Taean, Republic of Korea	11,000

coastlines. It is for this reason that some of the names listed may be unfamiliar. Exxon Valdez and Hebei Spirit are included for comparison although these incidents fall some way outside the group.

Number of Oil Spills

The incidence of large spills (>700 tons) is relatively low and detailed statistical analysis is rarely possible; consequently, emphasis is placed on identifying trends. Thus, it is apparent from Table 1.2 that the number of large spills has decreased significantly in the last 44 years during which records have been kept. The average number of major spills for the decade 2000–2009 is 3.5, one seventh of the average for years in the 1970s. Looking at this downward trend from another perspective, 54% of the large spills recorded occurred in the 1970s, and this percentage has decreased in each decade to 8% in the 2000s (Figure 1.12).

A decline can also be observed with medium-sized spills (7–700 tons) in Figure 1.4 and Table 1.23. Here, the average number of spills in the 2000s was close to 15, whereas in the 1990s, the average number of spills was almost double this number.

No large spills were recorded for 2012 but seven medium spills were recorded. Despite being higher than those seen in 2010 and 2011, this figure is still far below the averages for previous decades.

Background

ITOPF maintains a database of oil spills from tankers, combined carriers, and barges. This contains information on accidental spillages since 1970, except those resulting from acts of war.

It should be noted that the figures for the amount of oil spilt in an incident include all oil lost to the environment, including that which burnt or remained in a sunken vessel. There is considerable annual variation in both the incidence of oil spills and the amounts of oil lost. Consequently, the figures in the following tables and any averages derived from them should be viewed with an element of caution.

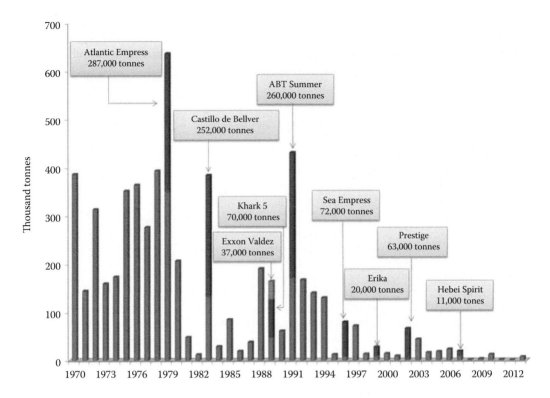

FIGURE 1.12   **(See color insert.)** Quantities of oil spilt >7 tonnes, 1970–2013 (rounded to the nearest thousand). (Courtesy of ITPOF, 2012.)

QUANTITIES OF OIL SPILT

The vast majority of spills are significant (i.e., less than 7 tons) and data on the number of incidents and quantity of oil spilt are incomplete due to the inconsistent reporting of smaller incidents worldwide.

Approximately 5.75 million tons of oil was lost as a result of tanker incidents from 1970 to 2013. However, as Figures 1.5 and 1.6 indicate, the volume of oil spilt from tankers demonstrates a significant improvement through the decades. Consistent with the reduction in the number of oil spills from tankers, the volume of oil spilt also shows a marked reduction. For instance, from Table 1.3 it is interesting to observe that an amount greater than the total quantity of oil spilt in the decade 2000–2009 (213,000 tons) was spilt in several single years in earlier decades.

The total amount of oil lost to the environment in 2013 was 7000 tons, the vast majority of which can be attributed to the three large spills (>700 tons) recorded during the year.

LARGE SPILLS

As demonstrated in Figures 1.8 and 1.12, when looking at the frequency and quantities of oil spilt, it should be noted that a few very large spills are responsible for a high percentage of oil spilt. For example, in more recent decades, the following can be seen:

- In the 1990s, there were 358 spills of 7 tons and over, resulting in 1,133,000 tons of oil lost; 73% of this amount was spilt in just 10 incidents.
- In the 2000s, there were 182 spills of 7 tons and over, resulting in 213,000 tons of oil lost; 53% of this amount was spilt in just 4 incidents.

TABLE 1.23
Oil Spills around the World

Spill/Vessel	Location	Dates	Min Tons	Max Tons	Authors
North Dakota pipeline spill	United States, North Dakota, Tioga	September 25–29, 2013	2810	2810	938, 939
Rayong oil spill	Thailand, Rayong/Ko Samet, Gulf of Thailand	July 27, 2013	43	163	940, 941
Cushing storage terminal spill	United States, Oklahoma, Cushing	May 18, 2013	340	340	942, 943
2013 Mayflower oil spill	United States, Arkansas, Mayflower	March 30, 2013	680	950	944
Magnolia refinery spill	United States, Arkansas, Magnolia	March 9, 2013	680	760	945, 946
Arthur Kill storage tank spill (Hurricane Sandy)	United States, New Jersey, Sewaren	October 29, 2012	1090	1130	947, 411
Sundre, Alberta oil spill	Canada, Sundre	June 8, 2012	410	410	948
Nigeria oil spill	Nigeria, Bonga Field	December 21, 2011	5500	5500	949
TK Bremen	France, Brittany, Erdeven	December 16, 2011	220	220	950
Campos Basin oil spill	Brazil, Campos Basin, Frade Field	November 7–15, 2011	89	400	951, 952
Rena oil spill	New Zealand, Tauranga, Bay of Plenty	October 5, 2011–August 2012	350	350	953, 954
North Sea oil spill	United Kingdom, North Sea, Gannet Alpha platform	August 10–13, 2011	216	216	955
2011 Yellowstone River oil spill	United States, Billings, Montana, Yellowstone River	July 1, 2011	105	140	956
Bohai Bay oil spill	China, Bohai Bay	June 4–19, 2011	204	204	957, 958
2011 Little Buffalo oil spill	Canada, Alberta	April 29, 2011	3800	3800	959, 960
Mumbai-Uran pipeline spill	India, Mumbai, Arabian Sea	January 21, 2011	40	55	961, 962
Fiume Santo power station	Italy, Sardinia, Porto Torres	January 11, 2011	15	15	963
Mumbai oil spill/MV MSC Chitra and MV Khalijia 3	India, Mumbai, Arabian Sea	August 7–9, 2010	400	800	964, 965, 966
Barataria Bay oil spill	United States, Barataria Bay, Gulf of Mexico	July 27, 2010–August 1, 2010	23	45	967, 441, 968, 970
Kalamazoo River oil spill	United States, Kalamazoo River, Calhoun County, Michigan	July 26, 2010	2800	3250	970, 971
Xingang Port oil spill	China, Yellow Sea	July 16–21, 2010	1500	90,000	972, 973
Jebel al-Zayt oil spill	Egypt, Red Sea	June 16–23, 2010	Unknown	Unknown	974
Red Butte Creek oil spill	United States, Salt Lake City, Utah	June 11–12, 2010	65	107	975, 442
Trans-Alaska Pipeline spill	United States, Anchorage, Alaska	May 25, 2010	400	1200	976
MT Bunga Kelana 3	Singapore, Singapore Strait	May 25, 2010	2000	2500	977, 978, 979
2010 ExxonMobil oil spill	Nigeria, Niger Delta	May 1, 2010	3246	95,500	980, 981, 982

(Continued)

TABLE 1.23 (*Continued*)
Oil Spills around the World

Spill/Vessel	Location	Dates	Min Tons	Max Tons	Authors
Deepwater Horizon	United States, Gulf of Mexico	April 20, 2010–July 15, 2010	492,000	627,000	983
2010 Great Barrier Reef oil spill/MV Shen Neng 1	Australia Great Keppel Island	April 3, 2010	3	4	984, 985, 986
2010 Port Arthur oil spill	United States, Port Arthur, Texas	January 23, 2010	1500	1500	987
Yellow River oil spill	China, Chishui River (Shaanxi)	January 5, 2010	130	130	988
Montara oil spill	Australia, Timor Sea	August 21, 2009	4000	30,000	989, 990
Full City oil spill	Norway, Rognsfjorden near Sastein south of Langesund	July 31, 2009	200	200	991
2009 Luderitz oil spill	Namibia, Southern coast	April 8, 2009	Unknown	Unknown	992
2009 Queensland oil spill	Australia, Queensland	March 10, 2009	230	260	993
West Cork oil spill	Ireland, Southern coast	February 2009	300	300	994
2008 New Orleans oil spill	United States, New Orleans, Louisiana	July 28, 2008	8800	8800	995
2007 Stafford oil spill	Norway, Norwegian Sea	December 12, 2007	4000	4000	996
2007 Korea oil spill	South Korea, Yellow Sea	December 7, 2007	10,800	10,800	997, 998
Kerch Strait oil spill	Ukraine Russia, Strait of Kerch	November 11, 2007	1000	1000	567
Cosco Busan oil spill	United States, San Francisco, California	November 7, 2007	188	188	1000
Kab 101	Mexico, Bay of Campeche	October 23, 2007–December 17, 2007	1869	1869	1001
Burnaby Oil spill	Canada, Burnaby, British Columbia	July 24, 2007	201	01	1002
Guimaraas oil spill	Philippines, Guimaras Strait	August 11, 2006	172	1540	1003
Jiyeh Power Station oil spill	Lebanon	July 14–15, 2006	20,000	30,000	1003
Citgo refinery oil spill	United States, Lake Charles, Louisiana	June 19, 2006	6500	6500	1004
Prudhoe Bay oil spill	United States, Alaska North Slope, Alaska	March 2, 2006	653	689	1005
Bass Enterprises (Hurricane Katrina)	United States, Cox Bay, Louisiana	August 30, 2005	12,000	12,000	1006
Shell (Hurricane Katrina)	United States, Pilottown, Louisiana	August 30, 2005	3400	3400	1006
Chevron (Hurricane Katrina	United States, Empire, Louisiana	August 30, 2005	3200	3200	1006
Murphy Oil U.S. refinery spill (Hurricane Katrina)	United States, Meraux and Chalmette, Louisiana	August 30, 2005	2660	3410	1006, 1007
Bass Enterprises (Hurricane Katrina)	United States, Pointe a la Hache, Louisiana	August 30, 2005	1500	1500	1006

(Continued)

TABLE 1.23 (*Continued*)
Oil Spills around the World

Spill/Vessel	Location	Dates	Min Tons	Max Tons	Authors
Chevron (Hurricane Katrina)	United States, Port Fourchon, Louisiana	August 30, 2005	170	170	1006
Venice Energy Services Company (Hurricane Katrina)	United States, Venice, Louisiana	August 30, 2005	81	81	1006
Shell Pipeline oil (Hurricane Katrina)	United States, Nairn, Louisiana	August 30, 2005	44	44	1006
Sundown Energy (Hurricane Katrina)	United States, West Potash, Louisiana	August 30, 2005	42	42	1006
MV Selendang Ayu	United States, Unalaska Island, Alaska	December 8, 2004	1560	1560	1008
Athos 1	United States, Delaware River, Paulsboro, New Jersey	November 26, 2004	860	860	1009
MP-80 Delta 20′ pipeline (Hurricane Ivan)	United States, Louisiana	September 16–19, 2004	963	963	1010
MP-69 Nakika 18′ and MP-151 Nakila 18′ pipeline (Hurricane Ivan)	United States, Louisiana	September 16, 2004–October 6, 2004	618	618	1010
Chevron-Texaco tank collapse (Hurricane Ivan)	United States, Louisiana	September 16–17, 2004	423	423	1010
Tasman Spirit	Pakistan, Karachi	July 28, 2003	28,000	30,000	1011, 1012
Bouchard No. 120	United States, Buzzards Bay, Bourne Massachusetts	April 27, 2003	320	320	1013
Prestige oil spill	Spain, Galicia	November 13, 2002	63,000	63,000	1014, 1015, 1016
Limburg (bombing)	Yemen, Gulf of Aden	October 6, 2002	12,200	12,200	1017, 1018
Manguinhos refinery	Brazil, Guanabara Bay, Rio de Janeiro	November 23, 2001	34	97	1019
Trans-Alaska Pipeline gunshot spill	United States, Alaska	October 4, 2001	932	932	1020
2001 Shell Ogbodo oil spill	Nigeria	June 25, 2001	9500	Unknown	1021
2001 Shell Ogoniland oil spill	Nigeria	May 2001	Unknown	Unknown	1022
Petrobras 36	Brazil, Roncador Oil Field, Campos Basin	March 15, 2001	274	274	332
Amorgos oil spill	Taiwan, Southern coast	January 14, 2001	1150	1150	1023
Jessica	Ecuador, Galapagos Islands	January 2001	568	568	901, 1024
Pine River	Canada, Chetwynd, British Columbia	August 1, 2000	850	850	1025
Project Deep spill	Norway, Helland-Hansen ridge	June 2000	100	100	1026
Treasure	South Africa, Cape Town	June 2000	1400	1400	901
Petrobras pipeline	Brazil, Guanabara Bay, Rio de Janeiro	January 2000	1100	1100	901, 1019

(Continued)

TABLE 1.23 (*Continued*)
Oil Spills around the World

Spill/Vessel	Location	Dates	Min Tons	Max Tons	Authors
Erika	France, Bay of Biscay	December 12, 1999	15,000	25,000	1008, 593
MV New Carissa	United States, Coos Bay, Oregon	February 4, 1999–March 9, 1999	230	230	1027
Mobil Nigeria oil spill	Nigeria	January 12, 1998	5500	5500	1006
Nakhodka	Japan, Sea of Japan	December 1997	6240	6240	1028
Julie N.	United States, Portland, Main	September 27, 1996	586	586	1029
Sea Empress	United Kingdom, Pembrokeshire	February 15, 1996	40,000	72,000	1008, 1014
North Cape	United States, Rhode Island	January 19, 1996	2500	2500	1030
Seki oil spill	United Arab Emirates	March 31, 1994	15,90	15,900	1008
Morris J. Berman oil spill	Puerto Rico	January 7, 1994	2600	23,600	1031
MV Braer	United Kingdom, Shetland	January 5, 1993	85,000	85,000	1014
Aegean Sea	Spain, A Coruna	December 3, 1922	74,000	74,000	1014
Katina P	Mozambique, Maputo	April 26, 1992	72,000	72,000	1014
Fergana Valley	Uzbekistan	March 2, 1992	285,000	285,000	1008
Kirki	Australia, Indian Ocean, off the coast of Western Australia	July 21, 1991	17,280	17,280	1032
ABT Summer	Angola, 700 nmi (1300 km; 810 mi) offshore	May 28, 1991	260,000	260,000	1014
MT Haven	Italy, Mediterranean Sea near Genoa	April 11, 1991	144,000	144,000	1014
Gulf War oil spill	Iraq, Persian Gulf	January 23, 1991	270,000	820,0900	1033, 1034
Mega Borg	United States, Gulf of Mexico, 57 mi (92 km) SE of Galveston, Texas	June 8, 1990	16,499	16,501	1035
American Trader	United State, Bolsa Chica State Beach, California	February 7, 1990	979	981	1014, 1036
Arthur Kill pipeline spill	United States, New Jersey, Sewaren	January 1, 1990	1840	1840	1037, 608
Khark 5	Spain, 350 nmi (650 km; 400 mi) off Las Palmas de Gran Canaria	December 19, 1989	70,000	80 m,000	1008, 1014
Presidente Rivera	United States, Delaware River, Marcus Hook, Pennsylvania	June 24, 1989	993	993	1039
Exxon Valdez	United States, Prince William Sound, Alaska	March 24, 1989	37,000	104,000	1014, 474
Odyssey	Canada, 700 nmi (1300 km; 810 mi) off Nova Scotia	November 10, 1988	132,000	132,000	1014
Ashland oil spill	United States, Floreffe, Pennsylvania	January 2, 1988	10,000	10,000	1040, 1041
Nova	Iran, Gulf of Iran, Kharg Island	December 6, 1985	70,000	70,000	1014
Grand Eagle	United States, Delaware River, Marcus Hook, Pennsylvania	September 28, 1985	1400	1400	1042

(Continued)

TABLE 1.23 (*Continued*)
Oil Spills around the World

Spill/Vessel	Location	Dates	Min Tons	Max Tons	Authors
SS Mobil Oil	United States, Columbia River, Longview, Washington	March 19, 1984	550	650	1043, 1044
Castillo de Bellver	South Africa, Saldanha Bay	August 6, 1983	252,000	252,000	1014
Nowruz field platform	Iran, Persian Gulf	February 4, 1983	260,000	260,000	1045
Tanio oil spill	France, Brittany	March 7, 1980	13,500	13,500	1046
Irenes Serenade	Greece, Pytlos	February 23, 1980	100,000	100,000	1014
MT Independenta	Turkey, Bosphorus	November 15, 1979	95,000	95,000	1014
Burmah Agate	United States, Galveston Bay, Texas	November 1, 1979	8440	8440	1047
Atlantic Empress/ Aegean Captain	Trinidad and Tobago	July 19, 1979	287,000	287,000	1014, 1048, 1049
Ixtoc I oil spill	Mexico, Bay of Campeche, Gulf of Mexico	June 3, 1979– March 23, 1980	454,000	480,000	1050, 1051
Betelgeuse	Ireland, Bantry Bay	January 8, 1979	64,000	64,000	1052
Amoco Cadiz	France, Brittany	March 16, 1978	223,000	227,000	1008, 1008, 1014, 1053, 1054
Trans-Alaska Pipeline sabotage by explosives	United States, Alaska	February 15, 1978	2162	2162	1055
Venpet/Venoil collision	South Africa, Cape St. Francis	December 16, 1977	26,600	30,500	
Ekofisk oil field	Norway, North Sea	April 22, 1977	27,600	27,6500	1053, 1056
Hawaiian Patriot	United States, 300 nmi (560 km; 350 mi) off Honolulu, Hawaii	February 26, 1977	95,000	95,000	1008, 1014
Borage	Taiwan, Northern coast	February 7, 1977	34,000	34,000	1057
Argo Merchant	United States, Nantucket island, Massachusetts	December 15, 1976	25,000	28,000	1058, 1059
NEPCO 140 oil spill	United States, Saint Lawrence River	June 23, 1976	1000	1000	1060, 1061
Urquiola	Spain, A Coruna	May 12, 1976	100,000	100,000	1014
Niger Delta	Nigeria, Niger Delta	1976–1996	258,000	328,000	1062
Corinthos	United States, Delaware River, Marcus Hook, Pennsylvania	January 31, 1975	36,000	36,000	
Jakob Maersk	Portugal, Oporto	January 29, 1975	88,000	88,000	1014
VLCC Metula	Chile, Strait of Magellan	August 9, 1974	50,000	60,000	1063
Sea Star	Iran, Gulf of Oman	December 19, 1972	115,000	115,000	1008, 1014
Oswego-Guardian/ Texanita collision	South Africa Stilbaai	August 21, 1972	10,m000	10,000	1063
Wafra	South Africa, Cape Agulhas	February 21, 1971	27,000	27,000	1064
Arizona Standard/ Oregon Standard collision	United States, San Francisco Bay	January 17, 1971	2700	2700	1065, 1066, 1067
Othello	Sweden, Tralhavet Bay	March 23, 1970	50,000	60,000	1008, 593
1969 Santa Barbara oil spill	United States, Santa Barbara California	January 28, 1969	10,000	14,000	1068

(Continued)

TABLE 1.23 (*Continued*)
Oil Spills around the World

Spill/Vessel	Location	Dates	Min Tons	Max Tons	Authors
Torrey Canyon	United Kingdom, Cornwall and Isles of Scilly	March 18, 1967	80,000	119,000	1008, 1014
African Queen oil spill	United States, Ocean City, Maryland	December 30, 1958	21,000	21,000	1069, 1070
Avila Beach pipeline	United States, Avila Beach, California	1950s–1996	1300	1300	1071
Guadalupe Oil Field	United States, Guadalupe, California	1950s–1994	29,000	29,000	1071
Greenpoint, Brooklyn oil spill	United States, Newtown Creek, Greenpoint, Brooklyn New York	1940s–1950s	55,200	97,400	1072
SS Frank H. Buck / SS President Coolidge collision	United States, San Francisco Bay, California	March 6, 1937	8870	8870	1065, 1073
Lakeview Gusher	United States, Kern County, California	March 14, 1910–September 10, 1911	1,230,000	1,230,000	1074
Thomas W. Lawson	United Kingdom, Isles of Scilly	December 14, 1907	7400	7400	1075

Therefore, the figures for a particular year may be severely distorted by a single large incident. This is clearly illustrated by incidents such as Atlantic Empress (1979), 287,000 tons spilt; Castillo de Bellver (1983), 252,000 tons spilt; and ABT Summer (1991), 260,000 tons spilt.

Causes of Spills

The causes and circumstances of oil spills are varied, but can have a significant effect on the final quantity spilt. The following analysis explores the incidence of spills of different sizes in terms of the operation that the vessel was undertaking at the time of the incident and the primary cause of the spill. For small- and medium-sized spills, operations have been grouped into Loading/Discharging, Bunkering, Other Operations, and Unknown Operations. Other Operations include activities such as ballasting, deballasting, and tank cleaning when the vessel is underway.

Reporting of larger spills tends to provide more information and greater accuracy, which has allowed further breakdown of vessel operations. Therefore, operations for larger spills have been grouped into Loading/Discharging, Bunkering, At Anchor (Inland/Restricted waters), At Anchor (Open water), Underway (Open water), Underway (Inland/Restricted waters), Other Operations, and Unknown Operations. The primary causes have been designated to Allisions/Collisions, Groundings, Hull Failures, Equipment Failures, Fire and Explosion, and Other/Unknown. Other causes include events such as heavy weather damage and human error. Spills where the relevant information is not available have been designated as Unknown.

Small- and medium-sized spills account for 95% of all the incidents recorded; a large percentage of these spills, 40% and 29%, respectively, occurred during loading and discharging operations which normally take place in ports and oil terminals (Figures 1.11 and 1.12). While the cause of these spills is largely unknown it can be seen that equipment and hull failures account for ~46% of these incidents for both size categories (Figures 1.11 and 1.12). Nevertheless, when considering other operations, there is a significant difference in the percentage of allisions, collisions, and groundings between these two size groups where we see the percentage increasing from 2% for smaller spills to 45% for medium spills (Figures 1.11 and 1.12).

Large spills account for the remaining 5% of all the incidents recorded and the occurrence of these incidents has significantly decreased over the past 44 years. From Figure 1.10, it can be seen that 50% of large spills occurred while the vessels were underway in open water; allisions, collisions, and groundings accounted for 59% of the causes for these spills (Figure 1.12). These same causes account for an even higher percentage of incidents when the vessel was underway in inland or restricted waters, being linked to some 98% of spills. Restricted water includes incidents that occurred in ports and harbors.

Perhaps, unsurprisingly activities during loading or discharging result in significantly more small- or medium-sized spills than large spills. However, large spills do still occur during loading and discharging, and from Figure 1.17 and Table 1.6, it can be seen that 57% of these incidents are caused by fires, explosions, and equipment failures.

Health Effects of the Gulf Oil Spill

According to Solomon and Janssen,[464] the oil spill in the Gulf of Mexico poses direct threat to human health from inhalation or dermal contact with the oil and dispersant chemicals, and indirect threat to seafood safety and mental health. Physicians should be familiar with health effects from oil spills to appropriately advise, diagnose, and treat patients who live and work along the Gulf Coast or wherever a major oil spill occurs.

Acute Health Effects from Oil and Dispersants

In Louisiana in the early months of the oil spill, more than 300 individuals, three-fourths of whom were cleanup workers, sought medical care for constitutional symptoms such as headaches, dizziness, nausea, vomiting, cough, respiratory distress, and chest pain. These symptoms are typical of acute exposure to hydrocarbons or hydrogen sulfide, but it is difficult to clinically distinguish toxic symptoms from other common illnesses.[465,466]

The U.S. EPA set up an air monitoring network to test for VOCs, PM, hydrogen sulfide, and naphthalene.

Skin contact with oil and dispersants causes defatting, resulting in dermatitis and secondary skin infections. Some individuals may develop a dermal hypersensitivity reaction, erythema, edema, burning sensations, or a follicular rash. Some hydrocarbons are phototoxic.

Potential Long-Term Health Risks

In the near term, various hydrocarbons from the oil will contaminate fish and shellfish. Although vertebrate marine life can clear PAHs from their system, these chemicals accumulate for years in invertebrates.[467] The Gulf provides about two-thirds of the oysters in the United States and is a major fishery for shrimp and crab. Trace amounts of cadmium, mercury, and lead occur in crude oil and can accumulate over time in fish tissues, potentially increasing future health hazards from consumption of large fin fish such as tuna and mackerel.

After the Exxon Valdez oil spill in 1989, a total of 1811 workers' compensation claims were filed by cleanup workers; most were for acute injuries but 15% were for respiratory problems and 2% for dermatitis.[468] No information is available in the peer-reviewed literature about longer-term health effects of this spill. A survey of the health status of workers 14 years after the cleanup found a greater prevalence of symptoms of chronic airway disease among workers with high oil exposures, as well as self-reports of neurological impairment and chemical sensitivity.[469]

Symptom surveys performed in the weeks or months following oil spills have reported a higher prevalence of headache, throat irritation, and sore or itchy eyes in exposed individuals compared with controls. Some studies have also reported modestly increased rates of diarrhea, nausea, vomiting, abdominal pain, rash, wheezing, cough, and chest pain.[470] One study of 6780 fishermen, which included 4271 oil spill cleanup workers, found a higher prevalence of lower respiratory tract symptoms 2 years after oil spill cleanup activities. The risk of lower respiratory tract symptoms increased with the intensity of exposure.[471]

A study of 858 individuals involved in the cleanup of the Prestige oil spill in Spain in 2002 investigated acute genetic toxicity in volunteers and workers. Increased DNA damage, as assessed by the comet assay, was found in volunteers, especially in those working on the beaches.[470] In the same study, workers had lower levels of CD4 cells, IL-2, IL-4, IL-10, and interferon compared with their own preexposure levels.

Studies following major oil spills in Alaska, Spain, Korea, and Wales have documented elevated rates of anxiety, depression, posttraumatic stress disorder, and psychological stress.[472] A mental health survey of 599 local residents 1 year after the Exxon Valdez spill found that exposed individuals were 3.6 times more likely to have anxiety disorder, 2.9 times more likely to have posttraumatic stress disorder, and 2.1 times more likely to score high on a depression index.[473] Adverse mental health effects were observed up to 6 years after the oil spill. Of course, this is not surprising since it has been shown that the same pathway for psychological stress tuna in the body is the same for detoxifying some oil toxics.

Clinicians should be aware of toxicity from exposures to oil and related chemicals. Patients presenting with constitutional symptoms should be asked about occupational exposures and location of residence. The physical examination should focus on the skin, respiratory tract, and neurological system, documenting any signs that could be associated with oil-related chemicals. Care consists primarily of documentation of signs and symptoms, evaluation to rule out or treat other potential causes of the symptoms, removal from exposure, and supportive care. Intradermal desensitization's for many of these toxics can help the chemically sensitive patients markedly in some cases as can sauna, intervenous nutrients, and immune modulators like autogenous lymphocytic factor and gamma globulin. The chemically sensitive patient can be devastated and incapacitated from the odors of the oil spill as we have seen along the Gulf Coast.

Preventory measure for those residents is that they should not fish in off-limit areas or where there is evidence of oil. Fish or shellfish with an oily odor should be discarded. Direct skin contact with contaminated water, oil, or tar balls should be avoided. If community residents notice a strong odor of oil or chemicals and are concerned about health effects, they should seek refuge in an air-conditioned environment. Interventions to address mental health in the local population should be incorporated into clinical and public health response efforts. Over the longer term, cohort studies of Gulf cleanup workers and local residents will greatly enhance the scientific data on the health sequelae of oil spills.

Corexit: The Dispersant for Oil Spills

The main ingredient in Corexit (the oil dispersant) is 2-butoxyethanol, which is toxic to blood, kidneys, liver, and the CNS, also causing cancer and birth defects. Corexit is mutagenic for bacteria, huge amounts of which live in the Gulf of Mexico. Corexit ruptures red blood cells and accumulates as it moves up the food chain. The EPA eventually conceded that Corexit is lethal for 50% of any group of test animals that comes in contact with it. Even the Department of Transportation classifies Corexit as "Class 6.1: Poisonous Material" for transportation purposes.

The risks of Corexit to humans, the fragile marsh ecosystems and marine life are potentially staggering. Ott[474] a marine toxicologist, has testified meeting people all over the Gulf who have shown symptoms including "headaches, dizziness, sore throats, burning eyes, rashes and blisters that go so deep, they are leaving scars."

Dispersants have never been used in such quantities before or at such depths in the ocean, or on open marshland. Dispersants are so dangerous because they accumulate up the food chain. Fiddler crabs absorb the toxins in their muscles and are then eaten by birds. Coyotes and feral pigs eat the bird corpses. Pelicans absorb the toxins from fish and even lightly oiled pelicans ingest the oil through their constant preening. Larger marine life like tuna, dolphins, and whales carry the greatest lethal loads. Stories have been told by fishermen finding vast, floating graveyards of birds, dolphins and whale corpses near the Macondo well site, which, they say, are secretly disposed of at night.

Oil on the surface is easier to see, easier to retrieve, easier to burn. One study shows that oil mixed with Corexit is 11 times as lethal as the oil alone.[475]

Dispersants are called dispersants because that is what they do. They disperse oil; they do not destroy it. Dispersants sink the oil below the surface, making it harder to see. On August 20, scientists produced new evidence of vast undersea plumes of oil driving for miles. Another team confirmed the discovery of a massive 22 mile subsea oil plume the size of Manhattan and, most dismayingly, very little evidence that the oil was being broken down by microbes.[475]

Pinetich confirmed that Coast Guard planes were flying out at night spraying Corexit on the water and land.[475]

Death by dispersants is slow and invisible. Death by dispersants wreaks its havoc over generations. Slow violence may be no less lethal and lasting.

In Barataria Bay, people suffer from cough. Workers have rashes, infected ears, and hands get blisters. When the southwind blows, lungs tighten and close. Some fishermen vomit, struggle to breathe, get dizzy, and/or suffer from diarrhea. Some have asthma, tachycardia, chests burning, and sore throats.

The slow violence of the oil spill comes on top of decades of slo-mo slaughter of the Gulf's marshes and ocean waters by three forces: industrial dumping, chemical contamination, and agricultural run-off; the forced engineering of the marshes by dredging and levees, and the tearing up of the vulnerable marshes by storms and hurricanes.

The Gulf is one of the richest and most diverse ecosystems in the hemisphere, our largest wetlands and 40% of our fishing grounds. But since the 1950s, decades of deregulation have turned the Gulf into the United States' largest industrial wasteland. If a gigantic hand emptied the Gulf like a basin of water, we would see a droned version of industrial New Jersey.

Ninety percent of all drilling for oil and gas in the United States takes place in the Gulf. On the map, the Gulf's water is marked with thousands of small, red blocks so thickly clustered. Each red square marks one of the 4000 platforms littering the Gulf, many of them abandoned and many leaking.

The Gulf also bears the brunt of agricultural pollution from the heartland: runoff and waste from Midwest cornfields, sewage plants, golf courses, factories, and nitrogen from fertilizer drain down the Mississippi into the Gulf every year. Through these damaged and vanishing marshes, massive watery superhighways have cut canals and passageways for the barges and huge ships on their way to the Gulf. Every straight line in the marshes is man-made. Every straight link has been forcibly dredged for flood control and shipping, the river and marshes forcibly re-engineered by levees and canals to stop flooding, thereby fatally closing off the silt and fresh water that the marshes needs to sustain themselves, and rendering them vulnerable to the yearly violence of the hurricanes.

The violence of Katrina was as great as the violence of the oil spill. Southern Louisiana is a half-drowned, shape-shifting, upside-down world, where boats float out of the treetops, and houses tilt out of the water.

DUST STORMS

Other less intensive wilderness areas are polluted by air currents coming from distal areas of spraying from hundreds to thousands of miles away. For example, West African dust comes via the trade winds to end up in Florida, Alabama, Mississippi, Louisiana, and Texas as well as in the opposite time of the year to the Amazon rainforest in South America.[219] This dust may contain bacteria, viruses, fungi, algae, various dirt particulates, radioactivity, pesticides, and particulates.[219] (Figure 1.13). The African dust comes into the United States from May to September. It seems to be loaded with toxics. Many chemically sensitive patients react to it.

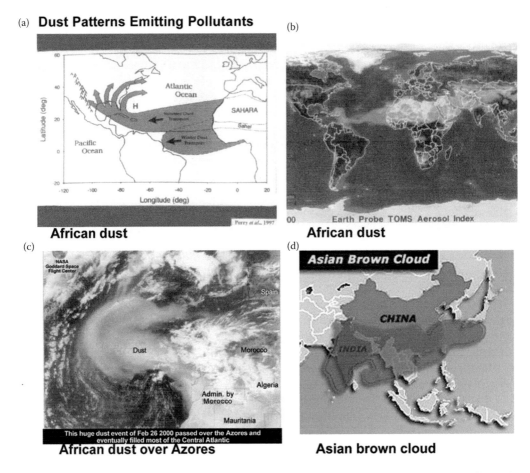

FIGURE 1.13   (See color insert.) African dust and Asian brown cloud patterns in 2005. The African dust comes via the trade winds and (goes) moves up the part of the United States east of the Rocky Mountains, over Bermuda, and on to England and Europe. The Gobi (Asian) dust goes across the Pacific and is usually stopped by the Rocky Mountains and distributed over California, Oregon, and Washington states. (Courtesy of NOAA—Gene Shinn.)

We have developed an analysis for it which works as a treatment.

The African dust stops on the eastern side of the Rocky Mountains and goes northeast going over the eastern United States and Canada on to England. The Gobi dust from Asia hits the states of California, Oregon, Washington, and Idaho. It carries many of the same substances as the African dust.

The Gobi dust comes in from the Western Gobi desert.

AIRBORNE AFRICAN SPRING DUST OVER THE EAST COAST OF PUERTO RICO INDUCES PROINFLAMMATORY AND OXIDANTS PROPERTIES IN HUMAN LUNG CELLS

Dust storm PM ≤ 2.5 collected during March 2004 was analyzed for metal content, oxidant capacity, and antioxidant response and interleukins expression. These parameters were measured in and after human bronchial epithelial cells exposure. Total Ozone Mapping Spectrometer aerosol index images, in conjunction with Puerto Rico Environmental Quality Board's data, were combined to define and establish African dust events (ADE) dates. PM filters were extracted with organic solvents hexane/acetone (1:1). Trace elements in the organic extracts were determined by inductively coupled plasma mass spectrometry and the oxidative capacity with the dithiothreitol assay. Cells were seeded onto a 96-well plate and exposed to the extracts. $PM_{2.5}$ ($\mu g/m^3$) showed a seasonal variation pattern, exhibiting high levels during spring and summer, 2004. The ADE extracts showed higher percentage of Cu, Pb, and V in addition to the high levels of Fe and Al when compared to non-ADE. The ADE and non-ADE $PM_{2.5}$ extracts contained similar oxidative capacity. The ADE extract-treated lysate exhibited a reduction in the total antioxidant capacity and glutathione concentrations. Secretions of IL-6 and IL-8 were significantly increased in cells exposed to extracts. The addition of a metal chelator increased antioxidant capacity and decreased the secretion of proinflammatory mediators in cells exposed to ADE extracts. African dust arriving from Puerto Rico increases local concentrations of trace elements in ambient $PM_{2.5}$, inducing inflammatory responses and reducing the antioxidant capacity of lung epithelial cells.

AFRICAN SPRING DUST STORMS ARRIVE TO PUERTO RICO CARRYING ENDOTOXINS THAT POTENTIATE PROINFLAMMATORY RESPONSES IN HUMAN LUNG CELLS

Airborne PM_{10} are "inhalable particles" composed of organic/inorganic compounds which can trigger inflammation processes. The Environmental Quality Board reports increment of PM_{10} in Puerto Rico when it receives the impact of African dust storms. They have found endotoxins (EN) in PM_{10} coming in these storm events as they reach the Puerto Rico coast. This study evaluates the proinflammatory contribution of ENX from ADE by means of IL-6 and IL-8 secretion using an *in vitro* model of human bronchial epithelial cells. A retrospective analysis of PM_{10} concentration and Total Ozone Mapping Spectrometer aerosol images were used to classify dates from the past March 2004 as ADE or non-ADE. ENX concentrations were measured in organic extracts of PM_{10} from ADE collected at a rural (Fajardo) and urban (Guaynabo) site in Puerto Rico. Cellular cytokine secretions and TLR mRNA expression were measured in cells exposed to these extracts. The highest ENX concentrations were obtained in PM from the urban site and these greatly partitioned into the organic extracts. ADE organic extracts stimulated IL-6 and IL-8 release from lung cells. Polymyxin B sulfate (EN inhibitor) decreased cytokine secretions in the ADE urban organic extract. Concomitantly, an increase in TLR2 mRNA was obtained with the ADE urban organic extract. These results highlight the importance of ENX as a preinflammatory mediator in PM_{10} from ADE. Overall, results suggest that ENX derived from ADE potentiate the effects of local anthropogenic material exacerbating bronchial proinflammatory response. The EHC-Dallas has developed an antigen for the African dust which has proved efficacious in treating people who were sensitive (Table 1.24).

In addition, much of the northern hemisphere and the top of the southern hemisphere are layered with methane gas (Figure 1.9).

Another recent example of rural emitters is the spraying of potatoes in Idaho, especially in the Bitterroot Valley where a significant amount of pesticides ends up in the mountains of eastern Montana and Wyoming[476] (Figure 1.14).

NUCLEAR LEAKS AND EXPLOSIONS

The United States and most of the world has standards for measuring leaks from nuclear power plants. As one can see, they are interspersed around the United States. The majority are in the Midwest and eastern United States.

The U.S. Nuclear Regulatory Commission (NRC) evaluates abnormal releases of tritium-contaminated water from nuclear power plants, particularly those that result in groundwater contamination.

This fact sheet provides a general overview of the health effects of tritium and the technical bases for the regulatory standards that the NRC uses to protect public health and safety, as well as the drinking water standards established by the U.S. EPA.

TABLE 1.24
Human Airborne Pathogens—African Dust

Agent	Disease
A. Bacteria	The "black plague" which killed off 1/4 of
Yersinia pestis	Europe's population in the fourteenth century
Bacillus anthracis	Anthrax
Mycobacterium tuberculosis	Tuberculosis
Legionella pneumophila	Legionnaires' disease
Bordetella pertussis	Whooping cough
Corynebacterium	Diphtheria
diphtheriae	Psittacosis
Chlamydia psittaci	Bacterial flu
Haemophilus influenza	Bacterial meningitis
Streptococcus pneumoniae	
Neisseria meningitidis	
B. Fungi	Cryptococcosis
Cryptococcus neoformans	Aspergillosis
Aspergillus sp.	Coccidiomycosis
Coccidioides immitis	Histoplasmosis
Histoplasma capsulatum	Blastomycosis
Blastomyces dermatitidis	
C. Virus	The "common cold"
Rhinoviruses	Viral flu
Influenza viruses	Chicken pox
Herpesvirus 3	Hantavirus pulmonary syndrome
Hantavirus	Smallpox
Poxvirus–variola virus	

Source: Gene Shinn—NOAA.

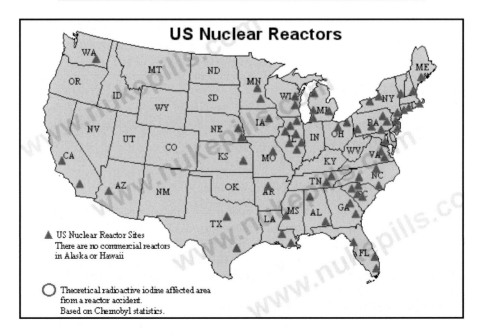

FIGURE 1.14   Nuclear reactor sites.

Tritium is a naturally occurring radioactive form of hydrogen that is produced in the atmosphere when cosmic rays collide with air molecules. As a result, tritium is found in very small or trace amounts in groundwater throughout the world. It is also a by-product of the production of electricity by nuclear power plants. Tritium emits a weak form of radiation, a low-energy beta particle similar to an electron. The tritium radiation does not travel very far in air and cannot penetrate the skin.[477]

Nuclear power plants have reported abnormal releases of water containing tritium, resulting in groundwater contamination.[477]

Most of the tritium produced in nuclear power plants stems from boron, absorbing neutrons from the plant's chain reaction. Nuclear reactors use boron, a good neutron absorber, to help control the chain reaction. Toward that end, boron either is added directly to the coolant water or is used in the control rods to control the chain reaction. Much smaller amounts of tritium can also be produced from the splitting of Uranium-235 in the reactor core, or when other chemicals (e.g., lithium or heavy water) in the coolant water absorb neutrons (NAS, 1996; UNSCEAR 1988).

Like normal hydrogen, tritium can bond with oxygen to form water. When this happens, the resulting water (tritiated water) is radioactive. Tritiated water (not be confused with heavy water) is chemically identical to normal water and the tritium cannot be filtered out of the water.[477]

Once tritium enters the body, it disperses quickly and is uniformly distributed throughout the soft tissues. Half of tritium is excreted within ~10 days after exposure.

Everyone is exposed to small amounts of tritium every day because it occurs naturally in the environment and the foods. Workers in federal weapons facilities; medical, biomedical, or university research facilities; or nuclear fuel cycle facilities may receive increased exposures to tritium.

Tritium is present naturally in the environment, and the radiation produced by natural tritium is identical to the radiation produced by tritium from nuclear power plants.

The radiation dose from tritium can be directly compared to the radiation dose from any other type of radiation, including natural background radiation and those received during medical procedures.

The tritium dose from nuclear power plants is much lower than the exposures attributable to natural background radiation and medical administrations.

Humans receive ~50% of their annual radiation dose from natural background radiation, 48% from medical procedures (e.g., x-rays), and 2% from consumer products. Doses from tritium and nuclear power plant effluents are a negligible contribution to the background radiation to which people are normally exposed, and they account for less than 0.1% of the total background dose (NCRP, 2009). As an example, assume that a residential drinking water well sample contains tritium at the level of 1600 pCi/L (a comparable tritium level was identified in a drinking water well near the Braidwood Station nuclear facility). The radiation dose from drinking water at this level for a full year (using EPA assumptions) is 0.3 mrem, which is at least 2000–5000 times lower than the dose from a medical procedure involving a full-body computed tomography (CT) scan (e.g., 500–1500 mrem from a CT scan). It is one thousand times lower than the approximate 300 mrem dose from natural background radiation. Fifty times lower than the dose from natural radioactivity (potassium) in the body (e.g., 15 mrem from potassium). Twelve times lower than the dose from a round-trip cross-country airplane flight (e.g., 4 mrem from Washington, DC to Los Angeles and back).

As low as reasonably achievable (ALARA) is a radiation safety principle for minimizing doses and releases of radioactive material by using all reasonable methods. In principle, no dose should be acceptable if it can be avoided or is without benefit.

A millirem (mrem) is a term used to describe how much radiation the body absorbs. For example, it is estimated that we receive a dose of 620/mrem every year from natural (e.g., radon) and human-made (e.g., medical) radiation sources.

The NRC's dose limits from radiation workers and the general publics are significantly lower than the levels of radiation exposure that cause health effects in humans, including a developing embryo or fetus. Although high doses and high dose rates may cause cancer in humans and genetic abnormalities in an embryo or fetus, public health data have not established the occurrence of these health risks following exposure to low doses and low-dose rates below about 10,000 mrem.

For additional comparison, a typical individual in the United States received an average annual radiation exposure of about 3410 mrem from natural sources (NCRP, 2009). Radon gas accounts for two-thirds of this exposure, while cosmic, terrestrial, and internal radiation account for the remainder. No adverse health effects have been discerned from doses arising from these levels of natural radiation exposure.

In addition, man-made sources of radiation from medical, commercial, and industrial activities contribute about another 310 mrem to our annual radiation exposure. One of the largest of these sources of exposure is CT scans, which account for about 150 mrem of the total from man-made sources. Other medical procedures together account for about another 150 mrem each year. In addition, some consumer products such as tobacco, fertilizer, welding rods, exit signs, luminous watch dials, and smoke detectors contribute about another 10 mrem to our annual radiation exposure.

For liquid effluents, including tritiated water, any licensee can demonstrate compliance with the 100 mrem per year dose standard by not exceeding the concentration values specified in Table 1.25 to 10 CFR Part 20. These concentration values if inhaled or ingested over the course of a year would produce a total effective dose of 50 mrem.

Picocurie (pCi) is a term used to describe how much radiation and, therefore, how much tritium is in the water. A pCi is a unit that can be directly measured by laboratory tests.

In 1976, EPA established a dose-based drinking water standard of 4 mrem per year to avoid the undesirable future contamination of public water supplies as a result of controllable human activities. In so doing, EPA set a maximum contaminant level of 20,000 pCi/L for tritium. This level is assumed to yield a dose of 4 mrem per year. If other similar radioactive materials are present in the drinking water, in addition to tritium, the sum of the annual dose from all radionuclides shall not exceed 4 mrem per year.

Since EPA developed the 1976 drinking water standard, scientists have improved the calculation methods to equate concentrations of tritium in drinking water (pCi/L) to radiation doses in people (mrem). In 1991, EPA calculated a tritium concentration to yield a 4 mrem per year dose as 60,900.

1. *Gastrointestinal*: This syndrome often follows absorbed doses of 6–30 Gy (600–3000 rad).[478] Nausea, vomiting, loss of appetite, and abdominal pain are usually seen within 2 hours. Vomiting in this time frame is a marker for whole-body exposures that are in the fatal range above 4 Gy. Without exotic treatment such as bone marrow transplant, death with this dose is common.[478] The death is generally more due to infection than gastrointestinal dysfunction.

2. *Neurovascular*: This syndrome typically occurs at absorbed doses greater than 30 Gy (3000 rad), though it may occur at 10 Gy (1000 rad).[478] It presents with neurological symptoms such as dizziness, headache, or decreased level of consciousness occurring within minutes to a few hours, and with an absence of vomiting. It is invariably fatal.[478]

The prodrome (early symptoms) of acute radiation sickness (ARS) typically includes nausea and vomiting, headaches, fatigue, fever, and short period of skin reddening.[478] These symptoms may occur at radiation doses as low as 35 rad (0.35 Gy). These symptoms are common to much illness and may not, by themselves, indicate ARS.[478]

Skin Changes

Cutaneous radiation syndrome (CRS) refers to the skin symptoms of radiation exposure.[479] Within a few hours after irradiation, a transient and inconsistent redness (associated with itching) can occur. Then, a latent phase may occur and last from a few days up to several weeks, when intense

TABLE 1.25

Average Effective Doses Received by Members of the Public in the U.S. From Commercial Nuclear Power Plant Radiological Effluent Releases

Year	Electrical Energy Produced (GW)	U.S. Population (1 × 10⁴)	Annual Effective Dose (mSv GW⁻¹ person⁻¹)						Total
			Gaseous Releases				Liquid Releases		
			F/A Gases	Total I-131	Tritium	Particulates	Tritium	F/D Gases	
1995	77.1	266,557	8.36×10^{-8}	1.95×10^{-10}	1.68×10^{-8}	1.28×10^{-9}	2.93×10^{-8}	2.90×10^{-8}	1.60×10^{-7}
1996	77.3	269,667	7.79×10^{-8}	2.75×10^{-10}	1.31×10^{-8}	1.10×10^{-9}	3.18×10^{-8}	2.89×10^{-8}	1.53×10^{-7}
1997	71.9	272,912	1.08×10^{-7}	1.29×10^{-10}	1.90×10^{-8}	1.47×10^{-9}	2.71×10^{-8}	1.22×10^{-8}	1.68×10^{-7}
1998	74.9	276,115	1.38×10^{-8}	2.80×10^{-10}	1.46×10^{-8}	2.66×10^{-9}	2.68×10^{-8}	1.37×10^{-8}	7.19×10^{-8}
1999	82.3	279,295	7.00×10^{-9}	1.75×10^{-10}	1.57×10^{-8}	3.06×10^{-10}	2.83×10^{-8}	1.10×10^{-8}	6.24×10^{-8}
2000	85.2	282,402	7.98×10^{-9}	1.80×10^{-10}	1.48×10^{-8}	1.08×10^{-9}	3.05×10^{-8}	1.07×10^{-8}	6.53×10^{-8}
2001	87.8	285,329	5.58×10^{-9}	9.21×10^{-11}	1.50×10^{-8}	8.57×10^{-10}	2.54×10^{-8}	7.97×10^{-9}	5.49×10^{-8}
2002	88.6	288,173	8.42×10^{-9}	1.95×10^{-10}	1.73×10^{-8}	6.62×10^{-10}	2.70×10^{-8}	1.96×10^{-8}	7.32×10^{-8}
2003	87.0	291,028	1.44×10^{-8}	3.79×10^{-10}	1.51×10^{-8}	3.04×10^{-9}	2.87×10^{-8}	1.15×10^{-8}	7.30×10^{-8}
2004	88.1	293,907	6.94×10^{-9}	2.67×10^{-10}	1.39×10^{-8}	2.07×10^{-10}	2.64×10^{-8}	6.38×10^{-9}	5.42×10^{-8}
2005	88.6	295,753	7.49×10^{-9}	9.78×10^{-11}	1.59×10^{-8}	5.11×10^{-9}	2.77×10^{-8}	5.99×10^{-9}	6.23×10^{-8}
2006	89.3	298,593	5.40×10^{-9}	9.84×10^{-11}	1.28×10^{-8}	4.24×10^{-10}	2.96×10^{-8}	6.18×10^{-9}	5.45×10^{-8}
2007	88.9	301,580	4.82×10^{-9}	1.09×10^{-10}	1.13×10^{-8}	9.48×10^{-9}	2.61×10^{-8}	4.95×10^{-9}	5.67×10^{-8}
2008	88.9	304,375	4.44×10^{-9}	1.03×10^{-10}	1.21×10^{-8}	1.85×10^{-9}	2.82×10^{-8}	1.01×10^{-8}	5.68×10^{-8}
2009	86.8	307,007	5.77×10^{-9}	7.31×10^{-11}	1.14×10^{-8}	3.32×10^{-10}	2.41×10^{-8}	1.41×10^{-8}	5.58×10^{-8}

reddening, blistering, and ulceration of the irradiated site are visible. In most cases, healing occurs by regenerative means; however, very large skin doses can cause permanent hair loss, damaged sebaceous and sweat glands, atrophy, fibrosis, decreased or increased skin pigmentation, and ulceration or necrosis of the exposed tissue.[479] Notably, as seen at Chernobyl, when skin is irradiated with high-energy beta particles, moist desquamation and similar early effects can heal, only to be followed by the collapse of the dermal vascular system after two months, resulting in the loss of the full thickness of the exposed skin.[480] This effect had been demonstrated previously with pig skin using high-energy beta sources at the Churchill Hospital Research Institute in Oxford.[481]

SPACEFLIGHT

During spaceflight, particularly flights beyond low Earth orbit, astronauts are exposed to both galactic cosmic radiation (GCR) and solar particle event (SPE) radiation. Evidence indicates past SPE radiation levels which would have been lethal for unprotected astronauts.[482] GCR levels which might lead to acute radiation poisoning are less well understood.[483]

PATHOPHYSIOLOGY

The most commonly used predictor of acute radiation symptoms is the whole-body absorbed dose. To help avoid confusion between these quantities, absorbed dose is measured in units of gray (Gy) or rad, while the others are measured in Sievert (Sv) or rem 1 rad = 0.01 Gy.[484]

In most of the acute exposure scenarios that lead to radiation sickness, the bulk of the radiation is external whole-body gamma, the case in which the absorbed equivalent and effective doses are all equal.

CHERNOBYL DISASTER

The Chernobyl disaster (Ukrainian, Chernobyl Catastrophe) was a catastrophic nuclear accident that occurred on April 26, 1986 at the Chernobyl Nuclear Power Plant in the Ukraine, which was under the direct jurisdiction of the central authorities of the Soviet Union. An explosion and fire released large quantities of radioactive particles into the atmosphere, which spread over much of the western USSR and Europe and around the Northern Hemisphere.

The Chernobyl disaster is widely considered to have been the worst nuclear power plant accident in history, and is one of only two classified as a level 7 event (the maximum classification) on the International Nuclear Event Scale (the other being the Fukushima Daiichi Japan nuclear disaster in 2011).[485]

According to official post-Soviet Data,[486,487] about 60% of the fallout landed in Belarus and the entire Northern Hemisphere (Table 1.26).

Rain was purposely seeded over 10,000 km^2 of the Belorussian SSR by the Soviet air force to remove radioactive particles from clouds heading toward highly populated areas. Heavy, black-colored rain fell on the city of Gomel.[488] Reports from Soviet and Western scientists indicate that Belarus received about 60% of the contamination that fell on the former Soviet Union. However, the 2006 TORCH report stated that half of the volatile particles had landed outside Ukraine, Belarus, and Russia. A large area in Russia to the south of Bryansk was also contaminated, as were parts of Northwestern Ukraine. Studies in surrounding countries indicate that over 1 million people could have been affected by radiation.[489]

RADIOACTIVE RELEASE

Iodine-131 and caesium-137 are responsible for most the radiation exposure received by the general population.[490]

TABLE 1.26

Level of Radioactivity in Various Countries after the Chernobyl Explosion

Country	37–185 kBq/m²		185–555 kBq/m²		555–1480 kBq/m²		>1480 kBq/m²	
	km²	% Country	km²	% Country	km²	% Country	km²	% Country
Belarus	29,900	14.4	10,200	4.9	4200	2.0	2200	1.1
Ukraine	37,000	6.2	3200	0.53	900	0.15	600	0.1
Russia	49,800	0.29	5700	0.03	2100	0.01	300	0.002
Sweden	12,000	2.7	–	–	–	–	–	–
Finland	11,500	3.4	–	–	–	–	–	–
Austria	8600	10.3	–	–	–	–	–	–
Norway	5200	1.3	–	–	–	–	–	–
Bulgaria	4800	4.3	–	–	–	–	–	–
Switzerland	1300	3.1	–	–	–	–	–	–
Greece	1200	0.91	–	–	–	–	–	–
Skrivebua	300	1.5	–	–	–	–	–	–
Italy	300	0.1	–	–	–	–	–	–
Moldova	60	0.2	–	–	–	–	–	–
Total	162,160 km²		19,100 km²		7200 km²		3100 km²	

Source: Wikipedia, https://en.wikipedia.org/wiki/Chernobyl_disaster.

The release of radioisotopes from the nuclear fuel was largely controlled by their boiling points, and the majority of the radioactivity present in the core was retained in the reactor.

All of the noble gases, including krypton and xenon, contained within the reactor were released immediately into the atmosphere by the first steam explosion.[490]

About 50%–60% of all core radioiodine in the reactor, containing about 1760 PBq (176 × 10¹⁶ Bq) which in mass units is 400 kg of iodine-131, was released, as a mixture of sublimed vapor, solid particles, and organic iodine compounds. Half-life is 8 days.[490]

About 20%–40% of all core caesium-137 was released, containing 85 PBq in all.[490,491] Cadmium was released in aerosol form; caesium-137 along with isotopes of strontium, are the two primary elements preventing the Chernobyl exclusion zone being reinhabited.[492] The caesium-137 activity represented by 8.5×10^{16} Bq would be produced by 24 kg of caesium-137.[107] Cs-137 has a half-life of 30 years.[490]

For tellurium-132, half-life of 78 hours, an estimated 1150 PBq was released.[490]

Xenon-133, the total radioactivity atmospheric release is estimated at 5200 PBq. Xe-133 has a half-life of 5 days.[490]

An early estimate for total nuclear fuel material released to the environment was 3 ± 0.5%. This corresponds to the atmospheric emission of 6 tons of fragmented fuel.[493]

Two sizes of particles were released: small particles of 0.3–1.5 μm (aerodynamic diameter) and large particles of 10 μm.

RADIATION LEVELS

The radiation levels in the worst-hit areas of the reactor building have been estimated to be 5.6 R/second (1.4 mA/kg), equivalent to more than 20,000 R/hour. A lethal dose is around 500 R (5Gy, 0.13 C/kg) over 5 hours, so in some areas, unprotected workers received fatal doses in less than a minute.

Most, including Akimov, died from radiation exposure within 3 weeks.[494]

EPA Raises Allowable Limits for Radioactive Particles

Meanwhile, back in the United States, Americans are shielded from the truth about the increasing amount of radioactive particles in their water and soil.

The EPA keeps the situation quiet by raising the allowable limits for radioactive particles in new guidelines. In fact, the president signed new protective action guides in 2013, raising allowable limits of radioactive particles.

The new limits allow long-term public exposure to radiation in amounts as high as 2000 mrem. According to PEER, this lax limit has the capability to increase a 1 in 10,000 person cancer rate to around 1 in 23 persons exposed over a 30-year period. This dramatic increase in the permissible radioactive levels in drinking water and soil following "radiological incidents" is reason for concern.

More concerning, is the contradictory language in the new standards. In Section 3.7, the EPA determines that the general public should be evacuated at levels beginning at 1000 mrem, yet further down, soil levels are found to be safe at 2000 mrem "for re-entry of some displaced individuals."

Residual Radioactivity in the Environment

Rivers, Lakes, and Reservoirs

The Chernobyl nuclear power plant is located next to the Pripyat River, which feeds into the Dnieper reservoir system one of the largest surface water systems in Europe, which at the time supplied water to Kiev's 2.4 million residents, and was still in spring flood when the accident occurred.[495] Guidelines for levels of radioiodine in drinking water were temporarily raised to 3700 Bq/L, allowing most water to be reported as safe,[496] and a year after the accident, it was announced that even the water of the Chernobyl plant's cooling pond was within acceptable norms. Despite this, 2 months after the disaster, the Kiev water supply was abruptly switched from the Dnieper to the Desna River.[495] Meanwhile, massive silt traps were constructed, along with an enormous 30-m-deep underground barrier to prevent groundwater from the destroyed reactor entering the Pripyat River.[495]

Bioaccumulation of radioactivity in fish[497] resulted in concentrations (both in Western Europe and in the former Soviet Union) that in many cases were significantly above guideline maximum levels for consumption.[496] Guideline maximum levels for radiocaesium in fish vary from country to country but are ~1000 Bq/kg in the European Union.[498] In the Kiev reservoir in the Ukraine, concentrations in fish were several thousand Bq/kg during the years after the accident.[497]

The contamination of fish caused short-term concern in parts of the United Kingdom and Germany and in the long term (years rather than months) in the affected areas of Ukraine, Belarus, and Russia as well as in parts of Scandinavia.[496]

Groundwater

Groundwater was not badly affected by the Chernobyl accident since radionuclides with short half-lives decayed away long before they could affect groundwater supplies, and longer-lived radionuclides such as radiocaesium and radiostrontium were absorbed to surface soils before they could transfer to groundwater.[499] However, significant transfers of radionuclides to groundwater have occurred from waste disposal sites in the 30 km (19 mi) exclusion zone around Chernobyl.

Flora and Fauna

After the disaster, 4 km^2 of pine forest directly downwind of the reactor turned reddish-brown and died, earning the name of the "Red Forest."[500] Some animals in the worst-hit areas also died or stopped reproducing. Most domestic animals were removed from the exclusion zone, but horses left on an island in the Pripyat River 6 km (4 mi) from the power plant died when their thyroid glands were destroyed by radiation doses of 150–200 Sv.[501] Some cattle on the same island died and those that survived were stunted because of thyroid damage. The next generation appeared to be normal.[501]

A robot sent into the reactor itself has returned with samples of black, melanin-rich radiotrophic fungi that are growing on the reactor's walls.[502]

Of the 440,350 wild boar killed in the 2010 hunting season, in Germany, over 1000 were found to be contaminated with levels of radiation above the permitted limit of 600 Bq/kg, due to residual radioactivity from Chernobyl.[503] Germany has "banned wild game meat because of contamination linked to radioactive mushrooms."[504]

The Norwegian Agricultural Authority reported that in 2009 a total of 18,000 livestock in Norway needed to be given uncontaminated feed for a period of time before slaughter in order to ensure that their meat was safe for human consumption. This was due to residual radioactivity from Chernobyl in the plants they graze on in the wild during the summer. The after-effects of Chernobyl were expected to be seen for a further 100 years, although the severity of the effects would decline over that period.[476] In Britain and Norway, as of 2011, "slaughter restrictions" remained for sheep raised on pasture contaminated by radiation fallout.[504]

Human Impact

Thyroid Cancer

Chernobyl Forum published a report in 2005 that revealed thyroid cancer among children to be one of the main health impacts from the Chernobyl accident. In that publication, more than 4000 cases were reported and that there was no evidence of an increase in solid cancers or leukemia. It said that there was an increase in psychological problems among the affected population.

On the death toll of the accident, the report states that 28 emergency workers (liquidators) died from acute radiation syndrome including beta burns and 15 patients died from thyroid cancer in the following years, and it roughly estimated that cancer deaths caused by Chernobyl may reach a total of about 4000 among the 5 million persons residing in the contaminated areas.

According to UNSCEAR, up to the year 2005, an excess of over 6000 cases of thyroid cancer have been reported. That is, over the estimated preaccident baseline thyroid cancer rate, more than 4000 casual cases of thyroid cancer have been reported in children and adolescents exposed at the time of the accident, a number that is expected to increase. They concluded that there is no other evidence of major health impacts from the radiation exposure.[505]

However, the risk of thyroid cancer associated with the Chernobyl accident is still high according to published studies.[506,507]

Other Health Disorders

Mettler[508] puts the number of worldwide cancer deaths outside the highly contaminated zone at "perhaps" 5000, for a total of 9000 Chernobyl-associated fatal cancers. The same report outlined studies based in data found in the Russian Registry from 1991 to 1998 that suggested that "of 61,000 Russian workers exposed to an average dose of 107 Sv, about 5% of all fatalities that occurred may have been due to radiation exposure."[509]

Deaths Due to Radiation Exposure

The number of potential deaths arising from the Chernobyl disaster is heavily debated. According to the Union of Concerned Scientists, the number of excess cancer deaths worldwide (including all contaminated areas) is ~27,000 based on the same LNT.[510]

Cytogenetic Examination of Persons Subjected to Radiation Exposure in Certain Regions of Ukraine

Ganina et al.[511] have summarized the results of cytogenetic studies of peripheral blood lymphocytes conducted in the institutions of Kiev and Kharkov in persons irradiated after the accident of the

Chernobyl NPP. The average level of chromosomal aberrations and the appearance of cytogenetic markers characteristic of their irradiation effect was higher in the examinees in comparison with the control. The increase in the number of aberrations in certain Kiev residents as well as the development of lymphogranulomatosis in some liquidators of the accident was accompanied by the reduction in the level of reparative DNA synthesis of blood lymphocytes.

Long-Term Radiation Damage to the Skin and Eye after Combined Beta and Gamma Radiation Exposure during the Reactor Accident in Chernobyl

According to Junk et al.,[512] 16 of these so called liquidators were repeatedly examined between 1991 and 1996. Their doses ranged from 0.35 to 9 Gy, partly confirmed by determination of chromosomal aberrations.

Four liquidators had posterior subcapsular opacifications in different degrees, one presented only after cataract extraction. One patient had dense corticonuclear cataracts and pseudoexfoliation-like changes. Three men had severe dry eye syndrome. Eight men had no ocular complications. Retinal radiation damages were absent. Fifteen liquidators suffered from severe chronic cutaneous radiation damage, which led to amputations in three cases.

Health Effects in Those with ARS from the Chernobyl Accident

According to Mettler et al.,[508] the Chernobyl accident resulted in almost one-third of the reported cases of ARS reported worldwide. Cases occurred among the plant employees and first responders but not among the evacuated populations or general population. The diagnosis of ARS was initially considered for 237 persons based on symptoms of nausea, vomiting, and diarrhea. Ultimately, the diagnosis of ARS was confirmed in 134 persons. There were 28 short-term deaths of which 95% occurred at whole-body doses in excess of 6.5 Gy. Underlying bone marrow failure was the main contributor to all deaths during the first 2 months. Allogeneic bone marrow transplantation was performed on 13 patients and an additional six received human fetal liver cells. All of these patients died except one individual who later was discovered to have recovered his own marrow and rejected the transplant. Two or three patients were felt to have died as a result of transplant complications. Skin doses exceeded bone marrow doses by a factor of 10–30, and at least 19 of the deaths were felt to be primarily due to infection from large area beta burns. Internal contamination was of relatively minor importance in treatment. By the end of 2001, an additional 14 ARS survivors died from various causes. Long-term treatment has included therapy for beta burn fibrosis and skin atrophy as well as for cataracts.

Bone Marrow Transplantation after the Chernobyl Nuclear Accident

According to Baranov et al.,[513] on April 26, 1986, an accident at the Chernobyl nuclear power station in the Soviet Union exposed about 200 people to large doses of total-body radiation. Thirteen persons exposed estimated total-body doses of 5.6–13.4 Gy received bone marrow transplants. Two transplant recipients, who received estimated doses of radiation of 5.6 and 8.7 Gy, are alive more than three years after the accident. The others died of various causes, including burns (the cause of death in five), interstitial pneumonitis (three), graft-versus-host disease (two), and acute renal failure and adult respiratory distress syndrome (one). There was hematopoietic (granulocytic) recovery in nine transplant recipients who could be evaluated, six of whom had transient partial engraftment before the recovery of their own bone marrow. Graft-versus-host disease was diagnosed clinically in four persons after exposure to radiation doses of 5.6–13.4 Gy; we do not know whether it is more likely after transient engraftment of transplanted stem cells. Because large doses of radiation affect multiple systems, bone marrow recovery does not necessarily ensure survival. Furthermore, the risk of graft-versus-host disease must be considered when the benefits of this treatment are being weighed.

ACUTE RADIATION SICKNESS: MORPHOLOGY OF CNS SYNDROME

According to Kamarad,[514] the present treatise is a report on the study of morphologic changes induced in the brain of laboratory animals by the exposure to supralethal doses of ionizing radiation. Most of the experiments were made with conventional female rats supplied by the firm Velaz. The animals were exposed to ^{60}Co gamma radiation doses within the range of 15–960 Gy. The material for study was sampled in the intervals from 15 minutes to 6 days after the irradiation had ended. Similar experiments, though on a smaller scale, were carried out with mice, rabbits, and dogs. The tissue samples were treated in current methods for the purposes of light microscopy, electron microscopy, and histochemistry. The signs of a cerebral edema dominate the light microscopical pattern of morphological changes during the first hours. The nerve cells show symptoms of acute swelling. There are small hemorrhages near some of the capillaries. In later periods, the nerve cells assume the nature of pyknomorphous neurons. The degree in which the changes are expressed however varies considerably. Dystrophic changes were also found for glial cells. Small hemorrhages are dispersed over all the areas of the brain. There are persisting signs of brain edema with dilated perivascular and pericellular spaces. The activities of the following enzymes were studied in histochemical examinations: acetylcholinesterase (ACE), nonspecific cholinesterase (CE), alkaline phosphatase (AP), acid phosphatase (AcP), ATP splitting enzyme (ATP), thiamine pyrophosphate (TPP), glycerol-3-phosphate dehydrogenase (GPDH), succinodehydrogenase (SDH), and acid nonspecific esterase (AE). A phase progress of activity changes was found for AP, CE, and ACE in the blood capillaries of the brain cortex after the exposure to the radiation doses of 50–200 Gy. The irradiation was first followed by elevation of their activity and then, in the intervals of 4–24 hours after irradiation, by a drop in their activity below the level obtained for the control animals (Table 1.27).

ENVIRONMENTAL RADIATION EXPOSURE

OUTCOME OF LOCAL RADIATION INJURIES: 14 YEARS OF FOLLOW-UP AFTER THE CHERNOBYL ACCIDENT

According to Gottlober et al.[515] in the Chernobyl nuclear power plant accident, 237 individuals initially suspected to have been significantly exposed to radiation during or in the immediate aftermath of the accident; the diagnosis of ARS could be confirmed in 134 cases on the basis of clinical symptoms. Of these, 54 patients suffered from CRS to varying degrees. Among the 28 patients who died from the immediate consequences of accidental radiation exposure, acute hematopoietic syndrome due to bone marrow failure was the primary cause of death only in a minority. In 16 of

TABLE 1.27

U.S. Average Exposure

Source	Exposure in mrem/year
Cosmic rays	45
External radiation from radioactive ores, etc.	60
Internal exposure from radioactive material ingested into the body	25
Diagnostic x-rays	70
Total	200

Source: Stewart C. 1977. *The Physics Teacher* 15:135. doi: http://dx.doi.org/10.1119/1.2339571.

Note: This does not include radon exposures which may be very high radiation units.

these 28 deaths, the primary cause was attributed to CRS. This report describes the characteristic cutaneous sequelae as well as associated clinical symptoms and diseases of 15 survivors of the Chernobyl accident with severe localized exposure who were systematically followed up by groups between 1991 and 2000. All patients presented with CRS of varying severity, showing xerosis, cutaneous telangiectasias and subungual splinter hemorrhages, hemangiomas and lymphangiomas, epidermal atrophy, disseminated keratoses, extensive dermal and subcutaneous fibrosis with partial ulcerations, and pigmentary changes including radiation lentigo. Surprisingly, no cutaneous malignancies have been detected so far in those areas that received large radiation exposures and developed keratosis; however, two patients first presented in 1999 with basal cell carcinomas on the nape of the neck and the right lower eyelid, areas that received lower exposures. During the follow-up period, two patients were lost due to death from myelodysplastic syndrome in 1995 and acute myelogenous leukemia in 1998, respectively. Other radiation-induced diseases such as dry eye syndrome (3/15), radiation cataract (5/15), xerostomia (4/15), and increased FSH levels (7/15) indicating impaired fertility were also documented. This study, which analyzes 14 years in the clinical course of a cohort of patients with a unique exposure pattern, corroborates the requirement for long-term, if not life-long, follow-up not only in atomic bomb survivors, but also after predominantly local radiation exposure.

INFECTION SYNDROME IN ARS PATIENTS SUBJECTED TO CHERNOBYL ACCIDENT

According to Ivanov et al.,[516] in spite of intensive antimicrobial prophylaxis and therapy, most patients with ARS I-IV severity grade (dose of 0.1–13.7 Gy) developed infections caused by bacteria, fungi, and viruses. Frequency and intensity of those infections were proportional to the radiation dose and severity grade of radiation sickness.

FUKUSHIMA DISASTER

According to Deagle,[517] the Fukushima Daiichi plant is one of the greatest environmental catastrophes in human history. The most pressing crisis at the moment is Cooling Pool 4, Reactor 1 lost containment before the tsunami from Sendai struck as it was located over a major fault line. Reactor 2 has proven criticality and loss of the corium below the reactor building. Reactor 3 is the MOX or Mixed Oxygen Plutonium hot reactor, with 38,000 times more dangerous radioactivity and touchy reactivity that detonated critical hydrogen ignited nuclear explosion of the cooling pool above the reactor, over many kilometers away. With millions of tons of moderate to highly radioactive water in sandy soil, subsidence and building structural integrity is a major challenge to maintain containment of cooling pool for the remaining materials that have not yet exited into the ground to interact with zirconium-mediated superheated tritium water generation. Apparently, now Pool 4 has leveled steam tubes going many kilometers into the ocean floor off Fukushima or toward Tokyo subway train tunnels. It would explain very high radiation readings even underground in the complex system of underground fault line that can transmit superheated radioactive steam underground to the largest metropolitan region of any city of Earth.

No ground penetrating radar or remote satellite site data have been collected and circulated to scientists or the public of the position underground of the nuclear melted corium of all four reactors. Millions of highly contaminated seawater has been released into the Pacific Ocean, and plans confirmed by Tepco and the Japanese government to prevent ocean floor superheated nuclear steam jet release of highly radioactive isotopes by concrete ocean floor covering of hundreds of miles has been released. A sea wall, tunneled DU-container corium catchers, Kevlar-spidersilk tents over each reactor, filtration systems to convert to solid radioactive waste, double-hulled ships to transport to a final deep trench ocean, or land mine facility have not been executed. Thus, by August 2012, ~61 controlled massive radiation air and water radioisotope releases have taken place, with billions of terabecquerels of radiation isotopes released into the Pacific ocean, and troposphere headed East to North America, and eventually entire Northern Hemisphere and then worldwide.

Our plants are now nuclear waste sites with Reactors 5 and 6 offline with many thousands of tons of 50+ years of highly enriched uranium, spent fuel with plutonium, and constant generation of tritanium laced superheated steam carrying cesium-134 with a 2-year short half-life, cesium-137 with a 40+ year half-life, and strontium-90 with similar half-life. The latter two isotopes carry a toxic load requiring four half-lives to reduce to approaching background if the reactions stop releasing isotopes. Plutonium generates a 24,800 year half-life and 100,000 year reductions to background, and U-238 has a 4.5 billion half-life requiring 18 billion years to background levels.

The multiple nuclear meltdowns at the Fukushima plants beginning on March 11, 2011, are releasing large amounts of airborne radioactivity that has spread throughout Japan and to other nations; thus, studies of contamination and health hazards are merited. In the United States, Fukushima fallout arrived just six days after the earthquake, tsunami, and meltdowns. Some samples of radioactivity in precipitation, air, water, and milk, taken by the U.S. government, showed levels hundreds of times above normal; however, the small number of samples prohibits any credible analysis of temporal trends and spatial comparisons. U.S. health officials report weekly deaths by age in 122 cities, about 25%–35% of the national total. Deaths rose 4.46% from 2010 to 2011 in the 14 weeks after the arrival of Japanese fallout, compared with a 2.34% increase in the prior 14 weeks. The number of infant deaths after Fukushima rose 1.80%, compared with a previous 8.37% decrease. Projecting these figures for the entire United States yields 13,983 total deaths and 822 infant deaths in excess of the expected. These preliminary data need to be followed up, especially in the light of similar preliminary U.S. mortality findings for 4 months after Chernobyl fallout arrived in 1986, which approximated final figures.

Mangano and Sherman[518] recently reported on an unusual rise in infant deaths in the northwestern United States for the 10-week period following the arrival of the airborne radioactive plume from the meltdowns at the Fukushima plants in norther Japan. This result suggested that radiation from Japan may have harmed Americans, thus meriting more research. They noted in the report that the results were preliminary, and the importance of updating the analysis as more health status data become available.[518]

Shortly after the report was issued, officials from British Columbia, Canada, proximate to the northwestern United States, announced that 21 residents had died of sudden infant death syndrome (SIDS) in the first half of 2011, compared with 16 SIDS deaths in all of the prior year. Moreover, the number of deaths from SIDS rose from 1 to 10 in the months of March, April, May, and June 2011 after Fukushima fallout arrived, compared with the same period in 2010.[519]

A recent conference concluded that 9000 persons worldwide survived with or died from cancer,[520] while a compendium of more than 5000 research papers put the excess death toll (from cancer and all other causes) at 985,000.[521]

In the United States, Chernobyl fallout was detected in the environment just 9 days after the meltdown. Gould and Sternglass[522] used EPA measurements of environmental radiation post-Chernobyl[523] and found elevated levels of radioactivity in air, water, and milk. For example, EPA data indicate that from May 13 to June 23, 1986, U.S. milk had 5.6 and 3.6 times more iodine-131 and cesium-137 than were recorded in May–June of 1985 (see Table 1.28). In some cities, especially those in the harder-hit Pacific Northwest, average concentrations were as much as 28 times the norms, while some individual samples were much higher.

Gould and Sternglass[522] also studied preliminary mortality data to analyze any potential impact from fallout. Using a 10% sample of all U.S. death certificates, they found that in a span of 4 months after Chernobyl (May–August 1986), total deaths in the United States rose 6% over the similar period in 1985 (see Table 1.29)[524] estimated deaths based on a 10% sample of death certificates, minus the New England states, for which data were incomplete at the time.

According to Mangano and Sherman,[518] eventually, final figures showed an increase of 2.3%, which exceeded the 0.2% decline in the first 4 months of the year.[525] The number of excess deaths

TABLE 1.28

Iodine-131 and Cesium-137 Concentrations in U.S. Milk, Spring 1985 versus Spring 1986

Date	Stations/ Measurements		Average	Times versus 1985
Iodine-131 Concentrations				
May 1 to June 30, 1985	55	103	2.53	–
May 13 to June 23, 1986	68	563	14.15	5.6
May 13 to June 23, 1986				
Boise, ID	1	8	71.00	28.1
Spokane, WA	1	9	56.44	22.3
Helena, MT	1	10	33.30	13.2
Rapid City, SD	1	10	31.90	12.6
Seattle, WA	1	9	30.67	12.1
Salt Lake City, UT	1	10	29.70	11.7
Portland, OR	1	7	24.00	9.5
Cesium-137 Concentrations				
May 1 to June 30, 1985	55	103	2.63	–
May 13 to June 23, 1986	68	563	9.47	3.6
May 13 to June 23, 1986				
Seattle, WA	1	9	39.33	15.0
Spokane, WA	1	9	29.44	11.2
Helena, MT	1	10	22.50	8.6
Boise, ID	1	8	21.38	8.2
Portland OR	1	7	21.14	8.0

Source: Mangano, J. J., J. D. Sherman. 2012. Unexpected mortality increase in the United States follows arrival of the radioactive plume from Fukushima: Is there a correlation? *Int. J. Health Ser.* 42(1): 47–64, 2012, Baywood Publishing Co., Inc. doi: http://dx.doi.org/10.2190/HS.42.1.f.

Note: Averages are in picocuries of iodine-131 and cesium-137 per liter of pasteurized milk. I-131 has a half-life of 8.05 days; Cs-137 has a half-life of 30 years.

or the difference between the actual and expected death total is 16,573. To date, the cause of this unusual pattern remains unknown, and no research testing hypotheses for causes other than Chernobyl have been published. This difference has a very high degree of statistical significance; there is a less than 1 in 10^9 probability that it occurred by random chance.

The change in deaths for infants was also analyzed. Preliminary data showed an increase of 3.1% in U.S. infant deaths in the first 4 months after Chernobyl, 1985 versus 1986. The final increase was 0.1%, compared with a 2.3% decline in 4 months before Chernobyl. The 1985–1986 differences in infant death rates were −2.9% (January–April) and +0.4% (May–August). These gaps amounted to excess infant deaths of 306 and 424, and differences were significant at $p < 0.08$ and $p < 0.055$.

The stillbirth, neonatal, and prenatal mortality increased in England and Wales within 11 months after Chernobyl's initial release,[526,527] and in Germany.[528] In two Ukrainian districts with increased levels of cesium-137 ground contamination, there was a significant increase in stillbirths.[529]

U.S. publications offered evidence that Americans may have suffered harm from Chernobyl, especially damage to fetuses and infants. Reports covered elevated levels of various radiation-related disorders, including newborn hypothyroidism,[530] infant leukemia,[531] and thyroid cancer among children.[532]

TABLE 1.29

Change in Total Infant Deaths, January–April and May–August, 1985–1986

	1985	1986	% change
Infant Deaths, Final			
January–April	13,473	13,169	−2.3%
May–August	12,788	12,800	+0.1%
Infant Deaths per 100,000, Final			
January–April	1123.55	1091.49	−2.9%
May–August	985.36	989.56	+0.4%
Total Deaths, Final			
January–April	737,963	736,418	−0.2%
May–August	657,311	672,569	+2.3%
May–August 1985 and 1986, Preliminary and Final Reported Deaths			
Total deaths, preliminary	65,377	69,271	+6.0%
Total deaths, final	657,311	672,569	+2.3%
Infant deaths, preliminary	1201	1239	+3.1%
Infant deaths, final	12,788	12,800	+0.1%

Source: Mangano, J. J., J. D. Sherman. 2012. Unexpected mortality increase in the United States follows arrival of the radioactive plume from Fukushima: Is there a correlation? *Int. J. Health Ser.* 42(1): 47–64, 2012, Baywood Publishing Co., Inc. doi: http://dx.doi.org/10.2190/HS.42.1.f.

Gould and Sternglass[522] showed that trends using preliminary data were rough approximations of the final data.

The EPA data cannot be used to assess the amount of time that Fukushima radiation existed in the U.S. environment or which areas of the nation received the highest amount of fallout. Anecdotal samples provide an abridged set of data. For example, iodine-131 in precipitation reached 242 and 390 pCi/L in Boise, Idaho, on March 22, hundreds of times greater than the typical value of about 2.0 pCi/L. The next highest value (200 pCi/L) was recorded in Kansas City, Kansas on March 29. The 10 highest values included diverse locations such as Salt Lake City, Utah (190 pCi/L), Jacksonville, Florida (150 pCi/L), and Boston, Massachusetts (92 pCi/L). Despite the paucity of data, it appears that radioactivity from Fukushima reached many, perhaps all, areas of the United States. Without more specific data, only the United States as a whole can be used to understand any potential changes in health status.

U.S. Total Deaths

During weeks 12–25, total deaths in 119 U.S. cities increased from 148,395 (2010) to 155,015 (2011), that is, 4.46%. This was nearly double the 2.34% rise in total deaths (142,006 to 145,324) in 104 cities for the prior 14 weeks, significant at $p < 0.000001$ (Table 1.2). This difference between actual and expected changes of +2.12%age points (+4.46%−2.34%) translates to 3286 "excess" deaths (155,015 × 0.02.12) nationwide.

According to Mangano and Sherman,[533] after March 19, 2011, total deaths were higher than a year earlier in 11 of the 14 weeks, with a 7.5% or greater increase in 4 of the weeks. The greatest rise occurred in weeks 12–20, with a 5.37% increase (96,900–102,108). In weeks 21–25, the increase was considerably lower, which was 2.74% (51,495–52,907). Whether this pattern will continue into the future or is temporary is not yet known (Tables 1.30 and 1.31).

TABLE 1.30

Changes in Reported Deaths, All Ages Weeks 12 to 25 and 14 Weeks Prior, 2010 versus 2011, 122 U.S. Cities

	Total Deaths					Total Deaths			
Week	2010	2011	No. (%)	Change	Week	2010	2011	No. (%)	Change
12	11,010	12,137	+1127	(+10.24)	50	10,323	10,702	+379	(+3.67)
13	11,097	11,739	+642	(+5.79)	51	7942	8839	+397	(+5.00)
14	11,075	12,052	+977	(+8.82)	52	8288	8194	−94	(−1.13)
15	10,712	10,928	+216	(+2.02)	1	11,557	11,804	+247	(+2.14)
16	10,940	10,743	−197	(−1.80)	2	11,299	10,775	−524	(−4.64)
17	10,549	10,826	+277	(+2.63)	3	10,110	10,689	+579	(+5.73)
18	10,637	11,251	+614	(+5.77)	4	10,832	10,420	−412	(−3.80)
19	10,389	11,300	+911	(+8.77)	5	10,524	10,295	−229	(−2.18)
20	10,491	11,132	+641	(+6.11)	6	9877	10,700	+823	(+8.33)
21	10,352	10,839	+487	(+2.77)	7	9802	10,952	+1.150	(+11.73)
22	9894	9538	−356	(−3.60)	8	10,198	10,762	+564	(+5.53)
23	10,781	10,770	−11	(−0.10)	9	10,586	10,779	+193	(+1.82)
24	10,178	10,981	+803	(+7.89)	10	10,699	10,639	−60	(−0.56)
25	10,290	10,779	+489	(+4.75)	11	9969	10,274	+305	(+3.06)
Total	148,395	155,015	+6620	(+4.46)*	Total	142,006	145,324	+3318	(+2.34)

Source: Sherman, J. D., J. Mangano. 2011. Is the dramatic increase in baby deaths in the U.S. a result of Fukushima fallout? *Counterpunch.*

Note: For weeks 12–25, actual number of deaths were available for 1653 (99.22%) in 2010 and 1650 (99.04%) in 2011 of the 119 cities for the 14 weeks. For weeks 50, 59, 52, and 1–11, actual number of deaths were available for 1445 (99.24%) in 2010 and 1443 (99.11%) in 2011 of the 104 cities for the 14 weeks.

* $p < 0.000001$.

U.S. Infant Deaths

The CDC weekly report provides reported deaths in the 122 participating cities for each of five age groups (<1, 1–24, 25–44, 45–64, and over 65). Of special interest to any analysis of potential health risks of environmental toxins are the fetus and infant, which are at greater risk than older children or adults. Thus, they examined trends for deaths of infants under 1-year old. The same cities used for total deaths are used here (Table 1.32). Infant death numbers are much smaller, accounting for just over 1% of total U.S. deaths in recent years.

Between 2010 and 2011, the total number of infant deaths for weeks 12–25 rose 1.80% (2674–2722), compared with a 8.37% decline (2520–2309) in the prior 14-week period. This difference was highly significant ($p < 0.0002$). In 8 of 14 weeks after March 19, 2011, an increase occurred from the year before, compared with just 4 of 14 weeks in the prior 14-week period. Some weeks had relatively large increases and decreases because the smaller number of infant deaths is subject to greater variability.

The 10.17% age point difference between actual and expected (+1.80% and −8.37%) means that 277 of the 2722 infant deaths (2772 × 0.1017) are "excess." Assuming that 30,000 U.S. infant deaths will occur in 2011 (577 per week), this means that 33.7% of deaths are reported (2722/14 = 194, or 33% of 577). Dividing 277 by 33.7% yields a projected 822 excess infant deaths in the United States in the 14 weeks after March 19, 2011.

Individual Locations

Deaths reported from U.S. cities with the largest populations and complete reporting in weeks 12–25 (2010 and 2011) and from the 14 previous week periods are given in Table 1.33 (all deaths)

TABLE 1.31

Changes in Reported Infant Deaths, Age under 1 Year Old: Weeks 12 to 25 and 14 Weeks Prior, 2010 versus 2011, 122 U.S. Cities

	Infant Deaths					Infant Deaths			
Week	2010	2011	No. (%)	Change	Week	2010	2011	No. (%)	Change
12	202	201	−1	(0.50)	50	177	202	+25	(+14.12)
13	182	210	+28	(+15.38)	51	150	129	−21	(−14.00)
14	189	198	+9	(+4.76)	52	120	113	−7	(−5.83)
15	208	163	−45	(−21.63)	1	198	158	−40	(−20.20)
16	186	188	+2	(+1.08)	2	193	177	−16	(−8.29)
17	177	200	+23	(+12.99)	3	206	158	−48	(−23.30)
18	200	196	−4	(−2.00)	4	207	148	−59	(−28,50)
19	172	214	+42	(+24.42)	5	177	178	+1	(+0.56)
20	221	224	+3	(+1.36)	6	174	173	−1	(−0.57)
21	183	196	+13	(+7.10)	7	165	188	+23	(+13.94)
22	173	152	−21	(−12.14)	8	191	158	−33	(−17.27)
23	295	174	−31	(−15.12)	9	192	174	−18	(−9.38)
24	194	191	−3	(−1.55)	10	189	165	−24	(−12.70)
25	182	215	+33	(+18.13)	11	181	188	+7	(+3.87)
Total	2674	2722	+48	(+1.80)*	Total	2520	2309	−211	(−8.37)

Source: Sherman, J. D., J. Mangano. 2011. Is the dramatic increase in baby deaths in the U.S. a result of Fukushima fallout? *Counterpunch.*

Note: For weeks 12–25, actual number of deaths were available for 1653 (99.22%) in 2010 and 1650 (99.04%) in 2011 of the 119 cities for the 14 weeks. For weeks 50–52 and 1–11, actual number of deaths were available for 1445 (99.24%) in 2010 and 1443 (99.11%) in 2011 of the 104 cities for the 14 weeks $*p < 0.0002$

TABLE 1.32

Changes in Reported Deaths, All Ages: Weeks 12 to 25, 2010 versus 2011 (versus 14 Weeks Prior) Most Populated U.S. Cities

City (Population Rank)	Total Deaths		No. (%) Change, 2010–2011			
	2010	2011	Weeks 12–25		Prior 14 weeks	
1. New York City	13,697	13,779	+82	(+0.60)	+1038	(+6.99)
2. Los Angeles	3440	3686	+246	(+7.15)	+44	(+1.17)
4. Houston	2291	2775	+484	(+21.13)	−1649	(−45.03)
6. Philadelphia	3708	4044	+336	(+9.06)	+207	(+5.42)
7. San Antonio	3489	3511	+22	(+0.63)	+222	(+6.32)
8. San Diego	2357	2220	−137	(−5.81)	+199	(+9.74)
Total	28,982	30,015	+1033	(+3.56)	+61	(+0.19)

Source: Mangano, J. J., J. D. Sherman. 2012. Unexpected mortality increase in the United States follows arrival of the radioactive plume from Fukushima: Is there a correlation? *Int. J. Health Ser.* 42(1): 47–64, 2012, Baywood Publishing Co., Inc. doi: http://dx.doi.org/10.2190/HS.42.1.f.

Note: Deaths reported for all weeks and cities except San Antonio (week ending December 26, 2009) and San Diego (week ending December 19, 2009).

TABLE 1.33

Changes in Reported Deaths, Age Under 1-Year Old: Weeks 12–25, 2010 versus 2011 (versus 14 Weeks Prior), Most Populated U.S. Cities

City (Population Rank)	Total Deaths		No. (%) Change, 2010–2011			
	2010	2011	Weeks 12–25		Prior 14 Weeks	
1. New York City	164	163	−1	(−0.61)	+32	(+20.92)
2. Los Angeles	74	58	−16	(−21.62)	−11	(−14.29)
4. Houston	105	117	+12	(+11.43)	−19	(−18.63)
6. Philadelphia	79	93	+14	(+17.22)	−7	(−7.14)
7. San Antonio	60	40	−20	(−33.33)	−8	(−14.29)
8. San Diego	37	33	−4	(−10.81)	+5	(+11.11)
Total	519	504	−15	(−2.89)	−8	(−1.51)

Source: Mangano, J. J., J. D. Sherman. 2012. Unexpected mortality increase in the United States follows arrival of the radioactive plume from Fukushima: Is there a correlation? *Int. J. Health Ser.* 42(1): 47–64, 2012, Baywood Publishing Co., Inc. doi: http://dx.doi.org/10.2190/HS.42.1.f.

Note: Deaths reported for all weeks and cities except San Antonio (week ending December 26, 2009) and San Diego (week ending December 19, 2009).

and Table 1.28 (infant deaths). Of the eight most populated cities, Chicago and Phoenix (third and fifth highest population) are omitted due to incomplete data.

For deaths of all ages, the U.S. 2010–2011 change of +3.56% in the 14 weeks after mid-March was well above the +0.19% change for the 14-week period before mid-March. This difference between the two changes of +3.37% age points was statistically significant at $p < 0.0001$.

Some elevated concentrations were found to be up to several hundred times the norm soon after the arrival of the Fukushima fallout, but no meaningful temporal trends and spatial patterns can be discerned from these data.

In the 14 weeks after the Fukushima fallout arrived in the United States, total deaths reported were 4.46% above the same period in 2010; in the 14 weeks before Fukushima, the increase from the prior year was just 2.34%. The gap in changes for infant deaths (+1.80% in the latter 14 weeks, −8.37% for the earlier 14 weeks) was even larger. Estimated "excess" deaths for the entire United States were projected to be 13,983 total deaths and 822 infant deaths.

Patterns of deaths among persons of all ages strongly reflect patterns among the elderly, who account for over two-thirds of all deaths. For the older population, explanations for excess deaths must be considered after exposure to higher levels of radioactive fallout. If cancer in some patients becomes active again, it may mean they already have cells carrying all but one of the three to our requisite mutations to express cancer. Exposure to radiation (or a toxic chemical) can provide the one final mutation to reactivate a quiescent tumor (Ide, C. 2011, personal communication, e-mail, July 28, 2011). Also, vulnerable are those elderly with depressed immune status, made worse by exposure to radiation.

The total of 155,015 U.S. deaths in the 14-week period after Fukushima, 2722 of which are infant deaths, represents a large database that are meaningful in a preliminary analysis of potential Fukushima effects.

The statistically significant difference in increased number of reported deaths (total and infant) for the 14-week period after Fukushima has an added dimension because of similar findings for the 4 months immediately after the Chernobyl meltdown in 1986, using a 10% sample of U.S. deaths. The post-Chernobyl increases, based on preliminary death data, were roughly comparable to the increases, calculated from final death data (Table 1.34). The preliminary versus final 1985–1986 change for the period May–August in total deaths was within 3.7%age points (+6.0% vs. +2.3%),

TABLE 1.34
Cities and Weeks Missing from Mortality Analysis

Weeks 12–25[a]

2010		2011	
3/27	El Paso, Texas	3/26	Worcester, Massachusetts
3/27	Somerville, Massachusetts	4/2	Duluth, Minnesota
3/27	Washington, DC	4/2	Minneapolis, Minnesota
4/3	St. Louis, Missouri	4/2	San Francisco, California
4/10	St. Louis, Missouri	4/2	St. Paul, Minnesota
4/10	San Jose, California	4/9	Duluth, Minnesota
4/17	San Jose, California	4/9	Minneapolis, Minnesota
4/17	San Jose California	4/9	St. Paul, Minnesota
5/15	Detroit, Michigan	4/16	Duluth, Minnesota
5/22	Long Beach, California	4/16	Minneapolis, Minnesota
5/22	San Jose, California	4/16	St. Paul, Minnesota
5/29	Jersey City, New Jersey	4/23	Tucson, Arizona
6/19	San Francisco, California	5/7	Charlotte, North Carolina
		6/11	Paterson, New Jersey
		6/18	Baton Rouge, Louisiana
		6/25	Shreveport, Louisiana
13/1666 = 0.78% missing		16/1666 = 0.96% missing	
1653/1666 = 99.22% reported		1650/1666 = 99.04% reported	

Weeks 50 (prior year)–11[b]

12/19	San Diego, California	12/18	Jersey City, New Jersey
12/26	Berkeley, California	12/18	Lansing, Michigan
12/26	El Paso, Texas	12/18	Paterson, New Jersey
12/26	Milwaukee, Wisconsin	12/18	Seattle, Washington
12/26	Newark, New Jersey	12/25	Houston, Texas
12/26	San Antonio, Texas	12/25	Seattle, Washington
1/2	Fort Wayne, Indiana	1/8	Columbus, Ohio
1/2	Jersey City, New Jersey	1/8	Somerville, Massachusetts
1/9	Cleveland, Ohio	1/22	New Haven, Connecticut
1/30	Columbus, Ohio	2/19	Columbus, Ohio
2/6	Kansas City, Missouri	2/19	Paterson, New Jersey
2/6	Seattle, Washington		
2/13	Jersey City, New Jersey		
13/1456 = 0.89% missing		11/1456 = 0.78% missing	
1442/1456 = 99.11% reported		1445/1456 = 99.22% reported	

Source: Mangano, J. J., J. D. Sherman. 2012. Unexpected mortality increase in the United States follows arrival of the radioactive plume from Fukushima: Is there a correlation? *Int. J. Health Ser.* 42(1): 47–64, 2012, Baywood Publishing Co., Inc. doi: http://dx.doi.org/10.2190/HS.42.1.f.

Note: Morbidity and Mortality Weekly Report indicated a "U" for unavailable.

[a] The analysis includes 119 cities (all 122 in the CDC report except Fort Worth, Texas; New Orleans, Louisiana; and Phoenix, Arizona). Of the 119 cities in the analysis, the mentioned weeks had no reported data ("U" for unavailable) by week ending.

[b] The analysis includes 104 cities (all 122 in the CDC report except Baton Rouge, Louisiana; Bridgeport, Connecticut; Camden, New Jersey; Charlotte, North Carolina; Chicago, Illinois; Cincinnati, Ohio; Detroit, Michigan; Fort Worth, Texas; Miami, Florida; New Orleans, Louisiana; Pasadena, California; Peoria, Illinois; Phoenix, Arizona; Pittsburgh, Pennsylvania; Rochester, New York; Renton, New Jersey; Washington, DC; and Wichita, Kansas). Of the 104 cities in the analysis, the mentioned weeks had no reported data ("U" for unavailable), by week ending.

and the count of infant deaths was within 3.0%age points (+3.1% vs. +0.1%). Thus, it is unlikely that, for Fukushima, final death counts would show results markedly different from the finding that more Americans, especially infants, died than expected in the 14-week period following arrival of the Fukushima fallout.

The 14-week excess death projections after mid-March 2011 (13,983 total, 822 infant) are relatively similar to actual excesses in May–August 1986 (16,573 total, 306 infant).

Recent assessments have suggested that the amount of radioactivity released from Fukushima equals or exceeds that released from Chernobyl. Given the continuing emission of radioisotopes from the melted reactors, the high density of population around the plant, and the close proximity to food sources, we can expect that morbidity and mortality will be high in Japan. The relative homogeneity of the Japanese population will allow for comparison of health consequences for people living in areas with lesser and greater levels of contamination, as has been done in areas affected by Chernobyl.[521]

Adverse health effects may also be expected in the United States, even though exposures have been far below those in Japan. Low-dose radiation exposure, previously assumed to be harmless, has been linked with elevated disease rates in children born to women who underwent pelvic x-rays while pregnant,[534] Americans exposed to atomic bomb fallout,[535] nuclear plant workers,[536] and, for leukemia, children exposed to very low doses after Chernobyl.[537] In addition, to physical diseases is loss of cognitive ability in adolescents following low-dose ionizing radiation *in utero*.[538]

The human fetus and infant are especially radiosensitive, given their rapid cell growth and cell division, as well as their small size that results in a proportionately larger dose. These exposures include x-ray, alpha, beta, and gamma radiation. Depending on the time of *in utero* radiation exposure, the result can be expressed as spontaneous abortion, premature birth, low birth weight, stillbirth, infant death, congenital malformations, and brain damage.

While this report concentrates on effects to humans, all life is sensitive to nuclear radiation exposure, including plants, fungi, insects spiders, birds, fish, and other animals.[1076] The best-studied group near Chernobyl (birds) shows a 50% percent decrease in species richness and a 66% drop in abundance in the most contaminated areas, compared with normal background in the same neighborhood.[1077]

More importantly, the findings reported by Mangano and Sherman[518] plus the disease patterns that developed after Chernobyl, indicate that public health personnel can anticipate and plan to put in place diagnostic and treatment procedures. Given the continued high levels of radioactive iodine, it is predicted that the incidence of thyroid disease, including thyroid insufficiency in newborns and thyroid cancer in children and adults, will increase.[521,541]

The health effects of exposure to radioactivity from the Fukushima meltdowns, both in Japan and around the world, will take a long time to fully assess. A quarter of a century after the Chernobyl disaster, and more than 60 years after the bombings of Hiroshima and Nagasaki, compilations of health casualties are still being updated (Tables 1.28, 1.29, 1.34, and 1.35).

GULF WAR

According to Haley et al.,[542] few medical conditions are as vexing as Gulf War illness (GWI) to the veterans who experience it, the physicians who are in charge with caring for the veterans, and the policy makers who determine the institutional attitudes and level of resources to be directed at the problem. In 1991, the U.S. military deployed 700,000 of the highest-performing members of the all-volunteer army to the Middle East for a 5-week air bombing campaign and a 5-day ground operation involving tank battles and little traditional combat. Yet, an estimated 25% of the force returned with a chronic, often disabling illness involving symptoms of multiple organ systems without obvious physical signs or laboratory abnormalities,[543] variously ascribed to fibromyalgia, somatization, deployment stress, chronic fatigue syndrome, adult-onset attention-deficit disorder, or simply multisymptom illness. Evidence from epidemiological and clinical studies suggests a chronic neurotoxic encephalopathy from exposure to cholinesterase-inhibiting chemicals,[543,544] which are seen in the chemically sensitive patients for years. A similar chronic illness has been

TABLE 1.35

Calculation of Significance of Differences in 2010 and 2011 Deaths

For example, in Table 1.30, the number of deaths rose by 4.46%, from 148,395 to 155,015, from weeks 12–25 in 2010 versus 2011. This is compared with a 2.34% increase from the prior 14-week period. The significance of difference between the two means (+2.34% versus +4.46%) was calculated using a *t*-test.

The formula $(O - E)/$SQRT (mean 1^2 + mean 2^2) was used, assuming

O = observed increase (1.0446)

E = expected increase (1.0234)

N_1 = number of deaths for weeks 12–25, 2011

N_2 = number of deaths for weeks 50–11, 2011

$$\text{Mean 1} = 1/(\text{SQRT } N_1) \times O = 1/(\text{SQRT } 155,015) \times 1.0446 = 0.002653$$
$$\text{Mean 2} = 1(\text{SQRT } N_2) \times E = 1/(\text{SQRT } 148,395) \times 1.0234 = 0.002657$$

The computations yield 0.0212/0.0037148, or a *z*-score of 5.71, which converts to a *p*-value of <0.000001 in any basic statistics table meaning there is less than a 1 in 1,000,000 chance that the difference occurred due to random chance.

Source: Mangano, J. J., J. D. Sherman. 2012. Unexpected mortality increase in the United States follows arrival of the radioactive plume from Fukushima: Is there a correlation? *Int. J. Health Ser.* 42(1): 47–64, 2012, Baywood Publishing Co., Inc. doi: http://dx.doi.org/10.2190/HS.42.1.f.

described in pesticide-exposed agricultural workers[545] and in survivors of the 1995 subway sarin attack in Tokyo, Japan.[546] Clearly, it is what has been described as chemical sensitivity.

Among the most troubling reports of the ill veterans are symptoms suggesting autonomic nervous system dysfunction which one also sees in chemical sensitivity. Ten thousand patients at the EHC-Dallas have measurable changes when studied for their chemical sensitivity. These include chronic fatigue, pathogen-free diarrhea, delayed gastric emptying and reflux, dizziness, light sensitivity, night sweats or inability to sweat, unrefreshing sleep, sexual dysfunction, and an unusually high rate of cholecystitis and cholecystectomy in atypically young male veterans.[543] A 2004 study by Haley et al.[544] measured autonomic function in 21 veterans who fit in a factor case definition of three syndrome variants and in 17 veteran control subjects (all male) who were matched by age, sex, and education, drawn from an epidemiological survey of a Naval Reserve unit.[547] Spectral analysis of 24-hour Holter electrocardiography demonstrated significant blunting of the normal nocturnal increase in high-frequency HRV (HF HRV), suggesting impaired central control of parasympathetic tone,[548] which has been recorded in chemically sensitive patients for years. But test results of baroreceptor function, sleep architecture by polysomnography, and sensor and motor nerve conduction were normal although some chemically sensitive patients have impaired sensory nerve condition or neurography. Stein et al.[549] reported reduced circadian variation in HF HRV among 12 veterans of the Gulf War (GW) meeting a modified case definition of multisymptom illness[550] recruited from a rheumatology clinic compared with 36 healthy civilian volunteers, but HF HRV reduction was present only in five female veterans and not in six male veterans with usable HRV measurements. In an evaluation of neuromuscular function in 49 ill British Gulf War veterans (GWV) and in 26 healthy controls, Sharief et al.[551] found no differences in quantitative test results of sensory detection thresholds, Valsalva and standing heart rate ratios, and thermoregulatory control of sweating; however, 24-hour HF HRV was not measured. None of these studies provided a thorough description of autonomic symptoms, and none was performed among a population-representative sample of veterans with the full spectrum of GWI symptoms. The three studies[548,549,551] are compatible with the possibility of a selective abnormality of central cholinergic parasympathetic control with preserved sympathetic adrenergic and cardiovagal baroreceptor function. Ninety-five percent of the people who have chemical sensitivity cannot sweat and thus some of the symptoms that can be corrected with environmental manipulation are not because of the ignoring of this act. Many chemically sensitive patients also have measurable sympathetic elevations along with their parasympathetic decrease which gives them a super adrenaline effect. There are several stages of the chemically sensitive problem and the GW patients may not have been exposed long enough to exhibit the increase in sympathetic effect.

Therefore, Haley et al.[547] designed a study to test this prestated hypothesis. They evaluated a population-representative sample of GWV meeting a validated case definition of GWI, with a control group and three syndrome variants representing the full spectrum of the condition.[552]

They studied 97 GW-era veterans, including 66 case veterans with GWI and 31 control veterans. The participants, randomly selected as a nested case–control study by a three-stage sample from the U.S. Military Health Survey, were representative of the entire GW-era veteran population. The 66 case veterans met the standardized factor case definition of GWI, which was previously validated in a clinical[552] and in a large nationally representative sample.[553] Specifically, they studied 21 veterans meeting the factor case definition of GW syndrome 1 (impaired cognition), 24 veterans with syndrome 2 (confusion-ataxia), and 21 veterans with syndrome 3 (central neuropathic pain). The 31 control veterans included 16 who did not meet the factor case definition of GWI but were deployed to the Kuwaiti theater of operations (deployed controls) and 15 who were in the military during the 1991 GW but were not deployed (nondeployed controls). The demographic characteristics and comorbidities of the final sample are given in Table 1.29.

All three GWI variant groups reported significantly more autonomic symptoms, assessed by the ASP, than the control group. The COMPASS scores were significantly elevated for all three syndrome groups compared with the controls and most elevated for syndrome 2. These data fit the pattern of the chemically sensitive that we have reported for years.

In the various symptom domains of the ASP, the syndrome 2 group had the highest autonomic symptom scores, but the pattern of symptom score elevations was similar among the three syndrome groups. The differences between cases and controls explained more variance ($R^2 \geq 0.20$) in the orthostatic intolerance, secretomotor, upper gastrointestinal dysmotility, sleep dysfunction, and urinary symptom domains and explained less variance ($R^2 < 0.20$) in the pupillomotor, autonomic constipation, vasomotor, male sexual dysfunction, and reflex syncope symptom domains, suggesting deficits related more to cholinergic than adrenergic autonomic systems. Moreover, the group difference on the male sexual dysfunction subscale was mainly due to erectile dysfunction, possibly related to parasympathetic cholinergic control, and not ejaculatory failure, a sympathetic adrenergic function (Table 1.36).

In objective autonomic tests, participants with GWI had significantly more evidence of autonomic deficits than the controls. The CASS varied significantly across the clinical groups ($p = 0.045$) and was higher in the syndrome 2 groups than in the controls ($p = 0.02$).

Compared with the controls, all three syndrome groups showed significantly reduced distal postganglionic sudomotor function, most significant in the foot, intermediate in the ankle and upper leg, and nonsignificant in the arm, indicating nerve length-related damage to the peripheral autonomic nervous system affecting the distal small cholinergic sudomotor fibers. In a multivariable linear model of sudomotor function in the foot controlling for age and race/ethnicity, the case–control difference was significant ($p = 0.02$) and did not vary by sex ($p = 0.78$ for group × sex interaction). Controlling for covariates did not alter these findings.

One of the big problems in the chemically sensitive patient is that the restoring of sweating appears to be necessary for recovery. At the EHC-Dallas, we have included sauna as a part of our prescription program for at least 20 years as sweating is essential for all recovery. We have treated 10,000 of our chemically sensitive and GW patients with sauna. This process appears to detoxify the micro, peripheral cholinergic nerves and rehabilitate their functions.

In contrast, no group differences were statistically significant in tests of tear production (Schirmer test), in sympathetic adrenergic function (including the BP responses to Valsalva maneuvers and tilt), or in any of the papillary measures.

The syndrome 2 and syndrome 3 groups had increased cooling detection threshold, which was statistically significant only for the syndrome 2 group. As other chemically sensitive patients, the GWI patients often are cold intolerant. None of the three syndrome groups differed significantly from controls on the heat pain threshold.

TABLE 1.36

Demographic and Comorbidity Measures in Controls and Gulf War Illness Variant Groups

Characteristic	Nondeployed Controls ($n = 15$)	Deployed Controls ($n = 16$)	Gulf War Illness Variant Group[a]			p Value[b]
			Syndrome 1 ($n = 21$)	Syndrome 2 ($n = 24$)	Syndrome 3 ($n = 21$)	
Age, mean (SD), year	51.9 (7.8)	47.8 (7.9)	48.2 (8.6)	49.8 (8.0)	51.0 (7.9)	0.42
Female sex no. (%)	3 (20)	3 (19)	7 (33)	7 (29)	4 (19)	0.78
Black race/ethnicity, no. (%)	2 (13)	4 (25)	3 (14)	4 (17)	3 (14)	0.91
Officer rank during the war, no. (%)	2 (13)	2 (13)	2 (10)	1 (4)	3 (14)	0.80
Education scale, mean (SD)	5.5 (1.7)	5.1 (1.8)	5.8 (1.8)	4.6 (1.6)	5.0 (2.0)	0.30
BMI, mean (SD)	30.1 (3.2)	29.6 (4.7)	29.0 (5.0)	28.4 (4.7)	30.7 (5.8)	0.66
Resting pulse rate, mean (SD), beats/min	75.9 (9.8)	75.9 (14.1)	75.4 (15.1)	73.3 (12.3)	74.4 (14.7)	0.80
Glomerular filtration rate from two 24-hour urine samples, mean (SD)	129 (42)	132 (35)	113 (35)	125 (23)	121 (31)	0.65
Taking anticholinergic medications or tricyclic antidepressants, no. (%)	1 (7)	0	2 (10)	3 (13)	1 (5)	0.62
Diabetes by history or glycated hemoglobin level ≥7% on admission, no. (%)	1 (7)	0	1 (5)	1 (4)	1 (5)	0.95
CDC definition of multisymptom illness, no. (%) MOS SF-12 t-score, mean (SD)	0	0	21 (100)	24 (100)	21 (100)	<001
Physical component	51.5 (9.4)	51.6 (7.7)	37.8 (12.3)	26.2 (7.6)	32.4 (.2)	<001
Mental component	57.8 (3.5)	58.4 (7.4)	34.5 (12.0)	39.6 (9.3)	45.6 (12.4)	<001
CDC definition of chronic fatigue syndrome, no. (%)	0	0	1 (5)	2 (8)	4 (19)	0.19
ACR survey Definition of fibromyalgia, no. (%) SCID diagnosis no. (%)	0	0	5 (24)	14 (58)	18 (86)	<001
Active major depressive disorder	0	0	5 (24)	1 (4)	3 (14)	0.04
Active alcohol abuse or dependence	3 (20)	1 (6)	6 (29)	10 (42)	5 (24)	0.15
Active drug abuse or dependence or admission urine test	2 (13)	2 (13)	4 (19)	5 (21)	1 (5)	0.58
CAPS diagnosis of active posttraumatic stress disorder, no. (%)[c]	0	0	8 (38)	9 (38)	5 (24)	0.002

[a] Syndrome 1 is impaired cognition, syndrome 2 is confusion-ataxia, and syndrome 3 is central neuropathic pain.

[b] By 5-group Fisher exact test or Wilcoxon rank sum test.

[c] Among 22 participants with PTSD by CAPS, the inciting event was a horrifying or life-threatening experience in seven of them (Haley et al., 2013).

Abbreviations: ACR, American College of Rheumatology; BMI, body mass index (calculated as weight in kilograms divided by height in meters square); CAPS, Clinician Administrated; PTSD, posttraumatic stress disorder scale; CDC, Centers for Disease Control and Prevention; MOS SF-12, Medical Outcomes Study 12-item Short Form Health Survey; SCID, Structured Clinical Interview for DSM-IV-R; S1 conversion factor; to convert glycated hemoglobin level to proportion of total hemoglobin, multiplied by 0.01.

From spectral analysis of 24-hour electrocardiogram monitoring, HF HRV increased normally at night in the control group but not in the three syndrome groups. In a repeated-measures mixed-effects linear model of log HF HRV, the case–control × day minus night interaction was statistically significant ($p < 0.001$), but the three-way interaction with sex was not ($p = 0.88$), indicating that the loss of circadian variation in the three syndrome groups compared with the controls was found in both men and women veterans. Controlling for the covariates did not alter these findings.

When analyzed by group, all three syndrome groups showed significant blunting or loss of the normal nocturnal increase. During the day, HF HRV of the syndrome 1 group did not differ from that of the controls, but the syndrome 2 group had significantly lower HF HRV than the controls, and the syndrome 3 group had significantly higher HF HRV than the controls, particularly during the morning hours.

HF HRV at night was moderately inversely correlated with the CASS index of objective autonomic test results ($r = -0.41$, $p < 0.001$). HF HRV during the day was weakly correlated with the CASS ($r = -0.22$, $p = 0.04$).

The COMPASS of all autonomic symptoms was inversely correlated with HF HRV and directly correlated with the CASS subscales. The correlation was highest with HF HRV during the day and with the CASS sudomotor subscale, and the correlation was lowest with the CASS cardiovagal and adrenergic subscales.

The individual symptom domains tended to be correlated with HF HRV or with the CASS sudomotor subscale but not both. Specifically, the vasomotor, secretomotor, upper gastrointestinal dysmotility, and pupillomotor symptom domains were most strongly correlated with the CASS sudomotor subscale. We have measured our 1000 chemically sensitive patients by pupillography and the Ishikawa method, showing autonomic changes in chemically sensitive patient's eyes. The orthostatic intolerance symptom domain was also correlated with the CASS sudomotor subscale, and it was the only symptom domain to be significantly correlated with the CASS adrenergic subscale. In contrast, the upper gastrointestinal dysmotility and sleep dysfunction symptom domains were most strongly associated with HF HRV at night, and the autonomic diarrhea, male sexual dysfunction, and urinary symptom domains were most strongly correlated with HF HRV during the day. Of the two components of male sexual dysfunction, erectile dysfunction, a parasympathetic function, was highly correlated with HF HRV during the day, while ejaculatory failure, an adrenergic function, was not. Like ejaculatory failure, reflex syncope was not associated with any of the objective autonomic measures, and these were the only autonomic symptom domains not associated with the three syndrome groups.

In a nested case–control sample drawn from a national survey in a large representative sample of the GW-era U.S. military population, this study found that a well-validated research case definition of GWI was strongly associated with standard scales of autonomic symptoms and with objective test of autonomic dysfunction. Autonomic symptom scores and objective test results were mostly abnormal compared with the controls in the syndrome 2 group. This reflects the findings of several prior studies in which syndrome 2 consistently was the most disabling[552,554] and had the most prominent abnormalities on various objective tests of brain function.[555–562]

The ASP autonomic symptom domains most strongly associated with the case definition tended to be those related predominantly to cholinergic autonomic control, and these symptoms domains tended to be most strongly associated with HF HRV measures or with the CASS sudomotor subscale but not with the CASS cardiovagal or adrenergic subscales. In the objective autonomic tests, the three syndrome groups differed mostly from controls on sudomotor testing (quantitative sudomotor axon reflex test). The degree of difference on the quantitative sudomotor axon reflex test was related to peripheral nerve length, typical of a length-dependent neuropathy of small-caliber, unmyelinated, peripheral nerve fibers. The increased cooling detection thresholds observed in the syndrome 2 group and the syndrome 3 group and described in a previous study[563] may also reflect underlying small-fiber impairment.

The autonomic nervous system impairment was most clearly demonstrated in the blunting of the normal rise in HF HRV at night. Because peripheral vagal baroreflex function was not significantly impaired, this abnormality of circadian variation in HF HRV suggests dysfunction in the CNS control of parasympathetic outflow just as Haley's study and ours showed. The sample size of this study was also sufficient to demonstrate significant, although more subtle, differences in HF HRV among the three syndrome groups during the day. Multivariable statistical analyses demonstrated that the objective findings of peripheral sudomotor neuropathy and impaired HF HRV were not explained by smoking, creatinine clearance, psychiatric comorbidity, diagnosis of heart disease, glycated hemoglobin level, officer rank during the war, indicators of deconditioning (BMI and resting pulse rate), or medications the participants were taking during the period of the study, including anticholinergic medications and tricyclic antidepressants.

According to Golomb,[544] the pattern of autonomic symptoms and objective test findings point predominantly to dysfunction of both central and peripheral cholinergic functions, possibly from neurotoxic damage to cholinergic neurons or receptors. This proposed explanation is compatible with prior studies[560,561] showing that, compared with control subjects, regional cerebral blood flow in veterans with GWI responds abnormally to cholinergic challenge with physostigmine, suggesting chronic alteration of cholinergic receptors in the brain. Experiments in rodents, undertaken to model the possible chronic effects of sarin in low doses to which GWV were exposed in the war, have identified persisting alterations of cholinergic receptors[564,565] and of autonomic responses.[566]

These findings and this explanation are compatible with a prior study[551] of neurologic function in ill GWV, which found no associations with tests of adrenergic autonomic function and nerve conduction investigations of large-caliber peripheral nerves but generally did not test for circadian variation in HF HRV. Haley's findings did not confirm the interaction of blunted circadian variation in HF HRV with sex (blunted in women but not in men) reported by Stein et al.[549] which may have resulted from their studying a small sample drawn from healthcare-seeking clients.

The robust sample size and external validity afforded by the nested case–control design drawn from a survey in a large population representative sample add greater confidence to the findings from prior small studies[549,555–561] performed in samples from single military units or from clinic volunteers. Particularly important for studying a disease defined by symptoms alone, the case definition of GWI used in this study is the only one that has been empirically validated by demonstrating a statistically good fit in the other GWV populations.[552,553] Its three syndrome variants provide homogeneous clinical groups to maximize statistical power and represent the full spectrum of the illness to determine whether autonomic dysfunction spans the entire spectrum or is limited to a part of it. The extensive work by Suarez et al.,[567] Low,[568] and Low et al.[569] in developing the ASP and the CASS testing systems, used in this study, provided validated measures of autonomic symptom domains and objective autonomic function testing. As in a previous study of autonomic symptoms measured by the ASP,[567] the validity of the veterans' symptom reports was supported by correlations of the COMPASS and its domains with the appropriate CASS subscales of objective autonomic test results.

The autonomic measures that differed between cases and controls in this study may prove useful in a strategy for clinical diagnosis of GWI. Of the objective tests used, the one showing the clearest discrimination among all three syndrome groups and the control group was the measurement of circadian variation in HF HRV. When tested with the repeated-measures mixed-effects linear model, which appropriately manages variance of the fixed and random effects, the group discrimination is extremely good. However, when HF HRV measurements in multiple epochs are combined to form a single measure of nighttime HF HRV for each participant, the resulting participant-level means display enough residual variance to reduce the usefulness in clinical diagnosis. Additional research should attempt to reformulate the measure of circadian variation in HF HRV to reduce the variance. Measures of the central nervous system mechanisms upstream from the autonomic dysfunction, such as neuroimaging or electroencephalography of brain function,[555–562] may also be combined with autonomic testing to improve clinical diagnosis. This ANS test has been performed for 20 years at the EHC-Dallas. It has proved very efficacious for dx and Rx using pupillography and HRV. Brain Triple-Camera SPECT scans have also been used in the chemically sensitive to confirm toxicity in over 1000 patients.

Perhaps the most important implications of the findings are those bearing on the long-standing debate about the nature of the GWI. These results confirm dysfunction among GWV of both central control of parasympathetic function and peripheral cholinergic autonomic nerves, further implicating underlying damage to the cholinergic components of the central and peripheral nervous systems.

Persian GWV used chemicals and medications that could be toxic if combined even at doses that are harmless alone.

GW and any other wars can cause massive contamination of the earth either in a stationary area involving many miles wide, or it can involve fluid area that are ever changing. However, exposures to troops and the civilian population the war gases and particulates can be devastating to both groups. According to Golomb, many areas of the body are involved including the cells and the energy producing mitochondria (Table 1.38). Areas of the body include the neurological, GI MS and CV systems[544] (Tables 1.37 through 1.43).

TABLE 1.37

Overview—According to Golomb

	GWI	OSMD	CMI
Dominant symptoms	Symptoms protean but focus on fatigue, cognitive–mood, musculoskeletal, also gastrointestinal, sleep, neurological	Symptoms protean but focus for MD on fatigue, cognitive–mood, musculoskeletal, also gastrointestinal, sleep, neurological	Symptoms protean with emphasis defined by the condition (fatigue for CFS; muscle for FM, GI, or IBS; CNS/"cognitive" for ASD; chemical sensitivity for MCS) but very high overlap
Symptom multiplicity/ heterogeneity	Symptoms multiplicity with high heterogeneity	Symptoms multiplicity with high heterogeneity	High heterogeneity of symptoms
Symptom latency	Variable latency to symptom onset	Variable latency to symptom onset	Variable latency to symptom onset
Exposure associations	Includes OPs/ acetylcholinesterase, inhibitors, paraoxonase gene variants, vaccines	Causes include OPs/ acetylcholinesterase inhibitors, paraoxonase gene variants, vaccines	Includes OPs/ acetylcholinesterase inhibitors, paraoxonase gene variants, vaccines
Objective findings	Includes autonomic dysfunction, reduced natural killer cell activity, coagulation	Include autonomic dysfunction, reduced natural killer cell activity, coagulation	Includes autonomic dysfunction, reduced natural killer cell activity[570,571]
	Activation, elevated autoimmune markers, elevated GGT, low paraoxonase activity	Activation, elevated autoimmune markers, elevated GGT, low paraoxonase activity	Coagulation activation,[572] elevated autoimmune markers,[573–821] elevated GGT,[575] low paraoxonase activity[576]
Related conditions	Includes CMI (except ASD). Also, includes hypertension, hearing loss, ALS	Includes CMI (extending to ASD). Also, includes hypertension, hearing loss, ALS	Includes hearing loss

Source: Golomb, B. A. 2012. Oxidative stress and mitochondrial injury in chronic multisymptom conditions from Gulf War illness to austism spectrum disorder. Gulf War Mitochondria. *Nature Preceedings*: hdl:10101/npre.2012.6847.1. Posted January 30, 2012.

TABLE 1.38
Predictions

	Observed with Oxidative Stress/ Mitochondrial Dysfunction	Preliminary Evidence or Comment
Other markers of oxidative stress and mitochondrial dysfunction will be elevated	Yes[796]	True for chronic fatigue syndrome,[579,580,784] a related condition that is elevated in GWV[618] (True for ASD)
Genetic risk markers related to mitochondrial function, antioxidant defense, energetic, and apoptosis will be identified	Yes, by definition	Gene associations related to mitochondrial function, energetic, and apoptosis have been reported for chronic fatigue syndrome,[582,583,761,812] a related condition that is elevated in GWV.[607,618,636] Deletions in genes for glutathione S-transferase enzymes (leading to loss of protection against oxidative stress) are strongly and significantly linked to multiple-chemical sensitivity.[584] Gene variants in paraoxonase have been observed in both GWI and ASD[a], and glutathione-related variants among others in ASD[585–587]
GWV will have increased rates of adverse effects with many medications and interventions because many adverse effects are mediated via oxidative stress and mitochondrial problems[577,588–590]	See comment. Examples of drugs with adverse effects mediated by oxidative stress include acetaminophen, aminoglycosides, fluoroquinolones, amiodarone, nonsteroidal anti-inflammatory agents, chemotherapeutics[588,590–605]	Increased drug adverse effects have been observed in irritable bowel syndrome,[606] a condition elevated in GWV[607] and linked to oxidative stress.[608] Regression reported by some parents following vaccinations in cases of ASD may be a consequence of impaired detoxification (such vaccination may boost the oxidative burden, however, and potentiate the process)
New oxidative stressor exposures—beyond medications and medical interventions, though those merit separate mention will have disproportionate adverse impact in exposed and particularly symptomatic GWV and CMI		Proxidant-antioxidant balance will be adversely affected, disadvantaging ability to defend against new oxidative stressors
Endothelial dysfunction will arise at elevated rates	Endothelial dysfunction is strongly linked to oxidative stress[609]	
Hepatic steatosis will develop at elevated rates, as will ectopic fat deposition in other locations	Hepatic steatosis relates strongly to oxidative stress[610,611]	
Low HDL and high triglycerides will emerge	These conditions (and all elements of metabolic syndrome) are linked to oxidative stress[612,613] and mitochondrial dysfunction[614]	

(Continued)

TABLE 1.38 (*Continued*)
Predictions

	Observed with Oxidative Stress/ Mitochondrial Dysfunction	Preliminary Evidence or Comment
Free fatty acids will be elevated	Elevated free fatty acids are linked to oxidative stress[615]	
Metabolic syndrome as a whole will arise at elevated rates	Metabolic syndrome is linked to oxidative stress[612,616] and mitochondrial dysfunction[614]	As above, weight gain and hypertension are already reported at elevated rates. Diabetes prevalence shows variable trends likely due to selection of diabetics out of deployment to high risk areas
Rates of diabetes will rise to first match then exceed rates in nondeployed (those with diabetes were disproportionately nondeployed)	Diabetes, like metabolic syndrome, is strongly linked to oxidative stress (as effect but possibly also cause)[617] and mitochondrial dysfunction[619,620]	This prediction is made despite mixed direction of trends in diabetes rates in published studies.[607,618] It is predicted that a clear increase will emerge
Rates of cardiovascular disease and will particularly peripheral arterial disease will emerge at an elevated rate as GWV age	These conditions, and especially peripheral arterial disease, are associated with oxidative stress[621–623] and mitochondrial dysfunction[624–626]	
Parkinson's disease will emerge at an elevated rate as GWV age	Parkinson's disease is linked to oxidative stress and mitochondrial dysfunction[578,632]	Like ALS (and Gulf War illness, Parkinson's disease bears an association to polymorphisms in paraoxonase and exposure to pesticides[627–631,821]
Elevated "depression" diagnoses will be found to disproportionately focus on somatic symptoms	Somatic symptoms in depression have been found to serve as markers for mitochondrial dysfunction.[627]	"Depression" has been reported to be elevated in GWV.[607] GWV have many somatic symptoms that will contribute to elevated scores in depression scales
"Age-related" hearing loss and tinnitus will be demonstrated to occur at elevated rates	[743,744,765,1100,1102]	GWV report physician-diagnosed tinnitus at elevated rates[607]
Other diagnoses linked to oxidative stress will occur at elevated rates		Some reports suggest increased cancer of some types[633] and cancer death in Gulf War veterans[634,635]
Exposed GWV who do not meet criteria for GWI will nonetheless show statistical abnormalities in markers of oxidative stress and sequelae of oxidative stress (perhaps intermediate between unexposed and those with GWI)		Asymptomatic persons with mt dysfunction at low heteroplasmy rates nonetheless show increased oxidative stress, proportional to the heteroplasmy level[796]

Source: Golomb, B. A. 2012. Oxidative stress and mitochondrial injury in chronic multisymptom conditions from Gulf War illness to austism spectrum disorder. Gulf War Mitochondria. *Nature Preceedings*: hdl:10101/npre.2012.6847.1. Posted January 30, 2012.

Note: GWI, Gulf War illness; GWV, Gulf War veterans; ALS, amyotrophic lateral sclerosis

[a]   Those with GWI have many somatic symptoms that will contribute to elevated scores in depression scales.

TABLE 1.39
Gulf War Associations

Associated Characteristic	Seen With Gulf War Illness (also other CMI)	Oxidative ↔mt Dysfunction
Exposure associations		
Acetylcholinesterase inhibitors strongly associated	Yes[544,636]	Yes[638,639]
Reactogenic vaccines also consistently associated	Anthrax vaccine associated,[636,640] vaccine adverse effects associated,[636,641] multiple vaccinations associated[636,642–644]	Reactogenic vaccines associated with OS,[847] anthrax vaccine among the most reactogenic of vaccines,[645] aluminum (vaccine adjuvants), mercury (thimerosal preservatives) linked OS, impaired antioxidant defense against other exposures, and MD[647–661]
Multiple other exposures are associated		
Symptom characteristics		
Brain and muscle dominate	Yes[550]	Yes[662]
Fatigue and fatigue with exertion prominent	Yes[550,607,618,663]	Yes[580,664,665,666]
Symptoms are protean spanning many domains	Yes[607,618,663]	Yes[1080]
Symptoms differ from person to person	Yes[550,607,618,663]	Yes[666,740,1081,1082]
Frequency to symptom onset variable, often prolonged, differs across individuals, and differs across symptoms within an individual	Yes[668]	Yes[667]
Individual symptoms associated		
Objective findings		
Routine labs generally unremarkable	Yes	Yes
PON genotype differences present	Yes. Other CMI add ASD,CFS	Yes
GGT elevated (marker of oxidative stress)	Yes[669,670] (other OS markers not examined). Other CMI	Yes[700,731]
PON1 activity reduced	Yes.[671,674,675] Other CMI	Yes[857,1083]
Natural killer cell activity reduced	Yes.[675,678] Other CMI	Yes[846,858,859,1084]
Heart rate variability blunted	Yes[548,549]	Yes[581,860]
Other autonomic abnormalities present	Yes.[681,684] Other CMI	Yes[720,739,1085]
Coagulation markers elevated	Yes.[685,689] Other CMI	Yes[646,861,862,1076] (OS promotes apoptosis,[690,864,,865] which activates coagulation pathways)[868]
Autoimmune markers elevated	Yes.[675,800] Other CMI[572–574] autism autoantibodies check	Yes. add cits[1086] May be partly adaptive[1087,1088]

Source: Golomb, B. A. 2012. Oxidative stress and mitochondrial injury in chronic multisymptom conditions from Gulf War illness to austism spectrum disorder. Gulf War Mitochondria. *Nature Preceedings*: hdl:10101/npre.2012.6847.1. Posted January 30, 2012.

Exposures: AChEI are particularly potent in inducing OS and MD[74]—and particularly strong consistent predictors of GWI. AChEI exposures, moreover, were also commonly recurrent when they occurred; and in addition, they cause MD by means beyond OS such as microtubule toxicity.[704,1089] The central role of OS in mediating AChEI.

TABLE 1.40

Associated Conditions Are Compatible with OSMD

Associated Conditions	Linked to GWV	Linked to OSMD
Chronic fatigue syndrome	Yes[607,618,636,705,805,1090]	Yes[579–580,583,682–683,686–688,1078]
Fibromyalgia	Yes[618,805,1090]	Yes[691–696]
Irritable bowel syndrome	Yes[607]	Yes[608]
Multiple-chemical sensitivity	Yes[607,618,636,663,705,1091–1092]	Yes[584]
Autism spectrum condition	No—different developmental timeline	Yes[576,697–699,702–703,794,1093–1095]
Hypertension	Yes[607,633,636,671–672]	Yes[619,768–770,1096–1097]
Weight gain	Yes[550,607,671]	Yes[612,614,616,776]
Amyotrophic lateral sclerosis	Yes[673,676–677]	Yes[772–773,1098–1099]
Hearing loss/tinnitus	Yes[607,618,636,836]	Yes[762–764,774,1082,1100–1103]
Fracture risk and reduced bone formation	Yes[679–680]	Yes[701,1104–1106]

Source: Golomb, B. A. 2012. Oxidative stress and mitochondrial injury in chronic multisymptom conditions from Gulf War illness to austism spectrum disorder. Gulf War Mitochondria. *Nature Preceedings*: hdl:10101/npre.2012.6847.1. Posted January 30, 2012.

TABLE 1.41

Frequency of Individual Symptoms within Gulf War Illness Symptom Profiles

Symptom Profiles	Symptom % within GWI Cases		
	Fatigue	Mood–Cognition Cluster	Musculoskeletal Cluster
All three symptoms (55.9)	Fatigue (100)	Memory problems (74.2)	Joint pain (94.3)
		Difficulty sleeping (70.8)	Joint stiffness (90.0)
		Moodiness (58.2)	Muscle pain (65.7)
		Difficulty with words (57.7)	
		Depression (56.3)	
		Anxiety (39.7)	
Fatigue + mood–cognition (24.8)	Fatigue (100)	Moodiness (86.4)	
		Difficulty sleeping (85.3)	
		Memory problems (73.4)	
		Depression (42.2)	
		Difficulty with words (26.4)	
		Anxiety	
Fatigue + musculoskeletal (0.4)	Fatigue (100)		Muscle pain (77 6)
			Joint stiffness (72.4)
			Joint pain (67.1)
Mood–cognition + musculoskeletal (19.0)		Memory problems (64.1)	Joint stiffness (92.4)
		Difficulty with words (44.8)	Joint pain (81.8)
		Difficulty sleeping (35.4)	Muscle pain (14.8)
		Moodiness (25.2)	
		Anxiety (12.2)	
		Depression (7.2)	

TABLE 1.42

Objective Autonomic and Quantitative Sensor Tests in Controls and Gulf War Illness Variant Groups[a]

	Controls Mean (SEM) (*n* = 31)	Gulf War Illness Variant Groups			*p* Value[b]
Variable		Syndrome 1 (*n* = 21)	Syndrome 2 (*n* = 23)	Syndrome 3 (*n* = 21)	
CASS	0.71 (0.27)	1.15 (0.32)	1.90 (0.31)[c]	0.57 (0.32)	0.045
OSART Sudomotor Quantitative Seat Production (µL)					
Foot	0.79 (0.07)	0.53 (0.08)[c]	0.40 (0.07)[d]	0.55 (0.08)[c]	0.055
Ankle	1.33 (0.12)	1.16 (0.16)	0.78 (0.15)[e]	0.92 (0.16)[c]	0.04
Upper leg	0.90 (0.09)	0.60 (0.11)	0.49 (0.10)[e]	0.68 (0.10)	0.02
Arm	1.09 (0.14)	1.01 (0.18)	0.96 (0.16)	1.34 (0.17)	0.24
Schrimer test tear production at 5 min (mm)	6.0 (1.2)	6.2 (1.5)	4.4 (1.4)	3.5 (1.5)	0.50
Ratio of expiration to inspiration for R-R intervals	1.25 (0.02)	1.23 (0.27)	1.25 (0.03)	1.24 (0.03)	0.78
Valsalva ratio	1.81 (0.05)	1.83 (0.64)	1.67 (0.06)	1.77 (0.06)	0.28
Change in systolic blood pressure from baseline at 3-minute tilt mmHg	0.12 (1.33)	2.70 (1.64)	0.67 (1.52)	−0.13 (1.60)	0.64
Maximum Papillary Constriction Velocity (mm/second)[f]					
Left eye	4.85 (0.17)	4.71 (0.21)	4.52 (0.20)	4.95 (0.21)	0.69
Right eye	4.96 (0.16)	4.58 (0.20)	4.51 (0.19)	4.95 (0.21)	0.29
Quantitative Sensory in the Dominant Hand					
Cooling Detection Threshold					
Just noticeable difference units	8.5 (0.7)	9.4 (0.8)	11.1 (0.8)[c]	10.7 (0.8)	0.12
Percentile	70.4 (4.4)	84.6 (5.2)	93.0 (5.0)[c]	86.8 (5.2)	0.13
Heat pain threshold					
Just noticeable difference units	23.0 (0.3)	22.5 (0.4)	22.7 (0.3)	22.3 (0.3)	0.38
Percentile	38.7 (5.0)	27.5 (6.2)	31.1 (5.8)	27.1 (6.0)	0.38
Basal corticotrophin level (pg/dL)	28.9 (2.9)	27.7 (3.4)	23.7 (2.7)	25.9 (3.2)	0.49
Basal cortisol level (µg/dL)	0.71 (0.08)	0.56 (0.08)	0.47 (0.06)	0.77 (0.11)	0.10

[a] Means (SEMs) are standardized for age, sex, and race/ethnicity (black versus other).

[b] By the Kruskal–Wallis nonparametric 4-group test.

[c] $p \leq 0.05$.

[d] $p \leq 0.001$ for difference from controls by Wilcoxon rank sum test. The sudomotor group differences remained significant after controlling for whether participants were taking anticholinergic medications or tricyclic antidepressants.

[e] $p \leq 0.01$.

[f] No significant group differences were observed in resting papillary diameter, dilation velocity, or constriction amplitude responses to 30-millisecond or 1-second light flash.

Abbreviations: CASS, Composite Autonomic Severity Score; QSART, Quantitative Sudomotor Axon Reflex Test.

SI conversion factors: To convert corticotrophin level per liter, multiply by 0.22; to convert cortisol level to nanomoles per liter, multiply by 27.588.

HEARING LOSS

Significant elevations in self-reported hearing loss after 1990 or 1991 in GWV versus control groups have been reported.[607,636,679,761] (However, obviously, even with military controls, there are uncertainties regarding noise exposure comparability. Additionally, formal testing has not yet been undertaken.) Hearing loss deemed "age-related" and "noise-related" is powerfully linked to OSMD.[762,763]

TABLE 1.43

Differences in Circadian Variation of Parasympathetic Cardiovagal Tone Measured by 24-Hour Holter Monitoring among Gulf War Illness Variant and Control Groups[a]

Group	Spectral Power of High-Frequency HRV Mean (SEM), ms²			
	Day 8:00 a.m. to 9:00 p.m.	Night 12:00 a.m. to 5:00 a.m.	Circadian Difference, Night Minus Day	p-value[b]
Model 1[c]				
Controls	135 (9)	226 (19)	91 (21)	<0.001
Cases	131 (6)	139 (8)	8 (10)	0.36
Controls minus cases	5 (10)	87 (22)	83 (25)	<0.001
Model 2[c]				
Controls	135 (9)	226 (19)	91 (21)	<0.001
Syndrome 1	133 (11)	125 (13)	8 (17)	0.60
Syndrome 2	106 (8)	129 (13)	23 (15)	0.07
Syndrome 3	160 (12)	165 (17)	4 (21)	0.82
Controls minus syndrome 1	2 (13)	101 (24)	99 (28)	<0.001
Controls minus syndrome 2	29 (11)	97 (24)	68 (27)	<0.001
Controls minus syndrome 3	−25 (15)	61 (27)	87 (31)	0.004

[a] Apparent discrepancies in reported differences are due to rounding.

[b] From repeated-measures mixed-effects linear model predicting log-transformed high-frequency HRV measured in 5-minute epochs every hour from the fixed effects of group, day minus night, and their interaction, with participants as random effects and the Dunett correction for multiple comparisons. Significance was not altered by controlling for age, sex, race/ethnicity, body mass index, officer rank during the war, glycated hemoglobin level, glomerular filtration rate, major depressive disorder active posttraumatic stress disorder, alcohol abuse, or dependence, smoking, and anticholinergic medication or tricyclic antidepressant use.

[c] Model 1 (all cases combined) tests the effects seen in Figure A given below. Model 2 (cases analyzed by Gulf War illness variant group) tests the effects seen in Figure B given below.

Abbreviation: HRV, heart rate variability.

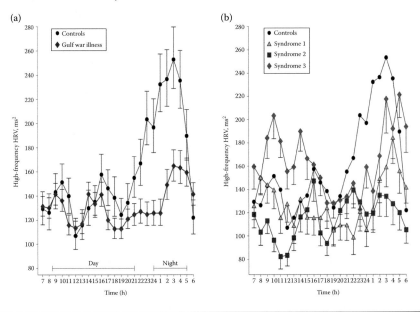

Accelerated hearing loss is common in MD,[706–708,721,722,732,742,764–767,1107] cited as among the most common symptoms of mitochondriopathy, together with fatigue and muscle symptoms.[743] And chemical exposures have been linked to both hair cell damage and noise-related hearing loss.[744,749]

Hypertension

Hypertension is found in a range of studies (Table 1.44).[604,605,634,674] Hypertension, too, is a condition with powerful relationship to OSMD.[758,759,768–770] Indeed, an evaluation of mitochondrial pedigrees estimated the fraction of patients with hypertension potentially due to mtDNA mutation involvement at 55% (95% CI 45%–65%).[771] Analogous to the GW situation, increased BP has been previously associated with environmental OS exposures. For instance, both arsenic and lead are reported to mediate their toxicity via OS[709–711]; and exposure to each arsenic (e.g., in the water supply)[712,713] and lead [709,710] have been linked to increased rates of hypertension. Hypertension and hearing loss are both common "age-related" conditions but have been seen with chemical sensitivity.

TABLE 1.44

Partial Spearman Rank Order Correlations of the Total COMPASS Score and Autonomic Symptom Profile Domains with Objective, Laboratory-Based Measures of Autonomic Function[a]

| Variable | Spectral Power of High-Frequency HRV | | CASS | | | |
	Night 12:00 a.m. to 5:00 a.m.	Day 8:00 a.m. to 9:00 p.m.	Total	Sudomotor	Cardiovagal	Adrenergic
Total COMPASS score	-0.20^b	-0.26^c	0.20^b	0.21^d	0.10	0.11
Autonomic Symptom Profile Domain						
Orthostatic intolerance	-0.17	-0.13	0.22^d	0.19^b	0.12	0.22^d
Vasomotor	-0.10	-0.14	0.14	0.22^d	-0.01	-0.02
Secretomotor	-0.12	-0.16	0.12	0.22^b	-0.04	-0.01
Upper gastrointestinal Dysmotility	-0.22^2	-0.21^d	0.28^c	0.26^c	0.16	0.10
Autonomic diarrhea	-0.12	-0.26^c	0.04	0.14	0.03	-0.13
Autonomic constipation	0.03	-0.05	0.04	0.01	0.15	0.01
Male sexual dysfunction	-0.13	-0.27^c	0.17	0.10	0.04	0.13
Erectile dysfunction	-0.16	-0.33^e	0.13	0.05	0.05	0.15
Ejaculatory failure	0.06	0.02	0.14	0.16	-0.05	-0.02
Urinary	-0.12	-0.31^c	0.12	0.11	0.03	0.05
Pupillomotor	-0.08	-0.18^b	0.15	0.23^d	0.06	-0.04
Sleep dysfunction	-0.23^d	-0.19^b	0.11	0.08	0.08	0.08
Reflex syncope	-0.04	0.06	0.06	0.08	0.06	0.09

[a] Partial Spearman rank order correlations are adjusted for age, sex, and race/ethnicity (black versus other).

[b] $p \leq 0.10$

[c] $p \leq 0.01$

[d] $p \leq 0.05$.

[e] $p \leq 0.005$.

Abbreviations: CASS, Composite Autonomic Severity Score; COMPASS, Composite Autonomic Symptom Scale; HRV, heart rate variability.

In contrast, amyotrophic lateral sclerosis (ALS) is an uncommon but serious age-related condition. ALS has been reported in several studies to have increased incidence in GWI (Tables 1.38 and 1.39). This condition has been conceptualized as resulting from "oxidative damage to mitochondrial DNA leading to the accumulation of mitochondrial DNA mutations"[714] in this case targeting the spinal cord compatible with the mechanism that is proposed for GWI more generally and other GWV-associated conditions. Extensive evidence links ALS to OS of the mitochondria OSMD.[715–719,723,724,728,772–774] Moreover, low concentrations and mutations of paraoxonase, central to organophosphate (AChEI) detoxification, have been linked to ALS[729,730,733,734] and GWI[671,674,735,775] (as well as to GWI-like multisymptom illness following organophosphate exposure outside the Gulf setting[736,737,741]), further propelling the case for OSMD in GWI. The mechanisms elucidated here (and previously elaborated in a different setting of exposure-induced ALS[745]), although spinal cord motor neurons are the primary condition defining target, MD in sporadic ALS should not be confined to spinal cord motor neurons but should (statistically) be evident in other tissues, particularly energetically demanding (and thus mitochondrially vulnerable) brain and muscle. Indeed, recent studies show that mitochondrial pathology in ALS extends to skeletal muscle[746–748,750–752] and symptoms extend to cognitive function in about half of cases.[753,754] Mounting evidence supports a connection of OSMD[612,614,615,754,755,776] to metabolic syndrome (each has been conceptualized as a unifying mechanism[755,776]), of which hypertension is one component. Consistent with this, studies have also reported increased incident weight gain in GWV versus controls.[607,663,671] Assessment for other elements of metabolic syndrome in GWV has not yet been undertaken, but increased metabolic syndrome represents a prediction of this model.

ANIMAL EXPERIMENTS

Experiments in animals have found that a combination of two or more substances used during the war far exceeds the danger of one individually. The results are the first to test the idea that a chemical synergy could be responsible for the GW syndrome, the unexplained mental and physical deterioration that many veterans have reported since returning home from the 1991 conflict.

They tested three chemicals used during the GW: pyridostigmine bromide, which was administered to protect against nerve gas exposure; DEET, an insect repellent; and permethrin, an insecticide. Chickens were used for the research because their bodies react to hazardous substances similarly to human bodies.

According to Abou-Donia et al.,[756] the key to the findings appears to be pyridostigmine bromide. The nerve gas pretreatment pill depletes about 85% of a liver enzyme that normally scavenges the body, deactivating particular toxins.[756]

After taking the drug, the individual has much more toxicity to DEET and permethrin.

The animals also suffered some of the same neurological problems seen in many of the veterans, including muscle weakness, diarrhea, and some tremors.

The chemicals had an additive effect: No hens died after being exposed to one substance, but groups exposed to two chemicals had a mortality of 20%–40%, and those exposed to three had 80% mortality.

SYMPTOMATOLOGY AMONG VETERANS: 10 YEARS AFTER DEPLOYMENT IN THE GULF WAR ILLNESS

Smith et al.[757] was to further elucidate the nature of illness in veterans of the 1990–1991 GW by examining the GWI definition advanced by the Centers for Disease Control and Prevention, which specified cases as having at least one symptom from two of the three factors: fatigue, mood–cognition, and musculoskeletal. Their methods involved a total of 311 male and female GW veterans drawn from across the nation, assessed in a survey-based study ~10 years after deployment. The results showed a total of 33.8% of the probability-weighted sample met GWI criteria. Multiple symptom profiles were found, with more than half of GWI cases endorsing a symptom on all the three factors and almost all cases endorsing at least one mood–cognition symptom. Their conclusion was that although the Centers for Disease Control and Prevention definition has some limitations that should be considered, it remains a useful tool for assessing the presence of illness in GW veterans.

Studies have examined symptoms in GW veterans in as few as 4 years[547,550] and as many as 8 years after deployment.[760] As reported in a study of GW veterans assessed 8 years after deployment,[636] veterans deployed to the GW theater report poorer general health than those deployed to Bosnia or those who served during the GW but were not deployed to the region of conflict. GW veterans also report higher rates of symptoms such as fatigue, mood disturbances, sleep problems, cognitive difficulties, and muscle pain than nondeployed peers.[777] Furthermore, there is some evidence for associations between self-reported exposures, such as use of pyridostigmine bromide, insect repellants and perceived threat regarding biological or chemical warfare, and reported illness symptomatology, as found in a study by Nisenbaum et al.,[778] which reported a rate of chronic multisymptom illness (CMI) of 46%. Continued research on the nature of GWI is needed to facilitate understanding of the prevalence of GW-associated health problems and to foster effective diagnoses and treatments for the population of veterans who served in the 1990–1991 GW.

The health of GW veterans, as measured by psychological distress, fatigue, and physical functioning, continues to be worse than that of nondeployed cohorts in general and non-GW deployed cohorts in particular.[672] A 10-year postdeployment follow-up of the National Health Survey of GW-era veterans and their families[779] examined the health of GW veterans in 2004 and 2005. Compared with their GW-era peers (who served in the military between September 1990 and May 1991 but did not serve in the Persian Gulf theater), GW veterans who were deployed to the Gulf region were more likely to have visited a clinic or hospital and fare worse on physical and mental health functioning.[780] This follow-up survey also examined the progression of unexplained multisymptom illness from 1995 to 2005, as defined by the presence of several different symptoms such as fatigue, muscle or joint pain, headaches, and memory problems, that persist for at least 6 months and are not adequately explained by a conventional medical diagnosis. In 2005, GW veterans reported a multisymptom illness rate of 36.5% compared with GW Era veterans' rate of 11.7%. Of those GW veterans with multisymptom illness, ~75% initially experienced symptoms between 1991 and 1995.

Notwithstanding the ambiguity surrounding the source and nature of GW veterans' health complaints,[781,782] researchers have explored the nature of GWI from a variety of perspectives and case definitions. For example, Lange et al.[783] focused on neuropsychological performance and determined that GW veterans with GWI, relative to GW veterans without health complaints, manifested cognitive deficits that could not be accounted for differences in psychiatric functioning. Several other studies have also examined neuropsychological symptoms in the context of GW deployment and GWI.[780,781] Others have targeted the possible role of toxin exposure,[782,784] the influence of conditioning,[785] and sex differences (or lack thereof) in health.[786] Additional examples include recent studies focused on a neurobiological basis for differences in semantic memory using functional magnetic resonance imaging,[787] and examinations of the psychophysiology of GWI in the context of immune networks.[788]

Although these and other investigations have shed light on the correlates of GWI, interpretation of these findings are complicated by the fact that studies have used different diagnostic criteria. For example, Lange et al.'s[779] case definition set forth two types of GWI: one characterized by chronic fatigue syndrome and other involving multiple-chemical sensitivity (MCS). Criteria for each type were taken from published case definitions. The chronic fatigue syndrome type required that a GW veteran report at least 6 months of extreme fatigue, accompanied by at least a 50% decrease in activity, and a minimum of seven (of 11) symptoms from a published case definition for chronic fatigue syndrome.[789] The MCS type, also based on a published case definition,[790] required sensitivity to at least five of eight specific chemicals or unusual sensitivity to daily chemicals, plus two (or more) lifestyle changes on account of the sensitivity. Haley et al.[547] derived their own subtypes of GWI by applying two series of factor analyses to generate six types of illness: impaired cognition, confusion-ataxia, arthomyoneuropathy, phobia-apraxia, fever-adenopathy, and weakness and incontinence. They defined a GWI case as meeting a high cutoff score based on a factor analysis-derived critical value for estimates of true factor scores on any of the six syndrome factors. Other researchers, however, have used still different diagnostic criteria. In the absence of a universal definition of GWI, these case definitions have varied considerably. Accordingly, GW veterans who meet criteria for one research team's definition of GWI may not be classified as cases under different criteria. For example, Haley et al.[547] pointed out that of the eight veterans in their sample who had received a physician's diagnosis of MCS and thus would likely correspond to Lange et al.'s[779] MCS subtype of GWI half of the group did not meet criteria for any of Haley et al.'s[547] six syndromes. Therefore, not only have studies examined varied potential exposures and perspectives, they have also applied varying case definitions to GWI. However, it is clear to us, who have been studying chemical sensitivity for 30 years, that all of these diagnosis variants are found in the chemically sensitive patient. The variability appears to be the route and dose of the toxics, the total body pollutant load, the biochemical individuality, and the genetic makeup of the individual. Thus, to the physicians and scientists at the EHC-Dallas, there is no mystery as to the varied symptoms and types of illness seen in the GW veterans.

Using the clinical approach, Fukuda and colleagues[550] reasoned that symptoms cardinal to GWI would meet the following three criteria: (1) they would be chronic, having lasted at least 6 months; (2) they would occur frequently in GW veterans, defined as endorsement by 25% or more of veterans in this sample; and (3) they would be more common in the sample's deployed veterans than in nondeployed veterans. Six symptoms met these criteria in the Air Force veteran sample and thus constituted the clinical case definition: fatigue, difficulty remembering or concentrating, moodiness, difficulty sleeping, joint pain, and joint stiffness.

To extend the number of clinically important symptoms, Fukuda et al.[550] next adopted a two-stage statistical approach. First, they split the sample in half randomly and performed an exploratory principal components analysis on all the 35 health symptoms in one subsample. Eight factors were retained for the subsequent confirmatory factor analysis (CFA) on the second subsample. This CFA revealed a two-factor solution: a factor labeled mood–cognition–fatigue (seven symptoms: depression, anxiety, moodiness, memory problems, fatigue, difficulty with words, and difficulty sleeping); and a factor labeled musculoskeletal (three symptoms: joint stiffness, joint pain, and muscle pain).

This study further examined the CDC case definition of GWI[550] by applying it to a national sample of veterans ~10 years after 1990–1991 GW deployment. Results after applying sampling weights were similar to rates reported in other large studies of GW veterans, and suggesting that more than a third of GW veterans meet criteria for GWI, with more than half of the cases endorsing a symptom on all the three factors. Furthermore, nearly all GWI cases endorsed at least one mood–cognition symptom.

Smith et al.[757] found that 55.9% of GWI cases in their study affirmed fatigue, at least one mood–cognition symptom and at least one musculoskeletal symptom, which was even higher than what was found in the study by Fukuda et al.[550] in which 41.8% reported at least one symptom from all the three clusters. The second most common symptom profile in both their study and the CDC study was fatigue and mood–cognition. The third most common pattern in both studies was musculoskeletal and mood cognition. Strikingly, 99.6% of GWI cases who endorsed fatigue and at least one musculoskeletal symptom also endorsed at least one mood–cognition symptom, meaning that less than 1% of our GWI cases did not endorse at least one mood–cognition symptom. Endorsing fatigue and at least one musculoskeletal symptom, but no mood–cognition symptoms, was also the least frequent RR symptom profile in Fukdua et al.'s[550] sample. In summary, although there were some differences with respect to the proportion of participants in each category, the relative ranking of the four symptom profiles was consistent across the studies.

Finally, Smith et al.[757] examined associations between the perception of having GWI and both GWI caseness and symptoms, as this information was not reported in the original Fukuda et al. article.[550] In a study by Chalder et al.,[644] which applied the CDC caseness criteria to a sample of British GWV, only 26.6% of veterans classified as cases under CDC criteria in fact believed they had GWI. In the present study, they found that 58.4% of veterans who were classified as cases believed they had GWI, and only 22.2% of veterans who did not meet the criteria believed that they had GWI. The overall pattern suggests that those who believed they had GWI were more likely to endorse symptoms and more likely to meet the caseness criteria for GWI than those who did not believe they were suffering from deployment-related illness.

MECHANISMS OF GWI

RNAS IN THE AREA OF PERSIAN GULF WAR VETERANS HAVE SEGMENTS HOMOLOGOUS TO CHROMOSOME 22q11.2

According to Urnovitz et al.,[791] reverse transcriptase PCR (RT-PCR) was used for polyribonucleotide assays with sera from deployed Persian GWV with the GW syndrome and a cohort of nonmilitary controls. Sera from veterans contained polyribonucleotides (amplicons) that were obtained by RT-PCR and that ranged in size from 200 to ca. 2000 bp. Sera from controls did not contain amplicons larger than 450 bp. DNA sequences were derived from two amplicons unique to veterans. These amplicons, which were 414 and 759 nucleotides, were unrelated to each other or to any sequence in gene bank database. The amplicons contained short segments that were homologous to regions of chromosome 22q11.2, an antigen-responsive hot spot for genetic rearrangements. Many of these short amplicon segments occurred near, between, or in chromosome 22q11.2 Alu sequences. These results suggest that genetic alterations in the 22q11.2 region, possibly induced by exposures led to pathogenesis of the GW syndrome. However, the data did not exclude the possibility that other chromosomes also may have been involved. Nonetheless, the detection of polyribonucleotides such as those reported here may have application to the laboratory diagnosis of chronic diseases that have a multifactorial etiology.

OXIDATIVE STRESS AND MITOCHONDRIAL DYSFUNCTION IN GWI AND OTHER CHEMICAL EXPOSURE

Excitotoxicity is another potential downstream mechanism. OS enhances excitotoxin effects, such as delayed calcium deregulation (DCD) which "precedes and predicts" cell death[791]; so does mitochondrial calcium accumulation.[791] Ca^{2+} combines with protein kinase A/C and when phosphorylated increases sensitivity up to 1000 times. Moreover, excitotoxins in turn cause OS and mitochondrial impairment, which is a major mediator of excitotoxin neurotoxicity.[792] The development of excitotoxic neurotoxicity leads to wide spread inability to tolerate normal environmental incitors such as food, mold, and other chemical toxicity and sensitivity preventing the patient from functioning well in society. This is because minute exposures, that is, perfumes, chemical cleaning agents, and various other odors of daily living will cause reactions. The resulting entity is chemical sensitivity.

Other sequelae of OS and MD further contribute to cell dysfunction, cell death, and symptoms but often show nonfunction with fatigue, weakness to ambient odors incapacitating others slowly.

Biochemical individuality in which some but not other exposed persons with apparently similar exposures have developed GWI (CMI)—emerges naturally from an OSMD conceptualization. Differences in genetic and nongenetic biological detoxification capability,[584,585,671,697,761,793–795] total OS load, and pro-oxidant/antioxidant balance,[585] prior inherited or acquired mitochondrial mutation load or heteroplasmy status,[796–799] heritable vulnerability to autoimmune disease, selective nutrient deficiency, and perhaps prior loss of cells in postmitotic organs provide individual differences in vulnerability to development of symptoms following Gulf (or civilian or other toxic)-associated OS exposures.

Routine laboratory tests are not classically abnormal in GWV (or CMI) or in OSMD patients. In each case, the objective finding has a demonstrated relation to OSMD (generally OS, which is more commonly tested). These include depressed paraoxonase (PON1),[671,674,775] increased gamma-glutamyl transferase (GGT),[669,670] reduced natural killer cell activity,[675,678] changes in HRV,[548,549] increased autoantibodies,[675,800] changes in blood complement levels, and increased coagulation activation.[685,689] Each has been reported in other CMI. Each is a documented consequence of OSMD. These findings are comparable to the findings of non-GW citizens and our other studies with chemical sensitivity. The EHC-Dallas has found most of these abnormalities in their chemically sensitive patients also including decrease in T-lymphocytes and often reduced gamma globulins and subsets.

In addition to symptoms, several conditions have been found to be elevated in GW veterans and others with toxic exposures. These include hearing loss, hypertension, and ALS. These conditions are also known to bear particularly strong relations to OSMD.

These findings are compatible with a common mechanism involving OSMD, targeting different tissues to varying degrees. Motor neurons are one possible (though relatively rare) target tissue, endgendering ALS when affected. However, other distributions of effect result in multisymptom conditions (GWI-CFS-spectrum conditions), metabolic syndrome features[801] hypersensitivity vasculitis, and a range of other conditions, which accompany one another at elevated rates.[705,802–804] Many chemically sensitive patients eventually develop cardiovascular and end-stage neurological entities such as cardiomyopathy, arteriosclerosis, PD, Alzheimer's disease, small vessel vasculitis, etc.

Patients with other CMI commonly have multiple "unexplained" symptoms spanning many domains. These conditions have substantial overlap with one another and with GWI[607,636,705,802–808] consistent with the hypothesis put forth here that common OSMD mechanisms target multiple domains, with factors like heteroplasmy (among others) producing differential vulnerability of potential target tissues.

According to Golumb[809] reported odds ratios for CFS range from ~4 to ~40 in GWV versus nondeployed controls, suggesting shared mechanisms at least for subsets of CFS. CFS patients show elevated OS,[682] an exaggerated prooxidant response to new OS[683] (which they propose may signify a preexisting adverse prooxidant: antioxidant balance), and activation of coagulation pathways.[670] Moreover, OS levels correlate with symptoms in chronic fatigue (CFS).[669] Evidence also favors a relation of CFS to MD: functional status in CFS correlates with carnitine levels[810,811]; and a subset of CFS cases show elevated lactate with exertion, and delayed ATP recovery after exercise, on magnetic resonance spectroscopy,[686] with OS believed to underlie the energetic effects.[579] Furthermore, an "ATP profile test" of mitochondrial function successfully (and completely) discriminated CFS cases, defined by the CDC criteria which require multisymptom illness (most similar to GWI).[618] Additionally, CFS patients have been reported to differ from controls in genetics related to mitochondrial function,[582] energetic,[582] and apoptosis.[812] Fibromyalgia and irritable bowel syndrome[607]—which are increased (~2–5-fold) in GWV—also bear evidence of a link to OSMD[691–694] (Tables 1.38 and 1.39). So does ASD.[576,585,794,813–815] Chemical sensitivity and electrical hypersensitivity have been linked to mutations in genes for glutathione-S-transferase (GST), which protects from OS by conjugating glutathione, detoxifying "a large range of compounds generated by reactive oxygen species induced damage to intracellular molecules."[584] It might be conjectured that apparent instances of exposure-triggered CS may entail exposure-triggered increased endogenous OS production (through mechanisms detailed above); and perhaps also exposure-triggered modifications in gene expression of key detoxifying enzymes.

CS sensitivity to chemicals—and also medication intolerance[816]—are significantly more common in GWV[607,618,636,663,705,805] and in overlap conditions.[802–804,817] Both chemical and drug adverse effects are commonly mediated through OSMD.[577,588–590] (CS like GWI and ASD cited elsewhere shows altered genetic profiles of PON.[671,738] This PON changes occur in chemically sensitive as shown in studies by Rea, Alter, and Organiziac. OSMD provides an account of why medication and vaccine adverse effects at the time of the Gulf War were associated with increased risk of developing GWI.[636,641,642,785] These adverse effects signal less favorable OSMD status at the time of exposure and/or greater OS stressor exposure, promoting OS dominance over antioxidant defenses, which may both predict and help mediate the development of multisymptom GWI in the setting of new OS exposure.

Other conditions have been linked to OSMD but have not (yet) been evaluated in GWI. An elevation in a number of these conditions in GWI represents a prediction of this theory. Some markers and objective conditions have been linked to GWI and OSMD, and at least one CMI, but have not been evaluated in other CMI. A prediction of this theory is that many, when examined in studies with sufficient power, will be seen in other CMI.

According to Golumb,[818] CMIs, including chronic fatigue syndrome, fibromyalgia, irritable bowel syndrome, chemical sensitivity, and the GWI, show strong overlap.[802–804,809] Autism spectrum disorder (ASD), despite little co-occurrence with GWI (due to military self-selection), encompasses multisymptom subsets bearing muscle, gastrointestinal, sleep, and other symptoms germane to

CMI. These are of OS and MD suggested to reflect a condition arising from similar mechanisms in a different developmental milieu. GWI entails a circumscribed set of experiences that may provide insights of relevance to these overlapping conditions.

According to Golomb,[818] GWI is compatible with a paradigm by which uncompensated exposure to oxidative/nitrative stressors accompanies and triggers MD, cell energy compromise, and multiple downstream effects such as vulnerability to autoantibodies. This promotes a profile of protean symptoms with variable latency emphasizing but not confined to energy-demanding postmitotic tissues, according with (and accounting for) known properties of multisystem overlap conditions. This advances understanding of GWI; health conditions attending GWI at elevated rates; and overlap conditions like chronic fatigue syndrome (CFS) and ASD, and chemical sensitivity providing prospects also linked to CMI.[572,573,819] Among the Gulf-era (August 1990–July 1991) non-Gulf deployed personnel, rates of "GWI" for those receiving military vaccines in that period OR 3.8 (95% CI 1.5–9.5) were intermediate between rates in nondeployed nonvaccinated (OR 1.0, the standard), and the Gulf deployed (OR 10.6%, 95% CI 4.9–23.1)[813] suggesting that vaccines bore a relation to illness irrespective of the Gulf setting.

Depleted uranium (bearing potential heavy metal and radioactive toxicity), paints, solvents, and fumes have also shown connections to illness in some epidemiological studies.[607,618,636,640,643] Additionally, pesticides exposures of non-AChEI classes also occurred.

Autoantibodies and colonization/infection with pathogens (below) and, as new OS exposures appear, to which existing OS and mitochondrial provide heightened vulnerability (due to adverse OS: antioxidant defense balance), OS may promote impaired gene expression related to detoxification, in part via alterations in DNA methylation. The subsequent total body pollutant loads will continue to hammer these deficient tendencies until they can trigger the symptoms and thus the illness just as any other chemical sensitivity individuals have.

Exposure Associations Causing Oxidative Stress Are Evident

According to Golomb,[544] a range of "unrelated" exposures are linked to GWI which can cause OS and MD. Acetylcholinesterase inhibitor (AChEI) exposures (organophosphates, as nerve agents, pesticides; and carbamates, as pesticides and pyridostigmine bromide nerve agent pretreatment pills), show especially strong and consistent links to health problems in GWV.[544] Moreover, AChEI shows a dose–response relationship to GWI (number of pyridostigmine bromide pills[544]; and proximity to the Khamisiyah munitions depot demolition (sarin nerve agent plume) is linked to the extent of brain atrophy and neuropsychological dysfunction in GWV.[820,821] Additional findings extend to genetic evidence such as peroxidase variants.[671] These support a causal association of AChEI to the GWI,[544] so mechanisms of toxicity by AChEI(s) are of special interest, (GWV/GWI(s) are also linked to reduced peroxidase activity levels[671,674]; however, low activity may be the effect and/or cause of paraoxonase[735,822] and other elements of organophosphate detoxification,[761] as well as low paraoxonase activity.[576] Our series of OS (i.e., nutrients and paraoxonase) has been quite impressive as shown by Alter and Organiziac. Peroxidase was definitely involved in some non-GW chemically sensitive patients who were exposed to natural gas, pesticides, formaldehyde, solvents, etc.

While AChEI show especially strong and consistent associations to GWI (and are also linked to other CMI), anthrax vaccine,[636,640,642,823] multiple vaccinations,[636,642–644,824] and adverse reactions to vaccinations[636,640,642] show generally consistent significant associations to GWI.

Chronic multisymptom illness has not traditionally been thought to include ASD, but multisymptoms cases of ASD may reflect manifestations of similar processes operating at a different developmental timepoint. ASD not uncommonly comprises multiple symptoms across a similar spectrum,[702,825–828] with purported links to similar exposure, and observed relations to OSMD.[586,697,699,783,794,829–835] (All ASD need not cohere with these principles.)

Accrued evidence now more vigorously supports a paradigm by which OS and MD conduce to one another, disposing to GWI or other CMI. These mechanisms may operate in some, many, or possibly most CMI. The GW setting has its distinctive constellation of OS exposures. However, the pathophysiological principle articulated, beyond their potential relevance to GWI, yield a new lens with which to review a range of important, interrelated health conditions (including but not confined to "overlap" CMI conditions often considered to be unexplained) and to understand their relationship to one another (in the military setting and outside of it).

MD (even persons with familial MD) may vary vastly in which symptoms are expressed—and in their timecourse of expression[667]—and an empiric feature of GWI and other CMI.[836] It is often presumed that symptoms, to relate to an exposure must arise during an exposure, and that the exposure must show acute toxicity. According to Golomb,[818] cancer and neurodegenerative disease, familiar disease conditions rather than symptoms, represent recognized exceptions.

GWI DOES NOT BEHAVE IN THIS FASHION

The GWI is characterized by variable latency to symptoms following Gulf exposures—with many new symptoms arising well after participation, and 40% of new symptoms reportedly arising more than a year after Gulf service.[668] Symptoms in MD are also characterized by variable latency to onset. MD produces (commonly) OS. OS triggers further mtDNA mutations and more MD. The severity of new mutations, and degree of heteroplasmy, determine the severity of OS production—and speed of progression. As mtDNA mutations and OS accrue, cells lose function or die, from energy depletion or OS-precipitated necrosis or apoptosis[837]—achieving phenotypic thresholds.[838,839] (See below for autoimmune predisposition.) Even in kindred with heritable mtDNA defects that involved neurological problems, "the age of onset of major neurological disturbance varied from 3 to 70 years."[667] The principles are similar whether initial mtDNA damage is heritable or acquired; however, acquired mtDNA mutations may be typified by multiple different mutations each in a low fraction,[798,840] which may particularly dispose to classical or "nonspecific" symptoms of MD, compatible with CMI. OS may predispose to autoantibodies and vulnerability to infection (below). Delayed symptoms may further arise from OS-promoted toxicity, which is underscored by findings that pretreatment (or immediate posttreatment) with antioxidants protects against AChEI-inducted lethality (and enhances recovery) in animals.[841–843] Anthrax vaccinations and multiple vaccinations are the next most strongly and consistently linked to GWI, in epidemiologic evidence.[844] These are tied, through aluminum-based adjuvants[652,653,656–658,660,843,845] and mercury (and other) preservatives,[659] to OS and MD—as well as inhibition of glutathione production, reducing antioxidant defense against other exposures.[656,659,846] Each additional exposure class presumptively inculpated in GWI is known to promote OS.[591,665,847–851]

GGT is an enzymatic antioxidant[852,853]: elevations serve as an early marker of OS[854] including AChEI exposure.[852,855] PON1 is an antioxidant enzyme (also specifically involved in organophosphate detoxification[856]) whose activity is depressed in settings of elevated OS.[857] OIB1 was depressed in GWV generally (relative to military controls)—and particularly so in those with GWI or more symptoms.[671,674,775] Natural killer activity is reduced with OS and increased with antioxidants.[846,858,859] Blunted HRV has been linked to OSMD.[581,860] Activation of the coagulation system relates to OS.[646,861–863] Both OS[690,864,865] and MD[866,867] each foster apoptosis which exposes phosphatidylserine at the cell surface, activating coagulation pathways.[868] Activation of the coagulation system has been repeatedly observed in the GWV.[685,689] OS also depresses vitamin D (vitD), vitD receptor expression, and mitochondrial vitD hydroxylase activities.[869,870] Low vitD and altered receptor function are linked to risk of autoimmune disease.[871–875]

According to Mostafalou[876] et al., on the other hand, ER stress and related pathways have been reported to be involved in cytotoxicity of some pesticides. Paraquat, a bipyridyl herbicide, which is suspected to increase the risk of PD following chronic exposures, has been reported to induce ER stress and trigger dopaminergic cell death by enhanced cleavage of a small ER cochaperone protein, p23, and inhibition of ERAD.[877] Elevated level of ER stress biomarkers like glucose-regulated protein 78 (GRP78), ER degradation-enhancing-α-mannosidase-like protein (EDEM), and C/EBP homologous protein (CHOP) has also been implicated in paraquat-induced toxicity in human neuroblastoma cells.

Further, paraquat-activated calpain and caspase 3 along with ER-induced cascade inositol-requiring protein 1 (IRE1)/apoptosis signal-regulating kinase 1 (ASK1)/c-Jun N-terminal kinase (JNK)[878] can be involved in GWI. In another study carried out on neuroblastoma cells rotenone-induced ER stress has become evident by increased phosphorylation of protein kinase RNA-like endoplasmic reticulum kinase (PERK), protein kinase RNA-activated (PKR), and eukaryotic initiation factor 2-α (eIF2α) as well as the expression of GRP78. Protein kinases A and C combined with Ca^{2+} and then phosphorylated can increase sensitivity up to 1000 times thus generating chemically sensitivity from these toxics. Moreover, rotenone activates glycogen synthase kinase 3β (GSK3β), and ER-related multifunctional serine/threonine kinase implicated in the pathogenesis of neurodegeneration.[879] Deltamethrin, a pyrethtoid pesticide, has been reported to induce apoptosis through ER stress pathway involving eIF2α calpain and caspase-12.[880] Induction of apoptosis by pyrrolidine dithiocarbamate (PDTC)/Cu complex, a widely used pesticide, has also been linked to the ER stress-associated signaling molecules, including GRP78, GRP94, caspase-12, activating transcription factor 4 (ATF4), and CHOP in lung epithelial cells.[881] Chloropicrin an aliphatic nitrate pesticide has been indicated to increase ER stress-related proteins, including GRP78, IRE1α, and CHOP/GADD 153 in human retinal pigment epithelial cells.[882] Some other pesticides belonging to the organochlorines (endosulfan), carbamates (formetanate, methomyl, pyrimicarb), and pyrethroids (bifenthrin) have been evaluated for their effects on stress proteins among which upregulation of the ER chaperone GRP78 and downregulation of the cytosolic chaperone HSP72/73 were significant. These effects can occur when ER is under stress and the UPR results in increased expression of ER chaperones and decreased protein synthesis in the cytosol.[883,884]

Protein Aggregation

Degradation according to Mostafalou et al.[876] of misfolded, damaged, or unneeded proteins is a fundamental biological process which has a crucial role in maintenance and regulation of cellular function. There are two major cellular mechanisms for protein degradation; ubiquitin-proteasome system (UPS) that mainly targets short-lived proteins by proteases, and autophagy that at most clears long-lived and poorly soluble proteins through the lysosomal machinery.[885] UPS is composed of ubiquitin for tagging and proteasomes for proteolysis of proteins, which are to be degraded. Deregulation of this system has been implicated in the pathogenesis of several chronic diseases, mostly neurodegeneration and cancers evidenced by decreased and increased proteasome activity, respectively.[886]

Environmental exposure to certain pesticides has been linked to proteasomal dysfunction in the development of neurogenerative diseases. The organochlorine pesticide dieldrin has been reported to decrease proteasome activity along with enhanced sensitivity to occurrence of apoptosis in dopaminergic neuronal cells.[887] Proteasome inhibition has also been shown in neuroblastoma cells exposed to rotenone, ziram, diethyldithiocarbamate, endosulfan, benomyl, and dieldrin.[888,889] Paraquat has also been noted to impair UPS given by decreased proteasome activity and increased ubiquitinated proteins in DJ-1-deficient mice and dopaminergic neurons.[890,891] Increased degradation of proteasome components has been presented as the mechanism of proteasome inhibition by rotenone and inducer of Parkinson.[892]

The lysosomal degradation pathway with autophagy is known as a self-digestion process by which cells not only get rid of misfolded proteins, damaged organelles, and infectious microorganisms but also provide nutrients during fasting. Defect of this process has found an emerging role in many human diseases such as cancer, neurodegeneration, diabetes, aging, and disorders of the liver, muscle, and heart.[893–895] There are a few reports on the involvement of defective autophagy in toxic effects of pesticides. Gonzalez-Polo[896] and colleagues showed a relationship between autophagy and paraquat-induced apoptosis in neuroblastoma cells in 2007.[896] This effect was confirmed in another study in which paraquat-induced autophagy was attributed to the occurrence of ER stress.[897] Lindane, a broad-spectrum organochlorine pesticide, has been reported to promote its toxicity through disruption of an autophagic process in primary rat hepatocytes[898] (Figure 1.3).

Taken together, chronic diseases discussed above are considered as the major disorders affecting public health in the twenty-first century. The relationship between these diseases and environmental exposures, particularly pesticides, increasingly continue to strengthen. Near to all studies carried out in the area of pesticides, and chronic diseases are categorized in the field of epidemiologic evidence or experimental investigation with mechanistic insight into the disease process. Some epidemiologic studies have been debated on their uncertainty in the elicitation of a definite conclusion because of some restrictions. However, existence of more than a few dozen reports on the association of one case like brain cancer with exposure to pesticide is enough to create concern even without finding a direct link. Abundance of evidence in this regard has promoted scientists to evaluate the mechanisms and other toxic chemicals by which pesticides develop chronic diseases. Although there remains a lot to do in this way, several mechanisms and pathways have been clarified for pesticide and other triggering agent-induced chronic diseases. It should not be forgotten that these mechanisms work alongside or sequentially rather than singly in most cases, or they even can potentiate effects in genetically susceptible individuals. However, the body of studies in this respect has become massive enough to consider pesticide exposure as a potential risk factor for developing chronic diseases. They are the number one triggers of chemical sensitivity along with a natural gas exposure. Considering chronic diseases as the most important global health problem, it is time to find a preventative approach in association with agrochemicals by logical reducing pesticide use or pesticide dependency and finding efficient alternatives for hazardous ones.

The exposures linked to GWI and other chemical sensitivities appear "unrelated" in chemical structure genetics and classical mechanism of action. However, they share common induction of toxicity via OSMD. Thus, AChEI toxicity and lethality are normally viewed in cholinergic terms. However, in fact they are mediated by OSMD (contributing to apoptosis)[638,639]: the salience of OSMD in their toxicity is underscored by the relation of their lethality to impaired glutathione mechanisms; and protection from OP lethality via preexposure or immediate postexposure to relevant antioxidants in experimental animal studies.[841–843] This favorable response is seen in the GW chemically sensitive patients who after exposure to toxics respond both orally and intravenously to oxidants like vitamin C, glutathione, multivitamins, and minerals.

High-dose nonindividualized vaccines, in contrast, are not known to inhibit AChE. However, these and other exposures linked to GWI, each exerts toxicity via OSMD. Further, the number of such exposures (crossing different classes) also predicted GWI[11]—and predicts greater OSMD.[847,848,899,900] These considerations begin to provide a framework, coupled with individual variabilities, for genesis of some cases of chemical sensitivity outside the GW setting. OS and MD clearly are part of the mechanisms that cause GWI.

According to Golomb,[901] one-fourth to one-third of U.S. and U.K. personnel deployed to the Persian Gulf in the 1990–1991 conflict exhibit GWI, established by excluding the fraction of nondeployed controls meeting the symptom portion of eligibility.[550,636,836,902,903] This is a staggering amount of injuries for the military. The foundation for GWI has been felt to elude physiological explanation[668,904] except for a few scientific clinicians working in the field of chemical sensitivity. GWI differs in exposure relations and symptom profiles from other postwar syndromes (e.g., posttraumatic stress disorder). This conflict had many exposures that were new (anthrax vaccine, depleted uranium, permethrin impregnated uniforms), unique, or comparatively unique (pyridostigmine bromide nerve agent pretreatment pills, oil fires, flea collar use by some, botulinum toxoid vaccine, nerve gas agent exposure resulting from ammunitions depot demolitions), and excessive (organophosphate and carbamate pesticide use). All of these toxics will increase the environmental total pollutant load and thus the total body pollutant loads. They are known to cause chemical sensitivity and surely accumulatively can cause an increase in total body pollutant load which will cause increase in hypersensitivity and thus an increase in chemical sensitivity.

OS and MD are closely intertwined, and each promotes the other. They evaluate characteristics of OSMD and GWI, to show that OSMD may underlie some, much, or most the excess of multisymptom illness (and neurodegenerative disease) reported in the GWV[618,636]—and civilians with CMI like chemical sensitivity.

About 26%–32% of GWV demonstrates chronic multisymptom health problems and thus has GWI apparently associated with participation[636,902] (i.e., the fraction bearing such problems, after subtracting what was "expected" based on nondeployed controls). The excess burden lies not in more persons with single or dual symptoms, or multiple mild symptoms, but in the added fraction bearing three or more symptoms of moderate or greater severity.[636] The 1990–1991 ground war lasted about 4 days; relatively few of the ~100,000 deployed U.S. veterans experienced combat or direct combat stressors. Though some effected veterans have brain dysfunction symptoms, most do not meet criteria for psychiatric illness, and stress-related exposures loose significance in multivariable models that adjust for chemical/environmental exposures (but not the converse).[836,903]

According to Golomb[901] and clinicians at the EHC-Dallas, GWI prominently features fatigue, muscle pain and weakness, and CNS symptoms (cognition, mood and personality change). The CDC case definition requires chronic symptoms in two of three domains of fatigue, cognitive–mood, and musculoskeletal.[902] Kansas criteria require symptoms in three of six domains—fatigue/sleep, pain (muscle-joint), cognitive–mood–neurological, gastrointestinal, respiratory, and skin[636]; these also must be multiple triggering agents.

An explanation focused on OS MD accounts for GWI, and other chronic multisymptom illness like chemical sensitivity. Put forth is a proposition by which exposures to oxidative stressors, in part via cumulative MD, in part via autoimmune effects in vulnerable individuals, in part via apoptosis/cell loss leading to coagulation activation and the spreading of chemical sensitivity, may increase the risk of a range of chronic health problems in GWV—including the multisymptom spectrum termed GWI—and other CMI especially chemical sensitivity. Such an account accords with known exposure relations of otherwise unlike character, explains symptoms with otherwise unexplained organ tropism, protean character, and variable timecourse to onset. It fits with the otherwise unexplained range of objective markers linked to these conditions that cross classical boundaries, resulting in chemical sensitivity. It explains observed associations to other health conditions of varying character and accounts for increases in multisymptom "overlap" conditions (and/or overlap of these syndromes with one another). A role for OSMD might be predicted on "first principles" (known pathophysiological effects of Gulf Exposures; and known clinical sequelae of these effects).[636] However, there is now direct evidence of a relation of OS and MD to each of the conditions to which GWI and chemical sensitivity relates, providing further triangulating support for a role for OS and MD extending to GWI and chemically sensitive.

OS also depresses vitamin D (vitD), vitD receptor expression, and mitochondrial vitD hydroxylase activities.[550,902] Lost vitD and altered receptor function are linked to risk of autoimmune disease[869–872,903] as well as other aspects of chemical sensitivity. Autoimmune markers are elevated in GWI,[873,874] as well as in other CMI. Vaccines have been linked to illness in GWV[550,642,675,821,875] and in some cases chronic fatigue. (They are also a politically and scientifically contentious proposed contributor to ASD). Reactogenic vaccines are a source of OS.[640] Additionally, vaccine adjuvants (based on aluminum—which is an oxidative stressor, as are components of vaccine preservatives and adjuvants) are expressly incorporated for the purpose of enhancing immune/antibody reactions—in principle to the intended administered antigen, but they may also adjuvant native protein and nonprotein substances. Adjuvant associated with vaccines remains resident in the body and may continue to exert adjuvant effects, promoting "autoimmune and/or other chemical sensitivity syndromes induced by adjuvants: "ASIA."[643,823,847,905,906] Low-dose preservative-free vaccine works so much better, having few complications. These have been given to over 230,000 chemically sensitive with little intolerances or complications. These have been given to over 20,000 chemically sensitive with few intolerances or complications. Low vitamin D activity (see above) is also linked to increased infection vulnerability.[907–911] These factors, coupled with EN deficits and OS-reduced NK activity,[873,912] may account for increased autoantibodies and evidence of a range of infectious agents (and antibodies to them), in GWI and associated exposures[873,913–916]—and other CMI[917–919] including ASD.[920–922] These contribute further to symptom heterogeneity and latency.

Excitotoxicity is another potential downstream mechanism. OS enhances excitotoxin effects, such as DCD which "precedes and predicts" cell death[791] so too does mitochondrial calcium accumulation.[791] Moreover, excitotoxins in turn cause OS and mitochondrial impairment, which is a major mediator of excitotoxin neurotoxicity.[792] The development of excitotoxic neurotoxicity leads to food, mold, and other chemical toxicity and sensitivity preventing the patient from functioning well in society because minute exposures, that is, perfumes, chemical cleaning agents, and various other odors of daily living will cause reactions that at times present the exposures.

REFERENCES

1. Pawankar, R., G. W. Canonica, S. T. Holgate, R. F. Lockey. WAO White Book on Allergy 2011–2012. Milwaukee, WI: World Allergy Organization; 2011. Accessed February 13, 2014. http://www.worldallergy.org/publications/wao_white_book.pdf

2. Ziska, L. et al. 2011. Recent warming by latitude associated with increased length of ragweed pollen season in central North America. *Proc. Natl. Acad. Sci. U.S.A.* 108:4248–4251.

3. Wolf, J., N. R. O'Neill, C. A. Rogers, M. L. Muilenberg, L. H. Ziska. 2010. Elevated atmospheric carbon dioxide concentrations amplify. *Alternaria alternata* sporulation and total antigen production. *Environ. Health Perspect.* 118:1223–1228.

4. Wayne, P., S. Foster, J. Connolly, F. Bazzaz, P. Epstein. 2002. Production of allergenic pollen by ragweed (*Ambrosia artemisiifolia* L.) is increased in CO_2-enriched atmospheres. *Ann. Allergy Asthma Immunol.* 88:279–282.

5. Arrhenius, S. 1896. On the influence of carbonic acid in the air upon the temperature of the ground. *Philos. Mag. J. Sci.* 41:237–276.

6. Wardman, A. E., D. Stefani, J. C. MacDonald. 2002. Thunderstorm-associated asthma or shortness of breath epidemic: A Canadian case report. *Can. Respir. J.* 9:267–270.

7. Packe, G. E., J. G. Ayres. 1985. Asthma outbreak during a thunderstorm. *Lancet* 2:199–204.

8. Porsbjerg, C., M. L. Linstow, S. C. Nepper-christensen, A. Rasmussen, J. Korsgaard, H. Nolte, V. Backer. 2002. Greenlandic population study group. Allergen sensitization and allergen exposure in Greenlander Inuit residing in Denmark and Greenland. *Respir. Med.* 96:736–744.

9. Sheffield, P. E., K. R. Weinberger, K. Ito, T. D. Matte, R. W. Mathes, G. S. Robinson, P. L. Kinney. 2011. The association of tree pollen concentration peaks and allergy medication sales in New York City: 2003–2008. *ISRN Allergy* 2011:537194.

10. Cakmak, S., R. E. Dales, R. T. Burnett, S. Judek, F. Coates, J. R. Brook. 2002. Effect of airborne allergens on emergency visits by children for conjunctivitis and rhinitis. *Lancet* 359:947–948.

11. Villeneuve, P. J., M. S. Doiron, D. Stieb, R. Dales, R. T. Burnett, R. Dugandzic. 2006. Is outdoor air pollution associated with physician visits for allergic rhinitis among the elderly in Toronto, Canada? *Allergy* 61:750–758.

12. Higgins, B. G., H. C. Francis, C. Yates, C. J. Warburton, A. M. Fletcher, C. A. Pickering, A. A. Woodcock. 2000. Environmental exposure to air pollution and allergens and peak flow changes. *Eur. Respir. J.* 16:61–66.

13. Boulet, L. P., H. Turcotte, M. Boutet, L. Montminy, M. Laviolette. 1993. Influence of natural antigenic exposure on expiratory flows, methacholine responsiveness, and airway inflammation in mild allergic asthma. *J. Allergy Clin. Immunol.* 91:883–893.

14. Darrow, L. A., J. Hess, C. A. Rogers, P. E. Tolbert, M. Klein, S. E. Sarnat. 2012. Ambient pollen concentrations and emergency department visits for asthma and wheeze. *J. Allergy Clin. Immunol.* 130:630–638.e4.

15. Héguy, L., M. Garneau, M. S. Goldberg, M. Raphoz, F. Guay, M. F. Valois. 2008. Associations between grass and weed pollen and emergency department visits for asthma among children in Montreal. *Environ. Res.* 106:203–211.

16. Zhong, W., L. Levin, T. Reponen, G. K. Hershey, A. Adhikari, R. Shukla, G. LeMasters. 2006. Analysis of short-term influences of ambient aeroallergens on pediatric asthma hospital visits. *Sci. Total Environ.* 370:330–336.

17. Erbas, B., M. Akram, S. C. Dharmage, R. Tham, M. Dennekamp, E. Newbigin, P. Taylor, M. L. K. Tang, M. J. Abramson. 2012. The role of seasonal grass pollen on childhood asthma emergency department presentations. *Clin. Exp. Allergy* 42:799–805.

18. Newson, R., D. Strachan, E. Archibald, J. Emberlin, P. Hardaker, C. Collier. 1997. Effect of thunderstorms and airborne grass pollen on the incidence of acute asthma in England, 1990–94. *Thorax* 52:680–685.

19. Alexis, N. E. et al. 2010. Low-level ozone exposure induces airways inflammation and modifies cell surface phenotypes in healthy humans. *Inhal. Toxicol.* 22:593–600.

20. Leikauf, G. D. 2002. Hazardous air pollutants and asthma. *Environ. Health Perspect.* 110:505–526.

21. Diaz-Sanchez, D., M. P. Garcia, M. Wang, M. Jyrala, A. Saxon. 1999. Nasal challenge with diesel exhaust particles can induce sensitization to a neoallergen in the human mucosa. *J. Allergy Clin. Immunol.* 104:1183–1188.

22. Jörres, R., D. Nowak, H. Magnussen. 1996. The effect of ozone exposure on allergen responsiveness in subjects with asthma or rhinitis. *Am. J. Respir. Crit. Care Med.* 153:56–64.

23. Brunekreef, B., G. Hoek, P. Fischer, F. T. Spieksma. 2000. Relation between airborne pollen concentrations and daily cardiovascular and respiratory-disease mortality. *Lancet* 355:1517–1518.

24. Rice, M. B., G. D. Thurston, J. R. Balmes, K. E. Pinkerton. 2014. Climate change. A global threat to cardiopulmonary health. *Am. J. Respir. Crit. Care Med.* 189 (5):512–519, Published online March 1, 2014. doi: 10.1164/rccm.201310-1924PP.

25. Duffy P. B., C. Tebaldi. 2012. Increasing prevalence of extreme summer temperatures in the U.S. *Clim. Change* 111:487–495.

26. Meehl G. A., C. Tebaldi. 2004. More intense, more frequent, and longer lasting heat waves in the 21st century. *Science* 305:994–997.

27. Fouillet, A., G. Rey, F. Laurent, G. Pavillon, S. Bellec, C. Guihenneuc-Jouyaux, J. Clavel, E. Jougla, D. Hémon. 2006. Excess mortality related to the August 2003 heat wave in France. *Int. Arch. Occup. Environ. Health* 80:16–24.

28. Stafoggia, M. et al. 2008. Factors affecting in-hospital heat-related mortality: A multi-city case-crossover analysis. *J. Epidemiol. Community Health* 62:209–215.

29. Medina-Ramón, M., A. Zanobetti, D. P. Cavanagh, J. Schwartz. 2006. Extreme temperatures and mortality: Assessing effect modification by personal characteristics and specific cause of death in a multi-city case-only analysis. *Environ. Health Perspect.* 114:1331–1336.

30. McMichael, A. J., R. E. Woodruff, S. Hales. 2006. Climate change and human health: Present and future risks. *Lancet* 367:859–869.

31. Curriero, F. C., K. S. Heiner, J. M. Samet, S. L. Zeger, L. Strug, J. A. Patz. 2002. Temperature and mortality in 11 cities of the eastern United States. *Am. J. Epidemiol.* 155:80–87.

32. Hayes, D. Jr., P. B. Collins, M. Khosravi, R. L. Lin, L. Y. Lee. 2012. Bronchoconstriction triggered by breathing hot humid air in patients with asthma: Role of cholinergic reflex. *Am. J. Respir. Crit. Care Med.* 185:1190–1196.

33. Aitken, M. L., J. J. Marini. 1985. Effect of heat delivery and extraction on airway conductance in normal and in asthmatic subjects. *Am. Rev. Respir. Dis.* 131:357–361.

34. Mireku, N., Y. Wang, J. Ager, R. C. Reddy, A. P. Baptist. 2009. Changes in weather and the effects on pediatric asthma exacerbations. *Ann. Allergy Asthma Immunol.* 103:220–224.

35. Lin, S., M. Luo, R. J. Walker, X. Liu, S. A. Hwang, R. Chinery. 2009. Extreme high temperatures and hospital admissions for respiratory and cardiovascular diseases. *Epidemiology* 20:738–746.

36. Bhaskaran, K., B. Armstrong, S. Hajat, A. Haines, P. Wilkinson, L. Smeeth. 2012. Heat and risk of myocardial infarction: Hourly level case-crossover analysis of MINAP database. *BMJ* 345:e8050.

37. Lim, Y. H., Y. C. Hong, H. Kim. 2012. Effects of diurnal temperature range on cardiovascular and respiratory hospital admissions in Korea. *Sci. Total Environ.* 417–418:55–60.

38. Shultz, J. M., J. Russell, Z. Espinel. 2005. Epidemiology of tropical cyclones: The dynamics of disaster, disease, and development. *Epidemiol. Rev.* 27:21–35.

39. National Oceanic and Atmospheric Administration (NOAA), National Climatic Data Center. 2011. Billion-dollar weather/climate disasters. Accessed February 13, 2014. http://www.ncdc.noaa.gov/billions/

40. Jenkins, J. L., M. McCarthy, G. Kelen, L. M. Sauer, T. Kirsch. 2009. Changes needed in the care for sheltered persons: A multistate analysis from Hurricane Katrina. *Am. J. Disaster Med.* 4:101–106.

41. IFRC (International Federation of Red Cross and Red Crescent Societies) World Disaster Report 2002. Geneva, Switzerland.

42. Parry, M. L., O. F. Canziani, J. P. Palutikof, P. J. van der Linden, C. E. Hanson. eds. 2007. *Contribution of Working Group II to the Fourth Assessment Report of the Intergovernmental Panel on Climate Change.* Cambridge, UK: Cambridge University Press.

43. Campbell-Lendrum, D. H., C. F. Corvalán, A. Prüss-Ustün. 2003. Climate change and human health — Risks and response. In *How Much Disease Could Climate Change Cause?* A. J. McMichael, D. H. Campbell-Lendrum, C. F. Corvalan, K. L. Ebi, A. K. Githeko, J. D. Scheraga, A. Woodward, eds., pp. 133–158. Geneva, Switzerland: World Health Organization.

44. Stanke, C., M. Kerac, C. Prudhomme, J. Medlock, V. Murray. 2013. Health effects of drought: A systematic review of the evidence. *PLoS Curr.* 5–5.

45. Cline, W. 2007. *Global Warming and Agriculture Impact Estimates by Country.* Washington, DC: Center for Global Development and Peterson Institute for International Economics.

46. Lozano, R. et al. 2012. Global and regional mortality from 235 causes of death for 20 age groups in 1990 and 2010: A systematic analysis for the Global Burden of Disease Study 2010. *Lancet* 380:2095–2128.

47. Stocker, T. F., D. Qin, G. K. Plattner, M. Tignor, S. K. Allen, J. Boschung, A. Nauels, Y. Xia, V. Bex, P. M. Midgley, eds., 2013. IPCC Working Group I. Summary for policymakers. In *Climate Change 2013: The Physical Science Basis. Contribution of Working Group I to the Fifth Assessment Report of the Intergovernmental Panel on Climate Change.* New York: Cambridge University Press.

48. Bond, T. C. et al. 2013. Bounding the role of black carbon in the climate system: A scientific assessment. *J. Geophys. Res. Atmos.* 118:5380–5552.

49. Nichols, J. L., E. O. Owens, S. J. Dutton, T. J. Luben. 2013. Systematic review of the effects of black carbon on cardiovascular disease among individuals with pre-existing disease. *Int. J. Public Health* 58:707–724.

50. Franco Suglia, S., A. Gryparis, J. Schwartz, R. J. Wright. 2008. Association between traffic-related black carbon exposure and lung function among urban women. *Environ. Health Perspect.* 116:1333–1337.

51. Gan, W. Q., J. M. FitzGerald, C. Carlsten, M. Sadatsafavi, M. Brauer. 2013. Associations of ambient air pollution with chronic obstructive pulmonary disease hospitalization and mortality. *Am. J. Respir. Crit. Care Med.* 187:721–727.

52. Smith, K. R. et al. 2009. Public health benefits of strategies to reduce greenhouse-gas emissions: Health implications of short-lived greenhouse pollutants. *Lancet* 374:2091–2103.

53. Lim, S. S. et al. 2012. A comparative risk assessment of burden of disease and injury attributable to 67 risk factors and risk factor clusters in 21 regions, 1990–2010: A systematic analysis for the Global Burden of Disease Study 2010. *Lancet* 380:2224–2260.

54. Marri, P. R., D. A. Stern, A. L. Wright, D. Billheimer, F. D. Martinez. 2013. Asthma-associated differences in microbial composition of induced sputum. *J. Allergy Clin. Immunol.* 131:346–352.e1–e3.

55. Cardenas, P. A., P. J. Cooper, M. J. Cox, M. Chico, C. Arias, M. F. Moffatt, W. O. Cookson. 2012. Upper airways microbiota in antibiotic-naïve wheezing and healthy infants from the tropics of rural Ecuador. *PLoS ONE* 7:e46803.

56. Hilty, M. et al. 2010. Disordered microbial communities in asthmatic airways. *PLoS ONE* 5:e8578.

57. Bisgaard, H. et al. 2007. Childhood asthma after bacterial colonization of the airway in neonates. *N. Engl. J. Med.* 357:1487–1495.

58. Vissing, N. H., B. L. K. Chawes, H. Bisgaard. 2013. Increased risk of pneumonia and bronchiolitis after bacterial colonization of the airways as neonates. *Am. J. Respir. Crit. Care Med.* 188:1246–1252.

59. Bisgaard, H., M. N. Hermansen, K. Bønnelykke, J. Stokholm, F. Baty, N. L. Skytt, J. Aniscenko, T. Kebadze, S. L. Johnston. 2010. Association of bacteria and viruses with wheezy episodes in young children: Prospective birth cohort study. *BMJ* 341:c4978.

60. Morris, A. et al. 2013. Lung HIV Microbiome Project. Comparison of the respiratory microbiome in healthy nonsmokers and smokers. *Am. J. Respir. Crit. Care Med.* 187:1067–1075.

61. Erb-Downward, J. R. et al. 2011. Analysis of the lung microbiome in the "healthy" smoker and in COPD. *PLoS ONE* 6:e16384.

62. Calışkan, M. et al. 2013. Rhinovirus wheezing illness and genetic risk of childhood-onset asthma. *N. Engl. J. Med.* 368:1398–1407.

63. Følsgaard, N. V., S. Schjørring, B. L. Chawes, M. A. Rasmussen, K. A. Krogfelt, S. Brix, H. Bisgaard. 2013. Pathogenic bacteria colonizing the airways in asymptomatic neonates stimulates topical inflammatory mediator release. *Am. J. Respir. Crit. Care Med.* 187:589–595.

64. Matsui, E. C., P. A. Eggleston, T. J. Buckley, J. A. Krishnan, P. N. Breysse, C. S. Rand, G. B. Diette. 2006. Household mouse allergen exposure and asthma morbidity in inner-city preschool children. *Ann. Allergy Asthma Immunol.* 97:514–520.

65. Dickey, J. H. 2011. Air pollution and primary care medicine. *Physicians for Social Responsibility.*

66. Chanlett, E. T. 1979. *Environmental Protection.* New York: McGraw Hill.

67. Schultz, E. S., O. Gruzieva, T. Bellander, M. Bottai, J. Hallberg, I. Kull, M. Svartengren, E. Melén, G. Pershagen. 2012. Traffic-related air pollution and lung function in children at 8 years of age: A birth cohort study. *Am. J. Respir. Crit. Care Med.* 186:1286–1291.

68. Noah, T. L., H. Zhou, H. Zhang, K. Horvath, C. Robinette, M. Kesic, M. Meyer, D. Diaz-Sanchez, I. Jaspers. 2012. Diesel exhaust exposure and nasal response to attenuated influenza in normal and allergic volunteers. *Am. J. Respir. Crit. Care Med.* 185:179–185.

69. Huang, W. et al. 2012. Inflammatory and oxidative stress responses of healthy young adults to changes in air quality during the Beijing Olympics. *Am. J. Respir. Crit. Care Med.* 186:1150–1159.

70. Rich, D. Q. et al. 2012. Association between changes in air pollution levels during the Beijing Olympics and biomarkers of inflammation and thrombosis in healthy young adults. *JAMA* 307:2068–2078.

71. Lin, W. et al. 2011. Acute respiratory inflammation in children and black carbon in ambient air before and during the 2008 Beijing Olympics. *Environ. Health Perspect.* 119:1507–1512.

72. Langrish, J. P. et al. 2012. Reducing personal exposure to particulate air pollution improves cardiovascular health in patients with coronary heart disease. *Environ. Health Perspect.* 120:367–372.

73. Søyseth, V., H. L. Johnsen, P. K. Henneberger, J. Kongerud. 2012. The incidence of work-related asthma-like symptoms and dust exposure in Norwegian smelters. *Am. J. Respir. Crit. Care Med.* 185:1280–1285.

74. Mehta, A. J. et al. 2012. SAPALDIA Team. Occupational exposure to dusts, gases, and fumes and incidence of chronic obstructive pulmonary disease in the Swiss Cohort Study on air pollution and lung and heart diseases in adults. *Am. J. Respir. Crit. Care Med* 185:1292–1300.

75. Dallas, M. L. et al. 2012. Carbon monoxide induces cardiac arrhythmia via induction of the late Na^+ current. *Am. J. Respir. Crit. Care Med.* 186:648–656.

76. Naveed, B. et al. 2012. Metabolic syndrome biomarkers predict lung function impairment: A nested case-control study. *Am. J. Respir. Crit. Care Med.* 185:392–399.

77. Van Hee, V. C., C. A. Pope 3rd. 2012. From Olympians to mere mortals: The indiscriminate, global challenges of air pollution. *Am. J. Respir. Crit. Care. Med.* 186:1076–1077.

78. Godish, T. 2003. *Air Quality.* 4th ed., Boca Raton, Florida: Lewis Books.

79. Brook, R. D. et al. 2004. Air pollution and cardiovascular disease: A statement for healthcare professionals from the expert panel on population and prevention science of the American Heart Association. *Circulation* 109:2655–2671.

80. Bloomer, B. J., J. W. Stehr, C. A. Piety, R. J. Salawitch, R. R. Dickerson. 2009. Observed relationships of ozone air pollution with temperature and emissions. *Geophys. Res. Lett.* 36:L09803.

81. Knowlton, K., J. E. Rosenthal, C. Hogrefe, B. Lynn, S. Gaffin, R. Goldberg, C. Rosenzweig, K. Civerolo, J. Y. Ku, P. L. Kinney. 2004. Assessing ozone-related health impacts under a changing climate. *Environ. Health Perspect.* 112:1557–1563.

82. Murazaki, K., P. Hess. 2006. How does climate change contribute to surface ozone change over the United States? *J. Geophys. Res.* 111:D05301.

83. Doherty, R. M. et al. 2009. Current and future climate- and air pollution-mediated impacts on human health. *Environ. Health* 8:S8.

84. Romieu, I. et al. 2012. Multicity study of air pollution and mortality in Latin America (the ESCALA study). *Res. Rep. Health Eff. Inst.* 171:5–86.

85. Peng, R. D. et al. 2013. Acute effects of ambient ozone on mortality in Europe and North America: Results from the APHENA study. *Air Qual. Atmos. Health* 6:445–453.

86. Song, H., W. Tan, X. Zhang. 2011. Ozone induces inflammation in bronchial epithelial cells. *J. Asthma.* 48:79–83.

87. Moore, K., R. Neugebauer, F. Lurmann, J. Hall, V. Brajer, S. Alcorn, I. Tager. 2008. Ambient ozone concentrations cause increased hospitalizations for asthma in children: An 18-year study in Southern California. *Environ. Health Perspect.* 116:1063–1070.

88. Glad, J. A., L. L. Brink, E. O. Talbott, P. C. Lee, X. Xu, M. Saul, J. Rager. 2012. The relationship of ambient ozone and PM(2.5) levels and asthma emergency department visits: Possible influence of gender and ethnicity. *Arch. Environ. Occup. Health* 67:103–108.

89. Babin. S., H. Burkom, R. Holtry, N. Tabernero, J. Davies-Cole, L. Stokes, K. Dehaan, D. Lee. 2008. Medicaid patient asthma-related acute care visits and their associations with ozone and particulates in Washington, DC, from 1994–2005. *Int. J. Environ. Health Res.* 18:209–221.

90. Babin, S. M., H. S. Burkom, R. S. Holtry, N. R. Tabernero, L. D. Stokes, J. O. Davies-Cole, K. DeHaan, D. H. Lee. 2007. Pediatric patient asthma-related emergency department visits and admissions in Washington, DC, from 2001–2004, and associations with air quality, socio-economic status and age group. *Environ. Health* 6:9.

91. Ko, F. W. S., W. Tam, T. W. Wong, D. P. S. Chan, A. H. Tung, C. K. W. Lai, D. S. C. Hui. 2007. Temporal relationship between air pollutants and hospital admissions for chronic obstructive pulmonary disease in Hong Kong. *Thorax* 62:780–785.

92. Brunekreef, B., S. T. Holgate. 2002. Air pollution and health. *Lancet* 360:1233–1242.

93. Jacquemin, B. et al. 2012. Epidemiological study on the Genetics and Environment of Asthma (EGEA). Air pollution and asthma control in the Epidemiological study on the genetics and environment of asthma. *J. Epidemiol. Community Health* 66:796–802.

94. Meng, Y. Y., M. Wilhelm, R. P. Rull, P. English, B. Ritz. 2007. Traffic and outdoor air pollution levels near residences and poorly controlled asthma in adults. *Ann. Allergy Asthma Immunol.* 98:455–463.

95. Thurston, G. D., M. Lippmann, M. B. Scott, J. M. Fine. 1997. Summertime haze air pollution and children with asthma. *Am. J. Respir. Crit. Care Med.* 155:654–660.

96. Alexeeff, S. E., A. A. Litonjua, H. Suh, D. Sparrow, P. S. Vokonas, J. Schwartz. 2007. Ozone exposure and lung function: Effect modified by obesity and airways hyperresponsiveness in the VA normative aging study. *Chest* 132:1890–1897.

97. Shore, S. A., Y. M. Rivera-Sanchez, I. N. Schwartzman, R. A. Johnston. 2003. Responses to ozone are increased in obese mice. *J. Appl. Physiol.* 95:938–945.

98. Akimoto, H. 2003. Global air quality and pollution. *Science* 302(5651):1716–1719.

99. Pryor, W. A., C. L. Squadrito, M. Friedman. 1995. A new mechanism for the toxicity of ozone. *Toxicol. Lett.* 82–83:287–293.

100. Pryor, W. A. 1994. Mechanisms of radical formation from reactions of ozone with target molecules in the lung. *Free Radic. Biol. Med.* 17:451–465.

101. Hollingsworth, J. W., S. R. Kleeberger, W. M. Foster. 2007. Ozone and pulmonary innate immunity. *Proc. Am. Thorac. Soc.* 4:240–246.

102. Guevara-Guzman, R., V. Arriaga, K. M. Kendrick, C. Bernal, X. Vega, O. F. Mercado-Gómez, S. Rivas-Arancibia. 2009. Estradiol prevents ozone-induced increases in brain lipid peroxidation and impaired social recognition memory in female rats. *Neuroscience* 159:940–950.

103. Pereyra-Munoz, N., C. Rugerio-Vargas, M. Angoa-Perez, G. Borgonio-Perez, D. Rivas-Arancibia. 2006. Oxidative damage in substantia nigra and striatum of rats chronically exposed to ozone. *J. Chem. Neuroanat.* 31:114–123.

104. Angoa-Perez, M., H. Jiang, A. Rodríguez, C. Lemin, R. A. Levine, S. Rivas-Arancibia. 2006. Estrogen counteracts ozone-induced oxidative stress and nigral neuronal death. *Neuroreport* 17:629–633.

105. Rivas-Arancibia, S., C. Dorado-Martínez, L. Colin-Barenque, K. M. Kendrick, C. de la Riva, R. Guevara-Guzmán. 2003. Effect of acute ozone exposure on locomotor behavior and striatal function. *Pharmacol. Biochem. Behav.* 74:891–900.

106. Avila-Costa, M. R., L. Coln-Barenque, T. I. Fortoul, J. P. Machado-Salas, J. Espinosa-Villanueva, C. Rugerio-Vargas, S. Rivas-Arancibia. 1999. Memory deterioration in an oxidative stress model and its correlation with cytological changes on rat hippocampus CA1. *Neurosci. Lett.* 270:107–109.

107. Gonzalez-Pina, R., C. Escalante-Membrillo, A. Alfaro-Rodriguez, A. Gonzalez-Maciel. 2008. Prenatal exposure to ozone disrupts cerebellar monoamine contents in newborn rats. *Neurochem. Res.* 33:912–918.

108. Araneda, S., L. Commin, M. Atlagich, K. Kitahama, V. H. Parraguez, J. M. Pequignot, Y. Dalmaz. 2008. VEGF overexpression in the astroglial cells of rat brainstem following ozone exposure. *Neurotoxicology* 29:920–927.

109. Finkelstein, M., M. Jerrett. 2007. A study of the relationships between Parkinson's disease and markers of traffic-derived environmental manganese air pollution in two Canadian cities. *Environ. Res.* 104(3):420–432.

110. Veronesi, B., G. Wei, J. Q. Zeng, M. Oortgiesen. 2003. Electrostatic charge activates inflammatory vanilloid (VR1) receptors. *Neurotoxicology* 24(3):463–473.

111. Gutner, U. A., L. B. Dundik, V. G. Korobko, Alice, V. Alessenko. 2005. The influence of tumor necrosis factor alpha on the processes of sphingomyelin cycle and lipid peroxidation in brain. *Zh Nevrol Psikhiatr Im S S Korsakova* 105:48–54.

112. Hermans, C., V. Deneys, E. Bergamaschi, A. Bernard. 2005. Effects of ambient ozone on the procoagulant status and systemic inflammatory response. *J. Thromb. Haemost.* 3:2102–2103.

113. Staal, J. B., R. A. de Bie, H. C. de Vet, J. Hildebrandt, P. Nelemans. 2009. Injection therapy for subacute and chronic low back pain: An updated Cochrane review. *Spine (Phila Pa 1976)* 34:49–59.

114. Fuccio, C., C. Luongo, P. Capodanno, C. Giordano, M. A. Scafuro, D. Siniscalco, B. Lettieri, F. Rossi, S. Maione, L. Berrino. 2009. A single subcutaneous injection of ozone prevents allodynia and decreases the over-expression of pro-inflammatory caspases in the orbito-frontal cortex of neuropathic mice. *Eur. J. Pharmacol.* 603:42–49.

115. Omaye, S. T. 2002. Metabolic modulation of carbon monoxide toxicity. *Toxicology* 180(2):139–150. doi: 10.1016/S0300-483X(02)00387-6. PMID 12324190.

116. Ryter, S. W., J. Alam, A. M. Choi. 2006. Heme oxygenase-1/carbon monoxide: From basic science to therapeutic applications. *Physiol. Rev.* 86:583–650.

117. Ryter, S. W., A. M. Choi. 2010. Heme oxygenase-1/carbon monoxide: Novel therapeutic strategies in critical care medicine. *Curr. Drug Targets* 11:1485–1494.

118. Motterlini, R., L. E. Otterbein. 2010. The therapeutic potential of carbon monoxide. *Nat. Rev. Drug discov.* 9:728–743.

119. USEPA. 2009. Integrated Science Assessment for Carbon Monoxide—Second External Review Draft.

120. Reboul, C., J. Thireau, G. Meyer, L. Andre, P. Obert, O. Cazorla, S. Richard. 2012. Carbon monoxide exposure in the urban environment: An insidious foe for the heart? *Respir. Physiol. Neurobiol.* 184:204–212.

121. ATSDR. 2012. Toxicological Profile for Carbon Monoxide. U.S. Dept. of Health and Human Services.

122. Samoli, E. et al. 2007. Short-term effects of carbon monoxide on mortality: An analysis within the APHEA project. *Environ. Health Perspect.* 115:1578–1583.

123. Tao, Y., L. Zhong, X. Huang, S. E. Lu, Y. Li, L. Dai, Y. Zhang, T. Zhu, W. Huang. 2011. Acute mortality effects of carbon monoxide in the Pearl River Delta of China. *Sci. Total Environ.* 410–411:34–40.

124. Schwartz, J., B. Coull. 2003. Control for confounding in the presence of measurement error in hierarchical models. *Biostatistics* 4:539–553.

125. HKEPD. 2012. Hong Kong Emission Inventory Report (EPD/TR 1/12).

126. Luo, Z., Y. Li, W. W. Nazaroff. 2010. Intake fraction of nonreactive motor vehicle exhaust in Hong Kong. *Atmos. Environ.* 44:1913–1918.

127. Hong Kong Census and Statistics Department. Hong Kong Demographic Census. 2008; Page 10 of 20 AJRCCM Articles in Press. Published on August 14, 2013 as 10.1164/rccm.201304-06760C.

128. The World Bank. 2012. Vehicles (per km of road). http://data.worldbank.org/indicator/IS.VEH.ROAD.K1

129. Nobre, L. S., J. D. Seixas, C. C. Romao, L. M. Saraiva. 2007. Antimicrobial action of carbon monoxide-releasing compounds. *Antimicrob. Agents Chemother.* 51:4303–4307.

130. Davidge, K. S., R. Motterlini, B. E. Mann, J. L. Wilson, R. K. Poole. 2009. Carbon monoxide in biology and microbiology: Surprising roles for the "Detroit perfume". *Adv. Microb. Physiol.* 56:85–167.

131. Chin, B. Y., L. E. Otterbein. 2009. Carbon monoxide is a poison… to microbes! CO as a bactericidal molecule. *Curr. Opin. Pharmacol.* 9:490–500.

132. Chung, S. W., S. R. Hall, M. A. Perrella. 2009. Role of haem oxygenase-1 in microbial host defense. *Cell Microbiol.* 11:199–207.

133. Wilson, J. L., H. E. Jesse, R. K. Poole, K. S. Davidge. 2012. Antibacterial effects of carbon monoxide. *Curr. Pharm. Biotechnol.* 13:760–768.

134. Ito, K., G. D. Thurston, R. A. Silverman. 2007. Characterization of PM2.5, gaseous pollutants, and meteorological interactions in the context of time-series health effects models. *J. Expo. Sci. Environ. Epidemiol.* 17:S45–S60.

135. Peel, J. L., P. E. Tolbert, M. Klein, K. B. Metzger, W. D. Flanders, K. Todd, J. A. Mulholland, P. B. Ryan, H. Frumkin. 2005. Ambient air pollution and respiratory emergency department visits. *Epidemiology* 16:164–174.

136. Tolbert, P. E., M. Klein, J. L. Peel, S. E. Sarnat, J. Sarnat. 2007. Multipollutant modeling issues in a study of ambient air quality and emergency department visits in Atlanta. *J. Expo. Sci. Environ. Epidemiol.* 17:S29–S35.

137. Bell, M. L., R. D. Peng, F. Dominici, J. M. Samet. 2009. Emergency hospital admissions for cardiovascular diseases and ambient levels of carbon monoxide: Results for 126 United States urban counties, 1999–2005. *Circulation* 120:949–955.

138. Otterbein, L. E., F. H. Bach, J. Alam, M. Soares, L. H. Tao, R. J. Davis, R. A. Flavell, A. M. Choi. 2000. Carbon monoxide has anti-inflammatory effects involving the mitogen-activated protein kinase pathway. *Nat. Med.* 6:422–428.

139. Otterbein, L. E., A. May, B. Y. Chin. 2005. Carbon monoxide increases macrophage bacterial clearance through Toll-like receptor (TLR)4 expression. *Cell. Mol. Biol.* 51:433–440.

140. Chung, S. W., X. Liu, A. A. Macias, R. M. Baron, M. A. Perrella. 2008. Heme oxygenase-1-derived carbon monoxide enhances the host defense response to microbial sepsis in mice. *J. Clin. Invest.* 118:239–247.

141. Desmard, M. et al. 2009. A carbon monoxide-releasing molecule (CORM-3) exerts bactericidal activity against pseudomonas aeruginosa and improves survival in an animal model of bacteraemia. *FASEB J.* 23:1023–1031.

142. Brouard, S., L. E. Otterbein, J. Anrather, E. Tobiasch, F. H. Bach, A. M. Choi, M. P. Soares. 2000. Carbon monoxide generated by heme oxygenase 1 suppresses endothelial cell apoptosis. *J. Exp. Med.* 192:1015–1026.

143. Zhang, X., P. Shan, J. Alam, R. J. Davis, R. A. Flavell, P. J. Lee. 2003. Carbon monoxide modulates Fas/Fas ligand, caspases, and Bcl-2 family proteins via the p38alpha mitogen-activated protein kinase pathway during ischemia-reperfusion lung injury. *J. Biol. Chem.* 278:22061–22070.

144. Dolinay, T., M. Szilasi, M. Liu, A. M. Choi. 2004. Inhaled carbon monoxide confers antiinflammatory effects against ventilator-induced lung injury. *Am. J. Respir. Crit. Care Med.* 170:613–620.

145. Bathoorn, E., D. J. Slebos, D. S. Postma, G. H. Koeter, A. J. van Oosterhout, M. van der Toorn, H. M. Boezen, H. A. Kerstjens. 2007. Anti-inflammatory effects of inhaled carbon monoxide in patients with COPD: A pilot study. *Eur. Respir. J.* 30:1131–1137.

146. Mitchell, L. A., M. M. Channell, C. M. Royer, S. W. Ryter, A. M. Choi, J. D. McDonald. 2010. Evaluation of inhaled carbon monoxide as an anti-inflammatory therapy in a nonhuman primate model of lung inflammation. *Am. J. Physiol. Lung Cell. Mol. Physiol.* 299:L891–L897.

147. Nemzek, J. A., C. Fry, O. Abatan. 2008. Low-dose carbon monoxide treatment attenuates early pulmonary neutrophil recruitment after acid aspiration. *Am. J. Physiol. Lung Cell Mol. Physiol.* 294:L644–L653.

148. Kim, D., A. Sass-Kortsak, J. T. Purdham, R. E. Dales, J. R. Brook. 2006. Associations between personal exposures and fixed-site ambient measurements of fine particulate matter, nitrogen dioxide, and carbon monoxide in Toronto, Canada. *J. Expo. Sci. Environ. Epidemiol.* 16:172–183.

149. Harrison, R. M., C. A. Thornton, R. G. Lawrence, D. Mark, R. P. Kinnersley, J. G. Ayres. 2002. Personal exposure monitoring of particulate matter, nitrogen dioxide, and carbon monoxide, including susceptible groups. *Occup. Environ. Med.* 59:671–679.

150. Godish, T. 1985. *Air Quality.* p. 29. Chelsea, MI: Lewis Publishers.

151. Langrish, J. P. et al. 2009. Beneficial cardiovascular effects of reducing exposure to particulate air pollution with a simple facemask. *Part. Fibre Toxicol.* 6:8. doi: [Online 13 March 2009]10.1186/1743-8977-6-8.

152. Grigg, J. 2012. Traffic-derived air pollution and lung function growth. *Am. J. Respir. Crit. Care Med.* 186:1208–1209.

153. Noah, T. L., H. Zhou, J. Monaco, K. Horvath, M. Herbst, I. Jaspers. 2012. *Am. J. Respir. Crit. Care Med.* 185(2):179–185. Published online January 15, 2012. doi: 10.1164/rccm.201103-0465OC.

154. Mena, M. A., F. Woll, J. Cok, J. C. Ferrufino, R. A. Accinelli. 2012. Histopathological lung changes in children due to biomass fuel. *Am. J. Respir. Crit. Care Med.* 185:687–688.

155. Calderón-Garcidueñas, L. et al. 2008. Air pollution, cognitive deficits and brain abnormalities: A pilot study with children and dogs. *Brain and Cognition* 68(2008):117–127. Journal Homepage: www.elsevier.com/locate/b&c.

156. Calderon-Garciduenas, L. et al. 2010. Urban air pollution: Influences on olfactory function and pathology in exposed children and young adults. *Exp. Toxicol. Pathol.* 62(1):91–102.

157. Calderón-Garcidueñas, L., G. Valencia-Salazar, A. Rodríguez-Alcaraz, T. M. Osnaya N. Gambling, A. Villarreal-Calderón, R. B. Devlin, J. L. Carson. 2001. Ultrastructural nasal pathology in children chronically and sequentially exposed to air pollutants. *Am. Respir. Crit. Care Med.* 24:132–138.

158. Calderón-Garcidueñas, L. et al. 2003. Respiratory damage in children exposed to urban pollution. *Pediatr. Pulmonol.* 36:148–161.

159. Calderón-Garcidueñas, L., M. Franco-Lira, R. Torres-Jardón, C. Henriquez-Roldán, G. Barragán-Mejía, G. Valencia-Salazar, A. González-Maciel, R. Reynoso-Robles, R. Villarreal-Calderón, W. Reed. 2007. Pediatric respiratory and systemic effects of chronic air pollution exposure: Nose, lung, heart, and brain pathology. *Toxicol. Pathol.* 35(1):154–162.

160. Calderón-Garcidueñas, L. et al. 2007. Elevated plasma endothelin-1 and pulmonary arterial pressure in children exposed to air pollution. *Environ. Health Perspect.* 115:1248–1253.

161. Calderón-Garcidueñas, L. et al. 2008. Systemic inflammation, endothelial dysfunction, and activation in clinically healthy children exposed to air pollutants. *Inhal. Toxicol.* 20:499–506.

162. Calderón-Garcidueñas, L. et al. 2008. Long-term air pollution exposure is associated with neuroinflammation, an altered innate immune response, disruption of the blood-brain-barrier, ultrafine particle deposition, and accumulation of amyloid beta 42 and alpha synuclein in children and young adults. *Toxicol. Pathol.* 36:289–310.

163. Calderón-Garcidueñas, L. et al. 2001. Canines as sentinel species for assessing chronic exposures to air pollutants: Part 1. Respiratory pathology. *Toxicol. Sci.* 61(2):342–355.

164. Calderón-Garcidueñas, L. et al. 2003. DNA damage in nasal and brain tissues of canines exposed to air pollutants is associated with evidence of chronic brain inflammation and neurodegeneration. *Toxicol. Pathol.* 31:524–538.

165. Jung, T., N. Bader, T. Grune. 2007. Lipofuscin: Formation, distribution, and metabolic consequences. *Ann. N. Y. Acad. Sci.* 1119:97–111.

166. Keller, J. N. 2006. Age-related neuropathology, cognitive decline, and Alzheimer's disease. *Ageing Res. Rev.* 5(1):1–13.

167. Corder, E. H., A. M. Saunders, W. J. Strittmatter, D. E. Schmechel, P. C. Gaskell, G. W. Small, A. D. Roses, J. L. Haines, M. A. Pericak-Vance. 1993. Gene dose of apolipoprotein E type 4 allele and the risk of Alzheimer's disease in late onset families. *Science* 261(5123):921–923.

168. Graves, A. B., J. D. Bowen, L. Rajaram, W. C. McCormick, S. M. McCurry, G. D. Schellenberg, E. B. Larson. 1999. Impaired olfaction as a marker for cognitive decline: Interaction with apolipoprotein E epsilon4 status. *Neurology* 53(7):1480–1487.

169. Kovács, T. 2004. Mechanisms of olfactory dysfunction in aging and neurodegenerative disorders. *Ageing Res. Rev.* 3:215–232.

170. Calhoun-Haney, R., C. Murphy. 2005. Apolipoprotein ε 4 is associated with more rapid decline in odor identification than in odor threshold or dementia rating scale scores. *Brain Cogn.* 58:178–182.

171. Handley, O. J., C. M. Morrison, C. Miles, A. J. Bayer. 2006. ApoE gene and familial risk of Alzheimer's disease as predictors of odour identification in older adults. *Neurobiol. Aging* 27:1425–1430.

172. Olofsson, J. K., S. Nordin, S. Wiens, M. Hedner, L. G. Nilsson, M. Larson. 2008. Odor identification impairment in carriers of ApoE-ε4 is independent of clinical dementia. *Neurobiol. Aging* 31(4):567–577.

173. Kozauer, A. N., M. M. Mielke, G. K. Chan, G. W. Rebock, C. G. Lyketsos. 2008. Apolipoprotein E genotype and lifetime cognitive decline. *Int. Psychogeriatr.* 20:109–123.

174. Secretaría del Medio Ambiente del Gobierno del Distrito Federal. Dirección General de Gestión Ambiental del Aire, Sistema de Monitoreo Atmosférico. Ciudad de México: 2006. La Calidad del Aire en la Zona Metropolitana del Valle de México, 1986–2005.

175. Secretaría del Medio Ambiente del Gobierno del Distrito Federal. SIMAT—Sistema de Monitoreo Atmosférico de la Ciudad de México. November, 2008. Available online at: http://www.sma.df.gob.mx/simat/

176. Vega, E., E. Reyes, H. Ruiz, J. García, G. Sánchez, G. Martínez-Villa, U. González, J. C. Chow, J. G. Watson. 2002. Analysis of $PM_{2.5}$ and PM_{10} in the atmosphere of Mexico City during 2000–2002. *J. Air Waste Manag. Assoc.* 54:786–798.

177. Doty, R. L., D. P. Perl, J. C. Steele, K. M. Chen, J. D. Pierce, P. Reyes, L. T. Kurland. 1991. Olfactory dysfunction in three neurodegenerative diseases. *Geriatrics* 46(Suppl 1):47–51.

178. Doty, R. L. 2003. Odor perception in neurodegenerative diseases and schizophrenia. In: *Handbook of Olfaction and Gustation*, R. L. Doty, ed., 2nd Edition, pp. 479–502. New York: Marcel Dekker.

179. Doty, R. L. 2008. The olfactory vector hypothesis of neurodegenerative disease: Is it viable? *Ann. Neurol.* 63:7–15.

180. Hawkes, C. 2003. Olfaction in neurodegenerative disorders. *Mov. Disord.* 18:364–372.

181. Strous, R. D., Y. Shoenfeld. 2006. To smell the immune system: Olfaction, autoimmunity and brain involvement. *Autoimmun. Rev.* 6:54–60.

182. Berendse, H. W., M. M. Ponsen. 2006. Detection of preclinical Parkinson's disease along the olfactory tract. *J. Neural. Transm. Suppl.* 70:321–325.

183. Tjalve, H., J. Henriksson. 1999. Uptake of metals in the brain via olfactory pathways. *Neurotoxicol.* 20:181–195.

184. Antunes, M., R. M. Bowler, R. L. Doty. 2007. San Francisco/Oakland Bay Bridge Welder Study: Olfactory function. *Neurol.* 69:1278–1284.

185. Pober, J. S., W. Min, J. R. Bradley. 2008. Mechanisms of endothelial dysfunction, injury, and death. *Ann. Rev. Pathol.* 4:71–95.

186. Mascagni, P., D. Consonni, G. Bregante, G. Chiappino, F. Toffoletto. 2003. Olfactory function in workers exposed to moderate airborne cadmium levels. *Neurotoxicology* 24:717–724.

187. Chen, L., R. A. Yokel, B. Henning, M. Toborek. 2008. Manufactured aluminum oxide nanoparticles decrease expression of tight junction proteins in brain vasculature. *J. Neuroimmune Pharmacol.* 3:286–295.

188. Linse, S., C. Cabaleiro-Lago, I. Lynch, S. Lindman, E. Thulin, S. E. Radford, K. A. Dawson. 2007. Nucleation of protein fibrillation by nanoparticles. *Proc. Natl. Acad. Sci. USA* 104:8691–8696.

189. Colvin, V. L., K. M. Kulinowski. 2007. Nanoparticles as catalysts for protein fibrillation. *Proc. Natl. Acad. Sci. USA* 104:8679–8680.

190. Cedervall, T., I. Lynch, M. Foy, T. Berggård, S. C. Donnelly, G. Cagney, S. Linse, K. A. Dawson. 2007. Detailed identification of plasma proteins adsorbed on copolymer nanoparticles. *Angew Chem. Int. Ed.* 46:5754–5756.

191. Cedervall, T., I. Lynch, S. Lindman, T. Berggård, E. Thulin, H. Nilsson, K. A. Dawson, S. Linse. 2007. Understanding the nanoparticle-protein corona using methods to quantify exchange rates and affinities of proteins for nanoparticles. *Proc. Natl. Acad. Sci. USA* 104:2050–2055.

192. Lynch, I., T. Cedervall, M. Lundqvist, C. Cabaleiro-Lago, S. Linse, K. A. Dawson. 2007. The nanoparticle-protein complex as a biological entity: A complex fluids and surface science challenge for the 21st century. *Adv. Colloid Interface Sci.* 134–135:167–174.

193. Selkoe D. J. 2002. Alzheimer's disease is a synaptic failure. *Science* 298:789–791.

194. Jellinger, K. A. 2003. Neuropathological spectrum of synucleopathies. *Movement Disorders* 8:S2–S12.
195. Calderón-Garcidueñas, L. et al. 2004. Brain inflammation and Alzheimer's-like pathology in individuals exposed to severe air pollution. *Toxicol. Pathol.* 32:650–658.
196. Doetsch, F., I. Caillé, D. A. Lim, J. M. García-Verdugo, A. Alvarez-Buylla. 1999. Subventricular zone astrocytes are neural ítem cells in the adult mammalian brain. *Cell* 97:703–716.
197. Bédard, A., A. Parent. 2004. Evidence of newly generated neurons in the human olfactory bulb. *Brain Res. Dev. Brain Res.* 151:159–168.
198. Alvarez-Buylla, A., D. A. Lim. 2004. For the long run: Maintaining germinal niches in the adult brain. *Neuron* 41:683–686.
199. Lledo, P. M., F. T. Merkle, A. Alvarez-Buylla. 2008. Origen and function of olfactory bulb interneuron diversity. *Cell* 31:392–400.
200. Petzold, G. C., D. F. Albeanu, T. F. Sato, V. N. Murthy. 2008. Coupling of neural activity to blood flow in olfactory glomeruli is mediated by astrocytic pathways. *Neuron* 58:897–910.
201. Elder, A. et al. 2006. Translocation of inhaled ultrafine manganese oxide particles to the central nervous system. *Environ. Health Perspect.* 114:1172–1178.
202. Donaldson, K. 2003. The biological effects of coarse and fine particulate matter. *Occup. Environ. Med.* 60:313–314.
203. Fang, G. C., Y. S. Wu, C. C. Wen, C. K. Lin, S. H. Huang, J. Y. Rau, C. P. Lin. 2005. Concentrations of nano and related ambient air pollutants at the traffic sampling site. *Toxicol. Ind. Health* 21:259–271.
204. Peters, A., B. Veronesi, L. Calderón-Garcidueñas, P. Gehr, L. C. Chen, M. Geiser, W. Reed, B. Rothen-Rutishauser, S. Schürch, H. Schulz. 2006. Translocation and potential neurological effects of fine and ultrafine particles: A critical update. *Part. Fiber Tox.* 3:1–13.
205. Geiser, M., B. Rothen-Rutishauser, N. Kapp, S. Schürch, W. Kreyling, H. Schulz, M. Semmler, V. Im Hof, J. Heyder, P. Gehr. 2005. Ultrafine particles cross cellular membranes by nonphagocytic mechanisms in lungs and in cultured cells. *Environ. Health Perspect.* 113(11):1555–1560.
206. Klein, J. 2007. Probing the interactions of proteins and nanoparticles. *Proc. Natl. Acad. Sci. U.S.A.* 104:2029–2030.
207. Hagens, W. I., A. G. Oomen, W. H. de Jong, F. R. Cassee. 2007. Sips AJAM. What do we (need to) know about the kinetic properties of nanoparticles in the body? *Reg. Toxicol. Pharmacol.* 49:217–229.
208. Des Rieux, A. E., G. E. Ragnarsson, E. Gullberg, V. Préat, Y. J. Schneider, P. Artursson. 2005. Transport of nanoparticles across an *in vitro* model of the human intestinal follicle associated epithelium. *Eur. J. Pharmacol. Sci.* 25:455–465.
209. Bennett, W. D., K. L. Zeman. 2005. Effect of race on fine particle deposition for oral and nasal breathing. *Inhal. Toxicol.* 17:641–648.
210. Hahn, I., P. W. Scherer, M. M. Mozell. 1993. Velocity profiles measured for airflow through a large-scale model of the human nasal cavity. *J. Appl. Physiol.* 75:2273–2287.
211. Schroeter, J. D., J. S. Kimbell, B. Asgharian. 2006. Analysis of particle deposition in the turbinate and olfactory regions using a human nasal computational fluid dynamics model. *J. Aerosol. Med.* 19:301–313.
212. Heegaard, P. M. H., U. Boas, D. E. Otzen. 2007. Dendrimer effects on peptide and protein fibrillation. *Macromol. Biosci.* 7:1047–1059.
213. Altman, J. 1969. Autoradiographic and histological studies of postnatal neurogenesis. IV. Cell proliferation and migration in the anterior forebrain, with special reference to persisting neurogenesis in the olfactory bulb. *J. Comp. Neurol.* 137:433–457.
214. Kaplan, M. S., J. W. Hinds. 1997. Neurogenesis in the adult rat: Electron microscopic analysis of light radioautographs. *Science* 197:1092–1094.
215. Shepherd, G. M., S. Charpak. 2008. The olfactory glomerulus: A model for neuro-glio-vascular biology. *Neuron* 58:827–829.
216. Mombaerts, P., F. Wang, C. Dulac, S. K. Chao, A. Nemes, M. Mendelsohn, J. Edmondson, R. Axel. 1996. Visualizing an olfactory sensory map. *Cell* 87:675–686.
217. Dickey, J. H. 2000. Part VII. Air pollution: Overview of sources and health effects. *Dis. Mon.* 46:566–589.
218. Wilkening, K. E., L. A. Barrie, M. Engle. 2000. Trans-Pacific air pollution. *Science* 290(5489):65–67.
219. Gyan, K., W. Henry, S. Lucille, A. Laloo, C. Lamsee-Ebanke, S. McKay, R. M. Antoine, M. A. Monteil. 2005. African dust clouds are associated with increased pediatric asthma accident and emergency admission on the Caribbean island of Trinidad. *Int. J. Biometeorol.* 49:371–376.
220. Rozenberg, M. 2003. Summary of PM2.5 produced by wintertime wood burning in 15 US cities. Available at http://burningissues.org

221. Awang, M. B., A. F. Rahman, W. Z. Adullah, R. Lazer, M. T. Majid. 2000. Air quality in Malaysia: Impacts, management issues and future challenges. *Respirology* 5:183–196.
222. Sapkota, A. J., M. Symons, J. Kleissl, L. Wang, M. B. Parlange, J. Ondov, P. N. Breysse, G. B. Diette, P. A. Eggleston, T. J. Buckley. 2005 Impact of the 2002 Canadian forest fires on particulate air pollution in Baltimore City. *Environ. Sci. Technol.* 39:24–32.
223. Solomon S., D. S. Battisti, S. C. Doney, K. Hayhoe, I. Held. 2011. *Climate Stabilization Targets: Emissions, Concentrations, and Impacts over Decades to Millennia.* Washington, D.C.: National Academy Press.
224. NASA. Fires and smoke in Russia. Earth Observatory 2010.
225. Henderson, S. B., F. H. Johnston. 2012. Measures of forest fire smoke exposure and their associations with respiratory health outcomes. *Curr. Opin. Allergy. Clin. Immunol.* 12:221–227.
226. Rappold, A. G. et al. 2011. Peat bog wildfire smoke exposure in rural North Carolina is associated with cardiopulmonary emergency department visits assessed through syndromic surveillance. *Environ. Health Perspect.* 119:1415–1420, http://dx.doi.org/10.1289/ehp.1003206 [online 27 Jun 2011].
227. Rappold, A. G., W. E. Cascio, V. J. Kilaru, S. L. Stone, L. M. Neas, R. B. Devlin, D. Diaz-Sanchez. 2012. Cardio-respiratory outcomes associated with exposure to wildfire smoke are modified by measures of community health. *Environ. Health* 11:71.
228. UNESCO World Water Development Report, 4th Edition, World Water Assessment Programme. 2012. Available from: http://www.unesco.org/new/en/natural-sciences/environment/water/wwap/wwdr/wwdr4-2012/
229. Goudie, A. S., N. J. Middleton. 1992. The changing frequency of dust storms through time. *Clim. Change* 20:197–225.
230. Ichinose, T. et al. 2008. Effects of Asian sand dust, Arizona sand dust, amorphous silica and aluminum oxide on allergic inflammation in the murine lung. *Inhal. Toxicol.* 20:685–694.
231. Murphy, S. A., K. A. BéruBé, F. D. Pooley, R. J. Richards. 1998. The response of lung epithelium to well characterised fine particles. *Life Sci.* 62:1789–1799.
232. Perez, L., A. Tobías, X. Querol, J. Pey, A. Alastuey, J. Díaz, J. Sunyer. 2012. Saharan dust, particulate matter and cause-specific mortality: A case-crossover study in Barcelona (Spain). *Environ. Int.* 48:150–155.
233. Chan, C. C., K. J. Chuang, W. J. Chen, W. T. Chang, C. T. Lee, C. M. Peng. 2008. Increasing cardiopulmonary emergency visits by long-range transported Asian dust storms in Taiwan. *Environ. Res.* 106:393–400.
234. Yang, C. Y., Y. S. Chen, H. F. Chiu, W. B. Goggins. 2005. Effects of Asian dust storm events on daily stroke admissions in Taipei, Taiwan. *Environ. Res.* 99:79–84.
235. Kanatani, K. T., I. Ito, W. K. Al-Delaimy, Y. Adachi, W. C. Mathews, J. W. Ramsdell. 2010. Toyama Asian Desert Dust and Asthma Study Team. Desert dust exposure is associated with increased risk of asthma hospitalization in children. *Am. J. Respir. Crit. Care Med.* 182:1475–1481.
236. Cheng, M. F., S. C. Ho, H. F. Chiu, T. N. Wu, P. S. Chen, C. Y. Yang. 2008. Consequences of exposure to Asian dust storm events on daily pneumonia hospital admissions in Taipei, Taiwan. *J. Toxicol. Environ. Health A.* 71:1295–1299.
237. Qian, Z., Q. He, H. M. Lin, L. Kong, C. M. Bentley, W. Liu, D. Zhou. 2008. High temperatures enhanced acute mortality effects of ambient particle pollution in the "oven" city of Wuhan, China. *Environ. Health Perspect.* 116:1172–1178.
238. Ren, C., G. M. Williams, S. Tong. 2006. Does particulate matter modify the association between temperature and cardio respiratory diseases? *Environ. Health Perspect.* 114:1690–1696.
239. Katsouyanni, K., A. Pantazopoulou, G. Touloumi, I. Tselepidaki, K. Moustris, D. Asimakopoulos, G. Poulopoulou, D. Trichopoulos. 1993. Evidence for interaction between air pollution and high temperature in the causation of excess mortality. *Arch. Environ. Health* 48:235–242.
240. Block, M., L. Calderon-Garciduenas. 2009. Air pollution: Mechanisms of neuroinflammation and CNS disease. *Trends Neurosci.* 32(9):506–516. doi: 10.1016/j.tins.2009.05.009.
241. Valavanidis, A., K. Fiotakis, T. Vlachogianni. 2008. Airborne particulate matter and human health: Toxicological assessment and importance of size and composition of particles for oxidative damage and carcinogenic mechanisms. *J. Environ. Sci. Health C. Environ. Carcinog. Ecotoxicol. Rev.* 26(4):339–362.
242. Nemmar, A., I. M. Inuwa. 2008. Diesel exhaust particles in blood trigger systemic and pulmonary morphological alterations. *Toxicol. Lett.* 176:20–30.
243. Oberdörster, G., Z. Sharp, V. Atudorei, A. Elder, R. Gelein, W. Kreyling, C. Cox. 2004. Translocation of inhaled ultrafine particles to the brain. *Inhal. Toxicol.* 16(6–7):437–445.

244. Wang, J. et al. 2008. Time-dependent translocation and potential impairment on central nervous system by intranasally instilled TiO(2) nanoparticles. *Toxicology* 254(1–2):82–90.

245. Wang, B. et al. 2007. Transport of intranasally instilled fine Fe$_2$O$_3$ particles into the brain: Microdistribution, chemical states, and histopathological observation. *Biol. Trace Elem. Res.* 118(3):233–243.

246. Calderón-Garcidueñas, L. et al. 2008. Long-term air pollution exposure is associated with neuroinflammation, an altered innate immune response, disruption of the blood-brain barrier, ultrafine particulate deposition, and accumulation of amyloid beta-42 and alpha-synuclein in children and young adults. *Toxicol. Pathol.* 36(2):289–310.

247. Rothen-Rutishauser, B., L. Mueller, F. Blank, C. Brandenberger, C. Muehlfeld, P. Gehr. 2008. A newly developed in vitro model of the human epithelial airway barrier to study the toxic potential of nanoparticles. *ALTEX* 25(3):191–196.

248. Block, M. L., L. Zecca, J. S. Hong. 2007. Review microglia-mediated neurotoxicity: uncovering the molecular mechanisms. *Nat. Rev. Neurosci.* 8(1):57–69.

249. Niwa, Y., Y. Hiura, H. Sawamura, N. Iwai. 2008. Inhalation exposure to carbon black induces inflammatory response in rats. *Circ. J.* 72(1):144–149.

250. Veronesi, B., C. de Haar, L. Lee, M. Oortgiesen. 2002. The surface charge of visible particulate matter predicts biological activation in human bronchial epithelial cells. *Toxicol. Appl. Pharmacol.* 178(3):144–154.

251. Long, T. C., J. Tajuba, P. Sama, N. Saleh, C. Swartz, J. Parker, S. Hester, G. V. Lowry, B. Veronesi. 2007. Nanosize titanium dioxide stimulates reactive oxygen species in brain microglia and damages neurons in vitro. *Environ. Health Perspect.* 115(11):1631–1637.

252. Silva, G. A. 2006. Neuroscience nanotechnology: Progress, opportunities and challenges. *Nat. Rev. Neurosci.* 7:65–74.

253. Mühlfeld, C., B. Rothen-Rutishauser, F. Blank, D. Vanhecke, M. Ochs, P. Gehr. 2008. Review Interactions of nanoparticles with pulmonary structures and cellular responses. *Am. J. Physiol. Lung. Cell Mol. Physiol.* 294(5):L817–L829.

254. Simkhovich, B. Z., M. T. Kleinman, R. A. Kloner. 2008. Review Air pollution and cardiovascular injury epidemiology, toxicology, and mechanisms. *J. Am. Coll. Cardiol.* 52(9):719–726.

255. Ma, J. Y., J. K. Ma. 2002. Review the dual effect of the particulate and organic components of diesel exhaust particles on the alteration of pulmonary immune/inflammatory responses and metabolic enzymes. *J. Environ. Sci. Health Environ. Carcinog. Ecotoxicol. Rev.* 20(2):117–147.

256. Burton, N. C., T. R. Guilarte. 2009. Review. Manganese neurotoxicity: Lessons learned from longitudinal studies in nonhuman primates. *Environ. Health Perspect.* 117(3):325–332.

257. Chen, H. et al. 2012. Abstract 9454: Risk of incident hypertension in relation to long-term exposure to ambient air pollution in Ontario, Canada. *Circulation* 126: A9454.

258. Brunekreef, B., B. Forsberg. 2005. Epidemiological evidence of effects of coarse airburne particles on health. *Eur. Respir. J.* 26: 309–318.

259. Jaward, F. M., S. N. Meijer, E. Steinnes, G. O. Thomas, K. C. Jones. 2004. Further studies on the latitudinal and temporal trends of persistent organic pollutants in Norwegian and UK background air. *Environ. Sci. Technol.* 38:2523–2530.

260. Naumova, Y. Y. et al. 2002. Polycyclic aromatic hydrocarbons in the indoor and outdoor air of 3 cities in US. *Environ Sci. Technol.* 36:2552–2559.

261. Oberdörster, G., Z. Sharp, V. Atudorei, A. C. P. Elder, R. Gelein, A. Lunts, W. Kreyling, C. Cox. 2002. Extrapulmonary translocation of ultrafine carbon particles following whole-body inhalation exposure of rats. *J. Toxicol. Environ. Health* 65(20):1531–1543.

262. MacNee, W., X. Y. Li, P. Gilmour, K. Donaldson. 2000. Systemic effect of particulate air pollution. *Inhal. Toxicol.* 12(Suppl 3):233–244.

263. Kreyling, W. G., M. Semmler, F. Erbe, P. Mayer, S. Takenaka, H. Schulz, G. Oberdörster, A. Ziesenis. 2002. Translocation of ultrafine insoluble iridium particles from lung epithelium to extrapulmonary organs is size dependent but very low. *J. Toxicol. Environ. Health. A.* 65(20):1513–1530.

264. Cassee, F. R., H. Muijser, E. Duistermaat, J. J. Freijer, K. B. Geerse, J. C. Marijnissen, J. H. Arts. 2002. Particle size-dependent total mass deposition in lung determines inhalation toxicity of cadmium chloride aerosols in rats. Application of a multiple path dosimetry model. *Arch. Toxicol.* 76:277–286.

265. Xia, T., P. Korge, J. N. Weiss, N. Li, M. I. Venkatesen, C. Sioutas, A. Nel. 2004. Quinones and aromatic chemical compounds in particulate matter induce mitochondrial dysfunction: Implications for ultrafine particle toxicity. *Environ. Health Perspect.* 112:1347–1358.

266. Wilson, M. R., J. H. Lightbody, K. Donaldson, J. Sales, V. Stone. 2002. Interactions between ultrafine particles and transition metals in vivo and in vitro. *Toxicol. Appl. Pharmacol.* 184:172–179.

267. Carty, C. L., U. Gehring, J. Cyrys, W. Bischof, J. Heinrich. 2003. Seasonal variability of endotoxin in ambient fine particulate matter. *J. Environ. Monit.* 5(6):953–958.

268. Kreyling, W. G., M. Semmler, W. Möller. 2004. Review. Dosimetry and toxicology of ultrafine particles. *J. Aerosol. Med.* 17(2):140–52.

269. Schins, R. P., J. H. Lightbody, P. J. Borm, T. Shi, K. Donaldson, V. Stone. 2004. Inflammatory effects of coarse and fine particulate matter in relation to chemical and biological constituents. *Toxicol. Appl. Pharmacol.* 195(1):1–11.

270. White, N., J. teWaterNaude, A. van der Walt, G. Ravenscroft, W. Roberts, R. Ehrlich. 2009. Meteorologically estimated exposure but not distance predicts asthma symptoms in schoolchildren in the environs of a petrochemical refinery: A cross-sectional study. *Environ. Health* 8:45. doi: 10.1186/1476-069X-8-45.

271. Rusconi, F. et al. 2011. Asthma symptoms, lung function, and markers of oxidative stress and inflammation in children exposed to oil refinery pollution. *2011 J. Asthma* 48(1):84–90. doi: 10.3109/02770903.2010.538106.

272. Berman, D. 2007. Pollen monitoring in South Africa. *Curr. Allergy Clin. Immunol.* 20:184–187.

273. City of Cape Town. 2002. *Northern Communities Air Monitoring Task Group (NCamtg).* Monthly Reports.

274. City of Cape Town. Air Quality Monitoring Network. Guidelines. http://web1.capetown.gov.za/web1/NewCityAirpol/Links/cmc_guidelines.asp

275. Smargiassi, A., T. Kosatsky, J. Hicks, C. Plante, B. Armstrong, P. J. Villeneuve, S. Goudreau. 2009. Risk of asthmatic episodes in children exposed to sulphur dioxide stack emissions from a refinery point source in Montreal, Canada. *Environ. Health Perspect.* 117:653–659.

276. Brunekreef, B., D. W. Dockery, M. Krzyzanowski. 1995. Epidemiologic studies on short-term effects of low levels of major ambient air pollution components. *Environ. Health Perspect.* 103(Suppl 2):3–13.

277. Sunyer, J. et al. 2003. Respiratory effects of sulphur dioxide: A hierarchical multicity analysis in the APHEA 2 study. *Occup. Environ. Med.* 60:e2.

278. City of Cape Town. 2003. Air Quality Monitoring Section, Scientific Services. Milnerton Air Quality Project. http://web1.capetown.gov.za/web1/NewCityAirpol/Reports/ncamtg/ncamtg.200301.pdf

279. Wicking-Baird, M. C., M. G. De Villiers, R. K. Dutkiewicz. *1997. Cape Town Brown Haze study.* In Report No. Gen 182. Cape Town: Energy Research Institute, University of Cape Town: 1–79.

280. Loyo-Berrios, N. I., R. Irizarry, J. G. Hennessey, X. G. Tao, G. Matanoski. 2007. Air pollution sources and childhood asthma attacks in Catano, Puerto Rico. *Am. J. Epidemiol.* 165:927–935.

281. Yang, C. Y., J. D. Wang, C. C. Chan, J. S. Hwang, P. C. Chen. 1998. Respiratory symptoms of primary school children living in a petrochemical polluted area in Taiwan. *Pediatr. Pulmonol.* 25:299–303.

282. Aekplakorn, W., D. Loomis, N. Vichit-Vadakan, C. Shy, S. Wongtim, P. Vitayonan. 2003. Acute effect of sulphur dioxide from a power plant on pulmonary function of children, Thailand. *Int. J. Epidemiol.* 32:854–861.

283. Wichmann, F. A., A. Muller, L. E. Busi, N. Cianni, L. Massolo, U. Schlink, A. Porta, P. D. Sly. 2009. Increased asthma and respiratory symptoms in children exposed to petrochemical pollution. *J. Allergy Clin. Immunol.* 123:632–638.

284. Eder, W., M. J. Ege, E. von Mutius. 2006. The asthma epidemic. *N. Engl. J. Med.* 355:2226–2235.

285. Morgenstern, V. et al. GINI Study Group, LISA Study Group. 2008. Atopic diseases, allergic sensitization, and exposure to traffic-related air pollution in children. *Am. J. Respir. Crit. Care Med.* 177:1331–1337.

286. D'Amato, G., G. Liccardi, M. D'Amato, S. Holgate. 2005. Environmental risk factors and allergic bronchial asthma. *Clin. Exp. Allergy* 35:1113–1124.

287. Deger, L., C. Plante, L. Jacques, S. Goudreau, S. Perron, J. Hicks, T. Kosatsky, A. Smargiassi. 2012. *Can. Respir. J.* 19(2); PMC3373279.

288. Charpin, D., J. P. Kleisbauer, J. Fondarai, B. Graland, A. Viala, F. Gouezo. 1988. Respiratory symptoms and air pollution changes in children: The Gardanne Coal-Basin Study. *Arch. Environ. Health* 43(1):22–27.

289. Dales, R. E., W. O. Spitzer, S. Suissa, M. T. Schechter, P. Tousignant, N. Steinmetz. 1989. Respiratory health of a population living downwind from natural gas refineries. *Am. Rev. Respir. Dis.* 139:595–600.

290. Forastiere, F., G. M. Corbo, P. Pistelli, P. Michelozzi, N. Agabiti, G. Brancato, G. Ciappi, C. A. Perucci. 1994. Bronchial responsiveness in children living in areas with different air pollution levels. *Arch. Environ. Health* 49:111–118.

291. Henry, R. L., R. Abramson, J. A. Adler, J. Wlodarcyzk, M. J. Hensley. 1991. Asthma in the vicinity of power stations: I. a prevalence study. *Pediatric. Pulmonol.* 11:127–133.

292. Halliday, J. A., R. L. Henry, R. G. Hankin, M. J. Hensley. 1993. Increased wheeze but not bronchial hyperreactivity near power stations. *J. Epidemiol. Commun. Health* 47:282–286.

293. Jacques, L., C. Plante, S. Goudreau, S. Perron, J. Hicks, T. Kosatsky, A. Smargiassi. *Rapport synthèse régional de l'étude sur la santé respiratoire des jeunes Montréalais de 6 mois à 12 ans.* Montréal: Direction de santé publique de l'Agence de la santé et des services sociaux de Montréal.

294. Bhopal, R. S., P. Phillimore, S. Moffatt, C. Foy. 1994. Is living near a coking works harmful to health? A study of industrial air pollution. *J. Epidemiol. Comm. Health* 48:237–247.

295. Ramadour, M., C. Burel, A. Lanteaume, D. Vervloet, D. Charpin. 2000. Prevalence of asthma and rhinitis in relation to long-term exposure to gaseous air pollutants. *Allergy* 55:1163–1169.

296. Ehrenberg, R. 2012. The facts behind the frack. *Science News* 20–25.

297. Johnson, J. 2013. Shaking up the fracking debate. *C & EN Chem. Eng.* 91(28):8.

298. van der Elst, M. J. 2013. Distant Quakes Trigger Tremors at U.S. Waste-Injection Sites, Says Study.

299. Johnson, J. 2013. Shaking up the fracking debate. *Chem. Engineer.* 91(28):8.

300. McFarland, E. 2012. Unconventional chemistry for unconventional natural gas. *Science* 338(6105):340–342.

301. B. P. Statistical Review of World Energy. 2012.

302. Blanc, P. D. 2012. Occupational and COPD: A brief review. *J. Asthma* 49:2–4.

303. Stamelou, M., K. Tuschl, W. K. Chong, A. K. Burroughs, P. B. Mills, K. P. Bhatia, P. T. Clayton. 2012. Dystonia with brain manganese accumulation resulting from SLC30A10 mutations: A new treatable disorder. *Mov. Disord.* 27(10):1317–1322.

304. Quadri, M. et al. 2012. Mutations in SLC30A10 cause parkinsonism and dystonia with hypermanganesemia, polycythemia, and chronic liver disease. *Am. J. Hum. Genet.* 90(3):467–477.

305. Tuschl, K. et al. 2012. Syndrome of hepatic cirrhosis, dystonia, polycythemia, and hypermanganesemia caused by mutations in SLC30A10, a manganese transporter in man. *Am. J. Hum. Genet.* 90(3):457–466.

306. Kalafova, A., J. Kovacik, M. Capcarova, A. Kolesarova, N. Lukac, R. Stawarz, G. Formicki, T. Laciak. 2012. Accumulation of zinc, nickel, lead and cadmium in some organs of rabbits after dietary nickel and zinc inclusion. *J. Environ. Sci. Health A Tox. Hazard. Subst. Environ. Eng.* 47(9):1234–1238. doi: 10.1080/10934529.2012.672073.

307. Klatka, J., M. Remer, R. Dobrowolski, W. Pietruszewska, A. Trojanowska, H. Siwiec, M. Charytanowicz. 2011. The content of cadmium, cobalt and nickel in laryngeal carcinoma. *Arch. Med. Sci.* 7(3):517–522. doi: 10.5114/aoms.2011.23422.

308. Gault, N., C. Sandre, J. L. Poncy, C. Moulin, J. L. Lefaix, C. Breson. 2010. Cobalt toxicity: Chemical and radiological combined effects on HaCaT keratinocyte cell line. *Toxicol. In Vitro* 24:92–98.

309. Barceloux, D. G. 1999. Nickel. *Clin. Toxicol.* 37(2):239–258.

310. Schroeder, W. H., M. Dobson, D. M. Kane. 1987. Toxic trace elements associated with airborne particulate matter: A review. *JAPCA* 37(11):1267–1287.

311. Claiborn, C. S., T. Larson, L. Sheppard. 2002. Testing the metals hypothesis in Spokane, Washington. *Environ. Health Perspect.* 110(Suppl 4):547–552.

312. Kowalczyk, G. S., G. E. Gordon, S. W. Rheingrover. 1982. Identification of atmospheric particulate sources in Washington, D.C. using chemical element balances. *Environ. Sci. Technol.* 16:79–90.

313. National Geographic Society. How Megafires Are Remaking American Forests. 1996–2015 *National Geogaphic.*

314. The Breath of the Black Dragon in Russia and China. 1988. *The New York Times.*

315. Srivastava, S., R. Haddad, G. Kleinman, C. A. Manthous. 1999. Erythema nodosum after smoke inhalation-induced bronchiolitis obliterans organizing pneumonia. *Crit. Care Med.* 27(6):1214–1216.

316. Megahed, M. A., F. Ghareeb, T. Kishk, A. El-Barah, H. Abou-Gereda, H. El-Fol, A. El-Sisy, A. M. Omran. 2008. Blood gases as an indicator of inhalation injury and prognosis in burn patients. *Ann. Burn Fire Disasters* 10(4):192–198.

317. Cohen, M. A., L. J. Guzzardi. 1983. Inhalation of products of combustion. *Ann. Emerg. Med.* 12(10):628–632.

318. Lee, L. T., C. H. Ho, T. C. Putti. 2014. Bronchiolitis obliterans organizing pneumonia following nitric acid fume exposure. *Occup. Med. (Lond.)* 64(2):136–138.

319. Jones, J., M. J. McMullen, J. Dougherty, 1987. Toxic smoke inhalation: Cyanide poisoning in fire victims. *Am. J. Emerg. Med.* 5(4):317–321.

320. Maantay, J. 2007. Asthma and air pollution in the Bronx: Methodological and data considerations in using GIS for environmental justice and health research. *Health Place* 13(1):32–56.

321. Stefanidou, M., S. Athanaselis. 2008. Health impacts of fire smoke inhalation. *Inhal. Toxicol.* 20(8):761–766. doi: 10.1080/08958370801975311.

322. Heimbach, D. M., J. F. Waeckerle. 1988. Inhalation injuries. *Ann. Emerg. Med.* 17(12):1316–1320.

323. Kao, H. W., L. Pare, R. Kim, A. N. Hasso. 2014. Toxic leukoencephalopathy with atypical MRI features following a lacquer thinner fire. *J. Clin. Neurosci.* 21(5):878–880. doi: 10.1016/j.jocn.2013.06.027.

324. CDC. 2011. *Chronic Disease Prevention and Health Promotion. Chronic Diseases and Health Promotion.* Atlanta, GA: U.S. Centers for Disease Control and Prevention.

325. CDC. 2007. *Fact Sheet: Wildfires.* Atlanta, GA: U.S. Centers for Disease Control and Prevention.

326. QFR Integration Panel. 2009. *Quadrennial Fire Review.* Washington, DC: U.S. Department of the Interior and U.S. Department of Agriculture.

327. National Interagency Fire Center. 2011. *Lightning Fires (by Geographic Area), Human Caused Fires (by Geographic Area).* Boise, ID: National Interagency Fire Center.

328. FAO. 2010. *Global Forest Resources Assessment 2010: Main Report.* Rome, Italy: Food and Agriculture Organization of the United Nations.

329. ESA. 2010. *Data User Element. ATSR World Fire Atlas, Algorithm #2, 2010 (Whole Year).* Paris, France: European Space Agency.

330. Weinhold, B. 2011. Fields and forests in flames: Vegetation smoke and human health. *Environ Health Perspective.* 119(9): a386–a393.

331. Williams, J., A. C. Hyde. 2011. Findings and implications from a coarse-scale global assessment of recent selected mega-fires. *Presented at Fifth International Wildland Fire Conference*, Sun City, South Africa, May 9–13, 2011.

332. Petrobras-36. 2008. Oil Rig Disasters. Retrieved May 21, 2010.

333. Alves, C. A., A. Vicente, C. Monteiro, C. Goncalves, M. Evtyugina, C. Pio. 2011. Emission of trace gases and organic components in smoke particles from a wildfire in a mixed-evergreen forest in Portugal. *Sci. Total Environ.* 409(8):1466–1475.

334. Samuelson, M., U. Cecilie Nygaard, M. Løvik. 2009. Particles from wood smoke and road traffic differently affect the innate immune system of the lung. *Inhal. Toxicol.* 21(11):943–951. PMID: 19552530.

335. Schreuder, A. B., T. V. Larson, L. Sheppard, C. S. Claiborn. 2006. Ambient woodsmoke and associated respiratory emergency department visits in Spokane, Washington. *Int. J. Occup. Environ. Health* 12(2):147–153. PMID: 16722195.

336. Johnston, F. H., R. S. Bailie, L. S. Pilotto, I. C. Hanigan. 2007. Ambient biomass smoke and cardio-respiratory hospital admissions in Darwin, Australia. *BMC Public Health* 7:240.

337. Henderson, S. B., M. Brauer, Y. C. Macnab, S. M. Kennedy. 2011. Three measures of forest fire smoke exposure and their associations with respiratory and cardiovascular health outcomes in a population-based cohort. *Environ. Health Perspect.* 119(9):1266–1271.

338. Delfino, R. J. et al. 2003. The relationship of respiratory and cardiovascular hospital admissions to the Southern California wildfires of 2003. *Occup. Environ. Med.* 66(3):189–197.

339. Johnston, F., I. Hanigan, S. Henderson, G. Morgan, D. Bowman. 2011. Extreme air pollution events from bushfires and dust storms and their association with mortality in Sydney, Australia 1994–2007. *Environ. Res.* 111(6):811–816.

340. Roberts, J. M. et al. 2011. Isocyanic acid in the atmosphere and its possible link to smoke-related health effects. *Proc. Natl. Acad. Sci. U S A* 108(22):8966–8971.

341. Nakayama Wong, L. S., H. H. Aung, M. W. Lamé, T. C. Wegesser, D. W. Wilson. 2011. Fine particulate matter from urban ambient and wildfire sources from California's San Joaquin Valley initiate differential inflammatory, oxidative stress, and xenobiotic responses in human bronchial epithelial cells. *Toxicol. In Vitro* 25(8):1895–1905.

342. Mueller, S. F., J. W. Mallard. 2011. Contributions of natural emissions to ozone and $PM_{2.5}$ as simulated by the community multiscale air quality (CMAQ) model. *Environ. Sci. Technol.* 45(11):4817–4823.

343. Woodruff, L. G., W. F. Cannon. 2010. Immediate and long-term fire effects on total mercury in forests soils of northeastern Minnesota. *Environ. Sci. Technol.* 44(14):5371–5376.

344. Burke, M. P. 2010. The effect of wildfire on soil mercury concentrations in Southern California watersheds. *Water Air Soil Water Pollut.* 212(1–4):369–385. http//dx.doi.org/10.1007/s11270-010-0351y

345. Naeher, L. P., G. L. Achtemeier, J. S. Glitzenstein, D. R. Streng, D. Macintosh. 2006. Real-time and time-integrated $PM_{2.5}$ and CO from prescribed burns in chipped and non-chipped plots: Firefighter and community exposure and health implications. *J. Expo. Sci. Environ. Epidemiol.* 16(4):351–361.

346. Lee, S., K. Baumann, J. J. Schauer, R. J. Sheesley, L. P. Naeher, S. Meinardi, D. R. Blake, E. S. Edgerton, A. G. Russell, M. Clements. 2005. Gaseous and particulate emissions from prescribed burning in Georgia. *Environ. Sci. Technol.* 39(23):9049–9056.

347. Robinson, M. S., M. Zhao, L. Zack, C. Brindley, L. Portz, M. Quarterman, X. Long, P. Herckes. 2011. Characterization of $PM_{2.5}$ collected during broadcast and slash-pile prescribed burns of predominately ponderosa pine forests in northern Arizona. *Atmos. Environ.* 45(12):2087–2094.

348. Bowman, D. M., F. H. Johnston. 2005. Wildfire smoke, fire management, and human health. *EcoHealth* 2(1):76–80.

349. EPA. 2011. *Particulate Matter. PM Standards.* Washington, DC: U.S. Environmental Protection Agency (updated July 6, 2011).

350. EPA. 2010. *CASAC Review of Policy Assessment for the Review of the PM NAAQS—Second External Review Draft.* Washington, DC: Clean Air Scientific Advisory Committee, U.S. Environmental Protection Agency.

351. De Vos, A. J., F. Reisen, A. Cook, B. Devine, P. Weinstein. 2009. Respiratory irritants in Australian bushfire smoke: Air toxics sampling in a smoke chamber and during prescribed burns. *Arch. Environ. Contam. Toxicol.* 56(3):380–388.

352. Incident Information System. 2011. Alligator River National Wildlife Refuge, Pains Bay Fire.

353. Incident Information System. 2011. N.C. Forest Service, Simmons Road.

354. Incident Information System. 2011. Great Dismal Swamp National Wildlife Refuge, Lateral West.

355. McCarty, J. L., S. Korontzi, C. O. Justice, T. Loboda. 2009. The spatial and temporal distribution of crop residue burning in the contiguous United States. *Sci. Total Environ.* 407(21):5701–5712.

356. McCarty, J. L. 2011. Remote sensing-based estimates of annual and seasonal emissions from crop residue burning in the contiguous United States. *J. Air Waste Manage. Assoc.* 61(1):22–34.

357. Mele, M., D. Servida, D. Lupis. 2012. Characterisation of sulphide-bearing waste-rock dumps using electrical resistivity imaging: The case study of the Rio Marina mining district (Elba Island, Italy). *Environ. Monit. Assess.* 185(7):5891–5907. doi: 10.1007/s10661-012-2993-2.

358. Morgan, R. 2006. Tips and Tricks for Recycling Old Computers. *SmartBiz.* Retrieved March 17, 2009.

359. Godri, K. J., S. T. Duggan, G. W. Fuller, T. Baker, D. Green, F. J. Kelly, I. S. Mudway. 2010. Particulate matter oxidative potential from waste transfer station activity. *Environ. Health Perspect.* 118(4):493–498.

360. Gil, Y., A. Kellerman. 1993. A multicriteria model for the location of solid waste transfer stations: The case of Ashdod, Israel. *GeoJournal* 29(4):377–384.

361. Fuller, G. W., T. Baker. 2001. *The Manor Road Air Pollution Study 2001.* London: King's College London.

362. Restrepo, C. et al. 2004. A comparison of ground-level air quality data with New York state department of environmental conservation monitoring stations data in South Bronx, New York. *Atmos. Environ.* 38(31):5295–5304.

363. Maciejczyk, P. B., J. H. Offenberg, J. Clemente, M. Blaustein, G. D. Thurston, L. Chi Chen. 2004. Ambient pollutant concentrations measured by a mobile laboratory in South Bronx, NY. *Atmos. Environ.* 38(31):5283–5294.

364. Fuller, G. W., T. D. Baker. 2008. *PM10 Source Apportionment at Bexley 4, Manor Road, Erith.* London: King's College London.

365. Sthiannopkao, S., M. H. Wong. 2013. Handling e-waste in developed and developing countries: Initiatives, practices, and consequences. *Sci. Total Environ.* 463–464:1147–53.

366. WEEE CRT and Monitor Recycling. 2009. Executiveblueprints.com. Retrieved November 8, 2012.

367. Romieu, I., F. Meneses, J. J. Sienra-Monge, J. Huerta, S. R. Velasco, M. C. White. 1995. Effects of urban air pollutants on emergency visits for childhood asthma in Mexico City. *Am. J. Epidemiol.* 141(6):546–553.

368. Schwartz, J., D. Slater, T. V. Larson, W. E. Pierson, J. Q. Koenig. 1993. Particulate air pollution and hospital emergency room visits for asthma in Seattle. *Am. Rev. Respir. Dis.* 147(4):826–831.

369. Studnicka, M., E. Hackl, J. Pischinger, C. Fangmeyer, N. Haschke, J. Kühr, R. Urbanek, M. Neumann, T. Frischer. 1997. Traffic-related NO2 and the prevalence of asthma and respiratory symptoms in seven year olds. *Eur. Respir. J.* 10(10):2275–2278.

370. Sunyer, J. et al. 1997. Urban air pollution and emergency admissions for asthma in four European cities: The APHEA project. *Thorax* 52(9):760–765.

371. Jackson, K. 1995. *The Encyclopedia of New York City.* New Haven, CT: Yale University Press.

372. Stohs, S. J., D. Bagchi. 1995. Oxidative mechanisms in the toxicity of metal ions. *Free Radic. Biol. Med.* 18(2):321–336.

373. Squadrito, G. L., R. Cueto, B. Dellinger, W. A. Pryor. 2001. Quinoid redox cycling as a mechanism for sustained free radical generation by inhaled airborne particulate matter. *Free Radic. Biol. Med.* 31(9):1132–1138.

374. Li, N., S. Kim, M. Wang, J. Froines, C. Sioutas, A. Nel. 2002. Use of a stratified oxidative stress model to study the biological effects of ambient concentrated and diesel exhaust particulate matter. *Inhal. Toxicol.* 14(5):459–486.

375. Nel, A. E., D. Diaz-Sanchez, N. Li. 2001. The role of particulate pollutants in pulmonary inflammation and asthma: Evidence for the involvement of organic chemicals and oxidative stress. *Curr. Opin. Pulm. Med.* 7(1):20–26.

376. Pourazar, J. et al. 2005. Diesel exhaust activates redox-sensitive transcription factors and kinases in human airways. *Am. J. Physiol. Lung Cell Mol. Physiol.* 289(5):L724–L730.

377. Prahalad, A. K., J. M. Soukup, J. Inmon, R. Willis, A. J. Ghio, S. Becker, J. E. Gallagher. 1999. Ambient air particles: Effects on cellular oxidant radical generation in relation to particulate elemental chemistry. *Toxicol. Appl. Pharmacol.* 158(2):81–91.

378. Künzli, N. et al. 2006. Comparison of oxidative properties, light absorbance, and total and elemental mass concentration of ambient PM2.5 collected at 20 European sites. *Environ. Health Perspect.* 114:684–690.

379. Mudway, I. S., N. Stenfors, S. T. Duggan, H. Roxborough, H. Zielinski, S. L. Marklund, A. Blomberg, A. J. Frew, T. Sandström, F. J. Kelly. 2004. An in vitro and in vivo investigation of the effects of diesel exhaust on human airway lining fluid antioxidants. *Arch. Biochem. Biophys.* 423(1):200–212.

380. Sternbeck, J., A. Sjödin, K. Andréasson. 2002. Metal emissions from road traffic and the influence of resuspension: Results from two tunnel studies. *Atmos. Environ.* 36(30):4735–4744.

381. Ayres, J. G. et al. 2008. Evaluating the toxicity of airborne particulate matter and nanoparticles by measuring oxidative stress potential—A workshop report and consensus statement. *Inhal. Toxicol.* 20(1):75–99.

382. O'Brien, N. 2012. Threat of Toxic Playgrounds. http://www.smh.com.au/national/threat-of-toxic-playgrounds-20120121-1qb5s.html?skin=text-only

383. Zuesse, E. 1981. Love canal: The truth seeps out. *Reason Magazine.*

384. Colten, C. E., P. N. Skinner. 1996. *The Road to Love Canal: Managing Industrial Waste Before EPA.* p. 153. Austin: University of Texas Press.

385. Levine, A. G. 1982. *Love Canal: Science, Politics and People.* p. 10. Lexington, MA: D.C. Heath and Company.

386. Blum, E. D. 2008. *Love Canal Revisited: Race, Class, and Gender in Environmental Activism.* p. 22. Kansas: University Press of Kansas.

387. Levine, A. G. 1982. *Love Canal: Science, Politics and People.* p. 9. Lexington, MA: D.C. Heath and Company.

388. Colten, C. E., P. N. Skinner. 1996. *The Road to Love Canal: Managing Industrial Waste Before EPA.* p. 157. Austin: University of Texas Press. 13.

389. Stroup, R. Free-Market Environmentalism (PDF), The Library of Economics and Liberty.

390. Levine, A. G. 1982. *Love Canal: Science, Politics and People.* p. 13. Lexington, MA: D.C. Heath and Company.

391. Blum, E. D. 2008. *Love Canal Revisited: Race, Class, and Gender in Environmental Activism.* Kansas: University Press of Kansas. p. 25.

392. Tyler Grable. 2011. The Love Canal Diaster.

393. Levine, A. G. 1982. *Love Canal: Science, Politics and People.* p. 14. Lexington, MA: D.C. Heath and Company.

394. Love Canal Protests Article ID WHEBN 0014578312. World Heritage Encyclopedia.

395. Blum, E. D. 2008. *Love Canal Revisited: Race, Class, and Gender in Environmental Activism.* p. 28. Kansas: University Press of Kansas.

396. Janerich D.T., et al. 1981. Cancer incidence in the Love Canal area. *Science* 212:1404–1407.

397. Ember, L. R. 1980. Uncertain science pushes Love Canal solutions to political, legal arenas. *Chem. Engg. News* 58: 22–29. 510.

398. Maugh, T. H. 1982. Health effects of exposure to toxic wastes. *Science.* 215:490–493; 215:643–647.

399. The Risks of Living Near Love Canal. 1982. Controversy and confusion follow a report that the Love Canal area is no more hazardous than areas elsewhere in Niagara Falls. *Science* 212: 808–809, 811.

400. Congressional Research Service, Report No. 83-160. 1983. *Liability for Injury Resulting from the Disposal of Hazardous Waste: Preliminary Bibliography on the 1983–1984, Intercollegiate Debate Resolution.*

401. National Research Council, Committee on Environmental Epidemiology. 1991. *Environmental Epidemiology, Vol. 1: Public Health and Hazardous Wastes, 196.* Washington: National Academy Press.

402. National Research Council, Committee on Environmental Epidemiology. 1991. *Environmental Epidemiology, Vol. 1: Public Health and Hazardous Wastes, 190–191.* Washington: National Academy Press.

403. National Research Council, Committee on Environmental Epidemiology. 1991. *Environmental Epidemiology, Vol. 1: Public Health and Hazardous Wastes, 165.* Washington: National Academy Press.

404. National Research Council, Committee on Environmental Epidemiology. 1991. *Environmental Epidemiology, Vol. 1: Public Health and Hazardous Wastes, 215.* Washington: National Academy Press.

405. New York State Department of Health—Love Canal. www.health.state.NY.US

406. U.S. v. Hooker Chemicals and Plastics Corp. 1994. 850 Federal Supplement, 993 (W.D.N.Y.).

407. Occidental to pay $129 Million in Love Canal Settlement. 1995. U.S. Department of Justice. Retrieved March 2, 2007.

408. Blum, E. D. 2008. *Love Canal Revisited: Race, Class, and Gender in Environmental Activism.* p. 29.449. Kansas: University Press of Kansas.

409. Levine, A. G. 1982. *Love Canal: Science, Politics and People.* p. 215. Lexington, MA: D.C. Heath and Company.

410. Jordan, M. 2003. *Hush Hush: The Dark Secrets of Scientific Research.* p. 108. Buffalo: Firefly Books.

411. Arthur Kill Oil Spill: Hurricane Sandy's Surge Dumps Diesel into New Jersey Waterway. 2012. *Huffington Post (USA).* Retrieved November 1, 2012.

412. Love Canal Follow-up Health Study: Project Report to ATSDR: Public Comment Draft. 2006. Albany: State of New York, Deparment of Health.

413. Levine, A. G. 1982. *Love Canal: Science, Politics and People.* p. 218. Lexington, MA: D.C. Heath and Company.

414. Donato, D. B., O. Nichols, H. Possingham, M. Moore, P. F. Ricci, B. N. Noller. 2007. A critical review of the effects of gold cyanide-bearing tailings solutions on wildlife. *Environ. Int.* 33(7):974–984.

415. Langdale, J. 2014. The Fukushima in Texas. http://www.texanstogether.org/node/7 http://www.texanstogether.org/content/incident-waste-pits.

416. Geraghty, E. M., H. G. Margolis, A. Kjemtrup, W. Reisen, P. Franks. 2013. Correlation between aerial insecticide spraying to interrupt West Nile virus transmission and emergency department visits in Sacramento County, California. *Public Health Rep.* 128(3):221–230.

417. Chung, W. M., C. M. Buseman, S. N. Joyner, S. M. Hughes, T. B. Fomby, J. P. Luby, R. W. Haley. 2013. The 2012 West Nile encephalitis epidemic in Dallas, Texas. *JAMA* 310(3):297–307. doi: 10.1001/jama.2013.8267.

418. Elnaiem, D. E. et al. 2008. Impact of aerial spraying of pyrethrin insecticide on culex pipiens and culex tarsalis (Diptera: Culicidae) abundance and west nile virus infection rates in an urban/suburban area of Sacramento County, California. *J. Med. Entomol.* 45(4):751–757

419. Demma, L. J. et al. 2005. Rocky mountain spotted fever from an unexpected tick vector in Arizona. *N. Engl. J. Med.* 353:587–594.

420. Chow, D. C., A. Grandinetti, E. Fernandez, A. J. Sutton, T. Elias, B. Brooks, E. K. Tam. 2010. Is volcanic air pollution associated with decreased heart-rate variability? *Heart Asia* 2(1):36–41.

421. Dockery, D. W. 2009. Health effects of particulate air pollution. *Ann. Epidemiol.* 19:257–63.

422. Schwartz, J. 1994. What are people dying of on high air pollution days? *Environ. Res.* 64:26–35.

423. Miller, K. A., D. S. Siscovick, L. Sheppard, K. Shepherd, J. H. Sullivan, G. L. Anderson, J. D. Kaufman. 2007. Long-term exposure to air pollution and incidence of cardiovascular events in women. *N. Engl. J. Med.* 356:447–458.

424. Liao, D., J. Cai, W. D. Rosamond, R. W. Barnes, R. G. Hutchinson, E. A. Whitsel, P. Rautaharju, G. Heiss. 1997. Cardiac autonomic function and incident coronary heart disease: A population-based case-cohort study. The ARIC Study. Atherosclerosis risk in communities study. *Am. J. Epidemiol.* 145:696–706.

425. Liao, D., G. W. Evans, L. E. Chambless, R. W. Barnes, P. Sorlie, R. J. Simpson Jr., G. Heiss. 1996. Population-based study of heart rate variability and prevalent myocardial infarction. The Atherosclerosis Risk in Communities Study. *J. Electrocardiol.* 29:189–198.

426. Tsuji, H., M. G. Larson, F. J. Venditti, Jr, E. S. Manders, J. C. Evans, C. L. Feldman, D. Levy. 1996. Impact of reduced heart rate variability on risk for cardiac events. The Framingham Heart Study. *Circulation* 94:2850–2855.

427. Gilligan, D. M., W. L. Chan, E. Sbarouni, P. Nihoyannopoulos, C. M. Oakley. 1993. Autonomic function in hypertrophic cardiomyopathy. *Br. Heart J.* 69:525–529.

428. Ghio, A. J., C. Kim, R. B. Devlin. 2000. Concentrated ambient air particles induce mild pulmonary inflammation in healthy human volunteers. *Am. J. Respir. Crit. Care Med.* 162(3 Pt 1):981–988.

429. Dockery, D. W., C. A. Pope3rd, R. E. Kanner, G. Martin Villegas, J. Schwartz. 1999. Daily changes in oxygen saturation and pulse rate associated with particulate air pollution and barometric pressure. *Res. Rep. Health Eff. Inst.* 83:1–19. Discussion 21–8.

430. Brook, R. D. 2008. Cardiovascular effects of air pollution. *Clin. Sci. (Lond.)* 115:175–187.

431. Hassing, C., M. Twickler, B. Brunekreef, F. R. Cassee, P. A. Doevendans, J. Kastelein, M. J. Cramer. 2009. Particulate air pollution, coronary heart disease and individual risk assessment: A general overview. *Eur. J. Cardiovasc. Prev. Rehabil.* 16:10–15.

432. Tunnicliffe, W. S., M. F. Hilton, R. M. Harrison, J. G. Ayres. 2001. The effect of sulphur dioxide exposure on indices of heart rate variability in normal and asthmatic adults. *Eur. Respir. J.* 17:604–608.

433. Liao, D., J. Creason, C. Shy, R. Williams, R. Watts, R. Zweidinger. 1999. Daily variation of particulate air pollution and poor cardiac autonomic control in the elderly. *Environ. Health Perspect.* 107:521–525.

434. Park, S. K., J. Schwartz, M. Weisskopf, D. Sparrow, P. S. Vokonas, R. O. Wright, B. Coull, H. Nie, H. Hu. 2006. Low-level lead exposure, metabolic syndrome, and heart rate variability: The VA Normative Aging Study. *Environ. Health Perspect.* 114:1718–1724.

435. Luttmann-Gibson, H., H. H. Suh, B. A. Coull, D. W. Dockery, S. E. Sarnat, J. Schwartz, P. H. Stone, D. R. Gold. 2006. Short-term effects of air pollution on heart rate variability in senior adults in Steubenville, Ohio. *J. Occup. Environ. Med.* 48:780–788.

436. Chan, C. C., K. J. Chuang, G. M. Shiao, L. Y. Lin. 2004. Personal exposure to submicrometer particles and heart rate variability in human subjects. *Environ. Health Perspect.* 112:1063–1067.

437. de Paula Santos, U. et al. 2005. Effects of air pollution on blood pressure and heart rate variability: A panel study of vehicular traffic controllers in the city of São Paulo, Brazil. *Eur. Heart J.* 26:193–200.

438. Longo, B. M., A. Rossignol, J. B. Green. 2008. Cardiorespiratory health effects associated with sulphurous volcanic air pollution. *Public Health* 122:809–820.

439. Longo, B. M., W. Yang. 2008. Acute bronchitis and volcanic air pollution: A community-based cohort study at Kilauea Volcano, Hawai'i, USA. *J. Toxicol. Environ. Health A* 71:1565–1571.

440. Tam, E. K., J. Kunimoto, S. J. Labrenz. 2007. Volcanic air pollution and respiratory symptoms in schoolchildren on the Big Island of Hawaii. *Proc. Am. Thor. Soc.* 238:A168.

441. Lin, R-G. II. 2010. Gulf oil spill: New spill in Gulf area after barge crashes into abandoned oil well. *The Los Angeles Times.* Retrieved July 28, 2010.

442. Jensen, D. P. 2010. Chevron: We won't be difficult on oil-spill cleanup costs. *The Salt Lake Tribune.* Retrieved June 18, 2010.

443. Gold, D. R., A. Litonjua, J. Schwartz, E. Lovett, A. Larson, B. Nearing, G. Allen, M. Verrier, R. Cherry, R. Verrier. 2000. Ambient pollution and heart rate variability. *Circulation* 101:1267–1273.

444. Vallejo, M., S. Ruiz, A. G. Hermosillo, V. H. Borja-Aburto, M. Cárdenas. 2006. Ambient fine particles modify heart rate variability in young healthy adults. *J. Expo. Sci. Environ. Epidemiol.* 16:125–130.

445. Loscalzo, J. 2004. Ozone—From environmental pollutant to atherogenic determinant. *N. Engl. J. Med.* 350:834–835.

446. Routledge, H. C., S. Manney, R. M. Harrison, J. G. Ayres, J. N. Townend. 2006. Effect of inhaled sulphur dioxide and carbon particles on heart rate variability and markers of inflammation and coagulation in human subjects. *Heart* 92:220–227.

447. Kobayashi, F., T. Watanabe, Y. Akamatsu, H. Furui, T. Tomita, R. Ohashi, J. Hayano. 2005. Acute effects of cigarette smoking on the heart rate variability of taxi drivers during work. *Scand. J. Work Environ. Health* 31:360–366.

448. Hayano, J., M. Yamada, Y. Sakakibara, T. Fujinami, K. Yokoyama, Y. Watanabe, K. Takata. 1990. Short- and long-term effects of cigarette smoking on heart rate variability. *Am. J. Cardiol.* 65:84–88.

449. Min, J. Y., K. B. Min, S. I. Cho, D. Paek. 2009. Combined effect of cigarette smoking and sulfur dioxide on heart rate variability. *Int. J. Cardiol.* 133:119–121.

450. Wheeler, A., A. Zanobetti, D. R. Gold, J. Schwartz, P. Stone, H. H. Suh. 2006. The relationship between ambient air pollution and heart rate variability differs for individuals with heart and pulmonary disease. *Environ. Health Perspect.* 114:560–566.

451. Hansell, A., C. Oppenheimer. 2004. Health hazards from volcanic gases: A systematic literature review. *Arch. Environ. Health* 59(12):628–639.

452. Ishigami, A., Y. Kikuchi, S. Iwasawa, Y. Nishiwaki, T. Takebayashi, S. Tanaka, K. Omae. 2008. Volcanic sulfur dioxide and acute respiratory symptoms on Miyakejima island. *Occup. Environ. Med.* 65(10):701–707. doi: 10.1136/oem.2007.033456.

453. Shinkura, R., C. Fujiyama, A. Suminori. 1999. Relationship between ambient sulfur dioxide levels and neonatal mortality near the Mt. Sakurajima volcano in Japan. *J. Epidemiol.* 9(5):344–349.

454. Horwell, C. J., B. J. Williamson, K. Donaldson, J. S. Le Blond, D. E. Damby, L. Bowen. 2012. The structure of volcanic cristobalite in relation to its toxicity; Relevance for the variable crystalline silica hazard. *Part. Fibre Toxicol.* 9:44. doi: 10.1186/1743-8977-9-44.

455. Wilson, M. R., V. Stone, R. T. Cullen, A. Searl, R. L. Maynard, K. Donaldson. 2000. In vitro toxicology of respirable Montserrat volcanic ash. *Occup. Environ. Med.* 57:727–733. doi: 10.1136/oem.57.11.727.

456. Housley, D. G., K. A. Bérubé, T. P. Jones, S. Anderson, F. D. Pooley, R. J. Richards. 2009. Pulmonary epithelial response in the rat lung to instilled Montserrat respirable dusts and their major mineral components. *Occup. Environ. Med.* 59:466–472.

457. Higuchi, K., C. Koriyama, S. Akiba. 2012. Increased mortality of respiratory diseases, including lung cancer, in the area with large amount of ashfall from Mount Sakurajima volcano. *J. Environ. Public Health* 2012:257831.

458. van Noorden, R. 2006. Mud volcano floods Java. news@nature.com. Retrieved October 18, 2006.

459. Choi, C. Q. What caused mud eruption. New study favors quake over drilling. NBC News.

460. Davies, R. J., S. A. Mathias, R. E. Swarbrick, M. J. Tingay. 2011. Probabilistic longevity estimate for the LUSI mud volcano, East Java. *J. Geol. Soc.* 168:517–523. doi: 10.1144/0016-76492010-129.

461. Porong turnpike safe to use during exodus. August 14, 2011.

462. Scalding mud volcano 'displacing thousands. Retrieved June 22, 2009.

463. Sidoarjo mud flow from NASA's Earth Observatory. Posted December 10, 2008.

464. Solomon, G. M., S. Janssen. 2010. JAMA report on health effects of the Gulf oil spill. *JAMA*. doi 10.1001/Jama 2010.1254.

465. Agency for Toxic Substances and Disease Registry (ATSDR). 1999. *Toxicological Profile for Total Petroleum Hydrocarbons (TPH).* Atlanta, GA: US Dept of Health and Human Services, Public Health Service.

466. National Toxicology Program. 2005. *Naphthalene. Report on Carcinogens.* 11th ed. Research Triangle Park, NC: US Dept of Health and Human Services, Public Health Service. http://ntp.niehs.nih.gov/ntp/roc/eleventh/profiles/s116znph.pdf. Accessed August 9, 2010.

467. Law, R. J., J. Hellou. 1999. Contamination of fish and shellfish following oil spill incidents. *Environ. Geosci.* 6(2):90–98.

468. Gorma, R. W., S. P. Berardinelli, T. R. Bender. 1991. *HETA 89-200 and 89-273-2111, Exxon/Valdez Alaska Oil Spill. Health Hazard Evaluation Report.* Cincinnati, OH: National Institute for Occupational Safety and Health.

469. O'Neill, A. K. 2003. Self-Reported Exposures and Health Status Among Workers From the Exxon Valdez Oil Spill: Cleanup [master's thesis]. New Haven, CT: Yale University.

470. Rodríguez-Trigo, G., J. P. Zock, I. Isidro Montes. 2007. [Health effects of exposure to oil spills]. *Arch. Bronconeumol.* 43(11):628–635.

471. Zock, J. P., G. Rodríguez-Trigo, F. Pozo-Rodríguez, J. A. Barberà, L. Bouso, Y. Torralba, J. M. Antó, F. P. Gómez, C. Fuster, H. Verea. 2007. SEPAR-Prestige Study Group. Prolonged respiratory symptoms in clean-up workers of the Prestige oil spill. *Am. J. Respir. Crit. Care Med.* 176(6):610–616.

472. Sabucedo, J. M., C. Arce, C. Senra, G. Seoane, I. Vázquez. 2010. Symptomatic profile and health-related quality of life of persons affected by the Prestige catastrophe. *Disasters* 34(3):809–820.

473. Palinkas, L. A., J. S. Petterson, J. Russell, M. A. Downs. 1993. Community patterns of psychiatric disorders after the Exxon Valdez oil spill. *Am. J. Psychiatry* 150(10):1517–1523.

474. Ott, R. 2010. How Much Oil Really Spilled From the Exxon Valdez? (audio/transcript). Interview with Brooke Gladstone. On The Media. National Public Radio. Retrieved June 29, 2010.

475. McClintock, A. 2010. Slow Violence and the BP Coverups. Counter Punch. Tells the Facts, Names the Names.

476. Fortsatt nedforing etter radioaktivitet i dyr som har vært på utmarksbeite – Statens landbruksforvaltning" (in Norwegian). SLF. June 30, 2010. Retrieved June 21, 2015.

477. Backgrounder on Tritium, Radiation Protection Limits, and Drinking Water Standards. U.S. NRC Library. http://www.nrc.gov/reading-rm/doc-collections/fact-sheets/tritium-radiation-fs.html.

478. Donnelly, E. H., J. B. Nemhauser, J. M. Smith, Z. N. Kazzi, E. B. Farfán, A. S. Chang, S. F. Naeem.2010. Acute radiation syndrome: Assessment and management. *South. Med. J.* 103(6): 541–546. doi: 10.1097/SMJ.0b013e3181ddd571. PMID 20710137.

479. Acute Radiation Syndrome: A Fact Sheet for Physicians. 2005. *Centers for Disease Control and Prevention.*

480. The medical handling of skin lesions following high level accidental irradiation. 1987. IAEA Advisory Group Meeting.

481. Wells, J., M. W. Charles. 1982. Non-uniform irradiation of skin: Criteria for limiting non-stochastic effects. *Proceedings of the Third International Symposium of the Society for Radiological Protection _Advances in Theory and Practice* 2: 537–542.

482. Superflares could kill unprotected astronauts. 2005. *New Scientist.*

483. National Research Council (U.S.). 2006. *Ad Hoc Committee on the Solar System Radiation Environment and NASA's Vision for Space Exploration. Space Radiation Hazards and the Vision for Space Exploration.* National Academies Press. ISBN 978-0-309-10264-3.

484. The Effects of Nuclear Weapons, Revised ed., US DOD 1962, p. 579.

485. Black, R. 2011. Fukushima: As Bad as Chernobyl? BBC. Retrieved August 20, 2011.

486. ICRIN Project. 2011. International Chernobyl Portal chernobyl.info. Retrieved 2011.

487. Environmental consequences of the Chernobyl accident and their remediation: Twenty years of experience. Report of the Chernobyl Forum Expert Group 'Environment' (PDF). 2006. Vienna: International Atomic Energy Agency. p. 180. Retrieved March 13, 2011.

488. Gray, R. 2007. How we made the Chernobyl rain. *Telegraph (London).* Retrieved November 27, 2009.

489. Chernobyl Accident 1986. 2015. World Nuclear Association. Retrieved April 21, 2015.

490. Chernobyl: Assessment of Radiological and Health Impact, 2002 update; Chapter II. 2002. The release, dispersion and deposition of radionuclides (PDF). OECD-NEA. Retrieved June 3, 2015.

491. *Unfall im japanischen Kernkraftwerk Fukushima. ZAMG.* 24 March 2011. Retrieved August 20, 2011.

492. Cesium-137: A Deadly Hazard. 2012. Large.stanford.edu. Retrieved on February 13, 2013.

493. Chernobyl, Ten Years On: Assessment of Radiological and Health Impact (PDF). 1995. OECD-NEA. Retrieved June 3, 2015.

494. Medvedev, G. 1989. *The Truth about Chernobyl* (Hardcover. First American edition published by Basic Books in 1991 ed.). VAAP.

495. Marples, D. R. 1988. *The Social Impact of the Chernobyl Disaster.* New York: St. Martin's Press.

496. *Chernobyl: Catastrophe and Consequences.* Springer, Berlin.

497. Kryshev, I. I. 1995. Radioactive contamination of aquatic ecosystems following the Chernobyl accident. *J. Environ. Radioactivity* 27(3):207. doi: 10.1016/0265-931X(94)00042-U.

498. EURATOM Council Regulations No. 3958/87, No. 994/89, No. 2218/89, No. 770/90.

499. Environmental consequences of the Chernobyl accident and their remediation (PDF). *IAEA,* Vienna.

500. Wildlife defies Chernobyl radiation, by Stefen Mulvey, *BBC News.*

501. The International Chernobyl Project Technical Report. 1991. IAEA, Vienna.

502. 'Radiation-Eating' Fungi Finding Could Trigger Recalculation Of Earth's Energy Balance And Help Feed Astronauts.

503. Jahre Tschernobyl: Deutsche Wildschweine immer noch verstrah Wissenschaft – WELT ONLINE, lt – Nachrichten. Die Welt (in German). 2011. Retrieved August 20, 2011.

504. Rossylyn, B. 2011. World's nuclear power industry in decline. *Canberra Times.*

505. "UNSCEAR – Chernobyl health effects". Unscear.org. Retrieved March 23, 2011.

506. Bogdanova, T. I., L. Y. Zurnadzhy E. Greenebaum, R. J. McConnell, J. Robbins, O. V. Epstein, V. A. Olijnyk, M. Hatch L. B. Zablotska, M. D Tronko. 2006. A cohort study of thyroid cancer and other thyroid diseases after the Chornobyl accident: Pathology analysis of thyroid cancer cases in Ukraine detected during the first screening (1998–2000). *Cancer* 11(107):2599–2566. doi: 10.1002/cncr.22321. PMC 2983485. PMID 17083123.

507. Dinets, A., M. Hulchiy, A. Sofiadis, M. Ghaderi, A. Höög, C. Larsson J. Zedenius. 2012. Clinical, Genetic and Immunohistochemical Characterization of 70 Ukrainian Adult Cases with Post-Chornobyl Papillary Thyroid Carcinoma. *Eur. J. Endocrinol.* 166(6):1049–1060. doi: 10.1530/EJE-12-0144. PMC 3361791. PMID 22457234.

508. Mettler, F. A. Jr, A. K. Gus'kova, I. Gusev. 2007. Health effects in those with acute radiation sickness from the Chernobyl accident. *Health Phys.* 93(5):462–469.

509. Chernobyl's Legacy: Health, Environmental and Socio-Economic Impacts (PDF). Chernobyl Forum assessment report. Chernobyl Forum. Retrieved April 21, 2012.

510. How Many Cancers Did Chernobyl Really Cause? UCSUSA.org. Retireved April 17, 2011.

511. Ganina, K. P. et al. 1994. A cytogenetic examination of persons subjected to radiation exposure in certain regions of Ukraine. *Tsitol. Genet.* 28(3):32–37.

512. Junk, A. K., P. Egner, P. Gottloeber, R. U. Peter, F. H. Stefani, A. M. Kellerer. 1999. Long-term radiation damage to the skin and eye after combined beta- and gamma- radiation exposure during the reactor accident in Chernobyl. *Klin Monbl Augenheilkd* 215(6):355–360.

513. Baranov, A. et al. 1989. Bone marrow transplantation after the Chernobyl nuclear accident. *N. Engl. J. Med.* 321:205–212. doi: 10.1056/NEJM198907273210401.

514. Kamarad, V. 1989. Acute radiation sickness — morphology of CNS syndrome. *Acta Univ. Palacki. Olomu. Fac. Med.* 121:7–144.

515. Gottlöber, P., M. Steinert, M. Weiss, V. Bebeshko, D. Belyi, N. Nadejina, F. H. Stefani, G. Wagemaker, T. M. Fliedner, R. U. Peter. 2001. The outcome of local radiation injuries: 14 years of follow-up after the Chernobyl accident. *Radiat. Res.* 155(3):409–416.

516. Ivanov, A. A. et al. 2005. Infection syndrome in acute radiation sickness patients subjected to Chernobyl accident. *Med. Tr. Prom. Ekol.* 3:1–7.

517. Dr Deagle, B. MD AAEM ACAM A4M. 2012. Fukushima Daiichi Nuclear Site Japanese and World Crisis. U.S. Homeland Security.

518. Mangano, J. J., J. D. Sherman. 2012. An unexpected mortality increase in the United States follows arrival of the radioactive plume from Fukushima: Is there a correlation? *Int. J. Health Ser.* 42(1): 47–64, 2012, Baywood Publishing Co., Inc. doi: http://dx.doi.org/10.2190/HS.42.1.f.

519. Fong, P. 2011. Sudden infant deaths on rise in B.C. *Toronto Star*, July 6, 2011. www.thestar.com/news/canada/article/1020924-sudden-infant-deaths-on-rise-in-b-c. Accessed August 4, 2011.

520. International Atomic Energy Agency. 2006. The Chernobyl Legacy: Health, Environment and Socio-Economic Impact and Recommendations to the Governments of Belarus, the Russian Federation, and Ukraine, 2nd Rev. Ed. Vienna. www.iaea.org/publications/booklets/Chernnobyl/Chernobyl.pdf. Accessed August 1, 2011.

521. Yablokov, A. V., V. B. Nesterenko, A. V. Nesterenko. 2009. *Chernobyl: Consequences of the Catastrophe for People and the Environment.* New York Academy of Sciences, New York.

522. Gould, J. M., E. J. Sternglass. 1988. Significant U.S. mortality increases after the Chernobyl accident. *Paper presented at Symposium on the Effects of Low Level Radiation in Humans*, Institute of Radiation Biology, University of Munich. February 27, 1988.

523. Office of Radiation Programs. Environmental Radiation Data, quarterly vols. U.S. Environmental Protection Agency. Montgomery AL, 1985 and 1986.

524. National Center for Health Statistics. Monthly Vital Statistics Reports, monthly vols. U.S. Department of Health and Human Services. Montgomery, AL, 1985–1987.

525. National Center for Health Statistics. 1986. Vital Statistics of the United States, final totals of U.S. deaths, annual vols. U.S. Department of Health and Human Services. Montgomery, AL.

526. Bentham, G. 1991. Chernobyl fallout and prenatal mortality in England and Wales. *Soc. Sci. Med.* 33(4):429–434.

527. Busby, C. C. 1995. *Wings of Death: Nuclear Contamination and Human Health.* Aberystwyth, UK: Green Audit Books.

528. Korblein, A., H. Kuchenoff. 1997. Perinatal mortality in Germany following the Chernobyl accident. *Rad. Env. Biophys* 36(1):3–7.

529. Kulakov, V. I., A. L. Sokur, A. L. Volobuev. 1993. Female reproductive function in areas affected by radiation after the Chernobyl power station accident. *Env. Health Perspect* 101:117–123.

530. Mangano, J. 1996. Chernobyl and hypothyroidism. *Lancet* 347:1482–1483.

531. Mangano, J. 1997. Childhood leukaemia in US may have risen due to fallout from Chernobyl. *BMJ* 314:1200.

532. Reid, W., J. Mangano. 1995. Thyroid cancer in the United States since the accident at Chernobyl. *BMJ* 311:511.

533. Sherman, J. D., J. Mangano. 2011. An unexpected rise in mortality increase in the U.S. follows arrival of radioactive plume from Fukushima, is there a correlation? *International Journal of Health Services.* 42(1).

534. Stewart, A. J., D. H. Webb. 1958. A survey of childhood malignancies. *BMJ* 1:1495–1508.

535. Institute of Medicine, Committee on Thyroid Screening Related to I-131 exposure, and National Research Council, Committee on Exposure of the American People from the Nevada Atomic Bomb Tests. 1999. *Exposure of the American People to Iodine-131 Exposure from Nevada Nuclear-Bomb Tests.* Washington, DC: National Academy Press.

536. Alvarez, R. 2000. *The Risks of Making Nuclear Weapons: A Review of the Health and Mortality Experience of U.S. Department of Energy Workers.* Washington, DC: Government Accountability Project.

537. Busby, C. C. 2009. Very low dose fetal exposure to Chernobyl contamination resulted in increases in infant leukemia in Europe and raises questions about current radiation risk models. *Int. J. Environ. Res. Public Health* 6(12):3105–3114. doi: 103390/ijerph60×.

538. Heiervang, K. S., S. Mednick, K. Sundet, B. R. Rund. 2010. Effect of low dose ionizing radiation exposure in utero on cognitive function in adolescence. *Scand. J. Psychol.* doi: 10.1111/j.1467-9450.2010.00814.x.

539. Hawkey, C. J. 1996. Non-steroidal anti-inflammatory drug gastropathy: Causes and treatment. *Scand. J. Gastroenterol. Suppl.* 220:124–127.

540. Maldonado, P. D., Barrera, I. Rivero, R. Mata, O. N. Medina-Campos, R. Hernández-Pando, J. Pedraza-Chaverrí. 2003. Antioxidant S-allylcysteine prevents gentamicin-induced oxidative stress and renal damage. *Free Radic. Biol. Med.* 35:317–324.

541. Sherman, J. D. 2000. *Life's Delicate Balance: Causes and Prevention of Breast Cancer*, pp. 57–66, 234–235. New York: Taylor & Francis.

542. Haley, R. W., E. Charuvastra, W. E. Shell, D. M. Buhner, W. W. Marshall, M. M. Biggs, S. C. Hopkins, G. I. Wolfe, S. Vernino. 2013. Cholinergic autonomic dysfunction in veterans with Gulf War illness. *JAMA Neurol.* 70(2):191–200. doi: 10.1001/jamaneurol.2013.596.

543. US Department of Veterans Affairs. 2012. Research Advisory Committee on Gulf War Veterans' Illnesses. http://www1.va.gov/rac-gwvi/. Accessed October 1, 2012.

544. Golomb, B. A. 2008. Acetylcholinesterase inhibitors and Gulf War illnesses. *Proc. Natl. Acad. Sci. U.S.A.* 105(11):4295–4300.

545. Ecobichon, D. J. 1994. Organophosphorus ester insecticides. In *Pesticides and Neurological Diseases*. Ecobichon, D. J., Joy, R. M., eds. 2nd ed., pp. 171–250. Boston, MA: CRC Press, Inc.

546. Yokoyama, K., S. Araki, K. Murata, M. Nishikitani, T. Okumura, S. Ishimatsu, N. Takasu. 1998. Chronic neurobehavioral and central and autonomic nervous system effects of Tokyo subway sarin poisoning. *J. Physiol. Paris* 92(3–4):317–323.

547. Haley, R. W., T. L. Kurt, J. Hom. 1997. Is there a Gulf War syndrome? Searching for syndromes by factor analysis of symptoms. *JAMA* 277(3):215–222.

548. Haley, R. W. et al. 2004. Blunted circadian variation in autonomic regulation of sinus node function in veterans with Gulf War syndrome. *Am. J. Med.* 117(7):469–478.

549. Stein, P. K., P. P. Domitrovich, K. Ambrose, A. Lyden, M. Fine, R. H. Gracely, D. J. Clauw. 2004. Sex effects on heart rate variability in fibromyalgia and Gulf War illness. *Arthritis Rheum.* 51(5):700–708.

550. Fukuda, K. et al. 1998. Chronic multisymptom illness affecting Air Force veterans of the Gulf War. *JAMA* 280(11):981–988.

551. Sharief, M. K., J. Priddin, R. S. Delamont, C. Unwin, M. R. Rose, A. David, S. Wessely. 2002. Neurophysiologic analysis of neuromuscular symptoms in UK Gulf War veterans: A controlled study. *Neurology* 59(10):1518–1525.

552. Iannacchione, V. G., J. A. Dever, C. M. Bann, K. A. Considine, D. Creel, C. P. Carson, H. Best, R. W. Haley. 2011. Validation of a research case definition of Gulf War illness in the 1991 US military population. *Neuroepidemiol.* 37(2):129–140.

553. Haley, R. W., G. D. Luk, F. Petty. 2001. Use of structural equation modeling to test the construct validity of a case definition of Gulf War syndrome: Invariance over developmental and validation samples, service branches and publicity. *Psychiatry Res.* 102(2):175–200.

554. Haley, R. W., A. M. Maddrey, H. K. Gershenfeld. 2002. Severely reduced functional status in veterans fitting a case definition of Gulf War syndrome. *Am. J. Public Health* 92(1):46–47.

555. Haley, R. W. et al. 1997. Evaluation of neurologic function in Gulf War veterans: A blinded case-control study. *JAMA* 277(3):223–230.

556. Hom, J., R. W. Haley, T. L. Kurt. 1997. Neuropsychological correlates of Gulf War syndrome. *Arch. Clin. Neuropsychol.* 12(6):531–544.

557. Roland, P. S., R. W. Haley, W. Yellin, K. Owens, A. G. Shoup. 2000. Vestibular dysfunction in Gulf War syndrome. *Otolaryngol. Head Neck Surg.* 122(3):319–329.

558. Haley, R. W., W. W. Marshall, G. G. McDonald, M. A. Daugherty, F. Petty, J. L. Fleckenstein. 2000. Brain abnormalities in Gulf War syndrome: Evaluation with ^{1}H MR spectroscopy. *Radiol.* 215(3):807–817.

559. Tillman, G. D., T. A. Green, T. C. Ferree, C. S. Calley, M. J. Maguire, R. Briggs, J. Hart Jr, R. W. Haley, M. A. Kraut. 2010. Impaired response inhibition in ill Gulf War veterans. *J. Neurol. Sci.* 297(1–2):1–5.

560. Haley, R. W., J. S. Spence, P. S. Carmack, R. F. Gunst, W. R. Schucany, F. Petty, M. D. Devous Sr, F. J. Bonte, M. H. Trivedi. 2009. Abnormal brain response to cholinergic challenge in chronic encephalopathy from the 1991 Gulf War. *Psychiatry Res.* 171(3):207–220.

561. Li, X. et al. 2011. Hippocampal dysfunction in Gulf War veterans: Investigation with ASL perfusion MR imaging and physostigmine challenge. *Radiology* 261(1):218–225.

562. Tillman, G. D., C. S. Calley, T. A. Green, V. I. Buhl, M. M. Biggs, J. S. Spence, R. W. Briggs, R. W. Haley, J. Hart, Jr., M. A. Kraut. 2012. Event-related potential patterns associated with hyperarousal in Gulf War illness syndrome groups. *Neurotoxicology.* 2012; 33(5):1096–1105.

563. Jamal, G. A., S. Hansen, F. Apartopoulos, A. Peden. 1996. The "Gulf War syndrome": Is there evidence of dysfunction in the nervous system? *J. Neurol. Neurosurg. Psychiatry* 60(4):449–451.

564. Jones, K. H., A. M. Dechkovskaia, E. A. Herrick, A. A. Abdel-Rahman, W. A. Khan, M. B. Abou-Donia. 2000. Subchronic effects following a single sarin exposure on blood-brain and blood-testes barrier permeability, acetylcholinesterase, and acetylcholine receptors in the central nervous system of rat: A dose-response study. *J. Toxicol. Environ. Health A* 61(8):695–707.

565. Henderson, R. F., E. B. Barr, W. B. Blackwell, C. R. Clark, C. Conn, R. Kalra. 2002. Response of rats to low levels of sarin. *Toxicol. Appl. Pharmacol.* 184(2):67–76.

566. Morris, M., M. P. Key, V. Farah. 2007. Sarin produces delayed cardiac and central autonomic changes. *Exp. Neurol.* 203(1):110–115.

567. Suarez, G. A., T. L. Opfer-Gehrking, K. P. Offord, E. J. Atkinson, P. C. O'Brien, P. A. Low. 1999. The Autonomic Symptom Profile: A new instrument to assess autonomic symptoms. *Neurol.* 52(3):523–528.

568. Low, P. A. 1993. Composite autonomic scoring scale for laboratory quantification of generalized autonomic failure. *Mayo Clin. Proc.* 68(8):748–752.

569. Low, P. A., J. C. Denq, T. L. Opfer-Gehrking, P. J. Dyck, P. C. O'Brien, J. M. Slezak. 1997. Effect of age and gender on sudomotor and cardiovagal function and blood pressure response to tilt in normal subjects. *Muscle Nerve* 20(12):1561–1568.

570. Patarca, R. 2001. Cytokines and chronic fatigue syndrome. *Ann. N. Y. Acad. Sci.* 933:185–200.

571. Brenu, E. W., M. L. van Driel, D. R. Staines, K. J. Ashton, S. B. Ramos, J. Keane, N. G. Klimas, S. M. Marshall-Gradisnik. 2011. Immunological abnormalities as potential biomarkers in chronic fatigue syndrome/myalgic encephalomyelitis. *J. Transl. Med.* 9:81.

572. Berg, D., L. H. Berg, J. Couvaras, H. Harrison. 1999. Chronic fatigue syndrome and/or fibromyalgia as a variation of antiphospholipid antibody syndrome: An explanatory model and approach to laboratory diagnosis. *Blood Coagul. Fibrinolysis* 10:435–438.

573. Ortega-Hernandez, O. D., Y. Shoenfeld. 2009. Infection, vaccination, and autoantibodies in chronic fatigue syndrome, cause or coincidence? *Ann. N. Y. Acad. Sci.* 1173:600–609.

574. Nancy, A. L., Y. Shoenfeld. 2008. Chronic fatigue syndrome with autoantibodies—The result of an augmented adjuvant effect of hepatitis-B vaccine and silicone implant. *Autoimmun. Rev.* 8(1):52–55

575. Menon, D. U. 2011. Biochemical screening for mitochondrial disease in patients with atuism spectrum disorder. In *AMFAR; 2011*; San Diego.

576. Pasca, S. P., B. Nemes, L. Vlase, C. E. Gagyi, E. Dronca, A. C. Miu, M. Dronca. 2006. High levels of homocysteine and low serum paraoxonase 1 arylesterase activity in children with autism. *Life Sci.* 78:2244–2248.

577. Tafazoli, S., P. J. O'Brien. 2005. Peroxidases: A role in the metabolism and side effects of drugs. *Drug Discov. Today* 10:617–625.

578. Shoffner, J. M., R. L. Watts, J. L. Juncos, A. Torroni, D. C. Wallace. 1991. Mitochondrial oxidative phosphorylation defects in Parkinson's disease. *Ann. Neurol.* 30:332–339.

579. Chaudhuri, A., P. O. Behan. 2004. In vivo magnetic resonance spectroscopy in chronic fatigue syndrome. *Prostaglandins Leukot. Essent. Fatty Acids* 71:181–183.

580. Myhill, S., N. E. Booth, J. McLaren-Howard. 2009. Chronic fatigue syndrome and mitochondrial dysfunction. *Int. J. Clin. Exp. Med.* 2:1–16.

581. Schwartz, J., S. K. Park, M. S. O'Neill, P. S. Vokonas, D. Sparrow, S. Weiss, K. Kelsey. 2005. Glutathione-S-transferase M1, obesity, statins, and autonomic effects of particles: Gene-by-drug-by-environment interaction. *Am. J. Respir. Crit. Care Med.* 172:1529–1533.

582. Whistler, T., E. R. Unger, R. Nisenbaum, S. D. Vernon. 2003. Integration of gene expression, clinical, and epidemiologic data to characterize Chronic Fatigue Syndrome. *J. Transl. Med.* 1:10.

583. Zhang, C., A. Baumer, I. R. Mackay, A. W. Linnane, P. Nagley. 1995. Unusual pattern of mitochondrial DNA deletions in skeletal muscle of an adult human with chronic fatigue syndrome. *Hum. Mol. Genet.* 4:751–754.

584. Schnakenberg, E., K. R. Fabig, M. Stanulla, N. Strobl, M. Lustig, N. Fabig, W. Schloo. 2007. A cross-sectional study of self-reported chemical-related sensitivity is associated with gene variants of drug-metabolizing enzymes. *Environ. Health* 6:6.

585. James, S. J. et al. 2006. Metabolic endophenotype and related genotypes are associated with oxidative stress in children with autism. *Am. J. Med. Genet. B Neuropsychiatr. Genet.* 141B:947–956.

586. James, S. J., S. Melnyk, S. Jernigan, A. Hubanks, S. Rose, D. W. Gaylor. 2008. Abnormal transmethyl-ation/transsulfuration metabolism and DNA hypomethylation among parents of children with autism. *J. Autism. Dev. Disord.* 38(10):1966–1975.

587. Williams, T. A., A. E. Mars, S. G. Buyske, E. S. Stenroos, R. Wang, M. F. Factura-Santiago, G. H. Lambert, W. G. Johnson. 2007. Risk of autistic disorder in affected offspring of mothers with a glutathi-one S-transferase P1 haplotype. *Arch. Pediatr. Adolesc. Med.* 161:356–361.

588. Tafazoli, S., D. D. Spehar, P. J. O'Brien. 2005. Oxidative stress mediated idiosyncratic drug toxicity. *Drug Metab. Rev.* 37:311–325.

589. Perez-Gomez, C., J. M. Segura, M. Blanca, M. Asenjo, J. M. Mates. 2000. Antioxidant activity levels and oxidative stress as blood markers of allergic response to drugs. *Biochem. Cell Biol.* 78:691–698.

590. Kass, G. E. 2006. Mitochondrial involvement in drug-induced hepatic injury. *Chem. Biol. Interact.* 163:145–159.

591. Agrawal, A., D. Chandra, R. K. Kale. 2001. Radiation induced oxidative stress: II studies in liver as a distant organ of tumor bearing mice. *Mol. Cell Biochem.* 224:9–17.

592. Abd El-Gawad, H. M., M. M. El-Sawalhi. 2004. Nitric oxide and oxidative stress in brain and heart of normal rats treated with doxorubicin: Role of aminoguanidine. *J. Biochem. Mol. Toxicol.* 18:69–77.

593. Abu-Qare, A. W., M. B. Abou-Donia. 2003. Combined exposure to DEET (N,N-diethyl-m-toluamide) and permethrin: Pharmacokinetics and toxicological effects. *J. Toxicol. Environ. Health B Crit. Rev.* 6:41–53.

594. Abushamaa. A. M., T. A. Sporn, R. J. Folz. 2002. Oxidative stress and inflammation contribute to lung toxicity after a common breast cancer chemotherapy regimen. *Am. J. Physiol. Lung Cell Mol. Physiol.* 283:L336–L345.

595. Bandyopadhyay, D., G. Ghosh, A. Bandyopadhyay, R. J. Reiter. 2004. Melatonin protects against piroxi-cam-induced gastric ulceration. *J. Pineal. Res.* 36:195–203.

596. Basivireddy, J., M. Jacob, K. A. Balasubramanian. 2005. Indomethacin induces free radical-mediated changes in renal brush border membranes. *Arch. Toxicol.* 79:441–450.

597. Basivireddy, J., M. Jacob, A. B. Pulimood, K. A. Balasubramanian. 2004. Indomethacin-induced renal damage: Role of oxygen free radicals. *Biochem. Pharmacol.* 67:587–599.

598. Boelsterli, U. A. 2002 Mechanisms of NSAID-induced hepatotoxicity: Focus on nimesulide. *Drug Saf.* 25:633–648.

599. Conklin, K. A. 2005. Coenzyme q10 for prevention of anthracycline-induced cardiotoxicity. *Integr. Cancer Ther.* 4:110–130.

600. Denicola, A., R. Radi. 2005. Peroxynitrite and drug-dependent toxicity. *Toxicol.* 208:273–288.

601. Goli, A. K., S. A. Goli, R. P. Byrd Jr., T. M. Roy. 2002. Simvastatin-induced lactic acidosis: A rare adverse reaction? *Clin. Pharmacol. Ther.* 72:461–464.

602. Naidu, P. S., A. Singh, S. K. Kulkarni. 2003. Quercetin, a bioflavonoid, attenuates haloperidol-induced orofacial dyskinesia. *Neuropharmacology* 44:1100–1106.

603. Perez de Hornedo, J., G. de Arriba, M. Calvino, S. Benito, T. Parra. 2007. Cyclosporin A causes oxida-tive stress and mitochondrial dysfunction in renal tubular cells. *Nefrologia.* 27:565–573.

604. Weyers, A. I., L. I. Ugnia, H. Garcia Ovando, N. B. Gorla. 2002. Ciprofloxacin increases hepatic and renal lipid hydroperoxides levels in mice. *Biocell.* 26:225–228.

605. Carbonera, D., A. Angrilli, G. F. Azzone. 1988. Mechanism of nitrofurantoin toxicity and oxidative stress in mitochondria. *Biochim. Biophys. Acta* 936:139–147.

606. Poitras, P., A. Gougeon, M. Binn, M. Bouin. 2008. Extra digestive manifestations of irritable bowel syndrome: Intolerance to drugs? *Dig. Dis. Sci.* 53:2168–2176.

607. Gray, G. C., R. J. Reed, K. S. Kaiser, T. C. Smith, V. M. Gastanaga. 2002. Self-reported symptoms and medical conditions among 11,868 Gulf War-era veterans: The Seabee Health Study. *Am. J. Epidemiol.* 155:1033–1044.

608. Maes, M. 2009. Inflammatory and oxidative and nitrosative stress pathways underpinning chronic fatigue, somatization and psychosomatic symptoms. *Curr. Opin. Psychiatry* 22:75–83.

609. Ashfaq, S., J. L. Abramson, D. P. Jones, S. D. Rhodes, W. S. Weintraub, W. C. Hooper, V. Vaccarino, R. W. Alexander, D. G. Harrison, A. A. Quyyumi. 2008. Endothelial function and aminothiol biomarkers of oxidative stress in healthy adults. *Hyperten.* 52:80–85.

610. Mitsuyoshi, H., Y. Itoh, T. Okanoue. 2006. Role of oxidative stress in non-alcoholic steatohepatitis. *Nippon. Rinsho.* 64:1077–1082.

611. Natarajan, S. K., C. E. Eapen, A. B. Pullimood, K. A. Balasubramanian. 2006. Oxidative stress in experimental liver microvesicular steatosis: Role of mitochondria and peroxisomes. *J. Gastroenterol. Hepatol.* 21:1240–1249.

612. Esposito, K., M. Ciotola, B. Schisano, L. Misso, G. Giannetti, A. Ceriello, D. Giugliano. 2006. Oxidative stress in the metabolic syndrome. *J. Endocrinol. Invest.* 29:791–795.

613. Grattagliano, I., V. O. Palmieri, P. Portincasa, A. Moschetta, G. Palasciano. 2007. Oxidative stress-induced risk factors associated with the metabolic syndrome: A unifying hypothesis. *J. Nutr. Biochem.* 19(8):491–504.

614. Weng, S. W. et al. 2005. Association of mitochondrial deoxyribonucleic acid 16189 variant (T->C transition) with metabolic syndrome in Chinese adults. *J. Clin. Endocrinol. Metab.* 90:5037–5040.

615. Tripathy, D., A. Aljada, P. Dandona. 2003. Free fatty acids (FFA) and endothelial dysfunction; role of increased oxidative stress and inflammation. – to: Steinberg et al. (2002) Vascular function, insulin resistance and fatty acids. *Diabetologia* 46:300–301.

616. Fujita, K., H. Nishizawa, T. Funahashi, I. Shimomura, M. Shimabukuro. 2006. Systemic oxidative stress is associated with visceral fat accumulation and the metabolic syndrome. *Circ. J.* 70:1437–1442.

617. Pereira, E. C., S. Ferderbar, M. C. Bertolami, A. A. Faludi, O. Monte, H. T. Xavier, T. V. Pereira, D. S. Abdalla. 2008. Biomarkers of oxidative stress and endothelial dysfunction in glucose intolerance and diabetes mellitus. *Clin. Biochem.* 41:1454–1460.

618. Steele, L. 2000. Prevalence and patterns of Gulf War illness in Kansas veterans: Association of symptoms with characteristics of person, place, and time of military service. *Am. J. Epidemiol.* 152:992–1002.

619. Lee, H. K., J. H. Song, C. S. Shin, D. J. Park, K. S. Park, K. U. Lee, C. S. Koh. 1998. Decreased mitochondrial DNA content in peripheral blood precedes the development of non-insulin-dependent diabetes mellitus. *Diabetes Res. Clin. Pract.* 42:161–167.

620. Lamson, D. W., S. M. Plaza. 2002. Mitochondrial factors in the pathogenesis of diabetes: A hypothesis for treatment. *Altern. Med. Rev.* 7:94–111.

621. Belch, J. J., I. R. Mackay, A. Hill, P. Jennings, P. McCollum. 1995. Oxidative stress is present in atherosclerotic peripheral arterial disease and further increased by diabetes mellitus. *Int. Angiol.* 14:385–388.

622. Loffredo, L., A. Marcoccia, P. Pignatelli, P. Andreozzi, M. C. Borgia1, R. Cangemi, F. Chiarotti, V. Francesco. 2007. Oxidative-stress-mediated arterial dysfunction in patients with peripheral arterial disease. *Eur. Heart J.* 28:608–612.

623. Mueller, T., B. Dieplinger, A. Gegenhuber, D. Haidinger, N. Schmid, N. Roth, F. Ebner, M. Landl, W. Poelz, M. Haltmayer. 2004. Serum total 8-iso-prostaglandin F2alpha: A new and independent predictor of peripheral arterial disease. *J. Vasc. Surg.* 40:768–773.

624. Bhat, H. K., W. R. Hiatt, C. L. Hoppel, E. P. Brass. 1999. Skeletal muscle mitochondrial DNA injury in patients with unilateral peripheral arterial disease. *Circulation* 99:807–812.

625. Hiatt, W. R. 2004. Carnitine and peripheral arterial disease. *Ann. N. Y. Acad. Sci.* 1033:92–98.

626. Makris, K. I., A. A. Nella, Z. Zhu, S. A. Swanson, G. P. Casale, T. L. Gutti, A. R. Judge, I. I. Pipinos. 2007. Mitochondriopathy of peripheral arterial disease. *Vascular* 15:336–343.

627. Gardner, A., R. G. Boles. 2008. Symptoms of somatization as a rapid screening tool for mitochondrial dysfunction in depression. *Biopsychosoc. Med.* 2:7.

628. Benmoyal-Segal, L. et al. 2005. Acetylcholinesterase/paraoxonase interactions increase the risk of insecticide-induced Parkinson's disease. *FASEB J.* 19:452–454.

629. Zintzaras, E., G. M. Hadjigeorgiou. 2004. Association of paraoxonase 1 gene polymorphisms with risk of Parkinson's disease: A meta-analysis. *J. Hum. Genet.* 49:474–481.

630. Carmine, A., S. Buervenich, O. Sydow, M. Anvret, L. Olson. 2002. Further evidence for an association of the paraoxonase 1 (PON1) Met-54 allele with Parkinson's disease. *Mov. Disord.* 17:764–766.

631. Akhmedova, S. N., A. K. Yakimovsky, E. I. Schwartz. 2001. Paraoxonase 1 Met--Leu 54 polymorphism is associated with Parkinson's disease. *J. Neurol. Sci.* 184:179–182.

632. Haas, R. H., F. Nasirian, K. Nakano, M. B. Ward, M. Pay, R. Hill, C. D. Shults. 1995. Low platelet mitochondrial complex I and complex II/III activity in early untreated Parkinson's disease. *Ann. Neurol.* 37:714–722.

633. McCauley, L., M. Lasarev, D. Sticker, D. Rischitelli, P. Spencer. 2002. Illness experience of Gulf War veterans possibly exposed to chemical warfare agents. *Am. J. Prev. Med.* 23:200.

634. Bullman, T. A., C. M. Mahan, H. K. Kang, W. F. Page. 2005. Mortality in US Army Gulf War veterans exposed to 1991 Khamisiyah chemical munitions destruction. *Am. J. Public Health* 95:1382–1388.

635. Barth, S. K., H. K. Kang, T. A. Bullman, M. T. Wallin. 2009. Neurological mortality among U.S. veterans of the Persian Gulf War: 13-year follow-up. *Am. J. Ind. Med.* 52:663–670.

636. Unwin, C., N. Blatchley, W. Coker, S. Ferry, M. Hotopf, L. Hull, K. Ismail, I. Palmer, A. David, S. Wessely. 1999. Health of UK servicemen who served in Persian Gulf War. *Lancet* 353:169–178.

637. El-Demerdash, F. M. 2001. Effects of selenium and mercury on the enzymatic activities and lipid peroxidation in brain, liver, and blood of rats. *J. Environ. Sci. Health B.* 36:489–499.

638. Milatovic, D., R. C. Gupta, M. Aschner. 2006. Anticholinesterase toxicity and oxidative stress. *Sci. World J.* 6:295–310.

639. Li, L., Y. Shou, J. L. Borowitz, G. E. Isom. 2001. Reactive oxygen species mediate pyridostigmine-induced neuronal apoptosis: Involvement of muscarinic and NMDA receptors. *Toxicol. Appl. Pharmacol.* 177:17–25.

640. Schumm, W. R. et al. 2002. Self-reported changes in subjective health and anthrax vaccination as reported by over 900 Persian Gulf War era veterans. *Psychol. Rep.* 90:639–653.

641. Schumm, W. R., E. J. Reppert, A. P. Jurich, S. R. Bollman, F. J. Webb, C. S. Castelo. 2002. Pyridostigmine bromide and the long-term subjective health status of a sample of over 700 male Reserve Component Gulf War era veterans. *Psychol. Rep.* 90:707–721.

642. Hotopf, M., A. David, L. Hull, K. Ismail, C. Unwin, S. Wessely. 2000. Role of vaccinations as risk factors for ill health in veterans of the Gulf war: Cross sectional study. *BMJ* 320:1363–1367.

643. Cherry, N., F. Creed, A. Silman, G. Dunn, D. Baxter, J. Smedley, S. Taylor, G. J. Macfarlane. 2001. Health and exposures of United Kingdom Gulf war veterans. Part II: The relation of health to exposure. *Occup. Environ. Med.* 58:299–306.

644. Chalder, T., M. Hotopf, C. Unwin, L. Hull, K. Ismail, A. David, S. Wessely. 2001. Prevalence of Gulf war veterans who believe they have Gulf war syndrome: Questionnaire study. *BMJ* 323:473–476.

645. Geier, M. R., D. A. Geier. 2004. Gastrointestinal adverse reactions following anthrax vaccination: An analysis of the Vaccine Adverse Events Reporting System (VAERS) database. *Hepatogastroenterology* 51:762–767.

646. Ceriello, A. 1993. Coagulation activation in diabetes mellitus: The role of hyperglycaemia and therapeutic prospects. *Diabetologia.* 36:1119–1125.

647. De Marchi, U., M. Mancon, V. Battaglia, S. Ceccon, P. Cardellini, A. Toninello. 2004. Influence of reactive oxygen species production by monoamine oxidase activity on aluminum-induced mitochondrial permeability transition. *Cell. Mol. Life Sci.* 61:2664–2671.

648. Gomez, M., J. L. Esparza, M. R. Nogues, M. Giralt, M. Cabre, J. L. Domingo. 2005. Pro-oxidant activity of aluminum in the rat hippocampus: Gene expression of antioxidant enzymes after melatonin administration. *Free Radic. Biol. Med.* 38:104–111.

649. Jyoti, A., D. Sharma. 2006. Neuroprotective role of *Bacopa monniera* extract against aluminium-induced oxidative stress in the hippocampus of rat brain. *Neurotoxicology* 27:451–457.

650. Katyal, R., B. Desigan, C. P. Sodhi, S. Ojha. 1997. Oral aluminum administration and oxidative injury. *Biol. Trace Elem. Res.* 57:125–130.

651. Lankoff, A., A. Banasik, A. Duma, E. Ochniak, H. Lisowska, T. Kuszewski, S. Góźdź, A. Wojcik. 2006. A comet assay study reveals that aluminium induces DNA damage and inhibits the repair of radiation-induced lesions in human peripheral blood lymphocytes. *Toxicol. Lett.* 161:27–36.

652. Mailloux, R., J. Lemire, V. Appanna. 2007. Aluminum-induced mitochondrial dysfunction leads to lipid accumulation in human hepatocytes: A link to obesity. *Cell Physiol. Biochem.* 20:627–638.

653. Murakami, K., M. Yoshino. 2004. Aluminum decreases the glutathione regeneration by the inhibition of NADP-isocitrate dehydrogenase in mitochondria. *J. Cell Biochem.* 93:1267–1271.

654. Nehru, B., P. Anand. 2005. Oxidative damage following chronic aluminium exposure in adult and pup rat brains. *J. Trace. Elem. Med. Biol.* 19:203–208.

655. Sargazi, M., A. Shenkin, N. B. Roberts. 2006. Aluminium-induced injury to kidney proximal tubular cells: Effects on markers of oxidative damage. *J. Trace Elem. Med. Biol.* 19:267–273.

656. Orihuela, D., V. Meichtry, N. Pregi, M. Pizarro. 2005. Short-term oral exposure to aluminium decreases glutathione intestinal levels and changes enzyme activities involved in its metabolism. *J. Inorg. Biochem.* 99:1871–1878.

657. Messer, R. L., P. E. Lockwood, W. Y. Tseng, K. Edwards, M. Shaw, G. B. Caughman, J. B. Lewis, J. C. Wataha. 2005. Mercury (II) alters mitochondrial activity of monocytes at sublethal doses via oxidative stress mechanisms. *J. Biomed. Mater. Res. B. Appl. Biomater.* 75:257–263.

658. Chen, C. et al. 2005. Increased oxidative DNA damage, as assessed by urinary 8-hydroxy-2′-deoxyguanosine concentrations, and serum redox status in persons exposed to mercury. *Clin. Chem.* 51:759–767.

659. Ueha-Ishibashi, T., Y. Oyama, H. Nakao, C. Umebayashi, Y. Nishizaki, T. Tatsuishi, K. Iwase, K. Murao, H. Seo. 2004. Effect of thimerosal, a preservative in vaccines, on intracellular Ca^{2+} concentration of rat cerebellar neurons. *Toxicology* 195:77–84.

660. Makani, S., S. Gollapudi, L. Yel, S. Chiplunkar, S. Gupta. 2002. Biochemical and molecular basis of thimerosal-induced apoptosis in T cells: A major role of mitochondrial pathway. *Genes Immun.* 3:270–278.

661. Pizzichini, M., M. Fonzi, L. Sugherini, L. Fonzi, A. Gasparoni, M. Comporti, A. Pompella. 2000. Release of mercury from dental amalgam and its influence on salivary antioxidant activity. *Bull Group Int. Rech. Sci. Stomatol. Odontol.* 42:94–100.

662. De Vivo, D. C., S. DiMauro. 1990. Mitochondrial defects of brain and muscle. *Biol. Neonate.* 58 Suppl 1:54–69.

663. Cherry, N., F. Creed, A. Silman, G. Dunn, D. Baxter, J. Smedley, S. Taylor, G. J. Macfarlane. 2001. Health and exposures of United Kingdom Gulf war veterans. Part I: The pattern and extent of ill health. *Occup. Environ. Med.* 58:291–298.

664. Flaherty, K. R., J. Wald, I. M. Weisman, R. J. Zeballos, M. A. Schork, M. Blaivas, M. Rubenfire, F. J. Martinez. 2001. Unexplained exertional limitation: Characterization of patients with a mitochondrial myopathy. *Am. J. Respir. Crit. Care Med.* 164:425–432.

665. Hooper, R. G., A. R. Thomas, R. A. Kearl. 1995. Mitochondrial enzyme deficiency causing exercise limitation in normal-appearing adults. *Chest* 107:317–322.

666. Chung, C. P., D. Titova, A. Oeser, M. Randels, I. Avalos, G. L. Milne, J. D. Morrow, C. M. Stein. 2009. Oxidative stress in fibromyalgia and its relationship to symptoms. *Clin. Rheumatol.* 28(4):435–438.

667. Crimmins, D., J. G. Morris, G. L. Walker, C. M. Sue, E. Byrne, S. Stevens, B. Jean-Francis, C. Yiannikas, R. Pamphlett. 1993. Mitochondrial encephalomyopathy: Variable clinical expression within a single kindred. *J. Neurol. Neurosurg. Psychiatry* 56:900–905.

668. Kroenke, K., P. Koslowe, M. Roy. 1998. Symptoms in 18,495 Persian Gulf War veterans. Latency of onset and lack of association with self-reported exposures. *J. Occup. Environ. Med.* 40:520–528.

669. Lee, H. A., A. J. Bale, R. Gabriel. 2005. Results of investigations on Gulf War veterans. *Clin. Med.* 5:166–172.

670. Ismail, K., K. Kent, R. Sherwood, L. Hull, P. Seed, A. S. David, S. Wessely. 2007. Chronic fatigue syndrome and related disorders in UK veterans of the Gulf War 1990-1991: Results from a two-phase cohort study. *Psychol. Med.* 38:953–961.

671. Haley, R. W., S. Billecke, B. N. La Du. 1999. Association of low PON1 type Q (type A) arylesterase activity with neurologic symptom complexes in Gulf War veterans. *Toxicol. Appl. Pharmacol.* 157:227–233.

672. Kang, H. K., C. M. Mahan, K. Y. Lee, C. A. Magee, F. M. Murphy. 2000. Illnesses among United States veterans of the Gulf War: A population-based survey of 30,000 veterans. *J. Occup. Environ. Med.* 42:491–501.

673. Coffman, C. J., R. D. Horner, S. C. Grambow, J. Lindquist. 2005. Estimating the occurrence of amyotrophic lateral sclerosis among Gulf War (1990-1991) veterans using capture-recapture methods. *Neuroepidemiology* 24:141–150.

674. Mackness, B., P. N. Durrington, M. I. Mackness. 2000. Low paraoxonase in Persian Gulf War Veterans self-reporting Gulf War Syndrome. *Biochem. Biophys. Res. Commun.* 276:729–733.

675. Vojdani, A., J. D. Thrasher. 2004. Cellular and humoral immune abnormalities in Gulf War veterans. *Environ. Health Perspect.* 112:840–846.

676. Haley, R. W. 2003. Excess incidence of ALS in young Gulf War veterans. *Neurology* 61:750–756.

677. Horner, R. D. et al. 2003. Occurrence of amyotrophic lateral sclerosis among Gulf War veterans. *Neurology* 61:742–749.

678. Whistler, T., M. A. Fletcher, W. Lonergan, X. R. Zeng, J. M. Lin, A. Laperriere, S. D. Vernon, N. G. Klimas. 2009. Impaired immune function in Gulf War illness. *BMC Med. Genomics.* 2:12.

679. Compston, J. E., S. Vedi, A. B. Stephen, S. Bord, A. R. Lyons, S. J. Hodges, B. E. Scammell. 2002. Reduced bone formation in UK Gulf War veterans: A bone histomorphometric study. *J. Clin. Pathol.* 55:897–899.

680. Gray, G. C., T. C. Smith, H. K. Kang, J. D. Knoke. 2000. Are Gulf War veterans suffering war-related illnesses? Federal and civilian hospitalizations examined, June 1991 to December 1994. *Am. J. Epidemiol.* 151:63–71.

681. Davis, S. D., S. F. Kator, J. A. Wonnett, B. L. Pappas, J. L. Sall. 2000. Neurally mediated hypotension in fatigued Gulf War veterans: A preliminary report. *Am. J. Med. Sci.* 319:89–95.

682. Jammes, Y., J. G. Steinberg, O. Mambrini, F. Bregeon, S. Delliaux. 2005. Chronic fatigue syndrome: Assessment of increased oxidative stress and altered muscle excitability in response to incremental exercise. *J. Intern. Med.* 257:299–310.

683. Manuel y Keenoy, B., G. Moorkens, J. Vertommen, I. De Leeuw. 2001. Antioxidant status and lipoprotein peroxidation in chronic fatigue syndrome. *Life Sci.* 68:2037–2049.

684. Sastre, A. 2003. Physiological and Genetic aspects of autonomic dysfunction in Gulf War Veterans. Research Presentation. In: *Meeting of the Research Advisory Committee on Gulf War Veterans' Illnesses (Public meeting)* June 16–17, 2003.

685. Hannan, K. L., D. E. Berg, W. Baumzweiger, H. H. Harrison, L. H. Berg, R. Ramirez, D. Nichols. 2000. Activation of the coagulation system in Gulf War Illness: A potential pathophysiologic link with chronic fatigue syndrome. A laboratory approach to diagnosis. *Blood Coagul. Fibrinolysis* 11:673–678.

686. Lane, R. J., M. C. Barrett, D. J. Taylor, G. J. Kemp, R. Lodi. 1998. Heterogeneity in chronic fatigue syndrome: Evidence from magnetic resonance spectroscopy of muscle. *Neuromuscul. Disord.* 8:204–209.

687. Land, J. M., G. J. Kemp, D. J. Taylor, S. J. Standing, G. K. Radda, B. Rajagopalan. 1993. Oral phosphate supplements reverse skeletal muscle abnormalities in a case of chronic fatigue with idiopathic renal hypophosphatemia. *Neuromuscul. Disord.* 3:223–225.

688. Barnes, P. R., D. J. Taylor, G. J. Kemp, G. K. Radda. 1993. Skeletal muscle bioenergetics in the chronic fatigue syndrome. *J. Neurol. Neurosurg. Psychiatry* 56:679–683.

689. Bach, R. 2009. Gulf War associated chronic coagulopathies update. In: *Meeting of the Research Advisory Committee on Gulf War Veterans Illnesses.* Boston University School of Public Health.

690. Sastre, J., F. V. Pallardo, J. Vina. 2000. Mitochondrial oxidative stress plays a key role in aging and apoptosis. *IUBMB Life* 49:427–435.

691. van de Glind, G., M. de Vries, R. Rodenburg, F. Hol, J. Smeitink, E. Morava. 2007. Resting muscle pain as the first clinical symptom in children carrying the MTTK A8344G mutation. *Eur. J. Paediatr. Neurol.* 11:243–246.

692. Benito-Leon, J., A. Berbel, J. Porta-Estessam, A. Martinez, J. Arenas. 1996. [Fibromyalgia in right half of the body as the onset of mitochondrial cytopathy. *Letter]. Rev. Neurol.* 24:1303–1304.

693. Villanova, M., E. Selvi, A. Malandrini, C. Casali, F. M. Santorelli, R. De Stefano, R. Marcolongo. 1999. Mitochondrial myopathy mimicking fibromyalgia syndrome. *Muscle Nerve* 22:289–291.

694. Bengtsson, A., K. G. Henriksson. 1989. The muscle in fibromyalgia--a review of Swedish studies. *J. Rheumatol. Suppl.* 19:144–149.

695. Ozgocmen, S., H. Ozyurt, S. Sogut, O. Akyol. 2006. Current concepts in the pathophysiology of fibromyalgia: The potential role of oxidative stress and nitric oxide. *Rheumatol. Int.* 26:585–597.

696. Pongratz, D. E., M. Spath. 1998. Morphologic aspects of fibromyalgia. *Z. Rheumatol.* 57(Suppl 2):47–51.

697. Chauhan, A., V. Chauhan. 2006. Oxidative stress in autism. *Pathophysiology* 13:171–181.

698. Blaylock. R. L. 2009. A possible central mechanism in autism spectrum disorders, part 2: Immunoexcitotoxicity. *Altern. Ther. Health Med.* 15:60–67.

699. Geier, D. A., J. K. Kern, C. R. Garver, J. B. Adams, T. Audhya, R. Nataf, M. R. Geier. 2009. Biomarkers of environmental toxicity and susceptibility in autism. *J. Neurol. Sci.* 280:101–108.

700. Banerjee, B. D., V. Seth, A. Bhattacharya, S. T. Pasha, A. K. Chakraborty. 1999. Biochemical effects of some pesticides on lipid peroxidation and free-radical scavengers. *Toxicol. Lett.* 107:33–47.

701. Compston, J. E., S. Vedi, A. B. Stephen, S. Bord, A. R. Lyons, S. J. Hodges, B. E. Scammell. 1999. Reduced bone formation after exposure to organophosphates. *Lancet* 354:1791–1792.

702. Poling, J. S., R. E. Frye, J. Shoffner, A. W. Zimmerman. 2006. Developmental regression and mitochondrial dysfunction in a child with autism. *J.Child Neurol.* 21:170–172.

703. Kern, J. K., A. M. Jones. 2006. Evidence of toxicity, oxidative stress, and neuronal insult in autism. *J. Toxicol. Environ. Health B. Crit. Rev.* 9:485–499.

704. Prendergast, M. A., R. L. Self, K. J. Smith, L. Ghayoumi, M. M. Mullins, T. R. Butler, J. J. Buccafusco, D. A. Gearhart, A. V. Terry Jr. 2007. Microtubule-associated targets in chlorpyrifos oxon hippocampal neurotoxicity. *Neuroscience* 146:330–339.

705. Thomas, H. V., N. J. Stimpson, A. L. Weightman, F. Dunstan, G. Lewis. 2006. Systematic review of multi-symptom conditions in Gulf War veterans. *Psychol. Med.* 36:735–747.

706. Hutchison, W. M., D. Thyagarajan, J. Poulton, D. R. Marchington, D. M. Kirby, S. S. M. Manji, H-H Dahl. 2005. Clinical and molecular features of encephalomyopathy due to the A3302G mutation in the mitochondrial tRNA (Leu(UUR)) gene. *Arch. Neurol.* 62:1920–1923.

707. Suzuki, S., Y. Hinokio, M. Ohtomo, Hirai, A. Hirai, M. Chiba, S. Kasuga, Y. Satoh, H. Akai, T. Toyota. 1998. The effects of coenzyme Q10 treatment on maternally inherited diabetes mellitus and deafness, and mitochondrial DNA 3243 (A to G) mutation. *Diabetologia* 41:584–588.

708. Tanji, K., J. Gamez, C. Cervera, F. Mearin, A. Ortega, J. de la Torre, J. Montoya, A. L. Andreu, S. DiMauro, E. Bonilla. 2003. The A8344G mutation in mitochondrial DNA associated with stroke-like episodes and gastrointestinal dysfunction. *Acta Neuropathol. (Berl)* 105:69–75.

709. Vaziri, N. D., Sica D. A. 2004. Lead-induced hypertension: Role of oxidative stress. *Curr. Hypertens. Rep.* 6:314–320.

710. Allen, T., S. V. Rana. 2003. Oxidative stress by inorganic arsenic: Modulation by thyroid hormones in rat. *Comp. Biochem. Physiol. C. Toxicol. Pharmacol.* 135:157–162.

711. Kwok, R. K. et al. 2007. Drinking water arsenic exposure and blood pressure in healthy women of reproductive age in Inner Mongolia, China. *Toxicol. Appl. Pharmacol.* 222:337–343.
712. Borthwick, G. M., M. A. Johnson, P. G., Ince P. J. Shaw, D. M. Turnbull. 1999. Mitochondrial enzyme activity in amyotrophic lateral sclerosis: Implications for the role of mitochondria in neuronal cell death. *Ann. Neurol.* 46:787–790.
713. Huang, Y. K., C. H. Tseng, Y. L. Huang, M. H. Yang, C. J. Chen, Y. M. Hsueh. 2007. Arsenic methylation capability and hypertension risk in subjects living in arseniasis-hyperendemic areas in southwestern Taiwan. *Toxicol. Appl. Pharmacol.* 218:135–142.
714. Aguirre, N., M. F. Beal, W. R. Matson, M. B. Bogdanov. 2005. Increased oxidative damage to DNA in an animal model of amyotrophic lateral sclerosis. *Free Radic. Res.* 39:383–388.
715. Albers, D. S., M. F. Beal. 2000. Mitochondrial dysfunction and oxidative stress in aging and neurodegenerative disease. *J. Neural. Transm. Suppl.* 59:133–154.
716. Barber, S. C., R. J. Mead, P. J. Shaw. 2006. Oxidative stress in ALS: A mechanism of neurodegeneration and a therapeutic target. *Biochim. Biophys. Acta* 1762:1051–1067.
717. Mancuso, M., F. Coppede, L. Migliore, G. Siciliano, L. Murri. 2006. Mitochondrial dysfunction, oxidative stress and neurodegeneration. *J. Alzheimers Dis.* 10:59–73.
718. Liu, R., B. Li, S. W. Flanagan, L. W. Oberley, D. Gozal, M. Qiu. 2002. Increased mitochondrial antioxidative activity or decreased oxygen free radical propagation prevent mutant SOD1-mediated motor neuron cell death and increase amyotrophic lateral sclerosis-like transgenic mouse survival. *J. Neurochem.* 80:488–500.
719. Mitsumoto, H. et al. 2008. Oxidative stress biomarkers in sporadic ALS. *Amyotroph. Lateral Scler.* 9:177–183.
720. Majamaa-Voltti, K., K. Majamaa, K. Peuhkurinen, T. H. Makikallio, H. V. Huikuri. 2004. Cardiovascular autonomic regulation in patients with 3243A > G mitochondrial DNA mutation. *Ann. Med.* 36:225–231.
721. Wortmann, S., R. J. Rodenburg, M. Huizing, F. J. Loupatty, T. de Koning, L. A. Kluijtmans, U. Engelke, R. Wevers, J. A. Smeitink, E. Morava. 2006. Association of 3-methylglutaconic aciduria with sensorineural deafness, encephalopathy, and Leigh-like syndrome (MEGDEL association) in four patients with a disorder of the oxidative phosphorylation. *Mol. Genet. Metab.* 88:47–52.
722. Wray, S. H., J. M. Provenzale, D. R. Johns, K. R. Thulborn. 1995. MR of the brain in mitochondrial myopathy. *AJNR. Am. J. Neuroradiol.* 16:1167–1173.
723. Murata, T., C. Ohtsuka, Y. Terayama. 2008. Increased mitochondrial oxidative damage and oxidative DNA damage contributes to the neurodegenerative process in sporadic amyotrophic lateral sclerosis. *Free Radic. Res.* 42:221–225.
724. Guegan, C., M. Vila, G. Rosoklija, A. P. Hays, S. Przedborski. 2001. Recruitment of the mitochondrial-dependent apoptotic pathway in amyotrophic lateral sclerosis. *J. Neurosci.* 21:6569–6576.
725. Kikuchi, H., A. Furuta, K. Nishioka, S. O. Suzuki, Y. Nakabeppu, T. Iwaki. 2002. Impairment of mitochondrial DNA repair enzymes against accumulation of 8-oxo-guanine in the spinal motor neurons of amyotrophic lateral sclerosis. *Acta Neuropathol. (Berl)* 103:408–414.
726. Kong, J., Z. Xu. 1998. Massive mitochondrial degeneration in motor neurons triggers the onset of amyotrophic lateral sclerosis in mice expressing a mutant SOD1. *J. Neurosci.* 18:3241–3250.
727. Wiedemann, F. R., G. Manfredi, C. Mawrin, M. F. Beal, E. A. Schon. 2002. Mitochondrial DNA and respiratory chain function in spinal cords of ALS patients. *J. Neurochem.* 80:616–625.
728. Cronin, S., M. J. Greenway, J. H. Prehn, O. Hardiman. 2007. Paraoxonase promoter and intronic variants modify risk of sporadic amyotrophic lateral sclerosis. *J. Neurol. Neurosurg. Psychiatry* 78:984–986.
729. Morahan, J. M., B. Yu, R. J. Trent, R. A. Pamphlett. 2007. A gene-environment study of the paraoxonase 1 gene and pesticides in amyotrophic lateral sclerosis. *Neurotoxicology* 28:532–540.
730. Slowik, A., B. Tomik, D. Partyka, W. Turaj, J. Pera, T. Dziedzic, P. Szermer, D. A. Figlewicz, A. Szczudlik. 2006. Paraoxonase-1 Q192R polymorphism and risk of sporadic amyotrophic lateral sclerosis. *Clin. Genet.* 69:358–359.
731. Whitfield, J. B. 2001. Gamma glutamyl transferase. *Crit. Rev. Clin. Lab. Sci.* 38:263–355.
732. Yuan, H. et al. 2005. Cosegregation of the G7444A mutation in the mitochondrial COI/tRNA(Ser(UCN)) genes with the 12S rRNA A1555G mutation in a Chinese family with aminoglycoside-induced and nonsyndromic hearing loss. *Am. J. Med. Genet. A* 138A:133–140.
733. Saeed, M., N. Siddique, W. Y. Hung, E. Usacheva, E. Liu, R. L. Sufit, S. L. Heller, J. L. Haines, M. Pericak-Vance, T. Siddique. 2006. Paraoxonase cluster polymorphisms are associated with sporadic ALS. *Neurology.* 67:771–776.

734. La Du, B. N., S. Billecke, C. Hsu, R. W. Haley. 2001. Broomfield CA. Serum paraoxonase (PON1) iso-zymes: The quantitative analysis of isozymes affecting individual sensitivity to environmental chemicals. *Drug Metab. Dispos.* 29:566–569.

735. Cherry, N., M. Mackness, P. Durrington, A. Povey, M. Dippnall, T. Smith, B. Mackness. 2002. Paraoxonase (PON1) polymorphisms in farmers attributing ill health to sheep a. dip. *Lancet* 359:763–764.

736. Mackness, B., P. Durrington, A. Povey, S. Thomson, M. Dippnall, M. Mackness, T. Smith, N. Cherry. 2003. Paraoxonase and susceptibility to organophosphorus poisoning in farmers dipping sheep. *Pharmacogenetics* 13:81–88.

737. Povey, A. C., M. I. Mackness, P. N. Durrington, M. Dippnall, A. E. Smith, B. Mackness, N. M. Cherry. 2005. Paraoxonase polymorphisms and self-reported chronic ill-health in farmers dipping sheep. *Occup. Med. (Lond)* 55:282–286.

738. McKeown-Eyssen, G., C. Baines, D. E. Cole, N. Riley, R. F. Tyndale, L. Marshall, V. Jazmaji. 2004. Case-control study of genotypes in multiple chemical sensitivity: CYP2D6, NAT1, NAT2, PON1, PON2 and MTHFR. *Int. J. Epidemiol.* 33:971–978.

739. Higashimoto, T., E. E. Baldwin, J. I. Gold, R. G. Boles. 2008. Reflex sympathetic dystrophy: Complex regional pain syndrome type I in children with mitochondrial disease and maternal inheritance. *Arch. Dis. Child* 93:390–397.

740. Zeviani, M., C. Antozzi. 1997. Mitochondrial disorders. *Mol. Hum. Reprod.* 3:133–148.

741. Golomb, B. A., E. K. Kwon, S. Koperski, M. A. Evans. 2009. Amyotrophic lateral sclerosis-like con-ditions in possible association with cholesterol-lowering drugs: An analysis of patient reports to the University of California, San Diego (UCSD) Statin Effects Study. *Drug Saf.* 32:649–661.

742. Fattal, O., K. Budur, A. J. Vaughan, K. Franco. 2006. Review of the literature on major mental disorders in adult patients with mitochondrial diseases. *Psychosomatics* 47:1–7.

743. Fechter, L. D., C. Gearhart, S. Fulton, J. Campbell, J. Fisher, K. Na, D. Cocker, A. Nelson-Miller, P. Moon, B. Pouyatos. 2007. JP-8 Jet Fuel Can Promote Auditory Impairment Resulting From Subsequent Noise Exposure in Rats. *Toxicol. Sci.* 98:510–525.

744. Nicotera, T. M., D. Ding, S. L. McFadden, D. Salvemini, R. Salvi. 2004. Paraquat-induced hair cell damage and protection with the superoxide dismutase mimetic m40403. *Audiol. Neurootol.* 9:353–362.

745. Dupuis, L., F. di Scala, F. Rene, M. de Tapia, H. Oudart, P. F. Pradat, V. Meininger, J. P. Loeffler. 2003. Up-regulation of mitochondrial uncoupling protein 3 reveals an early muscular metabolic defect in amyotrophic lateral sclerosis. *Faseb. J.* 17:2091–2093.

746. Dupuis, L., J. L. Gonzalez de Aguilar, A. Echaniz-Laguna, J. P. Loeffler. 2006. Mitochondrial dysfunc-tion in amyotrophic lateral sclerosis also affects skeletal muscle. *Muscle Nerve* 34:253–254.

747. Krasnianski, A., M. Deschauer, S. Neudecker, F. N. Gellerich, T. Müller, B. G. Schoser, M. Krasnianski, S. Zierz. 2005. Mitochondrial changes in skeletal muscle in amyotrophic lateral sclerosis and other neu-rogenic atrophies. *Brain* 128:1870–1876.

748. Vielhaber, S., C. Kornblum, H. J. Heinze, C. E. Elger, W. S. Kunz. 2005. Mitochondrial changes in skel-etal muscle in amyotrophic lateral sclerosis and other neurogenic atrophies--a comment. *Brain* 128:E38.

749. Dobrian, A. D., M. J. Davies, S. D. Schriver, T. J. Lauterio, R. L. Prewitt. 2001. Oxidative stress in a rat model of obesity-induced hypertension. *Hypertension* 37:554–560.

750. Vielhaber, S., A. Kudin, K. Winkler, F. Wiedemann, R. Schröder, H. Feistner, H. J. Heinze, C. E. Elger, W. S. Kunz. 2003. Is there mitochondrial dysfunction in amyotrophic lateral sclerosis skeletal muscle? *Ann. Neurol.* 53:686–687; author reply 687–688.

751. Echaniz-Laguna, A., J. Zoll, E. Ponsot, B. N'guessan, C. Tranchant, J. P. Loeffler, E. Lampert. 2006. Muscular mitochondrial function in amyotrophic lateral sclerosis is progressively altered as the disease develops: A temporal study in man. *Exp. Neurol.* 198:25–30.

752. Ringholz, G. M., S. H. Appel, M. Bradshaw, N. A. Cooke, D. M. Mosnik, P. E. Schulz. 2005. Prevalence and patterns of cognitive impairment in sporadic ALS. *Neurology* 65:586–590.

753. Wheaton, M. W., A. R. Salamone, D. M. Mosnik, R. O. McDonald, S. H. Appel, H. I. Schmolck, G. M. Ringholz, P. E. Schulz. 2007. Cognitive impairment in familial ALS. *Neurology* 69:1411–1417.

754. Miele, L., M. L. Gabrieli, A. Forgione, V. Vero, A. Gallo, E. Capristo. 2006. Oxidative stress in meta-bolic syndrome and nonalcoholic steatohepatitis. Is it possible a role for vitamins in clinical practice? *Recenti. Prog. Med.* 97:1–5.

755. Grattagliano, I., V. O. Palmieri, P. Portincasa, A. Moschetta, G. Palasciano. 2008. Oxidative stress-induced risk factors associated with the metabolic syndrome: A unifying hypothesis. *J. Nutr. Biochem.* 19:491–504.

756. Abou-Donia, M. B., K. R. Wilmarth, K. F. Jensen, F. W. Oehme, T. L. Kurt. 1996. Neurotoxicity resulting from co-exposure to pyridostigmine bromide, DEET, and permethrin: Implications of Gulf War chemical exposures. *J. Toxicol. Environ. Health* 48:35–56.

757. Smith, B. N., J. M. Wang, D. Vogt, K. Vickers, D. W. King, L. A. King. 2013. Gulf War illness: Symptomatology among veterans 10 years after deployment. *J. Occup. Environ. Med.* 55(1):104–110. doi: 10.1097/JOM.0b013e318270d709.

758. Cottone, S., G. Mule, E. Nardi, A. Vadalà, M. Guarneri, C. Briolotta, R. Arsena, A. Palermo, R. Riccobene, G. Cerasola. 2006. Relation of C-reactive protein to oxidative stress and to endothelial activation in essential hypertension. *Am. J. Hypertens.* 19:313–318.

759. Vaziri, N. D. 2002. Pathogenesis of lead-induced hypertension: Role of oxidative stress. *J. Hypertens. Suppl.* 20:S15–S20.

760. Hotopf, M., A. S. David, L. Hull, V. Nikalaou, C. Unwin, S. Wessely. 2003. Gulf war illness-better, worse, or just the same? A cohort study. *BMJ* 327:1370–1372.

761. Kaushik, N. et al. 2005. Gene expression in peripheral blood mononuclear cells from patients with chronic fatigue syndrome. *J. Clin. Pathol.* 58:826–832.

762. Manwaring, N., M. M. Jones, J. J. Wang, E. Rochtchina, C. Howard, P. Newall, P. Mitchell, C. M. Sue. 2007. Mitochondrial DNA haplogroups and age-related hearing loss. *Arch. Otolaryngol. Head Neck Surg.* 133:929–933.

763. Yamasoba, T., S. Someya, C. Yamada, R. Weindruch, T. A. Prolla, M. Tanokura. 2007. Role of mitochondrial dysfunction and mitochondrial DNA mutations in age-related hearing loss. *Hear Res.* 226:185–193.

764. Juhn, S. K., W. D. Ward. 1979. Alteration of oxidative enzymes (LDH and MDH) in perilymph after noise exposure. *Arch. Otorhinolaryngol.* 222:103–108.

765. Elverland, H. H., T. Torbergsen. 1991. Audiologic findings in a family with mitochondrial disorder. *Am. J. Otol.* 12:459–465.

766. Blondon, H., M. Polivka, F. Joly, B. Flourie, J. Mikol, B. Messing. 2005. Digestive smooth muscle mitochondrial myopathy in patients with mitochondrial-neuro-gastro-intestinal encephalomyopathy (MNGIE). *Gastroenterol. Clin. Biol.* 29:773–778.

767. Guillausseau, P. J. et al. 2001. Maternally inherited diabetes and deafness: A multicenter study. *Ann. Intern. Med.* 134:721–728.

768. Sun, F., J. Cui, H. Gavras, F. Schwartz. 2003. A novel class of tests for the detection of mitochondrial DNA-mutation involvement in diseases. *Am. J. Hum. Genet.* 72:1515–1526.

769. Watson, B., Jr., M. A. Khan, R. A. Desmond, S. Bergman. 2001. Mitochondrial DNA mutations in black Americans with hypertension-associated end-stage renal disease. *Am. J. Kidney Dis.* 38:529–536.

770. Arruda, W. O., L. F. Torres, A. Lombes, S. DiMauro, B. A. Cardoso, H. A. G. Teive, D. De Paola, R. R. Seixas. 1990. Mitochondrial myopathy and myoclonic epilepsy. *Arq. Neuropsiquiatr.* 48:32–43.

771. Petrobras P-36. 2008. Oil Rig Disasters. Retrieved May 21, 2010.

772. Ihara, Y., K. Nobukuni, H. Takata, T. Hayabara. 2005. Oxidative stress and metal content in blood and cerebrospinal fluid of amyotrophic lateral sclerosis patients with and without a Cu, Zn-superoxide dismutase mutation. *Neurol. Res.* 27:105–108.

773. Murata, T., C. Ohtsuka, Y. Terayama. 2008. Increased mitochondrial oxidative damage in patients with sporadic amyotrophic lateral sclerosis. *J. Neurol. Sci.* 267:66–69.

774. Chen, J. C., T. C. Tsai, C. S. Liu, C. T. Lu. 2007. Acute hearing loss in a patient with mitochondrial myopathy, encephalopathy, lactic acidosis and stroke-like episodes (MELAS). *Acta Neurol. Taiwan* 16:168–172.

775. Hotopf, M. et al. 2003. Paraoxonase in Persian Gulf War veterans. *J. Occup. Environ. Med.* 45:668–675.

776. Nicolson, G. L. 2007. Metabolic syndrome and mitochondrial function: Molecular replacement and antioxidant supplements to prevent membrane peroxidation and restore mitochondrial function. *J. Cell Biochem.* 100:1352–1369.

777. Barrett, D. H., G. C. Gray, B. N. Doebbeling, D. J. Clauw, W. C. Reeves. 2002. Prevalence of symptoms and symptom-based conditions among Gulf War veterans: Current status of research findings. *Epidemiol. Rev.* 24:218–227.

778. Nisenbaum, R., D. H. Barrett, M. Reyes, W. C. Reeves. 2000. Deployment stressors and a chronic multisymptom illness among Gulf War veterans. *J. Nerv. Ment. Dis.* 188:259–266.

779. Lange, G., L. A. Tiersky, J. DeLuca, J. B. Scharer, T. Policastro, N. Fiedler, J. E. Morgan, B. H. Natelson. 2001. Cognitive functioning in Gulf War Illness. *J. Clin. Exp. Neuropsychol.* 23:240–249.

780. Binder, L. M., D. Storzbach, K. A. Campbell, D. S. Rohlman, W. K. Anger. 2001. Neurobehavioral deficits associated with chronic fatigue syndrome in veterans with Gulf War unexplained illnesses. *J. Int. Neuropsychol. Soc.* 7:835–839.

781. Proctor, S. P., R. F. White, T. Heeren, F. Debes, B. Gloerfelt-Tarp, M. Appleyard, T. Ishoy, B. Guldager, P. Suadicani. 2003. Neuropsychological functioning in Danish Gulf War veterans. *J. Psychopathol. Behav. Assess* 25:85–93.

782. Friedl, K. E., S. J. Grate, S. P. Proctor. 2009. Neuropsychological issues in military deployments lessons observed in the DoD Gulf War Illnesses Research Program. *Mil. Med.* 174:335–346.

783. Chauhan, A., V. Chauhan, W. T. Brown, I. Cohen. 2004. Oxidative stress in autism: Increased lipid peroxidation and reduced serum levels of ceruloplasmin and transferrin--the antioxidant proteins. *Life Sci.* 75:2539–2549.

784. Nicolson, G. L., P. Berns, M. Y. Nasralla, J. Haier, N. L. Nicolson, M. Nass. 2003. GulfWar Illnesses: Chemical, biological and radiological exposures resulting in chronic fatiguing illnesses can be identified and treated. *J. Chronic Fatigue Syndrome* 11:135–154.

785. Ferguson, E., H. J. Cassaday. 1999. The Gulf War and illness by association. *Br. J. Psychol.* 90:459–475.

786. Unwin, C., M. Hotopf, L. Hull, K. Ismail, A. David, S. Wessely. 2002. Women in the Persian Gulf: Lack of gender differences in long-term health effects of service in United Kingdom Armed Forces in the 1991 Persian Gulf War. *Mil. Med.* 167:406–413.

787. Calley, C. S., M. A. Kraut, J. S. Spence, R. W. Briggs, R. W. Haley, J. Hart Jr. 2010. The neuroanatomic correlates of semantic memory deficits in patients with Gulf War illnesses: A pilot study. *Brain Imaging Behav.* 4:248–255.

788. Broderick, G., A. Kreitz, J. Fuite, M. A. Fletcher, S. D. Vernon, N. Klimas. 2011. A pilot study of immune network remodeling under challenge in Gulf War Illness. *Brain Behav. Immun.* 25:302–313.

789. Holmes, G. P. et al. 1988. Chronic fatigue syndrome: A working case definition. *Ann. Intern. Med.* 108:387–389.

790. Cullen, M. R. 1987. The worker with multiple chemical sensitivities: An overview. *Occup. Med.* 2:655–661.

791. Castilho, R. F., M. W. Ward, D. G. Nicholls. 1999. Oxidative stress, mitochondrial function, and acute glutamate excitotoxicity in cultured cerebellar granule cells. *J. Neurochem.* 72:1394–1401.

792. Singh, P., K. A. Mann, H. K. Mangat, G. Kaur. 2003. Prolonged glutamate excitotoxicity: Effects on mitochondrial antioxidants and antioxidant enzymes. *Mol. Cell Biochem.* 243:139–145.

793. Mackness, B., M. I. Mackness, S. Arrol, W. Turkie, P. N. Durrington. 1997. Effect of the molecular polymorphisms of human paraoxonase (PON1) on the rate of hydrolysis of paraoxon. *Br. J. Pharmacol* 122:265–268.

794. James, S. J., P. Cutler, S. Melnyk, S. Jernigan, L. Janak, D. W. Gaylor, J. A. Neubrander. 2004. Metabolic biomarkers of increased oxidative stress and impaired methylation capacity in children with autism. *Am. J. Clin. Nutr.* 80:1611–1617.

795. Sogut, S. et al. 2003. Changes in nitric oxide levels and antioxidant enzyme activities may have a role in the pathophysiological mechanisms involved in autism. *Clin. Chim. Acta* 331:111–117.

796. Canter, J. A., A. Eshaghian, J. Fessel, M. L. Summar, L. J. Roberts, J. D. Morrow, J. E. Sligh, J. L. Haines. 2005. Degree of heteroplasmy reflects oxidant damage in a large family with the mitochondrial DNA A8344G mutation. *Free Radic. Biol. Med.* 38:678–683.

797. Kirches, E., M. Michael, M. Warich-Kirches, T. Schneider, S. Weis, G. Krause, C. Mawrin, K. Dietzmann. 2001. Heterogeneous tissue distribution of a mitochondrial DNA polymorphism in heteroplasmic subjects without mitochondrial disorders. *J. Med. Genet.* 38:312–317.

798. Smigrodzki, R. M., S. M. Khan. 2005. Mitochondrial microheteroplasmy and a theory of aging and age-related disease. *Rejuvenation Res.* 8:172–198.

799. Schoeler, S., R. Szibor, F. N. Gellerich, T. Wartmann, C. Mawrin, K. Dietzmann, E. Kirches. 2005. Mitochondrial DNA deletions sensitize cells to apoptosis at low heteroplasmy levels. *Biochem. Biophys. Res. Commun.* 332:43–49.

800. Asa, P. B., Y. Cao, R. F. Garry. 2000. Antibodies to squalene in Gulf War syndrome. *Exp. Mol. Pathol.* 68:55–64.

801. Hopps, E., D. Noto, G. Caimi, M. R. Averna. 2010. A novel component of the metabolic syndrome: The oxidative stress. *Nutr. Metab. Cardiovasc. Dis.* 20:72–77.

802. Buchwald, D., D. Garrity. 1994. Comparison of patients with chronic fatigue syndrome, fibromyalgia, and multiple chemical sensitivities. *Arch. Intern. Med.* 154:2049–2053.

803. Brown, M. M., L. A. Jason. 2007. Functioning in individuals with chronic fatigue syndrome: Increased impairment with co-occurring multiple chemical sensitivity and fibromyalgia. *Dyn. Med.* 6:6.

804. Aaron, L. A., D. Buchwald. 2001. A review of the evidence for overlap among unexplained clinical conditions. *Ann. Intern Med.* 134:868–881.

805. Eisen, S. A. et al. 2005. Gulf War Study Participating Investigators. Gulf War veterans' health: Medical evaluation of a U.S. cohort. *Ann. Intern. Med.* 142:881–890.

806. Bourdette, D. N., L. A. McCauley, A. Barkhuizen, W. Johnston, M. Wynn, S. K. Joos, D. Storzbach, T. Shuell, D. Sticker. 2001. Symptom factor analysis, clinical findings, and functional status in a population-based case control study of Gulf War unexplained illness. *J. Occup. Environ. Med.* 43:1026–1040.

807. Baraniuk, J. N., B. Casado, H. Maibach, D. J. Clauw, L. K. Pannell, S. S. Hess. 2005. A Chronic Fatigue Syndrome - related proteome in human cerebrospinal fluid. *BMC. Neurol.* 5:22.

808. Ciccone, D. S., L. Weissman, B. H. Natelson. 2008. Chronic fatigue syndrome in male Gulf war veterans and civilians: A further test of the single syndrome hypothesis. *J. Health Psychol.* 13:529–536.

809. Frissora, C. L., K. L. Koch. 2005. Symptom overlap and comorbidity of irritable bowel syndrome with other conditions. *Curr. Gastroenterol. Rep.* 7:264–271.

810. Plioplys, A. V., S. Plioplys. 1995. Serum levels of carnitine in chronic fatigue syndrome: Clinical correlates. *Neuropsychobiology* 32:132–138.

811. Kuratsune, H., K. Yamaguti, M. Takahashi, H. Misaki, S. Tagawa, T. Kitani. 1994. Acylcarnitine deficiency in chronic fatigue syndrome. *Clin. Infect. Dis.* 18(Suppl 1):S62–7.

812. Fang, H., Q. Xie, R. Boneva, J. Fostel, R. Perkins, W. Tong. 2006. Gene expression profile exploration of a large dataset on chronic fatigue syndrome. *Pharmacogenomics* 7:429–440.

813. Deth, R., C. Muratore, J. Benzecry, V. A. Power-Charnitsky, M. Waly. 2008. How environmental and genetic factors combine to cause autism: A redox/methylation hypothesis. *Neurotoxicology* 29:190–201.

814. Dufault, R., R. Schnoll, W. J. Lukiw, B. Leblanc, C. Cornett, L. Patrick, D. Wallinga, S. G. Gilbert, R. Crider. 2009. Mercury exposure, nutritional deficiencies and metabolic disruptions may affect learning in children. *Behav. Brain Funct.* 5:44.

815. Geier, D. A., J. K. Kern, C. R. Garver, J. B. Adams, T. Audhya, M. R. Geier. 2008. A Prospective Study of Transsulfuration Biomarkers in Autistic Disorders. *Neurochem. Res.* 34:386–393.

816. Loevinger, B. L., D. Muller, C. Alonso, C. L. Coe. 2007. Metabolic syndrome in women with chronic pain. *Metabolism* 56:87–93.

817. Aaron, L., A. D. Buchwald. 2003. Chronic diffuse musculoskeletal pain, fibromyalgia and co-morbid unexplained clinical conditions. *Best Pract. Res. Clin. Rheumatol.* 17:563–574.

818. Golomb, B. A. 2002. Mitochondrial dysfunction. A mechanism of illness in Gulf War veterans? Written brief for Dept of Veterans Affairs Research Advisory Committee on Gulf War Illnesses.

819. Devanur, L. D., J. R. Kerr. 2006. Chronic fatigue syndrome. *J. Clin. Virol.* 37:139–150.

820. Proctor, S. P., K. J. Heaton, T. Heeren, R. F. White. 2006. Effects of sarin and cyclosarin exposure during the 1991 Gulf War on neurobehavioral functioning in US army veterans. *Neurotoxicology* 27:931–939.

821. Exley, C., L. Swarbrick, R. K. Gherardi, F. J. Authier. 2009. A role for the body burden of aluminium in vaccine-associated macrophagic myofasciitis and chronic fatigue syndrome. *Med. Hypotheses* 72:135–139.

822. D'Amelio, M. et al. 2005. Paraoxonase gene variants are associated with autism in North America, but not in Italy: Possible regional specificity in gene-environment interactions. *Mol. Psychiatry* 10:1006–1016.

823. Mahan, C. M., H. K. Kang, N. A. Dalager, J. M. Heller. 2004. Anthrax vaccination and self-reported symptoms, functional status, and medical conditions in the National Health Survey of Gulf War Era Veterans and Their Families. *Ann. Epidemiol.* 14:81–88.

824. Commonwealth Department of Veterans' Affairs. Australian Gulf War Veterans' Health Study 2003. http://www.dvagovau/media/publicat/2003/gulfwarhs/html/executive_summaryhtm 2003.

825. Liu, X., J. A. Hubbard, R. A. Fabes, J. B. Adam. 2006. Sleep disturbances and correlates of children with autism spectrum disorders. *Child Psychiatry Hum. Dev.* 37:179–191.

826. de Magistris, L. et al. 2010. Alterations of the intestinal barrier in patients with autism spectrum disorders and in their first-degree relatives. *J. Pediatr. Gastroenterol. Nutr.* 51:418–424.

827. Smith, R. A., H. Farnworth, B. Wright, V. Allgar. 2009. Are there more bowel symptoms in children with autism compared to normal children and children with other developmental and neurological disorders?: A case control study. *Autism* 13:343–355.

828. Jyonouchi, H., L. Geng, A. Ruby, C. Reddy, B. Zimmerman-Bier. 2005. Evaluation of an association between gastrointestinal symptoms and cytokine production against common dietary proteins in children with autism spectrum disorders. *J. Pediatr.* 146:605–610.

829. Correia, C. et al. 2006. Brief report: High frequency of biochemical markers for mitochondrial dysfunction in autism: No association with the mitochondrial aspartate/glutamate carrier SLC25A12 gene. *J. Autism Dev. Disord.* 36:1137–1140.

830. Ming, X., T. P. Stein, M. Brimacombe, W. G. Johnson, G. H. Lambert, G. C. Wagner. 2005. Increased excretion of a lipid peroxidation biomarker in autism. *Prostaglandins Leukot Essent. Fatty Acids* 73:379–384.

831. Zoroglu, S. S., F. Armutcu, S. Ozen, A. Gurel, E. Sivasli, O. Yetkin, I. Meram. 2004. Increased oxidative stress and altered activities of erythrocyte free radical scavenging enzymes in autism. *Eur. Arch. Psychiatry Clin. Neurosci.* 254:143–147.

832. Ramoz, N., J. G. Reichert, C. J. Smith, J. M. Silverman, I. N. Bespalova, K. L. Davis. 2004. Linkage and association of the mitochondrial aspartate/glutamate carrier SLC25A12 gene with autism. *Am. J. Psychiatry* 161:662–669.

833. Filipek, P. A., J. Juranek, M. T. Nguyen, C. Cummings, J. J. Gargus. 2004. Relative carnitine deficiency in autism. *J. Autism Dev. Disord.* 34:615–623.

834. Blaxill, M. F., L. Redwood, S. Bernard. 2004. Thimerosal and autism? A plausible hypothesis that should not be dismissed. *Med. Hypotheses* 62:788–794.

835. Lombard, J. 1998. Autism: A mitochondrial disorder? *Med. Hypotheses* 50:497–500.

836. Doebbeling, B. N., W. R. Clarke, D. Watson, J. C. Torner, R. F. Woolson, M. D. Voelker, D. H. Barrett, D. A. Schwartz. 2000. Is there a Persian Gulf War syndrome? Evidence from a large population-based survey of veterans and nondeployed controls. *Am. J. Med.* 108:695–704.

837. Odinokova, I. V., K. F. Sung, O. A. Mareninova, K. Hermann, I. Gukovsky, A. S. Gukovskaya. 2008. Mitochondrial mechanisms of death responses in pancreatitis. *J. Gastroenterol. Hepatol.* 23(Suppl 1):S25–S30.

838. Wei, Y. H. 1998. Mitochondrial DNA mutations and oxidative damage in aging and diseases: An emerging paradigm of gerontology and medicine. *Proc. Natl. Sci. Counc. Repub. China B* 22:55–67.

839. Rossignol, R., B. Faustin, C. Rocher, M. Malgat, J. P. Mazat, T. Letellier. 2003. Mitochondrial threshold effects. *Biochem. J.* 370:751–762.

840. Kovalenko, S. A., M. Tanaka, M. Yoneda, A. F. Iakovlev, T. Ozawa. 1996. Accumulation of somatic nucleotide substitutions in mitochondrial DNA associated with the 3243 A-to-G tRNA(leu)(UUR) mutation in encephalomyopathy and cardiomyopathy. *Biochem. Biophys. Res. Commun.* 222:201–207.

841. Pena-Llopis, S., M. D. Ferrando, J. B. Pena. 2002. Impaired glutathione redox status is associated with decreased survival in two organophosphate-poisoned marine bivalves. *Chemosphere* 47:485–497.

842. Pena-Llopis, S., M. D. Ferrando, J. B. Pena. 2003. Fish tolerance to organophosphate-induced oxidative stress is dependent on the glutathione metabolism and enhanced by N-acetylcysteine. *Aquat. Toxicol.* 65:337–360.

843. Pena-Llopis, S., M. D. Ferrando, J. B. Pena. 2003. Increased recovery of brain acetylcholinesterase activity in dichlorvos-intoxicated European eels Anguilla anguilla by bath treatment with N-acetylcysteine. *Dis. Aquat. Organ* 55:237–245.

844. Golomb, B. A. *A Review of the Scientific Literature as it Pertains to Gulf War Illnesses, Vol 3: Immunizations.* Santa Monica: RAND; in press.

845. Sharma, P., K. P. Mishra. 2006. Aluminum-induced maternal and developmental toxicity and oxidative stress in rat brain: Response to combined administration of Tiron and glutathione. *Reprod. Toxicol.* 21:313–321.

846. Droge, W., R. Breitkreutz. 2000. Glutathione and immune function. *Proc. Nutr. Soc.* 59:595–600.

847. Clapp, B. R., A. D. Hingorani, R. K. Kharbanda, V. Mohamed-Ali, J. W. Stephens, P. Vallance, R. J. MacAllister. 2004. Inflammation-induced endothelial dysfunction involves reduced nitric oxide bioavailability and increased oxidant stress. *Cardiovasc. Res.* 64:172–178.

848. Leonard, S. S., G. K. Harris, X. Shi. 2004. Metal-induced oxidative stress and signal transduction. *Free Radic. Biol. Med.* 37:1921–1942.

849. Ueha-Ishibashi, T., T. Tatsuishi, K. Iwase, H. Nakao, C. Umebayashi, Y. Nishizaki, Y. Nishimura, Y. Oyama, S. Hirama, Y. Okano. 2004. Property of thimerosal-induced decrease in cellular content of glutathione in rat thymocytes: A flow cytometric study with 5-chloromethylfluorescein diacetate. *Toxicol. In Vitro* 18:563–569.

850. Bagchi, D., M. Bagchi, E. Hassoun, J. Moser, S. J. Stohs. 1993. Effects of carbon tetrachloride, menadione, and paraquat on the urinary excretion of malondialdehyde, formaldehyde, acetaldehyde, and acetone in rats. *J. Biochem. Toxicol.* 8:101–106.

851. Bagchi, D., M. Bagchi, E. A. Hassoun, S. J. Stohs. 1995. In vitro and in vivo generation of reactive oxygen species, DNA damage and lactate dehydrogenase leakage by selected pesticides. *Toxicology* 104:129–140.

852. Sutcu, R., I. Altuntas, B. Yildirim, N. Karahan, H. Demirin, N. Delibas. 2006. The effects of subchronic methidathion toxicity on rat liver: Role of antioxidant vitamins C and E. *Cell Biol. Toxicol.* 22:221–227.

853. Jean, J. C., Y. Liu, L. A. Brown, R. E. Marc, E. Klings, M. Joyce-Brady. 2002. Gamma-glutamyl trans-ferase deficiency results in lung oxidant stress in normoxia. *Am. J. Physiol. Lung Cell Mol. Physiol.* 283:L766–L776.

854. Bo, S., R. Gambino, M. Durazzo, S. Guidi, E. Tiozzo, F. Ghione, L. Gentile, M. Cassader, G. F. Pagano. 2005. Associations between gamma-glutamyl transferase, metabolic abnormalities and inflammation in healthy subjects from a population-based cohort: a possible implication for oxidative stress. *World J. Gastroenterol.* 11:7109–7117.

855. Altuntas, I., N. Delibas, M. Demirci, I. Kilinc, N. Tamer. 2002. The effects of methidathion on lipid peroxidation and some liver enzymes: Role of vitamins E and C. *Arch. Toxicol.* 2002;76:470–473.

856. Mackness, B., P. N. Durrington, M. I. Mackness. Human serum paraoxonase. *Gen. Pharmacol.* 31:329–336.

857. Bajnok, L., I. Seres, Z. Varga, S. Jeges. 2008. Relationship of serum resistin level to traits of metabolic syndrome and serum paraoxonase 1 activity in a population with a broad range of body mass index. *Exp. Clin. Endocrinol. Diabetes* 116:592–599.

858. Nakamura, K., K. Matsunaga. 1998. Susceptibility of natural killer (NK) cells to reactive oxygen species (ROS) and their restoration by the mimics of superoxide dismutase (SOD). *Cancer Biother. Radiopharm.* 13:275–290.

859. Viora, M., M. G. Quaranta, E. Straface, R. Vari, R. Masella, W. Malorni. 2004. Redox imbalance and immune functions: Opposite effects of oxidized low-density lipoproteins and N-acetylcysteine. *Immunology* 104:431–438.

860. Manzella, D., M. Barbieri, E. Ragno, G. Paolisso. 2001. Chronic administration of pharmacologic doses of vitamin E improves the cardiac autonomic nervous system in patients with type 2 diabetes. *Am. J. Clin. Nutr.* 73:1052–1057.

861. Mezzano, D. et al. 2001. Inflammation, not hyperhomocysteinemia, is related to oxidative stress and hemostatic and endothelial dysfunction in uremia. *Kidney Int.* 60:1844–1850.

862. Ceriello, A., N. Bortolotti, E. Motz, S. Lizzio, B. Catone, R. Assaloni, L. Tonutti, C. Taboga. 2001. Red wine protects diabetic patients from meal-induced oxidative stress and thrombosis activation: A pleasant approach to the prevention of cardiovascular disease in diabetes. *Eur. J. Clin. Invest.* 31:322–328.

863. Pawlak, K., D. Pawlak, M. Mysliwiec. 2004. Extrinsic coagulation pathway activation and metallopro-teinase-2/TIMPs system are related to oxidative stress and atherosclerosis in hemodialysis patients. *Thromb. Haemost.* 92:646–653.

864. Schindowski, K., S. Leutner, S. Kressmann, A. Eckert, W. E. Muller. 2001. Age-related increase of oxidative stress-induced apoptosis in mice prevention by Ginkgo biloba extract (EGb761). *J. Neural. Transm.* 108:969–978.

865. Nishio, C., K. Yoshida, K. Nishiyama, H. Hatanaka, M. Yamada. 2000. Involvement of cystatin C in oxidative stress-induced apoptosis of cultured rat CNS neurons. *Brain Res.* 873:252–262.

866. Wolvetang, E. J., K. L. Johnson, K. Krauer, S. J. Ralph, A. W. Linnane. 1994. Mitochondrial respiratory chain inhibitors induce apoptosis. *FEBS Lett.* 339:40–44.

867. Xie, L., X. Zhu, Y. Hu, T. Li, Y. Gao, Y. Shi, S. Tang. 2008. Mitochondrial DNA oxidative damage triggers mitochondrial dysfunction and apoptosis in high glucose-induced HRECs. *Invest. Ophthalmol. Vis. Sci.* 49:4203–4209.

868. Reutelingsperger C. P., W. L. van Heerde, V. Annexin. 1997. The regulator of phosphatidylserine-cata-lyzed inflammation and coagulation during apoptosis. *Cell Mol. Life Sci.* 53:527–532.

869. Tissandie, E., Y. Gueguen, J. M. Lobaccaro, L. Grandcolas, P. Voisin, J. Aigueperse, P. Gourmelon, M. Souidi. 2007. In vivo effects of chronic contamination with depleted uranium on vitamin D3 metabo-lism in rat. *Biochim Biophys Acta* 1770:266–272.

870. Crivello, J. F. 1988. Oxidative stress limits vitamin D metabolism by bovine proximal tubule cells in vitro. *Arch Biochem Biophys* 262:471–480.

871. Adorini, L. 2002. Immunomodulatory effects of vitamin D receptor ligands in autoimmune diseases. *Int. Immunopharmacol.* 2:1017–1028.

872. Cantorna, M. T., B. D. Mahon. 2004. Mounting evidence for vitamin D as an environmental factor affecting autoimmune disease prevalence. *Exp. Biol. Med. (Maywood)* 229:1136–1142.

873. Holick, M. F. 2004. Sunlight and vitamin D for bone health and prevention of autoimmune diseases, cancers, and cardiovascular disease. *Am. J. Clin. Nutr.* 80:1678S–1688S.

874. Holick, M. F. 2005. Vitamin D: Important for prevention of osteoporosis, cardiovascular heart disease, type 1 diabetes, autoimmune diseases, and some cancers. *South Med. J.* 98:1024–1027.

875. Meehan, T. F., H. F. DeLuca. 2002. The vitamin D receptor is necessary for 1alpha,25-dihydroxyvitamin D(3) to suppress experimental autoimmune encephalomyelitis in mice. *Arch. Biochem. Biophys.* 408:200–204.

876. Mostafalou, S., M. Abdollahi. 2013. Pesticides and human chronic diseases: Evidences, mechanisms, and perspectives. *Toxicol. Appl. Pharmacol.* 268(2):157–177.

877. Chinta, S. J., A. Rane, K. S. Poksay, D. E. Bredesen, J. K. Andersen, R. V. Rao. 2008. Coupling endoplasmic reticulum stress to the cell death program in dopaminergic cells: Effect of paraquat. *Neuromolecular Med.* 10(4):333–342.

878. Yang, W., E. Tiffany-Castiglioni, H. C. Koh, I. H. Son. 2009. Paraquat activates the IRE1/ASK1/JNK cascade associated with apoptosis in human neuroblastoma SH-SY5Y cells. *Toxicol. Lett.* 191(2–3):203–210.

879. Chen, Y. Y., G. Chen, Z. Fan, J. Luo, Z. J. Ke. 2008. GSK3beta and endoplasmic reticulum stress mediate rotenone-induced death of SK-N-MC neuroblastoma cells. *Biochem. Pharmacol.* 76(1):128–138.

880. Hossain, M. M., J. R. Richardson. 2011. Mechanism of pyrethroid pesticide-induced apoptosis: Role of calpain and the ER stress pathway. *Toxicol. Sci.* 122(2):512–525.

881. Chen, Y. W. et al. 2010. Pyrrolidine dithiocarbamate (PDTC)/Cu complex induces lung epithelial cell apoptosis through mitochondria and ER-stress pathways. *Toxicol. Lett.* 199(3):333–340.

882. Pesonen, M., M. Pasanen, J. Loikkanen, A. Naukkarinen, M. Hemmila, H. Seulanto, T. Kuitunen, K. Vahakangas. 2012. Chloropicrin induces endoplasmic reticulum stress in human retinal pigment epithelial cells. *Toxicol. Lett.* 211(3):239–245.

883. Skandrani, D., Y. Gaubin, B. Beau, J. C. Murat, C. Vincent, F. Croute, 2006. Effect of selected insecticides on growth rate and stress protein expression in cultured human A549 and SH-SY5Y cells. *Toxicol. In Vitro* 20(8):1378–1386.

884. Skandrani, D., Y. Gaubin, C. Vincent, B. Beau, J. Claude Murat, J. P. Soleilhavoup, F. Croute, 2006. Relationship between toxicity of selected insecticides and expression of stress proteins (HSP, GRP) in cultured human cells: Effects of commercial formulations versus pure active molecules. *Biochim. Biophys. Acta* 1760(1):95–103.

885. Gies, E., I. Wilde, J. M. Winget, M. Brack, B. Rotblat, C. A. Novoa, A. D. Balgi, P. H. Sorensen, M. Roberge, T. Mayor. 2010. Niclosamide prevents the formation of large ubiquitin-containing aggregates caused by proteasome inhibition. *PLoS ONE* 5(12):e14410.

886. Paul, S. 2008. Dysfunction of the ubiquitin–proteasome system in multiple disease conditions: Therapeutic approaches. *Bioessays.* 30(11–12):1172–1184.

887. Sun, F., V. Anantharam, C. Latchoumycandane, A. Kanthasamy, A. G. Kanthasamy. 2005. Dieldrin induces ubiquitin–proteasome dysfunction in alpha-synuclein overexpressing dopaminergic neuronal cells and enhances susceptibility to apoptotic cell death. *J. Pharmacol. Exp. Ther* 315(1):69–79.

888. Chou, A. P., N. Maidment, R. Klintenberg, J. E. Casida, S. Li, A. G. Fitzmaurice, P. O. Fernagut, F. Mortazavi, M. F. Chesselet, J. M. Bronstein. 2008. Ziram causes dopaminergic cell damage by inhibiting E1 ligase of the proteasome. *J. Biol. Chem.* 283(50):34696–34703.

889. Wang, X. F., S. Li, A. P. Chou, J. M. Bronstein. 2006. Inhibitory effects of pesticides on proteasome activity: Implication in Parkinson's disease. *Neurobiol. Dis.* 23(1):198–205.

890. Yang, W., E. Tiffany-Castiglioni. 2007. The bipyridyl herbicide paraquat induces proteasome dysfunction in human neuroblastoma SH-SY5Y cells. *J. Toxicol. Environ. Health A* 70(21):1849–1857.

891. Yang, W., L. Chen, Y. Ding, X. Zhuang, U. J. Kang. 2007. Paraquat induces dopaminergic dysfunction and proteasome impairment in DJ-1-deficient mice. *Hum. Mol. Gene* 16(23):2900–2910.

892. Chou, A. P., S. Li, A. G. Fitzmaurice, J. M. Bronstein. 2010. Mechanisms of rotenone-induced proteasome inhibition. *Neurotoxicology* 31(4):367–372.

893. Gonzalez, C. D., M. S. Lee, P. Marchetti, M. Pietropaolo, R. Towns, M. I. Vaccaro, H. Watada, J. W. Wiley. 2011. The emerging role of autophagy in the pathophysiology of diabetes mellitus. *Autophagy* 7(1):2–11.

894. Levine, B., G. Kroemer. 2008. Autophagy in the pathogenesis of disease. *Cell* 132(1):27–42.

895. Shintani, T., D. J. Klionsky. 2004. Autophagy in health and disease: A double-edged sword. *Science* 306(5698):990–995.

896. Gonzalez-Polo, R. A., M. Niso-Santano, M. A. Ortiz-Ortiz, A. Gomez-Martin, J. M. Moran, L. Garcia-Rubio, J. Francisco-Morcillo, C. Zaragoza, G. Soler, J. M. Fuentes. 2007. Inhibition of paraquat-induced autophagy accelerates the apoptotic cell death in neuroblastoma SH-SY5Y cells. *Toxicol. Sci.* 97(2):448–458.

897. Niso-Santano, M., J. M. Bravo-San Pedro, R. Gomez-Sanchez, V. Climent, G. Soler, J. M. Fuentes, R. A. Gonzalez-Polo. 2011. ASK1 overexpression accelerates paraquat-induced autophagy via endoplasmic reticulum stress. *Toxicol. Sci.* 119(1):156–168.

898. Zucchini-Pascal, N., de Sousa, R. Rahmani. 2009. Lindane and cell death: At the crossroads between apoptosis, necrosis and autophagy. *Toxicology* 256(1–2):32–41.
899. Piotrowska, D., A. Dlugosz, J. Pajak. 2002. Antioxidative properties of coenzyme Q10 and vitamin E in exposure to xylene and gasoline and their mixture with methanol. *Acta Pol. Pharm.* 59:427–432.
900. Golomb, B. A. 2012. Oxidative stress and mitochondrial injury in chronic multisymptom conditions from Gulf War illness to austism spectrum disorder. Gulf War and Mitochondria. *Nature Preceedings*: hdl:10101/npre.2012.6847.1. Posted January 30, 2012.
901. Major Oil Spills. Retrieved November 2, 2008.
902. Binns, J. H. et al. 2004. Research Advisory Committee on Gulf War Veterans' Illnesses: Scientific Progress in Understanding Gulf War Veterans' Illnesses: Report and Recommendations. http://www1. va.gov/rac-gwvi/docs/ReportandRecommendations_2004.pdf
903. Binns, J. H. et al. 2008. *Gulf War Illness and the Health of Gulf War Veterans. Scientific Findings and Recommendations*. Washington DC: U.S. Government Printing Office.
904. Golomb, B. A. 2002. *Mitochondrial function and Gulf War Illnesses. Presentation to the Department of Veterans Affairs Research Advisory Committee on Gulf War Veterans' Illnesses*. Washington DC: November, 2002.
905. Bonnefont-Rousselot D., C. Chantalat-Auger, A. Teixeira, M. C. Jaudon, S. Pelletier, P. Cherin. 2004. Blood oxidative stress status in patients with macrophagic myofasciitis. *Biomed. Pharmacother.* 58:516–519.
906. Gherardi, R. K. 2003. Lessons from macrophagic myofasciitis: Towards definition of a vaccine adjuvantrelated syndrome. *Rev. Neurol. (Paris)* 159:162–164.
907. Gherardi, R. K. et al. 1998. Macrophagic myofascitis: An emerging entity. Group d'Etudes et Recherche sur les Maladies Musculaires Acquises et Dysimmunitaires (GERMMAD) de l'Association Francaise contre les Myopathies (AFM). *Lancet* 352:347–352.
908. Shoenfeld, Y., N. Agmon-Levin. 2011. 'ASIA' - Autoimmune/inflammatory syndrome induced by adjuvants. *J. Autoimmun.* 36:4–8.
909. Neaton, J. D., D. N. Wentworth, L. H. Kuller. 1997. Relationship of serum cholesterol and blood pressure with risk of death from AIDS [Abstract].
910. Jacobs, D. R. J., S. Sidney, K. Feingold, C. Iribarren. 1997. Inverse association between blood total cholesterol and HIV infection, AIDS, and AIDS death: Cause or effect? [Abstract].
911. Villamor, E. 2006. A potential role for vitamin D on HIV infection? *Nutr. Rev.* 64:226–233.
912. Ginde, A. A., J. M. Mansbach, C. A. Camargo Jr. 2009. Vitamin D, respiratory infections, and asthma. *Curr. Allergy. Asthma Rep.* 9:81–87.
913. Walker, V. P., R. L. Modlin. 2009. The Vitamin D Connection to Pediatric Infections and Immune Function. *Pediatr. Res.* 65:106R–113R.
914. Li, J. H. et al. 2006. [Study on association between vitamin D receptor gene polymorphisms and the outcomes of HBV infection]. *Zhonghua Yi Xue Yi Chuan Xue Za Zhi* 23:402–405.
915. Geier, M. R., D. A. Geier. 2004. A case-series of adverse events, positive re-challenge of symptoms, and events in identical twins following hepatitis B vaccination: Analysis of the Vaccine Adverse Event Reporting System (VAERS) database and literature review. *Clin. Exp. Rheumatol.* 22:749–755.
916. Asa, P. B., R. B. Wilson, R. F. Garry. 2002. Antibodies to squalene in recipients of anthrax vaccine. *Exp. Mol. Pathol.* 73:19–27.
917. Kerrison, J. B., D. Lounsbury, C. E. Thirkill, R. G. Lane, M. P. Schatz, R. M. Engler. 2002. Optic neuritis after anthrax vaccination. *Ophthalmology* 109:99–104.
918. Lane, R. G. et al. 2001. Optic neuritis following anthrax vaccination. *Iovs* 42:S326.
919. Hakariya, Y., H. Kuratsune. 2007. [Chronic fatigue syndrome: Biochemical examination of blood]. *Nippon. Rinsho.* 65:1071–1076.
920. Singh, V. K., W. H. Rivas. 2004. Detection of antinuclear and antilaminin antibodies in autistic children who received thimerosal-containing vaccines. *J. Biomed. Sci.* 11:607–610.
921. Singh, V. K. 2007. Thimerosal is unrelated to autoimmune autism. *Pediatr. Allergy Immunol.* 18:89.
922. Valicenti-McDermott, M. D., K. McVicar, H. J. Cohen, B. K. Wershil, S. Shinnar. 2008. Gastrointestinal symptoms in children with an autism spectrum disorder and language regression. *Pediatr. Neurol.* 39:392–398.
923. Mustafic, H. et al. 2012. Main air pollutants and myocardial infarction: A systematic review and meta-analysis. *JAMA* 307:713–721.
924. Pope, C. A.3rd, R. T. Burnett, D. Krewski, M. Jerrett, Y. Shi, E. E. Calle, M. J. Thun. 2009. Cardiovascular mortality and exposure to airborne fine particulate matter and cigarette smoke: Shape of the exposure-response relationship. *Circulation* 120:941–948.

925. Filleul, L. et al. 2006. The relation between temperature, ozone, and mortality in nine French cities during the heat wave of 2003. *Environ. Health Perspect.* 114:1344–1347.

926. Bravo-Alvarez, H. R., R. Torres-Jardón. 2002. Air pollution levels and trends in the México City metropolitan area. In *Urban Air Pollution and Forest: Resources at Risk in the Mexico City Air Basin Ecological Studies.* M. Fenn, L. de Bauer, T. Hernández, eds., vol. 156, pp. 121–159. New York: Springer-Verlag.

927. Molina, L. T. et al. 2007. Air quality in North America's most populous city – overview of the MCMA-2003 campaign. *Atmos. Chem. Phys.* 7:2447–2473.

928. Querol, X. et al. 2008. PM speciation and sources in Mexico during the MILAGRO-2006 Campaign. *Atmos. Chem. Phys.* 8:111–128.

929. Stone, E. A., D. C. Snyder, R. J. Sheesley, A. P. Sullivan, R. J. Weber, J. J. Schauer. 2008. Source apportionment of fine organic aerosol in Mexico City during the MILAGRO experiment 2006. *Atmos. Chem. Phys.* 8:1249–1259.

930. Dorman, D. C., M. F. Struve, M. W. Marshall, C. U. Parkinson, R. A. James, B. A. Wong. 2006. Tissue manganese concentrations in young male rhesus monkeys following subchronic manganese sulphate inhalation. *Toxicol. Sci.* 92:201–210.

931. Pall, M. L. 2013. Electromagnetic fields act via activation of voltage-gated calcium channels to produce beneficial or adverse effects. *J. Cell. Mol. Med.* 17(8):958–965.

932. Hänninen, O. O., R. O. Salonen, K. Koistinen, T. Lanki, L. Barregard, M. Jantunen. 2009. Population exposure to fine particles and estimated excess mortality in Finland from an East European wildfire episode. *J. Expo. Sci. Environ. Epidemiol.* 19:414–422.

933. Tin-Tin-Win-Shwe, D. Mitsushima, S. Yamamoto, A. Fukushima, T. Funabashi, T. Kobayashi, H. Fujimaki. 2008. Changes in neurotransmitter levels and proinflammatory cytokine mRNA expressions in the mice olfactory bulb following nanoparticle exposure. *Toxicol. Appl. Pharmacol.* 226(2):192–198.

934. Lucchini, R., L. Benedetti, S. Borghesi, S. Garattini, G. Parrinello, L. Alessio. 2003. Exposure to neurotoxic metals and prevalence of parkinsonian syndrome in the area of Brescia. *G. Ital. Med. Lav. Ergon.* 25 Suppl(3):88–89.

935. Wegesser, T. C., K. E. Pinkerton, J. A. Last. 2009. California wildfires of 2008: Coarse and fine particulate matter toxicity. *Environ. Health Perspect.* 117(6):893–897.

936. Weinhold, B. 2008. Ozone nation: EPA standard panned by the people. *Environ. Health Perspect.* 116(7):A302–A305.

937. Burke, M. P., T. S. Hogue, M. Ferreira, C. B. Mendez, B. Navarro, S. Lopez, J. A. Jay. 2010. The effect of wildfire on soil mercury concentrations in Southern California watersheds. *Water Air Soil Pollut.* 212(1–4):369–385.

938. Reuters, S. G. 2013. Corrosion may have led to North Dakota pipeline leak, regulators say. *NBC News.*

939. MacPherson, J. 2013. ND Farmer Finds Oil Spill While Harvesting Wheat. *ABC News.*

940. Oil spill threatens Rayong beaches. 2013. www.bangkokpost.com. *Bangkok Post.* Retrieved 31 July 2013.

941. No slick explanation for huge PTT oil spill. 2014. *Post Publishing PCL.* Retrieved November 16, 2014.

942. Enbridge spill at Cushing terminal mostly contained. 2013. Retrieved May 29, 2013.

943. Enbridge: Pipelines Operating Normally Following Cushing Spill. 2013. Retrieved May 29, 2013.

944. Exxon Oil Spill Could Be 40% Larger Than Company Estimates, EPA Figures Show. 2013. *InsideClimate News (USA).* Retrieved April 5, 2013.

945. Refiner Delek Cleaning Up 5,000-Barrel Spill in Arkansas Bayou. 2013. Retrieved May 29, 2013.

946. Cause of Mayflower Exxon-Mobil Oil Spill Still a Mystery. 2013. Retrieved May 29, 2013.

947. K Gallons of Diesel Fuel Leak in Arthur Kill. 2012. NBC (USA). Retrieved November 6, 2012.

948. Alberta Oil Spill: Up To 3,000 Barrels Spill Near Red Deer River Reports Plains Midstream Canada. 2012. *Huffington Post (Canada).* Retrieved June 15, 2012.

949. Vidal, J. 2011. *Nigeria on alert as Shell announces worst oil spill in a decade.* The GuardianLondon: Guardian Media Group. Retrieved December 22, 2011.

950. Oil leaks from cargo ship beached on French coast. 2011. Retrieved January 2, 2012.

951. Chevron Oil Spill Spurs Lawsuit to Freeze 17% of Brazil's Rigs. 2011. Retrieved January 2, 2012.

952. Brazil police to prove Chevron drilling, spill. 2011. *Reuters (Reuters).* Retrieved November 17, 2011.

953. Rena Owners Charged in New Zealand Grounding, Aft Section Sinks. 2012. *Environment News Service.* Retrieved January 18, 2013.

954. Bowen, M. 2013. Shipwreck, damaged reputations and a broke DOC. *Waikato Times.* Retrieved January 18, 2013.

955. Shell North Sea oil spill 'more than 200 tonnes'. 2011. *BBC (The Crown).* Retrieved August 15, 2011.

956. Ruptured pipeline sends oil coursing down the Yellowstone River. 2011. *Billings Gazette (Lee Enterprises)*. Retrieved July 2, 2011.

957. Brown, F. J. China Oil Spill Six Times Size of Singapore: Govt. 2011. (http://www.commondreams.org/headline/2011/07/15-3).

958. Jacobs, A. 2011. China Admits Extent of Spill From Oil Rig. *The New York Times*.

959. Alberta pipeline spill: Rainbow Pipeline spill near Peace River. 2011. *Calgary Herald (Lee Enterprises)*. Retrieved August 24, 2011.

960. Vanderklippe, N. 2011. Cost for oil companies pile up after spill. *The Globe and Mail*.

961. Green activists rap state for not being proactive. 2011. *Hindustan Times (HT Media Limited)*. Retrieved February 9, 2011.

962. Yogesh, N. Coast Guard ends op to control oil spill. 2011. *The Times of India* Bennett: Coleman & Co. Ltd.

963. Tiscali, R. 2011. Nuovo disastro ambientale nel polo industriale di Porto Torres, in pericolo il "Santuario dei Cetacei". *Tiscali (in Italian)*. Retrieved January 27, 2011.

964. Correspondent, NDTV. 2010. Oil leak off Mumbai coast has stopped: Coast Guard sources. NDTV. Retrieved August 12, 2010.

965. Dey, J. 2010. Ships collide near Mumbai. *Mid-Day (MiD DAY Infomedia Ltd.)*.

966. Tatke, S. 2011. Oil spill damage to soil irreversible: Report. *The Times of India (Bennett, Coleman & Co. Ltd.)*. Retrieved 24 January 2011.

967. The Associated Press. 2010. Louisiana Oil Geyser: 20-Foot Oil Leak Shooting Up In Plaquemines Parish After Hit By Tugboat. *The Huffington Post*. Retrieved July 27, 2010.

968. Crews work to shut-in damaged wellhead. 2010. *United States Coast Guard*. Retrieved August 2, 2010.

969. CNN wire staff. 2010. Leaking Barataria Bay oil well capped. *CNN*. Retrieved August 2, 2010.

970. Gallucci, J. 2010. Michigan Oil Spill Update: Oil in Kalamazoo River. *The Long Island Press*. Retrieved July 28, 2010.

971. Lambert, S. 2010. Air quality spurs evacuations in oil spill area. *The Battle Creek Enquirer*. Retrieved July 30, 2010.

972. The Associated Press. 2010. China Oil Spill Grows, Official Warns Of 'Severe Threat'. *The Huffington Post*. Retrieved July 22, 2010.

973. The Associated Press. 2010. China Oil Spill Far Bigger Than Stated, U.S. Expert Says. *The Huffington Post*. Retrieved July 31, 2010.

974. Kloosterman, K. 2010. Egypt Eco-Group HEPCA Reports Red Sea Spill is Capped, Beaches Cleaned. *Green Prophet*.

975. O'Donoghue A. J., J. Smith. 2010. Oil spill in Red Butte Creek threatens waters, wildlife". *The Deseret News*. Retrieved 14 June 2010.

976. AP News/Huffington Post. 2010. Alaska Oil Spill: Trans-Alaska Pipeline Shuts Down 800 Mile Area In North Slope. *AP/Huffington Post*. Retrieved July 29, 2010.

977. Oil leaks from tanker collision off Singapore. 2010. *BBC News*. Retrieved June 7, 2010.

978. Oil spill threatens Singapore coast. 2010. *ABC News*. Retrieved June 7, 2010.

979. Singapore closes popular beaches after oil spill hits coast. 2010. *The Hindu (Chennai, India)*. Retrieved June 7, 2010.

980. Mbachu, D. 2010. Exxon Nigerian Unit Oil Spill Caused by Corrosion. *BusinessWeek*. Retrieved June 11, 2010.

981. Brock, J. 2010. Africa's oil spills are far from U.S. media glare. 100,000 bpd of oil had leaked for a week from a pipeline that has since been mended. *Reuters*. Retrieved May 29, 2010.

982. Vidal, J. 2010. Nigeria's agony dwarfs the Gulf oil spill. The US and Europe ignore it. *The Observer (London)*. Retrieved June 1, 2010.

983. U.S. Coast Guard; U.S. Geological Survey. 2010. Deepwater Horizon MC252 Gulf Incident Oil Budget" (PDF). *National Oceanic and Atmospheric Administration*.

984. Coal carrier Shen Neng 1 oil spill dispersed, says Queensland Government. 2010. *The Herald and Weekly Times*. Retrieved June 7, 2010.

985. Battle to stabilise ship aground near Barrier Reef. 2010. *BBC News*. Retrieved June 7, 2010.

986. Chinese coal ship runs aground, leaks oil. 2010. United Press International. Retrieved June 7, 2010.

987. Gonzalez, A. 2010. Collision Causes Crude Oil Spill in Texas. *The Wall Street Journal*. Retrieved January 24, 2010.

988. Xeuquan, M. 2010. Diesel spill contaminates Yellow River tributaries. *Xinhua News*. Retrieved July 19, 2010.

989. WA oil spill 'one of Australia's worst'. 2009. *ABC News*. Archived from the original on 5 November 2009. Retrieved 5 November 2009.

990. Oil leaking 'five times faster' than thought. 2009. *ABC News*. Archived from the original on 5 November 2009. Retrieved November 5, 2009.

991. Reuters. 2009.

992. *The Namibian*. Archived from the original on June 7, 2011.

993. Oil spill: Qld beaches declared disaster zones. 2009. *ABC News (Australian Broadcasting Corporation)*. Retrieved July 14, 2010.

994. Siggins, L. 2009. Oil slick drifts towards Irish coast as polluter silence hurts clean-up efforts. *The Irish Times*. Retrieved February 18, 2009.

995. Kirkham, C., R. A. Vargas. 2008. Oil spill shuts down 80 miles of river. *New Orleans Times-Picayune*. pp. A1.

996. Oil Spill in North Sea Off Norway http://news.bbc.co.uk/1/hi/world/europe/7140645.stm.

997. Tanker oil spill off S Korea coast. 2007. *Al Jazeera English*. Retrieved November 16, 2008.

998. S Korea declares slick 'disaster'. 2007. *BBC News*. Retrieved November 16, 2008.

999. Fuel spill disaster reported in waters near Russia. 2007. *CNN International*. Retrieved November 16, 2008.

1000. Curiel, J., J. Kay, K. Fagan. November 9, 2007. Spill closes bay beaches as oil spreads, kills wildlife. *San Francisco Chronicle*. Retrieved November 16, 2008.

1001. Usumacinta and Kab 101 Blowout. Retrieved November 16, 2014.

1002. Burnaby Oil Spill. *Ministry of Environment (British Columbia)*. Retrieved 22 April 2012.

1003. Oil spills — Philippines, Indian Ocean and Lebanon. 2006. Greenpeace. Archived from the original on July 30, 2008. Retrieved November 16, 2008.

1004. CITGO Oil Spill (PDF). 2006. Louisiana Department of Environmental Quality. Retrieved November 16, 2008.

1005. Loy, W. 2006. Spill the largest in Slope's history. *Anchorage Daily News*. Retrieved November 16, 2008.

1006. Llano, M. 2005. 44 oil spills found in southeast Louisiana. *MSNBC*.

1007. Response and Prevention Branch Oil Team (May 2006). *Murphy Oil USA Refinery Spill, Chalmette & Meraux, LA Presentation (.PDF)*. U.S. Environmental Protection Agency, Region 6. Retrieved May 27, 2010.

1008. Oil Spill History. *The Mariner Group*. Retrieved November 2, 2008.

1009. University of Delaware Sea Grant Program. Athos 1 Oil Spill. Retrieved May 31, 2010.

1010. Research Planning, Inc. 2005. Preassessment Data Report, The MP-69/Hurricane Ivan Oil Discharges, Mississippi River Delta, Louisiana (pp. 10, 18) (PDF) (Report). Damage Assessment Center, National Oceanic and Atmospheric Administration.

1011. ITOPF. ITOPF Case History: Tasman Spirit. Retrieved November 16, 2014.

1012. van de Veen, H. 2004. "Saving Pakistan's Green Gold" (.PDF). *DGIS-ICD Programme, WWF International*. p. 19. Retrieved June 4, 2010.

1013. Buzzards Bay Oil Spill: Bouchard Barge No. 120. 2010. *Buzzards Bay National Estuary Program*. Retrieved June 4, 2010.

1014. Major Oil Spills. International Tanker Owners Pollution Federation. Retrieved November 2, 2008.

1015. Garcia, R. 2003. The Prestige: One year on, a continuing disaster (.PDF). *WWF-Spain*. Retrieved June 4, 2010.

1016. Wout Broekema. April 2015. *"Crisis-induced learning and issue politicization in the EU"*. Public Administration. doi: 10.1111/padm.12170.

1017. A Synopsis of the Terrorist Threat Facing the O&G Industry. Oil and Gas Industry Terrorism Monitor. Retrieved December 26, 2007.

1018. International Terrorism: The Threat. United Kingdom Home Office. Retrieved December 26, 2007.

1019. Oil spills at Guanabara Bay.

1020. *Trans-Alaska Pipeline Shot By A Drunk*. Retrieved November 16, 2014.

1021. The Land is Dead. 2001. Urhobo Historical Society.

1022. Alarm at oil spill in Ogoniland. 2001. BBC News.

1023. Cabinet frees Greek crew at the Taipei Times.

1024. Oil Spills at thinkquest.org.

1025. Pine River Oil Spill. *Ministry of Environment (British Columbia)*. Retrieved August 18, 2010.

1026. LaBelle, R. Technology Assessment and Research. *Minerals Management Service*. Retrieved June 21, 2010.

1027. Environmental Global Issues Map: New Carissa Oil Spill on the Oregon Coast. 1999. McGraw-Hill. Retrieved February 4, 2011.
1028. Nakhodka. Centre de Documentation de Recherche et d'Expérimentations. Retrieved June 1, 2010.
1029. How do oil spills impact Casco Bay? Report by the Casco Bay Estuary Partnership.
1030. Rhode Island Oil Spill Is More Serious Than Initially Thought. 1996. New York Times.
1031. Fact Sheet: Morris J. Berman Oil Spill (PDF). Retrieved January 5, 2010.
1032. Major Oil Spills in Australia: Kirki, Western Australia. 1991. Australian Maritime Safety Authority.
1033. Hosny, K., D. Al-Ajmi. 1993. Environmental impact of the Gulf War: An integrated preliminary assessment. *Environ. Manag.* 17(4):557–562. doi: 10.1007/BF02394670.
1034. Environmental Warfare. 1991. Persian Gulf War. Retrieved November 16, 2014.
1035. M/V Mega Borg. National Oceanic and Atmospheric Administration. Retrieved October 28, 2009.
1036. American Trader Oil Spill, California Office of Spill Prevention and Response.
1037. Dvarskas, A. 2008. Restoring Injured Natural Resources in the Harbor (PDF). The Tidal Exchange (New York - New Jersey Harbor Estuary Program) (22): p. 3. Retrieved November 12, 2012.
1038. Desvousges, W. H., R. W. Dunford, K. E. Mathews. 1992. Natural Resource Damages Valuation: Arthur Kill Oil Spill (PDF). Association of Environmental and Resource Economists Workshop, Snowbird, Utah. Retrieved November 12, 2012.
1039. Presidente Rivera Spill – June 24, 1989. 2004. University of Delaware Sea Grant Program. Retrieved June 2, 2010.
1040. Oil Spills report from the Air and Waste Management Association.
1041. Nightmare on the Monongahela. 1988. *Time Magazine.*
1042. 1985 Grand Eagle Oil Spill.University of Delaware Sea Grant Program. Retrieved 31 May 2010.
1043. Oil spills and near-misses in Northwest waters. 2002. *Seattle Post Intelligencer (Hearst Seattle Media, LLC).* Retrieved February 4, 2011.
1044. Helton, D., T. Penn. 1999. Putting response and natural resource damage costs in rerspective (PDF). International Oil Spill Conference: 21. Paper ID #114. Retrieved February 4, 2011.
1045. Oil Spills and Disasters. Retrieved November 16, 2008.
1046. ITOPF. ITOPF: TANIO. 1980. Retrieved November 16, 2014.
1047. Burmah Agate. National Oceanic and Atmospheric Administration. Retrieved November 16, 2008.
1048. Atlantic Empress. Centre de Documentation de Recherche et d'Expérimentations. Retrieved November 10, 2008.
1049. Tanker Incidents. Retrieved July 19, 2009.
1050. IXTOC I. National Oceanic and Atmospheric Administration. Retrieved November 3, 2008.
1051. Ixtoc 1 oil spill: Flaking of surface mousse in the Gulf of Mexico. Nature Publishing Group. Retrieved November 3, 2008.
1052. Betelgeuse. Centre de Documentation de Recherche et d'Expérimentations. Retrieved March 15, 2009.
1053. Amoco Cadiz. National Oceanic and Atmospheric Administration. Retrieved November 16, 2008.
1054. Amoco Cadiz. 2010. International Tanker Owners Pollution Federation. Retrieved May 30, 2010.
1055. The Trans-Alaska Pipeline. 2009. The Lay of the Land (The Center for Land Use Interpretation) 32. Retrieved July 28, 2010.
1056. Ekofisk Bravo. Oil Rig Disasters. 2008. Retrieved May 28, 2010.
1057. Fingas, M. 2000. *The Basics of Oil Spill Cleanup* 2nd ed., Boca Raton: Lewis Publishers.
1058. ITOPF. ITOPF: Argo Merchant. 1976. Retrieved November 16, 2014.
1059. Argo Merchant. National Oceanic and Atmospheric Administration. Retrieved November 16, 2008.
1060. McKinney, A. T. v. US – 30 (PDF). 1979. Retrieved July 1, 2009.
1061. Save The River Report (PDF). Retrieved July 1, 2009.
1062. Shell and the N15bn Oil Spill Judgement Debt. 2010. The Daily Independent (Lagos). Retrieved July 27, 2010.
1063. Devanney, J. 2010. *The Strange History of Tank Inerting (PDF).* Center for Tankship Excellence.
1064. http://www.incidentnews.gov/incident/6213.
1065. After 30 years, tankers safer but spills still a threat. 2001. The Associated Press. Retrieved May 28, 2010.
1066. Wood, R. H. 2006. *When Tankers Collide, A Preview.* AuthorHouse. Retrieved May 28, 2010.
1067. Huge oil spill in San Francisco Bay — tanker collision under Golden Gate bridge, California (1971)—on Newspapers.com. Newspapers.com. Retrieved June 25, 2015.
1068. Brief Oil and Gas History of Santa Barbara County from the County of Santa Barbara, California.
1069. The African Queen Shipwreck. 2010. ShipwreckExpo. Retrieved April 28, 2010.
1070. Howard (Delmar, Delaware). 2007. "African Queen". Delmar DustPan. Retrieved May 5, 2010.

1071. Le, P. 1999. Beach town forced to scrape away oil leak — and a chunk of its past. *Seattle Post-Intelligencer* (Hearst Seattle Media, LLC).

1072. Berman. R. 2005. Greenpoint, Maspeth Residents Lobby To Get 55-Year-Old Oil Spill Cleaned Up. *The New York Sun*. Retrieved June 2, 2010.

1073. Carter, H. R. 2003. Oil and California's Seabirds: An Overview (PDF). *Marine Ornithology* 31: p. 2. Retrieved June 2, 2010.

1074. Rintoul, W., S. F. Hodgson. 1990. Drilling Through Time: 75 Years with California's Division of Oil and Gas. Sacramento: Department of Conservation, Division of Oil and Gas pp. 13–15.

1075. Larn, R. 1992. *Shipwrecks of the Isles of Scilly*. Nairn: Thomas & Lochar.

1076. Moller, A. P., T. A. Mousseau. 2009. Reduced abundance of insects and spiders linked to radiation at Chernobyl 20 years after the accident. *Biol. Lett.* 5(3):356–359.

1077. Mousseau, T. A., A. P. Moller. 2011. Landscape portrait: A look at the impacts of radioactive contamination on Chernobyl's wildlife. *Bull. Atomic Sci.* 67(2):38–46.

1078. Kennedy, G., V. A. Spence, M. McLaren, A. Hill, C. Underwood, J. J. Belch. 2005. Oxidative stress levels are raised in chronic fatigue syndrome and are associated with clinical symptoms. *Free Radic. Biol. Med.* 39:584–589.

1079. Kondo, I., M. Yamamoto. 1998. Genetic polymorphism of paraoxonase 1 (PON1) and susceptibility to Parkinson's disease. *Brain Res.* 806:271–273.

1080. Smeitink, J. A. 2003. Mitochondrial disorders: Clinical presentation and diagnostic dilemmas. *J. Inherit. Metab. Dis.* 26:199–207.

1081. Fadic, R., D. R. Johns. 1996. Clinical spectrum of mitochondrial diseases. *Semin. Neurol.* 16:11–20.

1082. Jeyakumar, A., M. E. Williamson, T. M. Brickman, P. Krakovitz, S. Parikh. 2009. Otolaryngologic manifestations of mitochondrial cytopathies. *Am. J. Otolaryngol.* 30:162–165.

1083. Serhatlioglu, S., M. F. Gursu, F. Gulcu, H. Canatan, A. Godekmerdan. 2003. Levels of paraoxonase and arylesterase activities and malondialdehyde in workers exposed to ionizing radiation. *Cell Biochem. Funct.* 21:371–375.

1084. Wood, S. M., C. Beckham, A. Yosioka, H. Darban, R. R. Watson. 2000. Beta-carotene and selenium supplementation enhances immune response in aged humans. *Integr. Med.* 2:85–92.

1085. Momiyama, Y., Y. Suzuki, M. Ohtomo, Y. Atsumi, K. Matsuoka, F. Ohsuzu, M. Kimura. 2002. Cardiac autonomic nervous dysfunction in diabetic patients with a mitochondrial DNA mutation: Assessment by heart rate variability. *Diabetes Care* 25:2308–2313.

1086. Kalousova, M., L. Fialova, J. Skrha, T. Zima, J. Soukupová, I. M. Malbohan, S. Štípek. 2004. Oxidative stress, inflammation and autoimmune reaction in type 1 and type 2 diabetes mellitus. *Prague. Med. Rep.* 105:21–28.

1087. Resch, U., F. Tatzber, A. Budinsky, H. Sinzinger. 2006. Reduction of oxidative stress and modulation of autoantibodies against modified low-density lipoprotein after rosuvastatin therapy. *Br. J. Clin. Pharmacol.* 61:262–274.

1088. Traverso, N., S. Patriarca, E. Balbis, A. L. Furfaro, D. Cottalasso, M. A. Pronzato, P. Carlie, F. Botta, U. M. Marinari, L. Fontana. 2003. Anti malondialdehyde-adduct immunological response as a possible marker of successful aging. *Exp. Gerontol.* 38:1129–1135.

1089. Gearhart, D. A., D. W. Sickles, J. J. Buccafusco, M. A. Prendergast, A. V. Terry, Jr. 2007. Chlorpyrifos, chlorpyrifos-oxon, and diisopropylfluorophosphate inhibit kinesin-dependent microtubule motility. *Toxicol. Appl. Pharmacol.* 218:20–29.

1090. Self-reported illness and health status among Gulf War veterans. 1997. A population-based study. The Iowa Persian Gulf Study Group. *JAMA* 277:238–245.

1091. Bell, I. R., L. Warg-Damiani, C. M. Baldwin, M. E. Walsh, G. E. Schwartz. 1998. Self-reported chemical sensitivity and wartime chemical exposures in Gulf War veterans with and without decreased global health ratings. *Mil. Med.* 163:725–732.

1092. Reid, S., M. Hotopf, L. Hull, K. Ismail, C. Unwin, S. Wessely. 2001. Multiple chemical sensitivity and chronic fatigue syndrome in British Gulf War veterans. *Am. J. Epidemiol.* 153:604–609.

1093. Oliveira, G., L. Diogo, M. Grazina, P. Garcia, A. Ataíde, C. Marques, T. Miguel, L. Borges, A. M. Vicente, C. R. Oliveira. 2005. Mitochondrial dysfunction in autism spectrum disorders: A population-based study. *Dev. Med. Child. Neurol.* 47:185–189.

1094. Bradstreet, J. J., S. Smith, M. Baral, D. A. Rossignol. 2010. Biomarker-guided interventions of clinically relevant conditions associated with autism spectrum disorders and attention deficit hyperactivity disorder. *Altern. Med. Rev.* 15:15–32.

1095. Giulivi, C., Y. F. Zhang, A. Omanska-Klusck, C. Ross-Inta, S. Wong, Irva Hertz-Picciotto, F. Tassone, I. N. Pessah. 2010 Mitochondrial dysfunction in autism. *JAMA* 304:2389–2396.

1096. Johnstone, M. 1977. Mitochondrial calcium overload, a cause of essential hypertension. *Lancet* 1:650–651.

1097. Wilson, F. H. et al. 2004. A cluster of metabolic defects caused by mutation in a mitochondrial tRNA. *Science* 306:1190–1194.

1098. Bowling, A. C., J. B. Schulz, R. H. Brown, Jr., M. F. Beal. 1993. Superoxide dismutase activity, oxidative damage, and mitochondrial energy metabolism in familial and sporadic amyotrophic lateral sclerosis. *J. Neurochem.* 61:2322–2325.

1099. Ilieva, E.V., V. Ayala, M. Jove, E. Dalfó, D. Cacabelos, M. Povedano, M. Josep Bellmunt, I. Ferrer, R. Pamplona, M. Portero-Otín. 2007. Oxidative and endoplasmic reticulum stress interplay in sporadic amyotrophic lateral sclerosis. *Brain* 130:3111–3123.

1100. Van Campen. L. E., W. J. Murphy, J. R. Franks, P. I. Mathias, M. A. Toraason. 2002. Oxidative DNA damage is associated with intense noise exposure in the rat. *Hear Res.* 164:29–38.

1101. Bai, U., M. D. Seidman, R. Hinojosa, W. S. Quirk. 1997. Mitochondrial DNA deletions associated with aging and possibly presbycusis: A human archival temporal bone study. *Am. J. Otol.* 18:449–453.

1102. Seidman, M. D., N. Ahmad, D. Joshi, J. Seidman, S. Thawani, W. S. Quirk. 2004. Age-related hearing loss and its association with reactive oxygen species and mitochondrial DNA damage. *Acta Otolaryngol. Suppl.* 16–24.

1103. Seidman, M. D., M. J. Khan, U. Bai, N. Shirwany, W. S. Quirk. 2000. Biologic activity of mitochondrial metabolites on aging and age-related hearing loss. *Am. J. Otol.* 21:161–167.

1104. Ozgocmen, S., H. Kaya, E. Fadillioglu, R. Aydogan, Z. Yilmaz. 2006. Role of antioxidant systems, lipid peroxidation, and nitric oxide in postmenopausal osteoporosis. *Mol. Cell Biochem.* 295:45–52.

1105. Varanasi, S. S., R. M. Francis, C. E. Berger, S. S. Papiha, H. K. Datta. 1999. Mitochondrial DNA deletion associated oxidative stress and severe male osteoporosis. *Osteoporos. Int.* 10:143–149.

1106. Ochoa, J. J., J. L. Quiles, E. Planells, M. López-Frías, J. R. Huertas, J. Mataix. 2005. Lifelong supplementation with coenzyme Q10 protects from bone mineral density loss in rats during aging. *Fourth Conference of the International Coenzyme Q10 Association, Conference Proceedings 2005,* Los Angeles, 149–150.

1107. Sakaue, S., J. Ohmuro, T. Mishina, H. Miyazaki, E. Yamaguchi, M. Nishimura, M. Fujita, K. Nagashima, S. Tagami, Y. Kawakami. 2002. A case of diabetes, deafness, cardiomyopathy, and central sleep apnea: Novel mitochondrial DNA polymorphisms. *Tohoku. J. Exp. Med.* 196:203–211.

1108. Kang, H. K., B. Li, C. M. Mahan, S. A. Eisen, C. C. Engel. 2009. Health of US veterans of 1991 Gulf War: A follow-up survey in 10 years. *J. Occup. Environ. Med.* 51:401–410.

1109. Iversen, A., T. Chalder, S. Wessely. 2007. Gulf War Illness: Lessons from medically unexplained symptoms. *Clin. Psychol. Rev* 27:842–854.

1110. Haley, R. W. 2000. Will we solve the Gulf War syndrome puzzle by population survey or clinical research? *Am. J. Med.* 109:744–748.

1111. Urnovitz, H. B., J. J. Tuite, J. M. Higashida, W. H. Murphy. 1999. RNAs in the sera of Persian Gulf War veterans have segments homologous to chromosome 22q11.2. *Clin. Diagn. Lab. Immunol.* 6(3):330–335. PMCID: PMC103718.

1112. Haley, R. W., T. L. Kurt. 1997. Self-reported exposure to neurotoxic chemical combinations in the Gulf War. A .cross-sectional epidemiologic study. *JAMA* 277:231–237.

1113. Steele, J. 2003. 2 marines who balked at vaccine deployed. *San Diego Union Tribune.*

1114. Heaton, K. J., C. L. Palumbo, S. P. Proctor, R. J. Killiany, D. A. Yurgelun-Todd, R. F. White. 1991. Quantitative magnetic resonance brain imaging in US army veterans of the 1991 Gulf War potentially exposed to sarin and cyclosarin. *Neurotoxicology* 28:761–769.

1115. Pizzichini, M., M. Fonzi, L. Sugherini, L. Fonzi, M. Comporti, A. Gasparoni, A. Pompella. 2002. Release of mercury from dental amalgam and its influence on salivary antioxidant activity. *Sci. Total Environ.* 284:19–25.

1116. Stewart C. 1977. Radiation exposure in our daily lives. *The Physics Teacher.* 15:135. doi: http://dx.doi.org/10.1119/1.2339571.

1117. Jackson, R. B. et al. 2011. Methane contamination of drinking water accompanying gas-well drilling and hydraulic fracturing. *PNAS* 108:8172–8176.

2 Outdoor Air Pollution
Entry and Injury

INTRODUCTION

Pollutant entry and injury can take many pathways to cause chemical sensitivity and chronic degenerative disease. This volume in our series will introduce the pollutant entry to various organs and systems and how the body handles them. Pollutants include inorganic and organic chemicals, pesticides, natural gas, formaldehyde, molds, mycotoxins, terpenes, bacteria, viruses, electromagnetic field (EMF), etc. The body has three choices if it cannot reject the entry. It has to utilize, sequester, or detoxify the pollutant. The first three chapters deal with pollutant entry and often how the body initially deals with these entries, which are now legion. At times, the pollutants can be overwhelming, severely damaging the local region of entry like the cellular membranes and immediate tissue, or damage the region or at times the whole body. Depending upon the timing that the clinician sees the patient and the patient's ability to aid the physician can help the entry to be reversed without endogenous damage. At times, we are better with infectious disease in some areas but we as clinicians must do a better job at defining and reversing injury from molds, mycotoxins, toxic chemicals, and EMF before fatal end-organ damage occurs. The awareness of pollutant entry and injury can present the clinician the opportunity to prevent and at times completely reverse the disease before it becomes fatal.

MECHANISMS OF POLLUTANT ENTRY AND INJURY

Pollutant entry can be through nasal–brain, pulmonary, skin, GI, or GU tract. Mechanisms for environmental incitant changes in the body can be broken down into changes in the physiology of the brain and body's local anatomy, that is, membrane barrier leaks, physiology of the connective tissue, and the homeostatic, that is, local metabolism and how it handles oxidative stress (OS) and finally inflammation. Changes in physiology can be local, regional, central, or systemic as the incitant(s) enter and are dispersed throughout the body. The pollutant entry triggers the physiologic alarm system and the body increases its physiology to accommodate the foreign invader(s) in an effort to obtain homeostasis. These triggering mechanisms can be biological, chemical, or EMF stimulated. Once the body deals with the incitant(s), physiology by parking, eliminating, or neutralizing it, the metabolism equalizes homeostasis and returns to normal. The incitant(s) have been utilized, catabolized, or parked in some areas of the brain or other body parts or are systemic, going to the liver and kidney for further detoxification. If the incitant(s) persist, OS occurs while many physiologic changes occur. This process puts a strain on the nutrient pools and many changes in proteins, lipids, RNA, DNA, etc. occur. These incitants persist either in smaller or larger volumes, which trigger local response and then generalize system response, resulting in oxidative stress; if not controlled, inflammation occurs. Then, pathophysiological changes may occur, leading to local and/or general pathological process. It is up to the clinician and patient to stop the pollutant entry and reverse the metabolic process, which leads to the OS and inflammation before fixed-named disease occurs.

CENTRAL NERVOUS SYSTEM POLLUTANT INJURY

The brain handles pollutant entry a little differently than the rest of the body because toxics in the chemically sensitive and chronic degenerative diseases can go directly up the olfactory nerve and into the brain. It also goes into the brain to the prefrontal cortex instead of the limbic system as it does in a normal individual. The brain also handles waste management differently, making the chemically sensitive more vulnerable.

An example of how the brain demonstrates its ability to handle its waste is shown by Nedergaard[1]: This physiologic process is a prime example of neuroanatomy and physiology which differs from the rest of the body. The brain has just been found to have lymphatics but these physiologies have aberrations and other pathways to remove toxic fluids to join the lymphatics in the neck to eliminate wastes. This anatomy apparently disturbs the chemically sensitive physiology, making it more difficult to obtain and maintain homeostasis. It shows an intracellular and extracellular lymphatic pathway that is stressed by common pollutants and how it must be functioning and responding to incitant(s) entry. This particular physiology only shows the brain's anatomy and physiology plus both blood and lymphatics of the rest of the body are well known as to how they handle, metabolize, and park pollutants. The brain has drainage to the lymphatic system as described in the following paragraphs.

According to Nedergaard,[1] essentially all neurodegenerative diseases are associated with misaccumulation of cellular waste products, no matter the triggering agents, whether pesticide, solvents, mycotoxins, heavy metal, particulates, etc. Of these, misfolded or hyperphosphorylated proteins are among the most difficult for the brain to dispose. For example, tau- and beta-amyloid (Aβ) can accumulate as stable aggregates that are neurotoxic in conditions such as Alzheimer's disease (AD).[2] Intracellular proteasomal degradation and autophagy are considered the principal means for removing proteins in the central nervous system (CNS), and the dysfunction of each has been causally associated with neurodegeneration.[3] Yet, many cytosolic proteins are released into the interstitial space in the brain, suggesting that extracellular disposal routes may also eliminate waste.[4] As previously stated, Ca^{2+} attached to protein kinases A and C and then phosphorylated increases sensitivity up to 1000 times which makes hypersensitivity to pollutants such as molds, chemical toxics, mycotoxins, EMF, etc. an integral part of the clinical milieu telegraphing the problems the body has with the total environmental pollutant load. This hypersensitivity allows the clinician a set of obvious symptoms and signs that shows him/her the devastating effects of pollution and how it needs nutrition to counteract and repair pollutant entry and injury.

Throughout the body's tissue, bulk flow of the fluid between cells, into the blood or lymph, plays an important role in the removal of potentially toxic metabolic by-products. Lymphatic vessels are the principal means by which tissues eliminate excess fluid and proteins from the body, although the density of lymph vessels generally correlates with tissue metabolic rate.[5] Thus, it is puzzling because the high metabolic activity of neurons predicts the need for rapid elimination of their metabolic by-products. It was long thought that the movement of the cerebrospinal fluid (CSF), which is produced in the choroid plexus of the brain and flows through its ventricles and basal cisterns, constitutes a "sink" for waste products to diffuse from the brain, for eventual clearance to the general circulation. However, the large tissue distances in most of the brain prevent diffusion and bulk flow from making this process efficient. Albumin, for instance, would require more than 100 hours to diffuse through 1 cm of brain tissue.[6]

Two-photon imaging of live mice through a closed cranial window has since permitted the direct observation of CSF movement through the intact brain. This technique revealed that CSF is exchanged rapidly with interstitial fluid (ISF) in the brain by a highly organized, brain-wide pathway that consists of three serial elements: a para-arterial CSF influx route, a paravenous ISF clearance route, and an intracellular trans-astrocytic path that couples the two extracellular paravascular routes.[7] Specifically, CSF passes through the para-arterial space that surrounds arteries; the space is bound by the abluminal surface of the blood vessel and the apical processes of astrocytes. Water channels called aquaporin 4 (AQP4) on the vascular endfeet of astrocytes[8] facilitate convective flow out of the para-arterial space and into the interstitial space (Figure 2.1).

As CSF exchanges with ISF, vectorial convective fluxes drive waste products away from the arteries and toward the veins. ISF and its constituents then enter the paravenous space. As ISF exits the

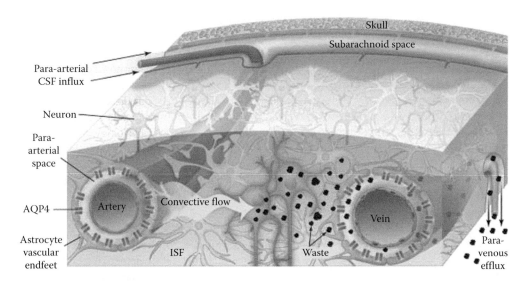

FIGURE 2.1 **(See color insert.)** ECF flowing outside the blood vessels in para-arterial spaces on the end-feet of astrocytes: The lymphatic system (glia water channels). (From Nedergaard, M. 2013. Neuroscience. Garbage truck of the brain. *Science* 340 (6140):1529–1530. Reprinted with permission from AAAS.)

brain through the paravenous route, it reaches the lymphatic vessels in the neck, and eventually returns its contents to the systemic circulation. Radio-labeled tracer studies indicate that 40%–80% of large proteins and solutes are removed from the brain through this macroscopic clearance pathway.[7]

CSF can also exit through the arachnoid villi, which extend through the outer protective membrane layer of the brain and allow CSF to exit to the bloodstream, as well as at sites along the cavity and craniospinal nerve roots.

Regardless of the route, its solutes and proteins ultimately reach the liver, where they are degraded. As such, the glymphatic system, so named for its dependence on glial water channels and its adoption of a clearance function similar to that of the peripheral lymphatic system, avoids the need for local protein processing and degradation. Instead, it facilitates transport to the same central excretion and recycling sites used by other peripheral tissues.

Studies of mice genetically engineered to lack AQP4 showed that fluid flux through the glymphatic pathway relies on specific expression of this water channel along the apical membrane of vascular endfeet of astrocytes.[7] When AQP4 is mislocated to the cell body of astrocytes or to astrocytic processes that do not abut the vasculature, as observed in traumatic brain injury or stroke,[9,10] clearance of soluble proteins through the glymphatic system declines substantially. This condition can cause much brain dysfunction and difficulty in restoring normal function.

An interesting question is whether the glymphatic system plays a role in spreading fibrillary tau aggregates through the interstitial space in neurodegenerative disease. The injection of brain extracts from mice containing an aggregation-prone form of human tau protein, into the brains of mice expressing wild-type human tau, induces self-assembly of the wild-type human tau into filaments. This results in the pathological spread of tau aggregates from the injection site to distant brain regions.[3,4,11] It severely disturbs homeostasis or at times makes it impossible.

Perhaps the most persuasive example of CSF recycling as the cause of dispersing the initial seeds of tau tangles is after traumatic brain injury. A large percentage of chemically sensitive patients have had previous head injuries which may be a factor in them developing their chemical sensitivity. As a result of axon damage, the tau concentration in CSF increases by as much as a factor of 40,000.[12] Consequently, as the heavily tau-laden CSF enters the brain tissue through the para-arterial space, it is taken up by cells closest to the paravascular boundary, thereby generating the typical paravascular predominance of tau-immunoreactive neurofibrillary tangles (NFT).[13] Similarly, glymphatic CSF influx may also act as a constant source for delivering Aβ, which could contribute to the growth of para-arterial deposits in cerebral amyloid angiopathy. In turn, the same para-arterial space that normally functions as a low-resistance influx path for CSF will narrow as the amyloid plaques enlarge, slowing glymphatic clearance and thus accelerating amyloid deposition.[14] Amyloid deposits from pollutant injury are seen in dogs and individuals living in Mexico City pollution.[15]

Such studies of the multiple pathways involved in glymphatic clearance may identify new targets for treating neurodegenerative diseases. For example, mislocation of AQP4 water channels may contribute to neurodegenerative disease progression. Thus, potentiating the insertion and activity of AQP4 channels in astrocytic vascular endfeet might mitigate or even reverse the course of protein-associated neurodegenerative disorders. The process of decreasing the total environmental pollutant load by living and working in five times less polluted building and fasting followed by a rotary diet may aid in this reversal.

Can the efficiency of glymphatic clearance be assessed? Preclinical analysis in rats shows that magnetic resonance imaging can provide a brain-wide map of both glymphatic influx and efflux, by which clearance kinetics can be derived and compared across subjects.[16,17] Triple-camera brain SPECT scans appear even more precise for the toxic expression. By extending this approach to humans, it may be possible to identify patients at risk for developing AD who would benefit from therapeutic intervention before symptomatic neurodegeneration ensues. We try to do this intervention on chemically sensitive patients who manifest cerebral confusion, mental abbreviations, short-term memory loss, and inability to stand on toes or walk a straight line. Similarly, this type of analysis might allow the monitoring of treatment responses, as well as the identification of environmental and genetic markers that predict enhanced susceptibility to glymphatic decline. Triggering agents must be found, compartmentalized, eliminated, or neutralized. Such an approach may also be suitable for victims of brain injury who develop chronic traumatic encephalopathy, which is characterized by paravascular tau tangles and premature neuronal degeneration[13] which then are triggered by low intensity, molds, mycotoxins, volatile organic hydrocarbons (HC), pesticides, formaldehydes, EMF, etc. There are currently no definitive diagnostics that identify susceptible individuals, and thus no means by which to achieve early clinical intervention. However, the chemically sensitive patient who has fuzzy thinking, short-term memory loss, brain fog, etc. may be the clinical symptoms which can be used for early intervention by removing the environmental triggering agents and thus removing the impediments to the egress of toxic cerebral flow. Thus, with reduction of the total body pollutant load, these neurodegenerative diseases may be prevented. Recognition that the brain, like all other organs, uses both local and organ-wide mechanisms for clearing interstitial protein waste may offer new insights into the pathophysiology and prophylaxis of neurodegeneration, as well as injuries and proteinopathies of the human CNS. Patients with long-term chemical sensitivity and chronic fatigue may fall into the category of Parkinson's disease (PD), multiple sclerosis, or AD or the chronic head injury modalities or all of the mentioned. When looking for optimum function and a reduction of acute and chronic brain dysfunction, their glymphatic system in the brain is plugged or narrowed distributing toxic fluid flow egress, causing their neurodegenerative problem.

OXIDATIVE STRESS RESPONSE OF EMF IN ADDITION TO CHEMICAL STRESS IN MEMBRANE AND INTRACELLULAR FUNCTION

The most important concept is how does the body respond to pollutant entry once it crosses or is involved with membrane changes.

Selye[18] described how the body responds and adapts to stressors of various types. This process occurs when the individual has demands on the homeostatic mechanisms.[18] This mechanism deals with each pollutant to bring the body's physiology to equilibrium. Chronic psychological stress has long been linked to a variety of morbidity and mortality end points but no one sees good anatomical and physiological proofs. However, pollutant and EMF stress of electrical impulses flow in brain

TABLE 2.1

Autonomic Nervous System Responses of 1000 Chemically Sensitive Patients

		Number of Patients
30% Sympathetic ↑ — Parasympathetic →		300
60% Sympathetic ↑ — Parasympathetic ↓		600
10% Sympathetic → — Parasympathetic ↓		100

Source: Environmental Health Center-Dallas.

and nerves is similar to psychological stress. It is difficult to separate the etiology of chronic pollutants and especially EMF exposure from psychological problems unless the clinician is aware of this fact and works in less polluted controlled environments. According to Didriksen,[19] there is a series of clinical psychological tests she and Butler[20] have developed to differentiate the psychological from the physical. The initial fight or flight reaction causes increased sympathetic nervous system and at times a decrease in parasympathetic activity as measured in over 1000 patients at the EHC-Dallas by heart rate variability and pupilography (Table 2.1).

The adrenal glands release epinephrine and norepinephrine into the bloodstream, either at higher levels or receive a block of the parasympathetic nervous system still resulting in an increase in functional adrenal response.

The adrenal glands also release corticosteroid hormones. We see these different patterns in the measurement of the heart rate variability for the autonomic NS response. We usually see in both the chemically sensitive and electrically sensitive patients either a sympathetic stimulation or asympathetic stimulation with a parasympathetic decrease, or occasionally we find a parasympathetic decrease only and with a sympathetic being normal. The latter gives a sympathetic output and thus an adrenalin response. In any of these situations, digestion stops, blood pressure and pulse rate increases, the heart pumps more blood to the muscles, and blood sugar levels increase. This acute response to EMF will mimic the psychological response syndrome because the physiology is similar without vasoconstriction, decrease in local fluid flow through the lymphatic, and cause local tissue hypoxia yielding local edema.

If stress is chronic, epinephrine and norepinephrine levels decline, but corticosteroid secretion continues at above normal levels. Chronic disturbance of the catecholamine or corticosteroid system by mycotoxin, food, chemical, or the electrical stimulation inevitably results in disease. *In vitro* studies of cellular stress show that heat shock or stress proteins are induced in cells by nonthermal EMFs.[21] These repair proteins can cause healing or damage repair, depending on their output.

MEMBRANE CHANGES WITH POLLUTANT ENTRY

Chemical pollutants, including EMFs, can also cause single- and double-strand DNA breaks,[22] increase permeability of the blood–brain barrier,[23] and cause influx of calcium into cells.[24] These aberrations can cause a multitude of problems one of which is the Ca^{2+} entry process. Leaks in the intracellular membrane occur by exposure to pollutants like NO, CO, SO_2, particulates, phenols, formaldehyde, natural gas, insecticides, molds, mycotoxins, bacteria, viruses, EMF, etc. With pollutant entry and injury, there is a decrease in tight junction proteins, evidence of individual cell damage, and upregulation of VCAM/ICA ratio in the vasculature all of which suggest failure of the physical barriers. This pollutant produces proinflammatory signals which may distribute reactive oxygen species (ROS), cytokines (CKs), and particulate matter (PM) to the tissue involved. The variable chemical and physiological characteristics of pollution are the activation of multiple pathways, which result in OS and inflammation. This influx of Ca^{2+} combines with protein kinases

A and C and when phosphorylated, it causes hypersensitivity up to 1000 times which can cause a vicious cycle and spreading of new sensitivities to multiple molds, foods, and chemicals which then can cause more pathology. It also can trigger the nitric oxide mechanisms reacting with hydrogen or superoxide nitrates, creating OS, inflammation, and disease process like neurodegeneration.[24]

The Ca^{2+} helps release a series of enzymes like protein kinases A and C, endonuclease, nitric oxide synthase, and endolymph protease. There is an almost instant change, releasing nitric oxide. Ca^{2+} also has a role in signal transduction, regulating energy output, cell metabolism, and pheno-typical expression of cell hosts.

An understanding of the complex biology of the effects of EMFs on human/higher animal biology inevitably must be derived from an understanding of the target or targets of such fields in the impacted cells and tissues. Despite this, no understanding has been forthcoming on what those targets are and how they may lead to the complex biological responses to EMFs composed of low-energy photons. According to Pall,[25] the great puzzle, here, is that these EMFs comprise low-energy photons, those with insufficient energy to individually influence the chemistry of the cell, raising the question of how nonthermal effects of such EMFs can possibly occur. Pall[25] has found that there is a substantial literature possibly pointing to the direct targets of such EMFs and it is the goal of his study to review that evidence as well as review how those targets may lead to the complex biology of EMF exposure.

According to Pall,[25] the role of increased intracellular Ca^{2+} following EMF exposure was already well documented more than 20 years ago when Walleczek[26] reviewed the role of changes in calcium signaling that were produced in response to EMF exposures. Other, more recent studies have confirmed the role of increased intracellular Ca^{2+} following EMF exposure. His review[26] included two studies[27,28] that showed that the L-type voltage-gated channel blocker, verapamil, could lower or block changes in response to EMFs. The properties of voltage-gated calcium channels (VGCCs) have been reviewed elsewhere.[29] Subsequently, extensive evidence has been published showing that the EMF exposure can act to produce excessive activity of the VGCCs in many cell types,[30–51] suggesting that these may be direct targets of EMF exposure. Many of these studies implicate specifically the L-type VGCCs such that various L-type calcium channel blockers can block responses to EMF exposure. However, other studies have shown lowered responses produced by other types of calcium channel blockers, including N-type and P/Q-type blockers, showing that other VGCCs may have important roles.[25] Diverse responses to EMFs are reported to be blocked by such calcium channel blockers, suggesting that most, if not all, EMF-mediated responses may be produced through VGCC stimulation.[25] VGCCs are essential to the responses produced by extremely low-frequency (including 50/60 Hz) EMFs and also to microwave frequency range EMFs, nanosecond EMF pulses, and static electrical and magnetic fields.

In a recent study, Pilla[52] showed that an increase in intracellular Ca^{2+} must have occurred almost immediately after EMF exposure, producing a Ca^{2+}/calmodulin-dependent increase in nitric oxide occurring in less than 5 seconds. Although Pilla[52] did not test whether VGCC stimulation was involved in his study, there are few alternatives that can produce such a rapid Ca^{2+} response, none of which has been implicated in EMF responses. Other studies, each involving VGCCs, also showed rapid Ca^{2+} increase following EMF exposures.[33,41,42,44,46] The rapidity of these responses rule out many types of regulatory interactions as being involved in producing the increased VGCC activity following EMF exposure and suggests, therefore, that VGCC stimulation in the plasma membrane is directly produced by EMF exposure.

According to Pall,[25] the increased intracellular Ca^{2+} produced by such VGCC activation may lead to multiple regulatory responses, including the increased nitric oxide levels produced through the action of the two Ca^{2+}/calmodulin-dependent nitric oxide synthases, nNOS, and eNOS. Increased nitric oxide levels typically act in a physiological context through increased synthesis of cGMP and subsequent activation of protein kinase G.[53,54] In contrast, in most pathophysiological contexts, nitric oxide reacts with superoxide to form peroxynitrite, a potent nonradical oxidant,[55,56] which can produce radical products, including hydroxyl radical and NO_2 radical.[57]

According to Pall,[25] as was noted above, most of the pathophysiological effects of nitric oxide are mediated through peroxynitrite elevation, resulting in consequent OS. There are many reviews and other studies implicating OS in generating pathophysiological effects of EMF exposure. In some of these studies, the rise in OS markers parallels the rise in nitric oxide, suggesting a peroxynitrite-mediated mechanism. Many toxics, including EMF, can trigger this mechanism.

Peroxynitrite elevation is usually measured through a marker of peroxynitrite-mediated protein nitration, 3-nitrotyrosine (3-N). There are four studies where 3-NT levels were measured before and after EMF exposure.[58–61] Each of these studies provides some evidence supporting the view that EMF exposure increases levels of peroxynitrite and therefore 3-NT levels.[58–61] Although these cannot be taken as definitive, when considered along with the evidence on OS and elevated nitric oxide production in response to EMF exposure, they strongly suggest a peroxynitrite-mediated mechanism of OS in response to EMFs.

According to Pall,[25] such a peroxynitrite-mediated mechanism may explain the many studies showing the single-stranded breaks in DNA, as shown by alkaline comet assays or the similar microgel electrophoresis assay, following EMF exposures in most such studies,[62–81] but not in all.[81–88] Some of the factors that are reported to influence whether such DNA single-strand breaks are detected after EMF exposure include the type of cell studied,[68,77] dosage of EMF exposure,[69] and the type of EMF exposure studied.[64,68] Exudative stress and free radicals have roles, both because there is a concomitant increase in OS and antioxidants (AOs) have been shown to greatly lower the generation of DNA single-strand breaks following EMF exposure[63,66,72,73] as has also been shown for peroxynitrite-mediated DNA breaks produced under other conditions. It has also been shown that one can block the generation of DNA single-strand breaks with nitric oxide synthase inhibitors.[73]

Peroxynitrite has been shown to produce single-strand DNA breaks,[89–91] a process that is inhibited by many but not all AOs.[90,91] It can be seen from this that the data on generation of single-strand DNA breaks, although quite limited, support a mechanism involving nitric oxide/peroxynitrite/free radical (OS). Although the data on the possible role of peroxynitrite in EMF-induced DNA single-strand breaks are limited, what data are available supports such a peroxynitrite role.

The EMFs composed of low-energy photons produce nonthermal biological changes, both pathophysiological and, in some cases, potentially therapeutic, in humans and higher animals.

It may be asked why we have evidence for the involvement of VGCCs in response to EMF exposure but no similar evidence for the involvement of voltage-gated sodium channels? Perhaps, the reason is that there are many important biological effects produced in increased intracellular Ca^{2+}, including but not limited to nitric oxide elevation, but much fewer are produced by elevated Na^+.

The possible role of peroxynitrite as opposed to protein kinase G in producing pathophysiological responses to EMF exposure raises the question of whether there are practical approaches to avoiding such responses? Typically, peroxynitrite levels can be highly elevated when both of its precursors, nitric oxide and superoxide, are high. Consequently, agents that lower nitric oxide synthase activity and agents that raise superoxide dismutases (SODs; the enzymes that degrade superoxide) such as phenolics and other Nrf2 activators that induce SOD activity,[92] as well as calcium channel blockers may be useful.

Although the various EMF exposures as well as static electrical field exposures can act to change the electrical voltage gradient across the plasma membrane and may, therefore, be expected to stimulate VGCCs through their voltage-gated properties, it may be surprising that static magnetic fields also act to activate VGCCs because static magnetic fields do not induce electrical changes on static objects. However, cells are far from static. Such phenomena as cell ruffling[93,94] may be relevant, where thin cytoplasmic sheets bounded on both sides by plasma membrane move rapidly. Such rapid movement of the electrically conducting cytoplasm may be expected to involve the electrical charge across the plasma membrane, thus potentially stimulating the VGCCs.

Earlier modeling of electrical effects across plasma membranes of EMF exposures suggested that such electrical effects were likely to be too small to explain EMF effects at levels reported to produce biological changes.[47] However, more recent and presumably more biologically plausible modeling have suggested that such electrical effects may be much more substantial[95–100] and may, therefore, act to directly stimulate VGCCs.

According to Pall, direct stimulation of VGCCs by partial depolarization across the plasma membrane is suggested by the following observations:

1. The very rapid, almost instantaneous increase in intracellular Ca^{2+} found in some studies following EMF exposure.[33,41,42,44,46,52] The rapidity here means that most, if not all indirect, regulatory effects can be ruled out.
2. The fact that not just L-type, but three additional classes of VGCCs are implicated in generating biological responses to EMF exposure, suggesting that their voltage-gated properties may be a key feature in their ability to respond to EMFs.
3. Most, if not all, EMF effects are blocked by VGCC channel blockers.
4. Modeling of EMF effects on living cells suggests that plasma membrane voltage changes may have key roles in such effects.[95–99] Saunders and Jefferys stated[101] that "it is well established that electric fields … or exposure to low frequency magnetic fields, will, if of sufficient magnitude, excite nerve tissue through their interactions with voltage gated ion channels." They further state[101] that this is achieved by direct effects on the electric dipole voltage sensor within the ion channel.

One question that is not answered by any of the available data is whether what is known as "dirty electricity,"[102–104] generated by rapid, in many cases, wave transients in EMF exposure, also acts by stimulating VGCCs. Such dirty electricity is inherent in any digital technology because digital technology is based on the use of such square wave transients and it may, therefore, be of special concern in this digital era, but there have been no tests of such dirty electricity that determine whether VGCCs have roles in response to such fields to our knowledge. The nanosecond pulses, which are essentially very brief, but high-intensity dirty electricity does act, at least in part, via VGCC stimulation, suggesting that dirty electricity may do likewise.

The only detailed alternative to the mechanism of nonthermal EMF effects discussed here, to our knowledge, is the hypothesis of Friedman et al.[105] and supported by Desai et al.[106] where the apparent initial response to EMF exposure was proposed to be NADH oxidase activation, leading to OS and downstream regulatory effects. Although they provide some correlative evidence for a possible role of NADH oxidase,[105] the only causal evidence is based on a presumed specific inhibitor of NADH oxidase, diphenyleneiodonium (DPI). However, DPI has been shown to be a nonspecific channel blocker,[107] clearly showing a lack of such specificity and suggesting that it may act, in part as a VGCC blocker. Consequently, a causal role for NADH oxidase in responses to EMF exposure must be considered to be undocumented.

In summary, the nonthermal actions of EMFs composed of low-energy photons have been a great puzzle because such photons are insufficiently energetic to directly influence the chemistry of cells. The current review provides support for a pathway of the biological action of ultralow-frequency and microwave EMF's nanosecond pulses and static electrical or magnetic fields: EMF activation of VGCCs leads to rapid elevation of intracellular Ca^{2+}, nitric oxide, and in some cases at least, peroxynitrite. Potentially therapeutic effects may be mediated through the Ca^{2+}/nitric oxide/cGMP/ protein kinase G pathway. Pathophysiological effects may be mediated through the Ca^{2+}; mediated effects may have roles as well, as suggested by Xu et al.[51] Certainly, biological, and chemical, particulates can trigger this mechanism, also resulting in OS.

Certainly, pacemakers, electroshock to restore proper rhythm, muscle stimulations, etc., work on the principle of activation of VGCC channels and the rapid change phenomena.

THERAPEUTIC EFFECT OF EMF ON BONE REPAIR

An example of a therapeutic effect for bone repair of electrical exposure in various medical situations includes increasing osteoblast differentiation and maturation and has been reviewed repeatedly by Becker and Marino.[108–119] The effects of EMF exposure on bone cannot be challenged although there is still considerable question about the best ways to apply this clinically.[108–119] Our focus here is to consider possible mechanisms of action. Multiple studies have implicated increased Ca^{2+} and nitric oxide in the EMF stimulation of bone growth[119–124]; they have also implicated increased cGMP and protein kinase G activity.[121,123,124] In addition, studies on other regulatory stimuli leading to increased bone growth have also implicated increased cGMP levels and protein kinase G in this response.[125–131] In summary, then, it can be seen from the above that there is a very well-documented action of EMFs in stimulating osteoblasts and bone growth.[132] The available data, although limited, support the action of the main pathway involved in physiological responses to Ca^{2+} and nitric oxide, namely, Ca^{2+}/nitric oxide/cGMP/protein kinase G in producing such stimulation.[25]

FREE RADICALS, OXYGEN, AND REACTIVE SPECIES INFLUENCING MEMBRANE AND INTRACELLULAR FUNCTION

According to Cornelli,[133] free radicals are defined as elements or complex molecules with an unpaired electron (e^-) in the external orbit. Among the 103 elements of the Mendelev table, 85 are free radicals. However, some of them have the tendency of donate electrons (e.g., Na, K, Cl, Co, Cu), whereas others (e.g., O or Fe) tend to capture electrons to compensate the unpaired orbital.

Consequently, the condition of being a free radical has to be followed by the tendency of the element (or molecule or compound) to donate or capture electrons, in other terms by the characteristic to be an oxidant or an AOS. One of the most important compounds related to oxidation is oxygen. The clinician sees this problem frequently in the practice of environmental medicine.

In the atomic oxygen (O), the 8 e^- rotates in five different orbitals represented as 1 s, 2 s, p_z which contains a couple of e^-each, and as $2p_x$, $2p_y$ which contain one e^-only. Since every element which has a single e^- (unpaired) in an orbital is defined as a "free radical," O by definition is a biradical.

Things do not change for the molecular oxygen O_2 (Figure 2.2) since the combination of the two atoms does not allow a compensation of the two extreme "combined orbitals" and consequently O_2 also remains a biradical and should be represented as $O_2{}^{\cdot\cdot}$. However, the convention is to use simply the symbol O_2.

According to Cornelli,[133] oxidation is a chemical process consisting of a loss of electrons, and theoretically every existing chemical entity can be oxidized; AOs are a very large and heterogeneous category of products that can donate electrons. These substances, including vitamins C, A,

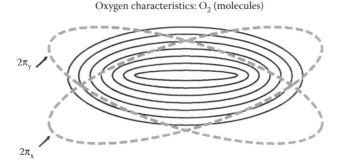

Oxygen characteristics: O_2 (molecules)

$2\pi_y$

$2\pi_x$

FIGURE 2.2 Oxygen with the unpaired orbital (dotted lines) which determine the biradical nature. (From Cornelli, U. 2007. Oxidation and antioxidants. Scientific basis of Physiological Regulating Medicine (P.R.M.). Seminar at Loyola University of Chicago.)

E, D, and B complexes, are frequently used by the clinician to counteract oxidative injury. The process to donate electrons is called reduction. At the moment that AOs donate electrons, they are called "reducents," and once that they have lost electrons, they become "oxidized." Consequently, the two processes, oxidation and reduction, are intimately connected. We use this process daily to counteract pollutant entry and injury.

In vitro, it is relatively easy to define if a compound behaves as an oxidant or AOS because the experimental conditions can be standardized; *in vivo*, this definition is sometimes controversial due to the presence of complex biological variables. However, the astute clinician develops a sense on when there is oxidative substances and injury in the body and when oxygen and nutrients need to be interjected into the clinical situation. This sense is extremely important when treating the chemically sensitive and EMF-sensitive patients.

In the simplest manner, in every living species, the balance between oxidation and AOs is fundamental for the life. It is homeostasis and in case oxidation processes prevail, the condition known as OS will be generated. This condition can be the cause of irreversible damages. It can also at times be reversed. It is needed to be avoided as much as possible by avoidance of pollutant entry and if entry occurs, neutralize it before irreversible, permanent metabolic and tissue damage occurs.

According to Cornelli,[133] as such, O_2 is constantly in search of electrons to compensate the two unpaired orbitals, and this is the essence of "oxidation." OS is caused by excess of oxidation and/or lack of antioxidated defense. OS is a temporary condition under strict control of antioxidant defense network which is represented by a variety of nutrients, enzymatic, and nonenzymatic systems (Table 2.2).

Starting as $O_2\cdot{}^-$, the final aim will be to become H_2O which can be achieved through many different steps, and each step will generate intermediates that are more oxidant than O_2 and are called ROS. A multitude of pollutants, including pesticides, natural gas, formaldehyde, phenols, molds, mycotoxins, EMF, and so on, can generate these reactive exposures.

It is known that O_2 is potentially toxic as was evident when it was used in premature infants, causing retrolental fibroplasias,[134] or in the artificial ventilation, causing pulmonary lesions[135] because of the formation of ROS.

The potential damage of O_2 is related to ROS, which are erroneously defined as "free radicals" since only some ROS are free radicals.

Dotted lines (Figure 2.2) indicate that only one e^- is present in the orbital and consequently the compound can be defined a free radical (and is represented with the dot on the right or on the left). However, even those ROS which are not free radicals have the capability to be strong oxidants (nonradical oxidants).

The capability to oxidize biological substrates is not a characteristic of ROS only, since a large group of substances defined as reactive species have this characteristic in common.

RS have been divided into ROS, reactive chlorine species (RCS), and reactive nitrogen species (RNS) (Table 2.3).

TABLE 2.2

Enzymes and Reactions in O_2 Quenching

$O_2{}^a$ Superoxide the O_2 is captured by superoxide dismutase (SOD) which "dismutates" $O_2\cdot$ into O_2 or H_2O_2

↓

H_2O_2 Fenton's reaction in the presence of transitions metals of metalloproteins (Fe, Cu, Zn)

↓

OH^a Catalase (mitochondria), peroxidase (cytoplasm)

↓

H_2O

[a] Dismutation is a biochemical process where an identical substrate is transformed into two different substances.

TABLE 2.3

Some of the Main Reactive Species (RS) Classified According to the Nature of the Substance, Free Radical, or Nonradicals, and Grouped by the Element which is Determining the Oxidation

Free Radicals	Formula	Nonradicals	Formula
Reactive Oxygen Species			
Oxygen	••	Singlet oxygen	$O_2{}^a$
Superoxide	$O_2{}^{•b}$	Hydrogen peroxide	H_2O_2
Hydroxyl	$OH^{•b}$	Ozone	O_3
Hydroperoxyl	$HO_2{}^{•b}$	Hypochlorous acid	HOCl
Peroxyl	$RO_2{}^•$	Hypobromous acid	HOBr
Alkoxyl	$RO^•$	Organic peroxides	ROOH
Carbonate	$CO_3{}^•$	Peroxynitrite	ONOO
Carbon dioxide	$CO_2{}^•$	Peroxynitrous acid	ONOOH
Reactive Chlorine Species			
		Nitryl chloride	NO_2Cl
		Chlorine gas	Cl_2
Reactive Nitrogen Species			
Nitric oxide	$NO^•$	Nitrous acid	HNO_2
Nitrogen dioxide	$NO_2{}^•$	Peroxynitrite	ONOO
		Peroxynitrous acid	ONOOH
		Alkyl peroxynitrite	ROONO
		Nitryl chloride	NO_2Cl

Note: RS are represented with a dot (with the exception of $O_2{}^{••}$, which is presented as O_2).

a Generated by sun radiation (UV).

b Intermediate step of the transformation (quenching) of O_2 into H_2O.

There are many other RS which can be represented as $C^•$ of $L^•$ of $R^•$ depending on the nature of the compound—carbon, lipidic, and generic radical, respectively. However, the entire body of RS in cells tends to be transformed into ROS. The reason of this transformation of RS into ROS is because the final product of the reaction of a ROS will be H_2O, which has an extremely low toxic value.

Some of the RS belong to two different categories since they are frequently placed in one category or the other. The presence of a large amount of RS in the body generates OS.

There are schematically the following three different pathways to generate OS: energetic, reactive, and metabolic.

ENERGETIC PATHWAY

The energetic pathway is related to the production of ATP and is developed in the mitochondria. The average caloric amount for human body functions is about 2100 kcal/day. A quantity of 300 M of ATP is produced (1 ATP = 7 kcal) to fulfill the needs, and 100 M of O_2 is necessary to produce this ATP.

(1) At least 1% of O_2 escapes the reaction of quenching in the form of one of the ROS, and oxidizes the closer substrates (leakage). (2) Since 100 M of O_2 is used to generate 300 M of ATP,

at least 3 M of ROS escapes the cascade from O_2 to H_2O. Four e^- are involved in this process, and ROS which are formed in each step can escape the process directed to the formation of water. This event is known as "leakage" and is proportional to the production of ATP.

This cascade indicates that an increase of SOD activity leads to a concomitant increase of H_2O_2 which can diffuse through biological membranes. Since all the reactions of Scheme I have to proceed concomitantly, a lack of coordination of the system may cause OS by leakage. At the same time, an exhaustion of catalase and/or peroxidase does not consent the final quenching of OH• into H_2O.

As an example, in Down's syndrome, SOD is very high because the gene for its code is in chromosome 21. These patients are easily under OS since all the quantity of H_2O_2 cannot be transformed efficiently into H_2O due to an alteration of the ratio SOD/catalase + peroxidase.[136]

In a cell producing energy, in case the quenching system (by nutrients) is not efficient or even in case of excessive production of ATP, it is possible to generate OS by leakage. Since this happens within the matrix of the mitochondria, they are the first structure to be damaged, and the energy production will be impaired. The patient develops a weakness and fatigue which is seen in most chemically sensitive and chronic degenerative patients.

This process is frequently seen in the chemically sensitive when overloaded by pollutants, such as pesticides, natural gas, formaldehyde, phenols, mold, mycotoxins, EMF, etc.

The cell will not produce the amount of ATP necessary for its normal activity and undergoes premature aging or apoptosis. The mitochondria are the main actors in the innate immunity. This process is usually and constantly in pollutant overload which puts an extra demand on them. Thus, more free radicals are generated.

REACTIVE PATHWAY

According to Cornelli,[133] the reactive pathway is related to the "oxidative burst" which is used by cells to kill bacteria or viruses or chemical toxins. In case of stimulation of a reactive cell (leukocytes, macrophages, etc.) by bacteria, viruses, oxidized lipoproteins, or other chemical and EMF stimulation, a large amount of O_2 will be produced through the activation of NADPH oxidase which is located on the cellular membrane of the cells.

In the cascade of the production of uric acid from xanthine, ROS are generated in the step from hypoxanthine to xanthine and in the following step from xanthine oxidase. Xanthine oxidase is considered the cause of the reperfusion damage.[137–139] Since during ischemia the availability of O_2 is extremely low, the tendency is to accumulate hypoxanthine locally. When suddenly the O_2 becomes available, a massive OS is developed by the sudden transformation of hypoxanthine to xanthine. This sudden burst of activity also occurs when a sudden release of an occluded blood vessel restores blood to a deprived area. The O_2 burst may occur after release of vascular and microvascular spasm. It has been shown that nonocclusive microvascular dysfunction in the heart can cause heart failure as bad as or worse than that of an occlusive valve disease. This may be partially due to the vessel spasm and relapse. The microvascular spasm is endemic in chemically sensitive patients when releases occur due to AOs, O_2 administration, or time; in a less polluted, controlled environment, the chemically sensitive patient may temporarily develop sensitivity and signs of ROS exposure and they can be neutralized by AOs, IV, Hz, and O_2. This apparently occurs in the chemically sensitive patient when the patient withdraws from pollutants, microvascular spasm opens up for the first time in weeks, months, or years. The chemically sensitive patient often misinterprets this as a new exposure, causing the patient to be ill. This condition is usually temporary for hours to days.

The enzymes producing ROS are localized in different parts of the cell and their metabolic formation is a very common process. Sensitivity to oxidation is a characteristic of a molecule. Lipids are extremely sensitive to oxidation and protein as well. Antiproteases, such as anticoagulant enzymes, are much more sensitive to the oxidation than proteases,[140,141] such as thrombin. The consequence of OS is the tendency to form a thrombus, resulting in occlusive vessel disease in the heart, lungs, legs, carotids, and brain. One sees this entity in advanced sensitivity to chemicals.

This brings to the attention the tendency of OS to facilitate the precipitation of acute ischemic episodes in case of cardiovascular disease, and also the help that can be derived from the use of AOs for prevention.

OS is also present in practically every woman under treatment with oral contraceptives since a consistent OS was shown in an experimental trial. The cause of this is not well defined, but the consequence can be the formation of superficial thrombosis which is one of the more frequent side effects of oral contraceptives.

Most Important Pathway: Metabolic Equilibrium

According to Cornelli,[133] since oxidation is a fundamental process for life, it is necessary to maintain equilibrium (homeostasis) between oxidation and AO capacity in every compartment of the body. This is extremely difficult with massive pollutant entry and injury as seen in chemical sensitivity. Usually, OS is a temporary condition and in case it becomes constant, it may generate a disease like chemical sensitivity, myocardial infarction, lupus, etc. The real problem is to understand when OS has to be counteracted to avoid the progression or the generation of a given disease. Chemical sensitivity is an example of this problem since these patients are constantly bombarded with odors and other exposures and hormones and chemicals that might not affect the average individual but will affect the wounded individuals. Chemical sensitivity will generate OS intermittently and in between cause low levels. OS is somewhat constant and can lead to fatal end-stage disease.

OS can seriously damage molecules such as lipids, DNA, proteins, etc. following an imbalance between production/presence of RS and AO defense. This consists of a pool of nonenzymatic AOs and enzymatic AOs which have to be present and be efficient in that part of the body where the oxidation is underway. Some examples may clarify the concept. Head injury will often make a chemically sensitive patient prone to OS exposure to the previously damaged area which cannot tolerate the volume of OS due to wound healing and lack of enzyme for neutralization. Sparse nutrients, including vitamin C, glutathione, taurine, multi B vitamins, and minerals in the area, will be insufficient to counteract the OS. Another example is a previous infection which leaves a wounded area and will make the patient prone to chemicals, developing chemical sensitivity because of not enough nutrients in that area to counter the new pollutant load.

Procollagen has to undergo an oxidation to become mature collagen. By oxidation, the lysine residue of procollagen becomes allysine and forms a bridge between two different trimers of procollagen. In case of OS, more residuals of lysine are oxidized to allysine and too many bridges are formed between procollagen trimers, and consequently the collagen becomes rigid and elastic. In this case, AOs may control the reaction and allow an efficient production of collagen, but once the rigidity occurs, they cannot enter sufficiently and rapid enough to counteract the oxidants.

It may be that OS acts as a defense mechanism against bacteria or virus, and in this case, OS is a protective mechanism. In case of blocking this reaction with AOs, a serious clinical problem can arise. Certain types of bacteria or even metastatic cells protect themselves with an efficient AO system; of course, at times, this system can break down, allowing the spread of the infection or cancer. However, it has not been our experience that nutrients spread infection or cancer. In fact, they usually counteract it.

The activation of macrophages through the oxidative burst is a protective mechanism. However, it is potentially damaging to the subendothelium, and in case of inappropriate control of oxidation, it can cause an initial injury which in time, if propagated by continued mold, chemical, or EMF injury, can cause inflammation and eventually atherosclerosis.

This ambivalence has generated criticism against AOs because they may interfere with the protection derived from oxidative processes. The intake of AOs, usually vitamin C and E, β-carotene and flavonoids, has been analyzed during clinical epidemiological studies which were focusing on some of them and the results were an alternation of positive and negative outcomes. This is where clinical judgment of when to use and when not to use is of extreme importance. It is the experience of the EHC-Dallas and EHC-Buffalo that AOs have been extremely positive when administered orally or by the intravenous route in the chemically sensitive and chronic degenerative disease patients after a big toxic exposure when one has undergone OS by pollutant overload. This nutrient administration has a positive protective effect. Administration of AO nutrients when taken chronically over many years has a positive effect.

OS has been implicated in many diseases, among which diabetes, cancer, cardiovascular and neurodegenerative diseases, and chemical sensitivity are the most common. With the increase of pollution, many other environmental sources such as ozone (O_3), carbon dioxide ($CO_2^\cdot$), carbon monoxide (CO), sulfur dioxide (SO_2), nitric oxide (NO/OONO) particulates are becoming very active partners for OS, and they are practically out of control in the chemically sensitive patient. Despite these threats to the equilibrium oxidation/AO defenses, OS was never measured in any of the epidemiological studies. In these conditions of epidemiological studies, it is hard to draw any valid conclusion on the benefit or not of AOs on the health status. Only when the individual studies give positive results in the face of OS, AOs can be evaluated.

Nobody would administer an antihypertensive drug to a patient with a normal blood pressure; however, AOs as well as removal of as much OS as possible works well as a preventative measure. The decrease in the total body pollutant load is always efficacious in the chemically sensitive patient, decreasing the amount of pesticides, solvents, car exhausts, etc. intake into the body to restore normal physiology and all the detoxification nutrients to build up in order to be ready for the next round of toxic insults.

Increased production of ROS and/or decreased capacity of AO defense can disrupt oxidative balance and result in damaging all components of the cell, including lipids, proteins, and DNA. Further, OS can disrupt various parts of cellular signaling because ROS are considered as one of the main messengers in redox signaling. However, the role of OS has been uncovered in induction and development of different kinds of human diseases, including chemical sensitivity, cancer, diabetes, neurodegeneration, atherosclerosis, schizophrenia, chronic fatigue syndrome, and renal and respiratory disorders.[142–146]

Furthermore, there is a huge body of literature on induction of OS by pesticides, and it has been implicated in development of health problems mediated by exposure to pesticides[147–150] especially in the generation of chemical and food sensitivity.[151–153] It has been revealed that pesticides can disturb oxidative homeostasis through direct or indirect pathways, including mitochondrial or extramitochondrial production of free radicals, thiol oxidation, and depletion of cellular AO reservoirs.[154–156]

This depletion allows for the inability to handle the myriad of odors coming into the chemically sensitive individual. This then triggers a cascade of altered physiology response causing weakness, fatigue, and sensitivity to other foods and chemicals, nutrient need occurs. Considering the OS as a powerful promoter of other cellular pathways involved in disease processes and as a unique attendant in inflammatory responses, it has been put in the spotlight of the most mechanistic studies regarding the association of pesticide's exposure with chronic disorders. OS has been implicated in the onset and progression of pesticide-induced PD.[157] In this regard, organochlorine pesticides have been reported to cause degeneration of dopaminergic neurons by an oxidative-dependent pathway in Parkinson's model.[158,159] Additionally, disrupting effects of organophosphates on glucose homeostasis have been reportedly linked to oxidative damages and inflammatory CKs and thought to be compensatory responses accompanied with reduced insulin signaling in insulin-sensitive organs such as liver, muscle, and adipose tissue.[160,161] As such, further disruption of glucose homeostasis in diabetic models of laboratory animals exposed to organophosphate insecticides has been associated with enhanced lipid peroxidation and decreased activity of AO enzymes.[162] OS has also been reported to be involved in nephrotoxicity of some pesticides, including diazinon, acephate, and paraquat.[163–165]

ENDOPLASMIC RETICULUM STRESS AND UNFOLDED PROTEIN RESPONSE

After membrane penetration, pollutant entry can damage the internal compartments of cells. The first compartment of secretary pathway endoplasmic reticulum (ER) is specialized for synthesis, folding, and delivery of proteins in addition to its fundamental role in the storage of calcium. Any disturbance in calcium homeostasis, redox regulation, and energy supply can cause perturbation of ER normal function resulting in accumulation of unfolded or misfolded proteins in this organelle, a situation which is called ER stress. Unfolded proteins occupy ER-resident chaperones, leading to the release of transmembrane ER protein kinases which activate a series of phosphorylation cascades resulting in increased expression of genes, which act as molecular chaperones to reestablish ER folding capacity or promote ER-associated degradation (ERAD) to remove misfolded proteins. This process is called unfolded protein response (UPR) aiming to adjust to the changing environment. Apparently, this process happens in the chemically sensitive patient because of the release of Ca^{2+} in the cell and protein kinases A and C, and then phosphorylated increases hypersensitivity up to 1000 times. It also releases a series of enzymes such as protein kinase, endonuclease, NO synthase, etc. as well as increasing the UPR.

In case of adaptation, which often occurs in chemical sensitivity, fails, ER stress results in the expression of genes involved in programmed cell death pathways or a hypersensitive response covering up the toxic damage until it is too late.[166] One sees the wasting syndrome in some chemically sensitive patients who are intolerant of most foods, therefore, losing weight and developing atrophied muscle in other tissues. Recent discoveries indicate that prolonged ER stress and UPR play an important role in the development of several human diseases, particularly chronic ones, including insulin resistance, diabetes,[167–169] PD, AD, ALS,[170–172] tumor formation, and a progression[173,174] of atherosclerosis, cardiomyopathy, chronic kidney diseases, and renal failure.[175,176]

On the other hand, ER stress and related pathways have been reported to be involved in cytotoxicity by some pesticides which can cause chemical sensitivity. Paraquat, a bipyridyl herbicide, which is suspected to increase the risk of PD following chronic exposures, has been reported to induce ER stress and trigger dopaminergic cell death by enhanced cleavage of a small ER cochaperone protein, p23, and inhibition of ERAD.[177] Also, some have developed UPR as their pesticide-induced chemical sensitivity progresses. Elevated levels of ER stress biomarkers like glucose-regulated protein 78 (GPR78), ER degradation enhancing-α-mannosidase-like protein (EDEM), and C/EBP homologous protein (CHOP) has also been implicated in paraquat-induced toxicity in human neuroblastoma cells. Further, paraquat activated calpain and caspase 3 along with ER-induced cascade inositol requiring protein 1 (IRE1)/apoptosis signal-regulating kinase 1 (ASK1)/c-Jun N-terminal kinase (JNK).[178]

In another study carried out on neuroblastoma cells, rotenone-induced ER stress has become evident by increased phosphorylation of protein kinase RNA-like ER kinase (PERK), protein kinase RNA-activated (PKR), and eukaryotic initiation factor 2-a (eIF2a) as well as the expression of GRP78. Moreover, rotenone activates glycogen synthase kinase 3β (GSK3β), an ER-related multifunctional serine/threonine kinase implicated in the pathogenesis of neurodegeneration.[179]

Deltamethrin, a pyrethroid pesticide, has been reported to induce apoptosis through ER stress pathway involving eIF2α calpain and caspase 12,[180] induction of apoptosis by pyrrolidine dithiocarbamate (PDT)/Cu complex, a widely used pesticide has also been linked to the ER stress-associated signaling molecules, including GRP78, GRP94, caspase-12, activating transcription factor 4 (ATF4), and CHOP in lung epithelial cells.[181] Chloropicrin, an aliphatic nitrate pesticide, has been indicated to increase ER stress-related proteins, including GRP78, IRE1α, and CHOP/GADD 153 in human retinal pigment epithelial cells.[182]

Some other pesticides belonging to the organochlorines (endosulfan), carbamates (formetanate, methomyl, pyrimicarb), and pyrethroids (bifentrin) have been evaluated for their effects on stress proteins among which upregulation of the ER chaperone GRP78 and downregulation of the cytosolic chaperone HSP72/73 were significant. These effects can occur when ER is under stress and the UPR results in increased expression of ER chaperones and decreased protein synthesis in the cytosol.[183,184] All of these are known to trigger or be involved in chemical sensitivity.

PROTEIN AGGREGATION

Degradation of misfolded, damaged, or unneeded proteins is a fundamental biological process which has a crucial role in maintenance and regulation of cellular function. There must be sufficient nutrients and in fact enzyme detoxidants pathway to assure regulation of detoxification. There are two major cellular mechanisms for protein degradation; ubiquitin proteasome system (UPS) that mainly targets short-lived proteins by proteases, and autophagy that mostly clears long-lived and poorly soluble proteins through the lysosomal machinery.[185]

UPS is composed of ubiquitin for tagging and proteasomes for proteolysis of proteins which are to be degraded. Deregulation of this system has been implicated in the pathogenesis of several chronic diseases, mostly neurodegeneration and cancers evidenced by decreased and increased proteasome activity, respectively.[186] Environmental exposure to certain pesticides has been linked to proteasomal dysfunction in development of neurodegenerative diseases. The organochlorine pesticide dieldrin has been reported to decrease proteasome activity along with enhanced sensitivity to occurrence of apoptosis in dopaminergic neuronal cells.[187] Proteasome inhibition has also been shown in neuroblastoma cells exposed to rotenone, ziram, diethyldithiocarbamate, endosulfan, benomyl, and dieldrin.[188,189] Paraquat has also been noted to impair UPS given by decreased proteasome activity and increased ubiquitinated proteins in DJ1 deficient mice and dopaminergic neurons.[190,191] Increased degradation of proteasome components has been presented as the mechanism of proteasome inhibition by rotenone, an inducer of PD.[192]

The lysosomal degradation pathway of autophagy is known as a self-digestion process by which cells not only get rid of misfolded proteins, damaged organelles, and infectious microorganisms, but also provide nutrients during fasting. Of course, fasting is essential in chemical sensitivity and is used frequently to clear pain, lack of energy, and brain dysfunction. The defect of this process has found an emerging role in many human diseases such as cancer, neurodegeneration, diabetes, aging, and disorders of the liver, muscle, and heart.[193–195] There are a few reports on the involvement of defective autophagy in toxic effects of pesticides. A relationship between autophagy and paraquat-induced apoptosis in neuroblastoma cells was shown by Gonzalez-Polo and colleagues in 2007.[196] This effect was confirmed in another study in which paraquat-induced autophagy was attributed to the occurrence of ER stress.[197] Lindane, a broad-spectrum organochlorine pesticide, has been reported to promote its toxicity through the disruption of an autophagic process in primary rat hepatocytes.[198] All of these substances have been shown to trigger chemical sensitivity.

OS causes neurodegeneration, atherosclerosis, schizophrenia, chronic fatigue syndrome, renal respiratory disorders, and chemical hypersensitivity.[142–146,151] On the other hand, there is a huge body of literature on induction of OS by pesticides and herbicides, and these have been implicated in the development of health problems mediated by exposure to pesticides.[147–151] It has been revealed that pesticides can disturb oxidative homeostasis through direct or indirect pathways, including mitochondrial or extra mitochondrial production of free radicals, thiol oxidation, and depletion of cellular AO reservoirs.[154–156] Considering the OS as a powerful promoter of other cellular pathways involved in disease process and a unique attendant in inflammatory response, it has been put in the spotlight of most mechanistic studies regarding the association of pesticide's exposure with chronic disorders.

OS has been implicated in the onset and progression of pesticide-induced PD.[157] Chemical sensitivity has been shown to have abundant OS as well as inflammation. Often, this OS is attributed to pesticide, natural gas, formaldehyde, and volatile organic HC exposure as well as other toxic chemicals when the total body pollutant load is exceeded. In this regard, organochlorine pesticides have been reported to cause the degeneration of dopaminergic neurons by an oxidative-dependent pathway in the Parkinson's model.[158,159] Additionally, disrupting effects of organophosphates on glucose homeostasis have been reportedly linked to oxidative damages and inflammatory CKs, and thought to be compensatory responses accompanied with reduced insulin signaling in insulin-sensitive organs such as liver, muscle, and adipose tissue.[160,161] As such, further disruption of glucose homeostasis in diabetic models of laboratory animals exposed to organophosphate insecticides have been associated with enhanced lipid peroxidation and decreased activity of AO enzymes.[162] We have seen this diabetic phenomenon not only triggered by OP insecticides but also triggered by phenol compounds like pure phenol and tricresyl phosphate. These appeared to simultaneously trigger the chemical sensitivity and diabetes mellitus.

A case report demonstrates this entity: An 8-year-old white diabetic female is insulin dependent. Diagnosis showed that she developed diabetes after exposure to aluminum and mercury. The patient was found to be sensitive to milk, wheat, gluten, and 24 other foods. She was also sensitive to molds, pesticides, and natural gas. Her T and B cells increased but her gamma globulin and substrate were normal. Total hemolytic complement decreased. The patient was placed on a rigid avoidance program for her food sensitivity, molds, and chemicals, and a rotary diversified diet avoiding the foods to which she was sensitive. A subcutaneous injection for neutralizing doses of foods and molds to which she was sensitive was done. She lost her need for insulin as her blood sugar returned to normal and has stayed stable. She is thriving on her treatment and the top of her class in reading and math.

MITOCHONDRIAL FUNCTION

Mitochondria are the powerhouses of the cell and contain their own genome. The majority of their constituent proteins is encoded by nuclear genes and translated in the cytosol. Harbauer et al. show that one of the main conducts for mitochondrial protein import is directly regulated by phosphorylation during mitosis and this in time promotes respiratory activity.[163] All human processes are provided by mitochondrial exhibition phosphorylation. Harbauer et al. identify a link between cell division cycle and mitochondrial protein transportation as a driver in this process.[163]

OS has also been reported to be involved in nephrotoxicity of some pesticides, including diazinon, acephate, and paraquat.[164–166] Mitochondria are a leading target of ROS[79,80] due to proximity to ROS production (much of which occurs in mitochondria),[79,81,82] such that mtDNA mutate at 10–1000 times the rate of nuclear DNA.[83,84] Since all mtDNA genes are germane to oxidative phosphorylation,[85–87] mtDNA damage with its ATP leaks and decrease in productions commonly hampers mitochondrial respiratory chain function which in turn further impairs cell energy production and often further increases ROS release.[77,78] Reduced energy and increased ROS each cause cell (and subcellular) dysfunction and can induce cell death by necrosis or apoptosis.[88–91,131] The chemically sensitive manifests this clinical situation by weakness and fatigue.

As shown in this volume under Gulf War veterans by Celum et al., as dynamic multifunctional organelles, mitochondria are the main source of ATP and ROS in the cell and have important roles in calcium homeostasis, synthesis of steroids and heme, metabolic cell signaling, and apoptosis. Abnormal function of the mitochondrial respiratory chain is the primary cause of imbalanced cellular energy homeostasis and has been widely studied in different types of human diseases most of all types of diabetes[199–202] and neurodegenerative disorders.[203] Perturbation of this organelle has been accepted as one of the crucial mechanisms of neurodegeneration since there is broad literature supporting mitochondrial involvement of proteins like α-synuclein, parkin, DJ-1, PINK1, APP, PS1 and 2, and SOD1 that have some known roles in major neurodegenerative disorders, including PD, AD, and ALS.[204] Some evidence even proposed the involvement of mitochondrial DNA and its alterations in development of these diseases.[205]

Parkinson's was almost the first disease in which the role of mitochondrial dysfunction was uncovered when the classical inhibitor of complex I electron transport chain, metabolite of MPTP, was reported to cause Parkinsonism in drug abusers.[206] In 2000, developing the symptoms of PD was also reported for broad-spectrum pesticide, rotenone whose mechanism of action is selective inhibition of complex I mitochondrial respiratory chain so that it has been widely used to create Parkinson's model in laboratory animals.[207] In this regard, interfering with mitochondrial respiratory chain functions has made a pattern in the development of different types of pesticides, and many agrochemicals are known to inhibit electron transport chain activity as their primary or secondary mechanism of action. Most of the pesticides interfering with mitochondrial respiratory chain activities are mainly inhibitors of complex I electron transport chain and some others partially inhibit complexes II, III, and V.[208] Moreover, a wide variety of pesticides has been known as uncouplers of mitochondrial oxidative phosphorylation.[209] This mechanism seems to play an important role in the chemically sensitive patient who has weakness and fatigue. Glyphosate herbicides (round-up ready) used extensively on wheat, soy, and cotton also damage the chemically sensitive and chronic degenerative disease patient.

Nevertheless, impairment of oxidative phosphorylation has been reported in exposure to a large number of pesticides, particularly neurotoxic agents through the inhibition of a biosynthetic pathway essential for mitochondrial function or extra mitochondrial generation of ROS.[210] Likewise, there is enough evidence on the role of mitochondrial dysfunction in pathophysiological features of diabetes, including insulin deficiency and insulin resistance. Pancreatic beta cell failure has been reported to be associated with mitochondrial dysfunction and can be caused by exposure to pesticides.[211]

On the other hand, exposure to pesticides inhibiting complex I and III mitochondrial respiratory chain can lead to a diminished oxygen consumption and cellular energy supply which in turn can result in reduced insulin signaling cascade. In this way, organochlorines, atrazine, and some dioxin-like pesticides, herbicides such as glyphosates have been shown to decrease mitochondrial capacity in the beta oxidation of fatty acids resulting in the accumulation of intracellular fat, a situation considered to develop obesity and insulin resistance.[212,213] Some chemically sensitive patients are obese probably through this mechanism as they are very sensitive to these pesticides. Once their load of pesticides is reduced and the total body load of toxics is reduced, they lose weight and decrease their chemical sensitivity.

Also, if the Ca^{2+} protein kinases A and C phosphorylation occurs, the patients develop hypersensitivity reactions. Additionally, the further increase in ROS that is a consequence of mtDNA damage can induce further mtDNA injury—advancing a cycle of OSMD, cell energy depletion, cell dysfunction, and potentially cell loss.[77,78,92] They can become hypersensitive to foods, molds, and other nonrelated toxics and nontoxic chemicals, thus increasing vulnerability to everyday exposure and living. We have seen this condition in many overexposed Gulf War Veterans and other chemically sensitive patients. (OS also promoted MD by inhibiting mitochondrial import of essential precursor proteins[93]). According to Golomb OS, adversely affecting the balance of OS to AO defense can increase vulnerability to and clinical consequences of new oxidative exposures which also produce weakness and fatigue as seen in chemically sensitive patients. When enough mitochondria are dysfunctioning or enough cells are dysfunctional or dead, symptoms such as weakness and fatigue or organ dysfunction emerge—mitochondrial "threshold effects." (OS may have further implications via effects on DNA methylation[95] and excitotoxicity,[95,96] which may be magnified in settings of low mitochondria EN production.[97,98]) It is reiterated that major exposures are known to produce toxicity via OSMD producing expectation of cell dysfunction and cell death. (Note that organophosphates further produce mitochondrial and energetic compromise through toxicity to microtubules,[99] interfering with mitochondrial biogenesis[100] and transport).[101] Mitochondria are dynamic rather than static organelles.[102,103]

OXIDATIVE SHIELDING (METABOLIC RESPONSE TO OXIDATIVE SHIELDING)

MITOCHONDRIA: INNATE IMMUNITY

An important mechanism involved in environmental incitant and triggering is oxidative shielding. ROS and chronic oxidative changes in membrane lipids and proteins found in many chronic diseases are not the result of accidental damage. According to Naviaux, these changes are the result of a highly evolved, stereotyped, and protein-catalyzed oxidative shielding response that all eukaryotes adopt when they are placed in a chemically, EMF, or microbiologically stressed environment.[214] The machinery of oxidative shielding evolved from pathways of innate immunity designed to protect the cell from attack and to limit the spread of infection. However, this response also protects against chemical and mycotoxicant and EMF exposure in the chemically sensitive and EMF-sensitive patient and will also generate ROS in addition to nutrient shielding.

Both OS and reductive stress trigger oxidative shielding. Functional and metabolic defects occur in the cell before the increase in ROS and oxidative changes. According to Naviaux, ROS are the response to the triggering of the disease, not the cause.[214] Environmental factors are the triggering agents of disease coupled with the hereditary defects. The environmental triggers have been shown throughout the body, the most common being natural gas, pesticides, mycotoxins, and car exhaust. These all need to be shielded.

Understand why cells choose to defend themselves from harm by intentionally making ROS such as superoxide and hydrogen peroxide and stiffening of the cell membrane to make it less permeable and vulnerable to microbiological, chemical, EMF attack are correlated with changes in environmental oxygen.[215]

The ability of cells to use oxygen to make ATP to detoxify and release it as a ROS for purposes of cell signaling and defense has been developed. One of the most ancient functions of mitochondria is cell defense. It is called metabolic response to cellular attack to injury or innate immunity.[216]

Mitochondrion plays a central role in innate immunity today. Most of the pathways of intermediary metabolism were developed during the anaerobic epoch of life's history on Earth and originally a defense mechanism even though the mitochondria are known as an energy producer damaged by pollutants in chemical sensitivity.

MITOCHONDRIA DYSFUNCTION

In chemical sensitivity, mitochondria malfunction yields weakness, fatigue, and brain dysfunction as well as peripheral neuropathy and small vessel vasculitis. Some evidence even proposed that the mitochondrial DNA and its alterations occur in the development of these diseases.[205] PD was almost the first disease in which the role of mitochondrial dysfunction was uncovered when the classical inhibitor of complex I electron transport chain, metabolite of MPTP, was reported to cause Parkinsonism in drug abusers.[206]

In 2000, developing the symptoms of Parkinson's was also as previously stated reported for a broad-spectrum pesticide, rotenone, whose mechanism of action is selective inhibition of complex I mitochondrial respiratory chain, so that it has been widely used to create Parkinson's model in laboratory animals.[207] In this regard, interfering with mitochondrial respiratory chain functions has made a pattern in the development of different types of pesticides, and many agrochemicals are known to inhibit electron transport chain activity as their primary or secondary mechanism of action. Most of the pesticides interfering with mitochondrial respiratory chain activities are mainly inhibitors of complex I electron transport chain and some others partially inhibit complexes II, III, and V.[208] Moreover, a wide variety of pesticides has been known as uncouplers of mitochondrial oxidative phosphorylation[209] but enhances the Ca^{2+} pathway to hypersensitivity.

Nevertheless, impairment of oxidative phosphorylation has been reported in the exposure to a large number of pesticides, particularly neurotoxic agents, through the inhibition of a biosynthetic pathway essential for mitochondrial function or extra-mitochondrial generation of ROS.[210] Likewise, there is enough evidence on the role of mitochondrial dysfunction in pathophysiological features of diabetes, including insulin deficiency and insulin resistance.

According to Naviaux, to understand why cells might choose to defend themselves from harm by intentionally making ROS, such as superoxide and hydrogen peroxide, and stiffening the cell membrane to make it less permeable and less vulnerable to attack, we need to start at the beginnings of life on our planet.[214] The great evolutionary pulses of metabolic and structural innovation of life on Earth can be correlated with changes in environmental oxygen.[215] In the beginning, all life on Earth was anaerobic and oxygen was toxic. The first cells to emerge in the Precambrian seas were anaerobic bacteria that made ATP by an oxygenic photosynthesis. This life chemistry dates to approximately 3.5 billion years ago (GYA).[217] Most of the pathways of intermediary metabolism that we know today were developed using this anaerobic epoch of life's history on Earth.

Isoprenyl and ubiquinol synthesis, fatty acid oxidation and synthesis, iron–sulfur cluster synthesis, glycolysis, carotenoid synthesis, the pentose phosphate pathway, the glyoxylate cycle, pyruvate dehydrogenase, cobalamin synthesis, heme synthesis, cytochromes, glutathione metabolism, electron transport, chemiosmotic proton-coupling for ATP synthesis, and both reductive and oxidative (reverse and forward) Krebs cycles all were present in the oldest bacteria known, the green sulfur bacteria.[218]

This rich ecology coevolved for a billion years before multicellularity took hold and expanded during the Cambrian approximately 0.54 GYA. The ability of cells to use oxygen to make ATP, detoxify it, and release it as ROS for purposes of cell signaling and defense were developed during this pivotal Precambrian epoch. The free radical theory of aging was proposed.[219]

MITOCHONDRIA, INNATE IMMUNITY, AND METABOLIC CELLULAR DEFENSE

The biochemical signature of an attack is a metabolic "steal" or diversion of electrons and resources such as nitrogen, phosphorus, iron, and copper. When limited cellular resources are used by predators and parasites, those resources are not available to the host cell. Mitochondria are uniquely equipped to detect and respond to this metabolic steal. When the local chemistry of the cell provides nutrients and resources in concentrations that are matched to mitochondrial metabolism, mitochondria will create a normal oxygen gradient of approximately 30 outside the cell to 0.2 torr in the mitochondrial matrix[220] (see above). When cellular resources are consumed by a parasite, a "metabolic mismatch" is produced.

Mitochondria have a proteome of approximately 1500 proteins.[221] Nearly 1000 of these proteins have catalytic functions in cell metabolism such as citrate synthase or malate dehydrogenase. Under normal physiologic conditions, the concentrations of thousands of nutrients and metabolic substrates in mitochondria are closely governed by the collective kinetic constants (K_m, K_{cat}, V, Hill coefficient, etc.) of all the enzymes responsible for transforming those metabolites. This has recently been computationally modeled in the Recon 1 and BiGG reconstructions of cell and organ metabolism.[222,223] Only the primary structure of an enzyme is genetically determined. The activity of an enzyme at any instant in time is determined by ambient metabolic conditions. The environmental triggering agents, for example, the K_m of citrate synthase for oxaloacetate is approximately 2 µM, but the enzyme is allosterically inhibited by ATP, NADH, acetyl-CoA, palmitoyl-CoA, and the product citric acid so the rate of converting oxaloacetate to citrate is changing minute to minute according to the condition of the cell.[224] When the concentrations of substrates are perturbed by viral or microbial infection, disease, toxin, or nutritional excess, mitochondria sense this as a metabolic mismatch between the optimum concentration of those metabolites for a given tissue and the actual concentration. Thus the chemically sensitive patient due to its varied metabolism responds differently at different times. At times, they have more resistance and other times are very vulnerable. This function at times makes treatment doses of antigens and nutrients difficult to deliver due to the need for varying doses. Of course, medications, nutrients, and interdermal neutralization at varying times are fixed doses and may not function at times of crises unless they are primed over weeks and months when the organism is stable.

This metabolic mismatch diverts electron flow away from mitochondria in the cell and decreases intramitochondrial electron flow, and mitochondrial oxygen consumption falls. When mitochondrial oxygen consumption (extraction) falls and the cell is still surrounded by 30 torr (2%–4%) oxygen supplied by capillaries, the concentration of oxygen in the cell rises sharply. When cellular oxygen rises, the redox of the cell rises and the chemistry of polymer assembly (DNA, RNA, lipid, protein, and carbohydrate synthesis) is ultimately stopped because the NADPH/NADP$^+$ ratio falls as the change in Gibbs chemical free energy of synthetic reactions becomes less negative (more positive changes in Gibbs chemical free energy are thermodynamically less favorable). Under these more oxidizing conditions, electrons are no longer available for carbon–carbon bond formation to build biomass for viral or intracellular bacterial replication. Electrons are instead abstracted by the rising tide of intracellular oxygen to make superoxide, other ROS, and RNS and form bonds between free thiols in amino acids such as cysteine, glutathione and peptides, to make disulfides (GSSG). The rising tide of intracellular oxygen also oxidized iron–sulfur clusters and redox-responsive sites in many proteins, inactivating proteins for macromolecular synthesis and activating proteins that shield the cell membrane from further attack. These include lipoxygenases and nuclear factor-kappa beta (NF-κβ),[225] NADPH oxidases,[226] redox-sensitive signaling systems in innate immunity such as the purinergic receptors,[227] and transcriptional regulators such as Keap1/Nrf2, and sirtuin-FoxO.[228] The net result of oxidative shielding in innate immunity is to limit the replication and prevent the exit of the invading pathogen or toxic substance. Once the limitation happens, the pathogen or toxin substance stays inert being encapsulated or is destroyed. We see this phenomena in the chemically sensitive patient who is exposed to an isolated toxic exposure. This shielding then renders the chemical harmless so homeostasis can be obtainable.

This phenomenon can be measured clinically when the PvO$_2$ will increase from 28 mm Hg often to 35–65 mm Hg level, indicating that oxygen is not being extracted by cell tissue as it is supposed to. As the shielding against the OS occurs, vascular spasm and shunting also occurs (see PvO$_2$).

According to Naviaux, oxidative shielding is a stereotyped response to cellular injury or attack.[214] To better understand the fundamental differences between the OS and the oxidative shielding perspectives, it is helpful to ask and answer a few questions from the viewpoint of these two different schools of thought.

Hostile, damaging, or unhealthy conditions surrounding the cell trigger the production of superoxide, hydrogen peroxide, and other ROS. ROS come from mitochondria and specialized enzyme systems in the cell.

The shielding school holds that the function of ROS is first, to protect the cell if possible, both as signaling molecules and by physically decreasing the cellular uptake, release, and exchange of potentially toxic pathogens or chemicals from and with the environment; and second, to actively kill the cell by apoptosis or necrosis when the local environmental conditions threaten to spread to neighboring cells and jeopardize the survival of the ROS which are an effect of disease, not the prime cause. The environmental triggering is the prime cause. In the shielding school, the organism is considered the ultimate unit of Darwinian selection. The fitness of an individual, in terms of its ability to reproduce, can be substantially increased by rapidly cutting off resources, walling off, or actively killing damaged or infected cells in a part of the body to the whole. Then, when fasting occurs in chemically sensitive damaged or dysfunctional cells, debris is phagocytized and the body is cleaned. This process has been performed in over 1000 chemically sensitive patients as part of their initial and energy treatment program; usually after a fast, chemically sensitive patients develop more energy and alertness as they clear out the deterrent.

Stress School Holds That the Function of ROS Is to Cause Cell Damage and Disease

The shielding school holds that because the prime cause of disease can ultimately be traced back to toxic exposure, microbial pathogen, unhealthy nutritional practices, nutrient loading, or unhealthy patterns of exercise, activity therapy should be directed at eliminating these causal factors. ROS production will naturally fall back to normal levels when physiologic balance is restored as we have shown in so many chemically sensitive patients we have treated.

The stress school holds that because ROS are the prime cause of disease, therapy should be directed at eliminating or normalizing ROS and ROS-related cell damage.

The scientific literature is ripe with cell culture and animal experiments showing apparent benefits of AO therapy and opinion papers that advocate AOs for treating everything from chemical sensitivity to diabetes to cancer and AD. When AOs alone are put to the test in randomized clinical trials, they generally fail or, worse, show evidence of unexpected harm in some authors' opinions. For example, in a meta-analysis of nine clinical trials that evaluated the benefit of treating type 2 diabetes with AOs such as α-tocopherol (vitamin E), there was no benefit.[229] Like many purified AO vitamins, vitamin E is a two-edged sword. The reasons for this are not entirely clear, but may relate to the fact that therapeutic dosing of purified micronutrients and AOs intervenes in regulatory pathways that produce biochemical symptoms associated with cell defense, but are not the actual cause of disease. Also, the hypersensitivity phenomena triggered by pollutant injury activates the Ca^{2+} protein kinases A and C when phosphorylated increases the environmental sensitivity 1000 times and the individuals who take them cannot tolerate nutrients. Vitamin E supplementation, alone or in combination with β-carotene, was shown to increase the risk of lung cancer in smokers.[230] Vitamin C supplementation was found to double the risk of cancer death in nonobese women (relative risk [RR] = 2.0; 95% CI = 1.12–3.58), while having no effect in obese women.[231] The SELECT clinical trial of vitamin E and selenium was terminated early because of an apparent increase in the risk of new onset diabetes in the selenium group and a 1.6-fold increased risk in prostate cancer in the vitamin E group.[232,233] If ROS are at the heart of cancer, diabetes, and heart disease, why are AOs so ineffective at preventing or treating these diseases? This statement is not entirely true since one of the prime prescriptions of chemical sensitivity and the chronic degenerative diseases is broad AO supplementation. This process is usually successful only when additional avoidance of some triggering agents and treatment of the hypersensitivity occur. This was not done in the studies just stated; therefore, their finding may not be valid in all cases.

Other data that may prove helpful in weighing the merits of the schools of oxidative shielding versus OS are the results of clinical trials in which a therapy recommended by the shielding school, for example, diet and exercise (which is known to stimulate ROS[234]), is directly compared with conventional medical intervention. When this is done in type 2 diabetes and its prodromal metabolic syndrome, diet and exercise are categorically superior to the best drug intervention. A recent meta-analysis of 13 clinical trials involving 3907 subjects found that the odds ratio for disease improvement with diet and exercise was 3.8 (95% CI = 2.5−5.9), but the odds ratios for disease improvement with drug treatment was 1.6 (95% CI = 1.0−2.5).[235] Diet and exercise can actually cure early type 2 diabetes while simultaneously reducing the risk of heart disease. In contrast, common drug interventions such as the thiazolidinedione insulin-sensitizing drug rosiglitazone will decrease diabetes, but increase the risk of heart failure.[236]

According to Naviaux, the stereotyped oxidative shielding response to danger and metabolic mismatch can be identified in all aerobic forms of life on Earth.[214] Even bacteria have it. For example, *Escherichia coli* rapidly generate superoxide and hydrogen peroxide in a manner reminiscent of mitochondria, by partially reducing oxygen at the site of NADH dehydrogenases and quinine acceptor sites along the inner membrane.[237] The magnitude of the response is regulated by nutrient availability, environmental toxin, and infection exposure.[238] It is noteworthy that ROS production by bacteria is highest under conditions of nutrient loading, similar to increased ROS production under nutrient loading in diabetes. Inhibitors of NADH dehydrogenase activity, such as the pesticides paraquat or rotenone, produce a rapid increase in ROS and mutation rates in the stressed bacteria[237] occurs. AO defenses in aerobic bacteria are coordinately upregulated by endogenously produced ROS by redox-reactive thiols on cysteines of peroxide-responsive OxyR and superoxide-sensitive SoxR transcription factors.

Plant cell ROS production leads to cross-linking of tyrosine-rich proteins in the cell wall.[239] Animal cells use many mechanisms, including the use of another tyrosine-rich protein, melanin, and the production of collagen scar tissue, to wall off the chronically disturbed or injured collection of cells. The initiating rise in intracellular oxygen that is caused by the failure of mitochondria to reduce oxygen to water is the hallmark of a metabolic "fever" or mismatch.

It is important to make the distinction between oxidative shielding and oxidative damage. When an oxidative shielding response is beneficial to the cell or the organism, then AO treatments designed to block or reverse it will have two effects: (1) There will be no effect on the primary cause of the cellular toxicity, for example, the viral infection, toxic exposure, or metabolic mismatch causing the cellular oxidative response and (2) chronic treatment may ultimately prove harmful because it inhibits the highly evolved protective and hermetic functions of protein-catalyzed oxidative shielding. However, we have not seen this happen with our regimen of vigorous AO nutrient supplementation except in acute exposure episodes where you cannot tell the difference between OS and shielding.

According to Naviaux, cell culture experiments have proved to be highly successful over the years in answering genetic questions.[214] However, cell culture experiments have not been as reliable and are often misleading in answering environmental and metabolic questions when the experiment is aimed at answering a question about multicellular development, organ function, or a whole animal phenotype. This happens because of four major differences between the metabolic conditions of cell culture and tissues. These can be briefly stated as the apoptosis, hyperoxia, cycling cell NADPH, and multicellularity problems.

According to Naviaux, mitochondria are the principal regulators of apoptosis.[240] This process lies at the heart of the developmental program of plants and animals that permits embryos to grow and remove cells that are no longer needed. Another essential function of apoptosis is the physical containment of injury or infection. Cells that become infected by viruses or other microbial pathogens initiate the program of apoptotic cell death to prevent the spread of infection. Many viruses and other microbes devote substantial genetic resources to thwart the infected cell's effort to commit suicide.[241] Evolution has preserved and refined the apoptotic program because it confers an increased fitness to the plant or animal during development and under attack. This can be seen as a form of cellular altruism without intent in which the death and removal of a few infected, injured, or obsolete cells increase the likelihood of survival of the organism. Protein-catalyzed ROS production and membrane and protein oxidation events precede the commitment to apoptosis in most cell types. These genetic and metabolic pathways have been selected over evolutionary time to increase the fitness of the organism. Ultimately, the oxidative shielding response confers evolutionary advantage for the organism. This advantage cannot be seen in cell culture because the death of cells in culture occurs without reference to the survival of the whole organism.

According to Naviaux, cells in culture are typically grown under ambient oxygen tensions of approximately 100 torr that result from diffusion from a 21% oxygen atmosphere at sea level.[214] They are not usually grown at the 2%–4% oxygen (15–30 torr) that is normal in tissues. Because all of the proteins involved in AO defense evolved under physiologic conditions of 15–30 torr oxygen, they typically have K_m values for oxygen in the at-to 30 torr range. Cell culture hyperoxia in the 30–100 torr range will naturally activate AO and prooxidant proteins that would otherwise be quiescent and substrate limited. This makes the interpretation of oxidative changes in cell culture clear. The measurement of a myriad of ROS such as superoxide and hydrogen peroxide and biomarkers of oxidation such as lipid peroxidation is technically simple in cultured cells. However, the judgment that these changes are deleterious in the context of the whole organism is biologically unsound.

Cycling cells have higher $NADPH/NADP^+$ ratios than postmitotic cells.[242] Cultured cells must double their biomass each day in preparation for division. Postmitotic cells in tissues do not increase in their biomass. Postmitotic cells direct electrons to NADH for cellular work, not NADPH for biomass production. This essential difference between growing and nongrowing cells must be grasped before the different roles of mitochondria in growing and nongrowing cells can be understood. The synthesis of lipids, proteins, DNA, and RNA requires the use of electrons carried by NADPH to make new carbon–carbon and other chemical bonds. NADPH is made in large amounts by the pentose phosphate pathway in which glucose 6-phosphate is used before entering glycolysis to make ribose for DNA and RNA synthesis and NADPH for macromolecular synthesis and glutathione metabolism.[243] When incoming electrons from glucose and other nutrients are directed to NADPH, those electrons are not available for NADH used in mitochondrial oxidative phosphorylation. The combined effect of increased NADPH and hyperoxia (21% O_2) in cell culture conspires to amplify superoxide and hydrogen peroxide production by NADPH oxidases, making the study of more subtle factors such as regulation of the pentose phosphate pathway by nitric oxide[244] and compartmental redox regulation during differentiation challenging or impossible.

According to Naviaux, in cell culture, investigators necessarily remove the normal connectedness of cells in tissues.[214] As a consequence, single cells in culture must be cell-autonomous, that is, they must synthesize everything they need for growth without reliance on supplies from other cells. This is not the case in somatic tissues. In tissues, distant and neighboring cells adopt complementary metabolic functions. It is wasteful for photoreceptor cells in the eye, for example, to express genes that are used to produce muscle contraction in the heart. Likewise, it is wasteful and potentially toxic for all somatic cells to make a particular hormone such as insulin or testosterone. In another example, the cells of the liver lobule clearly differentiate along the gradient of oxygen established between the high oxygen present in the vicinity of the hepatic artery in the portal triads where ornithine transcarbamoylase is expressed and the low oxygen present in center of the lobule surrounding the portal vein where ornithine aminotransferase is expressed.[245] Somatic cells epigenetically silence unused genes by DNA methylation and other processes. The process of DNA methylation is regulated by folate, B12, and S-adenosylmethionine metabolism which are also controlled by mitochondria.[246] The natural metabolic cooperativity among differentiated cells in the body is lost in cell culture. No longer is there any selective pressure for cells to cooperate as they do in tissues and organs. No longer can the death of a few cells be clearly identified in the context of its evolutionary function to decrease the probability of death of the organism under stress. It is easy to see how an investigator studying cells in a dish might think that active cell processes that cause cell death, such as apoptosis and necrosis, are "bad." However, it is the pathway's oxidative shielding, and occasionally cell death, that permits the organism to live on and reproduce under every changing condition of life on Earth.

CELL METABOLISM IS LIKE AN ECOSYSTEM

The chemical reactions of the cell take place in a myriad of discrete locations and compartments within the cell that are maintained in thermodynamic disequilibrium. This disequilibrium is changed more in the chemically sensitive and EMF-sensitive patient. Proteins and membranes in each of these compartments maintain the natural redox boundaries and oxygen gradients. Cell metabolism can be visualized intuitively as a coral reef ecosystem. The metabolic products of one compartment in the cell are used as resources by other compartments, just as one species of coral can provide resources for another species in the reef. Metabolism is a complex trophic web that stabilizes or destabilizes the differentiated function of the cell. Ultimately, the end products of metabolism are released from the cell into the blood and excreted in the urine, back into the external ecosystem. In both the coral reef and the microcosm of the cell, small-molecule metabolites and signaling molecules drive changes in gene expression, not the reverse. The success of transgenic and gene knockout experiments over the past 20 years has given scientists the impression that genes drive the evolution of metabolism. This is wrong. Rather, it is environmental nutrients and the small molecules of metabolism that drive the evolution of genes. The chemically sensitive patient is a great example of this phenomenon. In these patients, it appears that no matter what their genetic makeup is, the total environmental pollutant load and the specific environmental load are activated, they developed chemical sensitivity. However, the genes may divert their specific responses.

According to Naviaux, over evolutionary time, genes and gene expression patterns evolved to handle the resources provided by the environment.[246] These genes may cause the development of different responses, that is, GI upset in one set of patients, asthma in another and brain fog in another, cardiovascular dysfunction in others. Over shorter time periods of minutes to hours, and weeks to months, nutrients such as glucose, fats, and amino acids, and small molecules of metabolism are the forcing variables that induce the changes in enzyme activity and gene expression associated with feeding, fasting, and seasonal variations in nutrient availability. The amino acid leucine plays a central role in stimulating the master fuel regulator mammalian target of rapamycin (mTOR) and inhibiting AMP kinase and autophagy.[247]

Many intermediary metabolites act differently inside and outside the cell. This allows room for many functions to change or be faulty during the switch. Faulty switches may occur in the chemically sensitive patient, causing or altering the sensitivity. Inside the cell, they act as carbon skeletons for fat, protein, carbohydrate, DNA, and RNA synthesis. Outside the cell, they act as signaling molecules that bind cell receptors and alter gene expression. For example, ATP is an energy-carrying molecule inside the cell. Outside the cell, ATP is a "mitokine" and damage-associated molecular pattern[248] that binds ionotropic and metabotropic purinergic receptors, activating innate immunity and inflammatory pathways.[249] Succinate is a Krebs cycle intermediate inside the cell, but binds the G-protein-coupled receptor 91 (GPRC91) on the cell surface that can reverse the antiplatelet activity of aspirin.[250] In another example, citric acid inside the cell is the namesake of the "citric acid cycle," known more commonly as the Krebs cycle. Outside the cell, citrate is a mobile carbon source and barometer of nutrient availability. Citrate is taken into cells via a cell surface transporter called "I'm Not Dead Yet" (INDY) that when mutated leads to cellular citrate depletion and mimics the life-extending effects of caloric restriction.[251] These genetic manipulations illustrate the role of small molecule metabolites as being prime regulators of cell gene expression. The literature on this topic of metabolic regulation of gene expression is extensive (for a recent review, see Reference 252).

METABOLIC CONSEQUENCES OF NUTRIENT EXCESS

In 1929, Herbert Crabtree used mouse cancer cells to show that when glucose was added to a medium, oxygen consumption decreased.[253] Mitochondria were not yet identified as the oxygen-consuming particles, but the iron and cytochrome-containing respiratory catalyst to describe the site of oxygen consumption in cells[254] which was later discovered to be mitochondria. The Crabtree effect has been called the inverted Pasteur effect because in the Pasteur effect, exposure to oxygen was found to inhibit anaerobic glycolysis. The magnitude of the respiratory inhibition by glucose caused by the Crabtree effect varies between 5% and 50%[255] depending on the cell type and the concentration of glucose added. The Crabtree effect plays an important role in many conditions, including chemical sensitivity and diabetes, in which persistently high levels of calories and glucose produce a relative decrease in mitochondrial oxygen consumption, resulting in weakness and fatigue. There are several biochemical mechanisms that combine to produce the Crabtree effect under conditions of nutrient loading.[256] The most significant is the inhibitory effect of the cytosolically produced [ATP]/[ADP][Pk] ratio on mitochondrial ATP synthesis. This happens because mitochondrial oxidative phosphorylation requires cytosolic ADP and Pi to make ATP. When cytosolic ATP rises and ADFP falls, ADP becomes limiting in mitochondria and the excesses of cytosolic ATP inhibits the forward action of mitochondrial ATP synthase (complex V) by classic mechanisms of product inhibition. This induces a chemiosmotic backpressure of protons in the mitochondrial inner membrane space and hyperpolarizes the mitochondrial membrane, that is, makes the mitochondrial membrane potential ($\Delta\psi_m$) more negative. Excess electrons that enter mitochondria under these conditions cannot be used to make ATP because of the backpressure. The partial reduction of oxygen to superoxide and peroxide serves as a pressure release valve[257] that permits excess electrons to be dissipated and oxygen to be exported from the cell in the form of soluble hydrogen peroxide. All of these biophysical and thermodynamic consequences of nutrient loading result in a net decrease in mitochondrial oxygen consumption that we call the Crabtree effect. This effect explains why fasting periodically for 4–5 days helps right the metabolism's restoring energy to the chemically sensitive or chronic degenerative disease individual. With periodic fasting, even in skipping a meal or fasting for 1–2 days results in a return of energy and sharp brain function and elimination of weakness and fatigue.

Because mitochondria create the oxygen sink for the cell, when mitochondrial extraction of oxygen is decreased, cell and tissue oxygen levels rise, and the tissue extraction of oxygen from the blood falls. This is observed clinically as a decrease in the arteriovenous difference in pO_2 in the chemically sensitive patient, which results in weakness and brain dysfunction. The von Ardenne effect—PvO_2 increase is after 28 mm Hg at times over 50%–60%, resulting in tissue hypoxia and thus weakness and fatigue. Physiologically, this is interpreted as "wasted" oxygenation. Ultimately, this high tissue and venous oxygen results in the pruning of capillary beds and reductions in tissue vascularity, that is, peripheral vascular disease. Tissues then undergo OS and eventually inflammation. Over time, this leads to chronic tissue hypoxia, ischemia, and loss of organ function, to heart and kidney failure, and chronic neurodegenerative disease. Venous oxygen reflects this state when elevated over 28 mm Hg.

According to Naviaux, there is an ocean-scale analog to the cellular Crabtree effect.[246] When excessive amounts of nutrients are concentrated in agricultural fertilizer runoff and urban waste and carried downriver to the ocean, the metabolism of plankton in the sea is changed. Ultimately, this process creates seasonal and persistent "dead zones" of ocean hypoxia[258] that cannot support coral, fish, shellfish, or any eukaryotic life larger than a nematode or a few small snails. Repopulating these lost ecosystems can take years of concerted remediation. Excessive "calories" and nutrients injected into the ocean trigger an ecosystem-scale Crabtree effect, in a biphasic process that is similar to type II diabetes or food and chemical overload. First, there is an inhibition of anaerobic metabolism and a rapid increase in algal and cyanobacterial oxygenic photosynthesis to create plankton blooms. This occurs for the same metabolic reasons as in nutrient-loaded human cells; excess nutrients exceed the oxidative capacity of the cells and redirect these excess electrons to NADPH and biomass synthesis. In chemically sensitive patients, initial excess weight may develop with a few pounds to many generally. Nonphotosynthetic cells also shift to this more fermentative metabolism to facilitate rapid conversion of the new nutrient resources to biomass.

In diabetes, and some food and chemically sensitive patients, this shift to biosynthesis leads to organ hypertrophy and the accumulation of adipose tissue and intracellular fat which is used to park the myriad of toxic chemicals. The net result in the ocean is a transient increase in water oxygen because of photosynthesis and decreased oxygen utilization by heterotrophs. This metabolic shift is quantified by biological oceanographers as an increase in bacterial growth efficiency.[259] This first stage of hyperoxia is short-lived and rarely measured. This is similar to the situation in diabetic and chemical sensitivity and food-sensitive patient's tissues exposed to excessive nutrients. The second stage of the response to nutrient loading is a decrease in water oxygen. In the ocean, this occurs because the excess plankton biomass produced by the blooms dies and becomes fuel for other bacteria that extract oxygen from the water to process the dead biomass. Hypoxia results: In human tissues, chronic nutrient excess leads to tissue hypoxia because of capillary pruning that results from decreased mitochondrial oxygen consumption as described above, and from decreased arteriovenous differences in O_2. PvO_2 in the normal patient should be from 20 to 28 mm Hg, whereas in the chemically sensitive patient, the range is 30–70 mm Hg in over 1000 patients measured. This tissue vascular shunting has led to many aberrations of tissue function due to local hypoxia, including weakness, fatigue, and supersensitivity to chemicals, odors, foods, and molds. Initially, the tissue hypoxia from excess nutrient load is patchy, resulting in localized areas of ischemia and segments of dysfunction of various cells and organs. Later, the patches of organ hypoxia begin to merge and significant organ dysfunction occurs. The chemically sensitive patient has poor brain, heart, muscle, respiratory, and gastrointestinal malfunction. Examples of two tissue hypoxia and nutrient overloaded patients are as follows:

Patient 1: PvO_2—35 mm Hg. This 35-year-old white female had mild weight gain and an increase in odor sensitivity to phenol, perfume, car exhaust, weakness, and fatigue that would clear with the prescription of avoidance of pollutants, intradermal injection therapy, caloric restriction, and nutrient supplementation. A PvO_2 microvascular of tissue function is abnormal, taken from the antecubital fossa without using a tourniquet was 35 mm Hg. Supplementation with 6 L of O_2 for constant 2 hours/day using the von Ardenne technique over 18 days resulted in normalizing the PvO_2 to 26 mm Hg along with eliminating the fatigue and weakness. Caloric restriction by the rotary diet was as paramount as the O_2 therapy in creating strength and eliminating the weakness.

Patient 2: PvO_2—77 mm Hg. This 55-year-old white male developed severe chemical sensitivity with odor sensitivity to perfume, car exhaust, pesticides, formaldehyde, and numerous other chemicals, foods (weight gain of 20 lbs.) and mold. Two years ago, he became totally incapacitated, unable to work. He was treated with a massive avoidance procedure to his home by changing the gas furnace and stove, removing the carpets and sealing all the pressboard and plywood producing formaldehyde. He got on a rotary diet of organic food using limited calories, glass bottled spring water. He was better (having lost 20 lbs.) but still had severe weakness, fatigue, and intermittent brain dysfunction. He had difficulty in remembering with short-term memory loss and inability to grasp new ideas and carry out instructions. He was placed on oxygen therapy 8 L/minute for constant 2 hours/day for 54 days. As his PvO_2 steadily dropped from abnormality to 24 mm Hg over the 3-month period, he developed energy and cleared his brain dysfunction. He is now able to go out in society and function well normally. Not only oxygen delivered to the appropriate area but also the caloric restriction limited his nutrient overload, allowing the patient to function normally again through oxygenation and normal function of the tissue.

Redox Compartments and Oxygen Gradients in the Cell

The intracellular "ecosystem" of the eukaryotic cell comprises at least eight different organelle compartments, each with its nutritional state and own redox poise (Figure 2.1). These include: lysosomes,[260] smooth ER, rough ER,[261] the Golgi,[262] the cytosol,[263] peroxisomes,[264] the nucleus,[263] and the mitochondria. This ecosystem needs to always go toward homeostasis for optimum body function. These compartments are not in equilibrium because the proteins that maintain the redox in each compartment and the membranes that separate them are not diffusible.[265] The standard redox potentials of each of these compartments with regard to the glutathione complex (GSH/GSSG) have been measured.

In contrast to sharp boundaries of redox poise that define the different organelles of the cell, the concentrations of oxygen at any point in the cell is determined by oxygen diffusion along its gradient from the capillary to the mitochondrial matrix. With a little imagination, one can imagine that each organelle "swims" to a point in the cellular ecosystem that best meets its need for oxygen and nutrients. Excess nutrients can cause hypoxia by disturbing the microcirculation. The oxygen partial pressure of 40 torr in venous plasma, 30 torr in the pericellular space,[266] and 0.02–0.2 torr (25–250 nm) in mitochondria[267] can be conceptualized in an "oxygen well" or "target diagram" of the cell. When the measured glutathione redox complex is plotted against the log of the partial pressure of oxygen in torr, a linear regression can be calculated. The formula for this line is: GSH/GSSG redox (in mV) $=82.6 \times \log$ (oxygen in torr)-272. This connection between oxygen concentration at every point along the oxygen diffusion gradient and compartmental redox helps explain the profound effect that small changes in mitochondrial oxygen consumption, leading to increased dissolved oxygen concentrations throughout the extra mitochondrial compartments of the cell, can have on the metabolic and work performance of the cell. Indeed, the cell cycle has been characterized as a redox cycle.[268] Excess nutrients can influence these cells' anatomy and physiology so these are areas of hypoxia all over the body with patches eventually coalescing into large area of regional hypoxia. The chemically sensitive patients then do not function well, developing weakness and fatigue and loss of stamina and even brain function.

Cellular Thermodynamics and Work

Prigogine, described the mathematics of dissipative systems in which physical work and the capacity for self-organization can be extracted from the environment by maintaining a compartmentalized, collective chemical "distance" from thermodynamic equilibrium.[269] Mitochondria set a limit on the maximum free energy available for work by a cell by consuming oxygen and transforming metabolites. Excess nutrition dampens this performance. Highly aerobic mitochondria produce a deep oxygen gradient of nearly 150-fold, from 30 torr in the pericellular space to 0.2 torr[267] at the site of cytochrome c oxidase in the inner mitochondrial membrane. The depth of the oxygen sink creates the potential energy that acts like a coiled spring to drive the living clockwork of metabolism, development, differentiation, and organ function. Excess nutrition will alter the clockwork of metabolism and organ function.

Less active mitochondria maintain more shallow oxygen gradients and have a lower work capacity, but greater proliferative capacity. This is illustrated in Table 2.4. This occurs because electrons in the cytosol are redirected to NADPH and macromolecular synthesis and away from usage as NADH in mitochondria when oxygen consumption rates are lower. The ultimate energy currency of the cell is electrons that enter the cell in the form of the chemical bonds in the carbon skeletons of nutrients such as glucose, amino acids, and fatty acids. Mitochondrial oxygen consumption determines the depth of the oxygen sink and ultimately tips the redox balance of the cell either toward growth and proliferation or to differentiation and work. Energy is paramount with adequate oxygenation and limited caloric nutrition.

METABOLIC MEMORY AND EXERCISE

Short-duration physical or chemical stimuli produce long-term cellular effects by inducing kinetically linked chains of events that can be measured metabolically and by protein changes. This phenomenon is called metabolic memory. It is the result of post translational activation and inhibition and transcriptional activation and inhibition events that are initiated by the short-duration stimulus. Many examples are known. The most widely reported example is the long-term effect of short-term, strict metabolic management in patients with diabetes. Even after the management of diabetes is relaxed, long-term metabolic changes in insulin sensitivity and decreased incidence of vascular complications and end-organ disease are observed.[270] Once pollutants, including molds, food, and chemicals, are removed in the chemically sensitive space, the hypersensitivity will last in a way for weeks to months to years. This metabolic memory can be at times discouraging

---

TABLE 2.4
Compartmental Redox and Oxygen Tension in Mammalian Cells

Compartment	pH	Glutathione Redox, GSH/GSSG (mV)	Dissolved Oxygen (Torr)
Mitochondrial matrix	7.8–8.0	-330[263]	0.2[220,267]
Nucleus	7.6	-280[374]	0.8[a]
Peroxisomes	7.6	-270[264]	1[a]
Cytoplasm	7.3	-230[265]	3[a]
Rough ER	7.3	-185[261]	11[a]
Smooth ER	7.3	-160[265]	23[a]
Golgi	5.0[262]	-160	23[a]
Lysosomes	4.5	-160[260]	23[a]
Pericellular space	7.4	-150	30[375]
Venous plasma	7.3	-140[263]	40[376]

Note: Glutathione redox potentials vary between 10% and 15% according to growth conditions in single cells and vary up to 20% in different cell types. Plasma redox potentials vary between 5% and 10% in diurnal cycle and become up to 20 mV more oxidizing with age and disease.[374]

[a] Estimated from the regression equation: Log (pO$_2$ in torr) = mV redox + 272 + 82.6.

to the clinician and patients until it subsides. In the case of some chemically sensitive patients, this metabolic memory of the hypersensitivity and excess nutrition can reactivate upon pollutant exposure triggering adverse reactions causing the patient to be ill once again even though they have been apparently healthy.

Physical exercise is perhaps the best known method of inducing metabolic memory. Even a single session of exercise will produce an increase in basal metabolic rate for hours after the session.[271] Adaptive strength and cardiovascular benefits can be measured over days. Regular resistance training produces metabolic memory and reverses age-related changes in skeletal muscle over months.[271] The mechanisms of these adaptive changes to exercise seem to require the transient pulses of ROS that are produced.[234] In the toxic chemically sensitive patients, the autonomic nervous system is damaged. When the foods are removed to which the patient is sensitive, restoration of tolerance may occur in 1–6 months. This return to normal of the ANS may take a long time by objective measurement. This is true with chemical and mold avoidance. Metabolic memory can be a double-edge sword because here one has the memory of adverse reactions to ward off as the avoidance of toxics occurs.

ANTIOXIDANT THERAPY INHIBITS THE BENEFITS OF EXERCISE

What happens if the normal amounts of superoxide and hydrogen peroxide produced during exercise are inhibited by treatment with AOs? In a ground-breaking study in 2009, Ristow et al.[272] studied the effect of AO supplements (vitamin C at 1000 mg/day; vitamin E at 400 IU/day) on insulin sensitivity and markers such as plasma adiponectin and the master mitochondrial biogenesis regulator peroxisome proliferator-activated receptor-γ coactivator-1α (PGC-1α) after 1 month of exercise. They found that the subjects who exercised and did not take AO supplements had significant improvements in insulin sensitivity, adiponectin, and PGC-1α. AOs inhibited these metabolic benefits of exercise. Ristow et al.[272] proposed that mitochondrial hormesis or beneficial adaptation to stress requires transient OS to induce the downstream changes in nuclear gene expression that promote health and longevity.[273] However, AO supplementation has been found to be very efficacious for preventing and treating with prescription for chemical sensitivity and many degenerative diseases so the diabetic study finding may not be applicable in all kinetics of the situation. Many chemically sensitive patients cannot exercise or do so at a minimum and may be why the AOs work well in them. Also, the supplementation studies may have been done in healthy people who had adequate oxygenation and nutrition which would well bias this opinion.

CONCLUSIONS

ROS and oxidative changes in chronic disease are the symptoms of disease and not the cause. Triggering agents must be found and eliminated. This is the reason that less polluted environmental control units, housing, and work places are so effacious in treating and maintaining the chemically sensitive patient. Indeed, transient and regular stimulation of ROS production is required for mitochondrial hormesis and the beneficial physiologic adaptations associated with exercise and a diet rich in organic fruits and vegetables. Membrane lipid peroxidation, fibrosis, protein oxidation, and hundreds of other markers that were formerly cataloged as oxidative damage need to be understood as cellular oxidative shielding. The conserved pathways of oxidative shielding are protein-catalyzed reactions that evolved as the first step in innate immunity. They evolved to protect the cell from chemical and microbial threats in the environment. Both OS and reductive stress will trigger cellular oxidative shielding. Oxidative shielding takes many forms in different bacterial, plant, and animal phyla. All forms ultimately increase membrane rigidity, decrease membrane permeability, and inhibit cell division. This is temporarily a good thing for the cell overall, especially to the chemically sensitive patient who needs to shut out an influx of toxics. Systemwide conditions such as calorie restriction or nutrient loading modify the cellular response to stress. When stress coincides with excess of dietary nutrient cellular electrons are transferred preferentially to NADPH and not NADH. Synthesized ATP inhibits mitochondrial oxygen consumption via the Crabtree effect and chronic inflammation results. On the other hand, nonneutralizations of the chemically generated free individuals must be neutralized by AOs and a sufficient balance must be obtained, and supplementation is required to adequately counteract the toxics. This is seen constantly in the chemically sensitive patients where supplements and caloric restrictions are necessary.[274]

POLLUTION AND INFLAMMATION

According to Milani, inflammation is useful to the body to a point as it is aimed at the limitation, destruction, and elimination of etiologic agents (i.e., virus, bacteria, chemicals, EMF) or cellular detritus produced following tissue damage.[275] With Constant exposure to triggering agents and continued inflammation; if these agents are not removed, then the mechanism of chronic disease persists.

Peripheral memory traces of the event remains at the dendritic level, at the central level, and in the macrophages in the form of an electromagnetic template.[276] This template can be activated at any moment when an adverse incitant comes into the chemically sensitive patient. This is important because these substances or EMF imprints can cause and propagate inflammation. At times, they are activated by a small amount of antigen from molds, food, chemicals, or EMF resulting in full-blown illness. Therefore, when a prior injury or malady occurs, the body remembers it. This can then act as vulnerability for the nidus of a new exposure. Often, a series of these "cured" entities sets up the patient for chemical sensitivity and/or chronic degenerative disease.

Inflammation is an essential defensive phenomenon whose development and conditions are articulated by molecular events programmed according to an encoded procedure through mechanisms of convergent evolution: that is, (1) the Epstein–Barr virus contains a homologous gene to that of human IL-10 that encodes a product with similar activity to that of the natural CK. This makes it possible to see that the acquisition by the virus of the IL-10 gene during evolution has conferred on the virus the capacity to inhibit the immune response of the host and, consequently, a selective benefit for its own survival; (2) the interleukin-1 (IL-1) transduction mechanism is toll type; (3) IL-1α and IL-1β share the same ribbon-like structure folded at 12 points like the growth bonds of heparin and the Kunitz-type inhibitors of trypsin; (4) receptor similarity of a number of chemokines with the Duffy AG that mediates the penetration of *Plasmodium vivax* into erythrocytes. These examples of "molecular archaeology" demonstrate how the phylogenetic continuum is accomplished through progressive imperceptible transformations of the archaic genomes, but only for the essential functions—among them molecular defense and protection—the base-model (pattern) has remained essentially unchanged in comparison to the one that was active millions of years ago. However, these genes can backfire when an inappropriate triggering agent like pesticides, natural gas, EMF, food, and mold each enter the body in sufficient volume to trigger the memory which activates the molecular defense.

Tissue stress (infection, nonself, exo/endogenous toxicosis) of the inferior phyla turns into somatic stress involving complex apparatuses and systems in fish, reptiles, and birds, leaving the field open to the emotional stress specific to mammals that turns into a typical psychic and spiritual stress—reality because it is at the highest point of the evolutionary pyramid in man or animal because it is an alternative to tissue stress. However, tissue stress of inflammation is almost always a physical phenomenon which is triggered by environmental pollutants such as EMF, chemical, bacteria, virus, parasites, or other physical triggers.

The alerting of the nonspecific and specific, local and systemic immune system (IS) through neuroendocrine mediation creates the basis for the survival of the individual and the species. The *conditio sine qua non* for shaping by adapting it to the appropriate individual responses to internal and external requirements is necessary. It is necessary to decrease the total body pollutant load to decrease and eliminate the triggering agents in order to stop the inflammation. This concept is the key in treating chemical sensitivity.

The relationships between the human nervous system and IS are numerous[277]: Structural polymorphism, immaturity at birth, short- and long-term memory, amplification mechanisms of the afferent stimuli, control of the stressors in excess, auto-inhibition, local and remote effects, and various stereotyped responses occur.

The IS can be interpreted as a true mobile nervous system. The junction where stress, immunity, and pain are sorted is represented by the limbic brain which influences reactive behavior with the memory-affective-emotional dimension. However, the chemical sensitivity has a different olfactory pathway that goes to the prefrontal cortex and then to the limbic system. This is counter to normal person who has a pathway directly from the olfactory nerve to the limbic system.

Thus, it is the same with an almost identical genome, but is different, therefore, due to the individuality of the cultural, environmental, and emotional experiences.

Although there is a good discussion on inflammation of the aspects in disease, it is felt that an overall discussion of incitant entry from any cause and inflammation should be shown for the general and local body areas. Pathology prevails if inflammation is not reversed. It is clearly shown that nasal cerebral (neurovascular), respiratory, and dermal areas are the main avenue of air pollutant entry; some other routes are the gastrointestinal and genitourinary tracts. Excess pollutant entry which is constant will trigger inflammation.

Certainly, the neuro (through the olfactory area) and respiratory routes are the prime avenues for entry of the outdoor and indoor inhalant causes of OS and inflammation. The pathological changes seen in animals and patients are definite leading to end-stage disease, sensitivity, and pollutant exposure. These changes lead to chemical sensitivity and chronic degenerative disease.

CYTOKINES AND INFLAMMATION

According to Melani, CKs are peptides, a diverse group of signatory moleculism produced by different lines of cells of both the innate and specific adaptive IS.[277] These occur in response to a wide variety of inducing stimuli, mainly bacteria, virus, chemicals, particulates, EMF, and antigens that produce various responses depending on the cell types involved in inflammation and immunity. Examples are interleukins and lymphokines released from various cells like macrophages, lymphocytes, and leukocytes.

CKs have a para-endocrine function (transported by the blood in order to interact with the cells that have the receptors they can bind with). They can form prostaglandin E from arachidonic acid.

The functional characteristics of the CKs which are liberated in chemical sensitivity are illustrated schematically, but in essence, in Table 2.5. The second function combines four effects: (1) pleiotropism, the ability to affect more target cells, by inducing macrophages, leukocytes, and lymphocytes by attacking and attempting to destroy those that are damaged by bacteria, virus,

---

TABLE 2.5

Functions of Cytokines

1. CK secretion is a brief and self-limiting phenomenon.
2. CK secretion is pleotropic, attacking and defining infected target cells; antagonist, inhibiting macrophages and gamma globulin; redundant and inducing the protection of B lymphocytes; and synergistic by activating the major histocompatibility complex on many cell types.
3. CKs promote the synthesis and action of other CKs.
4. Local or systemic activity.
5. Necessity for target receptors on the target cells.
6. The target receptors are promoted by external signals to the cell.
7. The target cells respond to the CKs by modifying gene expression.

Source: Milani, L. 2007. Inflammation and physiological regulating medicine. *Physiol. Regul. Med.* 1:19–27.

chemical, EMF. This is the case of IL-4 (the response to the stimulation varies according to the cell type with which they have reacted through specific high-affinity receptors expressed on the surface of the target cells); this pleiotropism would explain the spreading phenomena seen in the untreated chemically sensitive patient, where more cells are involved and many are destroyed causing more and more foods and chemicals to be included in the triggering of chemical sensitivity. (2) Antagonism as with IFN-γ activating and IL-4 inhibiting macrophage functions; clinically, this would explain why the chemically sensitive patient cannot tolerate new chemical exposures. Here, gamma globulin might be suppressed due to weakness of the new B cells. This phenomenon is frequently seen in chemically sensitive patients who have low B cells and thus low gamma globulin. (3) Redundancy as with IL-2, IL-4, IL-5 which induce the proliferation of B lymphocytes and/or why multiple chemicals often can trigger the same inflammatory processes as seen frequently in the chemically sensitive patient. (4) Synergy as with IFN-γ and tumor necrosis factor-alpha (TNF-α) by activating the major histocompatibility complex (MHC) on many cell types. Again, in the chemically sensitive patient resulting in a spreading phenomenon due to concomitant low-dose antigen trigger augmenting the chemical sensitivity occurs.

An effect not sufficiently exploited is the synergy of action of the CKs (explosion of effects) in sequence (cascade of CKs). This phenomenon is seen clinically in the chemically sensitive patient where more exposure to untreated chemicals increase sensitivity which will make the chemically sensitive patient more vulnerable to another chemical exposure. This will often result in pan sensitivity for reaction to the majority of exposed chemicals. This will often render the patient incapacitated and unable to function in society. The CK reaction will proliferate, causing more and more inflammation due to the synergy of these triggered CKs.

An example of the synergy is the cause of the incitants that are not removed, resulting in nutrient deficiency. One hour after the inoculation of LPS (endotoxin from Gram-bacteria), a peak TNF-α concentration is obtained experimentally. While the TNF-α activity is becoming exhausted, the activity of IL-1 is boosted; as this declines, the activity of IL-12 increases,[278] propagating the inflammation.

This endotoxin can be generated by foods, mold, and chemicals in the respiratory and gastrointestinal tract in the chemically sensitive patient continuing to propagate the vulnerability to the food and chemical exposure to hypersensitivity.

The three CKs are secreted only by macrophages and NK cells. If these are constantly being stimulated, more inflammation will occur. The organic response is thereby optimized by a steady, secure, and effective plateau so that the host can adequately neutralize the effect of the LPS; however, extra AOs may be necessary. The phenomena appears to be true with the chemically sensitive patient, unless the triggering agents are removed when the clinician is looking for a stable intradermal endpoint in order to create treatment of food, mold, chemical, or neurotransmitter hypersensitivity. The clinician must first stabilize the patient's physiology by avoidance of pollutants, thus stabilizing CK output so the intradermal and AO-neutralization treatment will hold.

Individually, none of the three CKs are able to neutralize the LPS, even in greater than physiological concentrations. It is necessary for all three to be combined. We see this phenomena in the chemically sensitive patient who has widespread sensitivities to foods, mold, and chemicals triggered by the CKs. Though individual intradermal neutralization is necessary in the long-term composite administration of the neutralizing antigens, it is vital for long-term health and healing of the overall hypersensitivity because often one or two neutralizing antigens would not stop and quell the CKs reactions.

Physiologically, CKs are not stored in the cells; their synthesis requires the transcription of genes that have been silent until now and are activated after stimulation of the cell by environmental toxics. Such transcription activation is transitory but if constant, like in chronic inflammation, will cause nutrient depletion.

The mRNA that encodes the CKs are unstable. Consequently, the secretion of CKs is brief and self-limiting, so the intervention of more CKs "in relay" is necessary to support a biologically targeted effect (teleonomy of the natural phenomena). The clinician dealing with severe chemical sensitivity will see this phenomenon in that until the total body pollutant load is decreased, intradermal neutralization treatment cannot be accomplished because the specific treatment endpoints constantly change due to the unstable CKs. When the injections are administered, they reproduce patient's symptoms but then a proper dilution eliminates symptoms; the clinician can then give a treatment dilution that can be efficacious turning off the clinical reaction. Once the RNA is stabilized, the individual patient can then take treatment and do well. Thus, it only occurs with the combination of elimination of the triggering agents and the proper injection neutralizing dose. This is the importance for decreasing the total body pollutant load which is the most important modality to succeed by avoidance of pollutants in air, food, and water.

The vasoconstriction induced by adrenaline and the subsequent vasodilatation in which histamine, serotonin, and prostaglandins E2 and G2 are involved are equivalent to Selye's flight phase. The use of intradermal neutralization of histamine can reduce and at times eliminate the pollutant-induced microvasoconstriction allowing the environmentally sensitive patient temporary relief from the pollutant-triggered sensitivity. These patients can then reduce their sensitivity by eliminating pollutants that were in the cell creating dysfunction. The allopathic use of antihistamines and COX-2 inhibitors (cyclooxygenase lipoxygenase) inhibits the vasodilation by stopping passive hyperemia, diapedesis, and formation of exudates and phagocytosis with a resulting stand by state and toxicosis of the extracellular matrix (ECM) due to the accumulation of antigen detritus. The prolonged use of these drugs may result in chronic and autoimmune pathologies because of this phenomenon. The blood vessel inflammation turns into tissue inflammation, creating severe mitochondrial and cellular dysfunction as seen in chemical sensitivity. This phenomenon again is why elimination of the triggering agents of the CKs, intradermal neutralization of the responses, and nutrient supplementation is necessary in the chemically sensitive patient.

The biological division is nothing more than the watershed between angio- and histoinflammation. The sudden interruption of the phenomena following on Phase A can indicate temporary abolition of the symptoms, resetting the physiological course that is articulated by a strict, and predetermined timetable: A tissue that is not completely healed (end of Phase B) represents even after years a tissue of less resistance. This phenomenon is frequently observed on the chemically sensitive patient who often has a head injury (knocked out) and recovers without sequalae but later in life gets exposed to natural gas from a stove or heater or a pesticide exposure and develops cerebral chemical sensitivity. A serious irritation of the CNS occurs with a prodrome for various diseases like chemical sensitivity, lupus, vasculitis, arthritis, etc. This state even involves organs derived from different embryonic germ layers from which the damaged organ originates. This organ may be the site of the earlier pathology which discounts the prior injury phenomena. In actual fact, the recovery process is achieved when a balance is established between Th1 and Th2 immunity, regulated by Th3 immunity. The imbalance becomes established as a result of a functional deficit of the Th3 system.

No therapy is really effective if it does not respect the clock that millions of years have standardized. This is why the environmental treatment of avoidance, intradermal neutralization, nutrient supplementation, oxygen therapy, sauna, and immune modulation with autogenous lymphocytic factor, gamma globulin, etc. is so efficacious.

Proinflammatory CKs are IL-6, IL-8, IL-12, IL-17, IL-18 interferon gamma, neopterin, and the chemokines CXCL-12 and CXCI-13. In addition, lipoproteins are proinflammatory, including the VIsE. Pathophysiologic changes are associated with OS, excitotoxicity, changes in homocysteine metabolism, and altered tryptophan anabolism. CK producing cytotoxic inflammation are INF_2, leukotrienes, lipopolysaccharides, NF-κB, ROS, and CKs providing NOS. All these can be triggered from the macrophages, leukocytes, lymphocytes, often shown surrounding blood vessels biopsies releasing the substances triggered by a myriad of environmental incitants such as bacteria, virus, chemical, solvents, molds, mycotoxins, pesticides, natural gas, formaldehydes, phenols, EMF, etc.

TABLE 2.6

Outline Receptors, and Transmembrane Proteins with an External Part with Characteristic Receptors and an Internal Part with Boosters of the Cascade of Signals

Five Families

1. Type 1
   Four domains—α helix
   For IL-2, IL-6 proinflammatory
   For IL-4   anti-inflammatory
2. Type 2
   Similar to Type 1, without try-se-X-try-se
   For IL-10 proinflammatory $\rightarrow$ *STAT 3-type*
   Transduction
3. Receptors of the IgG superfamily characterized by extracellular IgG-like domains proinflammatory for IL-1α and β $\rightarrow$ toll-type transduction
4. TNF receptors high in cysteine. After attaching and becoming integrated with the ligand, they activate cytoplasmic proteins that promote apoptosis and/or stimulate gene expression for TNF proinflammatory $\rightarrow$ TRAF-type transduction
5. 7-Domain receptors: The mammalian genome codes for many receptors of this family. They mediate the chemotactic effect of the chemokines

Source: Milani, L. 2007. Inflammation and physiological regulating medicine. *Physiol. Regul. Med.* 1:19–27.

CKs receptors are transmembrane protein structures with an external part and an internal part that triggers the cascade of signals (transduction). Two molecules are attracted only if they resonate at the same frequency of oscillation.[279,280]

According to Milani, CKs receptors are divisible into five families in accordance with their three-dimensional morphology; each of them induces a different mode of transduction[277] (Table 2.6). Several receptors are coupled to others to control the amount of information, an interesting analogy is with the inhibitory corticospinal nervous tract blocking an excess of peripheral information, a type of protective relay that interrupts the circuit so as not to damage the apparatus. Clearly, when the chemically sensitive patients are overloaded with pollutants (i.e., car exhaust, natural gas, pesticides), they will trigger the CKs resulting in OS, inflammation, and an unstable metabolism.

A paradigmatic example is provided by IL-1 R2 (IL-1 Ra, IL-1 ra), present only in the B lymphocytes, which does not translate any activation signal; it is a real molecular trap, a decoy, or false receptor that blocks the excess IL-1 in order to limit and circumscribe the inflammation and prevent the B lymphocyte from immediately producing IgGs, thus allowing the inflammation to become activated.[281]

Anakinra, a recombinant IL-R2 etanercept and infliximab which blocks the TNF-α receptors have been introduced in the conventional therapy of rheumatoid arthritis and other inflammatory autoimmune pathologies. These drugs have opened up interesting therapeutic perspectives although the negative side effects are particularly impressive. We have found that avoidance and intradermal neutralization of molds, foods, and chemicals are very efficacious in treating the arthritis.

For anakinra: pain, bruises, bleeding at the injection site, frequently force the patients to discontinue treatment.[282] Other adverse reactions are headache and abdominal pain.[282] For etanercept and infliximab: Neutropenia, increased incidence of serious infections can occur. The receptors bind the CKs with high affinity and a constant dissociation of 10^{-10}–10^{-12} M. Consequently, to make a receptor perform its function, very low CK concentrations are sufficient because the number of receptors per cell is relatively low. In fact, the drug prescription for these entities is much better with the aforementioned environmental control which can eliminate the triggering agents and often the need for medication.

Besides the intrinsic characteristics, the concentrations of CKs are very important for therapeutic purposes as different concentrations induce different effects.

For example, low plasma concentrations of TNF-α and IL-1 (10^{-9} M) induce: (1) leukocyte activation, (2) secretion of IL-1, chemokines, and adhesion molecules (local proinflammatory effects); in moderate concentration: (1) fever (hypothalamic center for temperature regulation), (2) acute-phase proteins (from liver), (3) production of leukocytes (from bone marrow); at plasma concentrations ($\geq 10^{-7}$ M): septic shock with hypoglycemia, low endothelial resistance, and formation of thrombosis, low cardiac output. The effect of the different concentrations of a biological active principle had already been experimentally highlighted[283]: 10^{-5} M aconitine causes heart fibrillation; 10^{-7} M bradycardia; 10^{-18} M has no effect on a healthy heart and there is a normalization of the rhythm in the preintoxicated, isolated, and infused heart (*Anguilla anguilla Linn*). In a recent micro-autoradiographic receptor study,[284] it was shown that low-dose and low-tittered substances interact with the cell nucleus, while higher concentrations trigger a cellular response at the cytoplasm. These observations fit the use of intradermal specific dilution of the specific antigen neutralization for the triggering agents and neutralizing agents of the CKs.

Chronologically, the effects of low-dose immune-modulants have been reported by Poitevin et al.,[285] Wagner et al.,[286] Wagner,[287] Davenas et al.,[288] Poitevin et al.,[289] Daurat,[290] Enbergs and Arndt,[291] Enbergs,[292] Belon et al.,[293] Jaggi et al.,[294] Amadori et al., [295] and Rea et al.[296] Therefore, there is a sound scientific basis for the intradermal desensitization and neutralization process.

There is no receptor turnover since the receptor synthesis is regulated by appropriate external signals to the cell. This is one of the ways intradermal provocation neutralization apparently works when the neutralizing dose stops the reaction. The ligand CK and the specific receptor are neosynthesized only if required and simply do not exist when they are not needed, complying closely with the natural principle of parsimony.

It appears at times the inflammation is so chronic and intense that in the chemically sensitive patient, treatment is very difficult because the patient hardly tolerates even less polluted rooms, nutrients, and antigens. Some can even hardly tolerate any clothes.

AIR POLLUTION: NERVOUS SYSTEM AND INFLAMMATION

According to Block et al., Calderon-Garciduenas inflammation is increasingly recognized as a causal factor in the pathology and chronic nature of CNS diseases.[297] While diverse environmental factors have been implicated in neuroinflammation leading to CNS pathology, air pollution may rank as the most prevalent source of environmentally induced OS and inflammation.[298] Traditionally associated with increased risk for pulmonary[299] and cardiovascular disease,[300] air pollution is now also associated with diverse CNS diseases, including chemical sensitivity, AD, PD, stroke, myocardial infarction, and vasculitis.

With pollutant entry and injury, there is a decrease in tight junction proteins, evidence of endothelial cell damage, and upregulation of VCAM/ICAM in the cerebral vasculature, suggesting potential failure of the physical barrier. In addition, PM causes production of CKs and ROS in brain capillaries, which signal changes in transporter expression and function (e.g., P-glycoprotein, P-GP, and multidrug resistance-associated protein 2, MRP2) and a decrease in expression of various tight junction proteins. Thus, brain capillaries recognize air pollution and respond by regulating the physical and chemical barrier function and producing proinflammatory signals. In addition, this response may serve as a proinflammatory sensor and ultimately distribute ROS, CKs, and PM to the brain parenchyma, further contributing to CNS pathology.

VCAM-1

Vascular cell adhesion molecule-1 contains six or seven immunoglobulin domains, and is expressed on both large and small blood vessels only after the endothelial cells are stimulated by CKs.

The gene produces a cell surface sialoglycoprotein, a type I membrane protein that is a member of the IG superfamily.

The VCAM-1 protein mediates the adhesion of lymphocytes, monocyte, eosinophils, and basophils to vascular endothelium. It also functions in leukocyte–endothelial cell signal transduction.

Upregulation of VCAM-1 in endothelial cells by CKs occurs as a result of increased gene transcription (e.g., in response to TNF-α and IL-1).

ICAM-1

Intercellular adhesion molecule 1 (ICAM-1) (CD54, Cluster of Differentiation 54) is a protein in humans. This gene encodes a cell surface glycoprotein which is typically expressed on endothelial cells and cells of the IS. It binds to integrins of type CD11a/CD18 or CD11b/CD18 and is also exploited by rhinovirus as a receptor.[301]

ICAM-1 is a member of the immunoglobulin superfamily, the superfamily of proteins, including antibodies and T-cell receptors. ICAM-1 is a transmembrane protein possessing an amino-terminus extracellular domain, a single transmembrane domain, and a carboxy-terminus cytoplasmic domain. The structure of ICAM-1 is characterized by heavy glycosylation, and the protein's extracellular domain is composed of multiple loops created by disulfide bridges within the protein.

The protein encoded by this gene is a type of intercellular adhesion molecule continuously present in low concentrations in the membranes of leukocytes and endothelial cells. Upon CK stimulation, the concentrations greatly increase. ICAM-1 can be induced by IL-1 and tumor necrosis factor (TNF) and is expressed by the vascular endothelium, macrophages, and lymphocytes. When activated, leukocytes bind to endothelial cells via ICAM-1/LFA-1 and then transmigrate into tissues.[302]

According to Block and Calderon-Garciduenas et al.,[297] Table 2.7 shows an overview of the effects of air pollution in the brain. This table shows the neuroinflammatory and the inflammatory markers.

Air pollution is a multifaceted environmental toxin capable of assaulting the CNS through diverse pathways. Until recently, the mechanisms responsible for air pollution-induced pathology in the brain were unknown. However, despite the variable chemical and physical characteristics of air pollution and the consequent activation of multiple pathways, OS and inflammation are identified as common and basic mechanisms through which air pollution causes damage,[300] including CNS effects. Furthermore, while multiple cell types in the brain respond to exposure to air pollution, new reports indicate that microglia (brain immune cells) and brain capillaries may be critical actors responsible for cellular damage. In the experience of the EHC-Dallas and EHC-Buffalo, environmentally triggered vasculitis is common in the chemically sensitive patient, as have peripheral immune changes such as abnormal T and B cells, gamma globulin, and complements.

Symptoms associated with the proinflammatory cascade are due to the CKs IL-6, 8, 12, 17, 18, interferon gamma, neopterin, and chemokines CXCI 12 and 13. The microanatomy of pollutant injury has been shown on previous pages and will not be reflected here. Physical and neurological changes without inflammation were observed by Calderon-Garciduenas et al., in children and adults of Mexico City.[297] This led to serious brain involvement, including ischemic stroke.

A complex mixture of gases, PM, and chemicals present in outdoor and indoor air produces adverse health effects such as those seen in the chemically sensitive and chronic degenerative patients. Because the nasal cavity is a common portal of entry for such pollutants, the nasal olfactory and respiratory mucosa are vulnerable to damage and well-known targets for air pollutant-induced toxicity and carcinogenicity.[304–307] The nose–brain barrier depends on intact epithelia, including tight junctions and an intact xenobiotic metabolizing capacity.[308] Olfactory receptor cell dendrites are in direct contact with the environment, and, thus, pinocytosis and neuronal transport are likely routes of access to the CNS of potential toxins.[309] Olfactory receptor neurons project from the sensory epithelium to targets within the olfactory bulb, the first synaptic relay in the olfactory pathway.[309]

TABLE 2.7

Research Overview: Effects of Air Pollution on the Brain

Air Pollution Model	Experimental Model	Neuroinflammation and Pro-inflammatory Markers	Neuropatholgy and Behavior Changes	References
Particulate matter	Mouse	N/T	D Neuron damage in the substantia nigra	41
	Mouse	IL1-β, TNF-α, and INF-γ increase in Olfactory bulb	Change in neurotransmitters	113
	Mouse	Cytokine production JNK activation enhanced NF-κB expression	N/T	29,30
	Mouse	N/T	Changes in neurotransmitters	31
	Rat	N/T	Lipid peroxidation Decrease in exploratory behavior	32
	Cell culture	Microglial activation Superoxide production	DA neuron damage	58
	Cell culture	Microglial Activation TNF-α and IL-6 production	N/T	59
	Brain capillary culture	TNF-α and ROS Production C-Jun Phosphorylation	P-GP and MRP2 Increase tight Junction protein decrease	69
Ozone	Rat	N/T	Lipid peroxidation DA Neuron damage and death in substantia nigra, motor deficits	125–127
	Rat	N/T	Lipid peroxidation and impaired memory	124,128
	Rat	Astrocyte IL-6 and TNF-α increase at BBB	Increase in brainstem VEGF expression (adaptive repair response)	130
	Prenatal rat	N/T	DA, NA, DOPAC, and HVA decrease	129
	Cell culture	N/T	Astrocyte death	303
Nanoparticles	Cell culture	Microglial activation Superoxide production	DA neuron damage	70,116
	Cell culture	N/T	HBMEC toxicity, lower tight junction expression	68
	Mouse	N/T	Oxidative stress (brain) Lipid peroxidation	71–73
Chronic ambient air pollution	Human	COX₂, IL1-β, and iNOS, and CD14 increase	White matter lesions diffuse Aβ plaques, α-synuclein aggregation, BBB damage, cognitive deficits, and DNA damage	10,14,27,28,52,68
	Dog	iNOS, NF-κβ, and CD14 increase	White matter lesions diffuse Aβ plaques α-synuclein	11,12,28

Source: Reprinted from *Trends in Neurosciences*, 32, Black, M. L., L. Calderon-Garciduenas, Air pollution: Mechanisms of neuroinflammation and CNS disease, 506–516, Copyright 2009, with permission from Elsevier.

The mucociliary apparatus of the respiratory mucosa also functions as a barrier to protect against neuronal uptake and transport by trapping insoluble inhaled material in a layer of secretions that are in continuous movement toward the nasopharynx.[305] The contribution of air pollutant exposure to airway epithelial injury is well documented.

Healthy children and adult populations in Southwest Metropolitan Mexico City (SWMMC), an urban area characterized by significant daily concentrations of pollutants such as ozone, PM, and aldehydes, have shown extensive damage to the respiratory nasal epithelium.[310–313] Children in SWMMC display ultrastructural evidence of deficiencies in nasal epithelial junction integrity, cytoplasmic deposition of PM, and altered mucociliary defense mechanisms.[313] Canines living in SWMMC exhibit similar nasal respiratory lesions (Calderon-Garciduenas, unpublished observations), along with respiratory, bronchiolar, and myocardial pathology.[314,315] A sustained pulmonary inflammatory process is clearly seen in exposed canines,[315] and SWMC children show radiological and spirometric evidence of lung damage and CK imbalance.[316] Hyper and impaired olfaction, hyposmia, or anosmia is important early changes in neurodegenerative diseases, including AD and PD,[317–319] as well as in aging.[320,321] All layers of the olfactory bulb are affected in aging and AD, and olfaction is impaired in the early stages of AD.[318,322]

Aged canines are valuable models of aging.[323,324] Veterinarians have noticed geriatric behavioral changes in pet dogs, including decrements in attention and activity, wandering and disorientation, and disturbances of the sleep/wake cycle.[324,325] In aged dogs, Aβ accumulation correlates with cognitive dysfunction; plaques are of the diffuse subtype; and there is no neuritic involvement.[324] A threshold effect of plaque development was observed by Russell[326] in 103 laboratory-raised beagles. In dogs kept in outdoor kennels at Davis, California, and Fort Collins, Colorado, no plaques were apparent at ages younger than 10 years, but numbers progressively increased to 73% at ages 15–17.8 years.[326] Weigel[327] described in a cohort of 30 mongrel dogs a subpopulation with increased numbers of Aβ-positive diffuse plaques and concluded that only 43% of these mongrel dogs were susceptible to amyloidosis of that only the severely affected subpopulation was exposed to a factor or factors inducing this pathology. Fibers representing an early neuritic change that precedes tau hyperphosphorylation have been described by Satou et al.[328] in aging dogs.

This report describes early and progressive alterations in the nasal respiratory and olfactory mucosae, the olfactory bulb, and cortical and subcortical brain structures in healthy dogs in SWMC exposed daily to high levels of ambient air pollutants: canines from a comparable city, Tlaxcala, with low levels of pollution representing controls. Early changes included NF-κB—and inducible nitric oxide synthase (iNOS)-positive cells, vascular changes in cortical small arterioles and capillaries, apoptosis in glial and vascular smooth muscle cells and pericytes, cortical perineuronal satellitosis, and neuronal chromatolysis. These alternations were followed by reactive astrocytosis predominantly in cortical white matter and subapical regions, apolipoprotein E (APOE) immunoreactivity in abnormal lipid vacuoles in blood vessels, and astrocytic processes, nonneuritic plaques, and NFT.

Clinically healthy mongrel dogs from Tlaxcala and SWMC were studied. The selection of the two different cities was based on their concentrations of air pollutants and similar altitudes above sea level. Metropolitan Mexico City extends over 2000 km^2 and is located in an elevated valley, 2250 m above sea level. It is a megacity with 20 million residents and the associated production of air pollutants from automobiles, leakage of petroleum gas, and industrial activity. The climate is mild with year-round sunshine, light winds, and temperature inversions. Each of these factors contributes to create an environment in which complex photochemical reactions produce oxidant chemicals and other toxic compounds. Air quality data are provided by an automated surface network of 33 monitoring stations in and around MC; hourly, near-surface measurements are made of monitored pollutants, including ozone, PM_{10}, SO_2, NO_2, CO, and Pb. Mexico City's main pollutants are PM and ozone, with levels exceeding U.S. National Ambient Air Quality Standards (NAAQS) most of the year. The maximal concentrations of ozone precursors appear downwind of the emission zones toward the southern urban area, southwest and southeast MC.[329] According to Fast and Zhong,[330] the highest particle concentrations occur regularly in the vicinity of the peak ozone concentrations during the afternoon. Ozone concentrations as high as 0.48 ppm have been measured during severe air pollution[331]; the SWMC atmosphere is characterized by average maximal ozone daily concentrations of 0.250 ppm. An average of 4 ± 1 hours/day with ozone >0.08 ppm is recorded in SWMC year-round (83.9% of days).[329] NO_2 concentrations do not usually exceed the annual arithmetic mean of 0.053 ppm (4.6% of days), whereas SO_2 levels exceed the 24-hour primary standard of 0.14 ppm in the winter months. Both PM_{10} and $PM_{2.5}$ exceed their respective annual arithmetic means above the standards (annual NAAQS PM_{10} 78 $\mu g/m^3$ and $PM_{2.5}$ 21.6 $\mu g/m^3$ vs. standards of 50 $\mu g/m^3$ and 15 $\mu g/m^3$, respectively).[332,333] Other pollutants detected in SWMC include volatile organic compounds (VOC) such as linear and cyclic saturated and unsaturated HC; aromatic HC; aldehydes; ketones; esters; and acids and their halogenated derivatives.[334] Formaldehyde and acetaldehyde ambient values are in the range of 5.9–110 ppbv and 2–66.7 ppbv, respectively.[335] Mutagenic PM[336]; alkane HC[331]; benzene[337]; various metals such as vanadium, manganese, and chromium[338]; and peroxyacetyl nitrate[333] are also detected. Lichens absorb their nutrients from the atmosphere and can be used as sensitive monitors of airborne metals[339]; *Parmotrema arnoldii* accumulates lead, copper, and zinc in SWMC.[334] In addition, 500 metric tons of canine fecal materials are deposited daily on MC streets.[340] There is clearly a total environmental pollutant load that can be transferred to a total body pollutant load and that can cause and disturb the chemically sensitive patient.

The rationale behind selecting the SW geographical area in MC involved two major factors. First, the special distribution of pollutants such PM_{10}, O_3, SO_2, and NO_2 within the city reflects the higher concentrations of particulate and gaseous emissions in the northern part of the city where most industries are located. Ozone levels are higher in the south, a residential area, as a result of wind transport of the mass precursor pollutants emitted in the industrial northern and central regions. Second, their studies of healthy children and adults living in SWMC present evidence of nasal and pulmonary pathology, as well as serum CK imbalance in children.[316,341]

Tlaxcala was selected as the control city because its altitude is above sea level; Mexico City's atmospheric pollutant data were similar to that of MC, and studies in canines from this area have shown minimal pulmonary and cardiac pathology.[314,315] Tlaxcala is the capital city of the state of Tlaxcala, located 114 km east of Mexico City at 2252 m above sea level. It has a temperature climate, an average temperature year-round of 16°C, and 700 mm of annual rainfall. With 63,423 inhabitants, it is a city in compliance with current air pollution regulations.

Mexico City's atmospheric pollutant data were obtained from the available literature and a representative monitoring station located in the SW. Tlaxcala's data were obtained from the Subsecrataria de Ecologia SWMC data representing air pollution patterns corresponding to the ages of the dogs and tissue collection times (2000–2001) (Table 2.8).

According to Block et al., air pollution is a prevalent proinflammatory stimulus to the CNS that has been largely overlooked as a risk factor for neurodegenerative disease.[297] In the United States alone, an estimated 29 million people are exposed to PM_{10} and 88 million are exposed to $PM_{2.5}$.[315] Alarmingly, ultrafine PM < 200 $\mu g/m^3$ UFPM levels are unmonitored and unregulated in the United States, but exposure is estimated to be high. In addition, millions more are exposed to PM occupationally and in the setting of disasters, including war, fires, and the aftermath of terrorist attacks, such as the attack on the World Trade Center.[315] The diseases potentially affected by air pollution, such as chemical sensitivity, AD, and PD, are also widespread. Chemical sensitivity is the fastest-growing entity in the United States. At present, it is difficult to stop because of the massive contamination of air, food, and water. As the most prevalent neurodegenerative disease,[316] AD affects more than 4 million people in the United States and an estimated 27 million are affected worldwide.[310] PD is a devastating movement disorder and is the second most prevalent neurodegenerative disease,[316] affecting 1%–2% of the population over the age of 50.[311] Given these statistics,

TABLE 2.8

Physical Descriptions of Tlaxcala Control and W = SWMC Canines

Age	Control (Gender)	SWMMC (Gender)	Average Weight
24–48 hours	0	4 (2F/2M)[a]	275 ± 120 g
2–4 week	0	3 (1F/2M)[a]	554 ± 190 g
1 and 3 months	0	2 (M)[a]	460 g and 7 kg
8–12 months	2 (1F/1M)	2 (M)[a](F)	11.2 ± 2.4 kg
>1 year to <3 years	2 (1F/1M)	4 (2F/2M)	12.16 ± 5.74 kg
4–5 years	1 (F)	4 (2F/2M)	20.3 ± 5.2 kg
6–8 years	2 (F)	11 (7F/4M)[b]	22.0 ± 8.6 kg
11 and 12 years	1 (F)	2 (1F/1M)	37.33 ± 11.01 kg
Total	8	32	

Source: Subsecretaria de Ecologia. 2000–2001, Santa Rosa, Argentina.

[a] Animals raised at the animal facility outdoor/indoor kennel.

[b] Two males ages 6 and 7 also raised at the animal facility.

it is of significant concern that recent reports have linked air pollution to neuroinflammation and neuropathology associated with chemical sensitivity, AD, and PD.

The first studies exploring whether air pollution is culpable in neurodegenerative disease were investigated in animal (feral dog) populations naturally exposed to polluted urban environments.[342] Feral dogs living in regions of high pollution showed enhanced oxidative damage, premature presence of diffuse amyloid plaques, and a significant increase in DNA damage (apurinic/apyrimidinic sites) in olfactory bulbs, frontal, cortex, and hippocampus.[342,343] Further, dogs exposed to high concentrations of urban pollution show tissue damage and accumulated metals (nickel and vanadium) at target brain regions in a gradient fashion (olfactory mucosa > olfactory bulb > frontal cortex), implicating the nasal pathway as a key portal of entry.[342] In a striking similarity, both AD and PD share early pathology in the olfactory bulb, nuclei, and pathways, with olfactory deficits being one of the earliest findings in both diseases.[312] This work provided the first association between exposure to pollution and acceleration of neurodegenerative disease pathology.

Recently, these findings have now been confirmed and extended in humans and additional animal models. Analysis of brain tissue from individuals residing in highly polluted areas show an increase in CD-68, CD-163, and HLA-DR positive cells (indicating infiltrating monocytes or resident microglia activation), elevated proinflammatory markers (IL-1β, IL1-β; cyclooxygenase 2, COX_2), an increased in $A\beta_{42}$ deposition (hallmark disease protein of AD), blood–brain barrier (BBB) damage, endothelial cell activation,[313] and brain lesions in the prefrontal lobe.[340] Interestingly, upregulation of proinflammatory markers such as COX_2 and IL1-β, as well as the CD-14 marker for innate immune cells, were localized in frontal cortex, substantia nigra, and vagus nerves.[313] Further, animal studies have also shown that air pollution causes CK production,[344,345] increases MAP kinase signaling through JNK,[345] neurochemical changes,[332] lipid peroxidation,[346] behavior changes,[346] and enhanced NF-kβ expression.[344] Together, these studies clearly indicate that air pollution has effects on the CNS.

Abnormal filamentous protein aggregates and neuroinflammation are common denominators of both AD and PD.[347] While studies have yet to find a direct effect of air pollution on defined Lewy bodies (pathological hallmark of PD) or Aβ plaques (pathological hallmark of AD), exposure to urban air pollution has been shown to cause both neuroinflammation and accumulation of $A\beta_{42}$ (component of Aβ plaques) and α-synuclein (component of Lewy bodies) in target areas for AD and PD involvement.[313] As shown previously, for example, dogs exposed to high levels of air pollution show increased deposits of diffuse amyloid plaques, a decade earlier than their clean air counterpart residents.[342,343] Further, the accumulation of $A\beta_{42}$ and α-synuclein is reported to commence early in human childhood[313] with exposure to high concentrations of air pollution, supporting that air pollution may cause premature aging in the brain and/or instigate disease processes early in development. One plausible mechanism is that nanoparticles[348–350] and OS[308,324] modify aggregation and rate of protein fibrillation, potentially affecting soluble Aβ and α-synuclein. It is possible that these changes in protein aggregation associated with air pollution may mark early pathology in neurodegenerative disease processes. Some data are now coming in that long-term chemical sensitivity in patients damaged for 30–40 years do develop neurodegenerative disease in some case if they have suboptimal treatments.

It has also been proposed that environmental toxicants exert their effects at multiple points across human development to culminate in CNS disease, a theory labeled "the multiple hit hypothesis."[351] We see this phenomenon in the life time's history of the chemically sensitive in addition to chronic degenerative disease. Consistent with this premise, studies show that PM begins to impact the CNS early in childhood.[340] For example, MRI analyses have revealed structural damage (hyperintense white matter lesions) localized in the prefrontal cortex in children exposed to high concentrations of air pollution, which may be associated with cognitive dysfunction.[340] Notably, dogs exposed to the same air pollution also show frontal lesions with vascular/endothelial pathology and neuroinflammation.[340] Thus, young humans and animals may be particularly vulnerable to the inflammatory effects of air pollution and these effects may accumulate across an individual's lifespan.

While ischemic stroke,[314,352,353] multiple sclerosis (exposure to secondhand smoke promotes risk),[354] and PD[355] (manganese content in the air is linked to enhanced risk)[355] are currently the only CNS diseases with established increased epidemiological risk with air pollution exposure, it is likely that many other uninvestigated diseases have an even greater associated risk like chemical sensitivity. These risks may be distributed across the individual differences, in population susceptibility, as genetic predisposition may confer vulnerability to the CNS effects of air pollution, such as is the case with inherited $APOE_4$ allele carriers[313] in humans and APOE knockout mice.[333] However, given the high prevalence of AD and PD, the link between neuroinflammation and AD/PD pathogenesis, the established CNS pathology by air pollution, and the common high rate of human exposure to air pollution, extending both mechanistic and epidemiological studies to pursue the risks for other CNS diseases is of pressing concern to human health. Millions of people as they age have short-term memory loss, many of which if they are chemically sensitive show obliteration of the temporal lobes on Triple-camera brain SPECT scans. These findings are almost always attributed to pollutant injury over time. Simon et al.[356] have shown this on the brains of 100 chemically sensitive patients at the EHC-Dallas (Figures 2.3 and 2.4).

ISCHEMIC STROKE

According to Block et al., while it is well known that air pollution affects human health through cardiovascular and respiratory morbidity and mortality, it has only recently been shown that these deleterious effects extend to the brain.[297] The impact of air pollution upon the brain was first noted as an increase in ischemic stroke frequency found in individuals exposed to indoor coal fumes.[323] In the United States, stroke is the number one cause of adult disability and the third leading cause of death, behind only cancer and heart disease.[357] While the data on the association between cerebrovascular disease and ambient air pollution are limited, exposure to diverse air pollutants (e.g., PM, ozone, carbon monoxide, and nitrogen dioxide) in the ambient air is epidemiologically associated with enhanced risk for ischemic cerebrovascular events.[314,352,353] In fact, current reports demonstrate that enhanced risk for ischemic stroke correlates with air pollution, even in communities with relatively low pollutant concentrations (below current EPA safety standards).[314,341,353] While the mechanisms driving the pathology are somewhat unclear, ozone and PM have been shown to

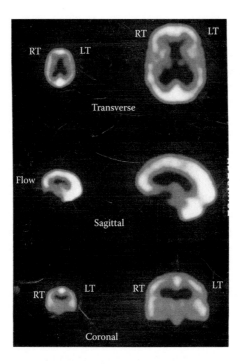

FIGURE 2.3   **(See color insert.)** Normal SPECT brain scan—smooth, uniform, distinct outlines, no rough edges or holes in cerebral hemispheres or abnormal temporal lobes.

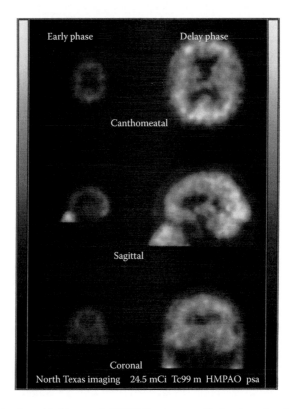

FIGURE 2.4   **(See color insert.)** Abnormal SPECT brain scan. Early phase barely visible, delayed phase holes in cerebrum, temporal lobes obliterate; no good defined lines.

TABLE 2.9

Variance Predicted by Age, Gender, and Residency, for WISC-R Subtests Suggesting an Effect of Residency N = 73

WISC-R Subset	Variance Explained (R^2)	F	p	Variance Explained Uniquely by Residency	t	p
Object assembly	0.433	17.591	<0.001	0.033	2.028	0.046
Picture arrangement	0.306	10.143	<0.001	0.038	1.945	0.056
Digit span	0.288	9.325	<0.001	0.065	2.529	0.014
Information	0.657	43.981	<0.001	0.029	2.396	0.019
Arithmetic	0.522	25.139	<0.001	0.033	2.196	0.031
Mazes	0.544	27.384	<0.001	0.020	1.733	0.088
Vocabulary	0.549	27.992	<0.001	0.019	1.682	0.097

Source: Calderón-Garcidueñas, L. et al. 2008. Air pollution, cognitive deficits and brain abnormalities: A pilot study with children and dogs. *Brain Cogn.* 68:117–127. http://englelab.gatech.edu/2008/calderongarciduenasetal2008.pdf

TABLE 2.10

Performance Age Compared to Chronological Age with Each Cohort for WISC-R

	Mexico City (N = 55)			Polotitlan (N = 18)		
	Mean Scale Age (SEM)	t	p	Mean Scale Age (SEM)	t	p
Chronological age	9.20 (0.30)	NA	NA	10.50(0.53)	NA	NA
Information	8.14 (0.30)	−2.3507	0.0190	9.94(0.72)	−0.5685	ns
Similarities	8.02 (0.32)	−2.60252	0.0094	8.97(0.73)	−1.53675	ns
Arithmetic	8.82 (0.27)	−0.86205	ns	10.51(0.71)	0.008872	ns
Vocabulary	7.86 (0.29)	−2.95074	0.0033	9.29(0.76)	−1.21902	ns
Comprehension	8.07 (0.24)	−2.4985	0.0127	9.04(0.45)	−1.46583	ns
Digit span	7.11 (0.18)	−4.60566	<0.001	8.53(0.65)	−1.98346	ns
Picture completion	8.67 (0.35)	−1.1675	ns	9.65(0.66)	−0.86389	ns
Picture arrangement	8.88 (0.31)	−0.71647	ns	11.29(0.88)	0.790057	ns
Block design	9.27 (0.36)	0.154673	ns	10.53(0.71)	0.027299	ns
Object assembly	8.11 (0.32)	−2.41858	0.0158	9.93(0.73)	−0.5819	ns
Coding	7.48 (0.31)	−3.79778	0.0002	8.79(0.77)	−1.72213	ns
Mazes	9.57 (0.49)	0.82379	ns	11.16(0.79)	0.661069	ns
Verbal IQ	7.79 (0.23)	−3.1259	0.0018	9.12(0.60)	−1.5282	ns
Performance IQ	8.46 (0.29)	−1.3828	ns	10.00(0.59)	−0.9143	ns
Full scale IQ	8.14 (0.25)	−2.2544	0.0024	9.59(0.57)	−0.9737	ns

Source: Calderón-Garcidueñas, L. et al. 2008. Air pollution, cognitive deficits and brain abnormalities: A pilot study with children and dogs. *Brain Cogn.* 68:117–127. http://englelab.gatech.edu/2008/calderongarciduenasetal2008.pdf

NA, not available.

TABLE 2.11

White Matter Lesions in Control and Mexico City Children MRI in Four Image Acquisition Sequences

Cohorts	Age/Gender	APOE	TLR4	WML/Total	Kruit Load Score[a]
Control	12F	3/3	AA	0	0
Control	12F	3/3	AA	0	0
Control	10M	3/3	AA	0	0
Control	9F	3/3	AA	0	0
Control	9M	3/4	AA	1	0.0042
Control	10F	4/4	AA	0	0
Control	8M	3/3	AA	0	0
Control	10F	3/3	AA	0	0
Control	16M	3/3	AA	0	0
Control	10F	3/3	AA	0	0
Control	10M	3/3	AA	0	0
Control	10F	3/3	AA	0	0
Control	13M	3/3	AA	0	0
MC	14F	3/3	GG	0	0
MC	17M	3/3	GG	3	0.0126
MC	18M	3/3	AA	1	0.0042
MC	11M	3/3	AA	1	0.0042
MC	9F	3/3	AA	7	0.0294
MC	10F	3/3	AA	3	0.0126
MC	8F	3/3	AA	9	0.0378
MC	11M	3/3	AA	1	0.0042
MC	12F	3/3	AA	0	0
MC	10M	3/3	AA	0	0
MC	12F	3/3	AA	0	0
MC	10F	3/3	AA	0	0
MC	8M	3/3	AA	0	0
MC	11F	3/3	AA	0	0
MC	12F	3/3	AA	1	0.0042
MC	10F	3/3	AA	0	0
MC	10M	3/3	AA	9	0.0378
MC	8M	2/3	AA	2	0.0084
MC	7F	3/3	AA	1	0.0042
MC	11M	3/3	AA	0	0
MC	7F	3/3	AA	3	0.0126
MC	11M	3/3	AA	1	0.0042
MC	10M	3/3	AA	0	0

Source: Calderón-Garcidueñas, L. et al. 2008. Air pollution, cognitive deficits and brain abnormalities: A pilot study with children and dogs. *Brain Cogn.* 68:117–127. http://englelab.gatech.edu/2008/calderongarciduenasetal2008.pdf

[a] Kruit et al.,[377]) score: The white matter lesions (WML) were defined as areas with high signal intensities on T2 weighted MRI: the count of WML was combined to get a quantitative measure of load by multiplying each lesion by a size-dependent constant: 0.0042 mL for 1 ($<$3 mm), 0.114 mL for 2 (4–10 mm), and 0.90 mL for 3($>$10 mm).

TABLE 2.12

White Matter Lesions in Three Mexico City Children with Repeated MRIs

MRI Date	Age/Gender	White Matter Lesions/Total	Kruit Score[a]
June 13, 2006	11M	1	0.0042
November 24, 2006	11M	1	0.0042
February 13, 2007	11M	1	0.0042
March 23, 2006	7F	2	0.0084
June 13, 2006[a]	7F	2	0.0084
November 24, 2006[a]	8F	2	0.0084
February 13, 2007[a]	8F	3	0.0126
June 13, 2006	11M	0	0
November 24, 2006	11M	1	0.0042
February 13, 2007	11M	1	0.0042

Source: Calderón-Garcidueñas, L. et al. 2008. Air pollution, cognitive deficits and brain abnormalities: A pilot study with children and dogs. *Brain Cogn.* 68:117–127. http://englelab.gatech.edu/2008/calderongarciduenasetal2008.pdf

[a] MRI shown in Figure 2.3.

TABLE 2.13

COX2, IL-1β, and GFAP mRNA in Frontal Cortex White Matter in Age-Matched Dogs from Mexico City and Control City

Groups	COX2/GAPDH[a]	IL-1β/GAPDH[a]	GFAP/GAPDH[a]
Control N:5	181.7 ± 44.75	746.2 ± 613.8	295503 ± 1161.45
Mexico City N:7	41764 ± 17152	4050 ± 1343	485135 ± 104243
	$p = 0.03$	$p = 0.01$	$p = 0.34$

Source: Calderón-Garcidueñas, L. et al. 2008. Air pollution, cognitive deficits and brain abnormalities: A pilot study with children and dogs. *Brain Cogn.* 68:117–127. http://englelab.gatech.edu/2008/calderongarciduenasetal2008.pdf

[a] Molecules per femtomol GAPDH rRNA.

rapidly modulate the expression of genes involved in key vasoregulatory pathways in the brain; with the food and water also being so contaminated, the total body pollutant load is exceeded, triggering the vasculitis and vasculopathy resulting in vasospasm and ischemic stroke, substantiating the idea that inhaled pollutants induce cerebrovascular effects.[358] However, in addition to a neurovascular impact, current reports also indicate that the effects of air pollution invade the brain parenchyma, causing pathology indicative of neurodegenerative disease. Clearly, the reduction of total body pollutant load is necessary to clear OS and inflammation. This reduction is necessary to have the body's physiology function well and at an optimum pace.

Cognitive dysfunction, gait abnormalities, falls, and depression occurred.[359–361] White matter lesions impair frontal lobe function[362] and indicate abnormalities of the subcortical fiber system.[363] Histopathology correlates in the elderly include enlarged Virchow–Robin spaces, degeneration of axons and myelin, and gliosis.[364,365] Progressive white matter hyperintensities in older adults are

TABLE 2.14

COX2, IL-1β, and GFAP mRNA in Frontal Cortex with White Matter Lesions by Brain MRI's versus Normal White Matter on MRI's in Mexico City Dogs

ID# DOG and Anatomical Area Sampled	COX2/ GAPDH[a]	IL-1β/GAPDH[a]	GFAP/GPDH[a]	WML by MRI	Differences between WML and/or Normal White Matter by MRI
1 FL2	101.3	280.8	53052	No	
1 FR2	91.3	502.4	380598	Yes	IL-1β 1.78-fold, GFAP 7.1-fold,
2 FL6	229.6	1217.0	168376	Yes	COX2 2.1-fold, IL-1β 2.24-fold
2 FR6	107.2	542.9	217355	No	
3 FL2	143.8	887.3	447983	No	
3 FR2	122.0	596.0	430648	No	COX2 1.17-fold, IL-1β 1.48-fold, GFAP 1.0-fold
4 FL1	133	9611	312843	No	
4 FL2	155	15927	1407132	Yes	IL-1β 1.9-fold, GFAP 2.86-fold
4 FL3	187	8351	491373	No	
4 FR3	36929	15900	1490285	Yes	COX2 197-fold, IL-1β 1.9-fold, GFAP 3.0-fold
5 FR2	138.2	1303.	291530	No	
5 FL2	72347	2122.7	531086	No	COX2 523.4-fold, IL-1β 1.62-fold, GFAP 1.82-fold
6 FL2	54.5	1063.6	31832	No	
6 FR2	274.3	3213.5	276814	No	COX2 5.03-fold, IL-1β 3.02-fold, GFAP 8.69-fold
7 FL	13014.5	1926	512403	Yes	COX2 11.7-fold, IL-1β 1.42-fold
7 FR	1105	1352	718854	No	

Source: Calderón-Garcidueñas, L. et al. 2008. Air pollution, cognitive deficits and brain abnormalities: A pilot study with children and dogs. *Brain Cogn.* 68:117–127. http://englelab.gatech.edu/2008/calderongarciduenasetal2008.pdf

[a] Molecules per femtomol GAPDH rRNA.

related to changes in regional cerebral blood flow.[366] Vascular changes predominantly involving subcortical areas (e.g., white matter, in basal ganglia, thalamus, and hippocampus) are seen in both AD and vascular dementia in patients, and in mixed dementia cases.[367] The common denominator for the hyperintense white matter lesions detected by brain MRI appears to be a vascular lesion with perivascular gliosis and enlarged Virchow–Robin spaces. Based on Calderon-Garciduenas's pilot results, it is suggested that the white matter lesions detected in 56.5% of Mexico City children tested represent the extreme of the vascular lesions with a breakdown of the BBB, and that the vascular pathology is likely of a diffuse nature as seen in young dogs.

In summary, clinically healthy children with no known risk factors for neurological or cognitive disorders residing in a highly polluted urban environment exhibited deficits in fluid cognition, memory, and executive functions relative to children living in a less polluted urban environment. In parallel, the number of the children living in the highly polluted city exhibited white matter hyperintense lesions in MRI, while only one child living in the less polluted city exhibited a single lesion. These white matter lesions along with the presence of more diffuse vascular pathology are likely to interrupt subcortical prefrontal cortex connections and other white matter tracts, potentially contributing to the cognitive dysfunction. Ultrafine PM reaching the frontal cortex in the highly exposed dogs and in young Mexico City adults[368] is likely contributing to the neuroinflammation.

In the United States, 158 million people live in areas where ozone exceeds the 8 hour standard, 29 million are exposed to PM_{10} and 88 million to $PM_{2.5}$.[369] Urban sites with high PM contributions from vehicles and industry[370] are highly visible polluted sources, although indoor pollution is also very important particularly for disadvantaged populations living in high-density multiunit dwellings in large urban areas.[371] The issue of air pollution causing cognitive deficits and brain structural changes in healthy children with all their potential consequences ought to be of major public importance. Alterations in measures of fluid intelligence and cognitive control predict school performance, complex learning, ability to control attention and avoid distraction, reading and listening comprehension, reasoning, and of key importance from the social point of view: the ability to block impulsive antisocial behavior.

MRI techniques have made it possible to study structural and metabolic brain development across age groups, including children,[372] and regional white matter alterations are related to decreases in performance on neuropsychological tests.[373] Triple-camera SPECT scans are even better to demonstrate pollutant altered brain dysfunction. Thus, as suggested by the interdisciplinary methodology of the present investigation, it is possible to comprehensively examine brain structural and functional changes and to determine the interrelationships between age, white matter changes, hippocampus measurements, cognitive function, and the cumulative doses of air pollutants. The work here presents a pioneering attempt to answer such urgent questions, and initial findings give encouragement that future, large-scale work in this area has great potential to give much needed answers. Clearly, pollutant overload causes chemical sensitivity and brain dysfunction (Tables 2.9 through 2.14).

REFERENCES

1. Nedergaard, M. 2013. Neuroscience. Garbage truck of the brain. *Science* 340 (6140):1529–1530.
2. Mucke, L., D. J. Selkoe. 2012. Neurotoxicity of amyloid β-protein: Synaptic and network dysfunction. *Cold Spring Harb. Perspect. Med.* 2 (7):a006338.
3. Frost, B., M. I. Diamond. 2010. Prion-like mechanisms in neurodegenerative diseases. *Nat. Rev. Neurosci.* 11 (3):155–159.
4. Walker, L. C., M. I. Diamond, K. E. Duff, B. T. Hyman. 2013. Mechanisms of protein seeding in neurodegenerative diseases. *JAMA Neurol.* 70 (3):304–310.
5. Loukas, M., S. S. Bellary, M. Kuklinski, J. Ferrauiola, A. Yadav, M. M. Shoja, K. Shaffer, R. S. Tubbs. 2011. The lymphatic system: A historical perspective. *Clin. Anat.* 24:807–881.
6. Cserr, H. F. 1971. Physiology of the choroid plexus. *Physiol. Rev.* 51 (2):273–311.
7. Iliff, J. J. et al. 2012. A paravascular pathway facilitates CSF flow through the brain parenchyma and the clearance of interstitial solutes, including amyloid β. *Sci. Transl. Med.* 4 (147):147ra111.
8. Nagelhus, E. A., T. M. Mathiisen, O. P. Ottersen. 2004. Aquaporin-4 in the central nervous system: Cellular and subcellular distribution and coexpression with KIR4.1. *Neuroscience* 129 (4):905–913.
9. Iliff, J. J., M. Nedergaard. 2013. Is there a cerebral lymphatic system? *Stroke* 44 (6 Suppl 1):S93–S95.
10. Ren, Z., J. J. Iliff, L. Yang, J. Yang, X. Chen, M. J. Chen, R. N. Giese, B. Wang X. Shi, M. Nedergaard. 2013. "Hit and Run" model of closed-skull traumatic brain injury (TBI) reveals complex patterns of post-traumatic AQP4 dysregulation. *J. Cereb. Blood Flow Metab.* 33 (6):834–845.
11. Clavaguera, F. et al. 2009. Transmission and spreading of tauopathy in transgenic mouse brain. *Nat. Cell Biol.* 11 (7):909–913.
12. Zemlan, F. P., E. C. Jauch, J. J. Mulcahhey, S. P. Gabbita, W. S. Rosenberg, S. G. Speciale, M. Zuccarello. 2002. C-tau biomarker of neuronal damage in severe brain injured patients: Association with elevated intracranial pressure and clinical outcome. *Brain Res.* 947:131–139.
13. Goldstein, L. E. et al. 2012. Chronic traumatic encephalopathy in blast-exposed military veterans and a blast neurotrauma mouse model. *Sci. Transl. Med.* 4 (134):134–160.
14. Weller, R. O., S. D. Preston, M. Subash, R. O. Carare. 2009. Cerebral amyloid angiopathy in the aetiology and immunotherapy of Alzheimer disease. *Alzheimers Res. Ther.* 1 (2):6–19.
15. Calderón-Garcidueñas, L. et al. 2012. Neuroinflammation, hyperphosphorylated tau, diffuse amyloid plaques, and down-regulation of the cellular prion protein in air pollution exposed children and young adults. *J. Alzheimers Dis.* 28:93–107.
16. Iliff, J. J., H. Lee, M. Yu, T. Feng, J. Logan, M. Nedergaard, H. Benveniste. 2013. Brain-wide pathway for waste clearance captured by contrast-enhanced MRI. *J. Clin. Inves.* 123 (3):1299–1309.

17. Yang, L., B. T. Kress, H. J. Weber, M. Thiyagarajan, B. Wang, R. Deane, H. Benveniste, J. Iliff, M. Nedergaard. 2013. Evaluating glymphatic pathway function utilizing clinically relevant intrathecal infusion of CSF tracer. *J. Transl. Med.* 11:107–116.

18. Selye, H. 1955. Stress and disease. *Science* 122:625–631.

19. Didriksen, N., A. Goven, J. R. Butler. 1985. Psychological stress: Effects on phagocytic immune functioning. *Clin. Ecol.* 4 (1):31–39.

20. Butler, J. R., J. I. Laseter, I. R. DeLeon. 1984. Pesticides and brain function changes in a controlled environment. *Clin. Ecol.* 2 (3):145–150.

21. Goodman, R., M. Blank. 2002. Insights into electromagnetic interaction mechanisms. *J. Cell. Physiol.* 192:16–22.

22. Phillips, J. L., N. P. Singh, H. Lai. 2009. Electromagnetic fields and DNA damage. *Pathophysiology* 16 (2–3):79–88.

23. Salford, L. G., A. Brun, K. Sturreson, J. L. Eberhardt, B. R. Persson. 1994. Permeability of the blood-brain barrier induced by 915 MHz electromagnetic radiation, continuous wave and modulated at 8, 16, 50 and 200 Hz. *Microsc. Res. Tech.* 27 (6):535–542.

24. Blackman, C. F., S. G. Benane, J. R. Rabinowitz, D. E. House, W. T. Joines. 1985. A role for the magnetic field in the radiation-induced efflux of calcium ions from brain tissue *in vitro*. *Bioelectromagnetics* 6 (4):327–337.

25. Pall, M. L. 2013. Electromagnetic fields act via activation of voltage-gated calcium channels to produce beneficial or adverse effects. *J. Cell. Mol. Med.* 17 (8):958–965.

26. Walleczek, J. 1992. Electromagnetic field effects on cells of the immune system: Role of calcium signaling. *FASEB J.* 6:3177–3185.

27. Cadossi, R., G. Emilia, G. Ceccherellil, G. Torelli. 1988. Lymphocytes and pulsed magnetic fields. In *Modern Bioelectricity*. A. Marino ed., pp. 451–496. New York: Dekker.

28. Papatheofanis, F. J. 1990. Use of calcium channel antagonists as magnetoprotective agents. *Radiat. Res.* 122:24–28.

29. Catterall, W. A. 2000. Structure and regulation of voltage-gated Ca^{2+} channels. *Annu. Rev. Cell. Dev. Biol.* 16:521–555.

30. Morgado-Valle, C., L. Verdugo-Díaz, D. E. García, C. Morales-Orozco, R. Drucker-Colín. 1998. The role of voltage-gated Ca^{2+} channels in neurite growth of cultured chromaffin cells induced by extremely low frequency (ELF) magnetic field stimulation. *Cell. Tissue Res.* 291:217–230.

31. Lorich, D. G., C. T. Brighton, R. Gupta, J. R. Corsetti, S. E. Levine, I. D. Gelb, R. Seldes, S. R. Pollack. 1998. Biochemical pathway mediating the response of bone cells to capacitive coupling. *Clin. Orthop. Relat. Res.* 350:246–256.

32. Gobba, F., D. Malagoli, E. Ottaviani. 2003. Effects of 50 Hz magnetic fields on fMLP-induced shape changes in invertebrate immunocytes: The role of calcium ion channels. *Bioelectromagnetics* 24:277–282.

33. Lisi, A., M. Ledda, E. Rosola, D. Pozzi, E. D'Emilia, L. Giuliani, A. Foletti, A. Modesti, S. J. Morris, S. Grimaldi. 2006. Extremely low frequency electromagnetic field exposure promotes differentiation of pituitary corticotrope-derived AtT20 D16 V cells. *Bioelectromagnetics* 27:641–651.

34. Piacentini, R., C. Ripoli, D. Mezzogori, G. B. Azzena, C. Grassi. 2008. Extremely low-frequency electromagnetic fields promote *in vitro* neurogenesis via upregulation of Ca(v)1-channel activity. *J. Cell. Physiol.* 215:129–139.

35. Morris, C. E., T. C. Skalak. 2008. Acute exposure to a moderate strength static magnetic field reduces edema formation in rats. *Am. J. Physiol. Heart Circ. Physiol.* 294:H50–H57.

36. Ghibelli, L. et al. 2006. NMR exposure sensitizes tumor cells to apoptosis. *Apoptosis* 11:359–365.

37. Fanelli, C., S. Coppola, R. Barone, C. Colussi, G. Gualandi, P. Volpe, L. Ghibelli. 1999. Magnetic fields increase cell survival by inhibiting apoptosis via modulation of Ca^{2+} influx. *FASEB J.* 13:95–102.

38. Jeong, J. H., C. Kum, H. J. Choi, E. S. Park, U. D. Sohn. 2006. Extremely low frequency magnetic field induces hyperalgesia in mice modulated by nitric oxide synthesis. *Life Sci.* 78:1407–1412.

39. Vernier, P. T., Y. Sun, M. T. Chen, M. A. Gundersen, G. L. Craviso. 2008. Nanosecond electric pulse-induced calcium entry into chromaffin cells. *Bioelectrochemistry* 73:1–4.

40. Kim, I. S., J. K. Song, Y. M. Son, T. H. Cho, T. H. Lee, S. S. Lim, S. J. Kim, S. J. Hwang. 2009. Novel effect of biphasic electric current on *in vitro* osteogenesis and cytokine production in human mesenchymal stromal cells. *Tissue Eng. Part A.* 15:2411–2422.

41. Höjevik, P., J. Sandblom, S. Galt, Y. Hamnerius. 1995. Ca^{2+} ion transport through patch-clamped cells exposed to magnetic fields. *Bioelectromagnetics* 16:33–40.

42. Barbier, E., B. Vetret, B. Dufy. 1996. Stimulation of Ca^{2+} influx in rat pituitary cells under exposure to a 50 Hz magnetic field. *Bioelectromagnetics.* 17:303–311.

43. Grassi, C., M. D'Ascenzo, A. Torsello, G. Martinotti, F. Wolf, A. Cittadini, G. B. Azzena. 2004. Effects of 50 Hz electromagnetic fields on voltage-gated Ca^{2+} channels and their role in modulation of neuroendocrine cell proliferation and death. *Cell. Calcium.* 35:307–315.

44. Craviso, G. L., S. Choe, P. Chatterjee, I. Chatterjee, P. T. Vernier. 2010. Nanosecond electric pulses: A novel stimulus for triggering Ca^{2+} influx into chromaffin cells via voltage-gated Ca^{2+}channels. *Cell. Mol. Neurobiol.* 30:1259–1265.

45. Marchionni, I., A. Paffi, M. Pellegrino, M. Liberti, F. Apollonio, R. Abeti, F. Fontana, G. D'Inzeo, M. Mazzanti. 2006. Comparison between low-level 50 Hz and 900 MHz electromagnetic stimulation on single channel ionic currents and on firing frequency in dorsal root ganglion isolated neurons. *Biochim. Biophys. Acta* 1758:597–605.

46. Rao, V. S., I. A. Titushkin, E. G. Moros, W. F. Pickard, H. S. Thatte, M. R. Cho. 2008. Nonthermal effects of radiofrequency-field exposure on calcium dynamics in stem cell-derived neuronal cells: Elucidation of calcium pathways. *Radiat. Res.* 169:319–329.

47. Adair, R. K., R. D. Astumian, J. C. Weaver. 1998. Detection of weak electric fields by sharks, rays, and skates. *Chaos* 8:576–587.

48. Constable, P. A. 2011. Nifedipine alters the light-rise of the electro-oculogram in man. *Graefes Arch. Clin. Exp. Ophthalmol.* 249:677–684.

49. Gmitrov, J., C. Ohkuba. 2002. Verapamil protective effect on natural and artificial magnetic field cardiovascular impact. *Bioelectromagnetics* 23 (7):531–541.

50. Kindzelskii, A. L., H. R. Petty. 2005. Ion channel clustering enhances weak electric field detection by neutrophils: Apparent role of SKF96365-sensitive cation channels and myeloperoxidase trafficking cellular responses. *Eur. Biophys. J.* 35:1–26.

51. Xu J., W. Wang, C. C. Clark, C. T. Brighton. 2009. Signal transduction in electrically stimulated articular chondrocytes involves translocation of extracellular calcium through voltage-gated channels. *Osteoarthritis Cartilage* 17:397–405.

52. Pilla, A. A. 2012. Electromagnetic fields instantaneously modulate nitric oxide signaling in challenged biological systems. *Biochem. Biophys. Res. Commun.* 426:330–333.

53. McDonald, L. J., F. Murad. 1996. Nitric oxide and cyclic GMP signaling. *Proc. Soc. Exp. Biol. Med.* 211:1–6.

54. Francis, S. H., J. L. Busch, J. D. Corbin, D. Sibley. 2010. cGMP-dependent protein kinases and cGMP phosphodiesterases in nitric oxide and cGMP action. *Pharmacol. Rev.* 62:525–563.

55. Pacher, P., J. S. Beckman, L. Liaudet. 2007. Nitric oxide and peroxynitrite in health and disease. *Physiol. Rev.* 87:315–424.

56. Pryor, W. A., G. L. Squadrito. 1995. The chemistry of peroxynitrite: A product from the reaction of nitric oxide with superoxide. *Am. J. Physiol.* 268:L699–L722.

57. Lymar, S. V., R. F. Khairutdinov, J. K. Hurst. 2003. Hydroxyl radical formation by O-O bond homolysis in peroxynitrous acid. *Inorg. Chem.* 42:5259–5266.

58. Guler, G., Z. Turkozer, A. Tomruk, N. Seyhan. 2008. The protective effects of N-acetyl-L-cysteine and epigallocatechin-3-gallate on electric field-induced hepatic oxidative stress. *Int. J. Radiat. Biol.* 84:669–680.

59. Sypniewska, R. K., N. J. Millenbaugh, J. L. Kiel, R. V. Blystone, H. N. Ringham, P. A. Mason, F. A. Witzmann. 2010. Protein changes in macrophages induced by plasma from rats exposed to 35 GHz millimeter waves. *Bioelectromagnetics* 31:656–663.

60. Grigoriev, Y. G., V. F. Mikhailov, A. A. Ivanov, V. N. Maltsev, A. M. Ulanova, N. M. Stavrakova, I. A. Nikolaeva, O. A. Grigoriev. 2010. Autoimmune processes after long-term low-level exposure to electromagnetic fields part 4. Oxidative intracellular stress response to the long-term rat exposure to nonthermal RF EMF. *Biophysics* 55:1054–1058.

61. Erdal, N., S. Gürgül, L. Tamer, L. Ayaz. 2008. Effects of long-term exposure of extremely low frequency magnetic field on oxidative/nitrosative stress in rat liver. *J. Radiat. Res.* 49:181–187.

62. Ahuja, Y. R., B. Vijayashree, R. Saran, E. L. Jayashri, J. K. Manoranjani, S. C. Bhargava. 1999. In vitro effects of low-level, low-frequency electromagnetic fields on DNA damage in human leucocytes by comet assay. *Indian J. Biochem. Biophys.* 36:318–322.

63. Amara, S., T. Douki, J. L. Ravanat, C. Garrel, P. Guiraud, A. Favier, M. Sakly, K. Ben Rhouma, H. Abdelmelek. 2007. Influence of a static magnetic field (250 mT) on the antioxidant response and DNA integrity in THP1 cells. *Phys. Med. Biol.* 52:889–898.

64. Focke, F., D. Schuermann, N. Kuster, P. Schär. 2010. DNA fragmentation in human fibroblasts under extremely low frequency electromagnetic field exposure. *Mutat. Res.* 683:74–83.

65. Franzellitti, S., P. Valbonesi, N. Ciancaglini, C. Biondi, A. Contin, F. Bersani, E. Fabbri. 2010. Transient DNA damage induced by high-frequency electromagnetic fields (GSM 1.8 GHz) in the human trophoblast HTR-8/SVneo cell line evaluated with the alkaline comet assay. *Mutat. Res.* 683:35–42.

66. Garaj-Vrhovac, V., G. Gajski, S. Pažanin, A. Sarolić, A. M. Domijan, D. Flajs, M. Peraica. 2011. Assessment of cytogenetic damage and oxidative stress in personnel occupationally exposed to the pulsed microwave radiation of marine radar equipment. *Int. J. Hyg. Environ. Health* 214:59–65.

67. Hong, R., Y. Zhang, Y. Liu, E. Q. Weng. 2005. Effects of extremely low frequency electromagnetic fields on DNA of testicular cells and sperm chromatin structure in mice. *Zhonghua Lao Dong Wei Sheng Zhi Ye Bing Za Zhi.* 23:414–417.

68. Ivancsits, S., E. Diem, A. Pilger, H. W. Rüdiger, O. Jahn. 2002. Induction of DNA strand breaks by intermittent exposure to extremely-low-frequency electromagnetic fields in human diploid fibroblasts. *Mutat. Res.* 519:1–13.

69. Ivancsits, S., E. Diem, O. Jahn, H. W. Rüdiger. 2003. Intermittent extremely low frequency electromagnetic fields cause DNA damage in a dose-dependent way. *Int. Arch. Occup. Environ. Health* 76:431–436.

70. Ivancsits, S., A. Pilger, E. Diem, O. Jahn, H. W. Rudiger. 2005. Cell-type specific genotoxic effects of intermittent extremely low-frequency electromagnetic fields. *Mutat. Res.* 583:184–188.

71. Kesari, K. K., J. Behari, S. Kumar. 2010. Mutagenic response of 2.45 GHz radiation exposure on rat brain. *Int. J. Radiat. Biol.* 86:334–343.

72. Lai, H., N. P. Singh. 1997. Melatonin and a spin-trap compound block radiofrequency electromagnetic radiation-induced DNA strand breaks in rat brain cells. *Bioelectromagnetics* 18:446–454.

73. Lai, H., N. P. Singh. 2004. Magnetic-field-induced DNA strand breaks in brain cells of the rat. *Environ. Health Perspect.* 112:687–694.

74. Lee, J. W., M. S. Kim, Y. J. Kim, Y. J. Choi, Y. Lee, H. W. Chung. 2011. Genotoxic effects of 3 T magnetic resonance imaging in cultured human lymphocytes. *Bioelectromagnetics* 32:535–542.

75. Paulraj, R., J. Behari. 2006. Single strand DNA breaks in rat brain cells exposed to microwave radiation. *Mutat. Res.* 596:76–80.

76. Romeo, S., L. Zeni, M. Sarti, A. Sannino, M. R. Scarfì, P. T. Vernier, O. Zeni. 2011. DNA electrophoretic migration patterns change after exposure of Jurkat cells to a single intense nanosecond electric pulse. *PLoS One* 6:e28419.

77. Schwarz, C., E. Kratochvil, A. Pilger, N. Kuster, F. Adlkofer, H. W. Rüdiger 2008. Radiofrequency electromagnetic fields (UMTS, 1,950 MHz) induce genotoxic effects *in vitro* in human fibroblasts but not in lymphocytes. *Int. Arch. Occup. Environ. Health* 81:755–767.

78. Svedenstål, B. M., K. J. Johanson, M. O. Mattsson, L. E. Paulsson. 1999. DNA damage, cell kinetics and ODC activities studied in CBA mice exposed to electromagnetic fields generated by transmission lines. *In Vivo* 13:507–513.

79. Svedenstål, B. M., K. J. Johanson, K. H. Mild. 2012. DNA damage induced in brain cells of CBA mice exposed to magnetic fields. *In Vivo* 13:551–552.

80. Trosić, I., I. Pavicić, S. Mlković-Kraus, M. Mladinić, D. Zeljezić. 2011. Effect of electromagnetic radiofrequency radiation on the rats' brain, liver and kidney cells measured by comet assay. *Coll. Antropol.* 35:1259–1264.

81. Burdak-Rothkamm, S., K. Rothkamm, M. Folkard, G. Patel, P. Hone, D. Lloyd, L. Ainsbury, K. M. Prise. 2009. DNA and chromosomal damage in response to intermittent extremely low-frequency magnetic fields. *Mutat. Res.* 672:82–89.

82. Fairbairn, D. W., K. L. O'Neill. 1994. The effect of electromagnetic field exposure on the formation of DNA single strand breaks in human cells. *Cell. Mol. Biol. (Noisy-le-grand)* 40:561–567.

83. Fiorani, M., O. Cantoni, P. Sestili, R. Conti, P. Nicolini, F. Vetrano, M. Dachà. 1992. Electric and/or magnetic field effects on DNA structure and function in cultured human cells. *Mutat. Res.* 282:25–29.

84. Malyapa, R. S., E. W. Ahern, W. L. Straub, E. G. Moros, W. F. Pickard, J. L. Roti Roti. 1997. Measurement of DNA damage after exposure to 2450 MHz electromagnetic radiation. *Radiat. Res.* 148:608–617.

85. McNamee, J. P., P. V. Bellier, V. Chauhan, G. B. Gajda, E. Lemay, A. Thansandote. 2005. Evaluating DNA damage in rodent brain after acute 60 Hz magnetic-field exposure. *Radiat. Res.* 164:791–797.

86. Scarfí, M. R., A. Sannino, A. Perrotta, M. Sarti, M. Mesirca, F. Bersani. 2005. Evaluation of genotoxic effects in human fibroblasts after intermittent exposure to 50 Hz electromagnetic fields: A confirmatory study. *Radiat. Res.* 164:270–276.

87. Stronati, L., A. Testa, P. Villani, C. Marino, G. Alovisolo, D. Conti, F. Russo, A. M. Fresegna, E. Cordelli. 2004. Absence of genotoxicity in human blood cells exposed to 50 Hz magnetic fields as assessed by comet assay, chromosome aberration, micronucleus, and sister chromatid exchange analyses. *Bioelectromagnetics* 25:41–48.

88. Testa, A., E. Cordelli, L. Stronati, G. Marino, A. Lovisolo, A. M. Fresegna, D. Conti, P. Villani. 2004. Evaluation of genotoxic effect of low level 50 Hz magnetic fields on human blood cells using different cytogenetic assays. *Bioelectromagnetics* 25:613–619.

89. Szabó, G., S. Bahrle. 2005. Role of nitrosative stress and poly(ADP-ribose) polymerase activation in myocardial reperfusion injury. *Curr. Vasc. Pharmacol.* 3:215–220.

90. Moon, H. K., E. S. Yang, J. W. Park. 2006. Protection of peroxynitrite-induced DNA damage by dietary antioxidants. *Arch. Pharm. Res.* 29:213–217.

91. Sakihama, Y., M. Maeda, M. Hashimoto, S. Tahara, Y. Hashidoko. 2012. Beetroot betalain inhibits peroxynitrite-mediated tyrosine nitration and DNA strand damage. *Free Radic. Res.* 46:93–99.

92. Hybertson, B. M., B. Gao, S. K. Bose, J. M. McCord. 2011. Oxidative stress in health and disease: The therapeutic potential of Nrf2 activation. *Mol. Aspects Med.* 32:234–246.

93. Ridley, A. J., H. F. Paterson, C. L. Johnston, D. Diekmann, A. Hall. 1992. The small GTP-binding protein rac regulates growth factor-induced membrane ruffling. *Cell* 70:401–410.

94. Wennström, S., P. Hawkins, F. Cooke, K. Hara, K. Yonezawa, M. Kasuga, T. Jackson, L. Claesson-Welsh, L. Stephens. 1994. Activation of phosphoinositide 3-kinase is required for PDGF-stimulated membrane ruffling. *Curr. Biol.* 4:385–393.

95. Joucla, S., B. Yvert. 2012. Modeling of extracellular neural stimulation: From basic understanding to MEA-based applications. *J. Physiol. Paris.* 106:146–158.

96. Pashut, T., S. Wolfus, A. Friedman, M. Lavidor, I. Bar-Gad, Y. Yeshurun, A. Korngreen. 2011. Mechanisms of magnetic stimulation of central nervous system neurons. *PLoS. Comput. Biol.* 7:e1002022.

97. Fatemi-Ardekani, A. 2008. Transcranial magnetic stimulation: Physics, electrophysiology, and applications. *Crit. Rev. Biomed. Eng.* 36:375–412.

98. Silva S., P. J. Basser, P. C. Miranda. 2008. Elucidating the mechanisms and loci of neuronal excitation by transcranial magnetic stimulation using a finite element model of a cortical sulcus. *Clin. Neurophysiol.* 119:2405–2413.

99. Radman, T., R. L. Ramos, J. C. Brumberg, M. Bikson. 2009. Role of cortical cell type and morphology in subthreshold and suprathreshold uniform electric field stimulation *in vitro*. *Brain Stimul.* 2:215–228.

100. Minelli, T. A., M. Balduzzo, F. F. Milone, V. Nofrate. 2007. Modeling cell dynamics under mobile phone radiation. *Nonlinear Dynamics Psychol. Life Sci.* 11:197–218.

101. Saunders, R. D., J. G. R. Jefferys. 2007. A neurobiological basis for ELF guidelines. *Health Phys.* 92:596–603.

102. Havas, M. 2008. Dirty electricity elevates blood sugar among electrically sensitive diabetics and may explain brittle diabetes. *Electromagn. Biol. Med.* 27:135–146.

103. Havas, M. 2006. Electromagnetic hypersensitivity: Biological effects of dirty electricity with emphasis on diabetes and multiple sclerosis. *Electromagn. Biol. Med.* 25:259–268.

104. de Vochta, F. 2010. "Dirty electricity": What, where, and should we care? *J. Expo. Sci. Environ. Epidemiol.* 20:399–405.

105. Friedman, J., S. Kraus, Y. Hauptman, Y. Schiff, R. Seger. 2007. Mechanism of short-term ERK activation by electromagnetic fields at mobile phone frequencies. *Biochem. J.* 405(Pt. 3):559–568.

106. Desai, N. R., K. K. Kesari, A. Agarwal. 2009. Pathophysiology of cell phone radiation: Oxidative stress and carcinogenesis with focus on the male reproductive system. *Reproduct. Biol. Endocrinol.* 7:114.

107. Wyatt, C. N., E. K. Weir, C. Peers. 1994. Diphenylamine iodonium blocks K^+ and Ca^{2+} currents in type I cells isolated from the rat carotid body. *Neurosci. Lett.* 172:63–66.

108. Ryabi, J. T. 1998. Clinical effects of electromagnetic fields on fracture healing. *Clin. Orthop. Relat. Res.* 355(Suppl. l):S205–S215.

109. Oishi, M., S. T. Onesti. 2000. Electrical bone graft stimulation for spinal fusion: A review. *Neurosurgery* 47:1041–1055.

110. Aaron, R. K., D. M. Ciombor, B. J. Simon. 2004. Treatment of nonunions with electric and electromagnetic fields. *Clin. Orthop. Relat. Res.* (419):21–29.

111. Goldstein, C., S. Sprague, B. A. Petrisor. 2010. Electrical stimulation for fracture healing: Current evidence. *J. Orthop. Trauma* 24(Suppl. l):S62–S65.

112. Demitriou, R., G. C. Babis. 2007. Biomaterial osseointegration enhancement with biophysical stimulation. *J. Musculoskelet. Neuronal. Interact.* 7 (3):253–265.

113. Griffin, X. L., F. Warner, M. Costa. 2008. The role of electromagnetic stimulation in the management of established non-union of long bone fractures: What is the evidence? *Injury* 39:419–429.

114. Huang, L. Q., H. C. He, C. Q. He, J. Chen, L. Yang. 2008. Clinical update of pulsed electromagnetic fields on osteoporosis. *Chin. Med. J.* 121:2095–2099.

115. Groah, S. L., A. M. Lichy, A. V. Libin, I. Ljungberg. 2010. Intensive electrical stimulation attenuates femoral bone loss in acute spinal cord injury. *PMR* 2:1080–1087.

116. Schidt-Rohlfing, B., J. Silny, K. Gavenis, N. Heussen. 2011. Electromagnetic fields, electric current and bone healing – what is the evidence? *Z. Orthop. Unfall.* 149:265–270.

117. Griffin, X. L., M. L. Costa, N. Parsons, N. Smith. 2011. Electromagnetic field stimulation for treating delayed union or non-union of long bone fractures in adults. *Cochrane Database Syst. Rev.* (4):CD008471.

118. Chalidis, B., N. Sachinis, A. Assiotis, G. Maccauro. 2011. Stimulation of bone formation and fracture healing with pulsed electromagnetic fields: Biologic responses and clinical implications. *Int. J. Immunopathol. Pharmacol.* 24 (1 Suppl. 2):17–20.

119. Zhong, C., T. F. Zhao, Z. J. Xu, R. X. He. 2012. Effects of electromagnetic fields on bone regeneration in experimental and clinical studies: A review of the literature. *Chin. Med. J.* 125:367–372.

120. Diniz, P., K. Soejima, G. Ito. 2002. Nitric oxide mediates the effects of pulsed electromagnetic field stimulation on the osteoblast proliferation and differentiation. *Nitric Oxide* 7:18–23.

121. Fitzsimmons, R. J., S. L. Gordon, J. Kronberg, T. Ganey, A. A. Pilla. 2008. A pulsing electric field (PEF) increases human chondrocyte proliferation through a transduction pathway involving nitric oxide signaling. *J. Orthop. Res.* 26:854–859.

122. Lin, H. Y., Y. J. Lin. 2011. In vitro effects of low frequency electromagnetic fields on osteoblast proliferation and maturation in an inflammatory environment. *Bioelectromagnetics* 32:552–560.

123. Cheng, G., Y. Zhai, K. Chen, J. Zhou, G. Han, R. Zhu, L. Ming, P. Song, J. Wang. 2011. Sinusoidal electromagnetic field stimulates rat osteoblast differentiation and maturation via activation of NO-cGMP-PKG pathway. *Nitric Oxide* 25:316–325.

124. Pilla, A., R. Fitzsimmons, D. Muehsam, J. Wu, C. Rohde, D. Casper. 2011. Electromagnetic fields as first messenger in biological signaling: Application to calmodulin-dependent signaling in tissue repair. *Biochim. Biophys. Acta* 1810:1236–1245.

125. Rangaswami, H., R. Schwappacher, T. Tran, G. C. Chan, S. Zhuang, G. R. Boss, R. B. Pilz. 2012. Protein kinase G and focal adhesion kinase converge on Src/Akt/β-catenin signaling module in osteoblast mechanotransduction. *J. Biol. Chem.* 287:21509–21519.

126. Marathe, N., H. Rangaswami, S. Zhuang, G. R. Boss, R. B. Pilz. 2012. Pro-survival effects of 17β-estradiol on osteocytes are mediated by nitric oxide/cGMP via differential actions of cGMP-dependent protein kinases I and II. *J. Biol. Chem.* 287:978–988.

127. Rangaswami, H. et al. 2010. Cyclic GMP and protein kinase G control a Src-containing mechanosome in osteoblasts. *Sci. Signal.* 3:ra91.

128. Rangaswami, H., N. Marathe, S. Zhuang, Y. Chen, J. C. Yeh, J. A. Frangos, G. R. Boss, R. B. Pilz. 2009. Type II cGMP-dependent protein kinase mediates osteoblast mechanotransduction. *J. Biol. Chem.* 284:14796–14808.

129. Saura, M., C. Tarin, C. Zaragoza. 2010. Recent insights into the implication of nitric oxide in osteoblast differentiation and proliferation during bone development. *Sci. World J.* 10:624–632.

130. Zaragoza, C., E. López-Rivera, C. García-Rama, M. Saura, A. Martínez-Ruíz, T. R. Lizarbe, F. Martín-de-Lara, S. Lamas. 2006. Cbfa-1 mediates nitric oxide regulation of MMP-13 in osteoblasts. *J. Cell. Sci.* 119:1896–1902.

131. Wang, D. H., Y. S. Hu, J. J. Du, Y. Y. Hu, W. D. Zhong, W. J. Qin. 2009. Ghrelin stimulates proliferation of human osteoblastic TE85 cells via NO/cGMP signaling pathway. *Endocrine* 35:112–117.

132. Becker, R. O., J. A. Spadaro, A. A. Marino. 1977. Clinical experiences with low intensity direct-current stimulation of bone-growth. *Clin. Orthop. Relat. Res.* 124:75–83.

133. Cornelli, U. 2007. Oxidation and antioxidants. Scientific basis of Physiological Regulating Medicine (P. R. M.). Seminar at Loyola University of Chicago.

134. Comroe, J. H., R. D. Dripps, P. R. Dumke, M. Deming. 1945. Oxygen toxicity. *JAMA* 128:707–710.

135. Nash, G., J. B. Blennerhasset, H. Pontoppidan. 1967. Pulmonary lesions associated with oxygen therapy and artificial ventilation. *N. Engl. J. Med.* 276:368–374.

136. Zitnanova, I., P. Korytar, O. I. Aruoma, M. Sustrová, I. Garaiová, J. Muchová, T. Kalnovicová, S. Pueschel, Z. Duracková. 2004. Uric acid and allantoin levels in Down syndrome: Antioxidant and oxidative mechanism? *Clin. Chico. Acta* 341:139–146.

137. Cicco, G., P. C. Panzera, G. Catalano, V. Memeo. 2005. Microcirculation and reperfusion injury in organ transplantation. *Adv. Exp. Med. Biol.* 566:563–573.

138. Campise, M., F. Bamonti, C. Novembrino, S. Ippolito, A. Tarantino, U. Corelli, S. Lonati, B. M. Cesana, C. Ponticelli. 2003. Oxidative stress in kidney transplantation. *Transplantation* 76:1474–1478.

139. Katz, M. A. 1986. The expanding role of oxygen free radicals in clinical medicine. *West. J. Med.* 144:441–446.

140. Grisham, M. B. 1994. Oxidants and free radicals in inflammatory bowel disease. *Lancet* 344:859–861.

141. Stadtman, E. R., C. N. Oliver. 1991. Metal -catalyzed oxidation of proteins. *J. Biol. Chem.* 266: 2005–2008.

142. Ahmad, R., A. K. Tripathi, P. Tripathi, R. Singh, S. Singh, R. K. Singh. 2010. Studies on lipid peroxidation and non-enzymatic antioxidant status as indices of oxidative stress in patients with chronic myeloid leukaemia. *Singapore Med. J.* 51 (2):110–115.

143. Ciobica, A., M. Padurariu, I. Dobrin, C. Stefanescu, R. Dobrin. 2011. Oxidative stress in schizophrenia: Focusing on the main markers. *Psychiatr. Danub.* 23 (3):237–245.

144. Fendri, C., A. Mechri, G. Khiari, A. Othman, A. Kerkeni, L. Gaha. 2006. Oxidative stress involvement in schizophrenia pathophysiology: A review. *Encéphale* 32 (2 Pt 1):244–252.

145. Lushchak, V. I., D. V. Gospodaryov. 2012. *Oxidative Stress and Diseases.* InTech, www.intechopen.com.

146. Nathan, F. M., V. A. Singh, A. Dhanoa, U. D. Palanisamy. 2011. Oxidative stress and antioxidant status in primary bone and soft tissue sarcoma. *BMC Cancer* 11:382.

147. Grosicka-Maciag, E. 2011. Biological consequences of oxidative stress induced by pesticides. *Postepy Hig. Med. Dosw.* 65:357–366.

148. Olgun, S., H. P. Misra. 2006. Pesticides induced oxidative stress in thymocytes. *Mol. Cell. Biochem.* 290:137–144.

149. Slaninova, A., A. Smutna, H. Modra, A. Svoboda. 2009. A review: Oxidative stress in fish induced by pesticides. *Neuro Endocrinol. Lett.* 30:2–12.

150. Soltaninejad, M. Abdollahi. 2009. Current opinion on the science of organophosphate pesticides and toxic stress: A systematic review. *Med. Sci. Monit.* 15 (3):RA75–RA90.

151. Rea, W. J., K. Patel. 2010. *Reversibility of Chronic Degenerative Disease and Hypersensitivity: Regulating Mechanisms of Chemical Sensitivity.* Boca Raton, FL: CRC Press.

152. Randolph, T. G. 1961. Human ecology and susceptibility to the chemical environment. *Ann Allergy* 19:518–540.

153. Dickey, L. D. 1976. *Clinical Ecology.* Fort Collins, CO: Clinical Ecology Publications.

154. Abdollahi, M., S. Mostafalou, S. Pournourmohammadi, and S. Shadnia. 2004. Oxidative stress and cholinesterase inhibition in saliva and plasma of rats following subchronic exposure to malathion. *Comp. Biochem. Physiol. C. Toxicol. Pharmacol.* 137 (1):29–34.

155. Braconi, D., Bernardini G., M. Fiorani, C. Azzolini, B. Marzocchi, F. Proietti, G. Collodel, A. Santucci. 2010. Oxidative damage induced by herbicides is mediated by thiol oxidation and hydroperoxides production. *Free Radic. Res.* 44 (8):891–906.

156. Mostafalou, S., M. Abdollahi, M. A. Eghbal, N. Saeedi Kouzehkonani. 2012. Protective effect of NAC against malathion-induced oxidative stress in freshly isolated rat hepatocytes. *Adv. Pharm. Bull.* 2 (1):79–88.

157. Singh, C., I. Ahmad, A. Kumar. 2007. Pesticides and metals induced Parkinson's disease: Involvement of free radicals and oxidative stress. *Cell. Mol. Biol. (Noisy-le-Grand)* 53 (5):19–28.

158. Kanthasamy, A. K. M., S. Kaul, S. V. Anantharam, A. G. Kanthasamy. 2002. A novel oxidative stress-dependent apoptotic pathway in pesticide-induced dopaminergic degeneration in PD models. *J. Neurochem.* 81:76.

159. Sharma-Wagner, S., A. P. Chokkalingam, H. S. Malker, B. J. Stone, J. K. McLaughlin, A. W. Hsing. 2000. Occupation and prostate cancer risk in Sweden. *J. Occup. Environ. Med.* 42 (5):517–525.

160. Mostafalou, S., M. A. Eghbal, A. Nili-Ahmadabadi, M. Baeeri, M. Abdollahi. 2012. Biochemical evidence on the potential role of organophosphates in hepatic glucose metabolism toward insulin resistance through inflammatory signaling and free radical pathways. *Toxicol. Ind. Health* 28 (9):840–851.

161. Teimouri, F., N. Amirkabirian, H. Esmaily, A. Mohammadirad, A. Aliahmadi, M. Abdollahi. 2006. Alteration of hepatic cells glucose metabolism as a non-cholinergic detoxication mechanism in counteracting diazinon-induced oxidative stress. *Hum. Exp. Toxicol.* 25 (12):697–703.

162. Begum, K., P. S. Rajini. 2011. Augmentation of hepatic and renal oxidative stress and disrupted glucose homeostasis by monocrotophos in streptozotocin-induced diabetic rats. *Chem. Biol. Interact.* 193 (3):240–245.

163. Harbauer, A. B., M. Opali Ska, C. Gerbeth, J. S. Herman, S. Rao, B. Schonfisch, B. Guiard, O. Schmidt, N. Pnaffer, C. Meisinger. 2014. Mitochondria. Cell cycle-dependent regulation of mitochondrial preprotein translocase. *Science* 346:1109–1113.

164. Poovala, V. S., V. K. Kanji, H. Tachikawa, A. K. Salahudeen. 1998. Role of oxidant stress and antioxidant protection in acephate-induced renal tubular cytotoxicity. *Toxicol. Sci.* 46 (2):403–409.

165. Shah, M. D., M. Iqbal. 2010. Diazinon-induced oxidative stress and renal dysfunction in rats. *Food Chem. Toxicol.* 48 (12):3345–3353.

166. Tomita, M., T. Okuyama, H. Katsuyama, T. Ishikawa. 2006. Paraquat-induced gene expression in rat kidney. *Arch. Toxicol.* 80 (10):687–693.

167. Xu, C., B. Bailly-Maitre, J. C. Reed. 2005. Endoplasmic reticulum stress: Cell life and death decisions. *J. Clin. Invest.* 115 (10):2656–2664.

168. Back, S. H., S. W. Kang, J. Han, H. T. Chung. 2012. Endoplasmic reticulum stress in the β-cell pathogenesis of type 2 diabetes. *Exp. Diabetes Res.* 2012:618396.

169. Kim, M. K., H. S. Kim, I. K. Lee, K. G. Park. 2012. Endoplasmic reticulum stress and insulin biosynthesis: A review. *Exp. Diabetes Res.* 2012:509437.

170. Scheuner, D., R. J. Kaufman. 2008. The unfolded protein response: A pathway that links insulin demand with beta-cell failure and diabetes. *Endocr. Rev.* 29 (3):317–333.

171. Doyle, K. M., D. Kennedy, A. M. Gorman, S. Gupta, S. J. Healy, A. Samali. 2011. Unfolded proteins and endoplasmic reticulum stress in neurodegenerative disorders. *J. Cell. Mol. Med.* 15 (10):2025–2039.

172. Lindholm, S., H. Wootz, L. Korhonen. 2006. ER stress and neurodegenerative diseases. *Cell Death Differ.* 13 (3):385–392.

173. Nassif, M., S. Matus, K. Castillo, C. Hetz. 2010. Amyotrophic lateral sclerosis pathogenesis: A journey through the secretory pathway. *Antioxid. Redox Signal.* 13 (12):1955–1989.

174. Koumenis, C. 2006. ER stress, hypoxia tolerance and tumor progression. *Curr. Mol. Med.* 6 (1):55–69.

175. Lee, A. S., L. M. Hendershot. 2006. ER stress and cancer. *Cancer Biol. Ther.* 5 (7):721–722.

176. Dickhout, J. G., R. E. Carlisle, R. C. Austin. 2011. Interrelationship between cardiac hypertrophy, heart failure, and chronic kidney disease: Endoplasmic reticulum stress as a mediator of pathogenesis. *Circ. Res.* 108 (5):629–642.

177. Tabas, I. 2010. The role of endoplasmic reticulum stress in the progression of atherosclerosis. *Circ. Res.* 107 (7):839–850.

178. Chinta, S. J., A. Rane, K. S. Poksay, D. E. Bredesen, J. K. Andersen, R. V. Rao. 2008. Coupling endoplasmic reticulum stress to the cell death program in dopaminergic cells: Effect of paraquat. *Neuromol. Med.* 10 (4):333–342.

179. Yang, W., E. Tiffany-Castiglioni, H. C. Koh, I. H. Son. 2009. Paraquat activates the IRE1/ASK1/JNK cascade associated with apoptosis in human neuroblastoma SH-SY5Y cells. *Toxicol. Lett.* 191 (2–3):203–210.

180. Chen, Y., G. Chen, Z. Fan, J. Luo, Z. J. Ke. 2008. GSK3beta and endoplasmic reticulum stress mediate rotenone-induced death of SK-N-MC neuroblastoma cells. *Biochem. Pharmacol.* 76 (1):128–138.

181. Hossain, M., J. R. Richardson. 2011. Mechanism of pyrethroid pesticide-induced apoptosis: Role of calpain and the ER stress pathway. *Toxicol. Sci.* 122 (2):512–525.

182. Chen, Y. W. et al. 2010. Pyrrolidine dithiocarbamate (PDTC)/Cu complex induces lung epithelial cell apoptosis through mitochondria and ER-stress pathways. *Toxicol. Lett.* 199 (3):333–340.

183. Pesonen, M., M. Pasanen, J. Loikkanen, A. Naukkarinen, M. Hemmila, H. Seulanto, T. Kuitunen, K. Vahakangas. 2012. Chloropicrin induces endoplasmic reticulum stress in human retinal pigment epithelial cells. *Toxicol. Lett.* 211 (3):239–245.

184. Skandrani, D., Y. Gaubin, B. Beau, J. C. Murat, C. Vincent, F. Croute. 2006. Effect of selected insecticides on growth rate and stress protein expression in cultured human A549 and SH-SY5Y cells. *Toxicol. In Vitro* 20 (8):1378–1386.

185. Skandrani, D., Y. Gaubin, C. Vincent, B. Beau, J. Claude Murat, J. P. Soleilhavoup, F. Croute. 2006. Relationship between toxicity of selected insecticides and expression of stress proteins (HSP, GRP) in cultured human cells: Effects of commercial formulations versus pure active molecules. *Biochim. Biophys. Acta* 1760 (1):95–103.

186. Gies, E., I. Wilde, J. M. Winget, M. Brack, B. Rotblat, C. A. Novoa, A. D. Balgi, P. H. Sorensen, M. Roberge, T. Mayor. 2010. Niclosamide prevents the formation of large ubiquitin-containing aggregates caused by proteasome inhibition. *PLoS One* 5 (12):e14410.

187. Paul, S. 2008. Dysfunction of the ubiquitin–proteasome system in multiple disease conditions: Therapeutic approaches. *Bioessays* 30 (11–12):1172–1184.

188. Sun, F., V. Anantharam, C. Latchoumycandane, A. Kanthasamy, A. G. Kanthasamy. 2005. Dieldrin induces ubiquitin–proteasome dysfunction in alpha-synuclein overexpressing dopaminergic neuronal cells and enhances susceptibility to apoptotic cell death. *J. Pharmacol. Exp. Ther.* 315 (1):69–79.

189. Chou, A. P., N. Maidment, R. Klintenberg, J. E. Casida, S. Li, A. G. Fitzmaurice, P. O. Fernagut, F. Mortazavi, M. F. Chesselet, J. M. Bronstein. Ziram causes dopaminergic cell damage by inhibiting E1 ligase of the proteasome. *J. Biol. Chem.* 283 (50):34696–34703.

190. Wang, X. F., S. Li, A. P. Chou, J. M. Bronstein. 2006. Inhibitory effects of pesticides on proteasome activity: Implication in Parkinson's disease. *Neurobiol. Dis.* 23:198–205.

191. Yang, W., E. Tiffany-Castiglioni. 2007. The bipyridyl herbicide paraquat induces proteasome dysfunction in human neuroblastoma SH-SY5Y cells. *J. Toxicol. Environ. Health A* 70 (21):1849–1857.

192. Yang, W., L. Chen, Y. Ding, X. Zhuang, U. J. Kang. 2007. Paraquat induces dopaminergic dysfunction and proteasome impairment in DJ-1-deficient mice. *Hum. Mol. Genet.* 16 (23):2900–2910.

193. Chou, A. P., S. Li, A. G. Fitzmaurice, J. M. Bronstein. 2010. Mechanisms of rotenone-induced proteasome inhibition. *Neurotoxicology* 31 (4):367–372.

194. Gonzalez, C. D., M. S. Lee, P. Marchetti, M. Pietropaolo, R. Towns, M. I. Vaccaro, H. Watada, J. W. Wiley. 2011. The emerging role of autophagy in the pathophysiology of diabetes mellitus. *Autophagy* 7 (1):2–11.

195. Levine, B., G. Kroemer. 2008. Autophagy in the pathogenesis of disease. *Cell* 132 (1):27–42.

196. Shintani, T., D. J. Klionsky. 2004. Autophagy in health and disease: A double-edged sword. *Science* 306 (5698):990–995.

197. Gonzalez-Polo, R. A., M. Niso-Santano, M. A. Ortiz-Ortiz, A. Gomez-Martin, J. M. Moran, L. Garcia-Rubio, J. Francisco-Morcillo, C. Zaragoza, G. Soler, J. M. Fuentes. 2007. Inhibition of paraquat-induced autophagy accelerates the apoptotic cell death in neuroblastoma SH-SY5Y cells. *Toxicol. Sci.* 97 (2):448–458.

198. Niso-Santano, M., J. M. Bravo-San Pedro, R. Gomez-Sanchez, V. Climent, G. Soler, J. M. Fuentes, R. A. Gonzalez-Polo. 2011. ASK1 overexpression accelerates paraquat-induced autophagy via endoplasmic reticulum stress. *Toxicol. Sci.* 119 (1):156–168.

199. Abdul-Ghani, M. A., R. A. DeFronzo. 2008. Mitochondrial dysfunction, insulin resistance, and type 2 diabetes mellitus. *Curr. Diab. Rep.* 8 (3):173–178.

200. Kim, J. A., Y. Wei, J. R. Sowers. 2008. Role of mitochondrial dysfunction in insulin resistance. *Circ. Res.* 102 (4):401–414.

201. Lowell, B. B., G. I. Shulman. 2005. Mitochondrial dysfunction and type 2 diabetes. *Science* 307 (5708):384–387.

202. Ma, Z. A., Z. Zhao, J. Turk. 2012. Mitochondrial dysfunction and beta-cell failure in type 2 diabetes mellitus. *Exp. Diabetes Res.* 2012:703538.

203. Johri, A. M. F. Beal. 2012. Mitochondrial dysfunction in neurodegenerative diseases. *J. Pharmacol. Exp. Ther.* 342 (3):619–630.

204. Martin, L. J. 2012. Biology of mitochondria in neurodegenerative diseases. *Prog. Mol. Biol. Transl. Sci.* 107:355–415.

205. Lin, M. T., M. F. Beal. 2006. Mitochondrial dysfunction and oxidative stress in neurodegenerative diseases. *Nature* 443 (7113):787–795.

206. Langston, J. W. 1996. The etiology of Parkinson's disease with emphasis on the MPTP story. *Neurology* 47 (6 Suppl. 3):S153–S160.

207. Caboni, P., T. B. Sherer, N. Zhang, G. Taylor, H. M. Na, J. T. Greenamyre, J. E. Casida. 2004. Rotenone, deguelin, their metabolites, and the rat model of Parkinson's disease. *Chem. Res. Toxicol.* 17 (11):1540–1548.

208. Gomez, C., M. J. Bandez, A. Navarro. 2007. Pesticides and impairment of mitochondrial function in relation with the parkinsonian syndrome. *Front. Biosci.* 12:1079–1093.

209. Ilivicky, J., J. E. Casida. 1969. Uncoupling action of 2,4-dinitrophenols, 2-trifluoromethylbenzimidazoles and certain other pesticide chemicals upon mitochondria from different sources and its relation to toxicity. *Biochem. Pharmacol.* 18 (6):1389–1401.

210. Ranjbar, A., M. H. Ghahremani, M. Sharifzadeh, A. Golestani, M. Ghazi-Khansari, M. Baeeri, M. Abdollahi. 2010. Protection by pentoxifylline of malathion-induced toxic stress and mitochondrial damage in rat brain. *Hum. Exp. Toxicol.* 29 (10):851–864.

211. Jamshidi, H. R., M. H. Ghahremani, S. N. Ostad, M. Sharifzadeh, A. R. Dehpour, M. Abdollahi. 2009. Effects of diazinon on the activity and gene expression of mitochondrial glutamate dehydrogenase from rat pancreatic Langerhans islets. *Pestic. Biochem. Physiol.* 93 (1):23–27.

212. Lee, H. K. 2011. Mitochondrial dysfunction and insulin resistance: The contribution of dioxin-like substances. *Diabetes Metab. J.* 35 (3):207–215.

213. Lim, S., S. Y. Ahn, I. C. Song, M. H. Chung, H. C. Jang, K. S. Park, K. U. Lee, Y. K. Pak, H. K. Lee. 2009. Chronic exposure to the herbicide, atrazine, causes mitochondrial dysfunction and insulin resistance. *PLoS One* 4 (4):e5186.

214. Naviaux, R. K. 2012. Oxidative shielding or oxidative stress? *J. Pharmacol. Exp. Ther.* 342 (3):608–618.

215. Holland, H. D. 2006. The oxygenation of the atmosphere and oceans. *Philos. Trans. R. Soc. Lond. B. Biol. Sci.* 361:909–915.

216. West, A. P., G. S. Shadel, S. Ghosh. 2011. Mitochondria in innate immune responses. *Nat. Rev. Immunol.* 11:389–402.

217. Calavier-Smith, T. 2006. Cell evolution and Earth history: Stasis and revolution. *Philos. Trans. R. Soc. Lond. B. Biol. Sci.* 361:969–1006.
218. Tang, K. H., R. E. Blankenship. 2010. Both forward and reserve TCA cycles operate in green sulfur bacteria. *J. Biol. Chem.* 285:35848–35854.
219. Harman, D. 1956. Aging: A theory based on free radical and radiation chemistry. *J. Gerontol.* 11:298–300.
220. Gnaiger, E., R. Steinlechner-Maran, G. Méndez, T. Eberl, R. Margreitter. 1995. Control of mitochondrial and cellular respiration by oxygen. *J. Bioenerg. Biomembr.* 27:583–596.
221. Pagliarini, D. J. et al. 2008. A mitochondrial protein compendium elucidates complex I disease biology. *Cell* 134:112–123.
222. Schellenberger J., J. O. Park, T. M. Conrad, B. Ø. Palsson, 2010. BiGG: A biochemical genetic and genomic knowledgebase of large scale metabolic reconstructions. *BMC Bioinformatics* 11:213.
223. Rolfsson, O., B. Ø. Palsson, I. Thiele. 2011. The human metabolic reconstruction Recon 1 directs hypotheses of novel human metabolic functions. *BMC Syst. Biol.* 5:155.
224. Shepherd, D., P. B. Garland. 1969. The kinetic properties of citrate synthase from rat liver mitochondria. *Biochem. J.* 114:597–610.
225. Serezani, C. H., C. Lewis, S. Jancar, M. Peters-Golden. 2011. Leukotriene B4 amplifies NF-κB activation in mouse macrophages by reducing SOCS1 inhibition of MyD88 expression. *J. Clin. Invest.* 121:671–682.
226. Jiang, F., Y. Zhang, G. J. Dusting. 2011. NADPH oxidase-mediated redox signaling: Roles in cellular stress response, stress tolerance, and tissue repair. *Pharmacol. Rev.* 63:218–242.
227. Hillmann, P., G. Y. Ko, A. Spinrath, A. Raulf, I. von Kügelgen, S. C. Wolff, R. A. Nicholas, E. Kostenis, H. D. Höltje, C. E. Müller. 2009. Key determinants of nucleotide-activated G protein-coupled P2Y(2) receptor function revealed by chemical and pharmacological experiments, mutagenesis and homology modeling. *J. Med. Chem.* 52:2762–2775.
228. Speciale, A., J. Chirafisi, A. Saija, F. Cimino. 2011. Nutritional antioxidants and adaptive cell responses: An update. *Curr. Mol. Med.* 11:770–789.
229. Suksomboon, N., N. Poolsup, S. Sinprasert. 2011. Effects of vitamin E supplementation on glycaemic control in type 2 diabetes: Systematic review of randomized controlled trials. *J. Clin. Pharm. Ther.* 36:53–63.
230. Alpha-Tocopherol, Beta Carotene Cancer Prevention Study Group. 1994. The effect of vitamin E and beta carotene on the incidence of lung cancer and other cancers in male smokers. *N. Eng. J. Med.* 330:1029–1035.
231. Lin J., N. R. Cook, C. Albert, E. Zaharris, J. M. Gaziano, M. Van Denburgh, J. E. Buring, J. E. Manson. 2009. Vitamins C and E and beta carotene supplementation and cancer risk: A randomized controlled trial. *J. Natl. Cancer. Inst.* 101:14–23.
232. Lippman, S. M. et al. 2009. Effect of selenium and vitamin E on risk of prostate cancer and other cancers: The Selenium and Vitamin E Cancer Prevention Trial (SELECT). *JAMA* 301:39–51.
233. Klein, E. A. et al. 2011. Vitamin E and the risk of prostate cancer: The Selenium and Vitamin E Cancer Prevention Trial (SELECT). *JAMA* 306:1549–1556.
234. Niess, A. M., P. Simon. 2007. Response and adaptation of skeletal muscle to exercise—The role of reactive oxygen species. *Front. Biosci.* 12:4826–4838.
235. Dunkley, A. J., K. Charles, L. J. Gray, J. Camosso-Stefinovic, M. J. Davies, K. Khunti. 2012. Effectiveness of interventions for reducing diabetes and cardiovascular disease risk in people with metabolic syndrome: Systematic review and mixed treatment comparison meta-analysis. *Diabetes. Obes. Metab.* 14:616–625.
236. DREAM Trial Investigators, Dagenais, G. R. et al. 2008. Effects of ramipril and rosiglitazone on cardiovascular and renal outcomes in people with impaired glucose tolerance or impaired fasting glucose: Results of the Diabetes REduction Assessment with ramipril and rosiglitazone Medication (DREAM) trial. *Diabetes Care* 31:1007–1014.
237. Cabiscol, E., E. Piulats, P. Echave, E. Herrero, J. Ros. 2000. Oxidative stress promotes specific protein damage in saccharomyces cerevisiae. *J. Biol. Chem.* 275:27393–27398.
238. González-Flecha, B., B. Demple. 1997. Transcriptional regulation of the Escherichia coli oxyR gene as a function of cell growth. *J. Bacteriol.* 179:6181–6186.
239. Bradley, D. J., P. Kjellbom, C. J. Lamb. 1992. Elicitor- and wound-induced oxidative cross-linking of a proline-rich plant cell wall protein: A novel, rapid defense response. *Cell* 70:21–30.
240. Karbowski, M. 2010. Mitochondria on guard: Role of mitochondrial fusion and fission in the regulation of apoptosis. *Adv. Exp. Med. Biol.* 687:131–142.
241. Galluzzi, L., C. Brenner, E. Morselli, Z. Touat, G. Kroemer. 2008. Viral control of mitochondrial apoptosis. *PLoS Pathog.* 4:e1000018.

242. Attene-Ramos, M. S., K. Kitiphongspattana, K. Ishii-Schrade, H. R. Gaskins. 2005. Temporal changes of multiple redox couples from proliferation to growth arrest in IEC-6 intestinal epithelial cells. *Am. J. Physiol. Cell Physiol.* 289:C1220–C1228.

243. Wamelink, M. M., E. A. Struys, C. Jakobs. 2008. The biochemistry, metabolism and inherited defects of the pentose phosphate pathway: A review. *J. Inherit. Metab. Dis.* 31:703–717.

244. Bolanos, J. P., M. Delgado-Esteban, A. Herrero-Mendez, S. Fernandez-Fernandez, A. Almeida. 2008. Regulation of glycolysis and pentose-phosphate pathway by nitric oxide: Impact on neuronal survival. *Biochim. Biophys. Acta* 1777:789–793.

245. Naviaux, R. K., K. A. McGowan. 2000. Organismal effects of mitochondrial dysfunction. *Hum. Reprod.* 15 (Suppl 2):44–56.

246. Naviaux, R. K. 2008. Mitochondrial control of epigenetics. *Cancer Biol. Ther.* 7:1191–1193.

247. Han, J. M., S. J. Jeong, M. C. Park, G. Kim, N. H. Kwon, H. K. Kim, S. H. Ha, S. H. Ryu, S. Kim. 2012. Leucyl-tRNA synthetase is an intracellular leucine sensor for the mTORC1-signaling pathway. *Cell* 149:410–424.

248. Zhang, Q., M. Raoof, Y. Chen, Y. Sumi, T. Sursal, W. Junger, K. Brohi, K. Itagaki, C. J. Hauser. 2010. Circulating mitochondrial DAMPs cause inflammatory responses to injury. *Nature* 464:104–107.

249. Marques-da-Silva, C., G. Burnstock, D. M. Ojcius, R. Coutinho-Silva. 2011. Purinergic receptor agonists modulate phagocytosis and clearance of apoptotic cells in macrophages. *Immunobiology* 216:1–11.

250. Spath, B., A. Hansen, C. Bokemeyer, F. Langer. 2012. Succinate reverses in-vitro platelet inhibition by acetylsalicylic acid and P2Y receptor antagonists. *Platelets* 23:60–68.

251. Birkenfeld, A. L. et al. 2011. Deletion of the mammalian INDY homolog mimics aspects of dietary restriction and protects against adiposity and insulin resistance in mice. *Cell Metab.* 14:184–195.

252. Buchakjian, M. R., S. Kornbluth. 2010. The engine driving the ship: Metabolic steering of cell proliferation and death. *Nat. Rev. Mol. Cell. Biol.* 11:715–727.

253. Crabtree, H. G. 1929. Observations on the carbohydrate metabolism of tumours. *Biochem. J.* 23:536–545.

254. Warburg, O. H., E. Negelein. 1928. Über den Einfluss der Wellenlänge auf die Verteilung des Atmungsferments. (Absorptionsspektrum des Atmungsferments.) [On the influence of wavelength on the activity of the respiratory ferment [in the presence of carbon monoxide]. *Biochemische Zeitschrift* 193:339–346.

255. Ibsen, K. H. 1961. The crabtree effect: A review. *Cancer Res.* 21:829–841.

256. Sussman, I., M. Erecińska, D. F. Wilson. 1980. Regulation of cellular energy metabolism: The crabtree effect. *Biochim. Biophys. Acta* 591:209–223.

257. Fisher-Wellman, K. H., P. D. Neufer. 2012. Linking mitochondrial bioenergetics to insulin resistance via redox biology. *Trends Endocrinol. Metab.* 23:142–153.

258. Diaz, R. J., R. Rosenberg. 2008. Spreading dead zones and consequences for marine ecosystems. *Science* 321:926–929.

259. Azam, F., F. Malfatti. 2007. Microbial structuring of marine ecosystems. *Nat. Rev. Microbiol.* 5:782–791.

260. Gille, L., H. Nohl. 2000. The existence of a lysosomal redox chain and the role of ubiquinone. *Arch. Biochem. Biophys.* 375:347–354.

261. Hwang, C., A. J. Sinskey, H. F. Lodish. 1992. Oxidized redox state of glutathione in the endoplasmic reticulum. *Science* 257:1496–1502.

262. Navas, P., I. Sun, F. L. Crane, D. M. Morré, D. J. Morré. 2010. Monoascorbate free radical-dependent oxidation-reduction reactions of liver golgi apparatus membranes. *J. Bioenerg. Biomembr.* 42:181–187.

263. Go, Y. M., D. P. Jones. 2008. Redox compartmentalization in eukaryotic cells. *Biochim. Biophys. Acta* 1780:1273–1290.

264. Yano, T., M. Oku, N. Akeyama, A. Itoyama, H. Yurimoto, S. Kuge, Y. Fujiki, Y. Sakai. 2010. A novel fluorescent sensor protein for visualization of redox states in the cytoplasm and in peroxisomes. *Mol. Cell. Biol.* 30:3758–3766.

265. Jones, D. P. 2010. Redox sensing: Orthogonal control in cell cycle and apoptosis signalling. *J. Intern. Med.* 268:432–448.

266. Pittman, R. N. 2011. Oxygen gradients in the microcirculation. *Acta Physiol. (Oxf.)* 202:311–322.

267. Scandurra, F. M., E. Gnaiger. 2010. Cell respiration under hypoxia: Facts and artefacts in mitochondrial oxygen kinetics. *Adv. Exp. Med. Biol.* 662:7–25.

268. Burhans, W. C., N. H. Heintz. 2009. The cell cycle is a redox cycle: Linking phasespecific targets to cell fate. *Free Radic. Biol. Med.* 47:1282–1293.

269. Prigogine, I. 1984. Oxidative shielding or oxidative stress. *J. Pharm. Exp. Ther.* 342(3).

270. Cooper, M. E. 2009. Metabolic memory: Implications for diabetic vascular complications. *Pediatr. Diabetes* 10:343–346.
271. LaForgia, J., R. T. Withers, C. J. Gore. 2006. Effects of exercise intensity and duration on the excess post-exercise oxygen consumption. *J. Sports Sci.* 24:1247–1264.
272. Ristow, M., K. Zarse, A. Oberbach, N. Klöting, M. Birringer, M. Kiehntopf, M. Stumvoll, C. R. Kahn, M. Blüher. 2009. Antioxidants prevent health-promoting effects of physical exercise in humans. *Proc. Natl. Acad. Sci. U S A* 106:8665–8670.
273. Ristow, M., S. Schmeisser. 2011. Extending life span by increasing oxidative stress. *Free Radic. Biol. Med.* 51:327–336.
274. Rea, W. J., R. Overberg, J. Bland, and the members of the American Academy of Environmental Medicine. 2010. *Reversibility of Chronic Degenerative Disease and Hypersensitivity. Vol. 1.* Boca Raton, FL: CRC Press, pp. 63–66.
275. Milani, L. 2007. Inflammation and physiological regulating medicine. *Physiol. Regul. Med.* 1:19–27.
276. Hull, J., M. Mc Arthur. 2003. A possible role of electromagnetic templates in macrophages memory. *Fund. Ist. Anat.* 427:211–219.
277. Milani, L. 2006. Dal fegato vaticinatore alla Nuova Tavola delle Omotossicosi. Dai Punti di Weihe al same-same-but-different nella terapia della steatoepatite non alcoolica. *La. Med. Biol.* 4:13–26.
278. Abbas, A. K., A. H. Lichtman, J. S. Pober. 2000. *Cellular and Molecular Immunology.* Philadelphia, PA: W. B. Saunders Company, p. 544.
279. Preparata, G. 1995. *Quantum Electrodynamic Coherence in Matter.* Singapore: World Scientific, pp. 199–210.
280. Preparata, G. 1997. Regimi coerenti in Fisica e Bio logic. Il problema Bella forma. *Rivista di Biologia/Biology Forum* 90:434–436.
281. Dinarello, C. A. 1996. Biologic basis for interleukin-1 in disease. *Blood* 87:2095–2147.
282. Cohen, S. 2002. Treatment of rheumatoid arthritis with anakinra, a recombinant human interleukin 1 receptor antagonist. *Arthritis Rheum.* 46:614–624.
283. Pennec, J. P., M. Aubin. 1984. Effect of Aconitum and Veratrum on the isolated perfused heart of common eel (*Anguilla anguilla*). *Comp. Biochem. Physiol.* 776:367–369.
284. Stumpf, W. E. 2005. Drug localization and targeting with receptor microscopic autoradiography. *J. Pharmacol. Toxicol. Methods* 51 (1):25–40.
285. Poitevin, B., M. Aubin, J. F. Royer. 1983. The effects of Belladonna and Ferrum phosphoricum on the chemuluminescence of human poly-morphonuclear neutrophils. *Ann. Homéop. Fr.* 3:5–12 (translated title from French).
286. Wagner, H., K. Jurcic, A. Doenicke, E. Rosenhuber. 1986. Actions of homeophatic preparations on fagocyte activity of granulocytes. In vitro tests and double blind controlled studies. *Arzneim. Forsch./Drug Res.* 36:1424–1425 (translated title from German).
287. Wagner, H. 1988. Studi immunologici *in vitro* e *in vivo* con farmaci vegetali a bassi dosaggi. *Rivista Italiana di Omotossicologica* 3:13–19.
288. Davenas, E. et al. 1988. Human basophil degranulation triggered by very diluted antiserum against IgE. *Nature* 333:816–818.
289. Poitevin, B., E. Davenas, J. Benveniste. 1988. In vitro immunological degranulation of human basophils is modulated by lung histamine and apis mellifica. *Brit. J. Clin. Pharmacol.* 25:439–444.
290. Daurat, V., P. Dorfman, M. Bastide. 1988. Attività immunomodulante di basse dosi di interferone α e β nel topo. *Biomed. Pharmacother.* 42:197–206 (translated title from French).
291. Enbergs, H., G. Arndt. 1993. Effects of different homeophatic potencies of Lachesis on lymphocyte cultures obtained from rabbit blood. *Biol. Tier.* 4 (translated title from German).
292. Enbergs, H. 1998. Efficacia dei farmaci omeopatici Suis ed Arnica comp.-Heel® sull'attività dei linfociti e dei fagociti. *La Med. Biol.* 3:5–14.
293. Belon, P., J. Cumps, M. Ennis, P. F. Mannaioni, M. Roberfroid, J. Sainte-Laudy, F. A. Wiegant. 2004. Histamine dilutions modulate basophil activation. *Inflamm. Res.* 53 (5):181–188.
294. Jäggi R., U. Würgler, F. Grandjean, M. Weiser. 2004. Doppia inibizione della 5-lipoossigenasi/cicloossigenasi con un farmaco omeopatico ricostituito. *Inflamm. Res.* 53 (4):150–157.
295. Amadori, M., B. Begni, L. Milani. 2007. Anti-inflammatory activity of low dose IFN-α. In vitro study on porcine leukocytes. *Physiol. Regulating Med.* 1:29–35.
296. Rea, W. J., S. D. Miller, C. Lee. 2010. *Reversibility of Chronic Degenerative Disease and Hypersensitivity. Vol. I.* Boca Raton, FL: CRC Press.
297. Block, M. L., L. Zecca, J. S. Hong. 2007. Microglia-mediated neurotoxicity: Uncovering the molecular mechanisms. *Nat. Rev. Neurosci.* 8:57–69.

298. Craig, L. et al. 2008. Air pollution and public health: A guidance document for risk managers. *J. Toxicol. Environ. Health A* 71:588–698.
299. Riedl, M. A. 2008. The effect of air pollution on asthma and allergy. *Curr. Allergy Asthma. Rep.* 8:139–146.
300. Mills, N. L., K. Donaldson, P. W. Hadoke, N. A. Boon, W. MacNee, F. R. Cassee, T. Sandström, A. Blomberg, D. E. Newby. 2009. Adverse cardiovascular effects of air pollution. *Nat. Clin. Pract. Cardiovasc. Med.* 6:36–44.
301. Genes and Mapped Phenotypes. 2008. *Nat Cen Biotech Information.* Bethasda, MD: U.S. National Library of Medicine.
302. Yang, L., R. M. Froio, T. E. Sciuto, A. M. Dvorak, R. Alon, F. W. Luscinskas. 2005. ICAM-1 regulates neutrophil adhesion and transcellular migration of TNF-alpha-activated vascular endothelium under flow. *Blood* 106 (2):584–592.
303. Iakimenko, I. L., E. P. Sidorik, A. S. Tsybulin. 2011. Metabolic changes in cells under electromagnetic radiation of mobile communication systems. *Ukr. Biokhim. Zh.* 83:20–28.
304. Henriksson, J., H. Tjalv. 2000. Manganese taken up into the CNS via the olfactory pathway in rats affects astrocytes. *Toxicol. Sci.* 55:392–398.
305. Morgan, K. T., T. M. Monticello. 1990. Airflow, gas deposition, and lesion distribution in the nasal passages. *Environ. Health Perspect.* 85:209–218.
306. Nakashima, T., M. Tanaka, M. Inamitsu, T. Uemura. 1991. Immunohistopathology of variations of human olfactory mucosa. *Eur. Arch. Otorhinolaryngol.* 248:370–375.
307. Paik, S. I., M. N. Lehman, A. M. Seiden, H. J. Duncan, D. V. Smith. 1992. Human olfactory mucosa. The influence of age and receptor distribution. *Arch. Otolaryngol. Head Neck Surg.* 118:731–738.
308. Dahl, A. R., J. L. Lewis. 1993. Respiratory tract uptake of inhalants and metabolism of xenobiotics. *Annu. Rev. Pharmacol. Toxicol.* 33:383–407.
309. Lin, D. M., J. Ngai. 1999. Development of the vertebrate main olfactory system. *Curr. Opin. Neurobiol.* 9:74–78.
310. Calderón-Garciduenas, L., A. Osorno-Velazquez, H. Bravo-Alvarez, R. Delgado-Chavez, R. Barrios-Marquez. 1992. Histopathological changes of the nasal mucosa in Southwest Metropolitan Mexico City. *Am. J. Pathol.* 140:225–232.
311. Calderón-Garciduenas L., N. Osnaya, A. Rodríguez-Alcaraz, A. Villarreal- Calderón. 1997. DNA damage in nasal respiratory epithelium from children exposed to urban pollution. *Environ. Mol. Mut.* 30:11–20.
312. Calderón-Garciduenas, L., A. Rodríguez-Alcaraz, A. Villarreal-Calderón, O. Lyght, D. Janszen, K. T. Morgan. 1998. Nasal epithelium as a sentinel for airborne environmental pollution. *Toxicol. Sci.* 46:352–364.
313. Calderón-Garciduenas, L., G. Valencia-Salazar, A. Rodríguez-Alcaraz, T. M. Gambling, R. García, N. Osnaya, A. Villarreal-Calderón, R. B. Devlin, J. L. Carson. 2001a. Ultrastructural nasal pathology in children chronically and sequentially exposed to air pollutants. *Am. J. Respir. Cell. Mol. Biol.* 24:132–138.
314. Calderón-Garciduenas, L., T. M. Gambling, H. Acuna, R. Garcia, N. Osnaya, S. Monroy, A. Villarreal-Calderón, J. Carson, H. S. Koren, R. B. Devlin. 2001c. Canines as sentinel species for assessing chronic exposures to air pollutants: Part 2. Cardiac pathology. *Toxicol. Sci.* 61:356–367.
315. Calderón-Garciduenas, L. et al. 2001b. Canines as sentinel species for assessing chronic exposures to air pollutants: Part 1.Respiratory pathology. *Toxicol. Sci.* 61:342–355.
316. Calderón-Garciduenas, L., A. Mora, L. A. Fordham, G. Valencia, C. J. Chung, A. Villarreal-Calderón, H. S. Koren, R. B. Devlin, M. J. Hazucha. 2001d. Lung damage and cytokine profile in children chronically exposed to air pollutants. *Am. J. Respir. Crit. Care Med.* 163:A884.
317. Hock, C., S. Golombowski, F. Muller-Spahn, O. Peschel, A. Riederer, A. Probst, E. Mandelkow, J. Unger. 1998. Histological markers in nasal mucosa of patients with Alzheimer's disease. *Eur. Neurol.* 40:31–36.
318. Kovacs, T., N. J. Cairns, P. L. Lantos. 1999. Beta-amyloid deposition and neurofibrillary tangle formation in the olfactory bulb in ageing and Alzheimer's disease. *Neuropath. Appl. Neurobiol.* 25:481–491.
319. Wszolek, Z. K., K. Markopoulou. 1998. Olfactory dysfunction in Parkinson's disease. *Clin. Neurosci.* 5:94–101.
320. Hirai, T., S. Kojima, A. Shimada, T. Umemura, M. Sakai, C. Itakura. 1996. Age-related changes in the olfactory system of dogs. *Neuropath. Appl. Neurobiol.* 22:531–539.
321. Hoffman, H. J., E. K. Ishii, R. H. MacTurk. 1998. Age-related changes in the prevalence of smell/taste problems among the United States adult population. Results of the 1994 disability supplement to the National Health Interview Survey (NHIS). *Ann. NY Acad. Sci.* 855:716–722.

322. Kovacs, T., N. J. Cairns, P. L. Lantos. 2001. Olfactory centres in Alzheimer's disease: Olfactory bulb is involved in early Braak's stages. *Neuroreport* 12:285–288.

323. Borras, D., I. Ferrer, M. Pumarola. 1999. Age-related changes in the brain of the dog. *Vet. Pathol.* 36:202–211.

324. Cummings, B. J., E. Head, W. Ruehl, N. W. Milgram, C. W. Cotman. 1996. Canine as an animal model of human aging and dementia. *Neurobiol. Aging* 17:259–268.

325. Ruehl, W. W., D. S. Bruyette, A. DePaoli, C. W. Cotman, N. W. Milgram, B. J. Cummings. 1995. Canine cognitive dysfunction as a model for human age-related cognitive decline, dementia and Alzheimer's disease: Clinical presentation, cognitive testing, pathology and response to 1-deprenyl therapy. *Prog. Brain Res.* 106:217–225.

326. Russell, M. J., M. Bobik, R. G. White, Y. Hou, S. A. Benjamin, J. W. Geddes. 1996. Age-specific onset of beta-amyloid in beagle brains. *Neurobiol. Aging* 17:269–273.

327. Wegiel J., H. M. Wisniewski, J. Dziewiatkowski, M. Tarnawski, A. Dziewiatkowska, J. Morys, Z. Soltysiak, K. S. Kim. 1996. Subpopulation of dogs with severe brain parenchymal beta amyloidosis distinguished with cluster analysis. *Brain Res.* 728:20–26.

328. Satou, T., B. J. Cummings, E. Head, K. A. Nielson, F. F. Khan, N. W. Milgram, P. Velazquez, D. H. Cribbs, A. J. Tenner, C. W. Cotman. 1997. The progression of beta-amyloid deposition in the frontal cortex of the ages canine. *Brain Res.* 774:35–43.

329. García-Gutierrez, A., M. Herrera-Hernandéz, H. Bravo-Alvarez. 1991. Campus ozone concentrations related to new blends in gasoline sold in Mexico City. A statistical analysis. *Air Waste Management Assoc.* A115-4.

330. Fast, D. J., S. Zhong. 1998. Metereological factors associated with inhomogeneous ozone concentrations with the Mexico Basin. *J. Geophysical. Res.* 103 (D15):18927–18946.

331. Blake, D. R., F. S. Rowland. 1995. Urban leakage of liquefied petroleum gas and its impact on Mexico city air quality. *Science* 269:953–956.

332. Cicero-Fernandéz, P., W. A. Thistlewaite, Y. I. Falcon, I. M. Guzman. 1993. TSP, PM10 and PM10/TSP ratios in the Mexico city metropolitan area: A temporal and spatial approach. *J. Exp. Anal. Environ. Epidemiol.* 3:1–14.

333. Edgerton, S. A. et al. 1999. Particulate air pollution in Mexico city: A collaborative research project. *J. Air Waste Manag. Assoc.* 49:1221–1229.

334. Los Alamos National Laboratory, US Department of Energy. 2001. library@lanl.gov. *Mexico City Air Quality Research Initiative* Vol II, LA-12699 UC-902 June 1994 pl-S9.

335. Baez, A. P., R. Belmont, H. Padilla. 1995. Measurements of formaldehyde and acetaldehyde in the atmosphere of Mexico city. *Environ. Pollut.* 89:163–167.

336. Villalobos-Pietrini, R., S. Blanco, S. Gomez-Arroyo. 1995. Mutagenicity assessment of airborne particles in Mexico city. *Atmospheric Environ.* 89:163–167.

337. Meneses, F., I. Romieu, M. Ramirez, S. Colome, K. Fung, D. Ashley, M. Hernandez-Avila. 1999. A survey of personal exposures to benzene in Mexico city. *Arch. Environ. Health* 54:359–363.

338. Riveros-Rosas, H., G. D. Pfeifer, D. R. Lynam, J. L. Pedroza, A. Julian-Sanchez, O. Canales, J. Garfias. 1997. Personal exposure to elements in Mexico city air. *Sci. Total Environ.* 198:79–96.

339. Villaclara, G., T. Cantoral. 1986. Avances en la investigación de liquenes epifitos como indicadores de contaminación atmosférica en el Valle de México. *Memorias del Curso IV Simposio Internacional sobre Biología de la Contaminación*, México DF, pp. 30–31.

340. Cano, D. 2001. *Heces caninas grave problema de salud*. Mexico City: El Universal, 17:4.

341. Calderón-Garciduenas, L. et al. 2000. Exposure to air pollution is associated with lung hyperinflation in healthy children and adolescents in southwest Mexico city. A pilot study. *Inhal. Toxicol.* 12:537–561.

342. Bennett, W. D., K. L. Zeman, C. W. Kang, M. S. Schechter. 1997. Extrathoracic deposition of inhaled, coarse particles (4.5 μm) in children vs. adults. *Ann. Occup. Hyg.* 41:497–502.

343. Bevilacqua, M. P., M. A. Gimbrone. 1987. Inducible endothelial functions in inflammation and coagulation. *Semin. Thromb. Hemost.* 13:425–433.

344. Chao, C. C., S. Hu, T. W. Moliter, E. G. Shaskan, P. K. Peterson. 1992. Activated microglia mediate cell injury via a nitric oxide mechanism. *J. Immunol.* 149:2736–2741.

345. Chao, S. E., R. S. Lee, S. H. Shih, J. K. Chen. 1998. Oxidized LDL promotes vascular endothelial cell pinocytosis via a prooxidation mechanism. *FASEB J.* 12:823–830.

346. Claudio L. 1996. Ultrastructural features of the blood–brain barrier in biopsy tissue from Alzheimer's disease patients. *Acta Neuropath.* 91:6–14.

347. Acarin, L., B. Gonzalez, B. Castellano. 2000. STAT3 and NFkappaB activation precedes glial reactivity in the excitotoxically injured young cortex but not in the corresponding distal thalamic nuclei. *J. Neuropathol. Exp. Neurol.* 59:151–163.

348. Clarke, R. W., B. Coull, U. Reinisch, P. Catalano, C. R. Killingsworth, P. Koutrakis, I. Kavouras, J. J. Godleski. 2000. Inhaled concentrated ambient particles are associated with hematologic and bronchioalveolar changes in canines. *Environ. Health Perspect.* 108:1179–1187.

349. Clemens, J. A. 2000. Cerebral ischemia: Gene activation, neuronal injury, and the protective role of antioxidants. *Free Radic. Biol. Med.* 28:1526–1531.

350. Corona, T., J. L. Rodrígues, E. Otero, L. Stopp. 1996. Multiple sclerosis in Mexico: Hospital cases at the National Institute of Neurology and Neurosurgery, Mexico city. *Neurología* 11:170–173.

351. de la Torre, J. C. 2000. Cerebral hypoperfusion, capillary degeneration, and development of Alzheimer disease. *Alzheimer Dis. Assoc. Discord.* 14:S72–S81.

352. Bravo, H., R. Camacho, G. Roy-Ocotla, R. Sosa, R. Torres. 1991. Analysis of the change in atmospheric urban formaldehyde and photochemistry activity as a result of using methyl-t-butyl ether (MTBE) as an additive in gasolines in the metropolitan area of Mexico city. *Atmos. Environ.* 25:285–288.

353. Bukowski, J. A., D. Wartenberg, M. Goldschmidt. 1998. Environmental causes for sinonasal cancers in pet dogs, and their usefulness as sentinels of indoor cancer risk. *J. Toxicol. Environ. Health A* 54:579–591.

354. Divine, K. K., J. L. Lewis, P. G. Grant, G. Bench. 1999. Quantitative particle-induced X-ray emission imaging of rat olfactory epithelium applied to the permeability of rat epithelium to inhaled aluminum. *Chem. Res. Toxicol.* 12:575–581.

355. Driscoll, K. E., J. M. Carter, D. G. Hassenbein, B. Howard. 1997. Cytokines and particle-induced inflammatory cell recruitment. *Environ. Health Perspect.* 105:1159–1164.

356. Simon, T. R., G. H. Ross, W. J. Rea, A. R. Johnson, D. C. Hickey. 1999. Neurotoxicity in single photon emission computed tomography brain scans of patients reporting chemical sensitivities. *Toxicol. Ind. Health* 15:415–420.

357. Brandli, O. 1996. Are inhaled dust particles harmful for our lungs? *Schweiz. Med. Wochenschr.* 126:2165–2174.

358. Behl, C., B. Moosmann, D. Manthey, S. Heck. 2000. The female sex hormone oestrogen as neuroprotectant: Activities at various levels. *Novartis Found Symp.* 230:221–234.

359. Breteler, M. M. et al. 1994. Cerebral white matter lesions, vascular risk factors, and cognitive function in a population-based study: The Rotterdam Study. *Neurology* 44:1246–1252.

360. Longstreth, W. T. Jr., T. A. Manolio, A. Arnoldm, G. L. Burke, N. Bryan, C. A. Jungreis, P. L. Enright, D. O'Leary, L. Fried. 1996. Clinical correlates of white matter findings on cranial magnetic resonance imaging of 3301 elderly people. The Cardiovascular Health Study. *Stroke* 27:1274–1282.

361. van Straaten, E. C. et al.; LADIS Group. 2006. Impact of white matter hyperintensities scoring method on correlations with clinical data: The LADIS study. *Stroke* 37:836–840.

362. Tullberg, M., E. Fletcher, C. DeCarli, D. Mungas, B. R. Reed, D. J. Harvey, M. W. Weiner, H. C. Chui, W. J. Jagust. 2004. White matter lesions impair frontal lobe function regardless of their location. *Neurology* 63:246–253.

363. Gootjes, L., S. J. Teipel, Y. Zebuhr, R. Schwarz, G. Leinsinger, P. Scheltens, H. J. Möller, H. Hampel. 2004. Regional distribution of white matter hyperintensities in vascular dementia, Alzheimer's disease and healthy aging. *Dement. Geriatr. Cogn. Disord.* 18:180–188.

364. Scarpelli, M., U. Salvolini, L. Diamanti, R. Montironi, L. Chiaromoni, M. Maricotti. 1994. MRI and pathological examination of post-mortem brains: The problem of white matter high signal areas. *Neuroradiology* 36:393–398.

365. Wahlund, L. O., F. Barkhof, F. Fazekas, L. Bronge, M. Augustin, M. Sjogren, A. Wallin, H. Ader, D. Leys, L. Pantoni, F. Pasquier, T. Erkinjuntti, P. Scheltens; European Task Force on Age-Related White Matter Changes. 2001. A new rating scale for age-related white matter changes applicable to MRI and CT. *Stroke* 32:1318–1322.

366. Kraut, M. A., L. L. Beason-Held, W. D. Elkins, S. M. Resnick. 2008. The impact of magnetic resonance imaging-detected white matter hyperintensities on longitudinal changes in regional cerebral blood flow. *J. Cereb. Blood Flow Metab.* 28:190–197.

367. Jellinger, K. A., J. Attems. 2007. Neuropathological evaluation of mixed dementia. *J. Neurol. Sci.* 257:80–87.

368. Calderón-Garciduenãs, L. et al. 2008. Long-term air pollution exposure is associated with neuroinflammation, an altered innate immune response, disruption of the blood-brain barrier, ultrafine particulate deposition, and accumulation of amyloid beta-42 and alpha-synuclein in children and young aduvalts. *Toxicol. Pathol.* 36:289–310.

369. U.S. Environmental Protection Agency. 2004. *Green Book: Particulate Matter Nonattainment Area Summary.* United States Evironmental Protection System.

370. Seagrave, J. et al. 2006. Lung toxicity of ambient particulate matter from southeastern U.S. sites with different contributing sources: Relationships between composition and effects. *Environ. Health Perspect.* 114:1387–1393.

371. Baxter, L. K., J. E. Clougherty, F. Laden, J. I. Levy. 2007. Predictors of concentrations of nitrogen dioxide, fine particulate matter, and particle constituents inside of lower socioeconomic status urban homes. *J. Expo. Sci. Environ. Epidemiol.* 17:433–444.

372. Evans, A. C. 2006. The NIH MRI study of normal brain development. *Neuroimage* 30:184–202.

373. Brickman, A. M., M. E. Zimmerman, R. H. Paul, S. M. Grieve, D. F. Tate, R. A. Cohen, L. M. Williams, C. R. Clark, E. Gordon. 2006. Regional white matter and neuropsychological functioning across the adult lifespan. *Biol. Psychiatry* 60:444–453.

374. Go, Y. M., E. P. Jones. 2011. Cysteine/cystine redox signaling in cardiovascular disease. *Free Radic Biol Med* 50:495–509.

375. Copp, S. W., L. F. Ferreira, K. F. Herspring, D. M. Hirai, B. S. Synder, D. C. Poole, T. I. Musch. 2009. The effects of antioxidants on microvascular oxygenation and blood flow in skeletal muscle of young rats. *Exp Physiol.* 94:961–971.

376. West, J. B. 2000. *Respiratory Physiology: The Essentials.* Lippincott, Philadelphia, PA.

377. Kruit, M. C. et al. 2004. Migraine as a risk factor for subclinical brain lesions. *J. Am. Med. Assoc.* 291:427–434.

3 Indoor Air Pollution

INTRODUCTION

Contaminated indoor air began with soot from open fires on the ceilings of prehistoric caves, tepees, and hogans. Later, during the times of the great plagues and tuberculosis epidemics, home air was very bad for health because of extremely poor ventilation. Coal- and wood-burning fireplaces emitted particulates and toxic fumes that were not dispersed. Instead, these pollutants contaminated residents, breaking down their mucosal resistance. With the passage of time and the development of civilization, changes in air cleanliness in the home resulted in the control of several diseases, such as tuberculosis, caused by indoor air pollution. However, indoor air in the twenty-first century has developed its own distinctive pollution problems. The use of rapidly disintegrating synthetic materials, fossil fuels, and pesticides coupled with the sealing of buildings in an attempt to conserve fuel for prevention of heat or cold loss has brought us back to dangerous conditions of indoor air contamination, with a resultant increase in chemical and electrical sensitivity. In the 1960s, Randolph[1] followed by Dickey[2] published the first descriptions of chemical sensitivity due to modern indoor air pollution. He pointed out that chemical sensitivity was exacerbated by modern indoor air pollution in the home and workplace, which was mostly invisible and of a toxic chemical nature. Three decades later, our studies at the EHC-Dallas[3] have produced both empirical and analytical data that support and confirm Randolph's work. Ryan et al.[4] and Sheldon et al.[5] have found that indoor pollution levels often exceed acceptable outdoor air standards.

Recently, a new wave of indoor pollutants has hit our homes and workplaces. These include inorganic pollutants, such as carbon monoxide and dioxide, nitrous oxides, ozone, and several others, and organic pollutants, such as pesticides, natural gases, formaldehyde (FA), solvents, terpenes, paints, mold, etc. Electromagnetic radiation has now become the greater problem indoors due to TVs, computers, cell phones, Wi-Fi, and smart meters. This new wave of indoor pollution is extremely serious since the primary effects of exposure to it are often seen on the nervous and cardiovascular systems, creating hypersensitivity, cancer, arteriosclerosis, and chronic degenerative neurological and cardiovascular disease.

SOURCES OF POLLUTION

Fifty percent of indoor air is generated from outside. An area of high outdoor air pollution will tend to increase indoor air pollution unless the building is so tight that there is no air exchange. In this case, even though outdoor air is not contributing to indoor air pollution, the levels generated from indoor sources, combined with inadequate ventilation, could still be sufficiently elevated to cause discomfort for the chemically sensitive and chronic degenerative disease patient.

Both outdoor air and its pollutants may infiltrate the indoor environment through windows, doors, cracks, and the ventilation system (Figure 3.1). Clean ambient outdoor air can infiltrate indoor air and prove beneficial by diluting indoor pollutants. Infiltration of polluted air, however, can be harmful by bringing outside toxins inside, thus increasing the total body load (burden) of the chemically sensitive individuals exposed to them. Areas near gas fracking and oil refineries are examples of the latter.

Most studies of pollutants entering the indoor environment from outdoor ambient air measure levels of the "criteria" pollutants for which National Ambient Air Quality Standards exist.[6] These pollutants are ozone, nitrogen oxides, carbon monoxide, sulfur dioxide, suspended particulates,

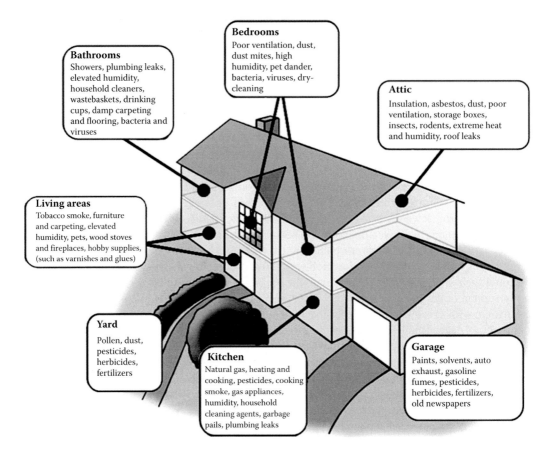

FIGURE 3.1 **(See color insert.)** Sources of indoor air pollution observed to exacerbate chemical sensitivity.

and lead (Chapters 1 and 4 of this volume). Other pollutants that originate outdoors, however, are also found in the indoor environment. These include respirable fraction particulates, trace metals, carbon dioxide, pollen and fungal spores, hydrogen sulfide, peroxyacetyl nitrate, polyaromatic hydrocarbons, pesticides, EMF emissions from Wi-Fi, smart meters, high-power lines, radon and radon daughter products, etc.

Pollutants generated from indoor sources may be similar. They include carbon monoxide, carbon dioxide, nitrogen oxides, oxidants, hydrocarbons, biological aerosols, molds, pesticides, hydrocarbon products, terpenes, EMF, and radon and radon daughter products as well as respirable particulates. Many of these pollutants may be found at higher levels indoors than outdoors. In addition, toxic volatile organic chemicals are seen in much greater numbers than outside, and these exacerbate chemical sensitivity.

Along with the infiltration of outdoor air contaminants, the generation of air contaminants from indoor sources also contributes to indoor air pollution. Typical indoor sources of air pollution are combustion (heating and cooling, coal, wood, oil, gas, electrical), consumer products (aerosol sprays, degreasers, hair dryers, room deodorants, insecticides), building materials (particle board containing FA, molds, and acrylic nitrite paints, concrete blocks, carpets, and glues), tobacco smoke, human body emissions (bacteria, odors, carbon dioxide), and house pets (bacteria, allergens). All of these sources contribute to total body pollutant load (burden) and can potentially disturb the human body's homeostatic mechanisms. The following review of sources of indoor air pollution will concentrate mainly on nonbiological and nonradioactive air pollutants (Table 3.1), although these latter types may also adversely affect the chemically sensitive by increasing total body load (burden).

TABLE 3.1
Environmental Gradients
(Least to Most Outgasing)

Stone
Ceramics
Steel
Iron
Hardwood
Copper
Aluminum
Fluorocarbons
Polyurethanes
Epoxies
Silicones
Polyvinyls
Polyethylenes
Polyesters

Though radon is known to increase total body load, its acute effects on the chemically sensitive are unknown but appear to be adverse. The reasons why so much emphasis in this chapter is placed on the organic pollutants are that they are very important in generating and exacerbating chemical sensitivity and often can be eliminated or decreased. The EMF has become a major problem and with awareness and measuring devices can be eliminated or decreased. Smart meters and Wi-Fi have to be shielded. Molds are specific for isolated contaminated buildings that have water leaks.

COMBUSTION

Most studies of air pollutants generated indoors particularly focus on emissions from gas, oil, or coal combustion. These, along with pesticides and tobacco smoke, have been found by physicians, including Randolph (Randolph, T. G. 1987, personal communication), Rea (Rea, W. J. 1987, unpublished data), Rapp (Rapp, D. J. 1987, personal communication), Kroker (Kroker, G. 1987, personal communication), Little (Little, C. H. 1987, personal communication), Monro (Monro, J. 1987, personal communication), and Maberly (Maberly, D. J. 1987, personal communication), to be the largest generators of indoor air pollution affecting the chemically sensitive. The emissions most often quantified are carbon monoxide and carbon dioxide, nitric oxide, and nitrogen dioxide, although there are several other natural gas fumes, such as methane, ethane, propane, butane, benzene, pentane, methylpentanes, cyclopentanes, hexanes, heptanes, octanes, ethylbenzene, toluene, xylene, etc., that may be just as, or more, important.

Inorganic and organic sources of combustion will be discussed individually (Figure 3.2).

Inorganic pollutants, including carbon dioxide, sulfur dioxides, nitrogen oxides, carbon monoxide, ozone, lead, particulates, and ammonia, cause symptom exacerbation in the chemically sensitive. Each will be discussed separately.

- Around 3 billion people cook and heat their homes using open fires and leaky stoves burning biomass (wood, animal dung, and crop waste) and coal.
- Nearly 2 million people die prematurely from illness attributable to indoor air pollution from household solid fuel use.
- Nearly 50% of pneumonia deaths among children under five are due to particulate matter (PM) inhaled from indoor air pollution.

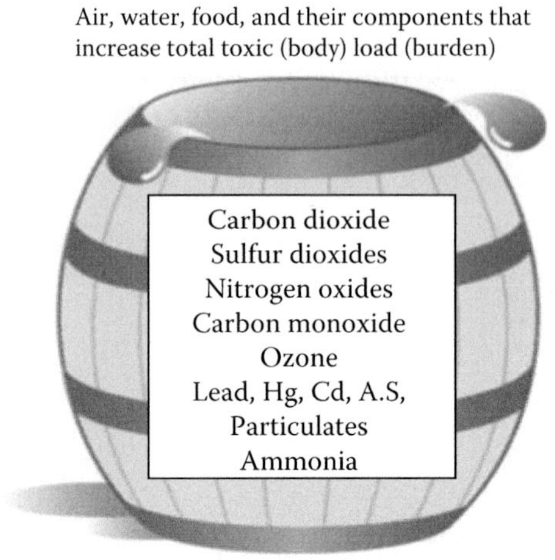

Air, water, food, and their components that
increase total toxic (body) load (burden)

Carbon dioxide
Sulfur dioxides
Nitrogen oxides
Carbon monoxide
Ozone
Lead, Hg, Cd, A.S,
Particulates
Ammonia

FIGURE 3.2   Sources of inorganic pollutants. A.S.: arsenic; Hg: Mercury; Cd: cadmium.

- More than 1 million people every year die from chronic obstructive respiratory disease (COPD) that develops due to exposure to such indoor air pollution.
- Both women and men exposed to heavy indoor smoke are 2–3 times more likely to develop COPD.
- Due to the vast chemical exposure, several people develop chemical sensitivity due to leaks from the gas cook stove.
- Others develop electrical sensitivity from the microwave oven, TV, computers, etc.

INDOOR AIR POLLUTION AND HOUSEHOLD ENERGY: THE FORGOTTEN 3 BILLION

Around 3 billion people still cook and heat their homes using solid fuels in open fires and leaky stoves. About 2.7 billion burn biomass (wood, animal dung, crop waste) and a further 0.4 billion use coal. Most are poor, and live in developing countries.

Such cooking and heating produces high levels of indoor air pollution with a range of health-damaging pollutants, including small soot particles that penetrate deep into the lungs. In poorly ventilated dwellings, indoor smoke can be 100 times higher than acceptable levels for small particles. Exposure is particularly high among women and young children, who spend the most time near the domestic hearth.

Nearly, 2 million people a year die prematurely from illness attributable to indoor air pollution due to solid fuel use (2004 data). Among these deaths, 44% are due to pneumonia, 54% from chronic obstructive pulmonary disease (COPD), and 2% from lung cancer.

Nearly half of deaths among children under 5 years old from acute lower respiratory infections (ALRI) are due to PM inhaled from indoor air pollution from household solid fuels.[247]

Many more people develop chemical, food, mold, and EMF sensitivity altering the brain and other physiological functions (Figure 3.3).

CONTRIBUTORS OF THE TOTAL ENVIRONMENTAL POLLUTANT LOAD IN THE TOTAL BODY POLLUTANT LOAD

Carbon dioxide: Carbon dioxide is generally found at higher levels indoors than outdoors. Respiration from occupants is the primary source of carbon dioxide in the indoor environment. Carbon dioxide is also a by-product of combustion. Petroleum-driven appliances are another source

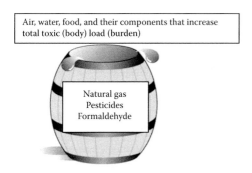

Air, water, food, and their components that increase total toxic (body) load (burden)

Natural gas
Pesticides
Formaldehyde

Air quality at home

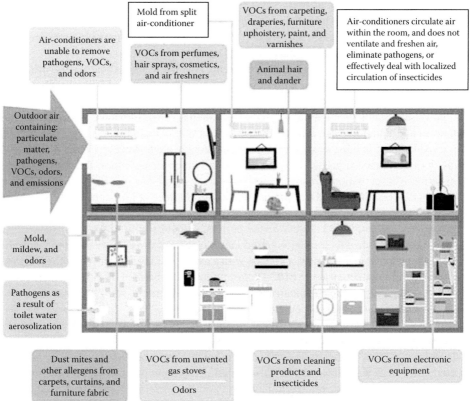

Mold from split air-conditioner

VOCs from carpeting, draperies, furniture upholstery, paint, and varnishes

Air-conditioners circulate air within the room, and does not ventilate and freshen air, eliminate pathogens, or effectively deal with localized circulation of insecticides

Air-conditioners are unable to remove pathogens, VOCs, and odors

VOCs from perfumes, hair sprays, cosmetics, and air freshners

Animal hair and dander

Outdoor air containing: particulate matter, pathogens, VOCs, odors, and emissions

Mold, mildew, and odors

Pathogens as a result of toilet water aerosolization

Dust mites and other allergens from carpets, curtains, and furniture fabric

VOCs from unvented gas stoves

Odors

VOCs from cleaning products and insecticides

VOCs from electronic equipment

FIGURE 3.3 (**See color insert.**) Air quality at home.

of carbon dioxide with the resultant indoor levels determined by the amount of gas burned and the rate of air exchange with outdoor air. Carbon dioxide is definitely produced from burning natural gas ($CH_4 + 2O_2 \rightarrow CO_2 + 2H_2O$), but it is not quantified when sources of indoor air pollution are surveyed because it is not considered toxic at concentrations typically found indoors. This assumption, however, may be unwarranted. We have noticed that chemically sensitive patients who are exposed to increasing levels of this pollutant in the Environmental Control Unit (ECU) experience a loss of vigor and mental acuity.

Measurements of carbon dioxide levels in a California high school with various ventilation rates were reported by Berks et al.[7] Carbon dioxide levels indoors and outdoors were similar (300–500 ppm) in the early morning hours before the occupants arrived. After 7 a.m., as people arrived at the school, the carbon dioxide levels climbed throughout the day until 3 p.m., when the occupants began to leave. The maximum indoor levels recorded during the day were about 1600 ppm with a ventilation rate of 2.5 ft³/minute per occupant. Throughout this study, outdoor levels of carbon dioxide remained fairly constant. After school ended, the indoor carbon dioxide levels fell exponentially back to outdoor levels by 9 p.m. Berks et al.[7] also found higher indoor carbon dioxide levels associated with lower forced-ventilation rates. Similar findings were reported by Edgar et al.[3] in our studies at the EHC-Dallas. Elevation of carbon dioxide levels occurred particularly in our first ECU where ventilation was not as good as in subsequent units. In these latter ECUs where efficient depollution devices were utilized, elevated carbon dioxide levels appeared to be much less of a problem. Although the presence of CO_2 in the environment is normally unobtrusive, we observed that the chemically sensitive do not function well when CO_2 levels in the ECU were elevated, even though these levels were not toxic.

Sulfur dioxides: Although sulfur dioxides do not create several problems inside homes, they have been known to contribute to indoor air pollution. Sources of sulfur dioxide in the home include gas and coal stoves, sewer gas leaks, and some of the seepage from outdoor air when present. Sulfur dioxides have been shown to exacerbate chemical sensitivity.

Two studies show sulfur dioxide levels in home. Andersen[8] found that on the average, indoor concentrations of sulfur dioxide in an unoccupied room with doors and windows closed were 51% of outdoor values in Arhus, Denmark.

In the United States, Spengler et al.[9] measured annual sulfur dioxide concentrations in several urban areas and found that the indoor/outdoor ratio was less than 1.0. Clearly, few problems with sulfur dioxide occur in most homes, unless they are coal heated. However, if the presence of sulfur dioxide does not increase problems associated with indoor air pollution, the chemically sensitive will experience exacerbation of their illness.

Nitrogen oxides: Nitrogen oxides pollute indoor air. Sources of nitrogen oxides in indoor air are outdoor infiltration and indoor gas appliances,[10–12] including hot water heaters and furnaces,[13] both convective- and radiant-type kerosene space heaters,[12–14] and gas-fired space heaters.[15] The major source of nitrogen oxide contamination of indoor air is the gas stove.[16,17] Wade et al.[17] speculate that a relatively high moisture content in a kitchen with a gas stove may further promote the formation of nitrogen oxides. In our series at the EHC-Dallas, pollutants generated by gas stoves are the primary offenders in indoor air for the chemically sensitive along with pesticides. These include methane gas as well as NO_2, CO, SO_4, and particulates.

Nitrogen oxide pollution of indoor air can be accentuated by failure to use heaters appropriately. Ritchie and Oatman[14] measured emissions from kerosene heaters and found that "safe threshold standards," which are neither safe nor real thresholds, were commonly exceeded when ventilation guidelines were not followed. They also found that the use of a unit 2.5 times larger than was required to heat a given area resulted in increased pollution levels that greatly surpassed American Society of Heating, Refrigerating and Air Conditioning Engineers (ASHRAE) standards. While using an appropriately sized heater with correct ventilation reduces the amount of air contamination caused by a kerosene heater, this practice does not eliminate pollution. At the EHC-Dallas, we have seen that several people fell ill by exposure to even minute levels of contamination produced by kerosene heaters, and there appear to be no safe levels of kerosene in indoor air.

Traynor et al.[15] found that some unvented gas-fired space heaters can emit levels of carbon dioxide and nitrogen dioxide that exceed existing guidelines for indoor air quality (IAQ). Our studies in the ECU showed very little nitrous oxides in the first environmental unit and almost none in the better ventilated units. These units clearly had better air than those examined by Traynor.[15]

Only a few studies have been published on the relationship between indoor and outdoor levels of nitrogen dioxide. Thompson et al.[18] found similar levels of nitrogen dioxide inside and outside. Spengler et al.[9] found the ratio of indoor to outdoor levels of nitrogen oxide was less than 1 in homes without gas stoves. Hawthorne et al.[19] measured indoor concentrations of nitrogen oxides in a bedroom situated over a garage and found that levels in this room increased after a car engine in the garage was operated for 3 minutes. We have seen a similar result with chemically sensitive patients being extremely ill by rising fumes. Under environmentally controlled conditions at the EHC-Dallas, Edgar et al.[3] found nitrous levels to be higher outside of the ECU, and nonexistent in the ECU when traffic was low. Nitrous oxides appear to be directly and strictly a function of outdoor fumes in this situation.

Studies comparing indoor and outdoor levels of nitrogen dioxide have produced various results. Thompson et al.,[18] for instance, found similar levels, except in air-conditioned buildings where indoor levels were found to be lower.

Carbon monoxide: Carbon monoxide is a pollutant commonly produced by combustion processes. Since combustion processes are involved with the working of gas-fueled appliances, these are largely responsible for indoor levels of carbon monoxide. Not only have gas stoves[10,20,21] heaters and furnaces[22] been shown to produce carbon monoxide, but the carbon monoxide they produce has also been shown to quickly diffuse throughout the house.[20] It dissipates mainly due to ventilation with outdoor air.[23] These appliances usually have to be removed from the homes of the chemically sensitive patients so that they function well.

Cigarette smoke is another common source of indoor carbon monoxide pollution.

Indoor levels of carbon monoxide can be increased by infiltration of contaminated outdoor air. Particularly, operating an automobile in an attached garage can increase indoor levels, as has been shown in studies of single-family dwellings[19] as well as business areas located adjacent to parking garages[24] underneath the building.

Carbon monoxide disturbs orderly oxidation and conjugation of xenobiotics in the chemically sensitive, resulting in enhanced chemical sensitivity.[25] It also binds to hemoglobin molecules, causing dysfunction.

Ozone: Several sources of ozone as an indoor air contaminant have been suggested. Hollowell et al.,[10] for example, attributed small increases of indoor air ozone concentrations to the use of electric stoves. The National Research Council[26] suggests that electric arcing from the electrostatic precipitator or UV radiation (document copier) may be a source of indoor air ozone contamination. We at the EHC-Dallas have determined that electrostatic depollution devices themselves may be sources of indoor ozone in addition to outside sources.

Our study conducted over a period of 6 months was carried out in a controlled ECU-type environment, using outgased and sealed plasterboard ceilings and walls and ceramic tile floors. The average concentration of ozone in this period was less than 0.05 ppm. However, fluctuations occurred to much greater levels.

Some of our employees complained of headaches, dryness of throat and mucous membranes of the nose and eyes, agitation, and other symptoms of ozone exposure. Detailed measurements carried out when these employees experienced symptoms showed that the ozone levels were suddenly increasing in four periods for several hours, peaking at 0.25, 0.20, 0.15, and 0.18 ppm levels, respectively. We identified the high-voltage unit of the electrostatic precipitator of the air filtering system in the office as the cause of the periodic increase in the ozone levels. The ozone contaminating the indoor air was generated by the electric sparks of the defective high-voltage unit. After this, source was eliminated, the ozone levels were reduced to the average values of less than 0.05 ppm, and the symptoms experienced by the personnel first subsided and, after a few weeks, disappeared completely. We also noted that the symptoms of our chemically sensitive patients who were brought into this area when levels of ozone were elevated were exacerbated, and their symptoms dissipated when the ozone decreased.

Generally, most of the research on the distribution, behavior, and fate of ozone indicate that infiltration of outdoor air into indoor air is the primary source of ozone in the indoor environment.[27] Ozone is a secondary pollutant generated by photochemical reactions involving nitrogen oxides, hydrocarbons, and sunlight.

Consistently, studies show a positive correlation between outdoor and indoor levels of ozone. Thompson et al.[18] found that indoor to outdoor ratios of ozone levels were less than 1 in a military hospital in southern California. This ratio increased by 30% in the late afternoon when the air-conditioning was in use; it increased by 50% when the air-conditioning was not running and the windows were open. Sabersky et al.[27] found an inverse relationship between the indoor-to-outdoor ratio of ozone and the "amount of indoor air." In 1984, Davies et al.[28] recorded simultaneous measurements of ozone both inside and outside an art gallery located in eastern England and found higher outdoor levels. At the EHC-Dallas, Edgar et al.[3] also found that the source of ozone air contamination in the ECUs was regularly contaminated outdoor air.

The decay rate of ozone is affected by a number of factors, including the type of indoor environment infiltrated, room temperature, room humidity, construction materials, type and use of air filters, room size, and furnishings[26,29] Sabersky et al.[27] found that indoor ozone levels decrease rapidly once outdoor infiltration was decreased by closing an area's doors and windows.

Ozone, a free radical itself, will help create other free radicals in the chemically sensitive, thus straining the antipollutant superoxide dismutase (SOD), glutathione peroxidase, and catalase enzymes.

Care must be taken when using an ozone generator to decrease indoor fume levels. Though the odor emitted from this device usually dissipates in a few hours, the ozone, as well as the toxic by-products, has been observed to linger for 1–2 weeks in some of our controlled environmental units.

Lead: Though it can enter from outside emissions, lead is rarely seen in homes. Only old homes with lead-based paints are still at risk from inside-generated pollutants. If ingested or inhaled in sufficient quantity, however, lead can cause and exacerbate chemical sensitivity (chapter on inorganics).

Halpern[30] measured indoor/outdoor ratios of lead particulate in several buildings in New York City. Indoor and outdoor air samples were taken simultaneously. Two of the sampling sites were in residential apartments, and two other sampling sites were in the American Museum of Natural History. For all four sites, the mean indoor/outdoor ratios were between 0.630 and 0.869. Significant differences were observed for the indoor/outdoor ratios of the respirable and nonrespirable samples between sites; a significant difference was observed for the indoor lead concentrations between the commercial and residential sites. Because ratios of indoor/outdoor pollution vary from site to site, the chemically sensitive must carefully investigate areas where they consider living and working.

Ammonia: Moschandreas et al.[31] measured the dispersion of ammonia from a commercially available cleaning agent in several different types of residences. In using 50 mL of a solution prepared from 100 mL of ammonia, Moschandreas et al.[31] found a range from a high of 3.09 ppm to a low of 0.091 ppm of ammonia in the first hour after cleaning the kitchen floor in the various residences he tested. The average first hour concentrations for all kitchens was 0.45 ppm. Ammonia will exacerbate chemical sensitivity, and therefore, commercial-strength cleaning agents that include ammonia ought not to be used in buildings where the chemically sensitive live and work. The chemically sensitive should also avoid areas around large commercial freezing and cooling devices as these also emit high levels of ammonia. At the EHC-Dallas, we have seen respiratory burns from reactive exposures to these sites (Figure 3.4).

Organic chemicals, especially those generated from gas, coal, kerosene and oil heat, pesticides, and products containing FA, are the prime offenders in indoor air that exacerbate chemical sensitivity. These are closely followed by the volatile organic chlorinated and nonchlorinated aliphatic and aromatic solvents. Each category will be discussed separately.

HYDROCARBONS

Hydrocarbons enter the indoor environment through a variety of sources. For instance, some hydrocarbons and their vapors are commonly found in building materials used to construct homes and businesses. Decane, xylene, undecane, 1,2,4-trimethylbenzene, propylbenzene, ethylbenzene, and nonane were identified in 20% of all samples of 32 construction materials tested for organic off-gassing properties.[32] Some other compounds that contaminate indoor air are toluene, butylacetate, and *o*-xylene, which may be introduced into the environment through sealing compounds, glues,

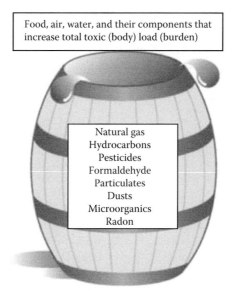

Food, air, water, and their components that increase total toxic (body) load (burden)

Natural gas
Hydrocarbons
Pesticides
Formaldehyde
Particulates
Dusts
Microorganics
Radon

FIGURE 3.4   Sources of organic pollutants.

cement, insulation foam, and paint. Also, solvent-based adhesives that contain toluene, styrene, and a variety of cyclic, branched, and normal alkanes, and are formulated for use in bonding carpets, vinyl floors, and subfloor assembly have been shown to emit significant amounts of organics.[33] Many of these are found in the blood of the chemically sensitive and will exacerbate their symptoms. Therefore, they should not be used in building materials with which the chemically sensitive will come in contact, and they should be removed from areas where the chemically sensitive are living and working. Natural gas heating seems to be a prime generator of many of the nonchlorinated hydrocarbons and is the primary generator along with pesticides of chemical sensitivity in the contaminated home.

TYPES OF HYDROCARBONS

The classifications for hydrocarbons, defined by the IUPAC nomenclature of organic chemistry, are as follows: methane, ethane, propane, butane, pentane, hexane, heptanes, octane, etc. Saturated hydrocarbons are the basis of petroleum fuels and are found as either linear or branched species. Natural gas (methane) is the number 1 inducer and propagator of chemical sensitivity, along with pesticides.

1. Saturated hydrocarbons (alkanes are the simplest of the hydrocarbon species and are composed entirely of single bonds and are saturated with hydrogen. The general formula for saturated hydrocarbons is C_nH_{2n+2} [assuming noncyclic structures]).[34] Hydrocarbons with the same molecular formula but different structural formulae are called structural isomers.[35] As given in the example of 3-methylhexane and its higher homologs, branched hydrocarbons can be chiral.[36] Chiral saturated hydrocarbons constitute the side chains of biomolecules such as chlorophyll and tocopherol.[37]
2. Unsaturated hydrocarbons have one or more double or triple bonds between carbon atoms. Those with double bond are called alkenes. Those with one double bond have the formula C_nH_{2n} (assuming noncyclic structures).[38] Those containing triple bonds are called alkynes, with general formula C_nH_{2n-2} (Table 3.2).[39]

TABLE 3.2

Simple Hydrocarbons and Their Variations

Number of Carbon Atoms	Alkane (Single Bond)	Alkene (Double Bond)	Alkyne (Triple Bond)	Cycloalkane	Alkadiene
1	Natural gas methane	–	–	–	–
2	Ethane	Ethene (ethylene)	Ethyne (acetylene)	–	–
3	Propane	Propene (propylene)	Propyne (methylacetylene)	Cyclopropane	Propadiene (allene)
4	Butane	Butene (butylene)	Butyne	Cyclobutane	Butadiene
5	Pentene	Pentene	Pentyne	Cyclopentane	Pentadiene (piperylene)
6	Hexane	Hexene	Hexyne	Cyclohexane	Hexadiene
7	Heptane	Heptene	Heptyne	Cycloheptane	Heptadiene
8	Octane	Octene	Octyne	Cyclooctane	Octadiene
9	Nonane	Nonene	Nonyne	Cyclononane	Nonadiene
10	Decane	Decene	Decyne	Cyclodecane	Decadiene

Common properties of hydrocarbons are the facts that they produce steam, carbon dioxide, and heat during combustion and that oxygen is required for combustion to take place. The simplest hydrocarbon, methane, burns as follows:

$$CH_4 + 2O_2 \rightarrow 2H_2O + CO_2 + Energy$$

In inadequate supply of air, CO gas and water vapor are formed:

$$2CH_4 + 3O_2 \rightarrow 2CO + 4H_2O$$

BURNING HYDROCARBONS

Hydrocarbons are currently the main source of the world's electric energy and heat sources (such as home heating) because of the energy produced when burned.[40] Often, this energy is used directly as heat such as in home heaters, which use either petroleum or natural gas. The hydrocarbon is burned and the heat is used to heat water, which is then circulated. A similar principle is used to create electric energy in power plants.

Another example of this property is propane:

$$C_3H_8 + 5O_2 \rightarrow 4H_2O + 3CO_2 + Energy$$
$$C_nH_{n+2} + (3n+1)/2O_2 \rightarrow (n+1)H_2O + nCO_2 + Energy$$

Burning of hydrocarbons is an example of an exothermic chemical reaction.

Hydrocarbons can also be burned with elemental fluorine, resulting in carbon tetrafluoride and hydrogen fluoride products.

GENERAL PROPERTIES

Because of differences in molecular structure, the empirical formula remains different between hydrocarbons; in linear, or "straight-run" alkanes, alkenes, and alkynes, the amount of bonded hydrogen lessens in alkenes and alkynes due to the "self-bonding" or catenation of carbon, preventing entire saturation of the hydrocarbon by the formation of double or triple bonds.

This inherent ability of hydrocarbons to bond to themselves is referred to as catenation and allows hydrocarbon to form more complex molecules, such as cyclohexane, and in rarer cases, arenes such as benzene. This ability comes from the fact that the bond character between carbon atoms is entirely nonpolar, in that the distribution of electrons between the two elements is somewhat even due to the same electronegativity values of the elements ($\sim$0.30), and does not result in the formation of an electrophile.

Generally, with catenation comes the loss of the total amount of bonded hydrocarbons and an increase in the amount of energy required for bond cleavage due to strain exerted upon the molecule; in molecules such as cyclohexane, this is referred to as ring strain, and occurs due to the "destabilized" spatial electron configuration of the atom.

In simple chemistry, as per valence bond theory, the carbon atom must follow the "4-hydrogen rule," which states that the maximum number of atoms available to bond with carbons equal to the number of electrons that are attracted into the outer shell of carbon. In terms of shells, carbon consists of an incomplete outer shell, which comprises four electrons, and thus has four electrons available for covalent or oxidative bonding.

Hydrocarbons are hydrophobic like lipids. Some hydrocarbons are also abundant in the solar system. Lakes of liquid methane and ethane have been found on Titan, Saturn's largest moon, confirmed by the Casssini–Huygens Mission.[35] Hydrocarbons are also abundant in nebulae, forming polycyclic aromatic hydrocarbon (PAH) compounds.

Sugie et al.[41] reported three cases of sudden death due to the inhalation of portable cooking stove fuel (case 1), cigarette lighter fuel (case 2), and liquefied petroleum gas (LPG) (case 3). Specimens of blood, urine, stomach contents, brain, heart, lung, liver, kidney, and fat were collected and analyzed for propylene, propane, isobutene, and n-butane by headspace gas chromatography (GCV). n-Butane was the major substance among the volatiles found in the tissues of cases 1 and 2, and propane was the major substance in case 3. A combination of the autopsy findings and the gas analysis results revealed that the cause of death was ventricular fibrillation induced by hard muscle exercise after gas inhalation in cases 1 and 2, and that the cause of death in case 3 might be hypoxia. It is possible that the victim in case 3 was under anesthetic toxicity of accumulated isobutene which is a minor component of liquefied petroleum gas.

According to Rossi et al.,[42] hydrocarbon inhalation is seldom chosen as a means to commit suicide. This practice is exclusively a prerogative of the prison population; it is, however, only exceptionally found in this environment. The two cases of lethal inhalation of propane/butane gas observed by Rossi et al. over a very short time occurred in this context. Toxicologic analyses were performed by means of GCV (had space) and revealed a propane/butane mixture in all specimens (heart blood, bile, and urine) except vitreous humor. Although fatal arrhythmia posthydrocarbon gas abuse is well known, the concentrations of the two hydrocarbons were sufficient to induce death by asphyxiation and were distributed (fairly) homogeneously in all biological fluids and organs examined, a parameter permitting one to assume that death occurred with a relatively short period of time. The absence of finding in vitreous humor and the trace amount in urine suggests that both men died very quickly.

According to Kim et al.,[43] smoke samples, in both gas and PM phases, of the three domestic stoves were collected using U.S. EPA modified method 5 and were analyzed for 17 PAH (HPLC0UV), acute toxicity (Microtox test), and mutagenicity (Ames test). The gas phase of smoke contributed > or = 95% of 17 PAH was from sawdust briquettes (260 mg/kg), but the highest emission of 11 genotoxic PAH was from kerosene (28 mg/kg). PM samples of kerosene smoke were not toxic. The total toxicity emission factor was the highest from sawdust, followed by kerosene and wood fuel. Smoke samples from the kerosene stove were not mutagenic. TA98 indicated the presence of both direct and indirect mutagenic activities in the gas phase. TA100 detected only direct mutagenic activities in both PM and gas phase samples. The higher mutagenicity emission factor was from wood fuel, $12 \times 10(6)$ (TA100-S9) and $2.8 \times 10(6)$ (TA98-S9). The low burning rate and high efficiency of a kerosene stove have resulted in the lowest PAH toxicity and mutagenicity emissions from daily cooking activities. The bioassays produced toxicity and mutagenicity results in correspondence with the PAH content of samples. The tests could be used for a quick assessment of potential health risks.

According to Lv and Zhu,[44] central ventilation and air-conditioner systems are widely utilized nowadays in public places for air exchange and temperature control, which significantly influences the transfer of pollutants between indoors and outdoors. To study the effect of central ventilation and air-conditioner systems on the concentration and health risk from airborne pollutants, a spatial and temporal survey was carried out using PAHs as agent pollutants. During the period when the central ventilation system operated without air-conditioning (AC-off period), concentrations of 2–4 ring PAHs in the model supermarket were dominated by outdoor levels, due to the good linearity between indoor air and outdoor air ($r(p) > 0.769$, $p < 0.05$), and the slopes (1.2–4.54) indicated that ventilating like the model supermarket increased the potential health risks from low-molecular-weight PAHs. During the period when the central ventilation and air-conditioner systems were working simultaneously (AC-on period), although the total levels of PAHs were increased, the concentrations and percentage of the particulate PAHs indoors declined significantly. The BaP equivalency (BaPeq) concentration indicated that utilization of air-conditioning reduced the health risks from PHs in the model supermarket.

According to Malouf and Wimberly,[45] living with natural gas can be a health hazard both for people who are healthy and for those who are already ill. It is especially risky for people who have weakened immune systems, including those who are asthmatic, allergic, or chemically sensitive. Gas appliances create a constant low-level exposure to gas which can cause or increase illnesses. Natural gas is a sensitizer, which means that exposure can lead to intolerance and adverse reactions both to it and other substances in our environment. It, along with pesticides, is the number 1 offending in the cause of chemical sensitivity.

The Lancet reported in 1996 that the use of domestic gas appliances, particularly gas stoves, was linked to increased asthma, respiratory illness, and impaired lung function, especially in young women. Women using gas stoves had double the respiratory problems of women cooking on electric stoves. The same study showed that using extractor fans which vented the cooking fumes outside did not reduce the adverse effects of gas.

The Canada Mortgage and Housing Corporation (CMHC) Clean Air Guide (1993) identified gas water heaters, furnaces, unvented space heaters, and cook stoves as significant contributors to chemical contamination in the home. They recommended that gas appliances be replaced with electrical ones to reduce indoor air pollution. In a combined series of studies of 47,000 patients, doctors found that "the most important sources of indoor pollution responsible for generating (environmental) illness were the gas cook stoves, hot water heaters, and furnaces" (Rea, W. J. of the Dallas Environmental Health Center).

"Traditionally natural gas is a pollutant chemical that can worsen both classical allergy and chemical sensitivity." (Dr. Gerald Ross Past President of the American Academy of Environmental Medicine in 1997.)

"For the chemically susceptible individual, this gas may be the worst form of fuel"[1]; studies found that when gas stoves were removed from the home of a person with chemical sensitivities, not only did their health improve but so did the health of all family members. Other studies have found that children living in homes with gas stoves had more than double the risk for respiratory symptoms, including asthma. Asthma patients who used a gas stove seven or more times a week were found to have doubled their risk of emergency room treatment. Infants who grow up in households with gas are almost twice as likely to develop childhood asthma than those who live with second-hand smoke. (Secondhand smoke itself doubles a child's risk of developing asthma.)

One of the principal products of gas combustion is water vapor. Cooking with gas or burning gas in any way without perfect venting generates considerable amounts of moisture. When this moisture remains inside a building, it is enough to be a significant contributor to molds. This excess moisture also provides better growing conditions for dust mites, viruses, and bacteria.

Natural gas brings harmful chemicals into homes through the methane it contains. Methane (which gives the flame its blue color as it does in propane) is an asphyxiant. It typically contains impurities and additives including radon and other radioactive materials, benzene, toluene, ethyl-benzene, and xylene (BTEX), organometallic compounds such as methylmercury, organoarsenic, and organolead. Mercaptan odorants are also added to natural gas so that it can be detected by scent before reaching explosive levels.

The components of the gas itself, as well as products of incomplete combustion, including nitrogen dioxide, carbon monoxide, and others, have health implications individually and synergistically, as they combine with each other and with other indoor pollutants.

Even taking all these precautions, when combustion gases leaving a chimney cool, they become heavier than air. Depending on wind conditions, they can reenter the living space. There is really no way at present to reduce the risk of gas appliances like stoves and clothes dryers. It is safest not to have any combustion at all inside the house.

Natural gas heatings in Nova Scotia have looked at whether there should be a gas pipeline and who should own it. But there has been no government assessment or public hearings into the health effects of home use of natural gas. Natural gas is not all bad news. Using gas to fire up the generators that produce electricity to heat homes and run appliances and in large industrial settings makes environmental and economic sense. Natural gas is a relatively clean burning fuel and it is less polluting of air than the coal and oil fuels we have traditionally burned.

But let us keep it far away from the air breathed inside houses, apartment buildings, and schools. If we consider healthcare costs and the impact of living with illness, bringing natural gas into homes is not a sensible choice.

According to Zang and Smith,[46] the nonmethane hydrocarbon emissions from several types of cookstoves commonly used in developing countries were measured in a pilot study conducted in Manila, the Philippines. Four types of fuel, that is, wood, charcoal, kerosene, and LPG, were tested. Because kerosene was burned in three different types of stoves, there were six fuel/stove combinations tested. Fifty-nine nonmethane hydrocarbons were identified frequently in emissions of these cookstoves, with emission ratios to CO_2 up to 5.3×10^{-3}. The emissions were quantitated with emission factors on both a mass basis (emissions/kg fuel) and a task basis (emissions/cooking task). On a task basis, combination of biomass fuels (wood and charcoal) generally produced higher emission factors than combustion of fossil fuels (kerosene and LPG). One type of kerosene stove (wick stove), however, still generated the greatest emissions of some individual and classes of hydrocarbons, indicating that emissions were dependent on not only fuel types but also combustion devices. Some hydrocarbons, for example, benzene, 1,3-butadiene, styrene, and xylenes, were of concern because of their carcinogenic properties. The lifetime risk from exposures to these compounds emitted from cookstoves was tentatively estimated by using a simple exposure model and published cancer potencies. These are all found in the breath analysis of some chemically sensitive patients. 1,3-butadiene is the number 1 or 2 toxic compound found in the chemically sensitive breath.

The age of a building may also contribute to the kind and amount of hydrocarbons present in its indoor air. Molhave et al.[32] found a significant difference in the overall chemical loading of indoor air, between new homes (those less than 3 years old) and old homes (those between 3 and 18 years). New homes had 15 times the concentrations of organic gases and vapors found in old homes[32] (Table 3.3). Also, 35–40 compounds were identified, on the average, in new homes, as compared with only 10–15 in the older dwellings. Toluene, α-pinene, and 3-xylene were the most frequently identified compounds in all the indoor air samples taken. However, decane and α-pinene were singularly prevalent in new homes, while toluene, 3-xylene, and ethanol were the common contaminants found in older structures.

TABLE 3.3

Difference in Organic Chemical Pollutants between New Homes (<3 Years) and Old Homes (3–18 Years)

	New	Old
Total organic gases	15[a]	1[a]
Number of types of organic gases	35–40	10–15

Source: Chemical Sensitivity Vol. II Page 695 Table 2. With permission.

[a] Total concentration of all gases.

The differences in concentrations and numbers of hydrocarbons found in the indoor air in this study suggest that contaminants from building materials may be gradually outgasing, and their concentrations in older homes may be diminishing and thus not detectable by present analytical methods. Also, while the frequent presence of toluene, 3-xylene, and ethanol may be the result of outgasing from a variety of building materials, these contaminants may, in fact, be present due to particular family activities that are carried on indoors or due to the presence of furnishings constructed from materials that also contain these contaminants. Furthermore, inadequate ventilation of newer homes constructed to be more energy efficient may be contributing to high pollution levels by not allowing dissipation of trapped contaminants. Given the ubiquitous nature of indoor air pollution, it is essential that the chemically sensitive be aware of potential sources of contamination in their building materials and furnishings and guard against contaminating their work and home environments.

Short-term, high levels of airborne contaminants may be introduced into the indoor environment through the use of consumer products such as cleaning products, aerosol sprays, paints, and cigarettes. The severity of pollution produced by these products depends on air ventilation rates, the exfiltration rate, and the reactivity of the gas in the room where the product is used. Clearly, to maintain optimum health, the chemically sensitive need to use less toxic cleaners, aerosols, and paints, and altogether avoid cigarette smoke.

A final source of hydrocarbons found in indoor air is pollution that is produced in the outdoors and is then able to seep inside. Benzo(*a*)pyrene concentrations in the ambient air, for instance, are primarily the result of emissions from transportation vehicles, electricity generation, coke production, and refuse burning.[47] Also, benzene and toluene may be present partially due to infiltration from outdoor air. Halogenated hydrocarbons may enter the indoor environment via clothes exposed to dry cleaning, spray cans, other cleaning materials, or chlorinated water sources. Eighty percent of the chemically sensitive patients seen at the EHC-Dallas have the dry cleaning solution tetrachloroethylene in their blood, and excessive or repeated exposure to this substance will increase their total body load (burden), and thus exacerbate their chemical sensitivity. It is clear that the chemically sensitive must decrease their exposure to toxic pollutants in order to function properly. For treatment, avoidance of these is altogether necessary.

Studies in the 1980s emphasized an ongoing problem with indoor air pollution. Pellizzari et al.,[48] for example, compared indoor and outdoor air samples and found that indoor air contained both larger numbers and higher levels of various volatile organic compounds (VOCs), many of which were found in the blood of the chemically sensitive. These findings suggest that sealing houses and buildings is not conducive to optimum health and certainly may stress the inhabitants' xenobiotic detoxification systems.

A qualitative study of organic chemicals in various homes in Chicago and Washington, DC[49] identified more than 250 different chemical compounds. Nearly all organic classes were found, including alkenes, alkynes, ketones, aromatics, chlorofluorocarbons, alcohols, aldehydes, esters, ethers, pesticides, and terpenes. The likely sources of these pollutants are human bioeffluents, food, house plants, perfumes, other household product, and, of course, building materials. With pollution sources being so common, it is easy to see how the chemically sensitive patient can become overloaded simply by living and working in his everyday environment. The symptoms then exacerbate, and final healing is prevented.

These studies complement our findings at the EHC-Dallas, which emphasize that current practices of building construction need to be changed. Much thought must be given to reducing toxic outgasing and creating environments that will enhance health and not precipitate chemical sensitivity.

Hawthorne et al.[19] measured selected volatile organics in 40 homes. They too found the presence of contaminants, including toluene and xylene, at levels generally greater that $20 \mu g/m^3$. They also identified benzene, tetrachloroethylene, lindane, naphthalene, some terpenes, phthalates, and siloxanes. Wallace[50] even showed higher levels of organics indoors versus outdoors in the heavy industrialized and chemical dump areas of New Jersey. Again, these studies graphically emphasize the ease with which indoor air pollution can increase as a result of an excessive number of indoor contaminants.

Pesticides: Pentachlorophenol (PCP) is extensively used in the treatment of wood products to control fungus growth and rotting. Ulsamer et al.[51] reported PCP levels in the air of log homes, ranging from less than $4 \mu g/m^3$ to $1000 \mu g/m^3$. Levels of PCP in conventional homes have not been measured in a large series, though isolated measurements of PCPs have been performed. We have seen some real disasters from the PCP-treated homes. Some whole families developed severe chemical sensitivity. Our experience with victims of PCP exposure leads us to advocate banning PCP from all building materials.

Products used to exterminate termites usually emit chloradane, heptachlor, and heptachlor epoxide into the ambient home air and will exacerbate chemical sensitivity. Although these are no longer marketed, they still have to be considered when evaluating pollution levels of an indoor environment because of their long (greater than 20 years) half-lives.

Routine use of organophosphate pesticides, some applied as frequently as once per month, has become a serious problem in several homes, office buildings, restaurants, etc. Organophosphates, pyrethroids, carbamates, and other pesticides used for pest control have now equaled petroleum-derived heat as the number 1 offender in indoor air pollution for the chemically sensitive. Not only must the chemically sensitive eliminate their contact with these substances, but they also must ensure that new ones that could create additional problems for them are not introduced into their homes or work environments. Nontoxic substances such as orthoboric acid suitable for pest control should be encouraged.

Other hydrocarbons, such as xylenes, toluenes, and other solvents are used routinely in house spraying as penetrators or vehicles for pesticides. Most of these VOCs have been found in the blood of the chemically sensitive in the parts per billion range and are known to exacerbate them.

"Inert" ingredients can be found in a variety of chemical products such as aerosol air fresheners, pan degreasers, and pesticides. Often, they are toxic hydrocarbons or other compounds such as DDT that, although banned for specific uses, have been allowed to remain in some of the products as inert ingredients since they are not specified as an active ingredient. These ingredients are often difficult to identify since contact with Washington, DC and the federal bureaucracy is essential to acquire information about them. Even then, information may not be accessible because of trade secrets laws. Routinely, however, several "inert" ingredients have been observed to markedly exacerbate the chemically sensitive who are often exposed to them inadvertently through aerosols. DDE, the breakdown products of DDT, have been found in the blood of several chemically sensitive patients. It is part of the total body pollutant load causing problems in the chemically sensitive. Since it has such a long half-life, it is still found in homes constructed in the 1950s until it was banned. The half-life is approximately 50 years, so it may be present for a patient's lifetime.

Organophosphorus (OP) insecticides are used worldwide in the control of agricultural, household, and veterinary pests. Dichlorvos (2,2-dichlorovinyl dimethyl phosphate) is a commonly used

OP insecticide. Study has shown that there are toxic effects of dichlorvos on the nuclei of freshly isolated human peripheral blood lymphocytes when incubated with 5, 10, 20, 80, and 100 microg/mL of dichlorvos. According to the results, dichlorvos induced micronuclei, decreased the mitotic and replication indexes. It is a genotoxic product causing chromosomal damage (an increase in micronucleus) and cell death (decrease in mitotic and replication indexes). This substance should never be used in the home. However, it is frequently used both in the homes and at work.

This is shown also in animal studies by Mansour and Mossa.[52] Their study showed the oxidative damage, biochemical and histopathological alterations in suckling rats whose mothers were exposed to the insecticide chlorpyrifos (CPF). Dams were administered CPF, via oral route. Doses equaled 0.01 mg/kg body weight (b.wt.; acceptable daily intake, ADI), 1.00 mg/kg b.wt. (no observed adverse effects level, NOAEL), and 1.35 mg/kg b.wt. (1/100 lethal dose [LD_{50}]) from postnatal day 1 until day 20 after delivery. At two high doses of CPF, the b.wt. gain and relative liver and kidney weight of suckling pups were significantly decreased. Exposure of the mothers to CPF caused increase in lipid peroxidation (LPO) and decrease in SOD and glutathione-S-transferase (GST) in lactating pups. CPF altered the level of the marker parameters related to the liver and kidneys. Consistent histological changes were found in the liver and kidneys of the subjected pups, especially at higher doses. The results suggested that the transfer of CPF intoxication through the mother's milk has resulted in oxidative stress and biochemical and histopathological alterations in the suckling pups. The data of this study may be considered as a contribution to the problem of lactational transfer of the relatively less persistent OP pesticides such as CPF. This finding is worldwide. This study showed the widespread use of pesticides, intoxication due to organophosphate insecticides is common in Turkey. OP compounds may cause late-onset distal polyneuropathy occurring 2 or more weeks after the acute exposure. An 18-year-old woman and a 22-year-old man were admitted to the hospital with weakness, paresthesia, and gait disturbances at 35 and 22 days, respectively, after ingesting dimethyl-2,2-dichloro vinyl phosphate (DDVP). Neurological examination revealed weakness, vibration sense loss, bilateral dropped foot, brisk deep tendon reflexes, and bilaterally positive Babinski sign. Electroneurography demonstrated distal motor polyneuropathy with segmental demyelination associated with axonal degeneration prominent in the distal parts of both lower extremities.

Another study has shown that bedbug control by pesticides is toxic and that other means for control can be used. The U.S. Environmental Protection Agency (EPA) wants to alert consumers that there has been an increase of individuals or companies who offer to control bedbugs with unrealistic promises of effectiveness or low cost. Because bedbug infestations are so difficult to control, there have been situations where pesticides that are not intended for indoor residential applications have been improperly used or applied at greater rates than the label allows. While controlling bedbugs is challenging, consumers should never use, or allow anyone else to use, a pesticide indoors that is intended for outdoor use, as indicated on the label. Using the wrong pesticide or using it incorrectly to treat for bedbugs can make the home owner, the family, and the pets sick. It can also make the home unsafe to live in—and may not solve the bedbug problem.

Bedbugs can cause itchy bites on people and pets. Unlike most public-health pests, however, bedbugs are not known to transmit or spread diseases. Pesticides are only one tool to use in getting rid of bedbugs. A comprehensive approach that includes prevention and nonchemical treatment of infestations is the best way to avoid or eliminate a bedbug problem. While more information can be found on EPA's website, a few examples of nonchemical methods of control include

- Removing clutter where bedbugs can hide
- Using mattress covers designed to contain bedbugs
- Sealing cracks and crevices
- Vacuuming rugs and upholstered furniture thoroughly and frequently, as well as vacuuming under beds (take the vacuum bag outside immediately and dispose in a sealed trash bag)
- Washing and drying clothing and bedsheets at high temperatures (heat can kill bedbugs)

- Placing clean clothes in sealable plastic bags when possible
- Being alert and monitoring for bedbugs so they can be treated before a major infestation occurs

This comprehensive method of pest control is called integrated pest management and includes a number of common sense control methods. If you need to use pesticides, follow these tips to ensure your safety and that the product works: However, do not use pesticides.

More information on IPM, bedbugs, and how to control them can be found in http://epa.gov/pesticides/bedbugs.

AFGHAN SCHOOL POISONINGS LINKED TO TOXIC CHEMICALS

Blood samples taken from Afghan schoolgirls who collapsed in apparent mass poisonings showed traces of toxic chemicals found in herbicides, pesticides, and nerve gas.

Suspicion has fallen on sympathizers of the Taliban, the hard-line Islamist militia that opposes education for women and prohibited girls from going to school when it was in power until being ousted by a 2001 U.S.-led invasion.

Poisonous levels of organophosphates were found in samples taken from girls sickened in incidents over the past 2 years. Forty-eight pupils and teachers at Kabul's Zabihullah Esmati High School and 60 students and teachers at the Totia Girls School were hospitalized after fainting or complaining of breathing problems, dizziness, and nausea. Students said that they began feeling unwell after being exposed to an unknown gas spreading through classrooms.

In addition to killing weeds and insects, organophosphates are the active ingredients of deadly nerve gases such as sarin and VX, and even low-level exposure can damage the nervous system.

Signs of organophosphate poisoning include headache, tiredness, upset stomach, and breathing trouble, all similar to the symptoms shown by the students and teachers at the Kabul schools (Figure 3.5).

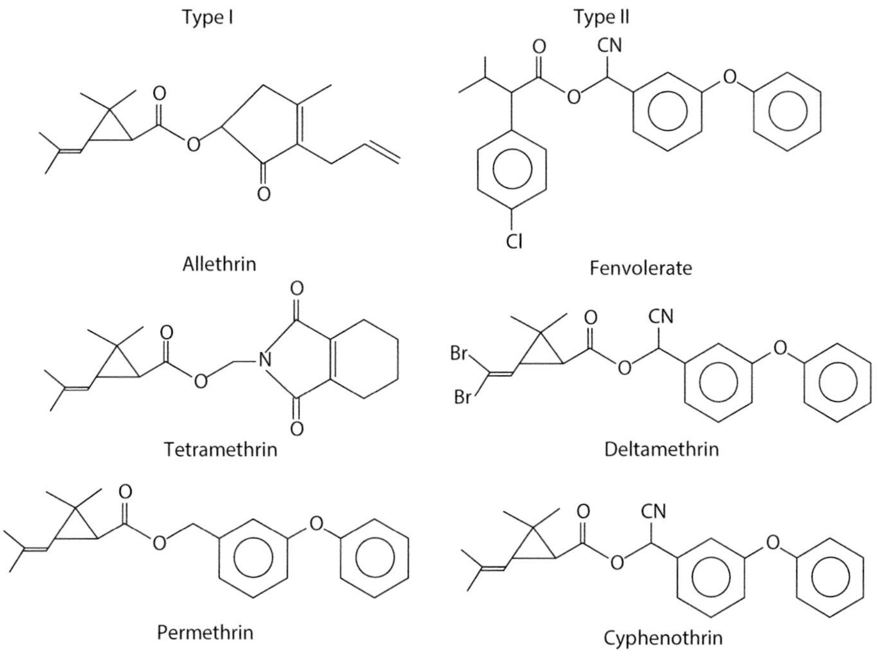

FIGURE 3.5 Pyrethroids.

Pyrethroids have been found in schools and animals—particularly in dogs that have been dewormed and kept inside. Dogs that have been poisoned with pyrethroids are extremely harmful when kept inside and sleeping with its owner.

Formaldehyde: FA is often used in building materials. Particularly, a glue composed of urea-formaldehyde is used to hold together the wood shavings that constitute chipboard (particle board). Owing to its composition, chipboard continually emanates FA into the indoor environment where it is often used for partitions, ceilings, floors, and furniture and can initiate and exacerbate chemical sensitivity. FA is a prime exacerbator of chemical sensitivity. Plywood and sheet rock have also been found to contain formaldehyde and eminate it.

Apparently, FA outgasing decreases over time. Hawthorne et al.[19] found that newer houses had higher levels of FA than did older homes. Wanner and Kuhn[53] found that the FA emitted from the building materials of new public buildings and homes constructed in Switzerland was half its original value after 12 months. Other studies, however, suggest that factors other than time play an important role in the amount of FA that is released into indoor air. Andersen et al.,[54] Godish et al.,[55] and Matthews et al.[56] found that room temperature, humidity, and ventilation affect FA outgasing. High concentrations of FA occur with high temperature, high humidity, and a low air exchange rate. Therefore, the chemically sensitive should avoid high temperature, high humidity, and low air exchange in order to maintain a minimally polluted indoor environment. They should also consider these factors when constructing new environments.

Sexton et al.[57] found that mobile homes had FA levels about twice as high as nonmanufactured residences. Since FA exposures have been a significant problem in initiating and exacerbating chemical sensitivity, the chemically sensitive should not live in mobile homes unless they are sealed to prevent outgasing or are constructed of nonpolluting metals, glass, and hardwood, and then sealed with aluminum wallpaper.

Formaldehyde: These are home substances that can contain FA (Table 3.4).

According to Golden,[58] FA is a well-studied chemical and effects from inhalation exposures have been extensively characterized in numerous controlled studies with human volunteers, including asthmatics and other sensitive individuals. They provide a rich database on exposure concentrations that can reliably produce the symptoms of sensory irritation. Although individuals can differ in their sensitivity to odor and eye irritation, the majority of authoritative reviews of the FA literature have concluded that an air concentration of 0.3 ppm will provide protection from eye irritation for virtually everyone. A weight of evidence-based FA exposure limit of 0.1 ppm (100 ppb) is recommended as an indoor air level for all individuals for odor detection and sensory irritation. It has recently been suggested by the International Agency for Research on Cancer (IARC), the National Toxicology Program (NTP), and the U.S. EPA that FA is causally associated with nasopharyngeal cancer (NPC) and leukemia. This has led U.S. EPA to conclude that irritation is not the most sensitive toxic endpoint and that carcinogenicity should dictate how to establish exposure limits for FA. In this review, a number of lines of reasoning and substantial scientific evidence are described and discussed, which leads to a conclusion that neither point of contact nor systemic effects of any type, including NPC or leukemia, are causally associated with exposure to FA. This conclusion supports the view that the equivocal epidemiology studies that suggest otherwise are almost certainly flawed by identified or yet to be unidentified confounding variables. Thus, this assessment concludes that an FA indoor air limit of 0.1 ppm should protect even particularly susceptible individuals from both irritation effects and any potential cancer hazard. Our experience with the severe chemically sensitive patient is below this limit. The environment must be FA free.

Toxic Effects of Formaldehyde on the Nervous System

According to Sonbgur et al.,[59] FA is found in the polluted atmosphere of cities, domestic air (e.g., paint, insulating materials, chipboard and plywood, fabrics, furniture, paper), cigarette smoke, etc.; therefore, everyone and particularly susceptible children may be exposed to FA. FA is also widely

TABLE 3.4
Products That Contain Formaldehyde

Brand	Category	Form	Percent
Aleenes School Glue	Arts and crafts	Liquid	<0.0030
Elmers Probond Exterior Wood Glue—09/14/2001—Old Product	Arts and crafts	Gel	<0.1
Eagle One Wax-As-U-Dry	Auto products	Pump spray	
Red Devil Speed Demon Acrylic Caulk, White	Home maintenance	Paste	
Red Devil Onetime Lightweight Spackling—02/18/2010	Home maintenance	Paste	
DAP Alex Fast Dry Acrylic Latex Caulk Plus Silicone	Home maintenance	Paste	
DAP Alex Plus Easy Caulk, White—04/27/2009	Home maintenance	Paste	
DAP AlexUltra 230 Premium Indoor and Outdoor Sealant, Clear with Microban Antimicrobial Product Prot	Home maintenance	Paste	0–0.1
DAP Alex Plus Acrylic Latex Caulk Plus Silicone, All Colors	Home maintenance	Paste	<0.02
DAP Dynaflex 230 Premium Indoor and Outdoor Sealant, All Colors—03/13/2009	Home maintenance	Paste	<0.02
DAP EnergySaver High Performance Air Leak and Gap Sealant—12/18/2009	Home maintenance	Paste	<0.02
DAP Kwik Seal Plus Easy Caulk High Gloss with Microban, All Colors	Home maintenance	Paste	<0.09
DAP Kwik Seal Plus Premium Kitchen and Bath Adhesive Caulk with Microban	Home maintenance	Paste	<0.08
DAP Kwik Seal Tub and Tile Adhesive Caulk, All Colors—05/23/2008	Home maintenance	Paste	<0.02
Phenoseal Laminate Repair Filler	Home maintenance	Paste	<0.02
Flood CWF Hardwoods, Clear Wood Finish for Hardwoods, Natural Tone	Home maintenance	Liquid	<0.1
Franklin Laminate Flooring Glue	Home maintenance	Paste	>0.01
Knauf Basement Wall Insulation	Home maintenance	Fiber	<0.1
Knauf Friendly Feel Duct Wrap, Unfaced and Faced	Home maintenance	Fiber	<0.1
Knauf FSK-Faced Residential Insulation	Home maintenance	Fiber	<0.1
Knauf Kraft-Faced Residential Insulation	Home maintenance	Fiber	<0.1
Knauf Wall Insulation	Home maintenance	Fiber	<0.1
Glidden Prime Coat Interior 100% Acrylic Multipurpose Stainkiller Primer Sealer, No. PC1000	Home maintenance	Liquid	<0.1
Red Devil Quickpaint Caulk Cartridge, White	Home maintenance	Paste	
Red Devil Wallpaper Seam Repair, Clear	Home maintenance	Paste	
Red Devil Onetime Lighten Up Lightweight Spackling	Home maintenance	Paste	
DAP Alex Plus Acrylic Latex Caulk Plus Silicone, Clear	Home maintenance	Paste	<0.06
DAP Alex Plus Easy Caulk, All Colors	Home maintenance	Paste	<0.009
DAP AlexUltra 230 Premium Indoor and Outdoor Sealant, All Colors with Microban Antimicrobial Product	Home maintenance	Paste	<0.02
DAP Dynaflex 230 Premium Indoor and Outdoor Sealant, Clear	Home maintenance	Paste	<0.06
DAP Elastopatch Smooth Flexible Patching Compound, Ready-to-Use	Home maintenance	Paste	<0.0001
DAP Fast N Final Lightweight Spackling, Ready-to-Use—03/17/2009	Home maintenance	Paste	<0.004
DAP Kwik Seal Plus Easy Caulk High Gloss with Microban, Clear	Home maintenance	Paste	0.1–1
DAP Kwik Seal Tub and Tile Adhesive Caulk, Clear	Home maintenance	Paste	<0.06
DAP Patch Stick Nail Hole and Crack Filler, Ready-to-Use—01/31/2006	Home maintenance	Paste	<0.004
DAP FRP Adhesive	Home maintenance	Paste	<0.02
Flood CWF Hardwoods, Clear Wood Finish for Hardwoods, Cedar Tone	Home maintenance	Liquid	<0.1

(Continued)

TABLE 3.4 (*Continued*)
Products That Contain Formaldehyde

Brand	Category	Form	Percent
Titebond II Premium Wood Glue	Home maintenance	Liquid	>0.01
Knauf Duct Liner EM	Home maintenance	Fiber	<0.1
Knauf Foil-Faced Residential Insulation	Home maintenance	Fiber	<0.1
Knauf Insulation Board	Home maintenance	Bard	<0.1
Knauf Sill Sealer	Home maintenance	Fiber	<0.1
Glidden Prime Coat Exteriors Multipurpose Latex Stainkiller Primer Sealer, No. PC3000	Home maintenance	Liquid	<0.01
DAP Latex Window Glazing Paste	Home maintenance	Paste	
Murphy Oil Soap Multi-Use Wood Cleaner with Orange Oil, Pump Spray—04/16/2012	Inside the home	Pump spray	
Elmers Probond Exterior Wood Glue—Old Product	Inside the home	Gel	<0.1
Fab 2X Spring Magic Liquid Detergent	Inside the home	Liquid	
Dynamo 2X Ultra Concentrated Laundry Detergent, Sunrise Fresh	Inside the home	Liquid	
Dynamo 2X Ultra Concentrated Laundry Detergent, Waterfall	Inside the home	Liquid	
Ajax 2X Ultra Liquid Detergent with Bleach Alternative	Inside the home	Liquid	
Quikrete Concrete Bonding Adhesive	Landscape/yard	Liquid	<0.1
Flood CWF-UV Clear Wood Finish, Gold Tone	Landscape/yard	Liquid	<0.1
Flood CWF UV5 Clear Wood Finish, Cedar	Landscape/yard	Liquid	<0.1
Quikrete Concrete Repair	Landscape/yard	Paste	<0.1
Flood CWF UV5 Clear Wood Finish, Natural	Landscape/yard	Liquid	<0.1
Tetra Pond Barley and Peat Extract	Landscape/yard	Liquid	<2.5
Global Keratin Hair Taming System with Juvexin, Light Wave	Personal care	Liquid	<0.2
Softsoap Body Wash, Pure Cashmere	Personal care	Liquid	
Softsoap Shea Butter Liquid Hand Soap	Personal care	Liquid	
Palmolive Aromatherapy Liquid Hand Soap	Personal care	Liquid	
Irish Spring Body Wash, Icy Blast	Personal care	Liquid	
Rejuvenol Chocolate Brazilian Keratin Treatment	Personal care	Liquid	1.0–2.0
Softsoap Liquid Hand Soap, Coconut and Warm Ginger	Personal care	Liquid	
Gerber Baby Wash With Lavender—15 Fl. Oz.	Personal care	Liquid	<0.01
Softsoap Body Wash, Ultra Rich Shea Butter	Personal care	Liquid	
Softsoap Advanced Moisture Cashmere Liquid Hand Soap	Personal care	Liquid	
Irish Spring Body Wash, Aloe	Personal care	Liquid	
Natures Miracle Ultra-Cleanse Gentle Dog Shampoo	Pet care	Liquid	
Hagen Tearless Shampoo for Cats	Pet care	Liquid	
Zodiac Organique 3 In 1 Beautifying Spray for Dogs	Pet care	Pump spray	0.1
Zodiac Organique Foam Shampoo for Cats	Pet care	Liquid	0.1
Tetra Aquarium AquaSafe for Goldfish	Pet care	Liquid	<2.5
Tetra Aquarium Plant FloraPride—08/17/2007	Pet care	Liquid	<2.5
Tetra Pond FloraFin	Pet care	Liquid	<2.5
Tetra Pond Fish Treatment	Pet care	Liquid	10.0–25.0
Hagen Flea and Tick Shampoo for Cats	Pet care	Liquid	
Tetra Plant Flora Pride Iron Intensive Fertilizer	Pet care	Liquid	<0.5
Zodiac Organique Foam Shampoo for Dogs	Pet care	Liquid	0.1
Tetra Aquarium Betta Safe	Pet care	Liquid	<2.5
Tetra Aquarium Aqua EasyBalance with Nitraban	Pet care	Liquid	<2.5
Tetra Aquarium Blackwater Extract	Pet care	Liquid	<2.5

used in industrial and medical settings and as a sterilizing agent, disinfectant, and preservative. Therefore, employees may be highly exposed to it in their settings. Of particular concern to the authors are anatomists and medical students, who can be highly exposed to FA vapor during dissection sessions. FA is toxic over a range of doses; chances of exposure and subsequent harmful effects are increased as (room) temperature increases, because of FA's volatility. Several studies have been conducted to evaluate the effects of FA during systemic and respiratory exposures in rats. This review compiles that literature and emphasizes the neurotoxic effects of FA on neuronal morphology, behavior, and biochemical parameters. The review includes the results of some of the authors' work related to FA neurotoxicity, and such neurotoxic effects from FA exposure were experimentally demonstrated. Moreover, the effectiveness of some of the antioxidants such as melatonin, fish omega-3, and CAPE was observed in the treatment of the harmful effects of FA. Despite the harmful effects from FA exposure, it is commonly used in the United States, Turkey, and elsewhere in dissection laboratories. Consequently, all anatomists must know and understand the effects of this toxic agent on organisms and the environment, and take precautions to avoid unnecessary exposure. The reviewed studies have indicated that FA has neurotoxic characteristics and systemic toxic effects. It is hypothesized that inhalation of FA, during the early postnatal period, is linked to some neurological diseases that occur in adults. Although complete prevention is impossible for laboratory workers and members of industries utilizing FA, certain precautions can be taken to decrease and/or prevent the toxic effects of FA.

Particulates: Suspended particulates in the indoor environment are a function of infiltration from the outdoor air and occupant activities such as cooking, vacuuming, and smoking. Yocom et al.[60] examined indoor and outdoor particulate levels for several different types of buildings in Hartford, Connecticut. Overall, their data showed indoor-to-outdoor ratios generally less than 1 for public buildings, office buildings, and single-family homes, assuming there were negligible sources from indoors. Daytime levels of particulates, both indoors and outdoors, were higher than nighttime levels because of the higher levels of human activity during the day. Also, for each of the different types of buildings, the winter indoor/outdoor particulate ratios were lower than during the other seasons, presumably due to reduced outdoor air ventilation. The chemically sensitive do better with lower particulate levels. Thus, it is advocated that cessation of activities that elevate this count. There are alternate methods of cleaning, such as water vacuuming. Elimination of carpets, use of protective hoods over stoves, and absolutely no indoor tobacco smoking are recommended.

The difficulty in assessing the influence of outdoor particulate levels on indoor particulate levels is due to the simultaneous presence of particulates from both sources. Andersen[8] reviewed previous studies on indoor/outdoor particulate monitoring, which showed indoor/outdoor ratios of about 0.4 for 1-hour averaging periods of suspended particulates. However, in studies with 24-hour samplings, the indoor/outdoor ratios ranged from 0.80 to 0.95. For his own research, he collected 150 paired samples of suspended PM simultaneously over 24-hour periods at distances of 1 m inside and 1 m outside a 135 m^3 room in the Technical School of Arrhus. All the windows and doors were closed, and only a minimal amount of human activity occurred each day. The indoor/outdoor ratios were less than 1 in almost 90% of the paired samples, and on average, the ratio was 0.69. Our measurements of particulates in the indoor air of our ECU are five times less than in uncontrolled indoor environments such as hospital rooms and corridors or private homes. Also, the quality of particulates in these areas is entirely different. These differences may be accounted for by our interior use of charcoal filters, natural paper, and ceramic fibers, in contrast to particulates generated for interior furnishings or building materials and exterior pollutants, such as synthetic materials or hydrocarbons from fuel and car exhaust.

Thompson et al.[18] measured suspended PM in several different types of buildings. Several compounds that are known to exacerbate chemical sensitivity were identified using GCV/mass spectrometry (MS).

A field survey of indoor respirable suspended particulates in the presence of smokers was recently performed.[61] Samples were obtained from inside and outside public areas with various ratios of smokers to nonsmokers. The ratios of indoor to outdoor respirable suspended-particulate levels ranged from 1.6 to 11.6 in the smoking sections of various indoor environments. The ratio of indoor to outdoor respirable particulates depends on factors such as smoker density, ventilation rates, and the amount of mixing of the indoor air. Our studies in the ECU have shown particulate levels to decrease over five times the levels found in areas of the hospital where cigarette smoke and synthetic pollutants were present. These lower levels markedly decrease symptoms of chemical sensitivity due to a decrease in total body load.

Cigarette and cigar smoking are usually considered a health hazard only to the smoker, but non-smokers's irritative and allergic responses to the smoke of both indicate that they can be adversely affected by the smoking of others. The products of cigarette smoke include a wide range of gaseous and particulate contaminants that exacerbate the chemically sensitive.

Smoke can be a significant source of air pollution in the indoor environment. In 1978, 53 million U.S. smokers consumed 615 billion cigarettes. Horn[62] estimated the average smoking rate to be two cigarettes per hour. For a chain smoker, as many as five cigarettes can be smoked within 1 hour. The chemically sensitive are grossly intolerant of smoke, which triggers a myriad of symptoms and usually stops them from working efficiently. Because of both particulate and gas emissions, smoke in the work environment often prevents the chemically sensitive from being able to perform adequately.

Heogg[63] found the emissions from burning cigarettes in a closed experimental chamber. He defined the smoke from the glowing end of the cigarette, as sidestream smoke, and the smoke leaving the mouthpiece of the cigarette as mainstream smoke. (S/M ratio—for various contaminants of cigarette combustion).

Heogg[63] found several toxic compounds, such as benzo(a)pyrene, have S/M ratios much greater than 1. Also, overall, sidestream smoke has quantitatively more contaminants than mainstream smoke. For carbon monoxide, the S/M ratio was 4.7. In measuring particulate size ranges, sidestream smoke never exceeded 2 μ at any time, and Hoegg theorized that mainstream particulates are also less than 2 μ in size. This study showed that smoking is a significant source of particulate and gaseous contaminants. From these contaminants, tar and nicotine are usually selected to characterize the relative toxicity of cigarette smoke. Tar is the amount of particulates produced corrected for water vapor. Nicotine, an alkaloid, is the largest fraction of the particulates produced. These high levels reported by Hoegg[63] emphasize that there is a marked increase of indoor contamination with cigarette smoking. All of these substances are known to exacerbate chemical sensitivity. Clearly, no cigarette smoking should be allowed in the homes or work areas of the chemically sensitive because even minute exposure has been observed to exacerbate symptoms.

Thompson et al.[18] measured suspended PM in several different types of buildings. The results of the indoor/outdoor particulate measurements in all the buildings were ratios less than 1, except for an elementary school that had no air ventilation system. The low ratios in other public and private buildings were attributed to air-conditioning with fiberglass filters and the use of particulate filters in the community hospital. The high ratio in the school was possibly caused by soil particles brought in on people's shoes. The presence of soil particles in indoor air is especially prevalent in the dry climates of the Southwest, and, although they can of themselves pose a threat to the chemically sensitive, this threat can be heightened if the soil particles contain pesticide or fuel particles.

Studies of indoor/outdoor ratios of suspended PM, reported by Yocom et al.,[60] are consistent with Thompson's findings. In 18 sets of paired indoor and outdoor data with 12-hour sampling periods, all sets except one showed indoor levels to be lower than outdoor levels. These studies were performed in several different types of buildings that were occupied by people. For organic PM, higher ratios on indoor/outdoor levels versus total suspended particulates were found. This higher ratio for organic particulates indicates the presence of indoor sources such as smoking and cooking, both of which produce odors that exacerbate chemical sensitivity. Indoor grilling and barbecuing, especially, produce excessive smoke that exacerbates the chemically sensitive.

Alsona et al.[64] reported on the characterization of particles in the indoor environment. They sought to determine the source and composition of particles in several rooms in different types of buildings. Measurements were carried out for the metals cadmium, iron, zinc, lead, and bromine with x-ray fluorescence. Measurements were frequently carried out on blank filters to obtain controls for their impurity content. They frequently contained iron, chromium, and copper, and occasionally manganese and zinc. The average indoor/outdoor ratios for the several different types of rooms were as follows: cadmium, 0.10; iron, 0.24; zinc, 0.41; lead, 0.42; and bromine, 0.36. By conducting several measurements on one room under six different conditions (i.e., plastic over windows, windows wide open, all surfaces covered with plastic, etc.), the authors were able to model the conditions influencing indoor particulate levels. They concluded that of the factors influencing dust concentrations in the indoor environment, the rate of deposition, and absorption on room surfaces is, to a point, more important than the leak rate constant and the resuspension of particulates, which only becomes important when the air is highly filtered before it enters the room. Again, the type of particulate is important to the chemically sensitive, since they might react to hydrocarbon-laden particulates, but not to cotton ones.

Several nanoparticles are found in indoor air. These are particulates of less than 200 nm. Their contents include silver, nickel, aluminum, chrome, cobalt, titanium, etc. These have been found to disturb neurologic, cardiovascular, respiratory, and other human body functions. They can be as devastating as the larger toxic particulates.

Lioy et al.[65] studies the indoor–outdoor relationships for organic PM. Overall, indoor levels were higher than outdoor levels, with mean indoor–outdoor concentration ratios for the three fractions as follows: dichloromethane, 1.6; cyclohexane, 1.29; and acetone, 0.92. All of these substances at these levels have been observed to exacerbate chemical sensitivity and show why indoor air must be decontaminated.

The new pollutant that will be found in the air is marijuana since it is being legalized in several states. The fumes from cannabis will become a problem for the United States and pulmonary individuals.

CLINICAL ASPECTS OF ORGANOPHOSPHATE-INDUCED DELAYED POLYNEUROPATHY

Organophosphate-induced delayed polyneuropathy (OPIDP) is a rare toxicity resulting from exposure to certain OP esters. It is characterized by distal degeneration of some axons of both the peripheral and central nervous systems (CNSs) occurring 1–4 weeks after single or short-term exposures. Cramping muscle pain in the lower limbs, distal numbness, and paresthesia occur, followed by progressive weakness, depression of deep tendon reflexes in the lower limbs and, in severe cases, in the upper limbs. Signs include high-stepping gait associated with bilateral foot drop and, in severe cases, quadriplegia with foot and wrist drop as well as pyramidal signs. In time, there might be significant recovery of the peripheral nerve function but, depending on the degree of pyramidal involvement, spastic ataxia may be a permanent outcome of severe OPIDP. Human and experimental data indicate that recovery is usually complete in the young. At onset, the electrophysiological changes include reduced amplitude of the compound muscle potential, increased distal latencies and normal or slightly reduced nerve conduction velocities. The progression of the disease, usually over a few days, may lead to nonexcitability of the nerve with electromyographical signs of denervation. Nerve biopsies have been performed in a few cases and showed axonal degeneration with secondary demyelination. Neuropathy target esterase (NTE) is thought to be the target of OPIDP initiation. The ratio of inhibitory powers for acetylcholinesterase and NTE represents the crucial guideline for the etiological attribution of OP-induced peripheral neuropathy. In fact, premarketing toxicity testing in animals selects OP insecticides with cholinergic toxicity potential much higher than that to result in OPIDP. Therefore, OPIDP may develop only after very large exposures to insecticides, causing severe cholinergic toxicity. However, this was not the case with certain triaryl phosphates (TAPs) that were not used as insecticides but as hydraulic fluids, lubricants, and plasticizers and do not result in cholinergic toxicity. Several thousand cases of OPIDP as a result of exposure to tri-ortho-cresyl phosphate have been reported, whereas the number of cases of OPIDP as a result of OP insecticide poisoning is much lower. In this article "Organophosphate-induced delayed polyneuropathy", they mainly discuss OP pesticide poisoning, particularly when caused by CPF, dichlorvos, isofenphos, methamidophos, mipafox, trichlorfon, trichlornat, phosphamidon/mevinphos, and by certain carbamates. They also discuss case reports where neuropathies were not convincingly attributed to fenthion, malathion, omethoate/dimethoate, parathion, and merphos. Finally, several observational studies on long-term, low-level exposures to OPs that sometimes reported mild, inconsistent, and unexplained changes of unclear significance in peripheral nerves are briefly discussed.

ACUTE AND DELAYED NEUROPATHY ON AIRPLANES THE AEROTOXIC SYNDROME

Paraoxon (PO); *p*-nitrophenyl valerate (PNV); phenyl valerate (PV); recombinant catalytic NTE esterase domain (rNEST); red blood cells (RBCs); rat liver microsomes (RLMs); triaryl phosphate (TAP); *tert*-butylphenyl phosphate (TBP); tri-cresyl phosphate (TCP); tri-(*p-tert*-butylphenyl) phosphate (TmBP); tri-ortho-cresyl phosphate (ToCP), 548-(*o*-cresyl) phosphate; and tri-(*p*-cresyl) phosphate (TpCP).

Since a new entity of indoor air pollution has occurred with toxic cabin air of airplanes, the aero toxic syndrome has occurred. It is probably another entity that mimics or is part of the chemical sensitivity syndrome.

HAZARDS IN JET CRAFT

Air quality is an important aviation problem. Problems arise from a number of factors, including

> *The problem of hypoxia*: Commercial flight levels typically range from 31,000 to 42,000 ft above sea level and the aircraft cabin is pressurized to an hypobaric environment equivalent to 8000 ft (2315 m). Hypoxia may interact adversely with chemical exposures.[66]
>
> *The problem of ventilation*: Studies indicate[67] that it is common that all modes of transport have ventilation rates less than current ASHRAE 62 guidelines for commercial buildings.[68] This finding, of itself, does not imply poor air quality. However, it suggests that initiatives to reduce air quality should be resisted.
>
> This indicates that opportunities to improve air quality should be encouraged. For example, a Canadian study of one aircraft type and airline found that 245 of 333 commercial flights did not satisfy the ASHRAE air ventilation criteria of 15 ft³/occupant, and that 18 of 33 flights had less than 10 ft³/occupant.[69]
>
> *The problem of contamination of air*: Chemical exposures in aircraft are not unheard of. The U.S. Aerospace Medical Association first expressed their concerns about the toxicity risks of cabin air contamination by hydraulics and lubricants.[70] The oils and hydraulics used in aircraft engines can be toxic, and specific ingredients of oils can be irritating, sensitizing (such as phenyl-alpha-naphthylamine; PAN) or neurotoxic (e.g., ortho-containing TAPs such as ToCP). If oil or hydraulic fluid leaks occur, this contamination may be in the form of unchanged material, degraded material from long use, combusted or pyrolized materials. These materials can contaminate aircraft cabin air in the form of gases, vapors, mists, and aerosols. Other risks have been identified more recently, either as part of the chemicals routinely used in maintaining airplanes,[71] or as products of the passengers or cargo.[67]
>
> *Problems of combustion and emergency situations*[72]: Passenger protective breathing equipment tests conducted by the U.K. Air Accidents Investigation Branch (AAIB) identify contaminants in combustion situations such as carbon monoxide, hydrogen cyanide, hydrogen fluoride, hydrogen chloride, nitrogen oxides, sulfur dioxide, ammonia, acrolein, and other hydrocarbon compounds.[73]

Notwithstanding normal operational activities or emergency situations, a range of other situations can arise whereby aircraft cabin air can be contaminated.[74] These include

1. Uptake of exhaust from other aircraft or on ground contamination sources
2. Application of deicing fluids
3. Hydraulic fluid leaks from a landing gear and other hydraulic systems
4. Excessive use of lubricants and preservative compounds in the cargo hold
5. Preservatives on the inside of aircraft skin
6. Large accumulations of dirt and brake dust may build up on inlet ducts, where auxiliary power units extract air from near the aircraft belly
7. Intake of oil and hydraulic fluid at sealing interfaces, around oil cooling fan gaskets, and in worn transitions
8. Oil contamination from synthetic turbine
9. Engine combustion products (e.g., defective fuel manifolds, seal failures, engine leaks)
10. Other air quality problems include ethanol and acetone, indicators of bioeffluents, and chemicals from consumer products.[75] One additional problem is the lower partial pressure of oxygen that is present in the cabins of planes flying at altitude.[66]

TRICRESYL PHOSPHATE

According to Winder,[76] TCP (CAS No. 1330-78-5) is also known as phosphoric acid, tris (methylphenyl) ester or tritolyl phosphate. TCP is a blend of 10 TCP isomer molecules, plus other structurally similar compounds, including phenolic and xylenolic compounds. TCP is a molecule comprising three cresyl (methylphenyl) groups linked to a phosphate group. The location of the methyl group in the cresyl group is critical for the expression of neurotoxicity, with ortho-, meta-, or para- prefixes that denote how far apart the hydroxyl and methyl groups are on the cresol molecule. Technically, there are 27 (3^3) different combinations of meta-, ortho-, and para-cresyl groups in TCP (Figure 3.3). Since the apparently different three-dimensional structures of the molecule are not chemically locked in place, they are not optical isomers. Therefore, structures with similar numbers of cresyl groups (such as ppm, pmp, and mpp) are considered the same molecules. This gets the apparent 27 structures down to the real 10 isomers conventionally described (Figure 3.6).

TCP is a compound with a toxicity typical of the OP compounds. Human toxicity to OP compounds has been known since at least 1899, when neurotoxicity to phosphocreosole (then used in the treatment of tuberculosis) was reported.[77] The study of OP toxicity is extensive, and is generally characterized by a toxicity of inhibition of the esterase enzymes, most particularly, cholinesterases[78] and neurotoxic esterases.[79] The mechanism of effect is phosphorylation.[80]

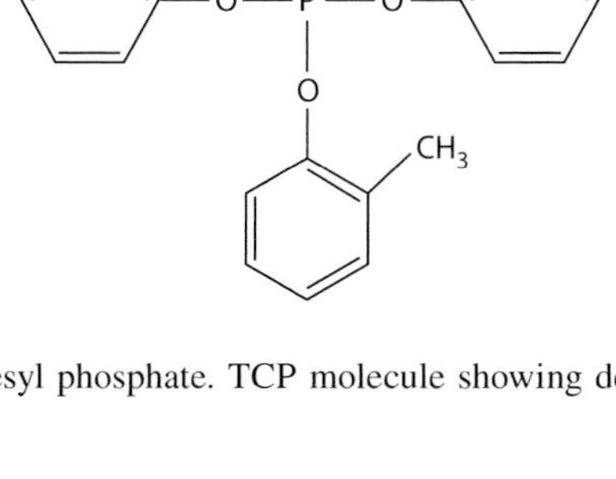

FIGURE 3.6   Structure of tricresyl phosphate. TCP molecule showing designation of *o*-, *m*-, and *p*-cresyl groups.

Signs of low-level intoxication include headache, vertigo, general weakness, drowsiness, lethargy, difficulty in concentration, slurred speech, confusion, emotional lability, and hypothermia.[81] The reversibility of such effects has been questioned.[82]

Signs of poisoning are usually foreshadowed by the development of early symptoms related to acetylcholine overflow and include salivation, lacrimation, conjunctivitis, visual impairment, nausea and vomiting, abdominal pains and cramps, diarrhea, parasympathomimetic effects on heart and circulation, fasciculations, and muscle twitches.[83] This is the basic site of inhibition for all OP molecules.[84,85]

A second reaction with certain OPs (including TCP) leads to further neurotoxic and neuropathological changes. This is inhibition of neurotoxic esterases which produces a progressive distal symmetrical sensorimotor mixed peripheral neuropathy, called organophosphorus-induced delayed neurotoxicity (OPIDN).[85,86] The mechanism of toxicity is now fairly well understood, as indeed are the OP structures which are predicted to cause OPIDN.[87]

OPIDN has a severe pathology. It is quite likely that such a severe condition would be presaged with a range of clinical and preclinical signs and symptoms. These have been reported extensively, and an "intermediate syndrome" was defined in 1987.[88]

More recently, chronic exposure to organophosphates has been associated with a range of neurological and neuropsychological effects.[89–93] Such symptoms (mainly neurological and neurobehavioral symptoms) may also be seen in exposed individuals who have been sufficiently fortunate in not having exposures that were excessive enough in intensity or duration to lead to clinical disease.

A distinct condition—chronic organophosphate neuropsychological disorder (COPIND)—has been described, of neurological and neuropsychological symptoms.[94] These include

1. Diffuse neuropsychological symptoms (headaches, mental fatigue, depression, anxiety, irritability)
2. Reduced concentration and impaired vigilance
3. Reduced information processing and psychomotor speed
4. Memory deficit and linguistic disturbances

COPIND may be seen in exposed individuals either following single or short-term exposures leading to signs of toxicity,[90] or long-term low-level repeated exposure with (often) no apparent signs of exposure.[92] The basic mechanism of effect is not known, although it is not believed to be related to the esterase inhibition properties of organophosphorus compounds. It is also not known if these symptoms are permanent.

In addition, since the introduction and extensive use of synthetic OP compounds in agriculture and industry half a century ago, several studies have reported long-term, persistent, chronic neurotoxicity symptoms in individuals as a result of acute exposure to high doses that cause acute cholinergic toxicity, or from long-term, low-level, subclinical doses of these chemicals.[95–97] The neuronal disorder that results from organophosphorus ester-induced chronic neurotoxicity (OPICN), which leads to long-term neurological and neurobehavioral deficits and has recently been linked to the effects being seen in aircrew despite OP exposures being too low to cause OPIDN.[98]

Furthermore, OPICN induced by low-level inhalation of organophosphates present in jet engine lubricating oils and the hydraulic fluids of aircraft could explain the long-term neurological deficits consistently reported by crewmembers and passengers, although organophosphate levels may have been too low to produce OPIDN.[99]

While the description above relates to the general toxicity of OPs, they are characteristic of exposure to TCP. The 10 isomers that make up TCP are toxicologically different, and it is well established that the ortho-containing isomers are the most toxic.[100–102] Of the 10 isomers of TCP, six contain at least one ortho-cresyl group; three mono-ortho (MOCP) isomers, two di-ortho (DOCP) isomers, and TOCP isomers. Other, similar ortho-containing chemicals, such as the xylenols and phenolics, are also present in commercial TCP formulations in small amounts. Manufacturers of

TABLE 3.5
Tricresyl Phosphate: Toxicity of Isomers

Isomer	Concentration (ppm)	Relative Toxicity	Equivalent Toxicity
TOCP	0.005	1	×1
DOCP	6	5	×30
MOCP	3070	10	×30,700
		Total	30,731

TCP have reduced the levels of ortho-cresyl and ortho-ethylphenyl isomers to reduce the potential for neurotoxicity of products containing TCP.[103] How much these refinements had removed the toxic impurities outlined above is not known. Indeed, toxicity was still being detected in commercially available products in 1988,[104] and questions have been raised about the lack of consistency between stated ingredient data and actual amounts of toxic isomers present in commercial formulations, and their impact on exposed individuals.[104]

In evidence to the Australian Senate Aviation Inquiry in 1999, Mobil USA noted that Mobil Jet Oil II contains less than 5 ppb (0.005 ppm) TOCP.[105] This is an impressively low amount, and suggests that the neurotoxic potential from a chemical containing such a low level would be vanishingly small.

According to Winder,[76] however, concentrations from other neurotoxic ingredients are not so readily available. In the Mobil USA evidence to the Australian Senate Aviation Inquiry, it became apparent that DOCPs were present in TCVP at a concentration of 6 ppm, and MOCPs were present at a concentration of 3070 ppm. As these ingredients are present in higher concentrations than TOCP, and have a significantly higher toxicity than TOCP, it is suggested that a statement of low TOCP content is misleading as it underestimates the toxicity of the OCP ingredients by a factor of 30,000 (Table 3.5).

TCP will also contain mixed esters of orthophosphoric acid with different cresyl radicals, of the be under mono- and di-cresyl types.[99] The important issue with this data is that the level of all ortho-cresyl phosphates should impact on the regulatory classification of materials containing TCP.

Occupational exposure standards must also not be applied to nonworkers, for example, passengers.

COMBUSTION AND PYROLYSIS PROCESSES

Further, an oil leak from an engine at high pressure and temperature may burn or pyrolize before it enters the cabin. This produces carbon-containing materials which, in the presence of energy and oxygen, produce the two oxides of carbon: carbon dioxide (CO_2) and carbon monoxide (CO). The first of these (CO_2) is produced in the presence of an abundance of oxygen, and the second CO is produced where stoichiometric concentrations of oxygen are lacking (usually in conditions of incomplete combustion). Both of these oxides are gases, one (carbon monoxide) is quite toxic at low concentrations causing toxic asphyxiation. Single or short-term exposure to CO is insufficient to cause asphyxiation but produces headache, dizziness, and nausea; long-term exposure can cause memory defects and CNS damage, among other effects.[106]

Several combustion and pyrolysis products are toxic. The toxic asphyxiants, such as carbon monoxide, have already been introduced above. Some thermal degradation products, such as acrolein and FA, are highly irritating. Others, such as oxides of nitrogen and phosgene, can produce delayed effects. Still others, such as PM (e.g., soot), can carry adsorbed gases deep into the respiratory tract where they may provoke a local reaction or be absorbed to produce systemic effects.

A leak of such an oil from an engine operating at altitude would see most of the oil pyrolize once it leaves the confined conditions of temperature and pressure operating in the engine. While it seems reasonable that any ingredients with suitable autoignition or degradation properties that allow such a transformation after release from the engine could be radically transformed, it is possible to speculate in only general terms about the cocktail of chemicals that could form. Presumably, it would include carbon dioxide, carbon monoxide, partially burned hydrocarbons (including irritating and toxic by-products, such as acrolein and other aldehydes and TCP (which is stable at high temperatures). These contaminants will be in gas, vapor, mist, and particulate forms. These contaminants could not be classified as being of low toxicity. The possible problems that might arise from exposure to such a cocktail cannot be dismissed without proper consideration.

CHEMICAL PRODUCTS USED IN AVIATION

According to Winder,[76] the aviation industry has used fuels, lubricants, hydraulic fluids, and other materials that can contain a range of toxic ingredients. Aircraft materials such as jet fuel, deicing fluids, engine oil, hydraulic fluids, and so on, contain a range of ingredients some of which are toxic.[107–110] Significant contaminants include aldehydes; aromatic hydrocarbons; aliphatic hydrocarbons; chlorinated, fluorinated, methylated, phosphate or nitrogen compounds; esters; and oxides (Tables 3.6 and 3.7).[104]

A range of aviation chemicals is shown in Table 3.8.

Inhalation is an important route of exposure, with exposure to uncovered skin being a second, less significant route (e.g., following exposure to oil mists or vapors). Ingestion is unlikely.

TABLE 3.6
Jet A Fuel Constitution

Constituent Composition		% Volume
Simple alkanes		53.7
Includes:		
Decane	16.5	
Undecane	36	
Methyl alkanes		3.77
Cycloalkanes		0.79
Monocyclic aromatic hydrocarbons		31.8
Includes:		
Benzene	0.02	
Butylbenzene	2	
1,2-Diethylbenzene	0.24	
1,2-Diethyl-3-propylbenzene	5.4	
1,4-Diethyl-2-ethylbenzene	0.2	
Ethylbenzene	0.02	
1-Methyl-4-propylbenzene	3.3	
Propylbenzene	3–5	
1,2,4,5-Tetramethylbenzene	9	
Toluene	Trace	
1,2,3-Trimethylbenzene	6.6	
Xylenes	0.07	
Polycyclic aromatic hydrocarbons		0.63
Includes:		
Naphthalene	0.14	
2-Methylnaphthalene	0.34	
1,3-Dimethylnaphthalene	0.15	

Source: Winder, C., J. C. Balouet. 2006. *Journal of Occupational Health and Safety – Australia and New Zealand* 17: 471–483.

TABLE 3.7
Jet A Fuel Constitution

Component	% Present
Saturated hydrocarbons (paraffins and cycloparaffins)	70%–80%
Aromatic hydrocarbons	17%–20%
Unsaturated hydrocarbons (olefins)	3%–6%

Source: Product Material Safety Data Sheet.

According to Winder,[76] a number of recently published studies reported acute or persisting biological or health effects such as human liver dysfunction, emotional dysfunction, abnormal electroencephalograms, shortened attention spans, decreased sensorimotor speed, and immune system dysfunction from single, short-term repeated exposure, or long-term repeated exposure of humans or animals to kerosene-based hydrocarbon fuels, to constituent chemicals of these fuels, or to fuel combustion products.[110–118] Other reports suggest that other aviation chemicals may be toxic.[104,119,120]

Occasionally, such exposures may be of a magnitude to induce symptoms of toxicity. In terms of toxicity, a growing number of aircrew are developing symptoms following both short-term and long-term repeated exposures.

The engine oils that are used in jet engines are precision oils that need to operate in extreme conditions. Some commercial jet oils have been in use as engine oils in aviation for decades. For example, Mobil USA note that Mobil Jet Oil II (a jet oil with close to half the market share) "has been essentially unchanged since its development in the early 1960s" and "most changes have involved slight revisions of the ester base stock due to changes in raw material availablility."[121]

Therefore, jet oils are specialized synthetic oils used in high-performance jet engines. They have an appreciable hazard based on toxic ingredients, but are safe in use by engineering personnel who handle the product routinely.

Aircraft engines that leak oil may expose others to the oils through uncontrolled exposure. Airplanes that use engines as a source of bleed air for cabin pressurization may have this source contaminated by the oil, if an engine leaks.

Using a typical commercial Jet Oil (Mobil, Jet Oil II), various sources such as the supplier's label on the cardboard box the cans are shipped in, the product Material Safety Data Bulletin (MSDB), and information from the manufacturer, list the following ingredients[104]:

1. Synthetic esters based in a mixture of 95% C_5–C_{10} fatty acid esters of pentaerythritol and dipentaerythritol;
2. 1% of a substituted diphenylamine;
3. 3% TCP (phosphoric acid, tris-methylphenyl) ester (CAS No. 1330-78-5);
4. 1% PAN (1-napthylamine, *N*-phenyl, CAS No. 90-30-2);
5. A last entry "ingredients partially unknown" is also noted on some documentation.

Of these ingredients, the most toxicologically significant components are the substituted diphenylamine, PAN, and TCP.

SUBSTITUTED DIPHENYLAMINE

According to Winder,[76] the substituted diphenylamine is variously reported as benzamine, 4-octyl-*N*-(4-octylphenyl) (CAS No. 101-67-7) or 0.1%–1% *N*-phenyl-benzeneamine, reaction product with 2,4,4-trimethylpentene (CAS No. 68411-46-1), and used as an antioxidant, in concentrations not greater than 1% (Figures 3.7 and 3.8).

TABLE 3.8
Aviation Chemicals

Product	Type	Ingredients	Formula
		Jet Fuels	
	Jet A and Jet A-1	A kerosene-based fuel, based on ASTM specification D1655	Varies, depending on manufacturer
	Jet B	A wide-cut blend of gasoline and kerosene, rarely used except in very cold conditions	Varies, depending on manufacturer
	Aviation gasoline		Varies, depending on manufacturer
		Aviation Fuel Additives	
	Antiknock additives	Tetraethyl lead (TEL)	
		Ethylene dibromide	
	Antioxidants	2,6-Di-tertiary-butyl-4-methyl phenol	
	Electrical conductivity/static dissipater additives	Stadis® 450	Proprietary mixture
	Corrosion inhibitor/lubricity improver	"DCI-4a"	Proprietary mixture
	Anti-icing additives	Diethylene glycol monomethylether	
	Metal deactivators	N,N'-disalicylidene-1,2-propane diamine	
	Biocides		
	Thermal stability improver additives	(Mainly military applications)—"+100"	Proprietary mixture
	Leak detection	Tracer A®	Proprietary mixture
		Lubricants, Based On	
	Mineral types		Proprietary mixtures
	Synthetic types		Proprietary mixtures
		Greases	
Speciality chemicals			
	Antiseize compounds		Proprietary mixtures
	Coolants		Proprietary mixtures
	Corrosion preventatives		Proprietary mixtures
	Damping fluids		Proprietary mixtures
	Deicing fluids		Proprietary mixtures
	Dry lubricants		Proprietary mixtures
	Instrument oils		Proprietary mixtures
	Lubricity agents		Proprietary mixtures
	Protectives		Proprietary mixtures
	Sealants, adhesives, epoxy resins		Proprietary mixtures
	Shock strut fluids		Proprietary mixtures
	Bonded parts		Proprietary mixtures

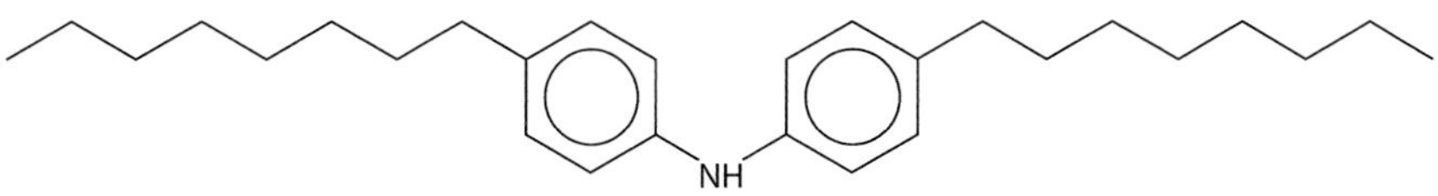

FIGURE 3.7 Benzamine, 4-octyl-*N*-(4-octylphenyl).

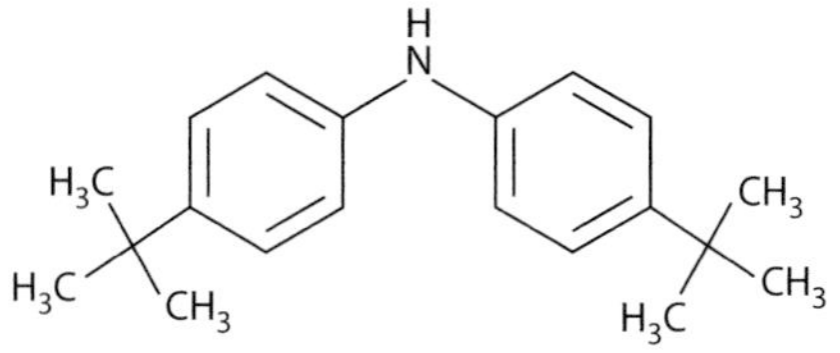

FIGURE 3.8 Substituted diphenylamines.

There is little toxicity data available for this ingredient, although it is not believed to be toxic by single exposure (no data on long-term exposure). The disclosure of this ingredient in hazard communication by identity probably relates to its environmental effects, such as poor biodegradability and toxicity to aquatic invertebrates.[122]

N-PHENYL-ALPHA-NAPHTHYLAMINE

According to Winder, *N*-phenyl-alpha-naphthylamine (CAS No. 90-30-2), also known as PAN, is a lipophilic solid used as an antioxidant in lubrication oils and as a protective agent in rubber products (Figure 3.2). In these products, the chemical acts as a radical scavenger in the auto-oxidation of polymers or lubricants. It is generally used in these products at a concentration of about 1% (its concentration in jet oils). The commercial product has a typical purity of about 99%. The impurities include *N*-phenyl-2-naphthylamine (CAS No. 135-88-6, 500 to below 5000 ppm), 1-naphthylamine (below 100–500 ppm), 2-naphthylamine (below 3–50 ppm), aniline (below 100–2500 ppm), 1-naphthol (below 5000 ppm), and 1,1-dinaphthylamine (below 1000 ppm) (Figure 3.9).

PAN is rapidly absorbed by mammalian systems and rapidly biotransformed.[123] Both urine and feces appear to be the main routes of excretion.[124]

By single dosing, PAN has a low toxicity, with LD_{50}s above 1 g/kg. The chemical has a similar mechanism of toxicity to several aromatic amines, of methemoglobin production. PAN is not irritating in primary skin and eye irritation studies. However, in a guinea pig maximization test, PAN was shown to be a strong skin sensitizer.[125] This result is supported by case studies in exposed workers.[126,127] At the concentration used (1%), Mobil Jet Oil II meets the cutoff criteria (1%) for classification as a hazardous substance in Australia for sensitization properties. Most genotoxicity studies report negative results, suggesting little genotoxicity potential.[124]

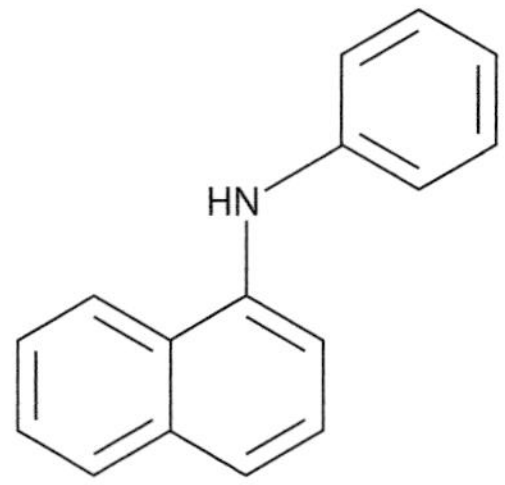

FIGURE 3.9 *N*-Phenyl-1-naphthylamine.

Most repeated dose toxicological studies focus on its potential carcinogenicity. An experimental study, using both PAN and the related compound, N-phenyl-2-naphthylamine, administered subcutaneously to mice found a heightened incidence of lung and kidney cancers.[128] The methodology used in this study makes evaluation of the results problematic (use of one gender, small sample sizes, limited number of dose groups, subcutaneous administration as an inappropriate route of exposure, and so on). A high incidence of various forms of cancer was also found among workers exposed to anti rust oil containing 0.5% PAN.[129] While these animal and human results offer only limited information, they are at least supportive of a mild carcinogenic effect.

According to Winder,[76] what emerges in the analysis of this information, is a pattern of symptoms related to local effects to exposure to an irritant, overlaid by the development of systemic symptoms in a number of human body systems, including nervous system, respiratory system, gastrointestinal system, and possibly immune system and cardiovascular system. These symptoms may be expressed specifically to systemic symptoms, or may be seen more generally, such as headache, behavioral change, or chronic fatigue.

The symptoms reported by exposed individuals as shown in Table 3.17 are sufficiently consistent to indicate the development of a discrete occupational health condition, and the term "aerotoxic syndrome" is introduced to describe it. The features of this syndrome are that it is associated with air crew exposure at altitude to atmospheric contaminants from engine oil or other aircraft fluids, temporarily juxtaposed by the development of a consistent symptomology, including short-term skin, gastrointestinal, respiratory, and nervous system effects, and long-term central nervous and immunological effects.

This syndrome may be reversible following brief exposures, but features have emerged of a chronic syndrome following significant exposures.[130–132]

More recent research has established a long-term syndrome of toxicological,[133,134] medical,[135,136] respiratory,[137] neuropsychological,[138] and psychological[139] effects.

On most jet turbine aircraft, unfiltered engine bleed air is fed into the cabin, providing oxygen and heat for those aboard.[140] Exposure of passengers and crew to some level of TAPs occurs in approximately 23% of monitored flights,[141,142] whereas higher levels of exposure can occur when engine seals wear or fail. Symptoms of aerotoxic syndrome resulting from such exposures can include extreme mental impairment,[143] an acute flight safety issue when crew exposure to contaminated air is significant. Material safety data sheets for synthetic jet lubricants list TAP contents of 1%–10%. Acute as well as long-term effects have been shown in the form of neurotoxicity resembling Parkinson's disease.

As stated previously, neurotoxicity of aromatic phosphate esters to humans was first reported in 1899 following the treatment of tuberculosis patients with phosphocreosote.[144] Studies in 1930 examining the cause of Ginger Jake paralysis, which affected 10,00–50,000 million individuals consuming extracts of ginger adulterated with TCP, identified ToCP as the paralytic agent.[145,146] Epidemic poisonings have since been associated with consumption of food adulterated with TCPs.[147–152] These problems are part of the organophosphate toxicity.

In the early 1950s, Aldridge reported that liver metabolism of ToCP was required to generate toxic metabolite(s).[78] In 1961, Casida et al.[153] reported the toxic metabolite of ToCP to be 2-(o-cresyl)-4H-1,3,2-benzodioxaphosphoran-2-one (CBDP or cyclic saligen cresyl phosphate), which has since been shown to be an inhibitor of several serine active-site esterases, including butyrylcholinesterase (BChE),[154] acetylcholinesterase (AChE),[155] carboxylesterase (CES),[156–158] and acyl peptide hydrolase (APH).[159] According to Baker et al., the in vitro role of microsomes in the metabolism of TAPs, including ToCP, was established by Sprague and Castles in 1985.[160] An analog of CBDP, phenyl saligenin phosphate,[161] is a potent inhibitor of NTE,[162] the inhibition and aging of which results in organophosphate (OP)-induced delayed neuropathy.[84] Toxic metabolites of other jet engine TAP additives, including those evaluated in Baker et al.'s study, have not yet been described in the literature.

The purpose of the present study was to develop an in vitro assay for assessing the inhibitory potential of TAPs using the biomarker esterase, BChE,[163] and to verify the in vitro results with in vivo exposures of mice. Mice were exposed by gavage to a commercial TCP mixed-isomer formulation,

Durad 125 (D125), and to two TAP found not to inhibit BChE with the *in vitro* bioactivation assay, tri-(*o-tert*-butylphenyl) phosphate (TpBP) and TpCP. The three compounds were compared for their ability to inhibit serine active-site enzymes from plasma, RBCs, liver, and brain. Finally, because the flavonoid compound naringenin has been shown to inhibit cytochromes P450,[164] they examined its effect on the bioactivation of D125.

Exposures of individuals aboard jet aircraft to aerosolized TAPs represent a serious health concern.[140,165–167] Because pressurization is necessary for proper engine seal function, exposure to aircraft engine lubricants containing TAPs occurs during "fume events," engine start-up/shutdown on the ground and throughout "uneventful" flights during normal acceleration or deceleration.[140–142] Exposures to aerosolized jet engine lubricants are poorly documented and are often overlooked by airline industries.[166] Boeing's new 787 "Dreamliner" does not use bleed air to condition the cabin.[168] For the foreseeable future, however, there will be thousands of aircraft still using bleed air to provide air for passengers and crew, with accompanying possibilities of TAP exposure. Therefore, it makes sense to develop lubricant formulations that are less toxic than current formulations.

Baker et al. describes a rapid *in vitro* assay for identifying potentially safer TAP lubricant additives and have validated the potential safety of some of these TAPs by *in vivo* exposure of mice. To date, almost all studies on the safety of TAP-containing compounds involved chronic exposure of chickens followed by evaluation of neuropathology and/or symptoms of organophosphate (OP)-induced delayed neuropathy[103,160,169–171] although rodents have also been used to examine the effect (s) of TAP exposure.[103,172] TAP bioactivation provided a rapid evaluation of 19 different parent compounds *in vitro*, using inhibition of BChE. None of the TAPs or commercial OP additive formulations inhibited BChE with both RLMs and NADPH implicating the cytochrome P450 superfamily in the bioactivation of the TAPs. Nine TAP formulations tested were not bioactivated at their limits of solubility (~20 µg/mL). Bioactivated ToCP produced the most potent BChE inhibition (IC_{50} values = 0.12–0.15 µg/mL, or ~330 nM). The D125 IC_{50} value was 0.36 µg/mL (±0.06). Human liver microsomes (University of Washington, School of Pharmacy Human Tissue Bank) also bioactivated TAPs in the presence of NADPH (not shown), but limited availability precluded their use for extensive analyses.

For *in vivo* validation, TpCP, TpBP, and D125 were administered to mice by gavage. Gavage exposure was determined in pilot studies to be a more appropriate route than dermal or IP exposure, and administration by aerosol was not feasible because of regulatory restrictions on inhalation exposures in our shared animal housing. D125 was chosen as a positive control for the *in vivo* studies, since it is used commercially and was also used as the *in vitro* control. TpCP and TpBP were selected because they generated no BChE inhibition *in vitro*. Further, others reported tri-p-substituted phenyl phosphates like TpCP to be less toxic than meta- and ortho-substituted TAPs, and chronic exposure studies using the hen model of organophosphate (OP)-induced delayed neuropathy reported relatively low toxicity of butylated TAP-containing formulations.[145] TpBP was especially interesting because none of the tert-butylated TAPs inhibited BChE *in vitro*, and TpBP exposures produced no BChE inhibition *in vivo*.

The efficacy of target enzyme inhibition is likely related to TAAP bulkiness or substituted aryl group(s) geometry, which may interfere with access to active-site serines.[173] TAPs with bulkier substitutions (e.g., TpBP and the tri-isopropylphenyl phosphates) were generally less inhibitory for esterases while bioactivated methyl-substituted TAPs were more efficient esterase inhibitors. However, the product(s) of bioactivated TpCP did not readily reach/bind to the BChE serine active site, but effectively inhibited the active-site serine of other enzymes (e.g., plasma and liver CESs and liver APH).

Different enzymes exhibit dramatically different sensitivities to inhibitory TAP metabolites. Consistent with the CES inhibition by TAPs in this study, Quistad and Casida reported the high sensitivity of CES to CDP inhibition.[162] APH, reported to be involved in cognition,[174,175] was inhibited *in vivo* by TAP metabolite(s). Inhibition and subsequent aging of NTE, a protein important for neuronal transport, may lead to paralysis if significantly inhibited following repeated exposure of animals to neurotoxic Ops.[84,176–179] The rNEST catalytic domain of NTE[180,181] was sensitive to CBDP (IC_{50} = 145 nM), although BChE was even more sensitive to CBDP (IC_{50} = 25 nM), in close agreement with the 30 nM IC_{50} of the related compound, phenyl saligenin cyclic phosphonate.[162] While CBDP was 16 times more effective at inhibiting BChE and rNEST, it was nonetheless a potent inhibitor of both enzymes. Exposure to this substance can cause illness in the humans exposed. This is especially true in the chemically sensitive patient who has high CBDP sensitivity.

Since it is clear from this study and interpretation of earlier studies of Aldridge with rat liver slices[78] that the P450 system is required for the conversion of TAPs into toxic metabolites, Baker et al. investigated whether naturally occurring inhibitors would block the conversion of TAPs to toxic metabolites. Naringenin, a compound found in grapefruit, inhibited the conversion of D125 into BChE inhibitor(s) in a concentration-dependent manner. The inhibition was observed at concentrations that fall well below the reported ~6 μM concentration of naringenin observed in plasma following ingestion of grapefruit juice.[182] Lu et al.[164] recently described the naringenin enantiomer-dependent inhibition of cytochromes CYP19, CYP2C9, CYP2C19, and CYP3A by the (R)- and (S)-enantiomers of naringenin. Additional research will be required to determine which of the P450 isomers are involved in the bioactivation of each of the TAPs and which naringenin enantiomer is the most potent inhibitor of the bioactivation of a specific TAP by a relevant P450 isozyme. While consumption of grapefruit juice following an exposure may block the conversion of TAP to toxic inhibitor, an important caveat comes from the observation that the microsomal/NADPH system is also involved in the inactivation of active metabolite(s) (data not shown). Aldridge[78] had observed in his earlier studies that incubation of ToCP with liver slices for extended periods of time decreased toxicity following bioactivation.

As normal neuronal function depends on several serine active-site enzymes, *in vitro* analysis of a representative panel of these enzymes would be informative. The *in vivo* data reported here suggest that such a panel should include, at least, APH, CES(s), and BChE. As rNEST is not stable over time and must be incorporated into lipid bilayers for functionality,[180] it would not yet be included in such a panel. The metabolites of TAPs that maximally inhibit the panel of enzymes would merit further toxicological testing. Availability of human cDNAs encoding additional enzymes should facilitate the generation of future screening panels.

In summary, *in vitro* testing of 19 TAPs for bioactivation into esterase inhibitors narrowed the focus of this study to three compounds for further *in vivo* testing. TpBP was significantly less inhibitory than TpCP or D125, suggesting that TpBP, or a similar compound based on its molecular characteristics should be a safer antiwear additive for jet engine lubricants, provided its performance characteristics meet those of similar TAP-containing formulations currently in use (e.g., D125). An inhibitory effect of the flavonoid naringenin on the bioactivation of D125 into BChE inhibitor(s) was also demonstrated; however, additional studies are required to determine if it might help modulate the effects of TAP exposures (Table 3.9).

According to Winder, the presence of contaminants in flight decks and passenger cabins of commercial jet aircraft should be considered an air safety, occupational health, and passenger health problem:

- Incidents involving leaks or engine oil and other aircraft materials into the passenger cabin of aircraft occur frequently and are "unofficially recognized through service bulletins, defect statistics reports, and other sources."
- The oils used in aircraft engines contain toxic ingredients which can cause irritation, sensitization, and neurotoxicity. This does not present a risk to crew or passengers as long as the oil stays in the engine. However, if the oil leaks out of the engine, contaminated bleed air may enter the air-conditioning system and cabin air. Where these leaks cause crew or passenger discomfort, irritation, or toxicity, this is a direct contravention of the U.S. Federal Aviation Authorities and the European Joint Aviation Authorities' airworthiness standards for aircraft ventilation (FAR/JAR 25.831).
- As indicated by manufacturer information and industry documentation, aviation targeting affected workers. Better attention further up the hierarchy might be more useful (Figure 3.10).

TABLE 3.9

Aerotoxic Syndrome: Short- and Long-Term Symptoms

Short-Term Exposure	Long-Term Exposure
• Neurotoxic symptoms: blurred or tunnel vision, nystagmus, disorientation, shaking and tremors, loss of balance and vertigo, seizures, loss of consciousness, paresthesia; • Neuropsychological or psychotoxic symptoms: memory impairment, headache, light-headedness, dizziness, confusion and feeling intoxicated • Gastrointestinal symptoms: nausea, vomiting • Respiratory symptoms: cough, breathing difficulties (shortness of breath), tightness in chest, respiratory failure requiring oxygen • Cardiovascular symptoms: increased heart rate and palpitations • Irritation of eyes, nose, and upper airways	• Neurotoxic symptoms: numbness (fingers, lips, limbs), paresthesia • Neuropsychological or psychotoxic symptoms: memory impairment, forgetfulness, lack of coordination, severe headaches, dizziness, sleep disorders • Gastrointestinal symptoms: salivation, nausea, vomiting, diarrhea • Respiratory symptoms: breathing difficulties (shortness of breath), tightness in chest, respiratory failure, susceptibility to upper respiratory tract infections • Cardiovascular symptoms: chest pain, increased heart rate and palpitations • Skin symptoms: skin itching and rashes, skin blisters (on uncovered body parts), hair loss • Irritation of eyes, nose, and upper airways • Sensitivity: signs of immunosuppression, chemical sensitivity leading to acquired or multiple chemical sensitivity • General: weakness and fatigue (leading to chronic fatigue), exhaustion, hot flashes, joint pain, muscle weakness, and pain

Rather than just responding to a problem reactively, this needs action on a number of fronts. According to Winder

1. Better-designed aircraft, engines, and APUs are needed that do not leak.
2. Better-designed aircraft environmental systems are needed that do not rely on bleed air.
3. Better and safer chemical products are needed to be used in this industry.
4. Standard, open, nonretributive systems for the reporting of leaks are needed.
5. Organizations in this industry need to acknowledge their occupational health and safety responsibilities as mandated by legislation and should develop and implement appropriate systems that allow those responsibilities to be met (because their existing systems do not).

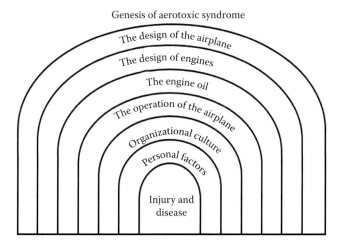

FIGURE 3.10 Genesis of aerotoxic syndrome.

TABLE 3.10
"No Odor" Residual Spray, "Pestgard"

Chemicals Identified in the Air above the Liquid

2-Hexene
2-Cyclohexene-1,3-methylbenzene
5-Methyl-1-hexene
1,1′-Oxybisisooctane
1-Decanol
1-Fluorododecane
Undecanal
5-Methyleneundecane
(Ethenyloxy)isooctane
N-(1-Phenylethylidene)methanamine
1-Octanol
(1,1-Dimethyl)cyclohexane
1,2-Diethylcyclobutane

6. All reports of leaks should be recorded and all such records should be openly available.
7. Risk assessments of exposures are needed that are inclusive, not exclusive, of workers and passengers.
8. Better health systems are needed that treat affected employees with sympathy and respect and not contempt.
9. Better models are needed for monitoring, diagnosis, treatment, rehabilitation, and compensation of affected workers. This is urgently needed for the legacy that already exists of pilots and flight attendants who have been affected, forced out of the industry, and have been in the wilderness ever since.
10. Research is needed into better engineering systems, less toxic chemicals, better diagnosis, better treatment, better risk assessments, and representative epidemiological surveys of employees in the industry. Proper medical and scientific research needs to be undertaken in order to help airline management and crew to better understand both the short- and long-term medical effects of being subjected to air contamination. This research must be independently funded and objectively reported. At best, it must be free of bias from vested interests that are so skillful at obscuring the issue (Tables 3.10 through 3.17).

VENTILATION

The obvious problems of indoor pollution have been recognized for several years. These include poor ventilation, large numbers of people in limited space, and endogenous polluting substances of furnishings and construction. Building codes that were initiated to deal with these problems require minimum ventilation for control of odor and combustion by-products, and these codes have become outdated as our technology has advanced. Little attention has been paid to the fact that up to 90% of an average individual's time is spent indoors. Randolph[1] suggested that a lesser amount of toxic materials be placed in the indoor environment in order to assure sufficient ventilation, since the amount of ventilation otherwise needed to clear these pollutants would be practically impossible to obtain. Implementation of this recommendation resulted in a decrease in total body (burden) load. Other researchers, including Dickey,[2] Rea,[183] Andersen,[8] Molhave et al.,[32] Spengler et al.,[9] Budiansky,[184] Repace et al.,[61] and Pellizzari et al.[185] have recognized, confirmed, and elaborated on Randolph's findings.[1] However, much of their information has gone unheeded by modern builders.

TABLE 3.11
Regular Odor Residual Spray,
"Pestgard"

Chemicals Identified in the Air above the Liquid

Acetamidoacetaldehyde

Methoxycyclobutane

Iodomethylbenzene

o-Xylene

Palmidrol

2-Phenylethylester benzoic acid

Benzoic acid derivative

1-Isocyano-4-methyl-benzene

1-Methylpropylbenzene

1-Ethyl-2,3-dimethylbenzene

4-Ethyl-1,2-dimethylbenzene

1-Ethyl-2,4-dimethylbenzene

1-Methyl-4-propanylbenzene

Naphthalene

Ventilation practices are also based on the assumption that outdoor air is fresh air. Sometimes, this assumption is true, but often outside air is full of pollutants that only exacerbate indoor problems (Chapter 2). Therefore, careful evaluation must be carried out as to when outdoor ventilation is needed or when only indoor recirculation is needed. If properly constructed, buildings in the twenty-first century should have the option of allowing outside air to come inside only upon demand (when outdoor pollution levels are low). The switch for letting in outdoor air should be easy to access and easy for the chemically sensitive to control.

Today, synthetic building materials, energy-efficient buildings, unvented gas heating and cooking appliances, and cleaning and personal care products enhance growing indoor air pollution, which tends to create and exacerbate chemical sensitivity. Technology has not kept up with the elimination of these pollutants. In fact, the new pollutant load of EMF has raised its ugly head making the total pollutant load much more of a problem.

In the past, it was common to express ventilation requirements per human occupant present in a space. Of course, the assumption underlying this practice was that the occupants were the only

TABLE 3.12
Chemicals Identified in the Actual Liquid

Permethrin

Toluene

9-Methyl-5-undecene

Dodecamethylcyclohexasiloxane

Pyrimidine siloxane derivative

Benzoic acid siloxane derivative

Trisiloxane derivative

Palmidrol

1-Fluorododecane

TABLE 3.13
Chemicals Identified in the Liquid Itself

Permethrin
p-Xylene
Cycloheptatrienylium bromide
1,1′-(1-Methyl-1,2-ethanediyl)benzene
1-Nitroethylbenzene
1,1-Dimethylpropylbenzene
Trisiloxane derivative
Tetrasiloxane derivative
o-Xylene
Palmidrol
1,4-Diethylbenzene
1-Nitroethylbenzene
1,3-Diethyl-*t*-methylbenzene
1-Ethyl-2,4-dimethylbenzene
1-Ethyl-2,3-dimethylbenzene
1,3-Diethyl-5-methylbenzene
1-Methyl-2-(2-propenyl)-benzene
Naphthalene
Cyclopropanecarboxylic acid derivative

TABLE 3.14
"Low Odor" Residual Spray, "Aireze"

Chemicals Identified in the Air above the Liquid
   Methylene chloride
   3-Ethyl-2,2-dimethyl-pentane
   1-Hexene
   5-Methyl-1-hexene
   1-Octanol
   3,7-Dimethyl-1-octene
   1,2,-Diethylcyclobutane
   Propylcyclopropane
   5-Methyleneundecane
Chemical Identified in the Actual Liquid
   Permethrin
   1,3-Dimethoxypropane
   Cycloheptatrienylium bromide
   1,2-Dimethylbenzene
   p-Xylene
   1-Ethyl-2-methylbenzene
   1,2,3-Trimethylbenzene
   1,1′-Oxybisoctane
   Siloxane derivative
   Benzyl benzoate
   2-Nitro-2-methylcyclohexanone
   2-(1-Methylpropyl)-cyclopentanone
   Palmidrol
   9-Methyl-(*Z*)-5-undecene
   2,2-Dimethylcyclohexanol
   Trisiloxane derivative
   Diethylphthalate

TABLE 3.15
In-Flight Spray, "Aerosol"

Chemicals Identified in the Air above the Liquid
  Acetic acid anhydride
  Fluorotrimethylsilane
  Hexamethylcyclotrisiloxane
  1,2-Dimethylbenzene
  1-Decanol
  6-Ethyl-1-heptanol
  2,4-Dimethyl-1-heptene
  1,1′-Bicycloheptyl
  1-Decanol
  Cyclohexane ethanol
  1-Nonyne
  Isoctanol
  Ethylidenecyclohexane
  (*E*)-2-Nonenal
  2-Propyl-2-pentanol
  (*E*)-2-Decenal
  Octamethyl-cyclotetrasiloxane
Chemicals Identified in the Liquid Itself
  Phenothrin
  (2-Bromoethyl)benzene
  Ethyl chrysanthemate

TABLE 3.16
Regular Odor Residual Spray, "Aireze"

Chemicals Identified in the Air above the Liquid
  4,5-Dimethyl-1-hexane
  3-Ethyl-2,2-dimethylpentane
  5-Methyl,1-hexane
  3,7-Dimethyl-1-octene
  1-Hexene
  5-Methyl-1-hexene
  1-Octanol
  2-Propyl-1-pentanol
Chemicals Identified in the Liquid Itself
  Permethrin
  1,3-Dimethylpropane
  Cycloheptatrienylium bromide
  1,2-Dimethylbenzene
  Diethylphthalate
  Benzyl benzoate
  Palmidrol
  1,1-Dimethylcyclohexane
  9-Methyl-(*Z*)-5-undecene
  3-Hexyl-1,1,2-trimethyl-*cis*-cyclobutane
  2-Pentyl-1-heptene
  1-Methoxynaphthalene

TABLE 3.17

Callington Aircraft Cabin Spray

Chemicals Identified in the Air above the Liquid
- Benzoic acid siloxane derivative
- Silane derivative
- Cyclotetrasiloxane derivative
- Tetramethylsilane

Chemicals Identified in the Liquid Itself
- Phenothrin
- 2-Bromoethylbenzene
- 1,2-Dimethylbenzene
- 1-Methoxy-3-methylbenzene

---

polluters and that outside air was fresh. Since Randolph[16] originally pointed out that building materials, inadequately cleaned ducts, furnishings, and maintenance procedures were the main polluters, the rest of science has had to reassess the early assumptions. The confirmed fact that materials as well as people are polluters is one foundation of this book.

When evaluating buildings for proper ventilation, one has to take into consideration that analytical instruments such as MS, GCV, and particulate counts are good evaluators, but that the human sensors must be the final arbiter of good air. Ecologists have long used a patient's nose and hands as sensors, enabling identification of less polluted environments through the sniff and touch technique. Bluyssen and Fanger[186] have crystallized this concept by suggesting the use of the "olfactory (OLF) unit" as a better way to evaluate and quantify the pollution of a building. The OLF unit is any pollution source required to cause the same dissatisfaction by the number of standard persons (OLFs) as the actual pollution source. For example, a carpet that outgases and causes inconvenience to an individual in a building is an OLF. The average chemically sensitive individual may have an exacerbated sense of smell. However, his perception of the OLF unit may be used to create ultraclean environments. Of course the OLF would not necessarily support the problem of EMF contamination. EMF meters and human sensors have to be used to evaluate and find the cause and sources of EMF exposure as well as EMF meters.

We,[187] along with Randolph,[1] Smith,[132] and Monro (Monro, J. 1987, personal communication) have found that, in addition to analytical equipment, the best way to evaluate buildings is to use emotionally stable, independent judges who have been sensitized to toxic hydrocarbons and have proven by challenge their efficacy in evaluating both safe and polluted buildings and objects. Using their senses, these judges can evaluate the building both when it is occupied and when it is not. Just as wine tasters use their taste buds or perfume testers use their sense of smell, these "sniffers" use not only their olfactory sense, but also other senses (e.g., vision and touch) to identify polluted areas. After analytical studies are performed, the sniffers can then evaluate whether a building has many pollutants for the existing ventilation system. This method is the final arbiter after use of analytical air analysis, particulate counters, GCV, and mass spectrometers. Emphasis should also be placed on the fact that though outside ventilation will dilute many pollutants, it may increase others, thus solving one problem but possibly creating another. No matter how good a ventilation system is, it will not overcome severely toxic emissions and extreme EMF frequencies. Evidence for this observation comes from our monitoring of synthetic indoor/outdoor carpeting. Although the carpeting remains in the outdoor air, the fumes it emits when exposed to direct sunlight are sufficient to cause illness in those chemically sensitive who are exposed to it. Also, outdoor areas that have been treated with pesticides are similarly able to produce fumes strong enough to injure the chemically sensitive. Obviously, if outdoor environments with ambient air are vulnerable to ongoing contamination as a result of the presence of chemical emitters, it is likely that indoor environments are at least equally vulnerable and must, therefore, be carefully managed with as few emitters as possible being brought inside. If EMF bases in the form of towers and generators, one has to get away from them to the same for 500 m to 2.2 km.

We and our chemically and electrically sensitive patients have used these sensory methods in evaluating over 30,000 buildings. Confirmed blood and room analytical levels, followed by individual inhaled challenges, also have proven this method to be efficacious in our hands. Observation of clearing of symptoms in 85% of our chemically and electrically sensitive patients when they lived in a less polluted environment further confirmed total environmental load pollutant reduction.

Similar methods were used to develop less polluted environmental units. Use of this OLF unit, and the EMF sensors in fact, led to the discovery that porcelain is the most inert substance for use in the homes of the chemically sensitive. It now provides a benchmark for other areas or materials needing evaluation. Aluminum and copper usually shields EMF.

Bluyssen and Fanger[186] published data quantifying these evaluations. Ventilation rates of tight buildings may be as low as 0.3 in exchanges per hour, whereas old buildings breathe up to 12 or more times per hour. Toxic chemicals, dusts, and molds may accumulate in air handling systems, and these may become a source of contamination that exacerbates chemical sensitivity.

CLINICAL EFFECTS OF INDOOR AIR POLLUTION

Andersen[8] and Molhave et al.[32] confirmed Randolph's[1] and Rea's[187] observations that the home is the most polluted place in our environment. They performed air analysis in new and older homes, detecting alkanes, alkylbenzenes, and terpenes in new homes up to 3 years of age. These were emanating mostly from building products.

In both Randolph's (Randolph, T. G. 1985, personal communication) and our combined series of 60,000 patients, the most important sources of indoor air pollution responsible for generating illness were the gas cook stove, hot water heaters, and furnaces. Followed by and almost equal to these were routine indoor pesticide and termite treatments. Now, EMF generating from electrical equipment, mobile phones, hair dryers, computers, and various other electrical computer rival the odor generators. Smart meters and Wi-Fi appear the worse. Wi-Fi from outdoors and smart meters are a growing problem.

Indoor contaminants that have been found to be associated with adverse health include aeroallergen, microorganisms, asbestos fibers, FA, pesticides, nitrogen dioxide, carbon monoxide, sulfur dioxide, particulates, radon decay products, and passive tobacco smoke. Newly indicated products include PCP for wood and leather treatment.

Over 30,000 different types of less polluted environments have been constructed under the supervision of the EHC-Dallas. They range from simple ridding of obvious chemical pollutants from the house to constructing ultrasophisticated hospital wings, office building, and patient's homes. Pictures of the original experimental chambers and rooms are shown in other chapters. Randolph[188] constructed rooms for 15 years before we started developing our first experimental chamber in 1976. First, metal sheds were used, followed by porcelain railers. Steel and aluminum studs were also used. Also, parallel studies were carried out, using iron studs, plaster, hardwood, sheetrock, etc.

Studies at the EHC-Dallas have confirmed that the most polluted place in our environment which most affects the chemically sensitive is the indoor environment. Because the clinical effects of polluted environments are significant for the chemically sensitive and the best prescription for exposure to a polluted environment is to reduce the number of contaminants present in it, we advocate environmental cleanup as an integral part of our management of chemical sensitivity.

REGULATION OF AIR POLLUTION

The American Conference of Governmental Industrial Hygienists has established guidelines that regulate certain pollutants in the industrial setting. The Threshold Limit Values (TLV) are officially considered to be safe for nearly all workers.[189] Because of wide variation in individual susceptibility, many workers may become ill at, or below the threshold limits. The 1970 Clean Air Act established National Ambient Air Quality Standards and provided for National Emission Standards for Hazardous Air Pollutants. Standards were set for six pollutants: carbon monoxide, sulfur dioxide, nitrogen oxides, ozone, particulates, and lead. There are no national standards for nonindustrial environments such as hospitals, schools, and private residences. Needless to say, all present standards appear inadequate for optimal health, as pointed out by Ziem et al.[190] Standards are arbitrary and based on little scientific evidence for individual health. Ziem et al.[190] have shown these standards to be of no value.

MODERN SOCIETY AND BUSINESS BUILDINGS

Many situations occur in business buildings of modern society. Several of these will be discussed. Some are in healthcare facilities:

1. Healthcare
2. Childcare and preschool
3. Nursing home
4. Entertainment
5. Shopping mall—restaurants
6. Offices
7. Schools
8. Flame retardants

MODERN SOCIETY AND WORK PLACES OR BUSINESS BUILDINGS

Toxic chemicals are all around us. Everyday products in our homes, workplaces, schools, stores, or places of worship are produced from chemicals. Chemicals selected for participant biomonitoring are specifically identified because they are emerging or known chemicals of concern, are known to be used in the healthcare setting, and have been associated with certain diseases whose incidences are on the rise, especially chemically sensitive. All of the 20 participating healthcare professions in a study according to Wilding.[191] had at least 24 individual chemicals in their body, and two participants had a high of 39 chemicals detected. Eighteen chemicals were detected in every single participant. There are several measures each of us can take to reduce our exposure, but it is important to note that we cannot shop, eat, or exercise our way out of this problem. Beyond individual or professional actions to avoid exposure, the most important thing every physician, nurse, or public health professional must do is advocate for change in how chemicals are managed in the United States.

The chemicals most common were as follows.

Bisphenol A

This is used to make rigid plastic polycarbonate (roughly 70% of bisphenol A [BPA]),[192] used in baby bottles, plastic water cooler bottles, kitchen appliances, CDs and DVDs, and shatter-proof "glass" applications, and to make epoxy resins (roughly 25% of BPA), including for linings of metal food and drink containers, printer toners and inks, industrial paints, dental sealants, and other products. Approximately 7 billion pounds of bisphenol A are manufactured every year.[193] BPA is an endocrine disruptor shown to induce health impacts identified in animal studies at the same levels found in people through biomonitoring by CDC and PSR.[194] Disorders associated with BPA exposure include miscarriages, infertility,[195,196] breast,[197] and prostate cancer,[198] altered brain development and function,[199] obesity,[200] heart disease,[201] diabetes, and thyroid dysfunction.[202]

Mercury

This is used widely in the healthcare setting, including in blood pressure gauges, thermometers, bougies, foley catheters, thermostats, fluorescent lights, switches, and dental amalgam. Spills and breaks can lead to direct exposure. Mercury is found in coal and released from power plants. Environmental mercury builds up through the aquatic food chain and is common in large fish (like tuna and swordfish). Mercury is a heavy metal and a neurotoxin that attacks the CNS and damages the brain. It can also pass from mother to the embryo and fetus, affecting brain development, resulting in mental retardation, abnormalities of fine motor skills, impaired visual-spatial perception, learning disabilities, attention deficit disorders, and hyperactivity.[203]

Perfluorinated Compounds

These are used in the manufacturing of protective coatings for carpets, stain- and grease-resistant clothing, paper coatings (like microwave popcorn bags), and nonstick pans. Our project tested for perfluorooctanoic acid (PFOA), perfluorononanoic acid (PFNA), perfluorodecanoic acid (PFDA), perfluorohexansulfonate (PFHxS), and perfluoroundecanoic acid (PFUnA).

All of these are breakdown chemicals for coatings, still in use. We also tested for perfluorooctanesulfonate (PFOS), which was an active ingredient in Scotchgard prior to 2000, and which has now been restricted by EPA. Perfluorinated compounds (PFCs) persist in people and wildlife[204] and have been linked to hormone and immune disruption in laboratory animals. PFC exposure can lead to liver and pancreatic tumors in animals, and can disrupt fetal development in humans.[205]

Phthalates

These are used as plasticizers and found in several consumer items such as cosmetics, hair spray, plastic products, and wood finishes. Many IV bags and tubing in the healthcare setting are preformed from PVC plastic which relies on phthalates to be flexible. Vinyl wallpaper may also contain phthalates. We tested for metabolites (chemicals after the human body has digested them) of five phthalates: dimethyl phthalate (DMP), diethyl phthalate (DEP), dibutyl phthalate (DBP), benzyl butyl phthalate (BzBP), and di(2-ethylhexyl) phthalate (DEHP), which has three metabolites. Low-level exposures affect the development of reproductive organs,[206] potentially causing adverse health effects in embryos, fetuses, and preterm babies. Polybrominated diphenylethers (PBDEs) are used as flame retardants in products like furniture, computers, electronic medical equipment, and mattresses. There are three primary commercial formulations of PBDEs, based on the number of bromine atoms attached to the molecule (called congeners). Two of the common commercial formulations, penta- and octa-BDE (with five and eight bromines, respectively), have been voluntarily phased out of U.S. production. Deca-BDE continues to be produced. PBDEs are toxic at low levels and persistent in the environment. PBDEs are associated with learning, memory, behavior disorders,[207] reproductive impairment, thyroid disruption, and cancer.[208]

Triclosan

This is used as a synthetic broad-spectrum antimicrobial agent in hundreds of products such as toothpaste, antibacterial soaps, cosmetics, fabrics, deodorants, and plastics. Triclosan is used primarily in the healthcare setting as a hand sterilizer. Triclosan can be converted to dioxin in sunlight or when heated.[209] This chemical is very stable over long periods of time and bioaccumulates in aquatic organisms and even in human breast milk. It can disrupt thyroid function[210] and can alter some hormone functions in humans,[211] though the health implications of this are still being explored (Figures 3.11 through 3.15).

Environmental Air Pollution in an Intensive Care Unit for Nephrology and Dialysis

According to Buemi et al.,[212] the quality indoor air depends on external pollutant concentrations and on internal sources, such as heating and air-conditioning systems, building materials, ventilation, cleaning products, personnel, and their activity. This study assessed environmental air pollution in

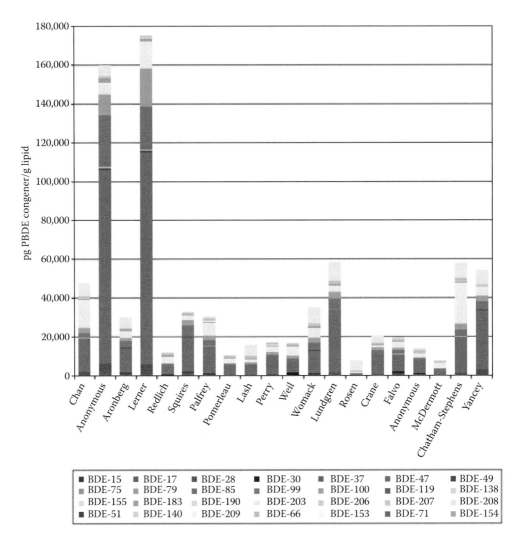

FIGURE 3.11   Polybrominated diphenyl ethers (PBDES).

an intensive care unit (ICU) for nephrology and dialysis. Air-dispersed particulate pollution was measured using a gravimetric method and spectroscopic photocorrelation. Microbiological pollution was evaluated by passive and active collection. Particulate concentrations exceeded recommended limits in some of the environments. There was a prevalence of small particles, which are the most harmful type of all. An overall evaluation of bacterial pollution showed low levels of contamination in some of the rooms. In none of the environments we were able to detect pathogens such as *Aspergillus fumigatus*, methicillin-resistant Staphylococci, or toxin-producing fungi.

Glutaraldehyde

Exposure of employees to glutaraldehyde: Glutaraldehyde is a toxic chemical that is used as a cold sterilant to disinfect and clean heat-sensitive medical, surgical, and dental equipment. It is found in products such as Cidex, Aldesen, Hospex, Sporicidin, Omnicide, Matricide, Wavicide, and others. Glutaraldehyde is also used as a tissue fixative in histology and pathology laboratories and as a hardening agent in the development of x-rays.

The National Institute for Occupational Safety and Health (NIOSH)[213] suggests ways in which healthcare workers may be exposed to glutaraldehyde, including (1) hospital staff who work in

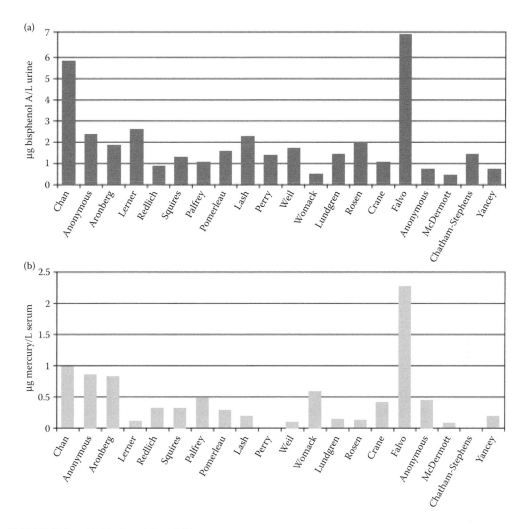

FIGURE 3.12 (a) Bisphenol A and (b) mercury.

areas with a cold sterilizing procedure that uses glutaraldehyde (e.g., gastroenterology or cardiology departments); (2) hospital staff who work in operating rooms, dialysis departments, endoscopy units, and ICUs, where glutaraldehyde formulations are used in infection control procedures; (3) central supply workers who use glutaraldehyde as a sterilant; (4) research technicians, researchers. and pharmacy personnel who either prepare the alkaline solutions or fix tissues in histology and pathology laboratories; (5) laboratory workers who sterilize bench tops with glutaraldehyde solutions; and (6) workers who develop x-rays.

Glutaraldehyde is used in a limited number of applications, rather than as a general disinfectant. Specific applications include use as a disinfecting agent for respiratory therapy equipment, bronchoscopes, physical therapy whirlpool tubs, surgical instruments, anesthesia equipment parts, x-ray tabletops, dialyzers, and dialysis treatment equipment.

Health Effects of Glutaraldehyde Exposure

Short-term (acute) effects: Contact with glutaraldehyde liquid and vapor can severely irritate the eyes, and at higher concentrations burns the skin. Breathing glutaraldehyde can irritate the nose, throat, and respiratory tract, causing coughing and wheezing, nausea, headaches, drowsiness, nosebleeds, and dizziness.

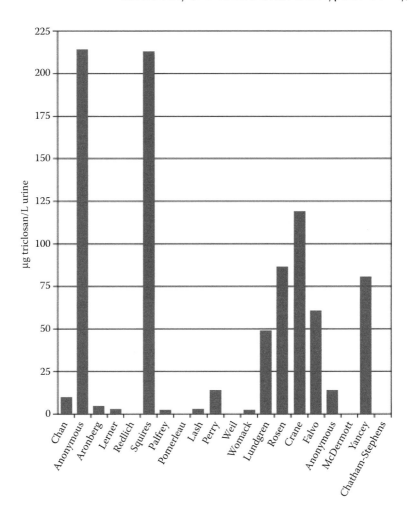

FIGURE 3.13 Triclosan.

Long-term (chronic) effects: Glutaraldehyde is a sensitizer. This means some workers will become very sensitive to glutaraldehyde and have strong reactions if they are exposed to even small amounts. Workers may get sudden asthma attacks with difficult breathing, wheezing, coughing, and tightness in the chest. Prolonged exposure can cause a skin allergy and chronic eczema, and afterwards, exposure to small amounts produces severe itching and skin rashes. It has been implicated as a possible cause of occupational asthma.

Limit Exposure to Glutaraldehyde through Work Practices, Engineering Controls, and Personal Protective Equipment

- Make sure that rooms in which glutaraldehyde is to be used are well ventilated and large enough to ensure adequate dilution of vapor, with a minimum air exchange rate of 10 air changes per hour. Ideally, install local exhaust ventilation such as properly functioning laboratory fume hoods (capture velocity of at least 100 ft/minute) to control vapor. Keep glutaraldehyde baths under a fume hood where possible. Use only enough glutaraldehyde to perform the required disinfecting procedure. Store glutaraldehyde in closed containers in well-ventilated areas. Airtight containers are available. Post signs to remind staff to replace lids after using product. Use specially designed, mobile, compact, disinfectant

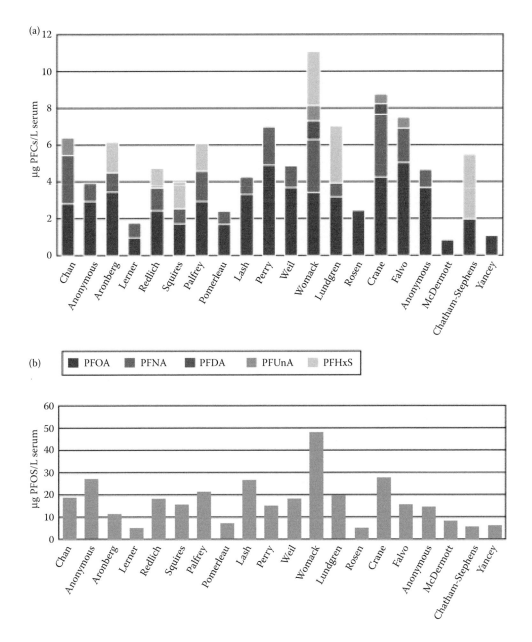

FIGURE 3.14 (a) Perfluorinated compounds and (b) perfluorooctanesulfonic acid (PFOS).

soaking stations to facilitate sterilization of heat-sensitive equipment such as endoscopes or GI scopes. These soaking stations provide an enclosed area for sterilizing trays, and remove fumes from glutaraldehyde and other disinfectants.

AIR POLLUTION AND CONTAMINANTS AT CHILDCARE AND PRESCHOOL FACILITIES IN CALIFORNIA

The Environmental Exposures in Early Childhood Education Environments study examined air pollution and contaminant levels in dust in family-based childcare and preschool facilities in California.[214] This study, which was conducted by researchers from the University of California,

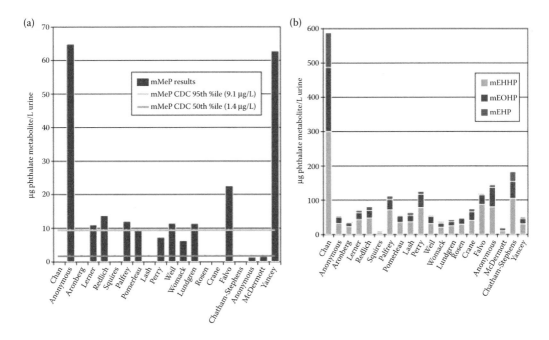

FIGURE 3.15   Phthalates. (a) Metabolite for dimethyl phthalate and (b) DEHP metabolites.

Berkeley and completed in 2012, is the first comprehensive study in childcare centers to measure a broad spectrum of pollutants, including several volatile organic chemicals, particles, and pesticides, and emerging pollutants such as flame retardants, phthalates, and PFCs.[214]

Understanding exposures in childcare and preschool environments is important because infants and young children spend as much as 10 hours per day, 5 days per week in childcare and preschool facilities. Children breathe more air per unit of b.wt. compared to adults and are also less developed immunologically, physiologically, and neurologically. Therefore, children may be more susceptible to the adverse effects of chemicals and toxins. Approximately 1 million children, 5 years or younger, attend childcare or preschool in California, which has the largest number of licensed childcare centers (49,000) in the United States; 80% of these are family-based centers located in homes. Additionally, 146,000 staff works in California's licensed childcare facilities.[214]

Aldehydes: FA levels in 87% of the facilities exceeded the California acute and chronic reference exposure guideline levels for noncancer health effects such as respiratory and sensory irritation (e.g., eyes, nose, throat, and lungs). In 2007, ARB implemented an Air Toxics Control Measure that limits FA emissions from building materials, furnishings, and other products made from pressed wood material such as plywood and particleboard. This should significantly reduce exposures in new homes in the future, but more actions are under consideration to further reduce FA exposures. Acetaldehyde levels did not exceed any California guidelines, but levels exceeded the U.S. guideline for respiratory and irritant effects in 30% of the facilities.[214]

Flame Retardants: Brominated flame retardants (PBDEs) can disrupt normal hormonal function and development, especially in infants and children. They can persist in the environment for years, especially indoors. The estimated nondietary ingestion of PBDEs (ingesting PBDEs that have been transferred from treated surfaces to the hands or objects that are mouthed) in children less than 1 year of age exceeded the U.S. EPA acceptable levels for PBDE-47 and PBDE-99 in 10% of the facilities.[214]

Particle Measurements: Indoor PM10[1] concentrations exceeded the level of the 24-hour California Ambient Air Quality Standard in 46% of the childcare and preschool facilities, and indoor $PM_{2.5}$ levels exceeded the level of the 24-hour National Ambient Air Quality Standard in 11%

of the facilities. While these measurements are not directly comparable to the standards because they were obtained over an 8–10-hour period, they indicate that potentially unhealthful exposures sometimes occur in day care facilities. Indoor ultrafine PM counts (the number of particles less than 0.1 μm in size) were highest in facilities where indoor cooking with gas occurred, and the counts were only weakly correlated with outdoor levels and traffic metrics.[214]

Metals in Floor Dust: Dust samples were analyzed for levels of metals such as lead and cadmium. Lead exposure estimates exceeded the age-adjusted California Proposition 65 no significant risk level (NSRL) benchmark based on carcinogenicity in 95% of facilities. However, the primary issue for childhood exposure to lead is developmental toxicity. As U.S. EPA believes there is no safe level of exposure to lead, there is no defined reference dose. However, the levels of lead in dust measured in this study are comparable to the typical levels found in homes, and it is unlikely that these levels significantly contribute to cases of childhood lead poisoning. Levels of cadmium did not exceed child dose estimates for the U.S. EPA's oral reference dose, the only health benchmark available for cadmium.[214]

STUDY FINDS REASONS TO IMPROVE INDOOR AIR QUALITY IN CHILDCARE FACILITIES

A first-of-its-kind study of the IAQ of 40 childcare centers in California finds that most concentrations of contaminants in the air are well within state and federal guidelines, although a few chemicals such as FA substantially exceeded guidelines.[215]

Although most of the VOCs that we commonly measure indoors are similar in childcare facilities and other indoor environments like homes and schools, Maddalena and McKone[216] findings suggest that there are a lot more chemicals in the air than is commonly measured. In addition to the target VOCs in their study, they identified over a 100 other VOCs in the air, many of which do not have reference exposure levels.

The study is the first to provide a detailed analysis of environmental contaminants and exposures for children in early childhood education facilities (ECE). ECE facilities include home-based childcare providers, private for profit or nonprofit preschools, and programs run by government agencies and religious institutions.[215]

They measured more than 40 VOCs in the air of these facilities; sources are cleaners and personal care products.

However, FA, acetaldehyde, chloroform, and benzene, or ethylbenzene exceeded child-specific Safe Harbor Levels. FA and acetaldehyde are known respiratory irritants and carcinogens.[215]

Children exhibit exploratory behaviors that place them in direct contact with contaminated surfaces, they are likely to be exposed to any contaminants present. Children have higher exposures because they breathe more air, eat more food, and drink more water per unit of b.wt compared to adults. They are also less developed immunologically, physiologically, and neurologically and therefore may be more susceptible to the adverse effects of chemicals and toxins."

FA concentrations in the air exceeded reference exposure levels in 35 of the facilities. It is typically emitted from furniture containing composite wood products like plywood, fiberboard, or particle board, but it can be emitted from other indoor sources, including carpets and carpet pads; paints and coatings; permanent press clothing, furniture fabrics, and draperies; personal care products; and indoor combustion sources such as gas ranges and fireplaces.[215]

Some of CARB's recommended strategies for reducing FA in the air include[215]

- Purchase products containing little or no FA
- Use ventilation systems and open windows
- Clean frequently to minimize dust, using a vacuum cleaner with a HEPA filter or a wet mop for hard surface floors

- Clean out cabinets and garages to eliminate older pesticides, solvents, and cleaning products that may leak, in order to help reduce indoor levels of pesticides and harmful chemicals
- Assure adequate ventilation to bring in outdoor air

FIFTY ARTICLES THAT THE IMPACT OF NURSING HOME AIR QUALITY ON PATIENT HEALTH AND WELLNESS

Nursing homes are great for elderly people who have a hard time living on their own, but a problem that happens sometimes in nursing homes is the quality of air, and this can cause some unwanted health problems for the elderly.[217] It is very important for nursing homes to constantly test the quality of air in their retirement centers to ensure the senior citizens who live there are breathing clean air.[217]

EXPOSURES TO ATMOSPHERIC EFFECTS IN THE ENTERTAINMENT INDUSTRY

According to Teschke et al.,[218] theatrical fogs are commonly used in the entertainment industry to create special atmospheric effects during filming and live productions. Exposures used oil- and glycol-based theatrical fogs to determine what fluids and effects were commonly used, to measure the size distributions of the aerosols, and to identify factors associated with personal exposure levels. In nonperformance jobs in a range of production types (television, film, live theater, and concerts), they measured airborne concentrations of inhalable aerosols, aldehydes, and PAHs, and collected observations about the sites and tasks performed. Both mineral oil and glycols were observed in use on about one-half the production days in the study. The most common effect produced was a generalized haze over the entire set. Mean personal inhalable aerosol concentrations were 0.70 mg/m^3 (range 0.02–4.1). The mean proportion of total aerosol mass less than 3.5 μm in aerodynamic diameter was 61%. Exposures were higher when mineral oils, rather than glycols, were used to generate fogs. Higher exposures were also associated with movie and television productions, with using more than one fog machine, with increased time spent in visible fog, and for those employed as "grips." Decreased exposures were associated with increasing room temperature, with increasing distance from fog machines, and for those employed as "sound technicians." Exposures to theatrical fogs are just beginning to be measured. It is important to consider these exposures in light of any health effects observed, since existing occupational exposure limits were developed in other industries where the aerosol composition differs from that of theatrical fogs.

Varughese et al.[219] studied 101 employees at 19 sites using fogs and measured personal fog exposures, across work shift lung function, and acute and chronic symptoms. Results were also compared to an external control population, studied previously.

Chronic work-related wheezing and chest tightness were significantly associated with increased cumulative exposure to fogs (mineral oil and glycols) over the previous 2 years. Acute cough and dry throat were associated with acute exposure to glycol-based fogs; increased acute upper airway symptoms were associated with overall increased fog aerosol. Lung function was significantly lower among those working closest to the fog source.

Mineral oil- and glycol-based fogs are associated with acute and chronic adverse effects on respiratory health among employees. Reducing exposure, through controls, substitution, and elimination where possible, is likely to reduce these effects.

IAQ IN RESTAURANTS WITH AND WITHOUT DESIGNATED SMOKING ROOMS

IAQ in restaurants was studied in two cities in northwest Ohio after clean indoor air ordinances had been enacted by Milz et al.[220] Carbon dioxide and ultrafine particles were measured in two restaurants in Toledo and two restaurants in Bowling Green. One restaurant in each city was smoke free, and one restaurant in each city contained a dedicated smoking room. A smoke free office space was also assessed as a reference site. Measurements were collected with data logging instrumentation simultaneously in both the designated smoking room, if present, and in the nonsmoking section. For smoke-free establishments, data logging instrumentation was also used. Carbon dioxide levels were elevated in all four restaurants, with only 32% of the measurements meeting the ASHRAE criterion level of 1000 ppm. Ultrafine particles currently do not have any formal standard or guideline. Statistically significant differences were evident between all four restaurants and the reference site. The largest differences were found between the two designated smoking rooms and the reference site ($p < 0.001$), with the mean levels in the smoking rooms up to 43 times higher than in the reference site. The results from this study indicate inadequate fresh air supply in all four restaurants, particularly in the designated smoking rooms, and the possibility that the designated smoking rooms were not containing the environmental tobacco smoke, based on the ultrafine particle concentrations measured in the nonsmoking areas of the smoking restaurants.

IAQ at Nine Shopping Malls in Hong Kong

Hong Kong is one of the most attractive shopping paradises in the world. Many local people and international tourists favor to spend their time in shopping malls in Hong Kong. Good IAQ is, therefore, very essential to shoppers. In order to characterize the IAQ in shopping malls, nine shopping malls in Hong Kong were selected for this study by Li et al.[221] The indoor air pollutants included carbon dioxide (CO_2), carbon monoxide (CO), total hydrocarbons (THC), FA (HCHO), respirable particulate matter (PM_{10}), and total bacteria count (TBC). More than 40% of the shopping malls had 1-hour average CO_2 levels above the 1000 ppm of the ASHRAE standard on both weekdays and weekends. Also, they had average weekday PM_{10} concentrations that exceeded the Hong Kong Indoor Air Quality Objective (HKIAQO). The highest indoor PM_{10} level at a mall was 380 $\mu g/m^3$. Of the malls surveyed, 30% had indoor airborne bacteria levels above 1000 cfu/m^3 set by the HKIAQO. The elevated indoor CO_2 and bacteria levels could result from high occupancy combined with insufficient ventilation. The increased PM_{10} levels could be probably attributed to illegal smoking inside these establishments. In comparison, the shopping malls that contained internal public transport drop-off areas, where vehicles were parked with idling engines and had major entry doors close to heavy traffic roads, had higher CO and PM_{10} indoor levels. In addition, the extensive use of cooking stoves without adequate ventilation inside food courts could increase indoor CO_2, CO, and PM_{10} levels.

Organic Compounds in Office Environments: Sensory Irritation, Odor, Measurements, and the Role of Reactive Chemistry

Sensory irritation and odor effects of organic compounds in indoor environments are reviewed by Wolkoff et al.[222] It is proposed to subdivide VOCs into four categories: (1) chemically nonreactive, (2) chemically "reactive," (3) biologically reactive (i.e., form chemical bonds to receptor sites in mucous membranes), and (4) toxic compounds. Chemically nonreactive VOCs are considered nonirritants at typical indoor air levels. However, compounds with low odor thresholds contribute to the overall perception of the IAQ. Reported sensory irritation may be the result of odor annoyance. It appears that odor thresholds for many VOCs probably are considerably lower than previously reported. This explains why many building materials persistently are perceived as odorous, although the concentrations of the detected organic compounds are close to or below their reported odor thresholds. Ozone reacts with certain alkenes to form a gas and aerosol phase of oxidation products, some of which are sensory irritants. However, all of the sensory irritating species have not yet been identified and whether the secondary aerosols (ultrafine and fine particles) contribute to sensory irritation requires investigation. Low relative humidity may exacerbate the sensory irritation impact. Practical implications: Certain odors, in addition to odor annoyance, may result in psychological effects and distraction from work. Some building materials continually cause perceivable odors, because the odor thresholds of the emitted compounds are low. Some oxidation products of alkenes (e.g., terpenes) may contribute to eye and airway symptoms under certain conditions and low relative humidity.

IAQ IMPACTS OF VENTILATION DUCTS: OZONE REMOVAL AND EMISSIONS OF VOLATILE ORGANIC COMPOUNDS

The concentrations of contaminants in the supply air of mechanically ventilated buildings may be altered by pollutant emissions from and interactions with duct materials. Morrison et al.[223] measured the emission rate of VOCs and aldehydes from materials typically found in ventilation ducts. The emission rate of VOCs per exposed surface area of materials was found to be low for some duct liners, but high for duct sealing caulk and a neoprene gasket. For a typical duct, the contribution to VOC concentrations is predicted to be only a few percent of common indoor levels. They exposed selected materials to approximately 100 ppb ozone and measured VOC emissions. Exposure to ozone increased the emission rates of aldehydes from a duct liner, duct sealing caulk, and neoprene gasket. The emission of aldehydes from these materials could increase indoor air concentrations by amounts that are as much as 20% of odor thresholds. They also measured the rate of ozone uptake on duct liners and galvanized sheet metal to predict how much ozone might be removed by a typical duct in ventilation systems. For exposure to a constant ozone mole fraction of 37 ppb, a lined duct would initially remove approximately 9% of the ozone, but over a period of 10 days of ozone removal efficiency would diminish to less than 4%. In an unlined duct, in which only galvanized sheet metal is exposed to the airstream, the removal efficiency would be much lower, approximately 0.02%. Therefore, ducts in ventilation systems are unlikely to be a major sink for ozone.

ISOLATION OF SULFUR-REDUCING AND SULFUR-OXIDIZING BACTERIA FOUND IN CONTAMINATED DRYWALL

Drywall from China has been reported to release sulfur-producing products which are corrosive to metals, result in noxious odors, and represent a significant health risk.[224] It has been reported that these emissions produce medical symptoms such as respiratory or asthma-type problems, sinusitis, gastrointestinal disorders, and vision problems in home owners and their household pets. They report here a method of identifying a causative agent for these emissions by sampling affected gypsum wallboard and subjecting those samples to real-time polymerase chain reaction (RT-PCR) studies. Specific DNA probes and primers have been designed and patented that detect a specific iron- and sulfur-reducing bacterium (i.e., *Thiobacillus ferrooxidans*). One hundred percent of affected drywall samples obtained from homes located in the southeastern United States tested positive for the presence of *T. ferrooxidans*. All negative controls consisting of unaffected wallboard and internal controls, *Geotrichum* sp., tested negative within our limits of detection.[224]

INDOOR AIR POLLUTION: IN THE KITCHEN

While the millions of deaths from well-known communicable diseases often make headlines, indoor air pollution remains a silent and unreported killer.[225] Rural women and children are the most at risk.[225]

Thick acrid smoke rising from stoves and fires inside homes is associated with around 1.6 million deaths per year in developing countries—that is one life lost every 20 seconds to the killer in the kitchen.[225]

Nearly half of the world continues to cook with solid fuels such as dung, wood, agricultural residues, and coal. Smoke from burning these fuels gives off a poisonous cocktail of particles and chemicals that bypass the human body's defenses and more than that doubles the risk of respiratory illnesses such as bronchitis and pneumonia.[225]

TABLE 3.18
Levels of Smoke in Home from Cooking

Pollutant	Emission (mg/m³)	Allowable Standard (mg/m³)
Carbon monoxide	150	10
Particles	3.3	0.1
Benzene	0.8	0.002
1,3-Butadiene	0.15	0.0003
Formaldehyde	0.7	0.1

Source: Based on the UNDP/DESA/WEC World Energy Assessment.

The indoor concentration of health-damaging pollutants from a typical wood-fired cooking stove creates carbon monoxide and other noxious fumes at anywhere between 7 and 500 times over the allowable limits.[225]

Day in day out, and for hours at a time, rural women and their children in particular are subjected to levels of smoke in their homes that far exceed international safety standards. The World Energy Assessment estimates that the amount of smoke from these fires is the equivalent of consuming two packs of cigarettes a day—and yet, these families are faced with what amounts to a nonchoice—not cooking using these fuels, or not eating.[225]

Note: Using 1 kg of wood/hour in 15 ACH 40 m³ kitchens emits, among other pollutants, the following (Table 3.18).

QUANTITATIVE ASSESSMENTS OF INDOOR AIR POLLUTION AND THE RISK OF CHILDHOOD ACUTE LEUKEMIA IN SHANGHAI

They investigated the association between indoor air pollutants and childhood acute leukemia (AL).[226] A total of 105 newly diagnosed cases and 105 1:1 gender-, age-, and hospital-matched controls were included. Measurements of indoor pollutants (including nitrogen dioxide [NO_2] and 17 types of VOCs) were taken with diffusive samplers for 64 pairs of cases and controls. Higher concentrations of NO_2 and almost half of VOCs were observed in the cases than in the controls, and were associated with the increased risk of childhood AL. The use of synthetic materials for wall decoration and furniture in bedroom was related to the risk of childhood AL. Renovating the house in the last 5 years, changing furniture in the last 5 years, closing the doors and windows overnight in the winter and/or summer, paternal smoking history, and outdoor pollutants affected VOC concentrations. Our results support the association between childhood AL and indoor air pollution.[226]

CHARACTERISTICS OF INDOOR GASEOUS AIR POLLUTANTS IN WINTER

There are several gaseous air pollutants found in indoor air. It is very important to precisely measure the concentration of these compounds in order to evaluate the risk to human health and to reduce their concentrations. According to Yamada et al.,[227] a diffusive sampling device is suitable for measurement of indoor air, because these are small and light, and can be used without a power supply for the pump. In this study, representative gaseous air pollutants in winter indoor and outdoor air were measured using diffusive sampling devices. Furthermore, the relationship between gaseous air pollutants, secondary formation mechanism, and the outbreak source were examined. The indoor concentrations of aldehydes, nitrogen dioxide, and ammonia were higher than outdoor concentrations. By contrast, indoor concentrations of ozone were lower than outdoor concentrations.

The indoor concentrations of nitrogen dioxide in 43% houses exceeded the maximum limit stated by environmental law (60 ppb). It was suggested that the main emission sources of nitrogen dioxide are kerosene and gas stoves. In addition, it was suggested that carbonyl compounds are formed by interactions between VOCs and ozone from outdoor air. Formic acid was estimated to be formed by the oxidation of FA with ozone, because a positive correlation between FA and formic acid, and an inverse correlation between FA and ozone, were observed in indoor air.

Infection

According to Curtis[228] of Environment International 2006, it has been well established that significantly higher rates of respiratory infection have been linked to indoor exposure to wood, coal, or dung burning or living in poorly ventilated buildings.[229,230] Recent research also suggests that high levels of outdoor air pollution may also increase risk of respiratory infections. A German study of 6000 croup cases found that increases in outdoor levels of total particulates and nitrogen dioxide levels of 10 and 70 $\mu g/m^3$ were associated with statistically significant 27% and 28% increases in croup, respectively.[231] Ecuadorian children exposed to higher levels of CO were found to have significantly more upper respiratory infections.[232] Studies in Finland and Turkey have found that childhood respiratory infections are about twice as common in cities with high air pollution levels as compared to less polluted areas.[233,234] Studies in Switzerland in 2013 by Stern et al.[235] in 366 infants showed significant increase after air pollutant exposures respiratory symptoms. Higher outdoor levels of PM_{10} and O_3 have been linked to significantly higher rates of hospital pneumonia admissions.[236,237] Higher daily levels of O_3 and SO_2 have been linked to significantly increased influenza admissions.[238] Higher outdoor dust exposure can increase risk of Coccidioidomyces infection in endemic areas.[239] A Nicaraguan study found that childhood diarrhea illness increased six fold in a community exposed to large quantities of volcanic ash containing large amounts of fluorides and toxic metals.[240]

RISK OF INDOOR AIRBORNE INFECTION TRANSMISSION ESTIMATED FROM CARBON DIOXIDE CONCENTRATION

The Wells–Riley equation, which is used to model the risk of airborne transmission of infectious diseases such as tuberculosis, is sometimes problematic because it assumes steady-state conditions and requires measurement of outdoor air supply rates, which are frequently difficult to measure and often vary with time.[241] An alternative equation is derived that avoids these problems by determining the fraction of inhaled air that has been exhaled previously by someone in the building (rebreathed fraction) using CO_2 concentration as a marker for exhaled-breath exposure. They also derive a nonsteady-state version of the Wells–Riley equation which is especially useful in poorly ventilated environments when outdoor air supply rates can be assumed constant. Finally, they derive the relationship between the average number of secondary cases infected by each primary case in a building and exposure to exhaled breath and demonstrate that there is likely to be an achievable critical rebreathed fraction of indoor air below which airborne propagation of common respiratory infections and influenza will not occur.[241]

EXPOSURE TO TRAFFIC-GENERATED AIR POLLUTANTS RESULTS IN DISRUPTION OF THE BLOOD–BRAIN BARRIER THROUGH ALTERED EXPRESSION OF TIGHT JUNCTION PROTEINS

In addition to its harmful effects in the pulmonary and cardiovascular systems, several recent studies have implicated environmental air pollution exposure in deleterious effects on the CNS, including neuroinflammation, stroke, and neurodegeneration.[242] We have reported that vascular oxidative stress, oxidized LDL (oxLDL), and matrix metalloproteinase (MMP) levels are significantly elevated in the systemic vasculature of atherosclerotic apolipoprotein KO (ApoE−/−) mice exposed to vehicular emissions; however, the effects of exposure in the cerebral vasculature have not yet been examined. Numerous recent epidemiological and laboratory studies show a positive correlation between exposure to high levels of air pollution and increased hospital admissions/occurrence of cerebrovascular events (e.g., stroke, transient ischemic attack), with significant elevations in resulting morbidity and mortality. To determine whether traffic-generated air pollutants mediate disruption of the blood–brain barrier (BBB) through altered expression of tight junction (TJ) protein expression, 10-week-old male ApoE−/− mice on a high-fat diet were randomly assigned to an inhalation exposure of either filtered air (FA: $n = 8$ per time point) or an exposure of 250 µg PM/m^3 diesel exhaust +50 µg PM/m^3 gasoline-mixed engine exhaust (ME: $n = 8$ per time point) for 6 hours/day for 7 or 30 days. Exposure to ME resulted in BBB integrity disruption as evidenced by increased FITC fluorescence in the brain, compared to FA controls, after systemic injection of FITC during exposures. Histological and molecular analysis showed a significant decrease in expression of BBB TJ proteins occluding and claudin-5 in cerebral vessels with ME exposure. Additionally, there was increased neurovascular MMP-2 and -9 activities shown by *in situ* zymography, and elevated cerebral iNOS expression, indicating neuroinflammation, in ME-exposed brains. Such findings indicate that inhalation exposure to traffic-generated air pollutants results in BBB disruption associated with increased MMP activity and decreased TJ protein expression.[242]

ROLE OF VENTILATION IN AIRBORNE TRANSMISSION OF INFECTIOUS AGENTS IN THE BUILT ENVIRONMENT: A MULTIDISCIPLINARY SYSTEMATIC REVIEW

There have been few recent studies demonstrating a definitive association between the transmission of airborne infections and the ventilation of buildings. The severe acute respiratory syndrome (SARS) epidemic in 2003 and current concerns about the risk of an avian influenza (H5N1) pandemic have prepare a review of this area timely. Li et al.[243] searched the major literature databases between 1960 and 2005, and then screened titles and abstracts, and finally selected 40 original studies based on a set of criteria. Li et al.[243] established a review panel comprising medical and engineering experts in the fields of microbiology, medicine, epidemiology, IAQ, building ventilation, etc. Most panel members had experience with research into the 2003 SARS epidemic. The panel systematically assessed 40 original studies through both individual assessment and a 2-day face-to-face consensus meeting. Ten of 40 studies reviewed were considered to be conclusive with regard to the association between building ventilation and the transmission of airborne infection. There is strong and sufficient evidence to demonstrate the association between ventilation, air movements in buildings, and the transmission/spread of infectious diseases such as measles, tuberculosis, chickenpox, influenza, smallpox, and SARS. There is insufficient data to specify and quantify the minimum ventilation requirements in hospitals, schools, offices, homes, and isolation rooms in relation to spread of infectious diseases via the airborne route.

FLAME RETARDANTS MAY CREATE DEADLIER FIRES

In one of the deadliest nightclub fires in American history, 100 people died at a rock concert in Rhode Island nearly a decade ago. But the biggest killer was not the flames; it was lethal gases released from burning sound-insulation foam and other plastics.

In a fatal bit of irony, attempts to snuff fires like this catastrophic one could be making some fires even more deadly.

New research suggests that chemicals—brominated and chlorinated flame retardants—that are added to upholstered furniture and other household items to stop the spread of flames increase emissions of two poisonous gases.

"According to Stec,[244] flame retardants have the undesirable effect of increasing the amounts of carbon monoxide and hydrogen cyanide released during combustion."

Two gases are by far the biggest killer in fires. They are responsible for 60%–80% of fire deaths, according to the National Fire Protection Association. During the Rhode Island fire, the levels of hydrogen cyanide and carbon monoxide were high enough to kill in less than 90 seconds. (There is no evidence, however, that flame retardants were involved; the nightclub's foam insulation reportedly was not treated with them.)

Flame retardants prepared from brominated or chlorinated chemicals are added to furniture cushions, carpet padding, children's car seats, plastics that encase electronics, and other consumer items. Under California standards adopted in the 1970s, foam inside furniture must withstand a 12-second exposure to a small, open flame, and much of the nation's furniture is manufactured with flame retardants to meet that standard.

But the researchers said in one experiment, nylon containing the flame retardant brominated polystyrene released six times more hydrogen cyanide when set afire than the same material containing a halogen-free flame retardant.

Hydrogen cyanide is 35 times more deadly than carbon monoxide, and during a fire it can kill in as little as 1 minute.

Both carbon monoxide and hydrogen cyanide are products of incomplete combustion. As a room on fire loses oxygen, combustion becomes less efficient and gases and smoke rapidly increase. Inhaling the toxic air becomes unavoidable for people trapped in a fire.

Brominated and chlorinated flame retardants work by interfering with combustion, which can increase the amount of the gases.

The new research focused on brominated polystyrene, a newer flame retardant manufactured by Albemarle Corporation and other companies. It is added to nylon for use in textiles, upholstery, and electrical connectors.

These newer compounds were designed to replace older flame retardants, mostly PBDEs, which have been banned since 2004 because they were building up in human bodies, including breast milk. PBDEs are still found in furniture manufactured before the bans.

PBDEs and other halogenated flame retardants were already known to produce other toxic chemicals when they burn, including highly toxic dioxins and furans.

Another replacement for PBDEs is called Tris (1,3-dichloroisopropyl) phosphate or TDCPP. Foam containing this chemical was shown to release high amounts of carbon monoxide and smoke during ignition, according to a 2000 study.

With or without fires, research suggests that flame retardants may have risks. PBDEs and other halogenated flame retardants have come under intense scrutiny in recent years. PBDEs have been linked in some studies of people and animals to impaired neurological development, reduced fertility, early onset of puberty, and altered thyroid hormones. This may also be toxic to the developing nervous system.

"It is estimated that escape times can be up to 15 times longer when flame retardants are present, providing increased survival chances," according to a statement from the European Brominated Flame Retardant Industry Panel, which includes Albemarle and Chemtura.

"Scientists have long pointed out that when flame retardants are included in upholstered furniture it slows or stops fires, thereby causing less burn, fewer flames, less smoke, and fewer toxic gases," he said. "This fact has been proven in large scale tests of upholstered furniture."

But a document signed by more than 200 scientists from 30 countries disputes that flame retardants have been proven effective. "Brominated and chlorinated flame retardants can increase fire toxicity, but their overall benefit in improving fire safety has not been proven," the 2010 statement says.

In the new research from the United Kingdom, some alternatives were found to create less toxic air than the halogenated flame retardants. Inorganic, or mineral-based, flame retardants had little effect on toxic gases released in a fire.

Each year, about 10,000 people die in fires in industrialized countries. On average, in the United States in 2010, someone died in a fire every 169 minutes, according to the National Fire Protection Association.

IAQ in Michigan Schools

IAQ parameters in 64 elementary and middle school classrooms in Michigan were examined for the purposes of assessing ventilation rates, levels of VOCs and bioaerosols, air quality differences within and between schools, and emission sources.[245] In each classroom, bioaerosols, VOCs, CO_2, relative humidity, and temperature were monitored over one workweek, and a comprehensive walk-though survey was completed. Ventilation rates were derived from CO_2 and occupancy data. Ventilation was poor in many of the tested classrooms, for example, CO_2 concentrations often exceeded 1000 ppm and sometimes 3000 ppm. Most VOCs had low concentrations (mean of individual species <4.5 $\mu g/m^3$); bioaerosol concentrations were moderate (<6500 count per m^3 indoors, $<41,000$ count per m^3 outdoors). The variability of CO_2, VOC, and bioaerosol concentrations within schools exceeded the variability between schools. These findings suggest that none of the sampled rooms were contaminated and no building-wide contamination sources were present. However, localized IAQ problems might remain in spaces where contaminant sources are concentrated and that are poorly ventilated.[245]

IAQ is a continuing concern for students, parents, teachers, and school staff, leading to several complaints regarding poor IAQ. Investigations of these complaints often include air sampling, which must be carefully conducted if representative data are to be collected. To better understand sampling results, investigators need to account for the variability of contaminants both within and between schools.[245]

IAQ, Ventilation and Health Symptoms in Schools: An Analysis of Existing Information

These studies reviewed the literature on IAQ, ventilation, and building-related health problems in schools and identified commonly reported building-related health symptoms involving schools until 1999.[246] They collected existing data on ventilation rates, carbon dioxide (CO_2) concentrations and symptom-relevant indoor air contaminants, and evaluated information on causal relationships between pollutant exposures and health symptoms. Reported ventilation and CO_2 data strongly indicate that ventilation is inadequate in many classrooms, possibly leading to health symptoms. Adequate ventilation should be a major focus of design or remediation efforts. Total VOCs, FA (HCHO), and microbiological contaminants are reported. Low HCHO concentrations were unlikely to cause acute irritant symptoms (<0.05 ppm), but possibly increased risks for allergen sensitivities, chronic irritation, and cancer. Reported microbiological contaminants included allergens in deposited dust, fungi, and bacteria. Levels of specific allergens were sufficient to cause symptoms in allergic occupants. Measurements of airborne bacteria and airborne and surface fungal spores were reported in schoolrooms. Asthma and "sick building syndrome" symptoms are commonly reported. The few studies investigating causal relationships between health symptoms and exposures to specific pollutants suggest that such symptoms in schools are related to exposures to VOCs, molds and microbial VOCs, and allergens.[246]

Exposure to Severe Urban Air Pollution Influences Cognitive Outcomes, Brain Volume, and Systemic Inflammation in Clinically Healthy Children

Exposure to severe air pollution produces neuroinflammation and structural brain alterations in children.[247] They tested whether patterns of brain growth, cognitive deficits, and white matter hyperintensities (WMH) are associated with exposures to severe air pollution. Baseline and 1 year follow-up measurements of global and regional brain MRI volumes, cognitive abilities (Wechsler Intelligence Scale for Children-Revised, WISC-R), and serum inflammatory mediators were collected in 20 Mexico City (MC) children (10 with WMH+, and 10 without, WMH− and 10 matched controls [CTL]) from a low-polluted city. There were significant differences in white matter volumes between CTL and MC children—both WMH$^+$ and WMH$^-$—in right parietal and bilateral temporal areas. Both WMH$^-$ and WMH$^+$ MC children showed progressive deficits, compared to CTL children, on the WISC-R Vocabulary and Digit Span subtests. The cognitive deficits in highly exposed children match the localization of the volumetric differences detected over the 1-year follow-up, since the deficits observed are consistent with impairment of parietal and temporal lobe functions. Regardless of the presence of prefrontal WMH, Mexico City children performed more poorly across a variety of cognitive tests, compared to CTL children, thus WMH$^+$ is likely only partially identifying underlying white matter pathology. Together these findings reveal that exposure to air pollution may perturb the trajectory of cerebral development and result in cognitive deficits during childhood.[247]

REFERENCES

1. Randolph, T. G. 1961. Human ecology and susceptibility to the chemical environment, Parts I and II. *Ann. Allergy* 19:518–540.
2. Dickey, L. D. 1976. *Clinical Ecology.* Springfield, IL: Charles C. Thomas.
3. Edgar, R. T., E. J. Fenyves, W. J. Rea. 1979. Air pollution analysis used in operating an environmental control unit. *Ann. Allergy* 42 (3):166–173.
4. Ryan, P. B., J. D. Spengler, R. Letz. 1983. The effects of kerosene heaters on indoor pollutant concentrations: A monitoring and modeling study. *Atmos. Environ.* 17:1339–1345.
5. Sheldon, L. S., L. C. Michael, E. D. Pellizzari, L. Wallace. 1987. Use of a portable gas chromatograph for identifying sources of volatile organics in indoor air. *Proceedings of the 4th International Conference on Indoor Air Quality and Climate*, Berlin, pp. 74–78.
6. Code of Federal Regulations. 1987. *40:50—National Primary and Secondary Ambient Air Quality Standards.* Washington, DC: U.S. Government Printing Office.
7. Berks, J. V., C. D. Hollowell, C. Lin, I. Turiel. 1979. *The Effects of Energy Efficient Ventilation Rates on Indoor Air Quality at a California High School.* Berkeley, CA: Lawrence Berkeley Laboratory, U.S. Department of Energy. Contract No. 7405ENG-48.
8. Andersen, I. 1972. Technical notes—Relationships between outdoor and indoor air pollution. *Atmos. Environ.* 6:275–278.
9. Spengler, J. D., B. G. Ferris, Jr., D. W. Dockery, F. Speizer. 1979. Sulfur dioxide and nitrogen dioxide levels inside and outside homes and the implications on health effects. *Environ. Sci. Technol.* 13:1276–1280.
10. Hollowell, C. D., R. J. Budnitz, G. W. Traynor. 1976. *Combustion-Generated Indoor Air Pollution.* Berkeley, CA: Lawrence Berkeley Laboratory, LBL-5918.
11. Palmes, E. D., C. Tomczyk, J. DiMatto. 1977. Average no. concentration in dwellings with gas or electric stoves. *Atmos. Environ.* 2:869–872.
12. Moschandreas, D. J., J. W. C. Stark, J. E. McFadden, S. S. Morse. 1978. Final Report, GEOMETEF-668, Contract No., 68-02-2294. Indoor Air Pollution in the Residential Environment, Vols. I and II, Washington, DC: U.S. Environmental Protection Agency, Enviromental Research Center, and U.S. Department of Housing and Urban Development, Office of Policy Development and Research. EPA 600/7-78/229A.
13. Yamanaka, S., H. Hirose, S. Takada. 1979. Nitrogen oxides emissions from domestic kerosene-fired and gas-fired appliances. *Atmos. Environ.* 13:407–412.
14. Ritchie, I. M., L. A. Oatman. 1983. Residential air pollution from kerosene heater. *J. Air Pollut. Control Assoc.* 33:879–881.
15. Traynor, G. M., J. R. Girman, M. G. Apte, P. D. White. 1985. Indoor air pollution due to emissions from unvented gas-fired space heaters. *J. Air Pollut. Control Assoc.* 35:231–237.
16. Randolph, T. G. 1962. *Human Ecology and Susceptibility to the Chemical Environment*, p. 70. Springfield, IL: Charles C. Thomas.
17. Wade, W. A., W. A. Cote, J. E. Yocom. 1975. A study of indoor air quality. *J. Air Pollut. Control Assoc.* 25:933–939.
18. Thompson, C. R., E. G. Hensel, G. Kats. 1973. Outdoor-indoor levels of six air pollutants. *J. Air Pollut. Control Assoc.* 23:881–886.
19. Hawthorne, A. R., R. B. Gammage, C. S. Dudney. 1986. An indoor air quality study of 4 east Tennessee homes. *Environ. Int.* 12:221–239.

20. Sterling, T. D., E. Sterling. 1979. Carbon monoxide levels in kitchens and homes with gas cooker. *J. Air. Pollut. Control Assoc.* 29:238–241.

21. Nagda, N. L., M. D. Koontz. 1985. Microenvironmental and total exposures to carbon monoxide for three population subgroups. *J. Air Pollut. Control Assoc.* 35:134–137.

22. Yates, M. W. 1967. A preliminary study of carbon monoxide gas in the home. *J. Environ. Health* 29:413–420.

23. Cote, W. A., W. A. Wade, J. E. Yocom. 1974. *A Study of Indoor Air Quality.* Washington, DC: U.S. Environmental Protection Agency. EPA-650/40-74-042.

24. Wallace, L. A. 1983. Carbon monoxide in air and breath of employees in an underground office. *J. Air Pollut. Control Assoc.* 33:680–682.

25. Rea, W. J. 1992. *Chemical Sensitivity.* Vol. 1. p. 47. Boca Raton, FL: Lewis Publishers.

26. National Research Council. 1981. *Indoor Pollutants.* Washington, DC: National Academy Press.

27. Sabersky, R. H., D. A. Sinema, F. H. Shair. 1973. Concentrations, decay rates, and removal of ozone and their relation to establishing clean indoor air. *Environ. Sci. Technol.* 7:347–881.

28. Davies, T. D., B. Ramer, G. Kaspyzok, A. C. Delany. 1984. Indoor/outdoor ozone concentrations at a contemporary art gallery. *J. Air Pollut. Control Assoc.* 31:135–137.302

29. Muller, F., L. Loeb, W. Mapes. 1973. Decomposition rates of ozone in living areas. *Environ. Sci. Technol.* 7:342–346.

30. Halpern, M. 1978. Indoor/outdoor air pollution exposure continuity relationships. *J. Air Pollut. Control Assoc.* 28:689–691.

31. Moschandreas, D. J., J. W. Stark, J. E. McFadden, S. S. Morse. 1978. *Indoor Air Pollution in the Residential Environment, Vol. I.* Geomet, EPA Contract No. 68-023-2294.

32. Molhave, L. et al. 1978. Indoor air pollution due to building materials. *International Indoor Climate Symposium*, Copenhagen, August 30–September 1, 1978.

33. Girman, J. R., A. T. Hodgson, A. S. Newton, A. W. Winkes. 1986. Emissions of volatile organic compounds from adhesives with indoor applications. *Environ. Int.* 12:317–321.

34. Silderberg, M. 2004. *Chemistry: The Molecular Nature of Matter and Change.* p. 623. New York: McGraw-Hill Companies.

35. Silderberg, M. 2004. *Chemistry: The Molecular Nature of Matter and Change.* p. 625. New York: McGraw-Hill Companies.

36. Silderberg, M. 2004. *Chemistry: The Molecular Nature of Matter and Change.* p. 627. New York: McGraw-Hill Companies.

37. Meierhenrich, U. Amino acids and the asymmetry of life. http://books.google.com/books?id=a2J23yPEaBQC&printsec=frontcover

38. Silderberg, M. 2004. *Chemistry: The Molecular Nature of Matter and Change.* p. 628. New York: McGraw-Hill Companies.

39. Silderberg, M. 2004. *Chemistry: The Molecular Nature of Matter and Change.* p. 631. New York: McGraw-Hill Companies.

40. Morgan, D. Lecture ENVIRO 100, World Coal, Coal and Electricity, University of Washington, May 11, 2008. http://www.worldcoal.org/coal/uses-of-coal/coal-electricity/, retrieved 07/03/2012.

41. Sugie, H. et al. 2004. Three cases of sudden death due to Butane or Propane gas inhalation: Analysis of tissues for gas components. *Forensic Sci. Int.* 143(203):211–214.

42. Rossi, R. et al. 2012. Two cases of acute propane/butane poisoning in prison. *J. Forensic Sci.* 57(3):832–834. doi: 10.1111/j.1556-4029.2011.02003.x. Epub December 8, 2011.

43. Kim, O. et al. 2002. Emission of polycyclic aromatic hydrocarbons, toxicity, and mutagenicity from domestic cooking using sawdust briquettes, wood, and kerosene. *Environ. Sci. Technol.* 36(5):833–839.

44. Lv, J., L. Zhu. 2013. Effect of central ventilation and air conditioner system on the concentration and health risk from airborne polycyclic aromatic hydrocarbons. *J. Environ. Sci. (China).* 25(3):531–536.

45. Malouf, A., D. Wimberly. 2000. http://www.Environmentalhealth.ca/summer01gas.html

46. Zhang, J., K. R. Smith. 1996. Hydrocarbon emissions and health risks from cookstoves in developing countries. *J. Expo. Anal. Environ. Epidemiol.* 6(2):147–161.

47. Bridbord, K., P. Brubaker, B. Gay, J. French. 1975. Exposure to halogenated hydrocarbons in the indoor environment. *Environ. Health Perspect.* 2:117–128.

48. Pellizzari, E. D., T. D. Hartwell, R. L. Perritt, C. M. Sparacino, L. S. Sheldon, H. S. Zelon, R. W. Whitmore, J. J. Breen, L. Wallace. 1986. Comparison of indoor and outdoor residential levels of volatile chemicals in five U.S. geographical areas. *Environ. Int.* 12:619–623.

49. Jarke, F. H., A. Dravnieks, S. Gordon. 1981. Organic contaminants in indoor air and their relation to outdoor contaminants. *ASHRAE Trans.* 87:750–762.

50. Wallace, L. A. 1987. *The Total Exposure Assessment Methodology (TEAM) Study: Summary and Analysis*, Vol. I. Washington, DC: U.S. Environmental Protection Agency. EPSA/600/6/87/002.

51. Ulsamer, A. G., K. C. Gupta, H. Kang. 1980. Organic indoor air pollutants. *Workshop on Indoor Air Quality Research Needs/Interagency Research Group on Indoor Air Quality*, U.S. Environmental Protection Agency, Washington, DC, December 3–5, 1980.

52. Mansour, S. A., A. H. Mossa. 2010. *Hum. Exp. Toxicol.* 29(2):77–92. doi: 10.1177/0960327109357276. Epub December 22, 2009.

53. Wanner, H. U., M. Kuhn. 1986. Indoor air pollution by building materials. *Environ. Int.* 12:311–315.

54. Andersen, L., G. R. Lundqvist, L. Molhave. 1975. Indoor air pollution due to chipboard used as a construction material. *Atmos. Environ.* 9:1121–1127.

55. Godish, T., J. Fell, P. Lincoln. 1984. FA levels in New Hampshire urea-formaldehyde foam insulated houses—Relationship to outdoor temperature. *J. Air Pollut. Control Assoc.* 34:1051–1052.

56. Matthews, T. G., K. W. Fung, B. J. Tromberg, A. R. Hawthorne. 1986. Impact of indoor environmental parameters on formaldehyde concentrations in unoccupied research houses. *J. Air Pollut. Control Assoc.* 36: 1244–1249.

57. Sexton, K., K. Liu, M. Petreas. 1986. Formaldehyde concentrations inside private residences: A mail-out approach to indoor air monitoring. *J. Air Pollut. Control Assoc.* 36:698–704.

58. Golden, R. 2011. Identifying an indoor air exposure limit for formaldehyde considering both irritation and cancer hazards. *Crit. Rev. Toxicol.* 41(8):672–721. doi: 10.3109/10408444.2011.

59. Sonbgur, A., O. A. Ozen, M. Sarislimaz. 2010. The toxic effects of formaldehyde on the nervous system. *Rev. Environ. Contam. Toxicol.* 203:105–118. doi: 10.1007/978-1-4419-1352-4_3.303

60. Yocom, J. E., W. L. Clink, W. A. Cote. 1971. Indoor/outdoor air quality relationships. *J. Air Pollut. Control Assoc.* 21:251–259.

61. Repace, J. L., W. R. Ott, L. A. Wallace. 1980. Total human exposure to air pollution. *73rd Annual Meeting Air Pollution Control Association*, Montreal, Canada.

62. Horn, D., S. Waingrow. 1968. Relationship of number of cigarettes smoked to 'tar' rating, *National Cancer Institute Monographs* 28:29–33.

63. Heogg, U. R. 1972. Cigarette smoke in closed spaces. *Environ. Health Perspect.* 2:117–128.

64. Alsona, J., B. L. Cohen, H. Rudolph, H. N. Jow, J. O. Frohliger. 1979. Indoor-outdoor relationships for airborne particulate matter of outdoor origin. *Atmos. Environ.*

65. Lioy, P. J., M. Avdenko, R. Harkov, T. Atherholt, J. Daisey. 1985. A pilot indoor-outdoor study of organic particulate matter and particulate mutagenicity. *J. Air Pollut. Control Assoc.* 35:653–657.

66. Balouet, J.-C., M. Kerguelen, C. Winder. 2001. Hazardous chemicals on Jet Aircraft A Case Study jet engine oils and aerotoxic syndrome. *Toxicology* 164, 164.

67. Spengler, J., H. Burge, T. Dumyahn, M. Muilenburg, D. Forester. 1997. *Environmental Survey on Aircraft and Ground Based Commercial Transportation Vehicles.* Boston, MA for commercial Airline Group. The Boeing Company Seattle, WA. May 31, 1997. Harvard School of Public Health.

68. ASHRAE. 1990. Ventilation for Acceptable Indoor Air Quality: ANSI/ASHRAE Standard 62. *American Society of Heating, Refrigerating and Air Conditioning Engineers.* Atlanta.

69. O'Donnell, A., G. Donnini, V. Nguyen. 1991. *ASHRAE J.* 42.

70. CAT, AMA. 1953. *Aviation Toxicology: An Introduction to the Subject and a Handbook of Data Committee of Aviation Toxicology.* Blakiston: Aero Medical Association.

71. Tupper, C. R. 1989. Chemical hazards in aeromedical aircraft. *Aviation, Space and Environmental Medicine* 60:73–75.

72. Smith, P. W., D. J. Lacefield, C. R. Crane. 1970. Toxicological findings in aircraft accident investigation. *Aerospace Medicine* 41:760–762.

73. Trimble, E. J. 1996. The management of aircraft passenger survival in fire. *Toxicology* 115, 41.

74. ASHRAE. 1999. Air Quality within Commercial Aircraft: ASHRAE Standard 161. American Society for Heating, Refrigeration, Air Conditioning and Energy, Atlanta.

75. Nagda, N. L., H. E. Rector. 2003. A critical review of reported air concentrations of organic compounds in aircraft cabins. *Indoor Air.* 13(3):292–301.

76. Winder, C., J. C. Balouet. 2006. Aircrew exposure to chemicals in aircraft: Irritation and toxicity symptoms of irritation and toxicity. *Journal of Occupational Health and Safety – Australia and New Zealand* 17: 471–483.

77. Echobion, D. J. 1993. Historical development. In *Pesticides and Neurological Diseases*, 2nd ed., D. J. Echobion, R. M. Joy, eds., Boca Raton, FL: CRC Press, pp. 2–19.

78. Aldridge, W. N. 1954. Tricresyl phosphates and cholinesterase. *Biochem. J.* 56:185–189.

79. Johnson, M. K. 1975. Structure-activity relationships for substrates and inhibitors of hen brain neurotoxic esterase. *Biochem. Pharmacol.* 24:797.

80. Earl, C. J., R. H. S. Thompson. 1952. Cholinesterase levels in the nervous system in tri-ortho-cresyl phosphate poisoning. *Brit. J. Pharmacol.* 7:685.

81. Eyer, P. 1995. Neuropsychopathological changes by organophosphorus compounds—A review. *Hum. Exp. Toxicol.* 14:857.

82. Kilburn, K. H. 1999. Evidence for chronic neurobehavioral impairment from chlorpyrifosa an organophosphate insecticides used indoors. *Environ. Epidemiol. Toxicol.* 1:153.

83. Minton, N. A., V. S. G. Murray. 1988. A review of organophosphate poisoning. *Med. Toxicol.* 3:350.

84. Johnson, M. K. 1975. Organophosphorus esters causing delayed neurotoxic effects: Mechanism of action and structure activity studies. *Arch Toxicol.* 34:259–288.

85. Metcalf, R. L. 1982. Historical perspective of organophosphorous ester-induced delayed neurotoxicity. *Neurotoxicology* 3:269.

86. Baron, R. L. 1981. Delayed neurotoxicity and other consequences of organophosphate esters. *Ann. Rev. Entolomol.* 26:29.

87. Johnson, M. K. 1990. Organophosphates and delayed neuropathy- Is NTE alive and well. *Toxicol. Appl. Pharmacol.* 102:385.

88. Senanayake, N., L. Karalliede. 1987. Neurotoxic effects of organophosphorus esters: An intermediate syndrome. *N. Engl. J. Med.* 316:761.

89. Dille, J. R., P. W. Smith. 1964. Central nervous system effects of chronic exposure to organophosphate insecticides. *Aerosp. Med.* 35:475.

90. Savage, E. P., T. F. Keefe, L. M. Mounce, J. A. Heaton, P. L. Burcar. 1988. Chronic neurological sequelae of acute organophosphorus pesticide intoxication. *Arch. Environ. Health* 43:38–45.

91. Rosenstock, L., M. Keifer, W. E. Daniell, R. McConnell, K. Claypoole. 1991. Chronic central nervous system effects of acute organophosphate pesticide intoxication. *Lancet* 338:225–227.

92. Steenland, M. 1996. Chronic neurological effects of organophosphate pesticides. *Brit. Med. J.* 312:1311.

93. UK DoH. 1999. Toxicology of Ops and the mechanisms involved. In *Organophosphates Committee on Toxicity of Chemicals in Food, Consumer Products and the Environment UK Department of Health.* London: HMSO.

94. Jamal, G. A. 1997. Neurological syndromes of organophosphorus compounds. *Adv. Drug React. Toxicol. Rev.* 16:133.

95. Gershon, S., F. B. Shaw. 1961. Psychiatric sequelae of chronic exposure to organophosphorous insecticides. *Lancet* 1:1371.

96. Metcalf, D. R., J. H. Y. Holmes. 1969. EEG, psychological and neurological alterations in humans with organophosphorous exposure. *Ann. NY Acad. Sci.* 160, 357.

97. Callender, T. J., L. Morrow, K. Subramanian. 1994. Evaluation of chronic neurological sequelae after acute pesticide exposure using SPECT brain scans. *J. Toxicol. Environ. Health* 41, 275.

98. Abou-Donia, M. B. 2004. *Arch. Environ.* Organophosphorus ester-induced chronic neurotoxicity. *Health* 58, 484.

99. Abou-Donia, M. 2005. *Contaminated Air Protection Conference: Proceedings of a Conference,* Imperial College, London, April 20–21, 2005. C. Winder, ed., BALPA/UNSW, Sydney, 59.

100. Smith, M. I., I. Elvove, P. J. Valaer, W. H. Frazier, G. E. Mallory. 1930. Pharmacologic and chemical studies of the cause of the so called ginger paralysis. *US Pub. Health Rep.* 45:1703.

101. Henschler, D., H. H. Bayer. 1958. Toxicologic studies of triphenyl phosphate, trixenyl phosphates, and triaryl phosphates from mixtures of homogenous phenols. *Arch. Exp. Pathol. Pharmacol.* 233:512.

102. Henschler, D. 1958. Die Trikresylphosphatvergiftung. Experimentelle Klärung von Problemen der Ätiologie und Pathogenese (Tricresyl phosphate poisoning. Experimental clarification of problems of etiology and pathogenesis). *Klin. Wochens.* 36:663.304

103. McCormick, D. L. et al. 1993. Reduction of tricresyl phosphate (TCP) Neurotoxicity by a modified manuracturing process. *Toxicologist* 13:122.

104. Winder, C., J. C. Balouet. 2002. Toxicity of Commercial Air Jets. *Environ. Res.* 89:146.

105. Mackerer, C. R., E. N. Ladov. 1999. Mobil USA Submission to the Australian Senate Inquiry into Air Safety—Bae 146 Cabin Air Quality.

106. WHO. 1986. *Early Detection of Occupational Diseases.* Geneva: World Health Organization, 154.

107. Healy, C. E., R. S. Nair, W. E. Ribelin, C. L. Bechtel. 1992. Subchronic rat inhalation study with Skydrol 500B-4 ire resistant hydraulic fluid. *Am. Ind. Hyg. Assoc. J.* 53:175–180.

108. Carpenter, H. M., D. J. Jenden, N. R. Shulman, J. R. Tureman. 1959. Toxicology of a triaryl phosphate oil: I Experimental toxicology. *AMA Arch. Ind. Health* 20:234–252.

109. Mattie, D. R., T. J. Hoeflich, C. E. Jones, M. L. Horton, R. E. Whitmire, C. S. Godin, C. D. Femming, M. E. Andesen. 1993. The comparative toxicity of operational air force hydraulic fluids. *Toxicol. Ind. Health* 9:995.

110. Hewstone, R. K. 1994. Environmental health aspects of lubricant additives. *Sci. Total Environ.* 156:243.

111. Stewart, P. A., J. S. Lee, D. E. Marano, R. Spirtas, C. D. Forbes, A. Blair. 1991. Retrospective cohort mortality study of workers at an aircraft maintenancefacility. II Exposures and their assessment. *Brit. J. Ind. Med.* 48:531.

112. Ritchie, G. D., K. R. Stiull, W. K. Alexander, A. F. Nordholm, C. L. Wilson, J.III. Rossi, D. R. Matrtie. 2001. A review of the neurotoxicity risk of selected hydrocarbon fuels. *J. Toxicol. Environ. Health B: Crit. Rev.* 4:223.

113. Kanikkannan, N., S. Burton, R. Patel, T. Jackson, M. S. Shaik, M. Singh. 2001. Percutaneous permeation and skin irritation of JP-8+100 jet fuel in a porcine model. *Toxicol. Lett.* 119:133.

114. Harris, D. T., D. Sakiestewa, D. Titone, R. F. Robledo, R. S. Young, M. Witten. 2001. Jet Fuel Induced Immunotoxicity. *Toxicol. Ind. Health* 16:261.

115. Kabbur, M. G., J. V. Rogers, P. G. Gunasekar, C. M. Garett, K. T. Geiss, W. W. Brinkley, J. N. McDougal. 2001. Effect of JP-8 jet fuel on molecular and biological parameters related to acute irritation. *Toxicol. Appl. Pharmacol.* 175:83.

116. Tu, R. H., C. S. Mitchell, G. G. Kay, T. H. Risby. 2004. Human exposure to the jet fuel, JP-8. *Aviat. Space Environ. Med.* 75:49.

117. Monteriro-Riviere, N. A., A. O. Inman, J. E. Riviere. 2004. Skin toxicity of jet fuels: Ultrastructural studies and the effects of substance. *Toxicol. Appl. Pharmacol.* 195:339.

118. Tesseraux, I. 2004. Risk factors of jet fuel combustion. *Toxicol. Lett.* 149:295.

119. Hobson, D. W., A. P. D'Addario, R. H. Bruner, D. E. Uddin. 1986. A subchronic dermal exposure study of diethylene glycol monomethyl ether and ethylene glycol monomethyl ether in the male guinea pig12. *Fund. Appl. Toxicol.* 6:339.

120. Geiss, K. T., J. M. Frazier. 2001. In vitro toxicities of experimental jet fuel system ice-inhibiting agents. *Sci. Total Environ.* 274:209.

121. Buck, W. H. 1999. Mobil Oil Corporation. 27 July.

122. ACC. 2001. *High Production Volume Chemical Submission. Substituted Diphenylamines.* Arlington, VA: American Chemistry Council. 18 December, 2001. http://www.epa.gov.gov/chemrtk/subdiapha/c13378.pdf

123. Miyazaki, K., S. Kawai, T. Sasayama, K. Iseki, T. Arita. 1987. Absorption, metabolism and excretion of N-phenyl-1-naphthylamine in rats. *Yakuzaigaku. Arch. Pract. Pharm.* 47:17, English abstract.

124. IPCS. 1998. *CICAD No 9: N-Phenyl-1-Naphthylamine.* Geneva: International Programme on Chemical Safety.

125. Boman, A., G. Hagelthorn, I. Jeansson, A.-T. Karberg, I. Rystedt, J. E. Wahlberg. 1980. Phenyl-alpha-naphthylamine—case report and guinea pig studies. *Cont. Dermat.* 6:299.

126. Kalimo, K., R. Jolanki, T. Estlander, L. Kanerva. 1989. Contact allergy to antioxidants in industrial greases. *Cont. Dermat.* 20:151.

127. Carmichael, A. J., I. S. Foulds. 1990. Isolated naphthylamine allergy to phenyl-alpha-naphthylamine. *Cont. Dermat.* 22:298.

128. Wang, H.-W., D. Wang, R.-W. Dzeng. 1984. Carcinogenicity of /V-phenyl-1-naphthylamme and JV-penyl-2-naphthylamine in mice. *Cancer Res.* 44:3098.

129. Jarvholm, B., B. Lavenius. 1981. A cohort study on cancer among workers exposed to an antirust oil. *Scand. J. Work Environ. Health* 7:179.

130. Balouet, J. C., C. Winder. 1999. *American Society of Testing and Materials (ASTM) Symposium on Air Quality and Comfort in Airliner Cabins*, New Orleans, USA.

131. Winder C. 2006. Hazardous chemicals on jet aircraft: Case study---jet engine oils and aerotoxic syndrome. *Curr Top Toxicol.* 3:65–88.

132. Smith, C. W. 1987. Eectrical snsitivities in alergy ptients. *Clinical Ecology* 4(3): 93–102.

133. Winder, C., S. Michaelis. 2005. Air quality in airplane cabins and similar enclosed spaces. In: *Handbook. Environmental Chemistry*, M. Hocking, ed., 4 Part H, p. 212. Springer Berlin Heidelberg.

134. van Netten, C. 2005. Air quality in airplane cabins and similar enclosed spaces. In: *Handbook. Environmental Chemistry*, M. Hocking, ed., 4 Part H, p. 193. Springer Berlin Heidelberg.

135. Harper, A. 2005. *Contaminated Air Protection Conference: Proceedings of a Conference*, Imperial College, London, April 20–21, 2005. C. Winder, ed., BALPA/UNSW, Sydney, 43.

136. Somers, M. 2005. *Contaminated Air Protection Conference: Proceedings of a Conference*, Imperial College, London, April 20–21, 2005. C. Winder, ed., UNSW, Sydney, 2005. 129.

137. Burdon, J., A. R. Glanvile. 2005. *Contaminated Air Protection Conference: Proceedings of a Conference*, Imperial College, London, April 20–21, 2005. C. Winder, ed., UNSW, Sydney, 53.

138. Heuser, G., O. Aguilera, S. Heuser, R. Gordon. 2005. *Contaminated Air Protection Conference: Proceedings of a Conference*, Imperial College, London, April 20–21, 2005. C. Winder, ed., UNSW, Sydney, 43.305

139. Coxon, L. 2002. Neuropsychological assessment of a group of BAe 146 aircraft crew members exposed to jet engine oil emissions. *J. Occup. Health Safety-Aust. NZ.* 18:313.

140. Michaelis, S. 2011. Contaminated aircraft cabin air. *J. Biol. Phys. Chem.* 11:132–145.

141. Crump, D., P. Harrison, C. Walton. 2011. *Aircraft Cabin Air Sampling Study; Part 1 of the Final Report Publisher.* Cranford (Bedfordshire), UK: Cranfied University.

142. Crump, D., P. Harrison, C. Walton. 2011. *Aircraft Cabin Air Sampling Study; Part 2 of the Final Report Publisher.* Cransfield (Bedfordshire), UK: Institute of Environment and Health.

143. Winder, C., J. C. Balouet. 2001. Aerotoxic syndrome. *Toxicology* 164:47–47.

144. Roger, H., Y. Poursines, M. Recordier. 1934. Polyneuritis after curative antitetanic serotherapy, with participation of the central nervous system and of the meninges (Anatomo-clinical observation). *Rev. Neurol-France* 1:1078–1088.

145. Abeyratne, R. 2002. Forensic aspects of the aerotoxic syndrome. *Med. Law.* 21:179–199.

146. Hale, M. A., J. A. Al-Seffar. 2009. Preliminary report on aerotoxic syndrome (AS) and the need for diagnostic neurophysiological tests. *Am. J. Electroneurodiagnostic Technol.* 49:260–279.

147. Smith, H. V., J. M. Spalding. 1959. Outbreak of paralysis in Morocco due to ortho-cresyl phosphate poisoning. *Lancet* 2:1019–1021.

148. Vasilescu, C., A. Florescu. 1980. Clinical and electrophysiological study of neuropathy after organophosphorus compounds poisoning. *Arch. Toxicol.* 43:305–315.

149. Susser, M., Z. Stein. 1957. An outbreak of tri-ortho-cresyl phosphate (T.O.C.P.) poisoning in Durban. *Br. J. Ind. Med.* 14:111–120.

150. Senanayake, N. 1981. Tri-cresyl phosphate neuropathy in Sri Lanka: A clinical and neurophysiological study with a three year follow up. *J. Neurol. Neurosurg. Psychiatry* 44:775–780.

151. Srivastava, A. K., M. Das, S. K. Khanna. 1990. An outbreak of tricresyl phosphate poisoning in Calcutta, India. *Food Chem. Toxicol.* 28:303–304.

152. Wang, D., Y. Tao, Z. Li. 1995. Toxic polyneuropathy due to flour contaminated with tricresyl phosphate in China. *J. Toxicol. Clin. Toxicol.* 33:373–374.

153. Casida, J. E., M. Eto, R. L. Baron. 1961. Biological activity of a trio-cresyl phosphate metabolite. *Nature* 191:1396–1397.

154. Clement, J. G. 1984. Importance of aliesterase as a detoxification mechanism for soman (Pinacolyl methylphosphonofluoridate) in mice. *Biochem. Pharmacol.* 33:3807–3811.

155. Boskovic, B. 1979. The influence of 2-/o-cresyl/-4 H-1:3:2-benzodioxa-phosphorin-2-oxide (CBDP) on organophosphate poisoning and its therapy. *Arch Toxicol.* 42:207–216.

156. Garrett, T. L., C. M. Rapp, R. D. Grubbs, J. J. Schlager, J. B. Lucot. 2010. A murine model for sarin exposure using the carboxylesterase inhibitor CBDP. *Neurotoxicology* 31:502–508.

157. Maxwell, D. M. 1992. The specificity of carboxylesterase protection against the toxicity of organophosphorus compounds. *Toxicol. Appl. Pharm.* 114:306–312.

158. Jimmerson, V. R., T. M. Shih, D. M. Maxwell, A. Kaminskis, R. B. Mailman. The effect of 2-(o-cresyl)-4H-1:3:2-benzodioxaphosphorin-2-oxide on tissue cholinesterase and carboxylesterase activities of the rat. *Fundam. App. Toxicol. (Official J. Soc. Toxicol.).* 13:568–575.

159. Quistad, G. B., R. Klintenberg, J. E. Casida. 2005. Blood acylpeptide hydrolase activity is a sensitive marker for exposure to some organophosphate toxicants. *Toxicol. Sci.* 86:291–299.

160. Sprague, G. L., T. R. Castles. 1985. Estimation of the delayed neurotoxic potential and potency for a series of triaryl phosphates using an in vitro test with metabolic activation. *Neurotoxicology* 6:79–86.

161. Kim, J. H., R. C. Stevens, M. J. Maccoss, D. R. Goodlett, A. Scherl, R. J. Richter, S. M. Suzuki, C. E. Furlong. 2010. Identification and characterization of biomarkers of organophosphorus exposures in humans. *Adv. Exp. Med. Biol.* 660:61–71.

162. Quistad, G. B., J. E. Casida. 2000. Sensitivity of blood-clotting factors and digestive enzymes to inhibition by organophosphorus pesticides. *J. Biochem. Mol. Toxicol.* 14:51–56.

163. Stefanidou, M., S. Athanaselis, H. Spiliopoulou. 2009. Butyrylcholinesterase: Biomarker for exposure to organophosphorus insecticides. *Intern. Med. J.* 39:57–60.

164. Lu, W. J., V. Ferlito, C. Xu, D. A. Flockhart, S. Caccamese. 2011. Enantiomers of naringenin as pleiotropic, stereoselective inhibitors of cytochrome P450 isoforms. *Chirality.* 23:891–896.

165. Marsillach, J., R. J. Richter, J. H. Kim, R. C. Stevens, M. J. MacCoss, D. Tomazela, S. M. Suzuki, L. M. Schopfer, O. Lockridge, C. E. Furlong. 2011. Biomarkers of organophosphorus (OP) exposures in humans. *Neurotoxicology* 32:656–660.

166. Murawski, J. T. L. International Conference Environmental System, Vol. 2011 Portland: Case study: Analysis of reported contaminated air events at one major US airline in 2009–2010.306

167. Liyasova, M., B. Li, L. M. Schopfer, F. Nachon, P. Masson, C. E. Furlong, O. Lockridge. 2011. Exposure to tri-o-cresyl phosphate detected in jet airplane passengers. *Toxicol. Appl. Pharm.* 256:337–347.

168. Sinnett, M. 2007. 787 No-bleed systems. *Aeromagazine* 4:1–4.

169. Weiner, M. L., B. S. Jortner. 1999. Organophosphate-induced delayed neurotoxicity of triarylphosphates. *Neurotoxicology* 20:653–673.

170. Durham, H. D., D. J. Ecobichon. 1984. The function of motor nerves innervating slow tonic skeletal muscle in hens with delayed neuropathy induced by tri-o-tolyl phosphate. *Can. J. Physiol. Pharmacol.* 62:1268–1273.

171. Carrington, C. D., H. R. Brown, M. B. Abou-Donia. 1988. Histopathological assessment of triphenyl phosphite neurotoxicity in the hen. *Neurotoxicology* 9:223–233.

172. Veronesi, B. 1984. A rodent model of organophosphorus-induced delayed neuropathy: Distribution of central (spinal cord) and peripheral nerve damage. *Neuropathol. Appl. Neurobiol.* 10:357–368.

173. Saboori, A. M., D. M. Lang, D. S. Newcombe. 1991. Structural requirements for the inhibition of human monocyte carboxylesterase by organophosphorus compounds. *Chem. Biol. Interact.* 80:327–338.

174. Richards, P. G., M. K. Johnson, D. E. Ray. 2000. Identification of acylpeptide hydrolase as a sensitive site for reaction with organophosphorus compounds and a potential target for cognitive enhancing drugs. *Mol. Pharmacol.* 58:577–583.

175. Pancetti, F., C. Olmos, A. Dagnino-Subiabre, C. Rozas, B. Morales. 2007. Noncholinesterase effects induced by organophosphate pesticides and their relationship to cognitive processes: Implication for the action of acylpeptide hydrolase. *J. Toxicol. Environ. Health B Crit. Rev.* 10:623–630.

176. Daughtrey, W., R. Biles, B. Jortner, M. Erlich. 1996. Subchronic delayed neurotoxicity evaluation of jet engine lubricants containing phosphorus additives. *Fundam. Appl. Toxicol.* 32:244–249.

177. Fioroni, F., A. Moretto, M. Lotti. 1995. Triphenylphosphite neuropathy in hens. *Arch. Toxicol.* 69:705–711.

178. Glynn, P. Axonal degeneration and neuropathy target esterase. *Arh. Hig. Rada. Toksikol.* 58:355–358.

179. Read, D. J., Y. Li, M. V. Chao, J. B. Cavanagh, P. Glynn. 2009. Neuropathy target esterase is required for adult vertebrate axon maintenance. *J. Neurosci. Official J. Soc. Neurosci.* 29:11594–11600.

180. Atkins, J., P. Glynn. 2000. Membrane association of and critical residues in the catalytic domain of human neuropathy target esterase. *J. Biol. Chem.* 275:24477–24483.

181. Glynn, P. 1999. Neuropathy target esterase. *Biochem. J.* 344(Pt 3):625–631.

182. Erlund, I., E. Meririnne, G. Alfthan, A. Aro. 2001. Plasma kinetics and urinary excretion of the flavanones naringenin and hesperetin in humans after ingestion of orange juice and grapefruit juice. *J. Nutrition* 131:235–241.

183. Rea, W. J. 1978. Environmentally triggered cardiac disease. *Ann. Allergy* 40:24.

184. Budiansky, S. 1980. Indoor air pollution. *Environ. Sci. Technol.* 14:1023–1027.

185. Pellizzari, E. D., T. D. Hartwell, R. L. Perritt, C. M. Sparacino, L. S. Sheldon, H. S. Zelon, R. W. Whitmore, J. J. Breen, L. Wallace. 1986. Comparison of indoor and outdoor residential levels of volatile chemicals in five U.S. geographical areas. *Environ. Int.* 12:619–623.

186. Bluyssen, P. M., P. O. Fanger. 1990. Addition of olfs from different pollution sources. In Indoor Air '90. *Procedings of 5th International Conference on Indoor Air Quality and Climate*, Toronto, July 29–August 3, 1990. D. S. Walkinshaw, ed., Vol. I, p. 569. Ottawa: Canada Mortgage and Housing Corporation.

187. Rea, W. J. 1976. Environmentally triggered thrombophlebitis. *Ann. Allergy* 37:101.

188. Randolph, T. G. 1964. The ecologic unit. Part I. *Hosp. Manage.* 97:45–47.

189. American Conference of Governmental Industrial Hygienists. 1981. *TLV's: Threshold Limit Values for Chemical Substances and Physical Agents in the Workroom Environment with Intended Changes for 1981*. Cincinnati, OH: ACGIH Publications Office.

190. Ziem, G. E., B. I. Castleman. 1989. Threshold limit values: Historical perspectives and current practice. *J. Occup. Med.* 31(11):910–918.

191. Wilding, B. C. 1991. Hazardous Chemicals in Health Care. Physicians for Responsibility.

192. Greiner, E., T. Kaelin, K. Nakamura. 2007. Bisphenol A. Report completed by SRI Consulting. Retrieved September 24, 2009. http://www.sriconsulting.com/CEH/Public/Reports/619.5000/

193. vom Saal, F. S. et al. 2007. Chapel Hill Bisphenol A Expert Panel Consensus Statement: Integration of mechanisms, effects in animals and potential impact to human health at current exposure levels. *Reprod. Toxicol.* 24:131–138. Retrieved September 28, 2009. http://www.environmentalhealthnews.org/newscience/2007/2007-0801bpaconsensus.pdf307

194. Myers, P. 2007. Synopsis comments on the Chapel Hill Bisphenol A Expert Panel Consensus Statement: Integration of mechanisms, effects in animals and potential impact to human health at current exposure levels. Retrieved September 28, 2009. http://www.environmentalhealthnews.org/newscience/2007/2007-0803chapelhillconsensus.html

195. Fernández, M., M. Bianchi, V. Lux-Lantos, C. Libertun. 2009. Neonatal exposure to bisphenol A alters reproductive parameters and gonadotropin releasing hormone signaling in female rats. *Environ. Health Perspect.* 117(5):757–762. Retrieved September 21, 2009. http://www.ehponline.org/members/2009/0800267/0800267.pdf

196. Muhlhauser, A., M. Susiarjo, C. Rubio, J. Griswold, G. Gorence, T. Hassold, P. A. Hunt. 2009. Bisphenol A effects on the growing mouse oocyte are influenced by diet. Retreived September 19, 2009. *Biol. Reprod.* doi: 10.1095/biolreprod.108.074815.

197. Jenkins, S., N. Raghuraman, I. Eltoum, M. Carpenter, J. Russo, C. Lamartiniere. 2009. Oral exposure to bisphenol A increases dimethylbenzanthracene-induced mammary cancer in rats. *Environ. Health Perspect.* 117(6):910–915. Retrieved September 21, 2009. http://www.ehponline.org/members/2009/11751/11751.pdf

198. Prin, G. S., L. Birch, W. T. Tang, S. M. Ho. 2007. Developmental estrogen exposures predispose to prostate carcinogenesis with aging. *Reprod. Toxicol.* 23(3):374–382.

199. Leranth, C., T. Hajszan, K. Szigeti-Buck, J. Bober, N. J. MacLusky. 2008. Bisphenol A prevents the synaptogenic response to estradiol in hippocampus and prefrontal cortex of ovariectomized nonhuman primates. *Proc. Nat. Acad. Sci.* 105:13705–13706. Retrieved September 21, 2009. http://www.pnas.org/content/105/37/14187.abstract?sid=5fd20951-d04a-4703-ba8a-c3ac855afab1.32 hazardous chemicals in health care

200. Hugo, E. R., T. D. Brandebourg, J. G. Woo, J. Loftus, J. Wesley-Alexander, N. Ben-Jonathan. 2008. Bisphenol A at environmentally relevant doses inhibits adiponectin release from human adipose tissue explants and adipocytes. *Environ. Health Perspect.* 116(12):1642–1647. Retrieved September 28, 2009. http://www.ehponline.org/members/2008/11537/11537.pdf

201. Lang I., T. Galloway, A. Scarlett, W. E. Henley, M. Depledge, R. B. Wallace, D. Melzer. 2008. Association of urinary Bisphenol A concentration with medical disorders and laboratory abnormalities in adults. *J. Am. Med. Assoc.* 300(11):1303–1310.

202. Heimeier, R., B. Das, D. R. Buchholz, Y. B. Shi. 2009. The xenoestrogen bisphenol A inhibits postembryonic vertebrate development by antagonizing gene regulation by thyroid hormone. *Endocrinology* 150(6):2964–2973.

203. CDC Morbidity and Mortality Weekly Report. 1999. Morbidity and Mortality Weekly Report 50(08)140. Blood and Hair Mercury Levels in Young Children and Women of Child Bearing Age-United States. 03 February, 2001.

204. Betts, K. S. 2007. Perfluoroalkyl acids: What is the evidence telling us? *Environ. Health Perspect.* 115(5): A250–A256. Retrieved September 28, 2009. http://www.ehponline.org/members/2007/115-5/focus.html

205. Washino, N. et al. 2009. Correlations between prenatal exposure to perfluorinated chemicals and reduced fetal growth. *Environ. Health Perspect.* 117(4):660–667. Retrieved September 18, 2009. http://www.pubmedcentral.nih.gov/articlerender.fcgi?tool=pmcentrez&artid=2679613

206. Kim, H. S., T. S. Kim, J. H. Shin, H. J. Moon, I. H. Kang, I. Y. Kim, J. Y. Oh, S. Y. Han. 2004. Neonatal exposure to di(n-butyl) phthalate (DBP) Alters male reproductive-tract development. *J. Toxicol. Environ. Health A* 67(23, 24):2045–2060.

207. Eriksson, P., E. Jakobsson, A. Fredriksson. 2001. Brominated flame retardants: A novel class of developmental neurotoxicants in our environment? *Environ. Health Perspect.* 109(9):903–908.

208. McDonald, T. A. 2002. A perspective on the potential health risk of PBDEs. *Chemosphere* 46, 745–755.

209. Kanetoshi, A., H. Ogawa, E. Katsura, H. Kaneshima. 1987. Chlorination of Irgasan DP300 and formation of dioxins from its chlorinated derivatives. *J. Chromatography* 389:139–153.

210. Zorrilla, L. M., E. K. Gibson, S. C. Jeffay, K. M. Crofton, W. R. Setzer, R. L. Cooper, T. E. Stoker. 2008. The effects of triclosan on puberty and thyroid hormones in male wistar rats. *Toxicol. Sci.* doi: 10.1093/toxsci/kfn225.

211. Calafat, A., X. Ye, L. Y. Wong, J. A. Reidy, L. L. Needham. 2008. Urinary concentrations of triclosan in the U.S. population: 2003–2004. *Environ. Health Perspect.* 116(3):303–307. Retrieved September 24, 2009. http://www.ehponline.org/members/2007/10768/10768.pdf

212. Buemi, M., F. Floccari, M. Nettò, A. Allegra, F. Grasso, G. Mondio, P. Perillo. 2000. Environmental Air pollution in an intensive care unit for nephrology and dialysis. *J. Nephrol.* 13(6):433–436.308

213. Occupational Safety and Health Administration. 2013. https://www.osha.gov/SLTC/etools/hospital/hazards/glutaraldehyde/glut.html

214. California Environmental Protection Agency, Air Resources Board. 2012. Air pollution and contaminants at child-care and preschool facilities in California. www.arb/ca.gov

215. Berkeley Lab, Environmental Energy Technologies Division (EETD). 2013. Study Finds Reasons to Improve Indoor Air Quality in Childcare Facilities. http://eetd.lbl.gov/news/article/25185/study-finds-reasons-to-improve-indoor-air-qual

216. Maddalena, R. and T. McKone. 2012. Lawrence berkeley national laboratory (berkeley lab). Study finds reasons to improve indoor air quality in childcare facilities.

217. NursingHomes.org. 2010. 50 Articles about the impact of nursing home air quality on patient health and wellness. http://www.nursinghomes.org/50-articles-about-the-impact-of-nursing-home-air-quali

218. Teschke, K., Y. Chow, C. van Netten, S. Varughese, S. M. Kennedy, M. Brauer. 2005. Exposures to atmospheric effects in the entertainment industry. *J. Occup. Environ. Hyg.* 2(5):277–284.

219. Varughese, S., K. Teschke, M. Brauer, Y. Chow, C. van Netten, S. M. Kennedy. 2005. Effects of theatrical smokes and fogs on respiratory health in the entertainment industry. *Am. J. Ind. Med.* 47(5):411–418.

220. Milz, S., F. Akbar-Khanzadeh, A. Ames, S. Spino, C. Tex, K. Lanza. 2007. Indoor Air quality in restaurants with and without designated smoking rooms. *J. Occup. Environ. Hyg.* 4(4):246–252.

221. Li, W. M., S. C. Lee, L. Y. Chan. 2001. Indoor air quality at nine shopping malls in Hong Kong. *Sci. Total Environ.* 273(1–3):27–40.

222. Wolkoff, P., C. K. Wilkins, P. A. Clausen, G. D. Nielsen. 2006. Organic compounds in office environments-sensory irritation, odor, measurements an d the role of reactive chemistry. *Indoor Air* 16(1):7–19.

223. Morrison, G. C., W. W. Nazaroff, J. A. Cano-Ruiz, A. T. Hodoson, M. P. Modera. 1998. Indoor air quality impacts of ventilation ducts: Ozone removal and emissions of volatile organic compounds. *J. Air Waste Manag. Assoc.* 48(10):941–952.

224. Hooper, D. G., J. Shane, D. C. Straus, K. H. Kilburn, V. Bolton, J. S. Sutton, F. T. Guilford. 2010. Isolation of sulfur reducing and oxidizing bacteria found in contaminated drywall. *Int. J. Mol. Sci.* 11, 647–655. doi: 10.3390/ijms11020647.

225. WHO/UNDP. 2004. 14 October. Indoor air pollution—The killer in the kitchen. http://www.who.mt/mediacentre/news/statements/2004/statement5/en/index.html

226. Gao, Y., Y. Zhang, M. Kamijima, K. Sakai, M. Khalequzzaman, T. Nakajima, R. Shir, X. Wang, D. Chen, X. Ji, K. Han, Y. Tian. 2014. Quantitative assessments of indoor air pollution and the risk of childhood acute leukemia in Shanghai. *Environmental Pollution-London then Barking* 187C:81–89.

227. Yamada, T., M. Ohta, S. Ucmiyami, Y. Inaba, S. Goto, N. Kunugita. 2010. Characteristics of indoor gaseous air pollutants in winter. *Journal of UOEH*, 32(3):245–255.

228. Curtis, S. 2006. Adverse health effects of outdoor air pollutants. *Environ. Int.* 32:815–830.

229. Brundage, J. F., R. M. Scott, W. M. Lednar, D. W. Smith, R. N. Miller. 1988. Building associated risk of febrile acute respiratory disease in Army trainees. *JAMA* 259:2108–2112.

230. Chauhan, A. J., S. I. Johnston. 2003. Air pollution and infection in respiratory illness. *Br. Med. Bull.* 68:95–112.

231. Schwartz, J., C. Spix, H. E. Wichman, E. Malin. 1991. Air pollution and acute respiratory illness in five German communities. *Environ. Res.* 56:1–14.

232. Estrella, B., R. Estrella, J. Oviedo, X. Narvaez, M. T. Reyes, M. Guitierrez, E. N. Naumova. 2005. Acute respiratory disease and carboxyhemoglobin status in school children in Quito, Ecuador. *Environ. Health Perspect.* 113:607–611.

233. Jaakkola, J. J., M. Paunio, M. Virtanen, O. P. Heinonen. 1991. Low-level air pollution and upper respiratory infections in children. *Am. J. Publ. Health* 81:1060–1063.

234. Keles, N., C. Ilicali. 1998. The impact of outdoor pollution on upper respiratory disease. *Rhinology* 36:24–27.

235. Stern, G., P. Latzin, M. Röösli, O. Fuchs, E. Proietti, C. Kuehni, U. Frey. 2013. A prospective study of the impact of air pollution on respiratory symptoms and infections in infants. *Am. J. Respir. Crit. Care Med.* 187:1341–1348.

236. Schwartz, J. 1994. PM10, ozone, and hospital admissions for the elderly in Minneapolis–St. Paul, Minnesota. *Arch. Environ. Health* 49:366–374.

237. Ye, F., W. T. Piver, M. Ando, C. J. Portier. 2001. Effects of temperature and air pollutants on cardiovascular and respiratory diseases for males and females older than 65 years of age in Tokyo, July and August 1980–1995. *Environ. Health Perspect.* 109:355–359.

238. Martins, L. C., M. Latorre, P. H. D. Saldiva, A. L. F. Braga. 2002. Air pollution and emergency room visits due to chronic lower respiratory diseases in the elderly: An ecological time-series study in São Paulo, Brazil. *J. Occup. Environ. Med.* 44:622–627.

239. Durry, E., D. Pappagianis, S. B. Werner, L. Hutwanger, R. K. Sun, R. Maure, M. M. McNeil, R. W. Pinner. 1997. Coccidioidomycosis in Tulare County, California, 1991: Reemergence of an endemic disease. *J. Med. Vet. Mycol.* 35:321–326.
240. Malilay, J., M. G. Real, A. Ramirez Vanegas, E. Noji, T. Sinks. 1996. Public health surveillance after a volcanic eruption: Lessons from Cerro Negro, Nicaragua, 1992. *Bull. Pam. Am. Health Organ* 30:218–226.
241. Rudnick, S. N., D. K. Milton. 2003. Risk of indoor airborne infection transmission estimated from carbon dioxide concentration. *Indoor Air* 13(3):237–245.
242. Lund, A. K., H. Oppenheim, JoAnn Lucero, L. Herber, J. McDonald. Abstract 15637: Exposure to Traffic-Generated Air Pollutants Results in Disruption of the Blood Brain Barrier through Altered Expression of Tight Junction Proteins.
243. Li, Y., G. M. Leung, J. W. Tang, X. Yang, C. V. H. Chao, J. Z. Lin, J. W. Lu, P. V. Nielson, J. Niu, H. Dian, A. C. Sleigh, H. J. J. Sa, J. Sandell, T. W. Wang, P. L. Vuea. 2007. Role of ventilation in airborne transmission of infectious agents in the build environment—A multidisciplinary systematic review. *Indoor Air* 17:2–18.
244. Stec, A. 2012. Flame retardants may create deadlier fires. *Sci. Am.* http://www.scientificamerican.com/article.cfm?id=flame-retardants-maycreat-deadlier–fires
245. Godwin, C., S. Batterman. 2007. Indoor air quality in Michigan schools. *Indoor Air* 17(2):109–121.
246. Daisey, J. M., W. J. Angell, M. G. Apte. 2003. Indoor air quality, ventilation and health symptoms in schools: An analysis of existing information. *Indoor Air* 13(1):53–64.
247. Calderon-Garciduenas, L. et al. 2011. Exposure to severe urban air pollution influences cognitive outcomes, brain volume and systemic inflammation in clinically healthy children. Journal homepage: www.elsevier.com/locate/b&c
248. WHO 2009. Updated 2016. Household Air Pollution and Health. Fact Sheet N292.

4 Inorganic Chemical Pollutants

The U.S. Environmental Protection Agency (EPA) has criteria inorganic outdoor air pollutants as follows: carbon monoxide (CO), nitrogen dioxide (NO_2), sulfur dioxide (SO_2), ozone (O_3), lead (Pb), and suspended particulate matter, which have widely variable chemical compositions (Table 4.1). For a large fraction of these criteria pollutants, well-defined limiting concentrations of ambient air quality standards have been established. However, these standards do not specify levels that are necessarily safe for all segments of the population. The chemically sensitive and chronic degenerative disease patients often cannot tolerate pollution levels which the government of the EPA says are safe (Figure 4.1).

In fact, in our opinion, pollutant concentrations may have been set too high for optimum health for any segment of the population and particularly, for the chemically sensitive and chronic degenerative disease patients. Of course, the mixtures of all of these pollutants found in the total environmental pollutant load, including the manmade and natural pollutants, are overwhelming to the individuals who develop chemical sensitivity and chronic degenerative disease.

CARBON MONOXIDE

Carbon monoxide (CO) is a colorless, tasteless, odorless gas that is formed due to incomplete combustion of carbon-based fuels. An ambient CO level greater than 100 ppm is considered toxic, and healthy individuals will start displaying severe clinical symptoms. Its toxicity is closely linked to its high affinity for hemoglobin, thus causing impaired oxygen delivery. Studies have also postulated a direct coronary effect, independent of the cellular hypoxia.[1]

In the outdoor environment, the major sources of carbon monoxide are petroleum and coal combustion from transportation and industry. Carbon monoxide may accumulate to dangerous levels when certain weather conditions are present in specific locations on earth. Due to its location adjacent to the eastern side of the Rocky Mountains and due to cold winter weather conditions with inversion, both of which combine to inhibit dispersion of pollutants, Denver, for example, is known for its high incidence of air pollution due to carbon monoxide. The other major indoor sources of carbon monoxide are unvented kerosene heaters, gas stoves, gas appliances, and cigarette smoking.

The well-known, acute effects of CO include cardiac effects (angina, ventricular arrhythmia), pulmonary effects (edema), visual effects (decreased light sensitivity, dark adaptation, tunnel vision), auditory effects (central hearing loss), neuropsychiatric effects (seizures, agitation, coma, depression, thermoregulation), dermatologic effects (bullae, alopecia, inhibition, sweat gland necrosis), and metabolic effects (lactic acidosis, myonecrosis, hyperglycemia, proteinuria).

Chronic effects involve the heart (decreased voltage, premature ventricular contractions, conduction block, lower defibrillatory threshold), neuropsychiatric functions (decreased cognitive ability, psychosis, agitation, depression, parkinsonism, incontinence), and hematologic functions (increased HB and HCT, increased erythropoietin, increased reticulocyte count, and disseminated intravascular coagulation). Such diffuse effects of carbon monoxide on the general population are inevitably intensified in the chemically sensitive and chronic degenerative disease, making this population particularly vulnerable to carbon monoxide at any concentration. These effects are due to the adverse responses seen in the enzyme detoxification systems that are already malfunctioning in the chemically sensitive and chronic degenerative diseased.

CO inhibits the cytochrome oxidase system (e.g., cytochrome A_3, cytochrome P-450) by binding to hemoproteins. It also inhibits most oxidation, degradation, and conjugation reactions which can be devastating for the chemically sensitive and chronic degenerative disease patients. Therefore, its intake

TABLE 4.1
Federal Ambient Air Quality Standards

Pollutant	Averaging Time	Primary Standard
Carbon monoxide	8 hours	9 ppm
	1 hour	35 ppm
Nitrogen dioxide	Annual average	0.05 ppm
Sulfur dioxide	Annual average	0.03 ppm
Suspended particulate matter	Annual geometric mean	75 ppm
Ozone	1 hour	0.12 ppm
Lead	3 months	1.5 $\mu g/m^3$

Source: Adapted from Godish, T. 1985. *Air Quality*, p. 217. Chelsea, MI: Lewis Publishers.

Note: These standards are for healthy humans. They are not based on long-term accumulation. No synergism is taken into account. No 24-hour, 7 day a week levels are pointed out. These federal standards are, therefore, invalid in the real world of constant exposure. They are presented so the physician will better understand their limited meaning when federal and local agencies use them as evidence of "good quality air."

into the body, even in low levels, may adversely affect detoxification systems and allow for the accumulation of toxic substances that are usually eliminated by these systems. The total body pollutant load increases. For the already vulnerable chemically sensitive, this physiological response of exposure to carbon monoxide results in exacerbation of signs and symptoms of their illness whatever they may be (Chapter 1).[2] The current exposure threshold limit value (TLV) for healthy people is 9 ppm for 8 hours and 35 ppm for 1 hour. No safe exposure threshold has been established for 7 days/week, 24 hours/day for people who are already damaged by disease or other toxic exposures such as the chemically sensitive or chronic degenerative disease. No agreed thresholds are present for mixtures in the normal population or the chemically sensitive or chronic degenerated patient, the thresholds are individual.

Most studies have focused on neurological and cardiac effects related to acute high-level CO exposures, such as accidents in domestic and industrial settings or intentional harm. However, there are additional significant CO sources in the form of industrial emissions, tobacco smoke, and

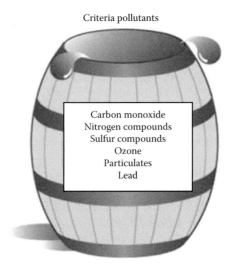

FIGURE 4.1 EPA criteria pollutants. (Rea, W.J. 1994. *Chemical Sensitivity, Volume II*, Page 713, Figure 1. With permission.)

traffic-related air pollution, as well as indoor biomass burning, used extensively in developing countries as the primary domestic energy. The EPA has set National Ambient Air Quality Standards, not to be exceeded more than once a year, at 35 ppm over a 1-hour average. Urban CO concentrations usually fluctuate between 2 and 40 ppm, but during periods of heavy traffic may well reach levels of 170 ppm.[3] Biomass combustion, however, can often climb to much higher levels, such as wildfires, wherein firefighters can be exposed to short, peak levels of 600–1000 ppm.[4] To put this in context of U.S. workplace exposure limits, the 8-hour time-weighted average exposure for CO is 50 ppm and for a short-term exposure (15 minutes), it is 200 ppm.

In a study by Dallas and colleagues, the mechanisms behind CO-induced arrhythmias were explored using isolated ventricular myocytes as well as an *in vivo* rat model.[5] The CO exposure levels chosen were 87 μM *in vitro* and 50 ppm *in vivo*, to simulate a high environmental exposure, according to the authors. The *in vitro* study demonstrated a nitrosylation of the cardiac sodium channel due to CO-induced increase in cellular NO, and thus an increase in the late Na^+ current. Myocytes were then exposed to an NO synthase (NOS) inhibitor, eliminating the previously observed CO effects providing further evidence of toxicity.

NITROGEN COMPOUNDS

The second major pollutants are the nitrous oxides. The most common of these are NO_2, N_2O, and NO. Many nitrogen compounds are known to harm the chemically sensitive and chronic degenerative disease patients and some may help them, especially NO. A few of the most common that can easily contribute to the total body pollutant load and thus increase chemical sensitivity are discussed in the following pages. Some of these compounds have been seen to induce chemical sensitivity. Most are detoxified by similar detoxification mechanisms; thus, their effects on the chemically sensitive may be cumulative.

NITROUS OXIDES

The nitrous oxides, nitrogen dioxide, and nitric oxide are discussed together, since they may occur together and may be converted to each other. All adversely affect the chemically sensitive though at times nitric oxide can be helpful as found in the NO/OONO reaction where the nitric oxide is favorable to the peroxynitrite molecule.

The major sources of nitrogen dioxide (NO_2) in outdoor air are coal and oil combustion, gas-fired transportation, and nitrogen fertilizers. For indoor air, these pollutants are generated in kerosene heaters, gas stoves, gas heaters, and arc welding. Nitric oxide (NO) and nitrous oxide (N_2O) are quickly converted to nitrogen dioxide at concentrations below 50 ppm. Therefore, high concentrations of NO may occur with low levels of NO_2, and as their levels drop, nitrogen dioxide appears (Table 4.2). The main health effect of NO is that it forms methemoglobin and subsequently acts on the nervous system. Animal experimentation indicates that NO is about one-fifth as toxic as NO_2 (assuming minimal contamination with NO_2 and no synergistic action, which may be quite unrealistic). Again, it should be emphasized that the data are limited, and levels may need to be much less due to synergisms and increased total load.

The TLV for NO is 25 ppm.[6] Again, this level does not apply to individual sensitivity for which there may be no safe limits.

The most frequent and significant N_2O respiratory effects seen at concentrations near or at ambient levels are altered lung function and symptomatic effects observed during controlled human exposure studies,[7] increased incidence of acute respiratory symptoms and illness seen in outdoor and indoor epidemiologic studies of homes using gas stoves,[8–11] and lung tissue damage and increased susceptibility to infection observed in animal toxicology studies.[12–14]

It is important to point out that controlled human exposure studies present conflicting and somewhat ambiguous results concerning respiratory effects of N_2O in both asthmatics and healthy

TABLE 4.2

Human Response to Short-Term NO$_2$ (Alone) Exposure

NO$_2$ Concentration (mg/m^3)	Exposure Time	Effect
0.23	Not reported	Odor threshold
0.14–0.50	Not reported	Threshold for dark adaptation
0.5–5.0	15 minutes	Increased airway resistance in asthmatics
11.3–15.2	5 minutes	Increased airway resistance in asthmatics and healthy adults
7.5–9.4	15 minutes	Decreases pulmonary diffusing capacity
9.4	5 minutes	Alveolar–arterial PO$_2$ difference

Source: U.S. DOE. 1986. *Indoor Air Quality Environmental Information Handbook: Radon.* Washington, DC: U.S. Department of Energy. DOE/PE/72013-2; Rea, W.J. 1994. *Chemical Sensitivity, Volume II*, Page 716, Table 2. With permission.

persons in concentrations in the range of 0.1–4.0 ppm NO$_2$ where NO$_2$ of 1 ppm equals, produces, or contains N$_2$O of 1.9 (1 ppm N$_2$O = 1.9 mg/m^3). Some studies report increased airway resistance or decreased lung function when bronchoconstricting agents are administered along with NO$_2$ exposure,[7,15,16] while others[15,17] show no statistically significant effects. One has to remember, however, that the negative studies were all performed while patients were in the masked state, without total reduction of body load. Because of this lack of consideration of deadaptation phenomenon in the study protocols, the results are probably inaccurate. The relationship of NO$_2$ exposure to respiratory effects is also relatively weak in recent indoor epidemiologic studies.[8–11,18] Animal studies substantiate an effect on immune dysfunction from NO$_2$ exposure,[13,14,19–21] but the difficulty of extrapolating these findings from animals to humans remains.

A 1977 and 2012 or 2013 study showed that workers exposed to nitrogen oxides below 2.8 ppm for 3–5 years had reduced levels of blood catalase values, which are often seen in the chemically sensitive. Also, chronic bronchitis and pulmonary emphysema were concluded to result from chronic N$_2$O exposure.[22] Exposure to nitrous gases such as those used in nitrous oxide freezing guns or anesthetics are known to cause impotency; skin flushing; destruction of methionine synthetase, B$_{12}$, and folic acid; bone marrow malfunction; cell-mediated immunity deregulation; liver dysfunction; neurological aberrations, including motor deficits; and reproductive abnormalities and deficiency with resultant chemical sensitivity and a spreading phenomenon.[23] Anaerobic bacteria of the intestine metabolize nitrous oxide through a reductive pathway. Free radicals are formed during this process and can produce toxic agents such as peroxidized lipids. Most of the toxic effects of NO$_2$ can be accounted for by the inactivation of methionine synthetase. In the chemically sensitive, failure of methylation is the primary abnormality of conjugation seen. Once this system malfunctions and toxic substances cease to be cleared, the spreading phenomenon is set in motion, and individuals become sensitive to substances such as phenol, chlorine, pesticides, and other toxic chemicals. Certainly, the chemically sensitive are vulnerable to this process, as is evidenced by the fact that the primary conjugation abnormality that they experience is methylation failure.

Epidemiological surveys have suggested that exposure to toxic amounts of nitrous oxide in the workplace can have significant health and reproductive consequences.[24] What follows is a classic case of chemical sensitivity due to nitrous oxide exposure.

Case Study: A very busy dermatologist began experiencing unusual fatigue, weakness, episodic flushing of the skin, and tachycardia about 2 years prior to presentation. These attacks of flushing progressed in intensity and frequency and were associated with itching of the skin as well.

Prior to arrival at the EHC-Dallas, he had developed intolerance to a variety of common inhalants, including cigarette smoke, vehicle exhaust, and perfumes. Contact with these produced difficulty breathing, headaches, tearing, and flushing spells, symptoms that became most intense while he was seeing patients in his office. He also began experiencing impotence and declining sexual ability.

As his illness progressed, this patient developed recurrent skin abscesses that required drainage. (He had suffered from cystic acne as a young man.) Cultures from these sites showed *Staphylococcus aureus*, *S. epidermidis*, Group B *Streptococcus*, *Proteus vulgaris*, and *P. mirabilis*.

After 1 year of progressing illness, he suddenly experienced a generalized anaphylactic reaction with shock, flushing, and laryngeal edema, apparently triggered by a cephalosporin antibiotic. More anaphylactic episodes followed with no apparent triggers detected. The flushing spells continued and became associated with chest pain, tachycardia, and palpitations. Verapamil was only marginally helpful for these cardiac symptoms. The progression of these symptoms, along with profound weakness, fatigue, and intolerance to both heat and cold, finally forced him to stop work. At the time of presentation, he complained of poor concentration and anxiety over his ill health and disability, but he was experiencing neither hallucinations nor irrational behavior.

Past history: His previous health had been robust, except for two surgical procedures: a rib resection for thoracic outlet syndrome and a lumbar disc decompression from which he recovered very quickly with no sequelae. He was a nondrinker and had not smoked for several years before the onset of this illness.

Physical exam: Heart rate was 60/minute and regular; BP was 15/80 mmHg; respiration was 16/minute; weight (dressed) was 62 lb. His general physical exam was normal except for facial erythema, cystic acne, and telangiectasis. He had a few petechial spots over his abdomen, and the skin on his hands was coarse and dry. Several infected furuncles were noted on his trunk. Neurological exam showed gross motor weakness, especially in the arms and hands. Cerebellar testing and gait appeared normal, as did his sensory exam. Mental state was also normal and appropriate. Cardiac and respiratory exam was normal. Additionally, no abdominal organomegaly was present. Medications were Vanceril for shortness of breath and, occasionally, diazepam.

Laboratory data: Extensive laboratory analysis revealed the following: Hgb = 14.1 g/dL: RBC = $4.38 \times 10^6/mm^3$; WBC = 4.60×10^3, with segs, 2990 (65%): lymphs, 1150 (25%); bands, 184 (4%); eosin, 92 (2%); platelets were 260,000; and the ESR ranged from 40 to 125.

Immunoglobulins were as follows: IgG = 991 mg/dL (normal: 54–1765 mg/dL); IgM = 133 mg/dL (normal: 42–250 mg/dL); IgA = 140 mg/dL (normal: 85–385 mg/dL); IgE (on RAST) = 7 IU/mL (normal: 15–150 IU/ML). ANA and antimitochondrial antibody (AMA) were both negative. Liver enzymes were mildly elevated: alkaline phosphatase = 117 μm/L (normal: 30–115 μm/L); SGPT = 63 μm/L (normal: 0–50 μm/L): LDH = 296 μm/L (normal: 100–225 μm/L). The SMAC was otherwise normal, including Cr = 1.0 mg/dL (normal: 0.7–1.4 mg/dL); glucose = 92 mg/dL (normal: 65–115 mg/dL).

Blood histamine levels were taken three times with readings of 5.0, 16.0, and 10.0 mcg/dL (control: 5.0–15.0). Urine histamine was 20 mcg/24 hours (control: 15–80). Blood serotonin was <22 ng/mL (control: 50–200). Hydroxyindole acetic acid (5-HIAA) levels were taken twice, with levels of 8.6 and 1.2 mg/24 hours (control: 1.0–7.0). Monoamine oxidase (MAO) was 20.2 nmol/10^8 plate/hour (control: 10.7–23.6). 17-Ketosteroids were done twice: 6.112 and 3.88 mcg/24 hours (control: 4–22).

Blood ammonia was high on three readings, at 170, 502, and 238 μmol/L (normal: 11–35). Blood acetaldehyde readings were 20 and 51.0 mcg/mL (normal: 0–2.0 mcg/mL). Thyroid function appeared normal, with T_4 = 10.4 mcg/dL (normal: 5–12 mcg/mL); T_3 uptake, 24% (normal: 22%–35%); T_7, 2.5 (normal: 1.1–4.2).

Red blood cell mineral analysis revealed several abnormalities: calcium = 9.58 mcg/mL (14–26 mcg/mL); copper = 1.24 ppm (normal: 0.56–0.88 ppm); iron = 890 ppm (normal: 910–1345 ppm); zinc = 12.20 ppm (normal: 6.20–10 ppm); and magnesium = 3.86 ppm (normal: 4.34–5.98 ppm).

A modified RAST was totally negative (class zero) for all foods tested, except lamb, which was class I. Total IgE on the RAST was reported as 7.

The erythrocyte superoxide dismutase (ESOD) was significantly depressed at 8.0 μ/mg Hb (C = 12–15). Glutathione (GSH) peroxidase was also reported to be low, at 2.08 μmol NADPH (C = 4.23–7.23). Lipid peroxide was at 2.63 nanomed/mL (C = 2.65–4.15).

Absolute T cells were significantly depressed at 907/mm³ (C = 1600–2000). Absolute B cells were 569 mm³ (C = 400–800). T_8 suppressors were decreased at 156/mm³ (C = 191–1512), and the T_4:T_8 ratio was elevated at 4.0. Blastogenesis with PHA 50 was also impaired (Table 4.3).

Skin biopsy of the area of flushing showed perivascular lymphocytic infiltrate, with no evidence of mastocytosis. The EKG showed tachycardia with left axis deviation and left anterior hemiblock. Holter monitor confirmed frequent premature atrial ventricular contractions.

Using Bionostics' case experience as our standard, we analyzed and interpreted data obtained from urine and plasma amino acid tests. We found the following: elevated plasma taurine—14 μmol/100 mL; normal urine levels; plasma methionine—low/normal; urine methionine—low; plasma cysteine—low; urine cysteine—low; and urine cystathionine—low. This overall pattern suggested disordered methionine metabolism. Retarded amino acid group transfer with multiple hyperaminoacidurias, mild hyperammonemia, and limited capacity for ammonia detoxification and mild ornithemia and glutamic acidemia suggested apparent functional deficiency in magnesium-activated enzymes (e.g., methionine synthetase).

Environmental evaluation: A careful environmental history revealed that the patient had purchased two nitrous oxide-powered cryotherapy units for his office about 6 months prior to the onset of symptoms. The patient reported that these units were used from 30 to 60 times per day in his very busy practice.

When the possibility of sensitivity to N_2O was entertained, the equipment was independently evaluated by an engineering company and found to be slowly leaking significant volumes of gas (even when not turned on) at an average flow of 18 L/ft per 3-hour period.

Environmental testing: This patient was tested in the environmental unit, a wing of the hospital that is specially designed to be less polluted. He was found to have developed various food and chemical sensitivities, including sensitivity to molds, terpenes, cigarette smoke, perfume, orris root, ethanol, house dust, fluogen, formaldehyde, and seven foods. Intradermal histamine skin testing with 0.01 mL of a 1:62,500 dilution reproduced flushing, headache, tachycardia, weakness, throat fullness, dizziness, and blurred vision. The histamine neutralizing dose was 20/7 (0.2 mL of 1:1,562,500 solution).

TABLE 4.3

Phagocytic Index and Killing Capacity in a 45-Year-Old White Male with Chemical Sensitivity

	Control	Patient
Blastogenesis Index		
PHA 50–stimulated blastogenesis	2257 cpm	933 cpm
Leukocyte Bacteriocidal Action		
Serratia marcescens	91%	84%
Staphylococcus aureus	71%	35%
Candida albicans	54%	30%
Leukocyte Phagocytic Action		
Serratia marcescens	98%	96%
Staphylococcus aureus	98%	93%
Candida albicans	92%	77%

Source: Rea, W.J. 1994. *Chemical Sensitivity, Volume II*, Page 716, Table 2. With permission.

TABLE 4.4

Double-Blind Inhaled Challenge: 45-Year-Old White Male after a Minimum of 5 Days Deadaptation in ECU with Total Load Reduced

	Substance	PPM	Reaction
Challenge 1	Placebo		No response
Challenge 2	N_2O	8	No response
Challenge 3	N_2O	80	Flushing, felt ill
Challenge 4	Placebo		No response
Challenge 5	N_2O	160	Marked flushing, felt ill, nausea, tachycardia

Source: Rea, W.J. 1994. *Chemical Sensitivity, Volume II*, Page 721, Table 4. With permission.

A double-blind inhaled challenge to nitrous oxide was performed whereby the patient was exposed for periods of 10 minute to either released N_2O. The patient was exposed to these concentrations along with two placebo challenges. The air was evacuated between exposures to prevent contamination. Three physicians monitored the patient's responses. The results are summarized in Table 4.4.

Tachycardia and flushing developed at 160 ppm, and at this point, the physicians feared the onset of the anaphylactic reaction that the patient had previously experienced. The test was, therefore, considered positive for significant nitrous oxide sensitivity and discontinued.

Long-term follow-up: This patient received appropriate ecologic treatment, including rotary diet, antigen therapy, and environmental control. Naturally, he continues to avoid as several pollutants as possible, especially nitrous oxide. He remains chemically sensitive, but is substantially improved with treatment.

Nitric oxide (NO) has been shown to form intrinsically in the body by using nitric oxide synthetase to convert arginine to NO. Nitric oxide causes free radicals because it is highly reactive.[25] Nitric oxide is found in the endothelium of blood vessels and is the substance that dilates them. It acts as a neurotransmitter affecting calcium channels and is necessary in macrophages to form nitrates and nitrites inducing inflammations. Also, Hibbs showed that nitric oxide killed tumor cells. Others have shown that nitric oxide kills adjacent neurons. Therefore, a fine line appears to exist between intrinsic NO and synthetic production with arginine conversion to NO. Imbalance of this system by pollutant injury may be another reason the chemically sensitive responds adversely. Pall has shown the values of NO at these ambient levels to change the NO/ONOO which can be extremely toxic.

Nitrous oxide and nitrogen dioxide have been shown to emanate from refineries such as the ones in Texas City, Galveston, etc. (Table 4.5).

NITRIC ACIDS

Nitric acids are used to make synthetic fertilizers and ammonia and hydrazines (Figure 4.2). Synthetic fertilizers contain nitrates made of nitric acids and can adversely affect the chemically sensitive who use these products. The negative effects of nitric acids are especially evident in farm country, where chemically sensitive patients typically do poorly.

HYDRAZINE–DIAZINE

Hydrazine (N_2H_4) is added to anticorrosion agents for heating oil tanks, boiler tubes, and borehole pipes. It has an ammonia odor, very unstable, and highly toxic. When combined with liquid oxygen, hydrazine is a valuable fuel for rocket propulsion. This reaction is accompanied by a large heat of combustion which is responsible for the high thrust. Hydrazine is often used as a foaming agent for rubber, thermoplastics, and other expanded products. The effect of hydrazines is due to the nitrogen

TABLE 4.5

NO$_x$ and NO$_2$ Ambient Air Monitoring Summary

Monitoring Location	Distance from BPTCR (Miles)	2009 (ppbv)		2010 (ppbv)	
		Max	Average	Max	Average
NO$_x$					
Texas City 34th St	1.8	115.9	6.77	95.6	6.01
Galveston 99th	8.3	76.8	4.53	108.6	4.14
Mustang Bayou	16	41.2	3.56	119.4	3.41
Seabrook Friendship Park	14.7	104.5	6.49	158.9	6.21
NO$_2$					
Texas City 34th St	1.8	41.0	5.68	43.6	5.41
Galveston 99th	8.3	43.9	3.99	43.7	3.66
Mustang Bayou	16	24.0	3.18	27.0	3.10
Seabrook Friendship Park	14.7	37.6	5.42	61.6	5.34

Source: Hosen, H. 1998, personal Communication.

gas liberated. Derivatives of hydrazine are important intermediates in the synthesis of special dyes, pharmaceutical products, and plastics. In particular, hydrazine plays an important part in the production of intermediates for the synthesis of polyamides such as nylon. Hydrazine also has a stabilizing effect on products made from natural rubber of styrene.

Hydroxylamine is sometimes prepared industrially by the reduction of salts of nitrous acid, HO—N=O, but mainly by the catalytic reduction of NO or HNO with hydrogen.[26]

The annual world production of hydroxylamine is several 100,000 tons. It has a very wide range of uses.

Once in the body, hydrazines are broken down to less toxic substances by either *oxidation* or *acetylation*. The conjugation reaction of acetylation can become overloaded and disturbed. Orderly food degradation is then disturbed, and results in food intolerance.

Ammonia

Ammonia (NH$_3$) is used in the cooling industry and farming. The greater part produced in industry is for fertilization of crops. High levels may be found in the air after artificial nitrogen fertilizing. It may also run off into underground water supplies. Excessive use of nitrates can cause acid rain.

Ammonia is formed naturally by the decay of animal and vegetable material that contains nitrogen in the form of protein. It is also formed as a product of metabolism of animals. In the manufacturing of nitrogen, water and methane (natural gas) are combined to get hydrogen ions which combine with nitrogen in the air to form ammonia.

Inhalation of high concentrations of ammonia causes temporary blindness and intolerable irritation of the eyes and the glottis. Large doses of ammonia can actually affect the cerebral energy metabolism in the brain.[27] Smaller doses cause irritation of the respiratory tract and conjunctivae. The major hazard of ammonia is to office workers from blueprinting and copying machines, to workers in the chemical industry where larger amounts of ammonia are used in the chemical processes, and to farmers exposed to fertilizers. The TLV for ammonia is 25 ppm, corresponding to about 18 mg/m^3.[28] Again, this value is probably too high for chronic exposures. Excess ammonia can overload the oxidative deamination mechanisms and create chemical sensitivity, as has been seen in the patients at the EHC-Dallas, giving both reactive airway disease and cerebral dysfunction. The catalytic oxidation of ammonia with atmospheric oxygen gives oxides of nitrogen which can easily be converted to nitric acid (Figure 4.3).

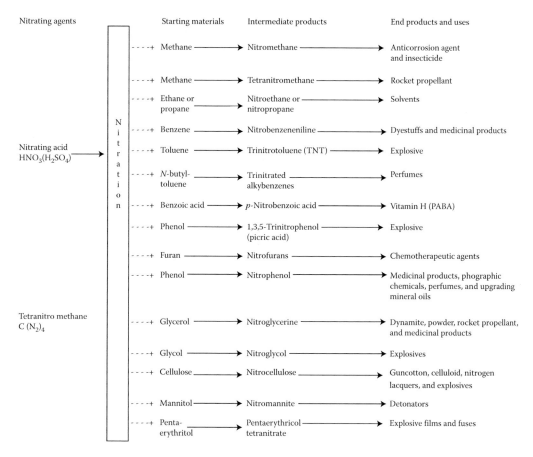

FIGURE 4.2 Some products made from nitro compounds able to exacerbate or benefit the chemically sensitive. (With permission from Hopp, V., I. Hennig. 1983. *Handbook of Applied Chemistry: Facts for Engineers, Scientists, Technicians, and Technical Managers*, Vol. IV, pp. 6–34. Washington, DC: Hemisphere Publishing; Rea, W.J. 1994. *Chemical Sensitivity, Volume II*, Page 722, Figure 2. With permission.)

SULFUR COMPOUNDS

Many sulfur compounds are known to cause and exacerbate chemical sensitivity. These are discussed together because their harmful effects are usually additive. Sometimes the reactions are violent and acutely precipitous, and sometimes they are chronic.

SULFUR AND SULFUR DIOXIDES

The main sources of sulfur dioxide in outdoor air are coal and oil combustion, transportation, sour gas fields, and refineries. Also, auto emission devices admit sulfur dioxides. Sulfuric acid is the largest quantity of inorganic substances produced by industry[29] (Figure 4.4). Sulfuric acids, along with sulfuric oxides, can account for acid rain (Figures 4.5 and 4.6). Acute exposure to sulfuric acids can be extremely toxic to humans.

Sulfur compounds can cause numerous problems, including severe allergic reactions and respiratory burns. One such compound, the volatile liquid, is carbon disulfide.

Studies of SO_2 at the Texas City Refinery shows that high levels vary during the year. The higher levels occur with the refinery flaring events but high levels persist all the time measured (Figure 4.7).

Many adverse clinical conditions are caused by sulfur compounds.

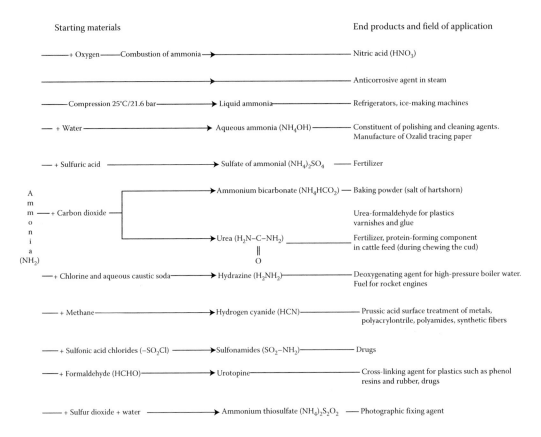

FIGURE 4.3 Products derived from ammonia. Many may adversely influence the chemically sensitive. (With permission from Hopp, V., I. Hennig. 1983. *Handbook of Applied Chemistry: Facts for Engineers, Scientists, Technicians, and Technical Managers*, Vol. II, pp. 3–17. Washington, DC: Hemisphere Publishing; Rea, W.J. 1994. *Chemical Sensitivity, Volume II*, page 724, figure 3. With permission.)

Asthmatic children are extremely susceptible to respiratory irritation from ambient air pollution, as discussed in this study. Severe asthma symptoms were observed following exposure to a +6-ppb incremented increase in daily 1-hour SO_2 maximum concentration (odds ratio [OR] = 2.36%, 95% CI: 1.16–4.81) and a +7-ppb incremented increase in daily 1-hour NO_2 maximum concentration (OR = 8.13%, 95% CI: 1.52–43.4).[30]

Smargiassi et al.[31] from Montreal showed that daytime SO_2 as the best prediction of asthma episodes.

Preliminary Air Dispersion Modeling conducted the preliminary recommendations for a class boundary would be based on parallels between reported sulfur dioxide emissions from the BP refinery in 2009 and sulfur dioxide epidemiological literature. Two peer-reviewed health studies determined a more than doubled risk in chemically sensitive children to asthma attacks or exacerbations based upon acute exposures to sulfur dioxide at concentrations greater than or equal to 50 $\mu g/m^3$. The plume generated by AERMOD using BP's reported emissions demonstrates the extent to which BP-specific air pollution is sufficient to cause an adverse respiratory response in chemically sensitive children in Texas City and La Marque. At each geographic location within the 50 $\mu g/m^3$ plume, there were at least seen instances in 2009 when the threshold was exceeded according to model predictions. Chemically sensitive children exposed to these levels are expected to suffer up to seven asthma attacks throughout the course of the modeled year as a result of BP's hazardous emissions. BP's reported emissions of sulfur dioxide were modeled for 2009 and 2010 for comparative analysis; however, 2009 was utilized from preliminary class boundary recommendation to avoid exclusion of past incurred exposure prior to 2010.

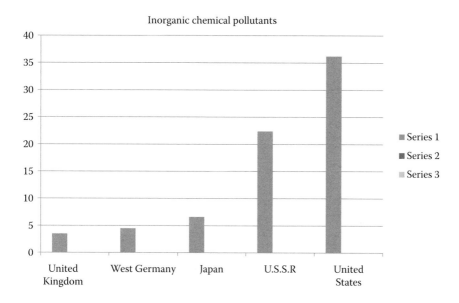

FIGURE 4.4   Sulfuric acid production—1979. Expressed as tons of H_2SO_4. (With permission from Hopp, V., I. Hennig. 1983. *Handbook of Applied Chemistry: Facts for Engineers, Scientists, Technicians, and Technical Managers*, Vol. II, pp. 5–8. Washington, DC: Hemisphere Publishing; Rea, W.J. 1994. *Chemical Sensitivity, Volume II*, Page 725, Figure 4. With permission.)

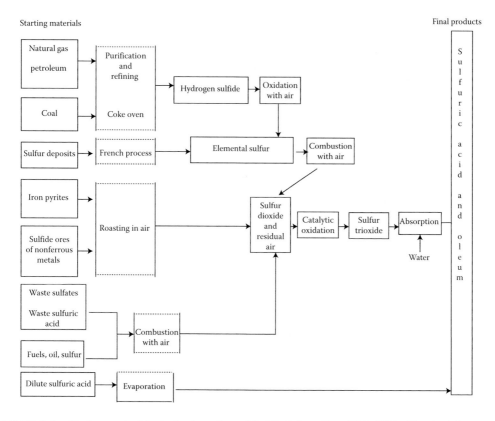

FIGURE 4.5   Starting materials to final products. Modified from Rea, W.J. 1994. *Chemical Sensitivity, Volume II*, Page 726, Figure 5. With permission.

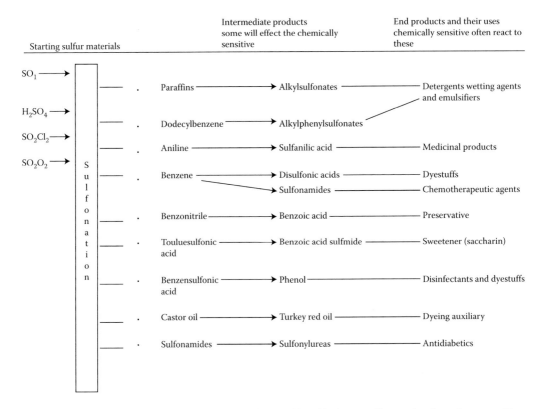

FIGURE 4.6 Summary of the manufacture of sulfuric acid and its intermediate and end products are able to influence the chemically sensitive. Some end up in the sulfur pool of the chemically sensitive, causing membrane binding of cytochrome P-450 and antibody reactions. (With permission from Hopp, V., I. Hennig. 1983. *Handbook of Applied Chemistry: Facts for Engineers, Scientists, Technicians, and Technical Managers*, Vol. IV, pp. 6–23; Vol. II, pp. 5–10. Washington, DC: Hemisphere Publishing; Rea, W.J. 1994. *Chemical Sensitivity, Volume II*, Page 727, Figure 5. With permission.)

The following materials are included in this section (Tables 4.6 and 4.7):

1. Proposed class boundary based on 2009 sulfur dioxide emissions reported to the TCEQ Emissions Inventory—seventh highest concentration at 50 $\mu g/m^3$ (Figure 4.8)
2. 2009 sulfur dioxide emissions reported to the TCEQ Emissions Inventory—highest and seventh highest concentration
3. 2009 volatile organic compound emissions reported to the TCEQ Emissions Inventory—highest and seventh highest concentration
4. 2010 sulfur dioxide emissions reported to the TCEQ Emissions Inventory—highest and seventh highest concentration
5. 2010 volatile organic compound emissions reported to the TCEQ Emissions Inventory—highest and seventh highest concentration

Winter Pollution

Short-term effect of winter air pollution on respiratory health of asthmatic children in Paris, France was seen. Winter air pollution's effect on childhood respiratory health in Paris was evaluated in this study. Changes in ambient air pollution were established as incremental increase of 50 $\mu g/m^3$ from

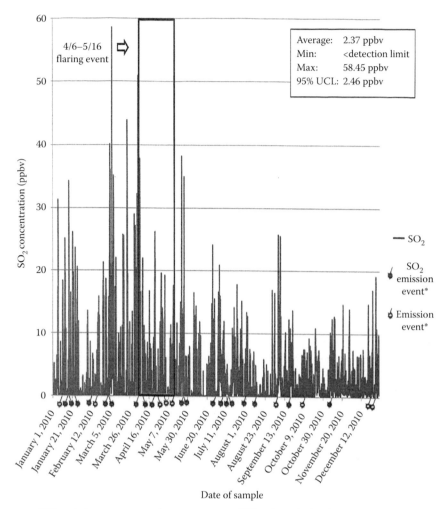

4/6–5/16
flaring event

Average:	2.37 ppbv
Min:	<detection limit
Max:	58.45 ppbv
95% UCL:	2.46 ppbv

— SO$_2$

SO$_2$
emission
event*

Emission
event*

Date of sample

*SO$_2$ emission event means there was a reported SO$_2$ release during the event.

FIGURE 4.7 2010 SO$_2$ detections at the Texas City Ball Park monitor. (Dr. Chen's Research Article Sulfur Dioxide and Volatile Organic Compound Esposure to a community in Texas City, Texas evaluated using Aermod and Empirical Monitoring Data. http://thescipub.com/html/10.,3844/ajessp.2012.622.632. With permission from Science Publications.)

daily minimum to maximum for each chemical, and resultant asthma attacks based on a number of symptom lag days were recorded. Significant associations were identified between same-day asthma attack and elevations in SO$_2$ (OR = 2.87%, 95% CI: 1.31–6.27) and NO$_2$ (OR = 2.18%, 95% CI: 1.10–4.32).[32]

There is controversy as to whether low levels of air pollution affect the symptoms and lung function in asthma. They addressed this by examining the short-term effects of winter air pollution on childhood asthma in Paris, France.

Segala et al.[32] performed a 6-month follow-up of 84 medically diagnosed asthmatic children classified into two groups of severity. The outcomes included incidence and prevalence of asthma attacks, symptoms and use of supplementary β$_2$-agonists, and peak expiratory flow (PEF) value

TABLE 4.6

Seven Highest SO$_2$ Concentrations Detected at Various Monitoring Locations 2010

SO$_2$ ppbv 1-Hour Maximum 2010

Maximum	Texas City Ball Park	Texas City 34th St.[a]	BP Texas City 31st St.	BP Texas City Onsite	BP Texas City Logan St.	2nd Avenue	Seabrook Friendship Park
First max	58	22	23	142	40	60	23
Second max	51	20	21	78	37	25	19
Third max	45	19	19	70	36	24	16
Fourth max	44	16	17	49	34	21	16
Fifth max	40	NA	17	40	33	NA	15
Sixth max	39	NA	16	35	29	NA	14
Seventh max	39	NA	16	35	28	NA	13

Source: Hosen, H. 1998, personal Communication.

[a] Texas City 34th St. and 2nd Avenue data are not publicly available. Data presented obtained from Valero monthly air monitoring reports.

NA: Data are not publicly available and have not been obtained at this time.

and its variability. The statistical analysis controlled the lack of independence between daily health outcomes, trends, and meteorology.

Air pollution was associated with an increase in reports and duration of asthma attacks and asthma attack for an increase of 50 µg/m^3 of sulfur dioxide (SO$_2$) on the same day (OR = 2.86). Maximum reduction in morning PEF (5%) and maximum increase in PEF variability (2%) were observed at a lag of 3 days for an increase of 50 µg/m^3 of SO$_2$ in the subgroup of mild asthmatics receiving no regular inhaled medication. In moderate asthmatic children, the duration of supplementary β$_2$-agonist use was strongly associated with air pollution.

The general pattern of these results provides evidence of the effect of the low levels of air pollution encountered in Western Europe on symptoms and lung function in childhood asthma.

Numerous studies conducted since 1980 have led to a better understanding of the health consequences of outdoor air pollution.[33] The presence of chemical contaminants in the air at relatively low concentrations, as is now usual in Western countries, shows harmful effects on subjects with

TABLE 4.7

SO$_2$ 1-Hour Maximums 2010 (µg/m^3)

Maximum	Texas City Ball Park	Texas City 34th St.[a]	BP Texas City 31st St.	BP Texas City Onsite	BP Texas City Logan St.	2nd Avenue	Seabrook Friendship Park
First max	153	58	59	371	106	157	60
Second max	133	52	55	203	98	65	49
Third max	117	50	50	183	95	63	42
Fourth max	115	42	45	129	88	55	42
Fifth max	105	NA	44	106	86	NA	39
Sixth max	103	NA	43	91	75	NA	36
Seventh max	101	NA	41	91	74	NA	34

Source: Hosen, H. 1998, personal Communication.

Note: 1 µg/m^3 = 0.3820313 ppbv.

[a] Texas City 34th St. and 2nd Avenue data are not publicly available. Data presented obtained from Valero monthly air monitoring reports.

NA: Data are not publicly available and have not been obtained at this time.

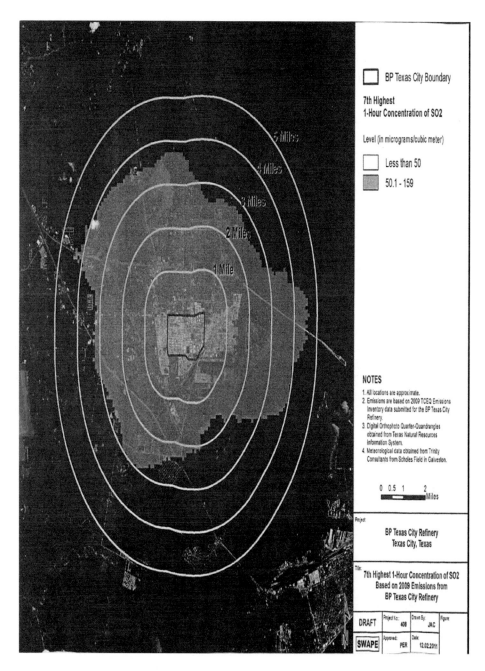

FIGURE 4.8 Seventh highest 1-hour concentration of SO₂ based on 2009 emissions from BP Texas City Refinery. (Dr. Chen's Research Article Sulfur Dioxide and Volatile Organic Compound Esposure to a community in Texas City, Texas evaluated using Aermod and Empirical Monitoring Data. http://thescipub.com/html/10.,3844/ajessp.2012.622.632. With permission from Science Publications.)

preexisting chronic respiratory disease,[34] especially children.[35] This has been observed for asthmatic subjects in controlled human exposure studies[33,36] and in various epidemiological studies using different methodologies. Several authors have studied the long-term effects of air pollution, comparing prevalence of asthma or bronchial hyperresponsiveness between areas with different air pollution levels.[37–39] Other studies have tested correlations between hospital visits for asthma and air pollutants.[40–44] Since hospital attendance for asthma reflects only severe asthma events, panel studies are used to evaluate the short-term health effect of air pollution on asthmatic adults,[45–48] asthmatic children,[49–53] or both.[54–56] These daily studies have given some controversial results, partly because they can be difficult to analyze,[57] and also because asthmatics can manage their own symptoms and pulmonary function by medication.[49] Moreover, most studies were conducted in North America or Northern Europe, and their results cannot be generalized to areas with different pollution and meteorological conditions.

The purpose of the present study was to examine the short-term effects of winter air pollution on the respiratory health of medically diagnosed asthmatic children. They used a panel study, controlling for the lack of independence of daily health outcomes and considering both maintenance and supplementary medications taken by the subjects.

Total incidence and prevalence rates of binary health outcomes over the study period and mean values of PEF variables are shown in Table 4.8 for the two groups of children. Both frequency and duration of asthma attacks and asthma-like symptoms were greater in moderate asthmatics than in mild asthmatics. The frequency and duration of respiratory infections were low in all children, whereas supplementary β_2 were used twice as often and for three times longer by mild than moderate asthmatics.

Temperature was negatively correlated with both incident and prevalent episodes of asthma and with prevalent episodes of nocturnal cough and shortness of breath. Temperature decrease was associated with PEF decrease. Humidity was positively correlated with both incident and prevalent episodes of wheezing and with incident episodes of shortness of breath and respiratory infections.

Association between pollutants and symptoms: Results in mild asthmatics are reported in Table 4.9 (incident episodes) and Table 4.10 (prevalent episodes). SO_2 was associated with both incident and prevalent episodes of asthma; use of supplementary β_2-agonists; incident episodes of nocturnal cough; prevalent episodes of shortness of breath; and respiratory infection. Associations between

---

TABLE 4.8

Frequency of Asthma Attacks, Symptoms, Respiratory Infections, and of Use of Supplementary β_2-Agonists

	Mild Asthmatics	Moderate Asthmatics
Asthma attacks[a]	0.7/2.0	1.7/3.6
Wheeze[a]	1.7/7.5	4.7/12.4
Nocturnal cough[a]	3.7/16.1	5.3/18.4
Shortness of breath[a]	2.3/9.1	5.6/18.3
Respiratory infections[a]	0.9/3.0	0.8/3.2
Supplementary β_2-agonists[a]	0.8/2.9	0.4/0.8
PEF am L/minute[b]	301.2 ± 80.6	302.2 ± 87.0
PEF var L/minute[b]	11.6 ± 1.7	14.1 ± 13.9

Source: Segala, C. et al. 2002. Short-term health effects of particulate and photochemical air pollution in asthmatic children. *Eur. Resp. J.* 20(4):899–906.

Mean values of morning peak expiratory low (PEF) and daily variability.

[a] Values are presented as incidence rate/prevalence rate, per 100 person days—days at risk[−1].

[b] Mean ± SD. Total incidence rate: (total number of incident episodes ×100)/(total number of person/days at risk); total prevalence rate: (total number of prevalent episodes ×100) (total number of person/days at risk). PEF am: morning PEF rate; PEF var: daily PEF variability.

TABLE 4.9

Odds Ratios (ORs) of the Effects of an Increase of 50 μg/m³ of Pollutants on Incident Episodes in Mild Asthmatics ($n = 43$)

Lag Days	SO$_2$	BS	PM$_{13}$	NO$_2$
Asthma				
0	2.86 (1.31–6.27)*	1.57 (0.79–3.12)	1.92 (0.88–4.21)⁺	2.33 (1.18–464)*
1	2.45 (1.01–5.92)*	1.35 (0.62–2.96)	1.30 (0.59–2.85)	1.51 (0.62–3.64)
2	1.40 (0.43–4.54)	–	–	–
3	1.52 (0.57–4.04)	–	1.39 (0.70–2.76)	–
4	2.33 (0.96–5.62)⁺	1.61 (0.81–3.20)	1.90 (0.79–4.59)	2.18 (1.10–4.32)*
Wheeze				
0	1.47 (0.90–2.41)	–	–	–
1	1.27 (0.48–3.38)	–	–	–
4	1.37 (0.57–3.32)	–	–	–
Nocturnal cough				
3	1.93 (1.18–3.15)*	1.65 (1.11–2.44)*	1.73 (1.17–2.57)*	1.62 (0.99–2.64)⁺
4	2.12 (1.43–3.13)*	1.86 (1.26–2.75)*	1.27 (0.95–1.71)	2.09 (1.28–3.42)*
Shortness of breath				
2	–	–	1.56 (086–2.80)	–
3	1.57 (0.79–3.11)	1.31 (0.73–2.36)	1.27 (0.64–2.51)	–
4	1.73 (0.79–3.78)	1.46 (0.74–2.91)	1.46 (0.74–2.91)	1.32 (0.60–2.89)
Respiratory infections				
1	1.52 (0.38–5.98)	–	1.46 (0.50–4.28)	–
2	1.66 (0.62–4.43)	–	1.36 (0.62–2.98)	–
3	2.39 (0.90–6.37)⁺	2.09 (0.96–4.58)⁺	2.50 (1.07–5.48)*	2.29 (1.05–5.02)*
4	1.80 (0.75–4.35)	2.06 (1.04–4.09)*	1.52 (0.63–3.66)	1.81 (0.83–3.96)
β$_2$-agonist				
3	1.58 (0.65–3.81)	1.41 (0.64–3.08)	–	−1.38 (0.77–2.48)
4	1.63 (1.00–2.66)*	1.41 (0.78–2.54)	–	–

Note: Each OR was obtained using a generalized estimating equations logistic model, adjusted for the effects of age, sex, weather data, and time trend terms. ORs <1.2 are omitted for brevity. The 95% confidence intervals are shown in parentheses.

⁺$p = 0.05$–0.10; *$p < 0.05$. (For further definitions, see legend to Table 4.2.)

health outcomes and the three other pollutants followed similar patterns, but the effects were weaker. Symptoms were more strongly associated with lagged (mostly lag 3 and 4 days time) than concurrent-day pollutant levels, except for asthma attack for which the risk for an increase of 50 μg/m³ of SO$_2$ was the highest on the same day: OR = 2.86%, 95% confidence interval (CI) (95% CI: 1.31–6.27).

No significant association was found at lag 5 or 6 days for incident episodes or at lag 6 days for prevalent episodes (not shown). In contrast, among moderate asthmatics (Table 4.11), associations between symptoms and pollutants were weaker, but prevalent use of supplementary β$_2$-agonists was strongly associated with each of the four pollutants on the same day and at lag 1, 2, and 3 days. The strongest risk was for an increase of 50 μg/m³ of SO$_2$ at lag 2 days: OR = 7.01%, 95% CI = 3.53–13.9.

Respiratory infections might confound the relationships between pollutants and health outcomes in asthmatic patients. They therefore reran all the models with respiratory infection as an additional explanatory variable. This slightly decreased the ORs but the effects remained significant independently of infection (data not shown).

TABLE 4.10

Odds Ratios (ORs) of the Effects of an Increase of 50 $\mu g/m^3$ of Pollutants on Prevalent Episodes in Mild Asthmatics ($n = 43$)

Lag Days	SO$_2$	BS	PM$_{13}$	NO$_2$
Asthma				
0	1.71 (1.15–2.53)*	1.32 (0.89–1.96)	1.32 (0.89–1.96)	1.31 (0.73–2.35)
1	1.55 (0.86–2.78)	1.21 (0.74–1.97)	–	–
4	1.23 (0.68–2.21)	–	–	1.20 (0.73–1.95)
Wheeze				
2	1.26 (0.77–2.06)	–	–	–
3	1.32 (0.81–2.15)	–	–	–
4	1.48 (0.90–2.41)+	1.23 (0.83–1.83)	–	–
Nocturnal cough				
4	1.32 (0.89–1.96)	1.27 (0.95–1.71)	–	1.28 (0.96–1.72)
Shortness of breath				
1	1.36 (0.92–2.01)	–	–	–
2	1.45 (0.98–2.14)*	1.20 (0.89–1.20)	1.22 (0.83–1.81)	–
3	1.52 (1.03–2.25)*	1.22 (0.91–1.64)	1.22 (0.82–1.80)	–
4	1.51 (1.02–2.24)*	1.25 (0.93–1.68)	1.25 (0.93–1.68)	–
5	1.23 (0.83–1.82)	–	–	–
Respiratory infections				
0	1.58 (0.72–3.46)	–	–	–
1	1.91 (0.79–4.62)	1.40 (0.70–2.77)	1.37 (0.69–2.72)	1.22 (0.61–2.41)
2	2.13 (0.97–4.67)*	1.54 (0.70–3.36)	1.66 (0.84–3.30)	1.23 (0.62–2.43)
3	2.09 (1.05–4.15)*	1.55 (0.86–3.07)	1.67 (0.93–3.00)+	1.52 (0.93–2.48)
4	2.05 (1.14–3.68)*	1.66 (1.02–2.71)*	1.47 (0.90–2.39)+	1.55 (1.04–2.29)*
5	1.40 (0.71–2.79)	1.35 (0.83–2.20)	1.23 (0.75–2.00)	1.23 (0.76–2.01)
β$_2$-agonist				
3	1.41 (0.78–2.53)	–	–	–
4	2.02 (1.02–4.01)*	1.21 (0.61–2.40)	–	–
5	1.96 (0.99–3.88)+	–	–	–

Note: Each OR was obtained using a generalized estimating equations logistic model, adjusted for the effects of age, sex, weather data, and time trend terms. ORs <1.23 are omitted for brevity. The 95% confidence intervals are shown in parentheses.

+$p = 0.05$–0.10; *$p < 0.05$. (For definitions, see legend to Table 4.2.)

Association between Pollutants and PEF Variables

There was no relationship between pollutants and PEF variables in either asthmatic group studies. Nevertheless, pollutants correlated slightly with these outcomes in the subgroup of 21 mild asthmatics with no inhaled steroids and no regularly scheduled β$_2$-agonists (Table 4.12). An increase of 50 $\mu g/m^3$ of one of the four pollutants resulted in a maximum decrease of 3%–5% in morning PEF (based on the group average of 300.6 L/minute). Lagged pollutants (mostly lag 3 and 4 days) were more strongly associated with PEF decrease than were concurrent day pollutant levels. Daily PEF variability increased by 1.9% for an increase of 50 $\mu m/m^3$ of SO$_2$ (maximum increase at lag 3 days). No relationship was found between PEF variability and the three other pollutants.

A smoke stack effect was seen in Texas City and LeMarque schools. This came from the refineries. This study shows the toxics that the children in the schools are breathing daily. This not only

TABLE 4.11
Odds Ratios (ORs) of the Effects of an Increase of 50 $\mu g/m^3$ of Pollutants in Moderate Asthmatics ($n = 41$)

Lag Days	SO$_2$	BS	PM$_{13}$	NO$_2$
		On Incident Episodes		
Asthma				
2	–	–	1.29 (0.79–2.10)	–
3	–	–	–	1.43 (0.80–2.58)
4	1.20 (0.55–2.62)	–	–	–
Wheeze				
0	–	–	–	1.35 (0.91–2.00)
3	1.23 (0.68–2.21)	1.26 (0.77–2.06)	1.26 (0.77–2.06)	1.37 (0.84–2.24)
4	–	–	1.23 (0.92–1.65)	–
Nocturnal cough				
2	1.34 (0.90–1.98)	1.22 (0.83–1.81)	–	1.54 (1.04–2.27)*
Shortness of breath				
4	–	–	–	1.24 (0.92–1.66)
Respiratory infections				
3	1.32 (0.37–4.71)	1.32 (0.60–2.90)	1.84 (0.76–4.45)	1.50 (0.62–3.63)
β_2-agonist				
0	–	1.65 (0.46–5.89)	1.97 (0.45–8.58)	1.80 (0.41–7.82)
4	–	–	–	1.28 (0.27–6.12)
		On Prevalent Episodes		
Asthma				
2	1.37 (0.76–2.47)	1.37 (0.92–2.03)	1.37 (0.93–2.03)	1.31 (0.80–2.13)
3	1.41 (0.86–2.30)	1.44 (0.97–2.13)+	1.23 (0.76–2.02)	1.64 (1.11–2.43)*
4	1.26 (0.77–2.06)	–	–	1.37 (0.84–2.23)
Wheeze				
3	–	–	–	1.26 (0.85–1.86)
4	1.31 (0.89–2.15)	–	–	1.26 (0.77–2.06)
5	1.21 (0.82–1.79)	–	–	–
Nocturnal cough				
4	1.23 (0.83–1.82)	1.22 (0.91–1.64)		
5	1.20 (0.90–1.62)	–	–	–
β_2-agonist				
0	3.67 (1.25–10.8)*	3.29 (1.36–7.95)*	4.73 (1.96–11.4)*	2.36 (1.08–5.17)*
1	4.60 (2.10–10.1)*	2.86 (1.59–5.15)*	5.29 (2.42–11.6)*	2.76 (1.69–4.51)*
2	7.01 (3.53–13.9)*	2.95 (1.99–4.36)*	4.44 (2.47–8.00)*	2.53 (1.27–5.02)*
3	4.74 (1.96–11.5)*	2.84 (1.58–5.12)*	2.85 (1.30–6.25)*	2.21 (0.83–5.90)+

Note: Each OR was obtained using a generalized estimating equations logistic model, adjusted for the effects of age, sex, weather data, and time trend terms. ORs <1.2 are omitted for brevity. The 95% confidence intervals are shown in parentheses. +$p = 0.05$–0.10; *$p < 0.05$. (For definitions, see legend to Table 4.2.)

means they are prone to be asthmatic but also severe toxicity. Thus, in the future, they may develop cancer, atheriosclerosis, and or neurovascular degenerative disease.

Segala et al.[32] have shown that moderately elevated air pollutants levels were associated in *mild asthmatic children* with increases in the incidence and duration of asthma attacks and asthma-like symptoms and with alterations of lung function as measured by reduction in PEF and increase

TABLE 4.12

Regression Coefficients[a] of the Effects of an Increase of 1 $\mu g/m^3$ of Pollutants on Peak Expiratory Flow (PEF) Variables in the Mild Asthmatic Group Taking No Corticosteroids and No Regularly Scheduled

	β_2-Agonist ($n = 21$)				
	Z-Transformed Morning PEF Values[b]			PEF Daily Variability % $\mu g^{-1} m^{3c}$	
Pollutant	Lag Days	β ($\pm$SE)	*p*-Value	β ($\pm$SE)	*p*-Value
SO$_2$	1	–		0.029 ± 0.015	0.06
	2	–		0.026 ± 0.022	NS
	3	-0.300 ± 0.163	0.06	0.038 ± 0.020	0.05
	4	-0.222 ± 0.163	NS	0.020 ± 0.018	NS
	5	–		0.035 ± 0.020	0.08
	6	–		0.035 ± 0.019	0.06
BS	3	-0.247 ± 0.145	0.09	0.022 ± 0.013	0.09
	4	-0.183 ± 0.117	NS	–	
PM$_{13}$	3	-0.181 ± 0.134	NS	–	
	4	-0.209 ± 0.108	0.05	–	
NO$_2$	3	-0.275 ± 0.150	0.06	–	
	4	-0.200 ± 0.157	NS	–	

Note: NS, not significant.

[a] Each parameter was obtained using a generalized estimating equations linear model, adjusted for the effects of age, sex, weather data, and time trend terms.

[b] Coefficients that correspond to a decrease of <3% in morning PEF for an increase of 50 $\mu g/m^3$ of pollutants are omitted for brevity.

[c] Coefficients that correspond to an increase of <1% in PEF variability for an increase of 50 $\mu g/m^3$ of pollutants are omitted for brevity.

in PEF variability. In moderately severe asthmatic children receiving daily treatment, both with inhaled steroids and inhaled β_2-agonists, only supplementary β_2-agonists use was strongly associated with air pollution. All these associations were observed at levels below the current acceptable standard air quality in a homogeneous group of 84 currently asthmatic children diagnosed by their hospital pulmonary pediatricians. Most previous panel studies of winter air pollution used a screening questionnaire to recruit children with chronic respiratory symptoms[49–52] without a medical diagnosis of asthma.

In the mild asthmatic group, air pollution was related both to daily symptom incidence and symptom duration and they observed that incidence tended to be associated with pollutants at shorter lags than prevalence. Most panel studies of asthmatic children have only described associations between symptom prevalence and air pollution.[49,50,52,53] The four pollutants were also associated with both incident and prevalent episodes of respiratory infections. Evidence of adverse effects of air pollution on respiratory illnesses has been related in several papers.[58–63] Since respiratory infections are related to asthma attacks,[64,65] they might have confounded the observed associations.[52] However, taking respiratory infections into account in the analysis did not substantially alter the association between pollutants and health outcomes. The reduction in PEF value and the increase of PEF variability were only reported in the subgroup of mild asthmatic children with no inhaled steroids and no regularly scheduled β_2-agonists, suggesting that anti-inflammatory treatment decreased the bronchial response to air pollution.

In the moderate asthmatic group, weaker associations between pollutants and asthma attacks or asthma-like symptoms were observed. This group is unlikely to be less susceptible to pollutants. It is possible that moderate asthmatics have a more efficient maintenance treatment and are better at managing their symptoms with supplementary medication. Indeed, the association between air pollution and supplement β_2-agonist use was strongest in the moderate asthmatic group. Pope et al.[49] similarly reported relatively weaker associations in a sample of asthmatic patients than in a school-based sample, except for the use of supplementary asthma medication.

Daily measurements of PEF have been used in several panels of asthmatic children. Morning[54] or evening measurements[49,50,53,56] or both[58] have been used to assess obstruction of proximal airways. They obtained the same pattern of results in this study by using evening PEF or mean value instead of morning PEF, but the effects were weaker (not shown). In this study, there was a significant training effect during the first days of the study and these days were, therefore, excluded from the analysis. Heterogeneity among individuals, which can introduce dependencies in the data[57] was taken into account by using daily mean Z-transformed peak flow values. They are not aware of any other panel study reporting relationships between air pollution and PEF variability in asthmatic children. Most of the children in this panel recorded three measurements every day. In a previous study, it was shown that three daily measurements (and possible two) are sufficient to assess bronchial lability in healthy adults.[66]

Weather changes have been reported to be triggers of respiratory symptoms in asthmatic children[64,67] and were indeed associated with health outcomes in their study. Therefore, all associations were adjusted for temperature and humidity. During a 6-month period, health outcomes, weather, and pollutant data show short-term and seasonal variations. Consequently, time trend variables, which are factors that may confound the associations between outcomes and environmental data, were taken into account in the analysis.

The use of stationary air pollution monitoring data to represent personal exposure is a weak point of this study, shared by most panel studies. Most of the child's time is spent indoors in winter. Nevertheless, studies comparing indoor and outdoor particulate concentrations have reported an average indoor/outdoor ratio of at least 0.5,[68,69] and some authors found that indoor NO_2 correlated highly with outdoor NO_2,[59] suggesting that outdoor pollution measurement is a reasonable proxy for personal exposure. Moreover, several authors have suggested that misclassification of exposure, if random, would result in a downward bias of the association between air pollution and health outcomes.[48,51,54]

The major local sources contributing to ambient air pollution in the Paris, France area are heating and automobile exhaust.[70] Although sulfur and particulate levels have decreased substantially over the last 30 years, the recent rise in vehicle traffic and the growing percentage of diesel engines[71] have, since 1985, contributed to an increase in emissions of nitrogen oxides, particulate matter, and volatile organic compounds. During the winter of 1992–1993, levels of pollutants, other than NO_2, were well below European Community (EC) and World Health Organization (WHO) standards. It is not clear from this data what component(s) was responsible for the observed health effects. Similar finding were observed for each of the four pollutants, in single pollutant models. However, the pollutants studied may only be indicators for more complex air pollution, some of pollutants not being measured in our study and because of the likely interactions between pollutants.[33,67]

The finding of associations between winter air pollutants and respiratory effects in asthmatic children is consistent with a previous study correlating hospital admissions for asthma and air pollution in Paris[72] and with published panel studies. A recent study of 83 African-American asthmatic children in Los Angeles[52] has associated shortness of breath, but not cough and wheeze with suspended particulates with an aerodynamic diameter of 10 μm (PM_{10}).

In the Utah Valley, Pope et al.[49] showed that PM_{10} was associated with an increase in reported upper and lower respiratory symptoms and asthma medication, and decreased PEF values in 34 symptomatic schoolchildren. In a second study,[50] children with chronic respiratory symptoms were estimated to report cough about twice as frequently for each 100 $\mu g/m^3$ increase in PM_{10}. In these three U.S. studies, no association was found with SO_2, as SO_2 levels were low. Likewise, in a panel of American children with persistent wheeze, Vedal et al.[54] failed to show any relationship between SO_2 and either respiratory illness or PEF levels. Recent panel studies in eastern Europe[53,56] reported a decrease in PEF and an increase in symptom score associated with relatively high levels of air pollution. In the Netherlands, Roemer et al.[51] followed 73 children with chronic respiratory symptoms during three winter months. He did not observe any significant association between pollution levels and incident episodes of either asthmatic symptoms or medications. In contrast, PM_{10}, black smoke, and SO_2 were associated with increased prevalent episodes of wheeze and bronchodilator use, and decreased morning and evening PEF. Forsberg et al.[55] studied a panel of three asthmatic patients, aged 9–71 years, living in Northern Sweden; shortness of breath was the only symptom that increased with increasing black smoke levels.

During this study period, NO_2 was the only pollutant to come close to the upper limit of the international guidelines (upper 24 hours value: 122 $\mu g/m^3$ vs. WHO 24 hours guideline value; 150 $\mu g/m^3$). NO_2 has been reported to be a risk factor for reduced lung function. In a repeated cross-sectional survey, weekly NO_2 concentrations were found to affect the lung function of children with asthmatic symptoms.[73] Evidence for the health effects of outdoor NO_2 on asthmatic symptoms is scarce.[74] NO_2 was not related to any of the health outcomes in the study of Roemer et al.[42] and in the study of Higgins et al.[48] the effect of NO_2 disappeared when SO_2 was included in regression models.

Any effect of pollution exposure on asthmatic symptoms and/or pulmonary function is not necessarily contemporaneous, and in this study, most of the significant associations between pollutants and health outcomes displayed a lag time. Previous panel studies have reported similar findings. Peters and coworkers[53,56] reported weak same-day effects and stronger cumulative effects of air pollution on asthmatic children for both PEF and symptoms. In the study of Roemer et al.,[51] weekly average pollution appeared to be more closely related than present day or previous day pollution to symptoms and PEF. Pope and Dockery[50] found that symptoms and PEF were more closely associated with 5 day moving average PM_{10} levels than concurrent day pollution, and suggested that the deficit in pulmonary function is immediate but continues to accumulate for several days.[49] This is consistent with previous studies of pollution episodes. Dassen et al.[75] reported that the maximal deficit in lung function of children was observed 2 weeks after an episode of maximal total suspended particle (TSP) concentration of 200–250 $\mu g/m^3$. Brunekreef et al.[76] reanalyzed data from a study published in 1982[77] and showed a stronger statistical association with the 5 day mean than the previous day mean TSP.

In conclusion, Segala et al.[32] have shown that prevailing levels of winter air pollution, which are below international air quality standards, had consistent and measurable effects on children with mild to moderate asthma. These effects lasted several days after exposure, suggesting a persistent inflammatory process. They also showed that moderate asthmatic patients could manage their bronchial responses to air pollution by treatment.

TAIWAN AND PETROCHEMICAL POLLUTED AREA

The health effects of environmental exposure to high levels of air pollution have been described and discussed extensively as shown in this chapter. Several studies have shown that poor ambient air quality is associated with increased prevalence of respiratory symptoms in children.[78–83] Development of the basic petrochemical industry in Taiwan started some 45 years ago in 1968. In all, 19 of 361 administrative counties in Taiwan have been classified as petrochemical industrial counties (PICs).[84] The pollutants emitted by the petrochemical industries included not only the vinyl chloride monomer and polycyclic aromatic hydrocarbons (PAHs) which have been recognized as environmental carcinogens, but also large quantities of criteria pollutants such as sulfur dioxide (SO_2), nitrogen dioxide (NO_2), and particulate matter (PM_{10}). An excess rate of liver cancer among males has been reported among those living in a PIC,[84] while the respiratory health/

PIC effects of petrochemical industry air emissions on the population in affected communities have not been well studied.

The objective of the present study was to determine whether or not there were adverse respiratory health outcomes in schoolchildren living close to petrochemical manufacturing facilities. This report characterizes the respiratory symptoms of schoolchildren both in Linyuan (petrochemical exposed area) and in a reference area (Taihsi) not in the immediate proximity of any petrochemical or other industrial emissions.

According to the pollution reports compiled since 1983 by the Environmental Protection Administration of Taiwan, nine serious air pollution events have occurred in these petrochemical counties between 1971 and 1990.[85]

Particulates, sulfur dioxide (SO_2) nitrogen dioxide (NO_2) and acid aerosols levels were significantly higher in the exposed area than in the reference area. The schoolchildren in the petrochemical area had significantly more upper respiratory symptoms and asthma compared with the children living in the control area. Although the association with known petrochemical air pollution is suggestive, this cross-sectional study cannot confirm a causal relation and further studies are needed.

The results show that children residing in Linyuan, the petrochemical-polluted area, had slightly more respiratory symptoms compared with the cohort living in Taihsi, an area with essentially no petrochemical or industrial pollution. The results are in agreement with the findings in the literature, and they indicate a higher prevalence of respiratory symptoms among children growing up in air polluted areas compared with children living in nonpolluted areas. Due to the limited population studied and the study design, the evidence can, however, not be considered as conclusive.

Other symptoms than respiratory have been found in other people. This case study and Figure 4.9 shows some of these.

Case Study: A 61-year-old man was assessed for a 4-year history of dizzy spells (which worsened 2 weeks prior to his arrival at the EHC-Dallas) and a 1-year history of frontal and sinus area headaches and passing out. His main symptom was episodes of smelling strong, unpleasant odors, which his doctors initially thought to be olfactory hallucinations. He had no auditory, gustatory, or visual disturbances. The patient would experience a strong unpleasant odor, feel as if he were drunk, and then become dizzy for 3–8 minutes. At first, he was convinced the order was being produced

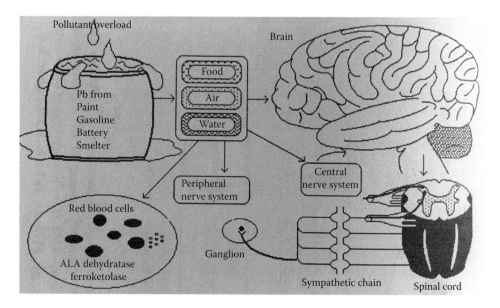

FIGURE 4.9 Lead injury to the nervous system and red blood cells. (From Rea, W.J. 1994. *Chemical Sensitivity, Volume II*, Page 728, Figure 6. With permission.)

from his car, but a careful evaluation revealed no problem with the vehicle. He also complained of inordinate fatigue and episodic flushing spells.

Results of an EEG suggested a temporal lobe abnormality, and he was worked up with several computerized tomographies (CT) and magnetic resonance imagining (MRI) scans for the brain. There was a suggestion of a mass on the first CT scan, but subsequent enhanced scans, MRI, and angiography were all normal.

His neurological exam was normal, and he had no convulsive seizures. He was thought to have a temporal-like seizure disorder wand was started on Dilantin and Xanax, which reduced, but did not stop, high sense of strong, unpleasant odors.

Occupational history revealed that he had worked for 37 years as an oil pumper and driller in the oil industry with chronic exposure to carbon disulfide (CS_2) gas that was emitted from wells and holding tanks. Part of his job had been opening these tanks and checking the levels of their contents. On four occasions, he had been found unconscious from exposure to these fumes, and on the last occasion, he had to be dragged away from the source of the gas before he was able to regain consciousness.

Measurement of the CS_2 concentration in the tanks at which this patient worked showed levels that ranged from a low of 100 ppm in a tank with many inhalation holes to the two highest readings of 29,000 and 55,000 ppm.

On admission to the Environmental Control Unit, he was placed in chemical isolation and fed nothing by mouth, except spring water, for 2 days. During this time, the sensation of the odd smell worsened (as is often the case when patients are first cleared of contaminants following chemical exposures), but by the time of discharge, the patient's headaches, joint pains, and smelling of this odor had subsided. Laboratory analysis showed normal immune parameters, except for slightly raised T suppressor cells at 1106/mm^3 (333–1070/mm^3). On the general volatile screening test, he was found to have tetrachloroethylene in his blood at 0.4 ppb. No other chemicals were found. The patient was exposed to CS_2 and all symptoms were reproduced. He has done well since avoiding this toxic substance.

Sulfur dioxide creates acid rain, which is a severe problem in some parts of the world, especially the northeastern United States and Canada and parts of western Europe.

In the form of bisulfate, sulfur dioxide has been used as a vegetable preservative. It is also used as a bleaching agent for apples, French fried potatoes, and asparagus, and as a preservative for dried fruits.[86]

The primary negative health effect of sulfur dioxide is irritation of the mucous membranes. Upper respiratory irritation and some nosebleeds have been seen in workers exposed to 10 ppm of SO_2.[87] At times, sulfur dioxide has been found to be lethal.[88]

Studies have set the odor threshold of sulfur dioxide as 3–5 ppm; the least concentration causing throat irritation is 8–12 ppm, while 20 ppm is the least concentration causing coughing or eye irritation in normal healthy adult males. The TLV for SO_2 is 5 ppm. Of course, these levels are much less for the chemically susceptible, and this chemical should not be used in foods.

Hydrogen Sulfide

Hydrogen sulfide (H_2S) has been reported to cause death in people who work with decaying organic materials such as fish, sewage, and manure.[89,90] H_2S causes asphyxiation by interfering with the use of oxygen in the cytochrome oxidase system, and when it interferes at a lesser degree, it causes increased chemical sensitivity.

Sulfur-containing conjugation occurs, causing deactivation of sulfurous compounds. This deactivation occurs either by H_2S combining with sulfates or through the GSH mechanism. Also, sulfur oxidation occurs through the oxidative mechanism, using the microsomal enzymes. Most of these processes turn lipophilic compounds into more water-soluble compounds or change the valence so they are less toxic, and when these processes are damaged by pollutant overload, chemical sensitivity is exacerbated.

Most problems resulting from exposure to sulfur compounds are due to excess environmental overload with malnutrition. However, some problems are the result of overload with metabolic genetic defects. There appears to be a group of people in the general population who are slow metabolizers of sulfur compounds.[2,91] This slow metabolism is probably due to a genetic deficiency, mainly of certain detoxification enzymes such as N-acetyl transferase.[2] This may partially explain why some chemically sensitive people have problems with sulfur in air, food, and water.

OZONE

Ozone is a specific air pollutant generated by photochemical reactions in the atmosphere and resulting from a combination of emissions of hydrocarbons, nitrogen oxides, and particulates by different combustion sources, particularly automobiles, electricity generating plants, high-voltage electric wires, ARC welding, and in airplanes at 30,000 feet. Ozone creates free radicals in the body, resulting in pulmonary and vascular damage[92,93] and in the chemically sensitive, exacerbating signs and symptoms. Ozone is a strong oxidant, and, at high levels (0.12 ppm), it can damage plants and be a respiratory irritant. It suppresses immunity, as evidenced by one study that showed significantly higher mortality in mice exposed to streptococcus after they had been exposed to ozone.[94] The immunosuppressive aspect of ozone is additive with other pollutants.[95] It has been shown to suppress the function of the pulmonary alveolar macrophages.[96] It also depresses T and B lymphocyte function and, to a lesser extent, neutrophil function.[97] Lymphocytes also develop chromosomal abnormalities following exposure to relatively low doses of ozone.[98]

Also, ozone can generate new antigenic species and might react with susceptible subgroups in proteins and other cellular components, to modify their structural and antigenic characteristics. Autoimmune reactions after ozone may explain some of the high incidences of autoantibodies in a subgroup of chemically sensitive. Ozone attacks polyunsaturated fatty acids such as in lipid membranes and sulfhydryl groups of proteins (especially enzymes), free amino acids (e.g., cysteines), and GSH.[99] It depletes the sulfhydryl content of the lung and cross-links the bases in DNA. It oxidized aromatic amino acids, especially tyrosine and phenylalanine, via their unsaturated rings.[99] Ozone breaks down products into toxic ozonides, which also causes tissue damage, especially to the phospholipids of the cell membranes.[100] Ozone can damage cytochrome enzymes of the pulmonary mixed-function oxidase (MFO) systems, resulting in increased chemical sensitivity.

Ozone acts as a protective layer high about the earth to filter radiation. Its absence in some areas (over Australia, for instance), due to excessive fluorocarbon use on the earth, has resulted in a marked increase in skin cancer. Other beneficial uses of ozone include the ozonation of water. The toxic effect of ozone on living tissues is beneficial during water sterilization because it kills the hazardous bacteria, viruses, and parasites. Its side products are mainly oxygen and thus also beneficial. Ozone has also been used as an oxidant to detoxify buildings that contain toxic substances and molds.

REVIEW OF OZONE AND ASTHMA

The aim of this study was to assess the association between asthma severity over a 12-month period and simultaneous home outdoor concentrations of air pollution. Findings of this evaluation demonstrated a strong correlation between the number of days with 8-hour average ozone concentration above 110 $\mu g/m^3$ (56 ppb) and asthma severity score (based on symptoms, frequency, treatment, etc.). Increase 8-hour average concentrations above this threshold resulted in a risk of increased asthma (OR = 2.53%, 95% CI: 1.69–3.79).[101]

This study examined the relationship of adverse asthma symptoms (bothersome or interfered with daily activities or sleep) to O_3 and PM_{10} in Southern California community in the air inversion zone with high O_3 and low PM. Asthmatic children and adolescents were evaluated for prevalence of symptoms, and it was found that children who normally exhibited symptoms on fewer than 20% of days were over twice as likely to on days with the difference of minimum to maximum 1-hour average reaching 58 ppb (OR = 2.15%, 95% CI: 1.04–4.44).[102]

Long-term relative risk (RR) of exposure to high versus low ambient ozone was considered in the analysis performed in this study. A 27-ppb ozone increment was determined between two populations for the 8-hour average, and 6-year and 20-year correlations with doctor-told asthma (DTA) were established. Between the two cohorts, males living in the higher ambient ozone region were at 2.09 (1.03–4.16) times the risk of being diagnosed with asthma as those in the control region while residing for 20 years. The 6-year baseline study evaluated at the beginning of the monitoring period demonstrated a RR of 2.03 (95% CI: 1.03–3) for males living in the elevated zone.[103]

Incremental effect of increased ambient ozone was determined in this study based on a population of nonsmoking adults over the course of 10 years. For a 10 ppb increase in ambient ozone concentration, males were found to be over three times at risk for development of asthma (RR = 3.12%, 95% CI: 1.61–5.85).[104]

Generation of ozone by traffic-related volatile organic compound air pollution is a considerable problem, and this review observed the prevalence of asthmatic hospitalizations during the period of decreased ozone in Atlanta during the 1996 Olympic Games in Atlanta, Georgia due to traffic restructuring. The study found that following a 24% reduction (from 81.3–58.6 ppb) in ambient ozone concentrations, the Medicaid database of asthma admissions to hospitals declined significantly, with an RR of 0.48 (95% CI: 0.44–0.86).[105]

ASTHMA—OCCUPATIONAL EXPOSURE—OZONE

Greer et al.[104] attempted to determine the association between occupational and air pollutant exposure with the development of adult asthma through the analysis of a standardized respiratory questionnaire administered to a cohort of 3914 nonsmoking adults in 1977 and again in 1987. Ambient air pollution concentrations were estimated over a 20-year period using monthly interpolations from fixed-site monitoring stations applied to zip code locations by month of residence and worksite. Secondhand smoke exposure was significantly associated with the development of asthma (RR = 1.45, CI = 1.21–1.75). Airways obstructive disease before age 16 was related to a marked increased risk (RR = 4.24, CI = 4.03–4.45). An increased risk of asthma was significantly associated with increased ambient concentrations of ozone exposure in men (RR = 3.12, CI = 1.61–5.85).[104]

In studying the development of asthma related to occupational and environmental exposures, smoking remains the major confounder. The few community-based epidemiologic studies examining occupational exposures[106–111] related to chronic obstructive pulmonary disease (COPD) and asthma have been summarized by Becklake.[112] Information on these effects related to environmental exposures in nonsmokers is lacking. In addition, increased attention has recently been placed on secondhand smoke exposure in the workplace.[113] Studying these effects in a Seventh-Day Adventist nonsmoking population in a long-term prospective study for which ambient community air pollution estimates were available has provided an opportunity to examine these factors as related to adult-onset asthma.

The regression coefficients and RRs for the variables comprising the final model are shown in Table 4.13. The variable "Years Worked with a Smoker through 1987" (YWS87) contained a CI that excludes one. Interestingly, "Obstructive Airways Disease Before Age Sixteen" (AODB16) is significant with a RR of 4.24. Even though the RR = 1.31 for mean ozone concentration exposure through 1987 (OX87) approaches statistical significance, the CI does include one. The variables "Years of Occupational Dust Exposure," "Years of Occupational Vapor Exposure," "Cumulative Occupational Asthmagenic Substance Exposure," and ambient mean TSP concentration all failed

TABLE 4.13

Multiple Logistic Regression for Cumulative Crude Incidence[a] of Asthma between 1977 and 1987

Variable[b]	Coefficient	Increment[c]	Relative Risk[d]	95% CI for Relative Risk
Definite Asthma by Reported Symptoms or Reported Physician Diagnosis Developed between 1977 and 1987 (AST87) (n = 3577, Incident Cases = 78)				
YWS87	0.038120*	10 year	1.45	1.21–1.80
OX87	0.275530	1 pphm[e]	1.31	0.96–1.78
AODB16	1.504500*	No or yes	4.24	4.03–4.45
Education	0.048769	4 year	1.21	0.85–1.71
Age	−0.018012	10 year	0.98	1.00–0.96
Gender	−0.289890	Male or female	0.75	1.23–0.46
Constant	−4.0270			
AST87: Sex-Specific Analysis, Men Only (n = 1305, Incident Cases = 27)				
YW87	0.041250**	10 year	1.50	1.12–2.01
OX87	1.1819000*	1 pphm	3.12	1.61–5.85
AODB16	2.0631000*	No or yes	7.01	3.07–14.60
Education	0.0987410	4 year	1.46	0.85–2.49
Age	0.0032417	10 year	1.0	0.97–1.04
Constant	−8.5669			
AST87: Sex-Specific Analysis, Women Only (n = 2272, Incident Cases = 51)				
YWS87	0.0412350**	10 year	1.50	1.17–1.92
OX87	−0.9656010	1 pphm	0.94	0.65–1.34
AODB16	1.2562000*	No or yes	3.36	1.72–6.38
Education	0.0146030	4 year	1.06	0.65–1.71
Age	−0.0280350[a]	10 year	0.97	0.95–1.00
Constant	−2.905			

Source: Greer, J. R., D. E. Abbey, R. J. Burchette. 1993. Asthma related to occupational and ambient air pollutants in non-smokers. *J. Occup. Environ. Med.* 4(5):909–915. http://journals.lww.com/joem/Abstract/1993/09000/Asthma_Related_to_Occupational_and_Ambient_Air.14.aspx

[a] Crude incident because information on those who died is missing.

[b] YWS87, years ever worked with a smoker through 1987; OX87, cumulative ambient ozone exposure through 1987; AODB 16, history of obstructive airways disease before age 16.

[c] Increment for computations of relative risks.

[d] Relative risk of increase in exposure of one increment, holding the other variables in the model constant.

[e] pphm, part per hundred million.

*$p < 0.001$; **$p < 0.01$; *** $p < 0.05$.

to reach 0.10 level of significance required to enter the model even when sex-specific analyses were done.

Further sex-specific analysis (Table 4.14) revealed a statistically significant RR for ozone in men of 3.12, but ozone was not significant at the 0.05 level in women. UWS87 and AODB16 remained significant in both genders, with RRs of 1.46 and 7.01 for men and 1.50 and 3.36 for women, respectively.

When sensitivity analyses were performed using "doctor-told asthma" as well as cases confirmed by medical records, AODB16 and YWS87 remained significant at the 0.05 level. Ozone

TABLE 4.14

Lung Function (SD) of Participants with and without Doctor Diagnosis of Asthma in 1993[a]

	Females		Males	
	Asthma ($n = 77$)	No Asthma ($n = 795$)	Asthma ($n = 47$)	No Asthma ($n = 472$)
FEV_1	87.9***	96.8	87.7**	98.4
(% predicted)[b]	(16.2)	(13.6)	(20.4)	(14.0)
FVC	91.4**	96.9	97.5	99.0
(% predicted)[b]	(14.6)	(13.4)	(18.1)	(13.4)
FEV_1VC	73.4**	75.9	67.2***	74.0
(%)	(8.1)	(6.0)	(11.5)	(6.9)
FEF_{25-75}	79.4***	97.1	76.5***	101.9
(% predicted)[b]	(32.5)	(31.6)	(44.4)	(38.8)
Bronchodilator response	5.0**	2.1	5.2**	2.1
(% change in FEV_1)[c]	(7.4)	(4.4)	(6.4)	(4.0)
PEF liability	12.0***	8.9	10.2*	8.1
(%)[d]	(6.5)	(5.3)	(6.2)	(4.4)

Source: Environ. Res. Long-term ambient ozone concentration and the incidence of asthma in non-smoking adults: The AHSMOG study. 80(2), McDonnell, W. F., D. E. Abbey, N. Nishino, M. D. Lebowitz. 110–121. Copyright Academic Press, 1999, with permission from Elsevier.

[a] Values are means. Differences between those with and without asthma tested using Student's *t* test.

[b] Predicted values derived from a healthy subset of this sample based upon age and height.

[c] Percentage increase above baseline FEV_1 following two puffs of inhaled albuterol.

[d] See Methods for full description of peak flow liability.

*$p \leq 0.05$; **$p \leq 0.01$; ***$p \leq 0.001$.

also remained in the model but was retained only at a 0.10 level of significance. Testing was also performed using physician-diagnosed asthma after age 18 as reported by questionnaire. A childhood history of colds, AODB6, and YWS87 were all highly significant. Further sensitivity testing using occupational exposures to both primary asthmagenic and secondary asthmagenic substances indicated that neither was significant.

Limitations of this cohort due to the use of self-reported data and interpolated ambient air pollution data have been discussed in detail elsewhere by Euler et al.[114] and Abbey et al.[115] Briefly, estimates of ambient ozone concentrations were interpolated from fixed-site monitoring stations taking into account the number of hours per day spent at worksite locations and home. Ozone levels at these stations were monitored on an hourly basis but direct measures were not made. Cumulative interpolated mean concentrations over a 2-year period for TSP and ozone have been demonstrated to have a Pearson correlation coefficient of 0.83 and 0.87, respectively, with actual monitored concentrations.[116]

Similar factors influence the collection of occupational exposure data that were solicited only on the 1987 questionnaire. Remote or low-level exposures would be more easily omitted. Due to the small number of incident cases of asthma and the small number of people reporting exposures other than environmental tobacco smoke (ETS) (661, 16.9% of the population), the power for detecting a RR greater than 1.5 for asthmagenic occupational exposures is <50%. Thus, they cannot conclude that a lack of statistical significance for other occupational exposures indicates a real lack of association.

One of the unique aspects of this population is that the average age at the time of enrollment was 56.5 years, and exposures and outcomes were recorded prospectively over the following 10-year period. Approximately two-thirds of the population had been exposed to long-term ambient concentrations of asthmagenic environmental pollutants. Of those exposed to asthmagenic substances on the job, 76% were men and 24% women. Due to the older average age of this population, it is possible that those sensitive to respiratory exposures may have migrated to occupations with minimum respiratory exposure before enrolling in this study: the healthy worker effect in reverse.

To correct for people developing asthma before 1977, they examined adult-onset asthma as an outcome that includes a self-reported physician diagnosis of asthma after age 18. The variables significantly associated with this outcome remained the same except for the addition of "childhood colds," a variable representing more than the average number of colds before age 7. The addition of childhood colds to the model is probably due to the earlier age of asthma diagnosis reported for this outcome variable.

Due to the lack of information on those that died between surveys, only an estimate of the crude incidence can be made. Excluding those who died, the estimated crude incidence of new cases of asthma for subjects over age 25 in 1976 was 2.1 per thousand per year, exactly the same incidence rate reported by the First National Health and Nutrition Examination Surveys (NHANES) (adjusted to the U.S. population) conducted between 1971 and 1984.[117] The Tecumseh[118] and Tucson[119] studies had similar rates, 2.0 per thousand per year for over age 24 and 4.0 per thousand per year for over age 19, respectively; however, all these populations included both smokers and nonsmokers.

Obstructive airways disease before "age 16" was highly predictive of asthma in all the models. These findings are similar to those found in the Tucson study using the same variable in regression analysis.[120,121] Impaired or decreased pulmonary function values consistently have been shown to predict COPD in other community-based studies in which pulmonary function testing was done.[106,120,121] A previous history of pulmonary disease appears to increase pulmonary susceptibility to respiratory exposures.

Asthma is generally considered an irreversible disease, but with certain occupationally induced forms resolution may occur after removal from the offending agent.[123] In 1987, Brooks and Kalica[124] reviewed the relationship between occupational exposures and COPD (focusing primarily on asthma) in an NHLBI workshop summary. The report suggests directions for future research and calls for better outcome definitions; however, ETS was not mentioned in this summary.[124] More than 200 different agents found in the working environment have been reported to cause occupational asthma.[125] Many of these substances occur in our population, but significant numbers are lacking to show a relationship.

In this population, ETS in the workplace is associated with the development of adult-onset asthma in both men and women. In fact, it is consistently associated with each of the asthma outcomes considered. ETS was the strongest occupationally related predictor of new onset asthma. Majedi et al.[126] have shown that passive smoking in the workplace is associated with decreased forced expiratory volume in 1 second, forced vital capacity, and forced midexpiratory flow rate (25–75) in nonsmokers. RRs associated with ETS reported here are consistent with those reported elsewhere.[113,127]

Long-term exposure to ozone was strongly associated with adult-onset asthma in men (RR = 3.12 for a 1 part per hundred million (pphm) incremental annual increase in mean concentration but not in women (RR = 0.94) in this population. Ozone is known to be a powerful oxidant that causes acute alveolar and bronchiolar inflammation with associated reductions in both forced expiratory volume in 1 second and forced midexpiratory flow rate (25–75).[128–130] These effects seem to be cumulative with repeated exposure and synergistic with other factors such as particulate matter, NO_2, and temperature.[131–133] However, ozone is highly volatile and is not stable in the indoor environment. This fact may explain why men appear to be more affected than women. A Student's t-test indicated that men were more likely to work in outdoor conditions than were women, an average of 18.6 versus 10.7 hours per week ($p < 0.01$) during the high-ozone season of June through September. This would increase their exposure to ozone and other pollutants shown to have synergistic effects on small airways.[122,133–135] Women are less likely to work in job settings where exposure to asthmagenic substances is likely to occur. Curiously, the coefficients for ozone and age in women were slightly negative but remained so close to zero that they may be considered insignificant. Approximately two-thirds of this population (64.5%) is female, which may dilute some of the effect of other occupational and outdoor environmental exposures.

Interestingly, TSP, which has been implicated in the genesis of asthma in other studies, was not a significant factor in the presence of ozone in this population. However, community ambient concentrations of the two pollutants are high correlated ($r = 0.74$), so we cannot rule out an association. Abbey et al.[116] have shown ambient concentrations of TSP in excess of 200 $\mu g/m^3$ to be significantly associated with development of new cases of asthma in this cohort.

In summary, workplace ETS is by far the most common preventable asthmagenic exposure in this population. This has practical public health implications due to the high prevalence of workplace ETS in this country. ETS is not as well recognized in the occupational setting as a potential respiratory irritant as many other less frequently encountered occupational exposures. A previous history of respiratory disease or symptoms strongly predicts the development of asthma. Common sense would suggest that these workers should avoid occupations associated with respiratory exposures, including ETS and ambient air pollutants. Long-term ozone exposure was also found to be a strong predictor of asthma in men but not in women. This is probably due to differences in time spent outdoors and the ability of ozone to potentiate other ambient and occupational respiratory irritants. With ever-increasing numbers of people exposed to photochemical pollutants, further work is needed to clarify the effects of ozone in combination with other pollutants in workplace and community environments.

Adult-Onset Long-Term Asthma and Ozone Air Pollution Indices

Monthly indices of ambient air pollutant concentrations measured at monitoring stations throughout California were interpolated to zip code centroids according to residence and work location histories, cumulated, and then averaged over time using methods described by Abbey et al.[116] Interpolations were not allowed to cross airflow boundaries or topographical obstructions of altitude greater than 250 m. The precision of interpolation methods has been evaluated and found to be very high with respect to cumulations over a 2-year period.[116] Pollutants included in these analyses included ozone, particles with an aerodynamic diameter ≤ 10 μm (PM_{10}), total suspended sulfates (SO_4), nitrogen dioxide (NO_2), and sulfur dioxide (SO_2). Prior to 1987, PM_{10} estimates were obtained using site- and season-specific regressions based on monitored TSPs, because PM_{10} was not monitored on a consistent statewide basis prior to this time.[136] In addition to mean concentration, alternative indices were used for ozone and PM_{10}. The 8-hour average ozone concentration between the hours of 9 a.m. and 5 p.m. was calculated and used as the primary exposure variable. The hours 9 a.m.–5 p.m. were chosen to correspond to usual hours at work as separate interpolations were used for home and work locations. Other indices included exceedance frequencies for a number of concentration cutoffs. Exceedance frequency was defined as the sum of hours for gaseous pollutants, or days for particulate pollutants, for which concentration was above a given cutoff. Cutoffs used for ozone were 60, 80, 100, 120, and 150 ppb. For PM_{10}, a cutoff of 100 $\mu g/m^3$ was used ($PM_{10}[100]$).

For 2881 of the 3091 participants, ambient ozone data were available for >80% of the months of the study. All primary analyses were conducted using the data from these 2881 individuals. A sensitivity analysis in which final models were rerun using the data from all 3091 individuals demonstrated similar results to those presented in this article.

The results from this prospective study indicate that the risk of developing adult-onset doctor-told asthma is higher for males living and working in areas with high ambient ozone concentrations. Although the numbers of cases are small, the crude and adjusted risks are similar for the upper two tertiles of ambient ozone concentration and are significantly larger than for the lower tertile of concentration. This, and the findings that development of DTA in males was most strongly associated with mean ozone concentration followed by 8-hour average ozone concentration followed by number of hours above 60 ppb, suggests that cumulative exposure to even low levels of ozone may be related to development of DTA.

The most likely explanation for not finding a similar ozone–DTA relationship in females is that ozone may be associated with DTA through promotion of the actions of other asthmogenic substances to which men have greater exposure than women either in the workplace or as the result of hobbies. This effect of ozone has been demonstrated in nonhuman primates exposed to platinum salts[137] and in other species (Ian Gilmour, personal communication). Furthermore, although the distributions of ambient ozone concentrations were similar for men and women, women actually received less exposure due to the considerably smaller time spent outdoors during the summers (Table 4.15). Other contributors to these differences may include gender differences in hormonal status[138] and diet[139] and in misclassification of asthma status which may have been greater in females than in males. Although large proportion of both male and female new asthma cases (85% and 94%, respectively) reported symptoms consistent with asthma, and lung function in both genders was consistent with reversible airway obstruction and increased peak flow lability compared to non-asthmatics, the degree of obstruction represented by FEV_1/FVC was considerably larger in males than females (Table 4.16), and only 27% of the new female cases reported use of asthma medication compared to 61% of the males.

The increased risk of development of DTA for males living in high ozone-areas could be due to one of two distinctly different processes; long-term exposure to ozone could contribute to induction of the basic pathophysiological events which constitute asthma or it could result in the exacerbation of existing mild or quiescent asthma which brings the participant to the attention of his physician resulting in a diagnosis. The first exploratory analysis, although limited in power, indicated that the ozone–DTA relationship as presented in Table 4.17 was not related to the presence or absence of symptoms consistent with asthma in 1977. It thus seems likely that ozone is associated with development of new cases of asthma. The second exploratory analysis, however, did suggest that living and working in a high ambient ozone environment was associated with an increased probability of

---

TABLE 4.15

Air Pollution Characteristics (1973–1993)[a] for Study Participants and Correlation of Other Pollutants with 8-Hour Average Ozone Concentration

Pollutant	Mean	Range	1[b]
Ozone 8-hour average concentration (ppb)	46.5	0.0[c]–74.9	–
Ozone mean concentration (ppb)	25.7	0.0–40.7	0.92 ($n = 2881$)[d]
PM_{10} mean concentration ($\mu g/m^3$)	50.3	0.0–83.8	0.88 ($n = 2735$)
PM_{10} (days/year when $PM_{10} > 199\ \mu g/m^3$)	30.2	0.0–150.7	0.68 ($n = 2735$)
SO_2 mean concentration (ppb)	4.9	0.0–10.5	0.25 ($n = 2111$)
SO_4 mean concentration ($\mu g/m^3$)	6.8	0.0–10.2	0.72 ($n = 2423$)
NO_2 mean concentration (ppb)	35.4	0.0–60.1	0.61 ($n = 2761$)

Source: *Environ. Res.* Long-term ambient ozone concentration and the incidence of asthma in non-smoking adults: The AHSMOG study. 80(2), McDonnell, W. F., D. E. Abbey, N. Nishino, M. D. Lebowitz. 110–121. Copyright Academic Press, 1999, with permission from Elsevier.

[a] SO_4 data were collected for the years 1977–1992.

[b] Correlation coefficient between 8-hour ozone average and each other pollutant over the years 1973–1992.

[c] Zero concentration assigned to a few individuals living in pristine area far from monitoring stations. Results from sensitivity analysis in which these individuals were excluded were similar to those results presented.

[d] Number of participants with values for both pollutants 1973–1992.

TABLE 4.16

Characteristics of Incident Cases of Doctor Diagnosis of Asthma Compared with Noncases[a]

Males				Females		
Cases (n = 32)	Noncases (n = 940)	p-Value	Variable	Cases (n = 79)	Noncases (n = 1707)	p-Value
55.2 (9.4)	54.2 (10.8)	0.592	Age (years as of April 1, 1977)	50.0 (11.3)	54.1 (11.2)	0.002
14.5 (3.6)	15.1 (3.1)	0.394	Education (years)	13.6 (2.7)	13.7 (2.4)	0.612
0%	4.8%	0.205	Resp. ill before age 16 (% yes)[b]	17.7%	6.4%	0.000
2.71 (0.97)	2.50 (0.81)	0.249	Childhood colds[c]	2.63 (1.04)	2.41 (0.88)	0.064
46.9%	28.2%	0.022	Smoke ever (% yes)	12.7%	11.2%	0.686
11.3 (13.6)	7.8 (12.0)	0.162	Years worked with smoker	7.4 (10.6)	4.6 (8.7)	0.023
13.5 (15.1)	7.7 (11.8)	0.039	Years lived with smoker	14.0 (16.1)	11.9 (15.2)	0.254
11.7 (17.7)	9.7 (14.8)	0.521	Years exposed fumes/dust	1.43(3.66)	1.40 (5.49)	0.938
16.9 (14.5)	18.4 (13.2)	0.567	Hours/week outdoor Summer (1977)	12.6 (12.8)	10.7 (9.2)	0.219
13.8 (10.6)	18.4 (12.6)	0.023	Hours/week outdoor Summer (1992)	11.4 (10.9)	10.6 (8.9)	0.527
50.7 (13.2)	46.2 (15.3)	0.068	Ozone 8-hour average (ppb)	44.4 (17.6)	46.7 (15.1)	0.253
51.6 (15.8)	50.5 (17.1)	0.711	PM_{10} mean $(\mu g/m^3)$[d]	48.5 (20.9)	50.2 (16.5)	0.484
32.7 (38.8)	31.1 (32.6)	0.825	PM_{10} {100] (days/year)[d]	32.5 (38.1)	29.2 (31.0)	0.466
7.16 (1.86)	6.73 (2.23)	0.253	SO_4 mean $(\mu g/m^3)$	6.37 (2.53)	6.85 (2.20)	0.132
4.8 (2.1)	4.9 (2.1)	0.956	SO_2 mean (ppb)	4.2 (2.1)	5.0 (2.2)	0.010

Source: *Environ. Res.* Long-term ambient ozone concentration and the incidence of asthma in nonsmoking adults: The AHSMOG study. 80(2), McDonnell, W. F., D. E. Abbey, N. Nishino, M. D. Lebowitz. 110–121. Copyright Academic Press, 1999, with permission from Elsevier.

Note: p-Values by t-test for continuous variable and x^2 test for categorical variables.

[a] Entries in table are means (SD) or expressed as the percentage of participants with a particular characteristic.

[b] Respiratory ill before age 16, bronchitis or pneumonia before age 16.

[c] Average number of colds compared with other children: 1, much less; 2, less; 3, about same; 4, more; 5 much more.

[d] Numbers of observations may be less than indicated at top of column due to missing data.

TABLE 4.17

Basic Principles of AF Management

- A stable rhythm is generally better than an unstable rhythm.
- Symptoms should drive decision-making.
- New-onset AF signals a high-risk period.
- Development of AF generally confers a worse prognosis in most serious diseases.
- Stroke risk must be considered.
- Safety should determine the initial antiarrhythmic drug chosen for rhythm control.
- Therapy for underlying conditions should be optimal and guideline based.

Source: Darby, A. E., J. P. Dimarco. 2012. Management of atrial fibrillation in patients with structural heart disease. *Circulation* 125(7):945–957. http://circ.ahajournals. org/content/125/7/945.short.

Note: AF indicates atrial fibrillation.

developing new symptoms (1977–1992) for both males and females who had reported a history of DTA in 1977, indicating that ozone may also be associated with exacerbation of existing asthma in both genders.

Both of these effects, induction of new asthma and exacerbation of existing asthma by ozone exposure, are biologically plausible. It is known that short-term experimental exposure of humans and animals to ozone results in a number of respiratory system effects, including epithelial cell damage and repair,[140] an inflammatory response,[140] increased epithelial permeability,[141] and increased nonspecific airway reactivity,[142,143] and it is known that long-term exposure of animals produces chronic airway inflammation and permanent or slowly resolving changes in the interstitial matrix of the lung.[144] Increased epithelial permeability to protein is consistent with increased access of inhaled antigen to cells of the immune system which could potentially contribute to either initial sensitization to or exacerbation of existing asthma. Changes in the interstitial matrix could potentially alter epithelial cell function[145] with possible effects upon airway responsiveness and inflammation.[146] Long-term exposure of primates,[147] mice,[148] and rats (Ian Gilmour, personal communication) to ozone has been shown to enhance sensitization to platinum, ovalbumin (OVA), and other foods, and house dust mite antigen, respectively. The increased nonspecific airway reactivity and increased response to inhaled antigen in asthmatics[149] following ozone exposure strongly suggest a role for at least short-term ozone exposure in the exacerbation of existing asthma.

Considerable epidemiologic evidence suggests that ozone exposure can exacerbate asthma, including relationships observed between short-term ozone exposure and medication use,[150] asthma attacks,[151,152] and emergency room admissions.[153,154] There has been a paucity of epidemiologic study of the role of long-term ozone exposure in incidence of asthma. Greer et al.[104] previously observed in the males of this cohort a relationship between long-term mean ambient ozone concentration and 10-year (1977–1987) development of "definite asthma" (required report of both DTA and symptoms) in those without "definite asthma" in 1977. Consistent with our current results, reanalysis of the 1977–1987 data reveals a significant ($p = 0.05$) relationship between 8-hour ozone concentration and development of DTA in 1987.

Most strengths and limitations of this study have been discussed in detail in other manuscripts[104,115,155] and will only be summarized here. Although the prospective nature of the study insures that all participants were free of DTA at the beginning of the period of observation, the long duration between questionnaires and our inability to ascertain the date of DTA for each participant prevented the authors from calculating only that exposure which occurred prior to asthma diagnosis. It is suspected that little bias would be introduced by this, however, as this cohort was generally residentially stable as evidenced by the high correlation ($r = 0.82$) between the mean 8-hour average ozone concentration for the baseline period (1973–1977) and the overall study period (1973–1992). To further test this they conducted a sensitivity analysis in which development of DTA (1977–1992) was regressed against ozone concentration measured during the study baseline period, 1973–1992. Using the ozone concentration data for the period 1973–1977 as the exposure variable, they observed a RR (9% CI of 2.03 (1.03–3.96) for a 27 ppb increment in 8-hour ozone concentration which is similar to that reported for the entire study period (2.09, 1.03–4.16) in Table 4.17. This suggests that the observed ozone–DTA relationship is unlikely to be biased to any great extent because some individuals developed DTA early in the study.

Bias in the estimates of the effects of ozone due to loss to follow-up is difficult to assess, but in this study, it most likely results in the underestimation of the true effect. Only 156 (2%) of the initial participants were untraceable in 1992. While asthma status of another 3050 (48%) individuals is unknown due to death or other reasons, ambient levels of ozone (1973–1992 or until time of death) for this group are known. Ozone concentrations for those remaining in the study were similar to those not participating for other reasons and lower than for the group that died during the study (Table 4.15). If incidence of asthma is related to mortality, the observed relationship between ozone and asthma would be biased toward the null. Another likely pattern of nonparticipation involves movement of those developing asthma from a high-ozone area to a cleaner area inside or outside the study area due to a lay perception that high levels of air pollution cause or exacerbate asthma. This would also result in an underestimation of effect.

Misclassification of exposure at the individual level is the result of both the interpolation of air pollution concentrations from surrounding monitoring stations to zip code centroids and the use of these estimates of outdoor concentration as measures of individual exposure.

Because ambient ozone concentration is strongly correlated with several other air pollutants, separation of the effects of the individual pollutants and assessment of contributions by more than one pollutant are problematic. In single-pollutant models and in the unadjusted data, however, ozone was more strongly associated with DTA than was any other monitored pollutant in males, and they evaluated the possibility of confounding measuring the effect that adding PM_{10}, SO_4, NO_2, SO_2 to the model had on the ozone coefficient. In no case was the ozone coefficient reduced by >10% in these two-pollutant models compared to the model containing ozone alone, although there was some evidence for multicollinearity in the model containing both ozone and PM_{10}. They had no measures of allergen exposure and cannot exclude the possibility of confounding by unmeasured environmental factors.

In summary, it was found that 8-hour average ambient ozone concentration (and other ozone metrics) averaged over a 20-year period was related to new reports of a doctor diagnosis of asthma over a period of 15 years in nonsmoking, adult males. They did not find a similar relationship between ozone and report of DTA in females. Their data suggest that this relationship in males may have been due to onset of new asthma although their data also show evidence of ozone-induced exacerbation of asthma symptoms in both males and females. Exposure to tobacco smoke either passively or through past smoking was related to a report of DTA in both males and females, and for females, younger age and a history of pneumonia or bronchitis before age 16 were also related to DTA. Further study of the role of long-term ozone exposure in the induction of new asthma is warranted with particular attention directed toward understanding of mechanisms and explanation of the observed gender differences.

OZONE NONSMOKER MALES

A prospective study of a cohort of 3091 nonsmokers, ages 27–87 years, to evaluate the association between long-term ambient ozone exposure and development of adult-onset asthma was performed. Over a 15 year period, 3.2% of males and 4.3% of females reported new doctor diagnoses of asthma. For males, it was observed a significant relationship between report of doctor diagnosis of asthma and 20-year mean 8-hour average ambient ozone concentration (RR = 2.09 for a 27 ppb increase in ozone concentration, 95% CI = 1.03–4.16). They observed no such relationship for females. Other variables significantly related to development of asthma were a history of ever-smoking for males (RR = 2.37%, 95% CI = 1.13–4.81), and for females, for a 7-year increment, 95% CI = 1.04–1.39), age (RR = 0.61 for a 16-year increment, 95% CI = 0.44–084), and a history of childhood pneumonia or bronchitis (RR = 2.96%, 95% CI = 1.678–5.03). Addition of other pollutants (PM_{10}, SO_4, NO_2, and SO_2) to the models did not diminish the relationship between ozone and asthma for males. These data suggest that long-term exposure to ambient ozone is associated with the development of asthma in adult males.

Incidence and prevalence of asthma in children, and to a lesser extent, in adults have been reported to be rising over the past several decades in many locations.[156–158] The reasons for the widespread increase in this multifactorial disease are unknown although suggested contributing factors include increased exposure to house dust mite or other antigens, changing patterns of viral infections, immunization with *Bordetella pertussis*, measles, and other vaccines, changes in diet exposure to new occupational agents, and increasing levels of air pollution. None of these is likely to be the sole cause of the increased prevalence and morbidity from asthma, although each of these is biologically plausible as a risk factor for developing asthma.

Although convention treats ozone as exacerbating asthma, evidence also suggests a role for long-term ozone exposure in the development of asthma for both humans and laboratory animals. Greer et al.[104] observed a relationship between the development of asthma and mean ambient ozone concentration over a period of 10 years in adult, male, nonsmoking Seventh-Day Adventists, but not in females. Biagini et al.[137] observed that 12-week exposures of nonhuman primates to a combination of ozone and platinum salts enhanced sensitization to platinum compared with exposure to platinum salts alone. Osebold et al.[148] observed that multiday exposures of mice to concentrations of ozone as low as 130 ppb ozone resulted in enhanced sensitization of mice to inhaled OVA. Similar adjuvant qualities of other pollutants have been noted.[159] The striking similarities between the effects[140,142,143] of short-term exposure of humans to ozone (e.g., airway inflammation and AHR and characteristics of asthma) also suggest a possible role for ozone in the pathogenesis of asthma.

The specific purpose of this longitudinal prospective study as to determine whether long-term residence and worksite location in areas of increased ambient ozone concentration was related to an increased incidence of asthma in nonsmoking adults. To test this hypothesis, they resurveyed the surviving members of the cohort reported upon by Greer et al.,[104] and they observed an association between the 20-year mean 8-hour average ambient ozone concentrations in the home and workplace locations and 15-year cumulative incidence of newly diagnosed cases of asthma in males, but not females. They also observed associations between tobacco smoke exposure and asthma incidence in both men and women.

OZONE AND PARTICLES

Experimental research in humans and animals points to the importance of adverse respiratory effects from short-term particle exposures and to the importance of proinflammatory effects of air pollutants, particularly O_3. However, particle averaging time has not been subjected to direct scientific evaluation, and there is a lack of epidemiological research examining both this issue and whether modification of air pollutant effects occurs with differences in asthma severity and anti-inflammatory medication use. The present study by Delfino et al.[102] examined the relationship of adverse asthma symptoms (bothersome or interfered with daily activities or sleep) to O_3 and particles <10 μm (PM_{10}) in a Southern California community in the air inversion zone (1200–2100 ft) with high O_3 and low PM ($r = 0.03$). A panel of 25 asthmatics 9–17 years of age were followed daily, August through October 1995 ($n = 1759$ person-days, excluding one subject without symptoms). Exposures included stationary outdoor hourly PM_{10} (highest 24-hour mean, 54 μg/m^3 vs. median of 1-hour maximums 56 μg/m^3) and O_3 (mean of 1-hour maximums 90 ppb, 5 days >120 ppb). Longitudinal regression analyses utilized the generalized estimating equations (GEE) model controlling for autocorrelation, day of week, outdoor fungi, and weather. Asthma symptoms were significantly associated with both outdoor O_3 and PM_{10} in single pollutant and co-regressions with 1-hour and 8-hour maximum PM_{10} having larger effects than the 24-hour mean. Subgroup analyses showed effects of current day PM_{10}. Maximums were strongest in 10 more frequently symptomatic (MS) children: the odds ratios (ORs) for adverse symptoms from 90th percentile increases were 2.24 (95% CI = 1.46–3.46) for 1-hour PM_{10} (47 μg/m^3); 1.82 (CI = 1.18–2.81) for 8-hour PM_{10} (36 μg/m^3; and 1.50 (CI = 0.80–2.80) for 24-hour PM_{10} (25 μg/m^3). Subgroup analyses also showed the effect of current day O_3 was strongest in 14 less frequently symptomatic (LS) children: the ORs were 2.15 (CI = 1.0–4.44) for 1-hour O_3 (58 ppb) and 1.92 (CI = 0.97–3.80) for 8-hour O_3 (46 ppb). Effects of 24-hour PM_{10} were seen in both groups, particularly with 5 day moving averages (ORs were 1.95 for MS and 4.03 for LS; $p = 0.05$). The largest effects were in seven LS children not on anti-inflammatory medications (5 day, 8-hour PM_{10}, 9.66 [CI = 2.80–33.21]; current day, 1-hour O_3, 4.14 [CI = 1.71–11.85]). Results suggest that examination of short-term particle excursions, medication use, and symptom severity in longitudinal studies of asthma yields sensitive measures of adverse respiratory effects of air pollution.

Air Pollution and Asthma Severity in Adults

Higher asthma severity score was significantly related to the 8-hour average of ozone during April–September (O_3^- 8 hour) and the number of days (O_3^- days) with 8-hour ozone averages above 110 µg/m^{-3} (for a 36-day increase), equivalent to the interquartile range (IQR), in O_3^- days, OR 2.22 (95% CI = 1.61–3.07 for one class difference in score). Adjustment for age, sex, smoking habits, occupational exposure, and educational level did not alter results. Asthma severity was unrelated to NO_2. Both exposure assessment methods and severity scores resulted in very similar findings. SO_2 correlated with severity but reached statistical significance only for the model-based assignment of exposure.

The observed associations between asthma severity and air pollution, in particular O_3 support the hypothesis that air pollution at levels far below current standards increases asthma severity.

Evidence of adverse effects of current air pollution on human health substantially increased in recent years.[160,161] Despite improvements in air quality in many regions of the world, primary and secondary pollutants from traffic and other sources of fossil fuel combustion such as particulate matter, diesel soot, or ozone remain of particular concern. Photochemical air pollution represented by ozone, oxides of nitrogen produced by vehicles, and respirable fine and ultrafine particulates are of interest owing to their toxic properties, and asthmatics are a particularly sensitive subgroup.[160] Associations between daily changes in air pollution and various acute respiratory outcomes including subclinical functional changes, symptoms, doctors or emergency room visits, hospitalizations, and death[3] have been reported among asthmatics.[162,163] Evidence of acute effects is based on several panel studies conducted in children, and to a lesser extent in adults. Greater susceptibility to acute effects of ambient air pollution in asthmatics with more severe asthma was observed in children[164] but was not consistent in adults.[165,166] A challenge and potential source of inconsistent results is the complex interrelation of asthma symptoms, its triggers and subjects' coping strategies though adaptation of treatment. As the typically moderate daily changes in air quality may lead to fluctuations in the expression of the disease, it is of interest to evaluate markers of asthma severity on a clinically relevant scale along the continuum between nonsymptomatic not regularly treated asthma and symptomatic asthma despite regular treatment.

The aim of the present study by Rage et al.[167] was to investigate the relations between individually assigned exposure to ambient air pollution and asthma severity assessed in two complementary ways. *First*, they use a clinically relevant score that integrates both symptoms and treatment. *Second*, they use a simpler score based on symptoms alone. They hypothesize that severity among adult asthmatics from the epidemiological study on the Genetics and Environment of Asthma, bronchial hyperresponsiveness, and atopy (EGEA) correlates with the average air quality at the residential location.

In the well-characterized sample of >300 adult asthmatics from the EDEA study, higher residential concentrations of O_3 were associated with more severe asthmas. The findings were very similar for the integrated score of clinical symptoms and treatment over the past 12 months and the novel five-level asthma symptom score. Moreover, results were not sensitive to the chosen exposure assessment approach nor to adjustment for age, sex, smoking habits, occupational exposure to asthmogens, and educations level. Results were also similar for asthmatics with or without treatment, and for smokers or nonsmokers. To the best of our knowledge, this is the first study using asthma severity scores to investigate effects of air pollution. As one score is anchored on symptoms and treatment, it better integrates the course of this disease where deteriorations of the state are usually coupled with adaptations in treatments among well-managed patients. The consistent associations observed in this study consolidate the findings. While several-panel studies and time-series studies suggest the course of asthma to be correlated with ambient oxidant concentrations in adults, the severity score is a promising integrated outcome.

The interpretation of the temporal nature of the observed association between O_3 and asthma severity is challenging and must be put in context of the study design. Depending on the assessment of outcomes and exposures, cross-sectional analyses may investigate not only long-term effects but also subacute or acute effects. Their questionnaires asked about the occurrence of symptoms and treatment in the last 12 months, thus results may be interpreted as a summary of all acute effects experienced during the past year. In this case, results are comparable to similar findings in panel studies showing asthma symptoms among adults to increase with atmospheric pollutants, both in North America and in Europe,[168] although some heterogeneity was observed in European cities. Deleterious effects of O_3 in moderate/severe adult asthmatics studies over 1 year have been reported from the Paris area.[163] The asthma severity score used in the present analysis includes frequency of attacks as well as symptoms between attacks and adaptive treatment. A complementary interpretation of the observed cross-sectional associations could be that asthma severity is increased as a consequence of chronic processes because of repeated long-term exposure. The fact that subjects who participated during winter showed similar associations with summertime O_3 concentrations as those participating during the summer period may be an indication of subacute or longer term effects of O_3 on asthma severity, as the O_3 seasons in France are by and large restricted to the summer period. However, a conclusive distinction of acute, subacute, or long-term effects of ambient O_3 exposure cannot be made with this cross-sectional approach nor in panel studies but would require large cohort studies. It would be particularly relevant to have repeated measurements at various seasons in large cohorts to disentangle subacute and chronic effects.

The associations between acute, subacute, and carryover chronic pathologies as a result of O_3 exposure is also not fully elucidated in experimental studies. Nevertheless, plausible biological mechanisms could explain the association of O_3 with asthma severity. The powerful oxidant capacity of inhaled O_3 is well known and could play a part for both acute and chronic effects by maintaining airway inflammation O_3 has also been shown to *favor a Th2 pattern*[169] and increase eosinophils,[170] but neither IgE nor eosinophils in our population were related to asthma severity.[171] Endogenous and exogenous determinants of susceptibility to the adverse effects of O_3 are most probably important and a source of random noise if not controlled in the analyses. Interactions of O_3 with genes involved in the regulation of oxidative stress, such as GSH S-transferases have already been observed in children,[172] and may have an important role in adults as well. Beyond acute effects, the pulmonary inflammatory response to inhaled O_3 and other oxidants, such as cigarette smoke, is a mechanism that could explain sustained effects of these environmental factors. Acute and chronic effects of air pollution may be interrelated, especially among asthmatics, as the repeated acute inflammatory effects may contribute to the chronic processes of airway remodeling and to severity of asthma.[173] The importance of the various inflammatory patterns in severe and persistent asthma has recently been underlined.[173] and further studies are needed to understand which pathways may be implicated, by combining environmental exposure, inflammatory markers and relevant genetic polymorphisms. Further studies should be conducted to improve exposure assessment in order to disentangle acute and chronic effects of air pollution. Information on the activity of the asthmatic disease over short periods, such as the last 15 days or 3 months should be collected as well. Indeed, the last recommendations of GINA, which focus on asthma control, will favor such data collection.[175]

In the first approach using the closest monitor, the maximum distance chosen between residential address and monitor was 40 km and this distance varies among studies, with some studies going as far as 80 km,[176] but most of our subjects (93%) lived within 10 km of a monitor. While this rather short distance minimizes the error in assigned exposure for homogeneously distributed pollutants such as O_3 or SO_2, errors are expected to be larger for spatially heterogeneous pollutants such as NO_2. We expect these errors to be nonsystematic, thus biasing associations toward the null.

The contrast in the assigned exposure was rather low in the case of NO_2 and SO_2, with respectively, a 1.5-fold and 1.8-fold change across the IQR of concentrations (31–45 and 15–27, respectively; closest monitor approach), thus affecting the statistical power to observe effects. In the case of O_3, power was clearly better with a 2.8-fold difference (IQR 20–56). The IFEN model resulted in similar contrasts for NO_2, whereas those for SO_2 were stronger (2.5-fold increase). This may explain why associations became significant in this model. IQR for O_3 was lower in the IFEN model (1.2-fold increase), nevertheless results remained statistically significant and support the interpretation that oxidant pollutants indicated by ambient O_3 affect asthma severity.

They found some evidence for heterogeneity of effects across centers with far smaller estimates in some cities. In both analyses performed adding center as a random effect or after exclusion of the centers, possibly driving the association in relation to the highest O_3 exposure, did not change the main estimate. However, owing to the limited sample size within cities, it is not possible to further elucidate whether effects of O_3 to be center-specific, driven, for example, by other environmental or population factors present in only a few locations, or whether *heterogeneity was a random finding.*

Based on other studies one may expect substantial correlations between ambient PM and NO_2,[177] thus explaining the O_3 findings with particles does not seem to be vary plausible in their study. Air conditioning was not assessed, but was not frequently used in France at the time of the survey. To what extent O_3 may be a marker of other constituents in the toxic mixture of ambient air cannot be answered with our study and the heterogeneity across centers may partly be explained by O_3 indicating in part different characteristics of air pollution across these regions.

In conclusion, they observed significant associations between ambient O_3 concentrations and asthma severity in adults. Results were consistent across two approaches of individual assignment of exposure as well as for two complementary markers of asthma severity. More studies are needed to elucidate the time sequence of pollution on asthma severity. But the present results add to the evidence of adverse effects of O_3 at levels far below current air quality standards among susceptible people—namely, those with asthma, supporting more stringent regulations of ambient O_3,[178] thought to be set to protect public health. The use of asthma severity scores to investigate the contribution of environmental factors to this complex and dynamic disease appears very promising.

Much has been published about pollutants causing respiratory disease. Now, data have recently been published about organic and inorganic chemicals causing cardiovascular disease. This will be elaborated in the following section.

CARDIOVASCULAR DISEASE

Pollutant exposure and subsequent injury to the immune and nonimmune detoxification systems, the hearts conducting system, or the intrinsic heart muscle frequently occur.

According to Darby and DiMarco,[179] atrial fibrillation (AF) is the most common sustained arrhythmia encountered by clinicians. The prevalence of AF increases with age, and the elderly are the fastest-growing subset of the population. They also have been the longest in years to be exposed to the increase in total environmental pollutant load. This phenomenon can be due to degeneration changes or injury. It has been estimated that there will be less than 12 million patients with AF in the United States within the next several decades.[180,181] These exposures may be triggered by carbon monoxide, nitrogen dioxide, sulfur dioxide, ozone, particulates, lead, mercury, etc., and other environmental substances like molds, food, chemicals, and electromagnetic impulses, especially inorganic pollutants.

AF may present in a wide variety of clinical conditions. The optimal management strategy for an individual patient with AF depends on the patient's underlying condition and whether incitants such as foods, molds, chemicals, and EMF can be neutralized or removed. In some patients, AF occurs in the absence of structural heart disease. The imbalance of the ANS and cardiac imbalance of the conducting system due to pollutant exposure must be considered. Clinical trials involving only or predominantly this type of AF may not be completely applicable to those with concomitant heart disorders since removal of environmental incitants and replacement of nutrients may be all that is necessary to correct the AF or dampen its effects. However, structural heart disease may influence both the approach to management (i.e., rate vs. rhythm control) and the treatment options available. For instance, fewer antiarrhythmic drugs are available for use in patients with heart failure (HF) as opposed to AF patients who have structurally normal hearts but abnormal conduction systems due to excess pollutant exposure. In addition, some patients with structural heart disease tolerate AF poorly, and the approach to these patients will differ from those with well-tolerated, minimally symptomatic AF. In any case, inorganic pollutants will have to be reduced in order for the patient to function well.

Several basic principles should be considered when management approaches are planned for any patient with AF (Table 4.18). First, no patient wants to be in AF or does better in AF than in native (i.e., untreated), stable sinus rhythm. Therefore, restoration and maintenance of sinus rhythm should be considered for every patient. In addition, a stable rhythm, even if that rhythm is persistent AF, is often better than an unstable rhythm with frequent and abrupt changes that may be highly symptomatic. An argument in favor of stability is suggested by data from the Atrial Fibrillation Follow-up Investigation of Rhythm Management (AFFIRM) trial. A substudy on mechanisms of death showed that the excess mortality associated with the rhythm control strategy in AFFIRM was not due to cardiac causes but rather was attributed largely to noncardiac illness[182] such as excess pollutant exposure and conduction injury. It seems possible that other critical illnesses as changes in the underlying rhythm, which in a vicious cycle further complicate the patient's problem (Figure 4.1).[183] As shown by Miyasaka and collegues[184,185] in studies from Olmstead County, Minnesota, the first episode of AF may be a time of particular concern because hospitalizations and mortality in the first few months after the first onset of AF are higher than in other periods. If the AF is triggered by pollutants these must be removed or neutralized. Most cardiac units are unaware when to manipulate the total environmental loads in the patient's behavior. These observations lead us to

---

TABLE 4.18

Estimated Logistic Regression Coefficients (β) and Relative (RR) of Developing Doctor Diagnosis of Asthma Associated with Increments in the Independent Variable for Males and Females

Variable	β (SE)	RR	Increment[a]	95% Confidence Interval
		Males		
Age (years)	0.0024 (0.0171)	1.04	16 years	0.61–1.74
Education (years)	−0.0290 (0.0637)	0.90	4 years	0.55–1.44
Ozone 8-hour average (ppb)	0.0277 (0.0135)*	2.09	27.0 ppb	1.03–4.16
Pneumonia/bronchitis Before age 16 (y/n)	−5.9809 (14.5151)	—[b]	Yes vs. no	—[b]
Smoke ever	0.8975 (0.3957)*	2.37	Yes vs. no	1.13–4.81
Constant	−4.7052 (1.5793)			
		Females		
Age (years)	−0.0331 (0.0109)**	0.61	16 years	0.44–0.84
Education (years)	−0.0473 (0.0538)	0.83	4 years	0.55–1.25
Ozone 8-hour average (ppb)	−0.0058 (0.0077)	0.86	27.0 ppb	0.58–1.26
Pneumonia/bronchitis Before age 16 (y/n)	1.1669 (0.3167)**	2.96	Yes vs. no	1.68–5.03
Years worked with smoker	0.0277 (0.0110)*	1.21	7 years	1.04–1/39
Constant	−1.7748 (1.0177			

Source: Environ. Res. Long-term ambient ozone concentration and the incidence of asthma in nonsmoking adults: The AHSMOG study. 80(2), McDonnell, W. F., D. E. Abbey, N. Nishino, M. D. Lebowitz. 110–121. Copyright Academic Press, 1999, with permission from Elsevier.

Note: Statistical significance calculated by likelihood ratio test (*, *p*-value <0.05; II, *p* < 0.01).

[a] Increment represents an interquartile range increase in each independent variable with the exception of yes/no variables.

[b] RR not estimated due to zeros in one cell. Parameter estimate for this variable is likely to be unstable. RR for ozone is unchanged when males with pneumonia or bronchitis before age 16 (*n* = 45) are excluded from the analysis.

believe that, in most patients, symptoms should be the major determinant behind choices between rhythm and rate control approaches.

Stroke is one of the more serious complications of AF. In all patients, stroke risk should be assessed, and the patient's specific disease state as well as more general risk factors including the $CHADS_2$ or CHA_2DS_2VASc scores need to be considered.[186,187] The patient's long-term prognosis must also be considered. Decisions made in an 85-year-old individual might well be inappropriate for someone in their 40s and 50s who would face years of treatment. However, pollutant reduction or removal or incitant neutralization must be considered in all treatment modalities for all ages. This removal includes biological inhalants (pollens, dust, and molds), food, chemicals, including metals, solvents, natural gas and pesticides, formaldehyde, and electromagnetic stimuli.

HEART FAILURE

AF and HF have been recognized as the two epidemics of modern cardiovascular medicine.[188] Both conditions frequently coexist because HF is a major risk factor for AF. The risk of AF increases 4.5- to 5.9-fold in the presence of HF, and HF is a more powerful risk factor for AF than advanced age, valvular heart disease, hypertension, diabetes mellitus, or prior myocardial infarction (MI).[189,190] AF prevalence increases as HF severity worsens. AF has been estimated to occur in 5%–10% of patients with mild HF, 10%–26% with moderate disease, and up to 50% with advanced HF.[191–194] Among acutely decompensated HF patients, 20%–35% will be in AF at presentation.[195] In nearly one-third, the AF will be of recent onset. Overall, patients with HF develop AF at a rate of 6%–8% per year, and AF is present in >15% of HF patients.

Controversy exists in regard to the prognostic significance of AF in HF. Although data suggest a worse prognosis for patients with HF and AF compared with those with HF but no AF, the complexities of both conditions make it difficult to determine whether AF is an independent risk factor or mortality or rather is indicative of disease severity. Certainly, if carbon monoxide or particulates persists causing the AF then it will increase the severity of the HF. If these pollutants can be reduced then both the AF and HF can be reduced.

RATE CONTROL

Adequate control of the ventricular response to AF improves symptoms by alleviating the negative hemodynamic effects of rapid rates. LV function may improve with adequate long-term rate control, particularly if the LV dysfunction is due to persistent tachycardia.[196] Recent guidelines suggest a goal heart rate of 80–100 bpm in managing acute episodes of AF.[197] Again decrease in the total body pollutant load and especially the criteria pollutants will aid in the reduction of HF. This is because of the ANS effect of pollutants which will decrease parasympathetic response and increase sympathetic influences resulting in increase of the rate.

RHYTHM CONTROL

Data from prospective randomized controlled trials demonstrating a survival advantage with pharmacological maintenance of sinus rhythm in HF are lacking. The AFIRM and RACE trials found that maintenance of sinus rhythm in mixed AF populations provided no benefit with a trend toward harm.[198,199]

A number of cardiac conditions predispose to the development of AF. Environmental triggers have been overlooked but clinical responses have shown that pollutants individually or in combination by virtue of a total environment pollutant can trigger the atrial fibrillation. A complex interaction often develops between AF and the arrhythmia substrate, and development of AF generally confers an adverse prognosis in most situations, primarily related to an increased risk of stroke. Increased exposure to ambient pollutant levels both indoor and outdoor with new onset AF may signal a period of particularly increased risk and should prompt careful evaluation and treatment. Here the clinician must decrease the total environmental and body pollutant load in order to stabilize the patient. Management of AF in the setting of concomitant cardiac disease primarily involves assessment of the stroke risk and anticoagulation as appropriate along with reasonable control of the ventricular response and the outdoor and indoor environment and mold, food, and chemical exposure. This means a detailed analysis of the outdoor and indoor environment in order to decrease the total body pollutant load. Decisions regarding rhythm control are largely dictated by symptoms. When pursued, rhythm control should initially be attempted pharmacologically, with safety primarily determining the agent chosen. However, the pollutant load should be reduced first. Catheter and surgical ablation are reserved as second-line therapies for patients in whom at least one antiarrhythmic drug has failed. Importantly, underlying diseases must be optimally managed with guideline-based therapies for AF treatments to be most effective.

The triggering of the arrhythmias should be evaluated as to air, food, and water contents and susceptibility. The clinician might be able to define triggering agents and eliminate or neutralize them in order to prevent AF and/or HF (Table 4.19).

A recent study by Mustafic et al.[200] has shown that each of the criteria pollutants from around the world except ozone are associated with MI. Ozone can certainly aggravate or contribute to the total body pollutant load, then causing arrhythmia with the combination of pollutants.

The potentially deleterious effect of episodes of high air pollution on health has been seen for >50 years. Poor health in the form of chemical EMF sensitivity and chronic degenerative disease have been described by Randolph, Dickey, and Rea for >40 years.[86,91,201]

Short-term exposure to high levels of air pollution may trigger MI, but this association remains unclear. However, Mustafic et al. have clarified this premise.[200]

To assess and quantify the association between short-term exposure and major air pollutants (ozone, carbon monoxide, nitrogen dioxide, sulfur dioxide, and particulate matter ≤ 10 μm [PM_{10}] and ≤ 2.5 μm [$PM_{2.5}$] in diameter) on MI risk, they studied numerous reports in a world review and found that EMBASE, Ovid MEDLINE in-process and other nonindexed citations, Ovid MEDLINE (between 1948 and November 28, 2011), and EBM Reviews-Cochrane Central Register of Controlled Trials and EBM Reviews-Cochrane Database of Systematic Reviews (between 2005 and November 28, 2011) were searched for a combination of keywords related to the type of exposure (air pollution, ozone, carbon monoxide, nitrogen dioxide, sulfur dioxide, PM_{10}, and $PM_{2.5}$) and to the type of outcome (MI, heart attack, acute coronary syndrome).[200]

According to Mustafic et al.,[200] two independent reviewers selected studies of any study design and in any language, using original data and investigating the association between short-term exposure (for up to 7 days) to one or more air pollutants and subsequent MI risk. Selection was performed from abstracts and titles and pursued by reviewing the full text of potentially eligible studies.

TABLE 4.19

Key Issues to Address in the Management of Acute AF Episodes in Patients with Heart Failure

- What is the hemodynamic status of the patient?
- Does the patient have an ICD or pacemaker?
- Does the patient have preserved or reduced systolic function at baseline?
- What is the duration of the AF episode?
- Is the patient already on drugs for anticoagulation and rate or rhythm control?
- What is the status of the pollutant generator for AF?

Source: Darby, A. E., J. P. Dimarco. 2012. Management of atrial fibrillation in patients with structural heart disease. *Circulation* 125(7):945–957. http://circ.ahajournals. org/content/125/7/945.short.

Note: AF indicates atrial fibrillation; ICD, implantable cardioverter-defibrillator.

Descriptive and quantitative information was extracted from each selected study. Using a random effects model, RRs and 95% CIs were calculated for each increment of 10 µg/m³ in pollutant concentration, with the exception of carbon monoxide, for which an increase of 1 mg/m³ was considered.

In industrialized countries, cardiovascular disease is the leading cause of mortality and is associated with significant morbidity.[202,203] These countries have high pollution levels. Since the 1990s, several epidemiological studies have demonstrated associations between air pollution levels and human health in terms of hospital admissions[204,205] and overall mortality, including respiratory[206] or cardiovascular mortality.[203] The senior author of this book has described the environmental triggers of specific vascular inflammation and cardiac triggers[91] for arrhythmias and HF (Vol. II) starting in the 1970s, etc., to the present. However, no other reported studies were performed under environmentally controlled conditions. However, the association between air pollution and near-term risk of MI remains controversial. Some studies have shown an association,[207,208] while other studies have found either no association[209,210] or association only for selected pollutants.[211,212] None have shown the effects of total body pollutant load because other than a few centers have correlated and studied it in the context of cardiovascular disease.

According to Mustafic et al.,[200] after a detailed screening of 117 studies, 34 studies were identified. All the main air pollutants with the exception of ozone, were significantly associated with an increase in MI risk (carbon monoxide: 1.048; 95% CI = 1.026–1.070; nitrogen dioxide: 1.011; 95% CI = 1.006–1.016; sulfur dioxide: 1.010; 95% CI = 1.003–1.017; PM_{10}: 1.006; 95% CI = 1.002–1.009; and $PM_{2.5}$: 1.025; 95% CI = 1.015–1.036). For ozone, the RR was 1.003 95% CI = 0.997–1.010, $p = 0.36$). Subgroup analyses provided results comparable with those of the overall analyses. Population attributable fractions ranged between 0.6% and 4.5% depending on the air pollutant.

In conclusion, all the main pollutants with the exception of ozone, were significantly associated with a near-term increase in MI risk.[200]

This meta-analysis is the first to our knowledge to assess the quality and magnitude of the associations between short-term exposure to major air pollutants and MI risk. Mustafic et al.[200] demonstrated a significant association between all analyzed pollutants, with the exception of ozone and MI risk.

The subgroup analyses were associated with lower heterogeneity and no significant publication bias, while yielding results comparable with those from the overall analysis. Thus, the findings are robust. We cannot rule out, however, that the absence of publications bias in the subgroups analyses is due to the reduced sample size. The significant associations observed in their study were consistent with evidence from experimental cellular, histological animal, and healthy volunteer studies.

A number of possible mechanisms for the associations reported herein have been suggested. The first potential mechanism is oxidative stress and/or inflammation.[202,213] Studies have shown that levels of inflammatory markers such as C-reactive protein[214] and cytokines are higher as a result of exposure to air pollution. The second potential mechanism is abnormal regulation of the cardiac autonomic nervous system.[202] resulting in a decrease parasympathetic nervous system and by an increase in adrenalin response with resultant tachycardia and/or arrhythmias. Several observational studies having linked high levels of air pollution with change in heart rate variability.[213]

The third possible mechanism is an increase in blood viscosity as a result of air pollution.[215] This association can promote thrombus formation,[216] accelerate the progression of atherosclerosis, and weaken the stability of atherosclerotic plaques or cause strokes or infarcts in the heart or other areas. A fourth potential mechanism is the air pollutants may increase vasoconstrictors such as endothelins.[217] The latter condition occurs in the microcells causing local tissue hypoxia which can result in arrhythmia and/or HF.

In addition, mechanisms including direct induction of cardiac ischemia by vasospasm[218] or direct arrhythmogenesis[219] have been evoked, although these were suggested from studies including women only. All these data from experimental studies strengthen the biological plausibility that exposure to air pollution may affect the risk of MI occurrence via multiple mechanisms.

Their findings regarding ozone differed compared with findings for other air pollutants. However, associations of ozone with health are difficult to estimate. Ozone is only one of several air components of the "photochemical cocktail" and the mechanisms of its formation and destruction are complex and varied.[220] It is well established that MI is less prevalent in the summer when temperature and ozone concentrations tend to be the highest.[221] Therefore, an adjustment for temperature is necessary. However, there was also a wide variability of approaches of adjustment for temperature, which led to variability in the RR estimates between exposure to ozone and MI risk. The idea advanced in some studies would be to limit the analysis to summer periods but the downfall of this approach is the dramatic reduction of the exposure period.[220,230] Moreover adjustment for temperature does not suffice because the mechanism of ozone formation is more closely dependent on solar radiation and brightness[220] and no study to our knowledge has ever adjusted for brightness.

They acknowledge that the magnitude of association is relatively small compared with those of classic MI risk factors, such as smoking, a pollutant, hypertension, or diabetes, which may have environmental triggers and which range from 2 to 3.[222] Nevertheless, the PAF of each pollutant is not negligible because the majority of the population, including young and disabled patients are exposed to air pollution, particularly in urban settings, and thus an improvement in air quality could have a significant effect on public health.

Potential limitations of their study need to be considered. First most studies have used a "single-pollutant" model in spite of possible interactions between pollutants. Few "multipollutant" models[209,223–225] have been used because they are difficult to implement and have not been validated. In addition, the application of an additive or multiplicative model requires a clear understanding of the nature of the relationship between exposure and disease, which is currently lacking. Thus, they have independently analyzed the association of each pollutant on the risk of MI without being able to evaluate the interactions between these pollutants.

In addition, heterogeneity in exposure ascertainment across studies exists. Some studies have considered the mean of concentration, other studies have used either peak or mean of concentration depending of the pollutant,[207,211,212,224,226–229] and the remaining studies have analyzed peak and mean of concentrations.[230,231] To the extent that the pathophysiological mechanisms are multiple, the dimension that is most likely to be involved in the risk of MI, between peak or mean of concentrations in pollutant, remains unclear. Additional limitations to inferences shown in their study relate to the observed statistical heterogeneity, publication bias, and the lack of validated quality scales for studies with time-series and case-crossover designs.

One strength of the study of Mustafic et al.[200] is the comprehensive nature of their search that spanned multiple databases and was not restricted to a particular publication, language or a single pollutant. In addition, subgroup analyses confirmed the robustness of the original results.

In conclusion, their meta-analysis is the first to our knowledge to evaluate the quality and magnitude of associations between short-term exposure to major air pollutants and the risk of MI. Mustafic et al.[200] demonstrated an increase in near-term risk of MI associated with short-term exposure to all major air pollutants, with the exception of ozone. Although the RRs were relatively low, the PAFs were not negligible because the majority of the population is exposed to air pollution in industrialized countries. Further research is needed to determine whether effective interventions that improve air quality are associated with a decreased incidence of MI.

LEUKOCYTE BEHAVIOR IN ATHEROSCLEROSIS, MI, AND HF AND VASCULAR SPASM

Cardiovascular diseases claim more lives worldwide than any other. Etiologically, the dominant trajectory involves atherosclerosis, a chronic inflammatory process of lipid-rich lesion growth in the vascular wall that can cause life-threatening MI. Those who survive MI can develop congestive

HF, a chronic condition of inadequate pump activity that is frequently fatal. Leukocytes are important participants in the various stages of cardiovascular disease progression and complication. The etiology of cardiovascular disease is environmental, including diet and water quality intake as well as food, chemical, and EMF sensitive air pollutants.

The immune system protects against pathogens such as viruses, bacteria, and parasitic worms, but its influence is much broader. The T and B lymphocyte, complement, and gamma globulin abnormalities are seen in chemical sensitivity and also may be found in AS. The system recognizes and responds to divergent environmental substances such as lead, mercury, carbon monoxide, sulfur dioxide, nitrous oxide, benzene, toluene, styrene, pesticides, particulates, and endogenous and exogenous compounds, that is, glutamate, aspartate, and vasopressin which triggers these aforementioned pollutants reaction. Various other endogenous substances and stimuli, as just shown and every known disease is at least partially associated with or dependent on immune function and nonimmune detoxification systems. Cardiovascular disease is no exception.

Over the past half century, advances in public health (emphasis on healthy diet, exercise, and smoking cessation), clinical cardiology (chest pain units, coronary stenting, and cardiac defibrillation), and scientific discoveries (lipid-lowering statins, angiotensin-converting enzyme inhibitors) have contributed to a steady decline in deaths from cardiovascular disease.[232] Despite these improvements, the disease is still responsible for 30% of deaths worldwide, surpassing all others, including cancer, and costing the global economy (in 2010) an estimated U.S. $863 billion. Much of this mortality and morbidity may have to do with the slow institution of Environmental Control Units, science and environmental techniques in order to eliminate and control pollutant entry and injury. Even after surviving MI or stroke, the likelihood of developing secondary complications, such as reinfarction or HF is high which increases costs through hospitalization and follow-up clinical care. The substitution or institution of environmental control techniques should and will decrease morbidity and mortality. The world population is rising, and it is estimated that by 2030, cardiovascular disease costs could increase to U.S. $1044 billion[233] or much more.

For several years after its recognition, atherosclerosis was thought to involve passive lipid deposition in the vessel wall. Today, we understand that atherosclerosis is a chronic oxidative stress and inflammatory disease driven by lipids, specifically low-density lipoproteins (LDLs) and leukocytes, and also these are triggered by the exposure to environmental incitants such as CO, Hg, N_2O, and OONO like other inorganic and organic chemicals and ultrafine particulates.[234] Neither atherosclerosis nor its complications adhere to a simple arithmetic of dietary lipid imbalance but rather comprise a syndrome in which environmental and genetic inputs disrupt biological systems directed by both the individual and total environmental pollutant load. In other words, lifestyle, age, hereditary factors, environmental exposures, and comorbidities disturb immune, digestive, endocrine, circulatory, and nervous systems, thereby altering immune function detoxification, metabolism, direct vessel wall disturbances, and many other processes while eliciting oxidative stress, inflammation, hypercholesterolemia, and hypertension. Atherosclerosis develops and causes MI or stroke when many things go wrong in many different ways. Particularly, the adverse environmental incitants are usually involved, resulting in vessel spasm or leaks with a series of mild hypoxic events leading to oxidative stress and chronic inflammation.

Leukocytes are keepers of the immune system: The various classes of myeloid and lymphoid cells that encompass the leukocyte repertoire recognize and eliminate pathogens and toxic chemicals, and molecular patterns perceived to be dangerous. They are supposed to eliminate environmentally triggered incitants but are often overwhelmed by their sheer volume and total toxicity. Working together, leukocytes can engender protective immunity and keep those functions and anatomy from harm. This is particularly true for the T and B lymphocytes. Yet leukocytes can also contribute to disease. Virtually every leukocyte class has been implicated in atherosclerosis and its complications, and their action is neither uniform nor hierarchial.[234] Some leukocytes are atherogenic, whereas others are atheroprotective; some sustain oxidative stress and inflammation after MI, yet others resolve it. The functional heterogeneity is a challenge but also an opportunity for therapeutic intervention because it suggests that specific disease-promoting functions can be targeted and those required for normal homeostasis can be spared. Avoidance of pollutants by reduction of the total body and specific pollutant load is usually necessary whereas replacement of nutrients involved in the detoxication function and repair mechanism is also essential for adequate prevention, detoxification, and repair to cells. Most of the latter processes are still ignored by the medical community.

The natural progression of atherosclerosis in the human involves the acquisition of specific features in the growing lesion. A key initiating process of atherosclerosis is the intimal retention of apolipoprotein (apo) B-containing lipoproteins in regions of disturbed blood flow and low shear stress[235] usually triggered by pollutants Pb, Hg, CO, N_2O, SO_2, benzene, methane, propane, butane, particulates, insecticides, natural gas, etc.[234] Lipid-rich macrophages, otherwise known as foam cells, appear early in the intima and can be identified in nearly 40% of newborns; they typically regress before the age of 2. The toxic load in the cord blood is seen in some patients. The existence of small pools of extracellular lipids in the intima is a feature of a preatheroma, whereas an easily discernible core of extracellular lipid marks an atheroma and contain multiple toxic substances. Increasingly complicated lesions are defined by fibrous thickenings usually triggered by pollutants, as are the appearance of fissures, hematoma, and thrombi; and calcification. By the age of 45%, 95% of people have some type of lesion. This lesion results from a lifetime exposure of environmental pollutant trying to sequester toxics. Problems occur if a lesion interferes with tissue oxygenation when either the lesion's size reduces blood flow or the lesion ruptures and occludes the vessel altogether. Of the two, lesions that rupture are far more dangerous. MI and stroke are sudden events that result from occlusion of vessels that oxygenate the heart and brain, respectively.[236]

MACROPHAGE

The macrophage as a protagonist for injury surely occurs. Macrophages are most numerous among leukocytes in any type of lesion and, with the possible exception of smooth muscle cells, the most prominent cellular contributors to the lesion's physical bulk.[237] In response to intimal lipid accumulation, disturbed blood flow, low shear stress, and other stimuli, endothelial cells permit monocytes (major precursors of macrophages) passage across the endothelium[238,239] to damage cardiovascular and neurological tissue. Newly infiltrated monocyte-derived macrophages recognize and ingest lipids that have accrued in the intima as a consequence of hypercholesterolemia. These lipids are accompanied by toxic inorganics and organic chemicals which may stimulate the process trying to detoxify or wall off the pollutants. Macrophages are specialized phagocytes that rely on different strategies to sense, internalize, and process the diverse lipid moieties they encounter.

Pattern recognition receptors (PRRs) expressed on the plasma membrane recognizes various native and oxidized lipoproteins and facilitates their uptake for lysosomal degradation.[240] Likewise, cytoplasmic sensors such as the NLRP3 inflammasomes respond to cholesterol crystals and release interleukin-1β (IL-1β), a major inflammatory cytokine.[241,242] The relative importance of specific sensors to the generation of foam cells and development of atherosclerosis continues to be debated: PRRs such as SR-A and CD36 are dispensable to foam-cell formation,[243] whereas the NLRP3 inflammasome influences atherosclerosis in one mouse model,[241] but not in another.[244]

Macrophage lipid uptake may be viewed as a protective potential healing response that backfires. Ingesting oxidized lipoproteins, as well as their imperceived total chemical content such as ingesting microbes, involves the scavenging of substances perceived to be dangerous, usually containing toxic inorganic and volatile organic chemicals. Thus, oxidative stress by pollutants occurs. After lipoprotein recognition and consequent ingestion, macrophages morph into foam cells, many of which eventually die and contribute to a large lipid core, a characteristic of lesions most vulnerable to rupture.[237] Surprisingly, foam-cell formation suppresses, rather than promotes, inflammatory gene expression.[245] Leukocytes may fuel an inflammatory cycle, but they also, in some incarnations, quench it.

Leukocytosis predicts cardiovascular events: Human and mouse blood contains at least two distinct monocyte subsets with differential migratory properties.[246] Mouse Ly-6C[high] monocytes share several properties with human CD16$^+$CD14$^+$ monocytes and are inflammatory. In response to hypercholesterolemia, the bone marrow and spleen overproduce Ly-6C^{high} monocytes that enter the circulation, contribute to excessive monocytosis, preferentially accumulate in lesions, and differentiate to macrophages. Ly-6C^{low} monocytes, which are thought to be primarily reparative, are similar to CD16$^+$CD14^{dim} human monocytes, patrol the vasculature, and infiltrate atheromata less frequently. If an overzealous immune system generates too many cells that contribute to pathology, then targeting the culprit subset may be atheroprotective.

Genetically engineered disruption of cholesterol metabolism defines the two major models of atherosclerosis; apolipoprotein E-deficient (ApoE$^+$) and LDL receptor (LDLR)-deficient mice develop two ApoE and other mice deficient in lipid-efflux proteins, such as the adenosine triphosphate (ATP)-binding cassette transporter 1 (ABCA1) and ATP-binding cassette transporter 1 (ABCAA1) and ATP-binding cassette subfamily G member 1 (ABCG1), have forged a mechanistic link between leukocyte and lipid biology. Trapped cholesterol in hematopoietic stem and progenitor cells (HSPCs) that lack the crucial cholesterol efflux machinery leads to the expression of the granulocyte-macrophage colony-stimulating factor (GM-CSF) and IL-3 common beta chain receptor on the plasma membrane contributes to excessive proliferation.[247,248] In other words, cholesterol efflux suppress proliferation. Concurrently, lipid-rich splenic phagocytes release IL-23, which induces a cascade that eventually liberates HSPCs from their medullary niches.[249] When HSPCs seed extramedullary sites, they encounter GM-CSF and IL-3.[250] The net effect is HSPC proliferation, extramedullary hematopoiesis, leukocytosis, and accelerated atherosclerosis.

Most humans are not ApoE, LDLR, ABCA1, or ABCG1 deficient; they are not impaired in handling cholesterol. But human cardiovascular disease does associate with leukocytosis,[251] perhaps a version of insufficient cholesterol handling rather than its complete breakdown. If so, then precise targeting of leukocyte-centric cholesterol pathways will be therapeutically desirable.

Macrophage Flux and Function

Macrophage flux involves monocyte migration across the endothelium, monocyte differentiation to macrophages, macrophage retention in the atheromata, exit, or death. The preferential accumulation of Ly-6C^{high} monocytes in the growing atheromata relies on chemokine-dependent signaling through CCR2-CCL2, CX3CR1-CX3CL1, and CCR5-CCL5,[252] and neutralizing these axes in mice almost abolishes atherosclerosis.[253,254] Upon accumulation and lipid ingestion, macrophages release netrin-1, a guidance molecule that binds to UNC5b on the plasma membrane and blocks the directed migration of macrophages out of the lesion.[255] In the absence of netrin-1, lesions are smaller. Lesions with large necrotic cores are most vulnerable. When one surveys, the peripheral blood counts differential in the chemically sensitive monocytes are usually decreased. This suggests that they are converting to macrophages in the tissue areas containing toxics.

A macrophage is not simply "a big eater," however, and it does not exist in isolation. Lesional macrophages are polyfunctional and interact with other leukocytes and nonleukocyte client cells. Macrophage polyfunctionality in the aorta represents either dedicated behavior of individually specialized cells (distinct macrophage subsets) or adaptive behavior elicited by the tissue environment (macrophage plasticity). Regardless of how division of labor is maintained, macrophages, as a cell population that accumulates lipids, secrete cytokines that attract other leukocytes, produce proteinases that digest the extracellular matrix, disturb smooth muscle cell function, and can influence endothelial-dependent vasodilatation.[237] Macrophages can also resolve inflammation and promote granulation tissue formation.[256]

Adaptive Immunity Not Only in Atherosclerosis But Also Other Inflammatory Vascular Diseases

Adaptive immunity is the immune system's arm that uses antigen specificity to generate potent defense and lost memory against specific pathogens important in atherosclerosis. Dendritic cells, which capture an antigen and present it to naïve T cells, reside in the aorta and affect progression of atherosclerosis,[257–259] possibly by interacting with T cells[260] previously activated in lymph nodes and tertiary lymphoid organs.[261] T cells are relatively rare in lesions. Even so, specific perturbations, most of T cell-associated cytokines, suggest that T helper (T_H)-1 and T_H17 cells are atherogenic, whereas T_H2 and regulatory T (T_{reg}) cells are protective.[262,263] T_H1 generated interferon (IFN)-γ, for example, activated macrophages and propagates inflammation, whereas T_{reg}-generated IL-10 and transforming growth factor (TGF)-β dampen inflammation. T-cells have been shown to be active in chemically sensitive vasculitis.

B cells, which are rare in lesions but more prevalent in the adventitia, can be both atheroprotective and atherogenic.[264,265] First be stimulated and increase in the blood. Then, as the disease progresses, they disappear from the blood being markedly decreased. These are caused by pollutant exposure of inorganic and organic toxics. The innate such as B1 B cells are atheroprotective, possibly because they produce natural immunoglobulin M (IgM) antibodies that mark lipids for Fc receptor-mediated removal. The adaptive B2 B cells on the other hand, contribute to disease, presumably by interacting with other leukocytes and/or secreting inflammatory cytokines.[264] Because cellular and molecular constituents implicated in adaptive immunity regulate atherosclerosis, they can be harnessed, at least experimentally, to alter disease progression. In the chemically sensitive, pollutant entry and injury can suppress or stimulate B cells levels, since they can cause chemical vasculitis, they also may trigger the A.S. vasculitis.

The generation of antigen specificity though genetic recombination defines adaptive immunity. In atherosclerosis, antibodies and CD4$^+$ T cells that react to lipid moieties such as oxLDL have been identified.[266,267] However, lymphocytes can secrete cytokines and proliferate in response to germline-encoded receptor signaling. Innate lymphoid cells, natural killer T cells (NK cells), tissue-resident γδT cells, and innate like B cells such as innate response activator (IRA) B cells share phenotypic features with their adaptive counterparts but differ in how they perceive and respond to molecular patterns.

Inflammatory professionals: Neutrophils, mast cells, and platelets are detectable in lesions and may influence atherosclerosis and its complications in important ways. Neutrophils, the inflammatory granulocytes, circulate in large numbers and accumulate early on at sites of injury or infection. Neutrophils also contain large quantities of myeloperoxidase, nicotinamide adenine dinucleotide phosphate (NADPH) oxidase, and lipoxygenases, which contribute to oxidative stress, a major determinant of endothelial cell dysfunction, lesion growth, and instability. Mast cells, best known for their role in allergy and anaphylaxis, promote atherosclerosis by releasing the contents of their protease-cytokine-autacoid-rich granules.[268] Platelets play an essential, dual role. During atherosclerosis, they adhere to the endothelium and help monocytes enter lesions.[269] During plaque rupture, they form the thrombus that causes ischemia of downstream tissue.[237] Thus, neutrophils, mast cells, and platelets all promote atherosclerosis by intensifying inflammation.

LEUKOCYTES IN MI AND HF

Small arteriosclerotic lesions that do not hinder blood flow are found in many people. They are certainly found in many chemically sensitive patients. Subclinical atherosclerosis manifests itself when lesions reduce tissue oxygen supply. Additional lesion growth and inward arterial remodeling gradually narrow the vessel diameter, thereby limiting blood flow. If coronary arterial stenosis reaches >80% downstream heart muscle becomes ischemic, especially when a high cardiac work load increases the oxygen demand. In contrast to atherosclerosis, where chronic low-grade stimulation by native and oxidized lipoproteins mobilizes leukocytes to the vessel wall, in MI, acutely dying myocytes elicit different triggers that nevertheless recruit similar classes of leukocytes. The population of macrophages[270] and dendritic cells[258] that reside in the healthy heart is quickly overwhelmed by inflammatory leukocytes.

Shortly after onset of ischemia, endothelial cells upregulate adhesion molecules that, along with released chemokines, trigger neutrophil extravasation. Rapid accumulation leads to an early neutrophil peak after injury.[256] In skin wounds, neutrophils protect against infection through phagocytosis of bacteria and release of reactive oxygen species (ROS). In the ischemic heart, neutrophils phagocytose dead tissue and release inflammatory mediators: an immunological misfire aimed at myocytes that survived the ischemic injury.

Aside from neutrophils, inflammatory Ly-6C^{high} monocytes are among the earliest responders. Distressed tissue expresses CCL2,[271] which attracts Ly-6C^{high} monocytes during the first several days after which the wounded heart switches to CX3CL:1-mediated recruitment of Ly-6C^{low} monocytes.[256] These inflammatory mediators include protease, which are tightly regulated to balance wound debridement with tissue destabilization, because unchecked proteolysis may cause infarct expansion or even rupture. During resolution of inflammation, reparative Ly-6C^{low} monocytes support angiogenesis and extracellular matrix synthesis by providing vascular endothelial growth factor (VEGF) and TGF-β.[256] Perhaps recruited monocytes influence a tissue in a manner that long-seeded, sessile macrophages no longer can.

With a short time delay and at lower numbers when compared to the infarct, monocytes also invade the nonischemic remote myocardium.[272] Here, myeloid cells may contribute to various processes: they may cause HF by facilitating ventricular dilation via proteolysis of the collagen matrix that lends mechanical stability to the heart; they may activate fibroblasts and promote interstitial myocardial fibrosis, they may harm myocytes through secretion of proapoptotic factors,

Lymphocytes are present in low numbers in the infarct and proliferate in draining lymph nodes shortly after ischemic injury.[273] CD4$^+$ T cell deficiency delays the transition from Ly-6C^{high} to Ly-6C^{low} monocyte presence and impairs healing of the heart. Likewise, depletion of dendritic cells disturbs resolution of inflammation.[274] These observations suggest a link to adaptive immunity, but it is unclear, given that MI is a form of sterile injury, whether any processed peptide antigens are recognized and presented. MI may be mobilizing elements of adaptive immunity without necessarily relying on its essential mechanisms.

The emerging picture positions leukocytes as both protective and harmful in MI. Ly-6C^{high} monocytes, for example, are required during the initial response to ischemia but can also be destructive if they persist in the infarct too long. Ly-6C^{low} monocytes, on the other hand, are probably essential to wound repair.[256,275] Optimal healing requires balance: Therapeutic strategies should therefore aim to recalibrate the leukocyte response toward optimal healing. *In vivo* RNA interference is one strategy that can selectively silence (CCR2) at defined time points, thus limiting the accumulation of Ly-6C^{high} monocytes in atherosclerotic plaque and the infracted myocardium.[276]

Leukocytes anchor system-wide mayhem after MI: Acute MI is a severe traumatic event that mobilizes multiple organ systems (Figure 4.3). A substantial number of the initially recruited monocytes derived from a reservoir in the splenic red pulp, where increased angiotensin-2 signaling triggers their mobilization within hours after injury.[277] For the first few days after infarction, leukocyte recruitment remains at astonishing levels.[275] To meet the demand, cell production increases in the bone marrow and the spleen. In the bone marrow, sympathetic nerves release noradrenaline, which binds to β$_3$ adrenergic receptors expressed by mesenchymal stem cells (MSCs).

These cells are part of a housekeeping team that regulates leukocyte progenitor cell activity in the bone marrow niche. In response to noradrenaline, MSCs withdraw the HSPC retention factor CXCL12 and liberate HSPCs into circulation. These cells then seed the spleen and amplify extramedullary myelopoiesis, enabling the organ to contribute monocytes beyond its baseline reservoir function. Local environmental changes in the spleen, including increased levels of IL-1β and stem cell factor (SCF/kit ligand), orchestrate the emergency cell production after MI.[275,278]

Regardless of how many leukocytes are needed in the infarcted myocardium, the activated endothelium that lines (unruptured) atherosclerotic plaques can recruit leukocytes that have become available in increased numbers as a result of the MI. This may partly explain why atherosclerotic lesions grow faster and develop a more advanced phenotype shortly after ischemic injury.[279] Since the inflammatory burst after MI generates proteolytic leukocytes, their "off-target" accumulation in atherosclerotic lesions may disrupt the fibrous cap, increasing the likelihood of reinfarction. Leukocyte activity post-MI should therefore be considered as a therapeutic target for secondary prevention.

Derailed infarct healing contributes to HF: Young and healthy humans, however, rarely suffer from MI. Atherosclerosis risk factors, and comorbidities such as diabetes and obesity many of which have an inflammatory component[280] typically precede ischemic injury. However, any pollutant overload such as the fumes of natural gas stoves and heaters, insecticides incidences, formaldehyde overload or CO, N_2O, SO_2 particulate, and mycotoxin exposure can increase inflammation. The smoldering systemic inflammation impedes infarct healing by interfering with the resolution of local inflammation and delaying the reparative phase.[281] Consequently, the infarct expands and the left ventricle dilates, ultimately leading to HF. This frequent syndrome, defined by the inability to pump sufficient quantities of oxygenated blood into peripheral tissues, manifests with shortness of breath and fluid retention and carries a mortality as high as 50%.[234] Data on leukocyte activity in the chronically failing myocardium are unavailable; however, inflammatory biomarkers, such a C-reactive protein and inflammatory mediators, such as the cytokines tumor necrosis factor-α (TNF-α) and IL-6, increase systemically in HF, and leukocytosis associates with disease progression.

Leukocytosis and inflammatory monocyte levels correlate with post-MI HF in patients.[282,283] After acute MI, the human bone marrow increases activity[284] and releases HSPCs into circulation,[285] possibly resulting in splenic proliferation.[278] Two monocyte subset peaks occur in the blood of patients with acute MI,[283] suggesting that the infracted human myocardium likewise mobilized monocyte subsets in distinct phases.

HALLMARKS OF LEUKOCYTE FUNCTION IN CARDIOVASCULAR DISEASE

The leukocyte system's role in cardiovascular disease has several prevailing features. First, the system appears to be maladaptive. The danger signal during atherosclerosis or after MI is unlikely to be a microbe but often is a mold, or the odor of specific chemicals, or a series of chemicals, yet leukocytes mobilize powerful antimicrobial and inflammatory molecules that cannot adequately handle either lipids or dying myocytes or the chemical pollutant load. Second, the system is heterarchical. Macrophage abundance in atherosclerosis does not imply hierarchy, and, indeed, other leukocytes such as dendritic cells may be acting in parallel. Third, the system is collaborative: Leukocytes communicate through processes that elicit activation, differentiation, degranulation, and transmigration. Fourth, the system is competitive in that selective ablation of various same-class leukocyte subsets often reveals opposing effects on atherosclerosis. Fifth, the system is pervasive. Leukocytes accumulate in vascular lesions or the myocardium, but they are produced in other tissues and circulate in the blood. Sixth, the system is integrated. Leukocytes do not operate in isolation but belong to network that connects organ systems (Figure 4.3).

Therapeutic approaches that target leukocytes to treat cardiovascular disease have not yet been realized, partly because the fundamental biology remains somewhat enigmatic.

PARTICULATES

"Particulates" (discussed in detail in Chapter 2), both chemical and physical, represent a broad class of substances found in the air in discrete particles, including liquid droplets, for example, sulfur oxides and nitrous oxides. In addition to these, the classification of particulates includes mainly allergens (e.g., pollens and dander), droplets, dust, pathogens (e.g., bacteria, viruses, and fungi), fibrous particles, particles generated by use of pressurized products, asbestos, tobacco smoke, fire retardants, and combustion products.[287]

Suspended particulates are those that hang in the air and are made up of silicates and other soil-derived minerals. They may reduce visibility, and because these are small (they are usually <5 μm in diameter and thus in a respirable range), they may be especially hazardous to health.

Particulates that can contribute to air pollution include silicates, soil-derived minerals, pollens, microorganisms, fibers, asbestos, tobacco smoke, titanium, and combustion products such as car and diesel exhausts.

The size of the particles determines their location and the magnitude of their impact. Size determines the surface area/total mass ratio, which increases with a decrease in particle size as shown in Chapter 2, particulate 10 μm, that is, sand and dirt of 2.5 ppbv, 250 μg/m^3 (fine), and 200 μ/m (ultrafine). This ratio becomes important in considering particle damage, since harmful chemical compounds (especially polynuclear aromatic hydrocarbons [PAH]) absorb onto the surface of particles which are then taken up by cells, with the particle acting as carrier. Other particles may of themselves be chemically reactive (e.g., asbestos, acid) and damage cells of the lungs through chemical interaction. Particulates from slag wool, rock wools, glass wools, filaments, and fibrous glass may have irritant effects. We have seen particles containing PAH, rock and glass wools, and asbestos severely trigger chemically sensitive individuals making their clinical course very difficult to measure and manage.

Particulates are often a combustion product. As combustion conditions affect the number, particle size, and chemical speciation of particles and because these conditions vary rapidly, it becomes very difficult to predict specific health effects resulting from exposure to particulate matter expressed as an average mass concentration. Respirable particles at concentrations of 2.5–250 μg/m^3 increase respiratory symptoms in compromised individuals.[287,288] Longer-term effects depend largely on interaction with cells whose damage is harder to classify. Ultrafine particulates of 200 μ/m can go almost anywhere in the body causing metabolic dysfunction and inflammation. They especially play havoc in the brain and heart.

Of concern in the health effects of respired particles is chemical or mechanical irritation of tissues, including nerve endings at the site of deposition, which may be particularly germane to chemical sensitivity, impairment of respiratory mechanics, aggravation of existing respiratory or cardiovascular disease, reduction in particle clearance and other host defense mechanisms, impact on host immune system, morphologic changes of lung tissues, carcinogenesis, and exacerbation of chemical sensitivity.

One can see that for the years of 2012 and 2013 that the particulates for outdoor air are about the same. Emissions from traffic are about the same and make up most of the air pollution.

The following are daily pollution counts in Dallas, Texas which may affect the chemically sensitive and EMF-sensitive patients (Tables 4.20 and 4.21):

Particulates can affect lung function. Particles that are not expelled from the nose by blowing or sneezing find their way into the respiratory tract. Soluble particulates enter the bloodstream through the lung. Insoluble ones may remain in the respiratory tract, sometimes for years. Some particulates such as dust, act as carriers for bacteria and viruses. Measles virus and Legionnaire's bacilli are common airborne pathogens transmitted this way. However, the most significant contribution to the health hazard of indoor particulates comes from tobacco smoke. Reactions to tobacco combustion products are very common especially among the chemically sensitive we have treated at the EHC-Dallas, where 95% are sensitive to tobacco smoke.

Those particulates included in the respirable particle class (<2.5 pm) present a risk to health greater than a comparable mass concentration of larger particles (>2.5 pm), since the smaller particles are breathed deep into the lungs, circumventing several respiratory defense mechanisms, and can deliver high concentrations of potentially harmful substances to a few cells that may then become severely damaged. Chemical sensitivity can be exacerbated by these small particles.

TABLE 4.20
Weather: Ambient Air Toxics for Dallas-Level Standard (January 2013)

Date	Temperature (°F)	Wind (mph)	CO (ppb)	SO$_2$ (ppb)	O$_3$ (ppb)	NO (ppb)	NO$_2$ (PPB)	O of N (ppb)	PM$_{2.5}$ (mcg/m^3)
1	46.4	8.2	0.2	0.1	18	1.6	9	9.7	11.23
2	39.9	7.1	1	2.9	20	128.2	29	158	16.71
3	48.3	8.1	1	3	35	136.	36.2	165	21.38
4	48.6	6.3	0.4	0.65	21	27	34.6	57.4	10.2
5	51.4	6.4	0.7	0.9	29	49.7	30.7	70.6	10.26
6	55	7	1.3	23.1	41	102.4	36.9	127.4	22.6
7	54.3	6.6	2	7.5	34	212.1	52.9	384	29.51
8	49.3	6.7	0.4	0.2	27	6.8	21.7	28.7	11.59
9	56.9	16.8	0.2	0.1	14	2.6	12.2	14.2	5.26
10	58	10.3	0.3	0.1	18	4.4	17.6	21	3.9
11	70.8	12.4	0.4	0.6	41	21.9	24.3	46.3	12.36
12	66.9	12.4	0.3	0.2	25	10.2	18.9	26.6	12.4
13	41.6	11	0.2	0	32	1.1	10.1	10.6	6.72
14	43.6	9.5	0.4	0.2	34	5.8	27.4	29.3	8.4
15	38.4	10.3	0.3	0.1	30	2.9	14.3	16	6.99
16	47.7	7.1	1.2	3.1	34	143.3	40.4	180.5	15.76
17	58.9	9.3	1.1	3.5	36	163.8	41.4	198	18.97
18	61.4	9.2	1.7	7.3	43	212.1	44	393	25.37
19	64.3	9	0.5	1.1	45	13.7	38.5	49.6	13.09
20	68.5	6.2	1.6	1.9	51	65.4	46.1	115.4	21.68
21	57.2	7.9	1.1	1.5	33	64.5	399	105.9	22.1
22	65.2	5.8	0.4	2.4	41	24.3	38.2	50.5	15.91
23	72.7	11.3	0.3	1.31	50	31.1	30.9	34.9	16.02
24	78.5	6.5	0.4	1	41	38.4	28.3	60.4	14.32
25	57.6	7	0.4	0.2	20	15	31.3	39.3	25.62
26	52	8.7	0.3	0	18	5.4	16.6	18.9	12.2
27	75.4	1.1	0.3	0.1	37	3.5	13.9	14.3	12.97
28	78.5	14.6	0.2	0.2	30	1.5	11.7	13.4	10.45
29	78.1	16.9	0.3	0.1	30	1.6	23.7	25.2	10.92
30	55.9	16.4	0.6	1.1	38	47.9	36.8	86.5	11.38
31	68.3	11.1	1	2.4	41	63.6	43.7	118.2	12.38

PM = particulate matter.
T: normal: 88–68°F, Wind: L: <7 mph, CO: H: >2 ppb, SO$_2$: H: >12 ppb, O$_3$: H: >75 ppb, NO: H: >200 ppb, NO$_2$: H: >22 ppb, O of N: H: >200 ppb, PM$_{2.5}$; H: >20 mcg/m^3 H or L January, 2013.

Titanium Dioxide: Subcategory of Particulates: Nanoparticles <200 nm

Titanium dioxide, a pesticide and chemical inert ingredient for which two exemptions from the requirement of a tolerance exists for its residues when used in pesticide formulations applied to growing crops and in pesticide formulations applied to animals. Titanium dioxide is a widely used inorganic white pigment that is produced from mined sources of titanium. It was formally thought to be inert. However, now new problems exist in the ultrafine particulate.

Titanium dioxide pigments are white inorganic pigments used primarily in the production of paints, printing inks, paper, and plastic products. Titanium dioxide is also used in several white or colored products, including foods, cosmetics, UV skin protection products, ceramics, fibers,

TABLE 4.21

Weather: Ambient Air Toxics for Dallas-Level Standard (January 2013)

Date	Temperature (°F)	Wind (mph)	CO (ppb)	SO$_2$ (ppb)	O$_3$ (ppb)	NO (ppb)	NO$_2$ (PPB)	O of N (ppb)	PM$_{2.5}$ (mcg/m^3)
1	57.9	11.4	0.3	0.9	34	1.4	15.8	14.4	7.46
2	52	8.8	0.6	1.4	32	60.4	31.2	81.2	9.1
3	58.5	12.7	1.2	4.9	32	200.3	32.7	210.3	15.19
4	60.8	6.2	1.6	4.8	24	1290.5	38.4	199.9	18.12
5	66.1	6	1.6	5.1	30	174.1	40.6	205.2	22.29
6	73.2	12.3	0.6	12.5	349	51.6	31.5	70.4	18.67
7	60.7	7.8	0.8	1.3	20	49.2	36.8	67.7	15.42
8	57.2	6.5	0.6	1.1	26	38	23.3	55.6	27.78
9	49.8	10.2	0.3	0.1	18	6.7	17.9	19.9	11.61
10	47	10.7	0.3	0.3	18	6.4	25.1	28.5	6.43
11	63.7	15.1	0.9	2.8	28	80.5	33.7	106.2	15.19
12	40.8	15.6	0.6	1.8	34	70.8	39.9	100.2	18.85
13	56.3	8.5	1.4	5.5	23	195.1	42.2	226.2	17.25
14	65.8	6.6	0.6	1.2	31	13.7	28.2	30.6	9.74
15	63.8	13.2	0.3	3	46	89.6	21.7	29.1	11.15
16	70.2	15.2	0.23	1	32	1.3	11	11.4	9.27
17	68	12.3	0.2	0.2	25	7.7	109.2	26.1	9.26
18	55.2	7.1	0.4	4.1	23	32.8	31.5	61.6	10.08
19	71.6	6.8	0.6	1.9	29	59.4	39.5	79.3	15.24
20	77.4	11.5	0.4	1.6	36	24.2	26.7	44.7	22.63
21	49.6	11.8	0.6	0.4	21	27.6	30.9	58.5	16.5
22	79.3	19.9	0.2	1.3	44	1.7	11	11	74.85
23	62	8	0.6	1.2	27	47.3	36.9	74.9	11.44
24	67	15.6	0.4	2.5	30	40.7	34.6	86.6	12.29
25	52.4	13.2	0.2	0	29	4.1	18	22.4	7.86
26	60.3	12.4	0.6	1.3	30	49.3	33	78.1	8.9
27	67.5	14.4	1	2.9	39	11.3	29.4	139.6	9.98
28	51.2	12.5	0.7	0.8		48.7	34.6	67.5	14.46
29	61.1	7.9	1.2	3		99.6	28.9	124	18.65
30	66.5	13.3	0.4	2.3	44	27.6	34.3	55.7	12.88
31	74.1	11.8	0.3	0.5	35	1.9	23.4	23.4	10.56

PM = particulate matter.

T: normal: 88–68°F, Wind: L: <7 mph, CO: H: >2 ppb, SO$_2$: H: >12 ppb, O$_3$: H: >75 ppb, NO: H: >200 ppb, NO$_2$: H: >22 ppb, O of N: H: >200 ppb, PM$_{2.5}$; H: >20 mcg/m^3 H or L January, 2012.

and rubber products. It is usually accepted as inert but as shown in the implant section can cause problems.

This hazard assessment relies upon peer-reviewed assessments of titanium dioxide performed by the European Commission Scientific Committee on Food (SCF), additives, flavorings, processing aids, and materials in contact with food. Based on its evaluation of the available data on titanium dioxide, JECFA concluded that the establishment of an acceptable daily intake was unnecessary. In its safety review of certain food colorants, the SCF reaffirmed an earlier determination regarding the use of titanium dioxide as a colorant in foodstuffs and concluded that titanium dioxide was acceptable for general food use without the need for establishment of an acceptable daily intake. In its most recent evaluation of titanium dioxide, EFSA concurred with the JECFA assessment of titanium dioxide and concluded that the use of titanium dioxide would not pose any safety concerns. Both the JECFA and EFSA evaluations of titanium dioxide noted there is no absorption or tissue storage of titanium dioxide. This has been counter to what we found in pure titanium implants and titanium alloy implants when in fact, both can become sensitive in specific individuals.

Titanium dioxide is not available as it is not absorbed via the gastrointestinal tract or through the skin. Inhalation exposure to high concentrations of titanium dioxide particles has been shown to result in pulmonary effects in rats, but these effects may be a rat-specific threshold phenomenon, possibly of little relevance to humans. Epidemiological data suggest that there is no carcinogenic effect associated with workplace exposure to titanium dioxide dust. Titanium dioxide is not carcinogenic in mice or rat dietary studies and no adverse effects were observed in chronic rat studies at concentrations up to 5% in the diet.[289]

Based on the insoluble nature of titanium dioxide in water and the low acute toxicity of titanium dioxide to freshwater fish, there are not any nontarget aquatic species risk concerns resulting from the use of titanium dioxide as an inert ingredient. Based on the lack of absorption, as well as no identified toxicological effects of concern in animal testing, there are no risk concerns for nontarget terrestrial organisms resulting from the use of titanium dioxide as an inert ingredient.

Taking into consideration all available information on titanium dioxide, it has been determined that there is a reasonable certainty that no harm to any population subgroup will result from aggregate exposure to titanium dioxide when considering dietary exposure and all other nonoccupational sources of pesticide exposure for which there is reliable information. However, we have seen several patients who developed a hypersensitivity to titanium and/or its alloy when preparing them for implants or for those who have implants already in them. Therefore, it is recommended that the exemptions from the requirement of a tolerance established for residues of titanium dioxide in/on raw agricultural commodities and animals can be considered reassessed as safe under section 408 (q) of the FFDCA.

The two tolerance exemptions for titanium dioxide being reassessed in this document are given in Table 4.22.

Additionally, under 40 CFR § 180.1195, titanium dioxide is exempted from the requirement of a tolerance for residues in or on growing crops, when used as an inert ingredient (UV protectant) in microencapsulated formulation of the insecticide lambda cyhalothrin at no more than 3.0% by weight of the formulation.[290] Since this tolerance exemption was established after August 3, 1996, it is not subject to the tolerance reassessment provision of FQPA.

TABLE 4.22

Tolerance Exemptions Being Reassessed in This Document

Tolerance Exemption Expression	40 CFR §	Use Pattern Pesticide	CAS Reg. No.	List Classification
Titanium dioxide (CAS Reg. No. 13463-67-7)	180,920[a]	Pigment/coloring agent in plastic bags used to wrap growing banana (preharvest), colorant on seeds for planting	13463-67-7	4B
Titanium dioxide (CAS Reg. No. 13463-67-7)	180,930[b]	Pigment/colorant in pesticide formulations for animal tag		

[a] Residues listed in 40 CFR § 180.920, formerly 40 CFR § 180.1001 (d), are exempted from the requirement of a tolerance when used as inert ingredients in pesticide formulations when applied to growing crops only.

[b] Residues listed in 40 CFR 180.930 (formerly 40 CFRS 180.1001(e)) are exempted from the requirement of a tolerance when used as inert ingredients in pesticide formulations when applied to animals.

Titanium dioxide is not dermally absorbed by humans.[291] Titanium dioxide is a frequently used compound in lung clearance studies, where a biologically inert substance is required; however, inhalation of high concentrations of fine or ultrafine titanium dioxide particles has been shown to result in pulmonary inflammation, fibrosis, and lung tumors in rats.[292] In contrast to the results in rats, inhalation effects were not observed in mice and hamsters and may be a rat-specific threshold phenomenon dependent upon lung overloading at high exposure concentrations and possibly of little relevance to humans. Epidemiological data suggest that there is no carcinogenic effect associated with workplace exposure to titanium dioxide dust.[293]

Based on the lack of absorption, history of safe use as a pigment and food additive, low toxicity, and lack of concern for human health effects, a safety factor analysis has not been used to assess the risks resulting from the use of titanium dioxide as a pesticide inert ingredient and an additional 10-fold safety factor for the protection of infants and children is unnecessary.

According to Rossi et al.,[294] nanotechnology and engineered nanomaterials (ENM) are here to stay. Recent evidence suggests that exposure to environmental particulate matter exacerbates symptoms of asthma. In the present study, they investigated the modulatory effects of titanium dioxide particle exposure in an experimental allergic asthma because it is so inert and thus can be used for the particulate evaluation.

Nonallergic (healthy) and OVA-sensitized (asthmatic) mice were exposed via inhalation to two different sizes of titanium dioxide particles, nanosized ($nTiO_2$) and fine ($ftiO_2$) for 2 hours a day, 3 days a week, for 4 weeks at a concentration of 10 mg/m^3. Different endpoints were analyzed to evaluate the immunological status of the mice.

Healthy mice elicited pulmonary neutrophilia accompanied by significantly increased chemokine CXCL5 expression when exposed to $nTiO_2$. Surprisingly, allergic pulmonary inflammation was dramatically suppressed in asthmatic mice which were exposed to $nTiO_2$ or $fTiO_2$ particles—that is, the levels of leucocytes, cytokines, chemokines, and antibodies characteristic to allergic asthma were substantially decreased.

Their results suggest that repeated airway exposure to TiO_2 particles modulates the airway inflammation depending on the immunological status of the exposed mice.

ULTRAFINE PARTICLES

The exploding market of nano-based products and nanotechnology as a whole have put the health professionals and regulatory authorities on alert. There is already growing evidence on the potential adverse health effects of ultrafine particles <200 nm on healthy individuals, but only part of the world's population can be categorized into this group. A large part of the population has impaired health conditions that will make them more susceptible to develop health problems from particulate exposure. This clearly is true for the chemically and electrically sensitive and chronic degenerative disease individual and especially susceptibility to nanoparticles of titanium and steel implants.

In industrialized countries, asthma, hypersensitivity, cardiovascular, neurodegeneration, and electromagnetic, and chemical sensitivity are increasingly prevalent.[294] According to the European Academy of Allergy and Clinical Immunology (EAACI), one in three children today is allergic and 30%–50% of them will develop asthma. It is estimated that by year 2015, half of all Europeans may be suffering from allergy[295] or chemical or electrical sensitivity. The studies are no different in the United States. Asthma is a product of both genetic predisposition and environmental pollution conditions. Children in wealthy countries are more likely to develop allergy-related asthma than children in poorer nations.[296] The hygiene hypothesis suggests that lack of intense infections due to improved hygiene, vaccination, and antibiotics has altered the immune system to improperly respond to neutral substances.[297] There also may be other reasons for this hypersensitivity. Approximately 80% of asthma cases today are caused by allergies but a growing number has developed nonallergic hypersensitivity causing chemical and electric hypersensitivity. Evidence already exists that environmental particulate matter, such as air pollutants and diesel exhaust particles, enhances airway, vascular, respiratory pesticides, hyperresponsiveness, and exacerbation of asthma as well as increases respiratory and cardiovascular mortality and morbidity.[298-300] The most susceptible population groups for these adverse health effects include elderly subjects with chronic cardiorespiratory disease, as well as children and asthmatic subjects of all ages. These studies do not even consider the neurological and vascular effects seen in a large number of the chemically sensitive and chronic degenerative disease population who have severe environmental perturbations. These changes in the chemically sensitive and chronic degenerative disease patients involve nanoparticles and small particles in their etiology. They do not necessarily involve the IGE or IgE mechanism; however, they involve the influx of intracellular Ca^{2+} across the cell membrane combining with protein kinase A and C being phosphorylated, which triggers their hypersensitivity up to 1000 times.

nTiO$_2$ and larger particles of titanium dioxide (TiO_2) are widely used in several fields of science and technology. According to the IAREC,[301] titanium dioxide accounts for 70% of the total production volume of pigments worldwide and is classified as possibly carcinogenic to humans. TiO_2 is used in various applications such as joints, coatings, UV protection, photocatalysis, sensing and electrochromics, photochromics, as well as food coloring.[302] Brightness and high refractive index are properties that have made TiO_2 the most widely used white pigment. Other properties of TiO_2 include chemical stability, low toxicity, and cheap price. Plain TiO_2 nanoparticles are often altered to be better and more specifically suit their use. Alterations can be made by doping TiO_2 with other elements or by modifying the surface with other semiconductor materials. TiO_2 mostly occurs as rutile, anatase, or brookite crystalline polymorphs (Figure 4.10). A large portion of the chemically and electrically sensitive and chronic degenerative disease patients are sensitive to titanium. Many patients with metal implants containing this substance are sensitive to titanium and/or its alloy.

Name	Fine TiO$_2$	Nano TiO$_2$
Morphology of particles	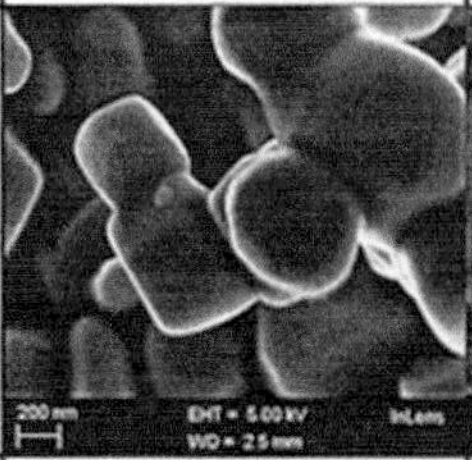	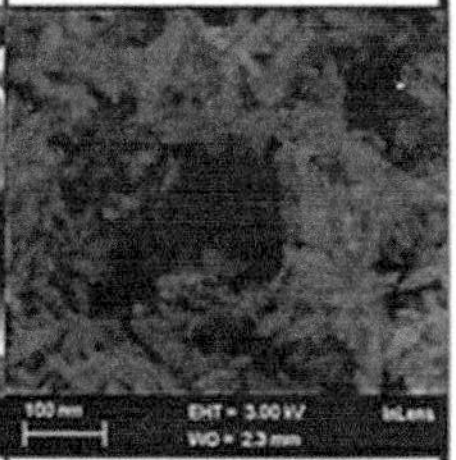
Vendor and product number	Sigma-Aldrich 224227	Sigma-Aldrich 637262
Particle size	<5 μm (by S-A)	10 × 40 nm (by S-A)
Specific surface area	2 m^2/g	132 m^2/g (130–190 m^2/g by S-A)
Phase structure	Rutile	Rutile
Composition	Ti, O	Ti, O SiO$_2$ coating (<5% by S-A)

FIGURE 4.10 Morphology of particles.

ANIMALS: SENSITIZATION AND EXPOSURE PROTOCOL

Following a 1-week acclimation period, 7-week-old female BALB/c/Sca mice (Scanbur AB, Soillentuna, Sweden) were randomized into two exposures and control groups (8 mice/group). Mice were sensitized intraperitoneally (IP) with 20 µg of OVA in alum (Sigma-Aldrich, St. Louis, Missouri) in 100 µL of phosphate-buffered saline (PBS) on days 1 and 14 of the experiment. Control group was given alum in 100 µL of PBS. Exposure groups were exposed three times a week for 2 hours for the duration of the 4 week experiment. The exposure concentration was 10 ± 2 mg/m^3 in all tests. This concentration was chosen to mimic occupational conditions where workers are exposed to concentrations of around 5 mg/m^3. On days 25–27, all mice were challenged with 1% OVA solution via the airways for 20 minutes administered using the ultrasonic nebulizer (DeVilbiss, Glendale Heights, Illinois).

Airway responsiveness was measured on day 28 using a single-chamber, whole-body plethysmograph system (Buxco, Troy, New York).[303] Briefly, mice were exposed to increasing concentrations (1, 3, 10, 30, and 100 mg/mL) of methacholine (MCh; Sigma Aldrich) in PBS delivered via an AeroSonic 5000 D ultrasonic nebulizer (DeVilbiss, ITW, Glendale Heights, Illinois). Before MCh exposure, the baseline is measured for 3 minutes. After baseline measurements, the MCh is nebulized for 1.5 minutes and airway reactivity is measured for 5 minutes per concentration. Lung reactivity parameters were expressed as Penh (enhanced pause) values. After measurement of lung responsiveness, the mice were sacrificed using an overdose of isoflurane and samples were collected for analysis.

SPLEEN CELL STIMULATIONS

Animal studies have shown sensitivity to titanium, for example, inhalation exposure to TiO$_2$ particles reduces leukocyte numbers and mucus secretion in the airways of asthmatic mice occur.

Asthmatic mice demonstrate increased numbers of eosinophils and lymphocytes in the airways compared to healthy controls. In healthy mice (PBS), there was a significant 4.6-fold increase in the influx of neutrophils following exposure to nTiO$_2$ (Figure 4.3), whereas the numbers of macrophages, eosinophils, and lymphocytes remain unaffected (Figure 4.11). Exposure to fTiO$_2$ had no effects on any cells in the BAL of healthy mice. Surprisingly, the numbers of eosinophils and lymphocytes, characteristic features of allergic inflammation, were dramatically reduced in asthmatic mice (OVA) after exposure to both nTiO$_2$ and fTiO$_2$. Macrophages were reduced in half following nTiO$_2$ and increased 1.7-fold following fTiO$_2$ exposure in asthmatic mice. Changes in numbers of pulmonary neutrophils remained nonsignificant.

Goblet cell hyperplasia in the lungs is a common feature of allergic asthma and mucus-secreting PAS+ goblet cells are usually not present in bronchioles and smaller conducting airways of mice.[304] Healthy mice showed clear lungs with no mucus-secreting cells, whereas PAS+ cells were abundant in the bronchial epithelium of allergic mice. Both TiO$_2$ particles caused a drastic reduction in the numbers of PAS+ cells in the allergic mice (nTiO$_2$ and D fTiO$_2$). Both exposed groups showed a statistically significant decrease in goblet cell numbers in the epithelium after the particle exposure (Figure 4.12).

AIRWAY REACTIVITY TO INHALED MCH SIGNIFICANTLY AFFECTED BY PARTICLE EXPOSURE

Airway hyperresponsiveness, a hallmark of asthma, was measured by airway reactivity to increased doses of inhaled MCh. Exposure of OVA sensitized and challenged mice to NaNoTiO$_2$ reduced AHR to the level of healthy mice. On the contrary, exposure to fTiO$_2$ (Figure 4.13) slightly increased the reactivity of the lungs, showing modest exacerbation of asthmatic symptoms. Rossi et al.[294] also exposed PBS groups to TiO$_2$ particles (data not shown) but no difference on airway reactivity to inhaled MCh was found between them and unexposed PBS groups.

Particle exposure results in a dramatic inhibition of proinflammatory, regulatory, and Th2 cytokines in the lungs of asthmatic mice.

The mRNA expression of proinflammatory cytokines, IL-1β, and TNF-α, was downregulated after particle exposure to about one-half and one-third, respectively, in asthmatic mice when compared to the nonexposed control. IL-1β and TNF-α levels were also reduced in half in healthy (PBS) mice following exposure to fTiO$_2$. Similarly Th2 type cytokines IL-4 and IL-13, which are present in asthmatic but not in healthy mice, were significantly diminished after exposure to both nTiO$_2$. To examine effects of particle exposure on the regulatory machinery, they measured mRNA expression of major suppressive cytokine IL-10 and Foxp3, a marker of T$_{reg}$ cells. fTiO$_2$ exposure reduced IL-10 levels by 2.5-fold and Foxp3 levels by 4.5-fold. nTiO$_2$ exposure again reduced IL-10 levels by over eight fold and Foxp3 levels by 2.3-fold (Figure 4.14). They also looked at if suppression in cytokine expression could be seen at the protein level. Reduction in the protein levels of both TNF-α and IL-13 in the BAL from asthmatic mice exposed to TiO$_2$ particles was observed with statistical significance (one-way ANOVA) in IL-13 levels.

The same suppression phenomenon that was seen in cytokines could be seen with all chemokines examined. mRNA expression of proinflammatory C–C motif chemokine 3 (CCL3) and neutrophil attracting CXCL5 and CXCL2 was decreased in asthmatic mice after exposure to both used particles. In healthy mice exposure to nTiO$_2$ caused an almost five fold elevation of CXCL5 levels, corresponding to high levels of neutrophils seen in the BALF of the same mice.

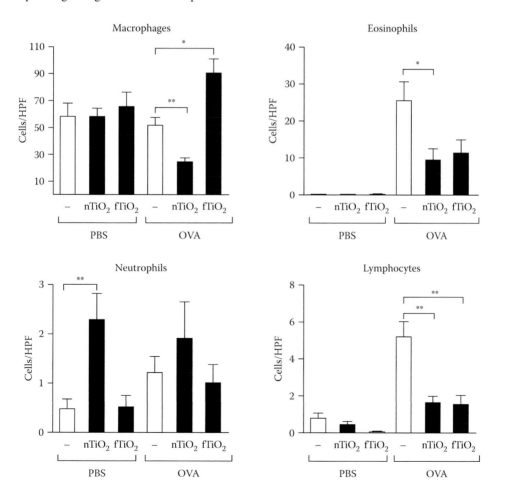

FIGURE 4.11 Macrophages, eosinophils, neutrophils, lymphocytes.

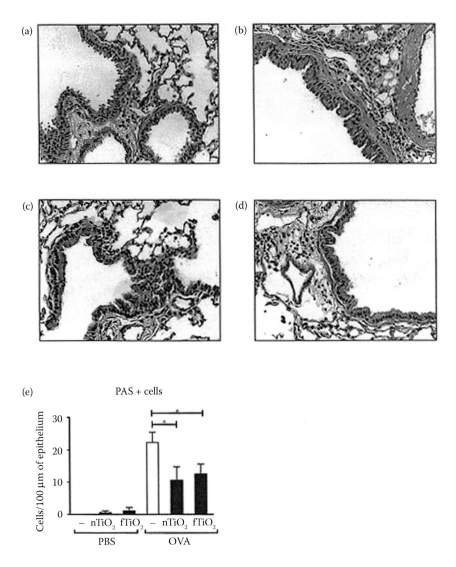

FIGURE 4.12 PAS + cells.

Inhibition of cytokine production in OVA-stimulated spleen cells and reduction in OVA-specific IgE levels suggests systemic immune suppression following particle exposure in asthmatic mice.

To evaluate possible systemic effects of particle exposure, they also examined spleen cells from asthmatic nTiO$_2$-exposed mice. Spleen cells were either stimulated with OVA or left untreated. OVA stimulated cells express TNF-α and IL-13 as expected, but when the mice had been exposed to nTiO$_2$, the protein levels were reduced amply. These findings suggest that there is indeed a systemic response that can be shown from the spleen cells.

To investigate effects of particle exposure on circulating antibodies, they examined the allergen-specific IgE and IgG2a levels (Figure 4.15). OVA-sensitized mice show high levels of OVA-specific IgE but exposure to fTiO$_2$ reduces the levels of OVA-specific IgE significantly. On the contrary, no significant changes in the levels of OVA-specific IgE could be seen after exposure to nTiO$_2$ particles. Levels of OVA-specific IgG2a were low and unaffected by particle exposure.

Initial particle sizes of particles used in the study by Rossi et al.[294] are for fTiO$_2$ 10.40 nm. Aerosolized particles in their experiment occurred as agglomerates. Specific surface area of nTiO$_2$

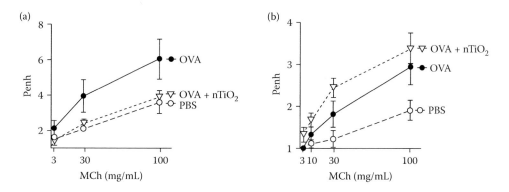

FIGURE 4.13 OVA measurements.

is 132 m²/g while it is only 2 m²/g for fTiO₂ (Figure 4.10). The aerodynamic number size distributions indicate that nTiO₂ dispersed in air using the solid particle dispenser occurred mostly as agglomerates of 1 nm at a number concentration of 69,000 cm⁻³, whereas fTiO₂ distribution consist mainly of agglomerates of 0.1–2 μm as measured using electronic low-pressure impactor. It can be concluded that in particle number concentration, most fTiO₂ are below 1 μm in size but particle

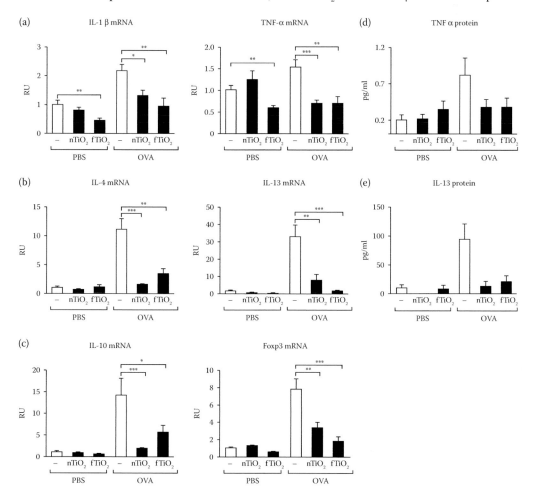

FIGURE 4.14 IL-1β mRNA, TNF-α mRNA, TNF-α protein, etc.

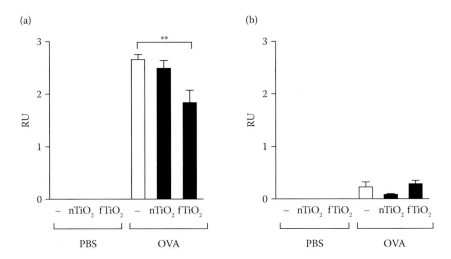

FIGURE 4.15   (a) OVA IgE and (b) OVA IgG2a.

mass concentration relies on over 1 μm in particles. Analysis of the hydroxyl radical formation capacity using the benzoic acid probe showed that neither of the used particles produced ˙OH radicals in a systematic dose–response pattern.[305]

Rossi et al.[294] reported recently that repeated inhalation exposure to silica coated rutile titanium dioxide nanoparticles (nTiO₂ induces pulmonary neutrophilia accompanied by expression of relevant cytokines and chemokines in healthy mice).[305] Out of five different TiO₂ particles, this was the only one that was slightly toxic. The purpose of the present study was to examine immunomodulatory effects of inhalation exposure to different-sized particles, nTiO₂ and fTiO₂ in OVA-sensitized, allergic mice. Interestingly, inhalation exposure to both nTiO₂ and fTiO₂ caused local and systemic inhibition of several features of experimental asthma. Their results indicate that particle exposure can modulate airway inflammation and AHR in quite distinct ways depending on the immune status of the animals. However it has also been observed at the EHC-Dallas and Buffalo that the neurological and vascular systems can be involved in the chemically sensitive and chronic degenerative disease patient. It appears that exposure to titanium and the particulate will trigger the sensitivity. This is certainly true by intradermal and/or oral exchange.

Present results obtained from healthy mice were in line with results from their previous study. Exposure to nTiO₂ particles caused an influx of pulmonary neutrophils and an expression of neutrophil attracting chemokine CXCL5. When healthy mice inhaled fTiO₂ the mRNA expression of two proinflammatory cytokines, TNFn-a and IL-1β, respectively, was suppressed. There have been a limited number of relevant studies done with inhalation and the results have been contradictory. Some studies have reported pulmonary neutrophilia after exposure to TiO₂ nanoparticles whereas others have not.[293,306] Comparison of these ENM is difficult due to different or insufficient methods of particle characterization. There are also few cases of inhalation exposure reported in humans reporting that inhalation of titanium dioxide may cause metal fume fever[307] or respiratory symptoms accompanied by reduction in pulmonary function.[308] This situation can occur in some chemically sensitive and chronic degenerative disease patients. However, much of their problems appear from titanium and titanium alloy implants (i.e., jaw, hip, etc.).

Epidemiological studies have shown that underlying respiratory disease may critically affect the severity of the symptoms when exposed to particulate air pollution.[298–300] The most susceptible population groups for these adverse effects include especially asthmatic subjects of all ages and chemically sensitive and chronic degenerative disease patients. In the present study, they examined whether the asthmatic mice were more susceptible to develop airway inflammation in response to exposure to TiO_2 nanoparticles when compared to healthy mice. Their surprise exposure to $fTiO_2$ and $nTiO_2$ significantly downregulated Th2-type inflammation in allergic mice by preventing the infiltration of eosinophils and lymphocytes to the lungs, inhibiting the expression of Th2 cytokines in the BAL as well as decreasing the numbers of mucus-producing goblet cells in the airway epithelium. To find out whether the observed suppression was also a systemic phenomenon, they stimulated spleen cells from the asthmatic mice with OVA. Stimulated cells derived from asthmatic mice readily expressed TNF-α and IL-13 protein, but cells from asthmatic mice that had been exposed to $nTiO_2$ lacked expression of these proteins suggesting that suppression was indeed a systemic effect.

Increased AHR to inhaled methacholine (MCh) is one of the hallmarks of allergic asthma. It was of interest that different-sized TiO_2 particles acted differently on AHR in the present study. Exposure to $nTiO_2$ reduced OVA-induced AHR to the baseline level of nonsensitized mice whereas exposure to $fTiO_2$ did not have any suppressive effect—actually, $fTiO_2$-exposed asthmatic mice exhibited slightly higher levels of AHR compared to asthmatic mice without $fTiO_2$ exposure. Since IL-13 is known to be closely involved in the development of AHR, it can be speculated that reduction of AHR seen in $nTiO_2$-exposed mice may at least partly be explained by diminished levels of IL-13 in the airways. On the other hand, $fTiO_2$-exposed mice also demonstrated reduced levels of IL-13 mRNA and protein in the airways but their AHR was not suppressed. Thus, yet unidentified factors regulating AHR are likely to play an important role in the modulation of AHR responses during TiO_2 particle exposure. Th2 cytokines IL-13 and IL-4 also control mucus production and their suppression may explain the clear-cut reduction of goblet cells in the airway epithelia. It is worth mentioning that some differences in the absolute values of Penh were observed in PBS and OVA groups between the two experiments. It should be emphasized that although the scale of Penh values differed between the two experiments, the relative difference between PBS and OVA groups was almost identical. It can therefore quite reliably be concluded that the particles studied exhibited different effects on airway reactivity in relation to PBS and OVA groups in these study settings. This differentiation between NTO_2 and FTO_2 may be of value in the treatment of hypersensitivity of the chemical state. If only the NTO_2 can be differentiated for antigen production, the clinician might be able to quell the hypersensitivity reaction reducing clinical inflammatory responses.

Suppression of inflammation similar to the one seen in the present study has been previously reported in the context of exposure to soot and iron oxide,[309] oak dust,[310] cigarette smoke,[311] and fullerenes.[312] Exposure of asthmatic mice to oak dust resulted in suppression of airway reactivity, IL-13, IFN-γ, CXCLr, CXCL2/3, and neutrophils. Thatcher et al.[311] reported reduction in eosinophil numbers, PAS+ cells, IL-5, IL-4, and total IgE. Fullerene exposure caused inhibition of anaphylaxis. In contrast to present findings Larsen et al.[313] reported that TiO_2 nanoparticles exhibited a strong adjuvant effect on the development of Th2 dominant immune response in the OVA allergic asthma model. The particles were delivered IP, which is an unnatural exposure route for nanoparticles in real life except in titanium and alloy implants. In the Rossi et al.[294] study, they examined the effects of airway exposure to TiO_2 particles, which better mimics the real-life exposure scenario. It is important to note that unlike the particles that people more often get exposed to such as air pollutants and mold, the particles they studied were free of bioactive organic matter. Organic matter contains pathogen-associated molecular patterns that activate innate immunity and cause an enhanced response in allergic mice. In line with this, they reported previously[314] that mold exposure together with allergen sensitization caused dramatically enhanced and qualitatively different pulmonary inflammation. The present results demonstrate that exposure to microbe-free TiO_2 particles may not increase Th2-associated airway inflammation and allergic AHR. It should be noted, however, that asthmatic symptoms are not always Th2 associated and therefore responses of exposure to TiO_2 particles in patients with non IgE asthma may differ from the present study. The clinical studies on the chemically sensitive patients would show that hypersensitivity exists.

It has been hypothesized by Rossi et al.[294] that anti-inflammatory Th2 response caused by allergen sensitization may be suppressed by the competing proinflammatory response elicited by

TiO$_2$ exposure. On the other hand, it has been suggested that T-cell dysfunction results in systemic immune suppression in mice exposed to multiwalled carbon nanotubes.[315] This T8 cell depression seen in the chemically sensitive must alter this response to the hypersensitivity stage as seen in several chemically sensitive patients. Also in the case of cigarette smoke exposure, reduced T helper function was considered as one possible reason for the suppression of allergic symptoms. Furthermore, consensus exists that Foxp3+ T$_{reg}$ cells are able to control the inflammation thus preventing overactive inflammatory process that harms hosts' own tissue. Rossi et al.[294] therefore also investigated whether the exposure to TiO$_2$ particles induces elevated levels of Foxp3, a marker of T$_{reg}$ ells, as well as regulatory cytokine IL-10. Expression levels of Foxp3 and IL-10 were, however, significantly inhibited in asthmatic mice by the particle exposure excluding the possibility that suppression was mediated mainly via T$_{reg}$ cells and regulatory cytokines.

Obviously, assessing risks associated with particle exposure is complicated. Rossi's et al.[294] study accentuates that attention has to be paid not only to various characteristics of particles but to various health conditions of people being exposed to them. We see that in the chemically sensitive and chronic degenerative patients who definitely react to ultrafine particulate exposure. An interesting study emphasizes Rossi et al.[294] results where pregnancy of healthy mice enhanced lung inflammatory responses to otherwise inert TiO$_2$ particles and caused increased allergic susceptibility in their offspring.[316] Still very little is known about the physicochemical characteristics which are associated with harmful toxicological potential of nanoparticles. In the present studies, the inflammatory potential was not associated with particle size, but very little information of the cause of the particulates has been given. Even though results slightly varied between the two TiO$_2$ examined the main mechanisms induced by particle exposure in the context of allergic asthma was suppression of Th2 type inflammation. Further studies are needed to provide a better foundation for easier and more reliable assessment and management of risks of nTiO$_2$ and larger particles. Nanoparticles of titanium dioxide may eventually be used to calm down AHR. Eventually, this may lead to problems. However, it has been shown at the EHC-Dallas and Buffalo that intradermal neutralization of titanium will at times stop the titanium sensitivity and calm the hypersensitive response.

Another angle that has not been discussed is the sensitization of titanium by the OVA effects on the nanoparticles. Clearly, 80% of the chemically sensitive patient's reactions also have food and mold sensitivity. These reactions will clearly be a problem in quelling TiO$_2$ reactions. This combination of sensitivity may make a vicious cycle of either hypersensitivity reactions or inflammation. In the patient exposed to nanoparticles, oxidative stress may occur as many react with a hypersensitivity response which can be void of inflammation, but as the disease progresses, inflammation may be processed, compounding the problem. Then, as seen in the chemically sensitive and chronic degenerative disease patient, we have a vicious cycle of hypersensitivity reactions to foods, molds, and ultrafine particulates and inflammation which will eventually lead to end-organ failure.

Pure titanium can be used for jaw and teeth replacements and other body implants such as knees, shoulders, etc.

Titanium alloys are also substances for these problems. They contain nickel, cobalt, chrome, molybdenum, iron, and at times other metals. Titanium dioxide is ubiquitous in other environments. There is more sensitivity to reactivity among the titanium alloys then the pure titanium. However, some chemically sensitive patients react to the pure titanium. Nickle is a predominant sensitizer in the titanium alloy. This compound may in combination with the titanium and other minerals increase the hypersensitivity propensity in the alloy.

LEAD

One of the oldest-known environmental pollutants is lead. Although actions have been taken for centuries to prevent lead poisoning, lead contamination pervades the modern environment.[317] Our prehistoric ancestors had 100–1000 times less lead in their bodies than the typical American of today. None was found in their bones.

High doses of lead ultimately result in lead encephalopathy, permanent neurological defects, anemia, and death. Low dosages of lead cause permanent neuropsychological defects and behavior disorders as well as chemical sensitivity. No demonstrably safe level of lead has been identified.

Lead is abundant in the earth's crust, with average concentrations between 10 and 20 mg/kg in the soil. The greatest natural sources are volcanic activity and geochemical weathering. It is estimated that the natural emissions of lead are about 19,000 tons. However, anthropogenic processes such as painting, addition of lead to petrol, battery manufacturing, etc. are important processes responsible for the environmental presence of lead.[318] Once lead particles go into the air, they are removed by deposition, transferred to the surface, and rapidly distributed in water or sediments according to the pH of dissolved salts.[318] Therefore, lead has become one of the most common environmental contaminants resulting from external sources. This metal is recognized as a common environmental and occupational health hazard[319] because of numerous industrial activities that favor its wide distribution. Human beings usually have lead in their organism,[320] which, upon sufficient exposure and/or accumulation in the body,[321,322] can exert adverse effects. Although having no physiological function, its toxic effects on humans and animals have long been known, affecting almost all organs and systems in the human body.

The effects of lead on human health depend on plasma levels and on the duration of exposure. Blood lead levels up to 29 µg/dL (1–1.4 µM) led to a 46% increase in all-cause mortality, a 39% increase in circulatory mortality, and a 68% increase in cancer mortality.[323] In addition, chronic exposure to low levels of lead causes hypertension in animals and humans.[322,323] Vupputuri et al.,[324] when reevaluating the results of the Third National Health and Nutrition Examination Survey,[325] reported a positive correlation between plasma lead concentration and arterial pressure in black men and women.

The limit of blood lead concentration recommended by the Agency for Toxic Substances and Disease Registry[319] is 60 µg/dL in occupationally exposed adults. However, an increase in arterial pressure has been reported for individuals with blood lead concentrations of 31.4 and 53.5 µg/dL.[324–326] Previous studies on lead toxicity have reported 42.5 ± 2.3 and 58.7 µg/dL,[327,328] blood concentrations that are similar to those found in the occupationally exposed population. In Brazil (Ministerio do Trablho; Norma Regulamentadora No. 7), the reference values for blood lead concentrations have been established at 40 µg/dL for unexposed persons and at 60 µg/dL for exposed persons.

A close relationship between lead exposure and hypertension has been reported in experimental studies on animals and in epidemiological reports.[320] Lead-induced hypertension is reported to result from the inhibition of NKA[328] and from the reduced bioavailability of NO plus an increased endothelial release of endothelin.[329,330] Free radicals reducing NO bioavailability[331] and depletion of antioxidant reserves[320,332] or their upregulation[333] have also been reported. Peripheral or central nervous mechanisms, such as the increase of sympathetic nerve activity, the reduction of baroreflex sensitivity, and the reduction of parasympathetic tone,[322] are also involved in lead-induced hypertension. In addition, Carmignani et al.[321,330] reported increased myocardial inotropism and increased ACE activity in rats exposed to 60 ppm lead acetate for 10 months.

Previous studies have shown that possible mechanisms involved in lead-induced hypertension are due to alterations in vascular tone.[320,328] Changes in vascular reactivity have not been extensively described in the presence of low lead concentrations and in the initial stages of lead exposure. However, studies have shown that chronic exposure to low lead concentrations induces aorta vasoconstriction.[334] On the other hand, chronic exposure to lead (100 ppm for 10 months) decreased the contractile response induced by 5-hydroxytryptamine (t-HT) in the aorta of lead-treated rats.[335] These effects could be mediated by increased production of ROS and vasoconstrictor prostanoids of the cyclooxygenase (COX) pathway.[328,336]

POLLUTION FROM HEAVY METALS DEVASTATES FARMLAND IN CHINA

The are several sources of Pb and they have now been shown to contaminate the soil when their generators are near good farm land.

Most mainlanders are familiar with air pollution, thanks to the thick smog that frequently envelops their cities, but many are unaware of the pollution affecting the ground beneath their feet. In China, air pollution can devastate the farmland. This also may be true in other parts of the world, including the United States.

It is estimated that >10% of mainland farmland in China was polluted and that about 12 million tons of grain was contaminated by heavy metals every year.

Shuhao[337] showed that soil pollutants included heavy metals, pesticides, and organic matter, with heavy metals—mainly cadmium, arsenic, chromium, and lead—as the main pollutants on Mainland China.

Industrial discharges exhaust fumes and solid industrial waste contributed the most to heavy metal contamination of soil, also adding that the abuse of fertilizer was also a problem.

"The effective utilization rate of fertilizer in the mainland is only 30%." "The rest of the nutrients end up in underground water. Some of the excess nitrogen fertilizer, the most commonly used, becomes nitrate-nitrogen—a cancer-causing chemical—and phosphate fertilizer contains heavy metals, since it is made from phosphate rock."

In parts of Baiyin, in Gansu province, and Taotou, in Inner Mongolia, which are notorious for heavy metal pollution, several residents have suffered mysterious bone aches and deaths from cancer.

Closer to home, studies have shown a similar condition in U.S. soil such as seen in Frisco, Texas.

Exide Technologies, shown at dusk two days before the smelter's shutdown on November 30, 2012, has a buffer zone of vacant land separating it from other properties. Even so, residents want to make sure the lead cleanup will be complete (Figure 4.16).

Many applauded the city of Frisco, Texas earlier this year for its agreement with Exide Technologies that ended operations at the company's nearly 50-year-old lead smelter.

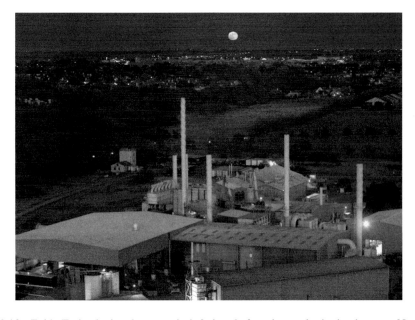

FIGURE 4.16 Exide Technologies shown at dusk 2 days before the smelter's shutdown on November 30, 2012.

Decontamination and demolition of the plant, which closed on November 30, 2012, started earlier. The question now is whether this Dallas, Texas suburb will get the cleanup right so it can move beyond its smelter past, something West Dallas has not been able to do in the decades since the RSR Corporation smelter closed in 1984.

There are reasons for optimism in Frisco. The city has seen less widespread contamination from the smelter's operations than West Dallas did from the smelter there. Fewer people lived near the Frisco plant in the early years when emissions were largely unregulated.

Frisco also benefited from Exide's buffer of vacant land between its operations and the surrounding neighborhood. Most of the contamination has been found on company property in the land-buffered soil. The buffer and less density made a huge difference because most of the lead contamination was found in its immediate buffered soil.

That was not the case in West Dallas. Hundreds of residential yards surrounding the RSR smelter were included in extensive cleanups in the 1980s and again in the 1990s after tests showed lead contamination well above federal standards. Today, the West Dallas smelter's former home along busy Singleton Boulevard is a vacant lot surrounded by brick walls and chain-link fences.

Some fear that will be Frisco's future with the Exide property, which is surrounded by some of the city's prime locations, including Frisco Square, the Museum of the American Railroad, Frisco High School, and the future 275-acre Grand Park.

In West Dallas, the plant's closure was spurred by air pollution and soil contamination that resulted in a large number of children with lead poisoning. Frisco, on the other hand, has not seen high levels of lead exposure among children who have been tested. Instead, its plant shutdown was driven more by economics.

Exide's cleanup in the coming months will target areas with contaminated soil. Other than the levels at the plant itself, testing shows the highest lead levels are on the 180 acres of Exide property that is being purchased by the Frisco Economic Development Corporation and the Frisco Community Development Corporation Cleanup will remove any soils with lead levels exceeding 250 ppm.

But plenty of questions remain. One of the biggest revolves around the plant's landfill. A state inspection last year found hazardous levels of lead and cadmium in Exide's nonhazardous landfill. Exide determined procedures for treating the industrial waste were not followed in 2010 and 2011.

In a plan approved by the Texas Commission on Environmental Quality, Exide plans to treat the waste in its active landfill cells until it meets standards and then dispose of it again. Once the landfill reaches capacity, it will be capped and covered.

Some have called for the landfill waste to be carted away. But others say that carries more risk than leaving the waste in place, covering it, and fencing off the area.

Other concerns revolve around contamination identified along Stewart Creek, which runs through the plant property, and the city's plans to build Grand Park with multiple lakes downstream from Exide. Groundwater issues must also be addressed.

Frisco was a farming town of about 1500 people when city officials celebrated the groundbreaking of an oxide manufacturing plant near downtown in 1964. Battery recycling, which melted lead in a process of smelting, began at the plant in 1969. For years, it was the city's largest employer.

Scrutiny began in late 2008 when Exide proposed to increase production at the same time that an area around the plant failed to meet the federal air quality standard for lead, which had been tightened 10-fold. Exide had been working on $20 million in improvements to reduce its lead emissions when the deal with the city of Frisco was announced in late May 2012.

Residents in West Dallas say their neighborhood is still contaminated with lead from its former smelter. Crushed battery chips from the smelter, often a sign of lead contamination, still turn up in people's yards. Frisco is also still finding battery chips.

In 1992, the city discovered that chunks of black plastic from the old batteries had been used as the base for the parking lot at Bicentennial Park and nearby Sunset Drive. This was the same year that federal officials were searching properties in West Dallas for contaminated battery chips.

Frisco and company officials did an extensive search at the time to find any other sited with battery chips and clean them up. Last year, state and federal inspections found battery chips along Stewart Creek. In September 2011, during site work for the new home of the Museum of the American Railroad, more battery chips were found in an old road bed. Tests showed lead levels in the soil of up to 2150 ppm.

Exide will reimburse the city for the cleanup costs on the railroad museum property. It also has an agreement with the city to pay for any future contamination that can be traced to its operations. Unlike in West Dallas, there are no plans in Frisco to test residential yards.

Two years ago, the EPA tested 13 public areas such as parks and schools within a mile of Exide. None of the samples had levels exceeding the agency's residential cleanup standard of 400 ppm.

The highest level found in the EPA's samples was 256 ppm at the Frisco ISD Child Development Center, a day care center for children of district employees.

Back in the 1980s during the first cleanup, lead exposure was acceptable as long as children's blood lead levels did not exceed 30. The U.S. Centers for Disease Control and Prevention now uses a level of 5 ppm and above to identify children exposed to lead so that action can be taken to reduce further exposure. But even that standard has its critics because scientists have found health effects at the lowest levels that can be measured.

Initial cleanup at that time focused on areas with soil lead levels greater than 1000 ppm. Today's standard for residential soil is 400 ppm. But there is mounting evidence that the standard is outdated because it does not protect children from harm.

As cleanup around Exide's plant continues, no one knows what science will reveal in the future about lead's dangers. So residents want the most thorough cleanup possible.

Common sources of lead contamination for the human environment are leaded paint, water, copper leaded pipes, food, dust soil, air, gasoline, batteries and battery factories, and lead smelters. The most important sources of lead contamination for the general population are food and city air. Food is contaminated by lead in air and soil and through solder in cans. High levels of lead have appeared quite frequently in milk and fruit juice when these drinks were contained in cans with a leaded seam.[338]

Studies based on assumed average daily diets for infants and the average level of lead in each food commodity group found that children receive a higher exposure of lead per kilogram of body weight as compared with adults. This finding, coupled with the fact that infants and young children have a higher rate of absorption of lead via the gastrointestinal tract, indicates the increased risk for children from environmental lead poisoning.[317]

Lead inhibits the activities of at least two enzymes (ALA dehydratase and ferrochelatase) concerned with the synthesis of heme in the red blood cells.[317] Typical features of lead toxicity are usually indicated by hypochromic anemia, increased free erythrocyte protoporphyrin, and excessive urinary excretion of ALA and coprotoporphyrin with near normal concentrations of PBG.[317] Lead also destroys the GSH replenishing system, which is devastating to the chemically sensitive who usually have initial low levels. This destruction may mean that there is not enough reduced GSH or its enzymes available for inactivation of nucleophiles and electrophiles or form conjugation reactions to occur. Then the chemically sensitive patient may not be able to detoxify other toxic chemicals, thus exacerbating their illness. A spreading phenomenon of increased sensitivity to other toxic substances then occurs. This inability to detoxify may explain why some patients who have normal serum lead develop chemical sensitivity when they are exposed to high levels of lead.

At the EHC-Dallas, we have seen 10 such cases of chemical sensitivity that developed in patients with normal lead levels. Their clinical history was exposure to high levels of lead at work followed by elevated lead levels in the blood that subsequently returned to normal. Following these events, these patients developed their chemical sensitivity, which continued to persist for years.

Lead is absorbed at different rates by different age groups. Animal studies by Forbes and Regina[339] and Taylor et al.,[340] and human studies by Schultz and Smith[341] indicate that absorption rates are significantly higher in the very young as compared with any other age group. The peak incidence of the toxic effects of lead was found to be from 2 to 3 years of age.[342] These effects were primarily in the neurological system.

The low dietary ingestion of calcium or iron (20% of recommended levels) by rates significantly increased their predisposition to lead toxicity.[340] Decreasing the calcium concentration of the diet was also found to increase susceptibility to lead toxicity in the dog, horse, and pig.[340] Iron deficiency, combined with lead exposure, acts synergistically to impair hemoglobin synthesis.[343] A milk diet has been linked with dramatic increases (33–57 times) in lead absorption principally due to greatly increased absorption of lead via the intestine.[344] Cigarette smoke contributes to the body's exposure to lead.[345]

LEVELS OF LEAD

Two hundred and ten smokers have been found to have about twice the levels of lead as those detected in the rib bones of nonsmokers.[345]

Populations with high risk of lead toxicity include children of 0–2 years old, children in day care centers, elementary school populations, and people with income below the poverty level.[346] Lead in gas station attendants who become chemically sensitive may be a significant factor in their illnesses. At present, according to most authorities, there are no safe levels of lead in the blood.

Lead can have very long activity; low concentrations of lead can cause neurobehavioral and learning problems.[91] Lead can be an enduring disrupting chemical.

DEREGULATION OF BDNF-TrkB SIGNALING IN DEVELOPING HIPPOCAMPAL NEURONS BY Pb^{2+}: IMPLICATIONS FOR AN ENVIRONMENTAL BASIS OF NEURODEVELOPMENTAL DISORDERS

Deregulation of synaptic development and function has been implicated in the pathophysiology of neurodegenerative disorders and mental diseases. A neurotrophin that has an important function in neuronal and synaptic development is brain-derived neurotrophic factor (BDNF). Stansfield et al.[347] examined the effects of lead (Pb^{2+}) exposure on BDNF-tropomyosin-related kinase B (TrkB) signaling during the period of synaptogenesis in cultured neurons derived from embryonic rat hippocampi. They show that Pb^{2+} exposure decreases BDNF gene and protein expression, and it may also alter the transport of BDNF vesicles to sites of release by altering Huntington phosphorylation and protein levels. Combined, these effects of Pb^{2+} resulted in decreased concentrations of extracellular mature BDNF (mBDNF). The effect of Pb^{2+} on BDNF gene expression was associated with a specific decrease in calcium-sensitive exon IV transcript levels and reduced phosphorylation and protein expression of the transcriptional repressor methyl-CpG-binding protein (MeCP2). TrkB protein levels and the autophosphorylation at tyrosine 816 were significantly decreased by Pb^{2+} exposure with a concomitant increase in p^{75} neurotrophin receptor ($p75^{NTR}$) levels and altered TrkB-$p75^{NTR}$ colocalization. Finally, phosphorylation of Synapsin I, a presynaptic target of BDNF-TrkB signaling, was significantly decreased by Pb^{2+} exposure with no effect on total Synapsin I protein levels. This effect of Pb^{2+} exposure on Synapsin I phosphorylation may help explain the impairment in vesicular release documented by Stansfield et al.[347] previously. Lead exposure during synaptogenesis alters vesicular proteins and impairs vesicular release.

The potential role of N-methyl-D-aspartate receptor (NMDAR)-dependent BDNF signaling[347] because it controls vesicle movement from the reserve pool to the readily releasable pool (RRP). In summary, the present study demonstrates that Pb^{2+} exposure during the period of synaptogenesis of hippocampal neurons in culture disrupts multiple synaptic processes regulated by BDNF-TrkB signaling with long-term consequences for synaptic function and neuronal development.

There is growing evidence that neurodevelopmental disorders such as autism spectrum disorders and schizophrenia are likely the result of genetic and environmental factors that come together in early life to produce neurological and mental dysfunction. Early-life Pb^{2+} exposure has been implicated as an environmental risk factor for mental disease.[348,349] However, although a great deal of work has examined the genetics of behavior and brain chemistry changes in subjects with mental disease and in animal models of mental disorders, there is a lack of knowledge in understanding mechanisms by which environmental factors have negative impact on brain development and neurological function. Among environmental pollutants, lead (Pb^{2+}) is a known neurotoxicant that has been recognized as a major public health problem, not only in the United States[350–352] but also on a global scale.[353–356] Childhood Pb^{2+} exposure has toxic effects on the brain manifested as impaired cognitive function,[357,358] intellectual capacity,[359,360] and end-of-grade performance[351] even at exposure levels below the current Centers for Disease Control level of concern.[357–359,361,362] The molecular mechanisms(s) by which Pb^{2+} exposure produces these changes are now beginning to emerge, and Stansfield et al.[347] are developing a working model that takes into consideration previously published observations and the most recent understanding on the effects of Pb^{2+} on both presynaptic and postsynaptic aspects of developing synapses.[352,363]

Using diverse experimental methods, studies in the early 1990s showed that Pb^{2+} is a potent noncompetitive antagonist of the NMDAR.[364–367] Pb^{2+} exposure during brain development was also shown to alter NMDAR composition[368–370] and modifies downstream signaling in the rat hippocampus.[352,371] Specifically, Pb^{2+} exposure reduces cAMP response-element binding (CREB) phosphorylation and binding activity in the nucleus.[371,372] CREB is a transcription factor whose activity is controlled by phosphorylation at multiple sites by several kinases, including the Ca^{2+}/calmodulin-dependent protein kinase II (CaMKII),[373] an enzyme whose activity and protein levels are reduced as a result of developmental Pb^{2+} exposure.[352] CREB activation regulates transcription of BDNF,[374–376] suggesting that Pb^{2+}-induced impairments in CREB activation alter BDNF transcription and thus negatively modulate a number of neuronal pathways, including presynaptic and postsynaptic targets.

Recent studies from Stansfield et al.[347] laboratory have demonstrated that exposure of hippocampal neurons to Pb^{2+} during the period of synaptogenesis decreases cellular proBDNF protein and extracellular levels of mBDNF.[363] The same study also showed that in the presynaptic active zone, Pb^{2+} exposure decreased the levels of the presynaptic vesicular proteins, synaptophysin (Syn) and snyaptobrevin (Syb), and impaired vesicular release. Specifically, it decreased a pool of fast-releasing vesicles, which is likely represented by the readily RRP.[363] They also found that some of the effects produced by Pb^{2+} exposure were similar to those produced by the NMDAR antagonist, APV, implicating a direct involvement of NMDAR inhibition. Finally, the Pb^{2+}-induced decrease of vesicular proteins and impaired vesicular release were fully mitigated by the exogenous addition of BDNF during the last 24 hour of Pb^{2+} exposure.[363] Together, those studies demonstrate that inhibition of NMDAR-dependent BDNF signaling by Pb^{2+} decreases levels of the vesicular proteins Syn and Syb, impairs synaptic vesicle mobilization, and vesicular release. The present work sought to further elucidate mechanism(s) by which Pb^{2+} exposure during the period of rapid synapse formation of hippocampal neurons in culture modifies BDNF-TrkB signaling and impairs synaptic function.

EFFECT OF Pb^{2+} EXPOSURE ON CELLULAR PROBDNF AND EXTRACELLULAR MBDNF CONCENTRATIONS

Primary hippocampal neurons were grown in culture and exposed to vehicle, 1 or 2 μM Pb^{2+} for 5 days during the period of synaptogenesis (DIV7–12). This experimental paradigm allowed the authors to target the specific effects of Pb^{2+} exposure on developing synapses. The concentrations of Pb^{2+} used in the present study are noncytotoxic as determined by a live/dead cytoxicity/viability assay and are relevant to concentrations found in the brain of rats with exposure levels similar to those in pediatric populations.[363,377]

They have previously reported that hippocampal neurons exposed to Pb^{2+} during the same period of development (DIV7–12) reduce level of the presynaptic vesicular proteins (Syn and Syb) and impair vesicular release, effects that were mitigated by the addition of BDNF during the last 24 hour of Pb^{2+} exposure.[363] They further showed that whole-cell levels of proBDNF protein and extracellular levels of mBDNF were reduced by Pb^{2+}.[363] To further confirm and extend these previous findings, they used immunofluorescent confocal imaging to measure proBDNF protein expression in dendrites (defined by MAP2 labeling) from hippocampal neurons exposed to Pb^{2+}. Consistent with their previous results, they found significant reductions in dendritic proBDNF levels that were apparent throughout the length of the dendrites ($n = 5$ independent trials, $F_{2, 689} = 50.04, p < 0.05$). Western blots confirmed that whole-cell proBDNF protein levels were significantly decreased by exposure to 1 and 2 μM Pb^{2+} ($n = 4$ independent trials, $F_{2, 8} = 10.39, p < 0.05$). In addition, extracellular levels of BDNF measured by ELISA were also significantly reduced by Pb^{2+} ($F_{2, 18} = 14.32$, $p < 0.001$).

To assess the possibility that proBDNF was reduced at sites of release in dendritic spines, they examined the juxtaposition of proBDNF with postsynaptic density protein-95 (PSD95). PSD95 is a scaffolding protein that interacts with the NMDAR on dendritic spines and serves as a marker of the postsynaptic compartment. Their data show that Pb^{2+} significantly reduced proBDNF-PSD95 juxtaposition by ca. 15%–35% ($n = 5$ independent trials, $F_{2, 81} = 7.914, p < 0.001$) and increased the percent of PSD95 that is expressed alone by 1%–25% ($n = 4$ independent trials, $F_{2, 66} = 4.009$, $p < 0.05$) without affecting PSD95 puncta density ($n = 5$ independent trials, $F_{2, 76} = 0.58, p > 0.05$). These data indicate that proBDNF levels at putative sites of release in dendritic spines are decreased by Pb^{2+} exposure. In general, the results presented above support and extend our previous findings[364] that hippocampal neurons exposed to Pb^{2+} during synaptogenesis exhibit decreased intracellular levels of proBDNF protein and this effect is present along the entire length of dendrites resulting in reduced levels of mBDNF in the extracellular media.

Based on these observations, they hypothesized that the effects of Pb^{2+} exposure on cellular proBDNF protein levels may be due to changes in BDNF gene expression. To this aim, we examined the effects of Pb^{2+} exposure on exon-specific BDNF messenger RNA (mRNA) transcripts using q-rtPCR. They found that of all BDNF exons examined, Pb^{2+} exposure significantly reduced exon IV (calcium sensitive) and exon IX (coding exon) mRNA transcript levels without affecting exon I or II transcripts ($n = 12$ independent experiments, exon IV: $F_{2, 29} = 4.080, p < 0.05$; exon IX: $F_{2, 54} = 6.187, p < 0.05$). These findings indicate a selective effect of Pb^{2+} exposure on Ca^{2+}-sensitive exon IV[378] whose transcriptional activation is modulated by Ca^{2+} entry via NMDAR channels.[379] The results indicate that Pb^{2+}-induced reductions in proBDNF protein levels may be the result of a specific effect on BDNF exon IV transcription.

MeCP2 2 Protein Levels and Phosphorylation Are Reduced by Pb²⁺ Exposure in the Absence of BDNF Promoter-Specific CpG Methylation Changes

To determine whether epigenetic mechanisms were involved in the reduction of exon IV mRNA transcription, they measured methylation of cytosine–guanine (CpG) units on promoter regions of exon IV and IX. They found no effect of Pb^{2+} exposure on methylation of the CpG units in the promoter regions of exon IV and IX ($p > 0.05$ for all units, suggesting that methylation of exon-specific promoters is not associated with transcription changes under their experimental conditions.

They also examined the levels of MeCP2 and phosphorylation at serine 421 (pS421MeCP2) because MeCP2 is responsible for transcriptional silencing,[380,381] and it specifically regulates BDNF exon IV transcription.[382,383] In the absence of activity-dependent Ca^{2+} influx, the BDNF exon IV promoter is tightly bound to MeCP2. Upon Ca^{2+} influx via NMDAR or voltage-gated calcium channel (VGCC), MeCP2 is phosphorylated at S421[384] inactivating its repressor function, allowing for the transcription of BDNF exon IV.[385–389] To test this hypothesis, they performed immunofluorescent confocal imaging and found significant reductions in the nuclear intensity of pS421MeCP2 and total MeCP2 (tMeCP2) in Pb^{2+}-exposed hippocampal neurons relative to vehicle control ($n = 5$ independent trials, $F_{2, 143} = 4.829$, $p < 0.05$ and $n = 5$ independent trails, $F_{2, 114} = 11.78$, $p < 0.05$, respectively). Western blots confirmed that pS421MeCP2 and tMeCP2 protein levels were significantly reduced by Pb^{2+} exposure ($n = 4$ independent trials, $F_{2, 9} = 19.29$, $p < 0.05$ and $n = 4$ independent trials, $F_{2, 9} = 5.24$, $p < 0.05$, respectively). In addition, the ratio of pS421MeCP2 to tMeCP2 protein measured by Western blot in the same gel was reduced by ~50% by Pb^{2+} ($n = 4$ independent trials, $F_{2, 9} = 12.0$, $p < 0.05$). These data indicate that Pb^{2+} exposure alters one of the epigenetic mechanisms responsible for transcriptional activation of the BDNF gene. That is, Pb^{2+} exposure, by reducing the phosphorylation of MeCP2 at S421, may remain bound to exon IV preventing transcription. This effect may be responsible for the reduced levels of BDNF exon IV transcripts and proBDNF protein measured in Pb^{2+}-exposed hippocampal neuron cultures. Studies to examine the direct binding of MeCP2 to the BDNF exon IV are currently being planned.

Pb²⁺ Exposure Alters Huntington Protein Levels and Phosphorylation Implications for BDNF Vesicle Transport

They have previously shown[363] and have confirmed in the present study that mBDNF in the extracellular fluid was reduced in hippocampal neurons exposed to Pb^{2+}. This effect could be the result of several factors: (1) Pb^{2+} may reduce BDNF gene and protein expression, (2) Pb^{2+} could also affect the transport of BDNF vesicles along microtubules to sites of release, and (3) Pb^{2+} may impair BDNF vesicle release. They have already shown that Pb^{2+} decreases BDNF gene and protein expression. Pb^{2+} may also affect the transport of BDNF along dendrites because it was found reduced proBDNF levels along the entire length of the dendrite in neurons exposed to Pb^{2+}. To further examine this possibility, they assessed the effect of Pb^{2+} exposure on the Huntington (Htt) protein and phosphorylation. Studies have shown that the Htt protein is involved in the transport of BDNF vesicles along microtubules,[390] and it controls the transport of vesicles in both an anterograde and retrograde fashion.[390,391] When Htt is phosphorylated at serine 421 (pS421Htt), anterograde transport is facilitated, and in the absence or reduced phosphorylation at S421, retrograde transport is favored.[391]

TrkB Protein Levels and Autophosphorylation Are Reduced by Pb²⁺ Exposure

The results described so far offer putative mechanism(s) that may be responsible for the reductions in intracellular and dendritic proBDNF protein levels and extracellular mBDNF in Pb^{2+}-exposed hippocampal neurons during synaptogenesis. They hypothesized that the decrease in the levels of extracellular mBDNF as a result of Pb^{2+} exposure may alter the expression of TrkB, the cognate receptor for mBDNF.

Using immunofluorescent confocal imaging an whole-cell Western blotting, they observed significant reductions in both TrkB activation as measured by phosphorylation at Y816 (average gray value: $n = 5$ independent trials, $F_{2, 56} = 4.307$, $p < 0.01$; $n = 4$ independent trials, $F_{2, 9} = 22.97$, $p < 0.001$, respectively) and total TrkB (tTrkB) protein levels (total gray value: $n = 5$ independent trials, $F_{2, 67} = 8.325$, $p < 0.05$; integrated intensity: $n =$ independent trials, $F_{2, 63} = <0.001$; $n = 11.38$, $p < 0.001$; $n = 4$ independent trials, $F_{2, 12} = 6.397$, $p < 0.05$, respectively) (ca. 30%–40%). Western blot confirmed that both pY816TrkB and tTrkB protein levels were significantly reduced by Pb^{2+}. Moreover, the ratio of pY816TrkB to tTrkB determined in the same gel was also significantly reduced (ca. 30%–60%) by Pb^{2+} ($n = r$ independent trials, $F_{2, 9} = 8.035$, $p < 0.001$. It should be noted that in the Western blot results, the decrease in pY816TrkB was dose dependent with the effect of 2 μM Pb^{2+} being greater than that of 1 μM Pb^{2+}. Taken together, these data suggest that Pb^{2+} exposure decreases TrkB protein levels and TrkB activation as measured by receptor autophosphorylation at Y816.

PB^{2+} EXPOSURE DECREASES SYNAPSIN I PHOSPHORYLATION WITH NO CHANGE IN TOTAL PROTEIN LEVELS

Based on the results presented above, it was important to determine if the decrease in Y8167TrkB phosphorylation had a functional downstream effect. Studies have shown that a well-characterized downstream target of BDNF-TrkB signaling in the presynaptic compartment is phosphorylation of Synapsin I.[392]

p75^{NTR} PROTEIN LEVELS AND COLOCALIZATION WITH TrkB ARE ALTERED BY PB^{2+} EXPOSURE

The present work provides compelling evidence that Pb^{2+} exposure during synaptogenesis of hippocampal neurons in culture dysregulates DNF-TrkB signaling, altering presynaptic function. The first series of experiments confirms and extends the previous findings[363] of reduced cellular proBDNF protein expression and this effect is observed along the entire length of the dendrites. Stansfield et al.[347] also confirmed decreased extracellular mBDNF in hippocampal neurons exposed to Pb^{2+}.[363] Extending these findings, they provide preliminary evidence that the reductions in extracellular levels of mBDNF may not only be the result of reduced BDNF gene and protein expression but it may also involve impairment of BDNF vesicle transport to sites of release in dendritic spines. The latter is based on the findings that Htt phosphorylation at S5421, a phosphorylation site on Htt that is known to modulate anterograde transport of BDNF vesicles,[391] was significantly reduced by Pb^{2+} exposure.

Htt appears to have two cellular functions: one as a transcription factor to facilitate BDNF synthesis[393] and a second as a regulator of BDNF vesicle transport.[394] Other studies have also demonstrated a role of pS421 Htt in neuronal survival and in N-methyl-D-aspartate (NMDA) excitotoxicity with increased pS421Htt being prosurvival and reduced pS421Htt enhancing cell death.[395] Thus, it is possible that Pb^{2+}-exposed hippocampal neuronal cultures express significantly lower levels of pS421Htt, and a pS421Htt/tHtt ratio may have impaired transport of BDNF vesicles and be more susceptible to excitotoxicy and/or apoptotic insults.

Additional support for the role of Htt in BDNF synthesis and transport comes from studies with the neurodegenerative disorder. Huntington's disease (HD) is the result of a cytosine–adenine–guanine repeat expansion in the gene encoding the Htt protein. HD patients express reduced serum and brain BDNF levels.[396] BDNF transcription is increased by Htt and decreased by mutant Htt,[397,398] and BDNF expression is impaired in HD mice.[397] Furthermore, neurons expressing the mutant Htt protein exhibit impairments in BDNF vesicle transport and treatments that increase the phosphorylation of S421 in mutant Htt rescue the defect in BDNF transport.[391] These studies implicate an essential role of the Htt protein and its phosphorylation at S421 in the regulation of BDNF synthesis and transport.

To investigate putative mechanism(s) by which Pb^{2+} exposure decreased cellular proBDNF protein levels, Stansfield et al.[347] analyzed exon-specific BDNF transcripts using q-rtPCR. Their results indicate that Pb^{2+} exposure resulted in a specific reduction of BDNF exon IV and IX mRNA transcripts with no change in the expression of exons I and II. It is known that NMDAR activation[374,379,399,400] upregulates BDNF transcripts containing exon IV via Ca^{2+}-dependent CREB transcription,[376,382] and NMDAR antagonists decrease BDNF exon IV expression.[401] Because Pb^{2+} is known to be a potent inhibitor of the NMDAR,[402,403] the present finding lends support to the hypothesis that the effects of Pb^{2+} on BDNF gene expression may be mediated via NMDAR inhibition.

They then investigated whether Pb^{2+} exposure resulted in epigenetic dysregulation of BDNF exons IV and IX by examining exon-specific promoter DNA methylation. Their results revealed no significant treatment effect on average DNA methylation levels across BDNF promoters or at individual CpG units, including the cyclic adenosine monophosphate response element (represented as CpG unit #1 of BDNF exon IV). Thus, under their experimental conditions, Pb^{2+} exposure does not affect exon IV or IX promoter methylation. However, it is known that exon IV BDNF mRNA transcription is specifically regulated by the transcriptional silencer, MeCP2. Activity-dependent Ca^{2+} influx phosphorylates MeCP2 at S421, inactivating its repressor function and allowing for the transcription of BDNF exon IV.[382,384,404,405] Here, they show that pS421MeCP2, tMeCP2 expression, and the pS421MeCP2/tMeCP2 ratio are significantly decreased by Pb^{2+} exposure. These data suggest that in the presence of Pb^{2+}, MeCP2 maintains its repressor function and prevents BDNF exon IV transcription. The implications of their present findings are best described by a recent report indicating that monkeys exposed to moderate levels of Pb^{2+} during the first year of life express reduced levels of brain MeCP2 protein in aging (23 years of age).[406] Therefore the modifications in MeCP2 protein expression and phosphorylation that they have found in hippocampal neurons exposed to Pb^{2+} during the period of synaptogenesis may have long-term consequences throughout the life span.

Altered BDF transcripts have been reported in Rett syndrome patients, a neurodevelopmental disorder characterized by mutations of MeCP2,[407,408] and BDNF levels are decreased in the brain of MeCP2 mutant mice.[409,410] Other studies have shown that reduced phosphorylation of MeCP2 at S421 reduces dendritic branching and alters the morphology of dendritic spines,[384] effects that have also been observed in the Pb^{2+}-exposed brain.[411,422] They should note that the phosphorylation of MeCP2 at S421 is selective for CaMKII and no other kinases,[384] and they have previously shown that CaMKII activity and protein levels are significantly reduced in the hippocampus of rats exposed to Pb^{2+} during development.[372] Because MeCP2 is a master regulator of transcription, the present findings suggest that the transcriptional activity of other genes whose promoters are regulated by MeCP2 may also be affected by Pb^{2+} exposure.

The next series of experiments was performed to link the postsynaptic modifications induced by Pb^{2+} with presynaptic mechanisms regulated by BDNF-TrkB signaling (Figure 4.17). BDNF released from dendritic spines activates TrkB downstream pathways, including MAPK PI3K, and PLCγ.[411] It is thought that mBDNF modulates synaptic neurotransmission by presynaptic TrkB activation,[412] and it has been shown that BDNF-induced neurotransmitter release is partially blocked by TrkB inactivation.[413,414] Their data reveal significant reductions in tTrkB protein expression by Pb^{2+} as well as reductions in TrkB autophosphorylation at Y816. Phosphorylation of TrkB at Y816 has been directly linked with PLCγ activation and mobilization of intracellular Ca^{2+}, release of presynaptic BDNF and glutamate,[412,413] and activation of CaMKII-CREB.[414,415] Furthermore, TrkB coupling to PLCγ signaling via Y816 phosphorylation is essential for long-term potentiation (LTP) in the hippocampus[416] and associative learning.[417] These results provide a putative mechanism by which a Pb^{2+}-induced impairment in the coupling of TrkB activation with downstream Ca^{2+} and CaMKII signaling can inhibit LTP and learning. Relevant to this observation, animals exposed to Pb^{2} during development express deficits in hippocampal LTP and spatial learning as young adults.[418] These new findings provide important mechanistic insights to help explain Pb^{2+} effects on synaptic plasticity and learning.

Studies by Jovanovic et al.[392,419] have shown that glutamate and gamma-aminobutyric acid (GABA) release are linked to presynaptic BDNF-TrkB signaling via MAPK phosphorylation of Synapsis I at sites 4/5 (serine 62/67). Synapsin I is a phosphoprotein that is essential for synaptic vesicle trafficking and in the phosphorylated state, it releases vesicles bound to act in filaments allowing their movement from the reserve pool to the RRP (docked vesicle).[420] Their data revealed that Pb^{2+} exposure reduces Synapsin I phosphorylation at serine 62/67 with no change in total Synapsin I protein levels. This novel finding provides a potential explanation to their previous observation[400] that Pb^{2+} exposure specifically decreases a pool of vesicles with fast-releasing kinetics, which are most likely representative of the RRP (docked vesicles). They are currently performing

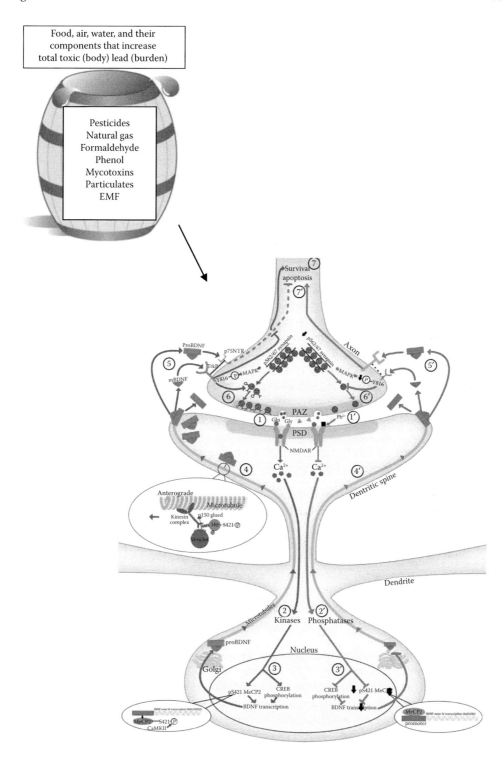

FIGURE 4.17 **(See color insert.)** Bidirectional communication of presynaptic and postsynaptic elements of the synapse defines their survival or retraction during development. On the left side of the same synapse, they define the function of normal synapses, whereas on the right side, they show the components that are affected by Pb^{2+}-induced effects in order to reduce the size of the figure. The green arrows denote normal function, whereas the red arrows indicate impaired function.

experiments to determine the number of vesicles in the reserve and RRP (docked vesicles) using electron microscopy in order to test this novel finding. Synapsin I phosphorylation at serine 62/67 modulates vesicle movement from the reserve pool to the RRP in a Ca^{2+}-independent manner, affecting both glutamatergic and GABAergic transmitter release.[392,419] These observations are consistent with and support their working model that the effects of Pb^{2+} on vesicular release are due to presynaptic changes independent of Pb^{2+} effects on calcium-sensitive proteins or VGCCs and can account for Pb^{2+} effects on both glutamatergic and GABAergic transmission.[400]

Lastly, the present studies provide evidence that Pb^{2+} exposure during hippocampal neuron synaptogenesis increases *p75NTR* expression and alters the equilibrium of TrkB/p75NTR colocalization. Activation of p75NTR by proBDNF can have a negative impact on dendritic morphology and spine number of hippocampal pyramidal neurons,[421] an effect that has been documented in the hippocampus of Pb^{2+}-exposed rats.[422] Overexpression of p75NTR in pyramidal neurons of wild-type mice resulted in reduced dendritic length and spine density,[421] and application of cleavage-resistant proBDNF decreased dendritic spine numbers in cultured neurons.[423] Conversely, deletion of the p75NTR results in increased sine density and complexity[421,423] in hippocampal pyramidal neurons. The findings of Stansfield et al. provide a putative mechanism by which developmental Pb^{2+} exposure results in reduction in dendritic arborization and dendritic spine density.[422] Finally, because p75NTR activation induces apoptosis, the increase in p75NTR protein observed, coupled with a decrease in TrkB protein, suggests that Pb^{2+}-exposed neuronal cultures may be more susceptible to apoptosis.

In summary, bidirectional communication between neurons is essential for the formation, strengthening, and maintenance of synaptic connections. The working model present here provides evidence that Pb^{2+} exposure disrupts synaptic development and function by altering BDNF-TrkB trans-synaptic signaling with subsequent changes in synaptic proteins and impairment in synaptic function. These effects are likely to alter synaptic maturation and the disruption of neurodevelopmental processes that may underlie the cognitive and behavioral deficits in Pb^{2+}-intoxicated children.

INTERACTION OF STRESS, LEAD BURDEN, AND AGE ON COGNITION IN OLDER MEN: THE VA NORMATIVE AGING STUDY

Cognitive decline has been associated with aging, and as the U.S. population shifts to a more elderly population, there is growing concern about the implications of cognitive dysfunction. However, cognitive decline varies widely across ages, which suggests that it may not be just a natural consequence of aging but may be linked to multiple risk factors.[424]

The relationship between lead and cognitive impairment has been documented extensively in children and in occupationally exposed populations.[425–429] Previous studies by Peters et al. and others have also shown an inverse association in bone lead levels as well as blood lead levels with cognition and changes in cognition over time among nonoccupationally exposed older men and older women.[430–433] Levels of lead in blood represent acute exposure and levels in bone represent cumulative exposure.

Psychological stress (hereafter referred to as stress) has also been associated with decrements in short-term memory and attention.[434–436] However, stress itself is not uniformly negative,[437] and under some conditions may result in improved learning and memory.[438] In general, stressful events may result in negative emotional states, such as depression and anxiety, which in turn may exert lasting effects on physiologic processes that influence disease states or enhance vulnerability to other environmental factors (e.g., lead). The negative emotional response to life events (stressors) results when one perceives or appraises these events as overwhelming their ability to cope.[439,440] In response, physiologic systems may operate at higher or lower levels relative to normal homeostasis. The resulting long-term damage of unchecked accommodation of defensive processes (e.g., neural, immune, endocrine) is conceptualized as allostatic load.[441–443]

Exposure to both lead and stress often co-occur and potentially operate through overlapping biologic pathways of action (e.g., the hypothalamic–pituitary–adrenal [HPA] axis with disrupted release of glucocorticoid [e.g., cortisol]). Recent laboratory studies have demonstrated that stress (restraint, cold, and novelty) modifies the neurotoxic effects of lead; moreover, lead and stress may have a combined effect in the absence of the effect of each alone.[437,444,445] Laboratory studies also show that the interactive effect is not limited to early development, a finding that indicates longer-term vulnerability.[446,447] In a recent human study, Glass et al.[448] found joint effects between neighborhood psychosocial hazards and cumulative lead exposure on cognitive function in older adults.

In this study, they did a cross-sectional examination of the modifying potential of stress on the relation of cumulative and acute lead exposures as predictors of cognition in a cohort of older men from the Normative Aging Study (NAS). They previously reported an association between lead and cognition[449–451] and an interaction of lead and age on cognition in this cohort.[451] They hypothesized that high stress would lower the scores on the Mini-Mental State Examination (MMSE; Psychological Assessment Resources, Lutz, Florida) and modify the lead–MMSE association and that the combined elevation of lead and stress would modify the relationship between age and cognitive impairment.

ANALYSIS

They first assessed the relationship between each of the stress measures and the MMSE. They next considered the modifying effect of stress in age by fitting a model that included the main effects of stress and age plus an interaction term of stress times age predicting the MMSE score.

They then assessed the interactive relationship between lead and stress by testing a model that included the main effects of lead and stress plus an interaction term of lead times stress to predict MMSE score. They log-transformed the lead measures to address the influence of extreme values. They modeled the association by IQR of log lead concentrations (approximately a twofold increase): blood lead (0.69 log units), patella lead (0.78 log units), and tibia lead (0.77 log units). They also checked their results by modeling untransformed lead values after using the extreme studentized deviation (ESD) many-outlier method to remove extreme outliers.[452] Finally, they assessed the relationship of lead–stress combinations as modifiers of the relationship between age and MMSE score. For these analyses, they dichotomized lead measures by their median: 5 μg/dL for blood lead, 26 μg/g for patella lead, and 19 μg/g for tibia lead; and created the following four groups: high stress and high lead, high stress and low lead, low stress and high lead, and low stress and low lead. They then ran the analyses with the main effects of lead–stress groups and age and interaction terms of lead–stress group times age to predict MMSE score.

In this cohort of older men, increased self-report of stress was related to lower cognition. Moreover, an inverse association with blood lead and MMSE was more pronounced among those who reported higher perceived stress using the PSS than among those who reported lower perceived stress. In addition, the combination of perceived stress and lead modified the relationship between age and cognition. This study corroborates laboratory studies and one other human study that indicated lead and stress interact to affect cognitive function[437,448] and further supports the theory that cognitive impairment is not singularly a result of aging but due to risk factors working in every concert.

Previous studies have reported that heterogeneity in cognition is especially pronounced in the elderly compared with younger adults.[455] Sapolsky et al.[453] reported that stress exposure over the life course, likely mediated through disrupted stress hormones, significantly affect the aging process. Their group and others have reported a relationship between biomarkers of lead and cognition as well as a negative interaction between lead and age on cognition in older adults.[430,432,433] To the best of our knowledge, this is among the first studies to assess the interaction of lead and stress on cognition in older men and the first to investigate the combined association of lead and stress as a modifier of the relationship between age and cognition.

Aging has been associated with an increase in oxidative stress and elevated glucocorticoids.[453,454] It has also been associated with impaired plasticity of the HPA axis in experimental studies and appears to predict negative effects of stress.[441,454] The outcome of chronic stress and aging on brain function shows similarities; however, stress and aging seem to impact cognition via different underlying mechanisms.[454] To add to the complexity, there is a paradox in stress–aging interactions: Although some evidence suggests that vulnerability to stress can increase with age, other data indicate that the threshold of tolerance to stress may increase with age.[454]

As proposed by Cory-Slechta and others,[437] the interactive effect of lead and stress may follow a multihit model. Lead and stress can both work through the activation of the HPA axis, which results in the release of a cascade of hormones such as cortisol. Disruption of the optimal balance of these stress hormones may enhance central nervous system vulnerability if they present insults on the same system of the brain via different mechanisms, overwhelming the ability of the system to maintain homeostasis.[437]

They observed some differences in the relationship between the two stress measures on cognition and their interactive relationship with lead. They found a significant negative relationship between the most stressful life event measure and MMSE score and a marginal negative relationship with PSS. In addition, even though the direction of the associations was the same, only PSS showed significant interaction with lead in association with MMSE. The most stressful life event rating assesses a stressful event judged by the respondent to have a negative impact, whereas the perceived stress measures the individual's perception of the current demands exceeding the ability to cope.[456] These measures, although correlated, may measure different constructs (i.e., may have independent relationships with disease risk and be mediated by different processes).[456] In a study looking at the stress relationship with the common cold, Cohen et al.[456] proposed that (1) measures such as the life events measure may pick up acute or direct effects, whereas the PSS may be indicative of dispositional affect (i.e., an overall predictable way of responding to situations) and that (2) the former may drive the development of symptoms whereas the latter may be related to increased susceptibility.

They also found a difference between the interactive association of stress and lead among the measures of lead exposure; a significant interaction with blood lead, marginal interaction with patella lead, and no interaction with tibia lead. Of note, there were substantially fewer bone lead measures than blood lead. However, Peters et al.[461] results for blood lead remained significant after they restricted the blood analyses to those with only bone lead measurements (data not shown). In a previous study in this cohort that looked at the cross-sectional relationship between lead and elevated MMSE, Wright et al.[451] observed a significant inverse relationship with blood and patella lead but not with tibia lead. These authors also found interactive relationships between blood and patella lead with age predicting elevated MMSE.[451] The relationship with blood and patella lead is consistent with the theory that bone lead is chronically released into blood, that mobilization rate in aging differs by bone type, and that this mobilized lead contributes to acceleration in cognitive decline.[451] Stress has been found to mobilize bone lead stores in animals.[457] In human studies, cortisol decreased mineral density and increased bone loss.[458–460] Of interest, the effect of cortisol differs by sex and was observed to affect trabecular (e.g., patella) bone in older men.[459,460] The differential effect of cortisol by sex may partially explain significant results found by Glass et al.[448] between neighborhood hazards and tibia lead (only tibia lead tested) on cognitive function in a mixed sample of adults. In addition, the contrasting results may reflect a difference in the measure of stress or the limitation of the MMSE used in their study to differentiate between domains of cognitive function that may be associated with different lead exposure measures.[450]

The combined effect of lead and stress is of particular concern, because HPA axis dysfunction has been linked to a myriad of disorders in addition to cognitive impairment, including cardiovascular and metabolic diseases and psychiatric disorders.[437] Indeed, they showed the interactive association of lead and stress on blood pressure and the prospective risk of hypertension in this same cohort.[461] It is also relevant in the context of low socioeconomic populations where the prevalence of these disorders is high and stress and lead tend to co-occur. Thus, the public health implications may be significant, given the possibility of improved neurobehavioral performance after reducing blood lead, which has been shown in several studies,[426,429,462,463] and stress.[463]

They note a number of limitations that may be addressed in future research. This study is cross-sectional, so temporality cannot be established. It is conceivable that deficits in cognitive function could be a source of stress or produce stressful experiences. As eluded to earlier in the discussion, use of the MMSE may be considered a limited assessment of cognition; however, the strength of the MMSE is that it is a general measure that is widely used and understood. They evaluated relationships using two measures of stress and three measures of lead exposure, raising the question of multiple comparisons. However, they chose to make these comparisons because of reported differences between the stress and lead exposure measures in their relationship with disease. In addition, although they controlled for a number of risk factors, there is the risk of omitted or inadequately controlled confounders. In addition, this study was not conducted in a low socioeconomic population where there is a greater likelihood of dual exposure to stress and lead. Finally, there are noted differences in the association of stress with cognition and in the interactive effect among males and females (at least in laboratory studies).[437,445,464] This finding suggests the need to look more closely at sex differences and the relationships found in their study.

In summary, their results show that stress is associated with lower cognition and modifies the relationship of age to cognition among community-dwelling older adult males. Furthermore, stress negatively modifies the relationship of blood lead and cognition, and combined high lead and high stress negatively modify the association of age with cognition.

NONCRITERIA POLLUTANTS

In addition to the criteria pollutants, a large number of inorganic chemicals might produce, under special conditions of weather, location, and combination, serious problems in both the outdoor and indoor environment. These contaminants are usually not found in significant quantities in the air, except near sources producing large amounts of pollution, such as industrial plants, waste disposal sites, highways, etc. Also, some inorganic contaminants, for example, mercury and copper, can be found in food and water.

Inorganic air pollutants can be metals or their oxides (such as mercury, arsenic, cadmium, beryllium, iron, zinc, copper, and nickel), mineral fibers (such as sand [SiO_2], glass and silica fibers, asbestos, etc.), inorganic gases (such as chlorine, bromine, iodine, fluorine, potassium, and sodium hydroxide), fumes of inorganic acids (such as hydrochloric acid [HCl]), and cyanide (CN). Also, a number of familiar metals have been incriminated; among them are cobalt, chromium, aluminum, and platinum (Figure 4.18). At the EHC-Dallas, all of these pollutants have been observed to exacerbate or induce chemical sensitivity. Each will be discussed separately.

MERCURY

Mercury in its elemental form is a liquid that is vaporized upon heating. It is a component of fossil fuel and is found in airborne emissions from fossil fuel burning factions. It travels through the environment via several pathways, including air, food, and water and bioaccumulation occurs from these routes.[465]

Inorganic mercury released into the environment is converted by microorganistic activity to methylmercury (MeHg), a persistent polluter that is soluble in a dispose tissue and passed up the food chain. It has been shown that melting of the polar ice caps each summer releases 200 tons of mercury which rains down over the earth. As a result, predator fish are significantly contaminated with MeHg than those that feed on plants and benthic organisms, that is, which fish have lower Hg levels than trout, walleye, or pike all of which are predatory[465] (see Hg in Chapter 2).

Ambient Mercury

Mercury is worthy of note in this context because of its high toxicity and great mobility in ecosystems. Mercury is known to exert its effects by combining with SH groups,[466,467] which are essential for the normal function of several proteins that constitute enzymes, ion channels, or receptors.[465,467] These effects include inhibition of ATP hydrolysis and Na^+- and Ca^{2+}-ATPase activity.[468,469]

Noncriteria pollutants

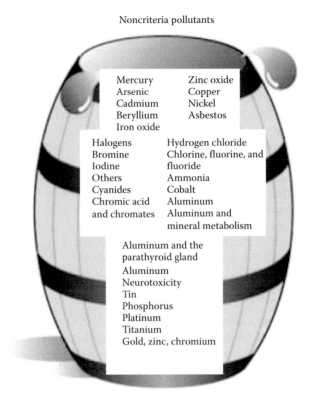

Mercury	Zinc oxide
Arsenic	Copper
Cadmium	Nickel
Beryllium	Asbestos
Iron oxide	

Halogens	Hydrogen chloride
Bromine	Chlorine, fluorine, and
Iodine	fluoride
Others	Ammonia
Cyanides	Cobalt
Chromic acid	Aluminum
and chromates	Aluminum and
	mineral metabolism

Aluminum and the
parathyroid gland
Aluminum
Neurotoxicity
Tin
Phosphorus
Platinum
Titanium
Gold, zinc, chromium

FIGURE 4.18 (**See color insert.**) Noncriteria pollutants.

The U.S. EPA recommends the reference blood concentration of mercury to be below that considered without adverse effects, which is 5.8 ng/mL.[470] However, in unexposed populations taken as controls, blood mercury concentration was reported to be 2.73 ng/mL in New York City adults and 1 ng/mL in China.[471,472] For many years, mercury was used in diuretics or as an ingredient of antiseptics.[466] However, after mercurials were replaced with more specific treatments, signs of mercury intoxication have become rare.[473] However, in the past decade, mercury intoxication and poisoning attained high levels[474–476] as a result of environmental pollution. The Minamata Bay episode resulting from industrial plastic disposal, the ingestion of contaminated wheat seeds in Guatemala, Iraq, and Pakistan, and contamination from metallic mercury used in gold mining in Brazil are examples of this problem.[476,477] Human toxicological data about MeHg poisoning show that symptoms of toxic effects appear at a concentration of mercury in blood of 0.1 μg/mL and death occurs at concentrations above 3 μg/mL.[474] It has also been reported that professional exposure to mercury vapor and the release of mercury from or during the removal of amalgam dental fillings increases the blood and plasma concentration of the metal.[478–480] After exposure to mercury vapor, blood concentrations attain 18 nM,[480] and after exposure to dental amalgam fillings and their removal, plasma concentration attains 5 nM.[479] Another important mechanism of exposure is fish consumption. Mercury attains 5.65 ng/mL among regular fish consumers[470,471] and levels of 7–10 ng/mL among exposed workers.

Recently, more attention has been paid to the toxic effects of mercury on the cardiovascular system and their association with hypertension, carotid atherosclerosis, MI, and coronary heart disease.[481–483] In the cardiovascular system, acute mercury exposure promotes reduction of myocardial force development[484] and inhibition of myosin ATPase activity.[484] Chronic exposure to this metal increases vascular resistance[485,486] and induces hypertension.[481]

Functional integrity of the endothelium is crucial for the maintenance of blood flow and antithrombotic capacity because the endothelium releases humoral factors that control relaxation and

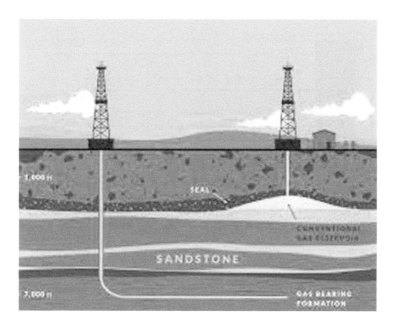

FIGURE 1.6 Horizontal drilling—fracking.

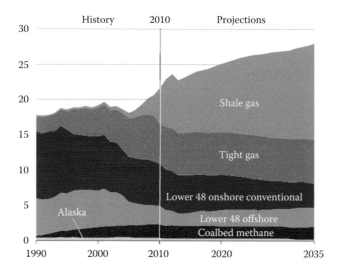

FIGURE 1.7 Changing production sources. Worldwide, about half of the known natural gas is in "conventional," highly permeable geologic formations, often together with liquid petroleum. The other half is the "unconventional gas" found in more diffuse, low-permeability geologic formations. In the United States, convention gas production peaked in the 1990s and today represents less than half of the annual U.S. gas production. (From E.I.A, Annual Energy Outlook 2012. Report Number DOE/EIA-0383, U.S. Energy Information Administration: Washington, DC.)

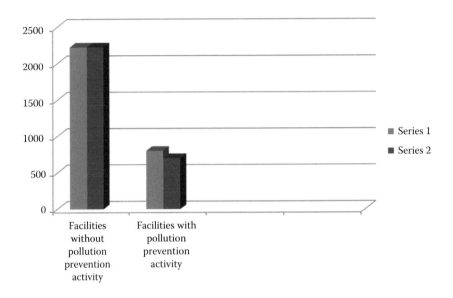

FIGURE 1.8 Series 1 is year 2002, Series 2 is year 2004. Amounts represent millions of 1 kg.

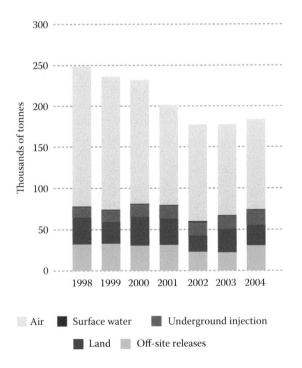

FIGURE 1.9 Releases of carcinogens and developmental/reproductive toxicants. (From Canadian and U.S. data.)

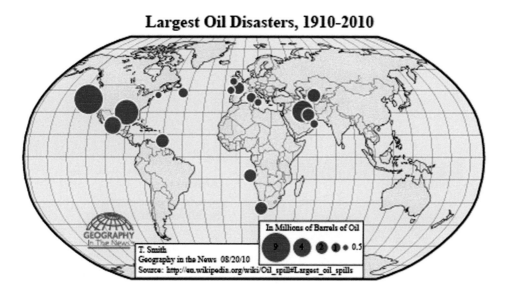

FIGURE 1.10 Largest oil disasters, 1910–2010.

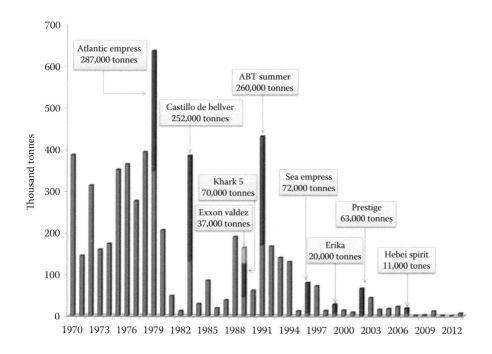

FIGURE 1.12 Quantities of oil spilt >7 tonnes, 1970–2013 (rounded to the nearest thousand). (Courtesy of ITPOF, 2012.)

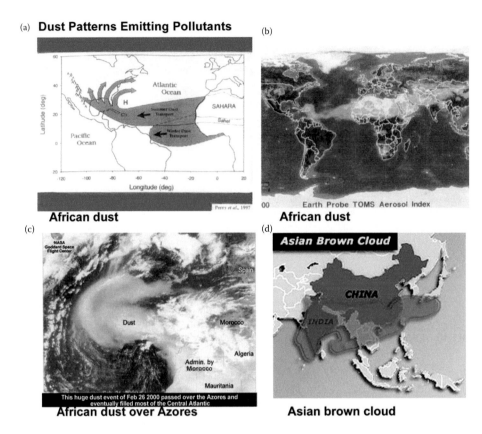

FIGURE 1.13 African dust and Asian brown cloud patterns in 2005. The African dust comes via the trade winds and (goes) moves up the part of the United States east of the Rocky Mountains, over Bermuda, and on to England and Europe. The Gobi (Asian) dust goes across the Pacific and is usually stopped by the Rocky Mountains and distributed over California, Oregon, and Washington states. (Courtesy of NOAA—Gene Shinn.)

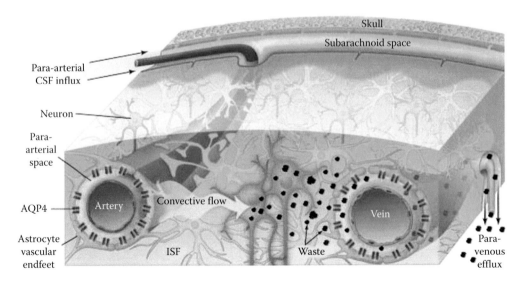

FIGURE 2.1 ECF flowing outside the blood vessels in para-arterial spaces on the endfeet of astrocytes: The lymphatic system (glia water channels). (From Nedergaard, M. 2013. Neuroscience. Garbage truck of the brain. *Science* 340 (6140):1529–1530. Reprinted with permission from AAAS.)

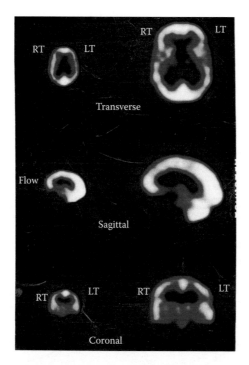

FIGURE 2.3 Normal SPECT brain scan—smooth, uniform, distinct outlines, no rough edges or holes in cerebral hemispheres or abnormal temporal lobes.

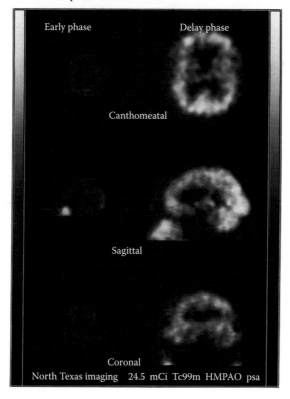

FIGURE 2.4 Abnormal SPECT brain scan. Early phase barely visible, delayed phase holes in cerebrum, temporal lobes obliterate; no good defined lines.

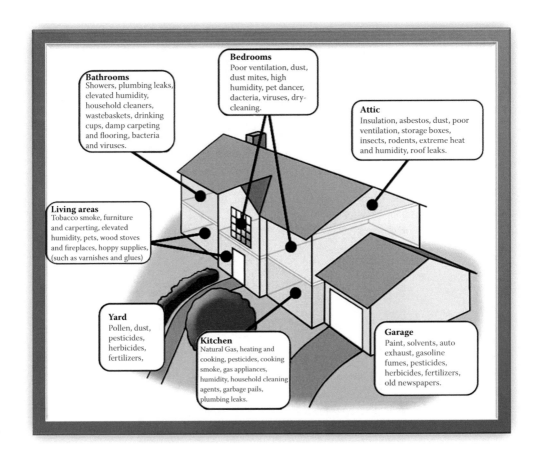

FIGURE 3.1 Sources of indoor air pollution observed to exacerbate chemical sensitivity.

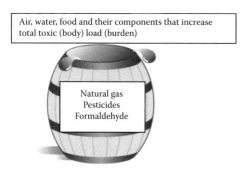

Air, water, food and their components that increase total toxic (body) load (burden)

Natural gas
Pesticides
Formaldehyde

Air quality at home

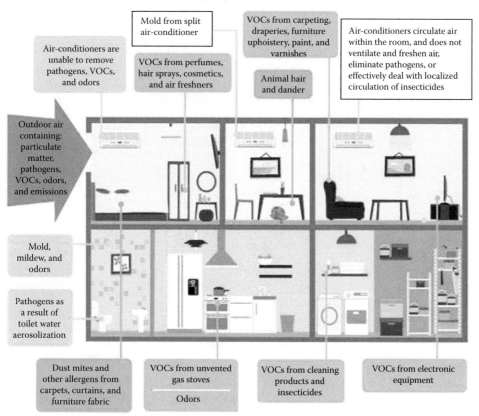

Mold from split air-conditioner

VOCs from carpeting, draperies, furniture upholstery, paint, and varnishes

Air-conditioners are unable to remove pathogens, VOCs, and odors

VOCs from perfumes, hair sprays, cosmetics, and air freshners

Air-conditioners circulate air within the room, and does not ventilate and freshen air, eliminate pathogens, or effectively deal with localized circulation of insecticides

Animal hair and dander

Outdoor air containing: particulate matter, pathogens, VOCs, odors, and emissions

Mold, mildew, and odors

Pathogens as a result of toilet water aerosolization

Dust mites and other allergens from carpets, curtains, and furniture fabric

VOCs from unvented gas stoves

Odors

VOCs from cleaning products and insecticides

VOCs from electronic equipment

FIGURE 3.3 Air quality at home.

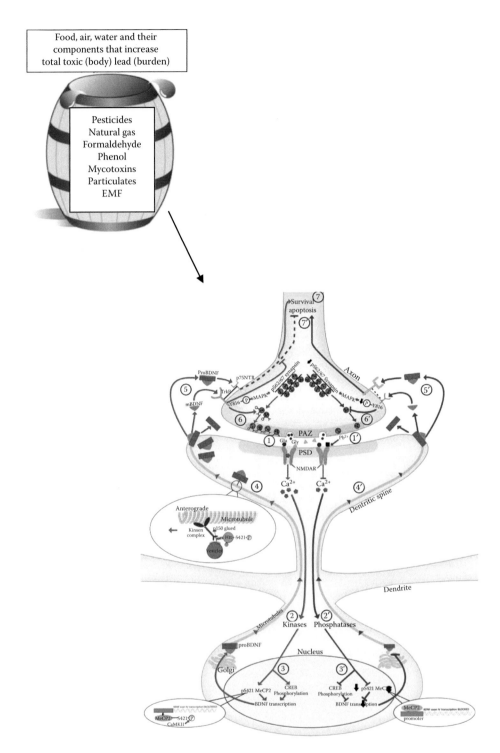

FIGURE 4.17 Bidirectional communication of presynaptic and postsynaptic elements of the synapse defines their survival or retraction during development. On the left side of the same synapse, they define the function of normal synapses, whereas on the right side, they show the components that are affected by Pb^{2+}-induced effects in order to reduce the size of the figure. The green arrows denote normal function, whereas the red arrows indicate impaired function.

Noncriteria pollutants

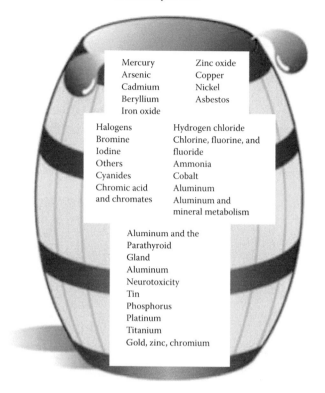

Mercury	Zinc oxide
Arsenic	Copper
Cadmium	Nickel
Beryllium	Asbestos
Iron oxide	

Halogens	Hydrogen chloride
Bromine	Chlorine, fluorine, and
Iodine	fluoride
Others	Ammonia
Cyanides	Cobalt
Chromic acid	Aluminum
and chromates	Aluminum and
	mineral metabolism

Aluminum and the
Parathyroid
Gland
Aluminum
Neurotoxicity
Tin
Phosphorus
Platinum
Titanium
Gold, zinc, chromium

FIGURE 4.18 Noncriteria pollutants.

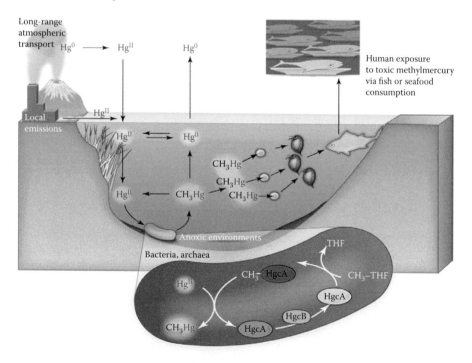

FIGURE 4.19 Mercury geochemical cycle. (From Poulain, A. J., T. Barkay. 2013. Cracking the mercury methylation code. *Science* 339(6125)1280–1281. With Permission from AAAS.)

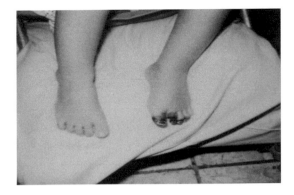

FIGURE 7.20 Four-year-old white female. After exposure to lawn pesticides, gangrene of foot developed.

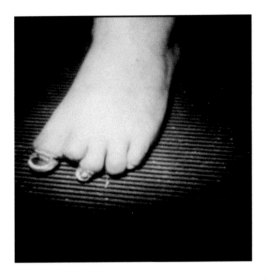

FIGURE 7.21 Four-year-old white female. After ECU treatment: minimal loss of toes; foot and leg intact.

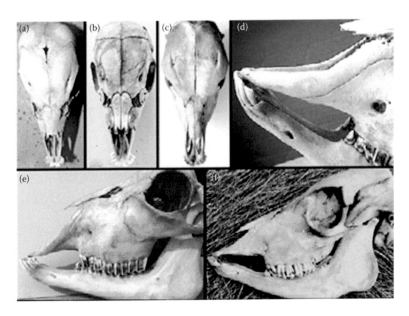

FIGURE 7.31 Brachygnathia superior and wide lower incisors on ruminant species. (a) White-tailed deer fawn skull. (b) Mule deer fawn skull. (c) Elk calf skull. (d) Adult male bighorn sheep skull, showing short narrow premaxillary bone. (e) Domestic beef calf skull. (f) Skull of an adult male domestic goat.

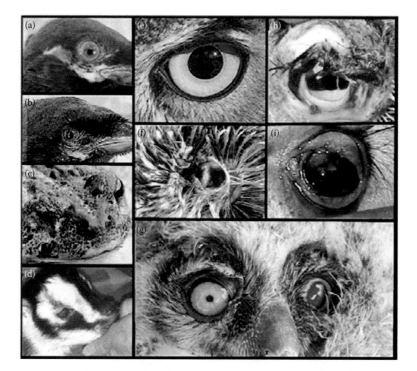

FIGURE 7.32 Recent eye malformations in vertebrates. (a) Black-billed magpie fledgling showing a normal-sized eye. (b) Blind black-billed magpie fledgling right eye, both eyes were underdeveloped. (c) Adult 2014 western toad with right eye not formed and left eye normal. (d) Pygmy goat born in 2015 with small eye, malformed external ear and BS. (e) The normal left eye and eyelids of a Great Horned Owl (GHOW). (f) Underdeveloped left eye with malformed eyelids and pupil on 2014 hatch year GHOW. (g) Face of a 2013 fledgling GHOW showing the malformed left pupil and malformed eyelids on both eyes. (h) The malformed left pupil and eyelids of another 2014 hatch year GHOW. (i) The inflamed conjunctiva of a female WTD fawn after exposure to environmental toxins.

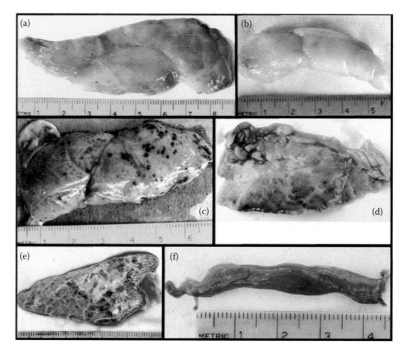

FIGURE 7.33 Newborn white-tailed deer thymus conditions. (a and b) Normal thymus color and shape. (c and d) Thymus with red spots throughout. (e) Odd shaped, mostly red thymus. (f) Undersized thymus, red throughout.

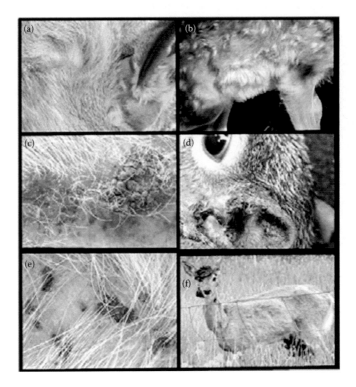

FIGURE 7.34 Skin disorders on wild and domestic mammals. (a) Large blisters at the base of the right ear on a male WTD fawn, born 2013. (b) Hair loss on shoulders, sides, and hind legs of a female WTD fawn after exposure to environmental toxins, born 2003. (c) Male WTD fawn inner ear skin with chemical blistering, born 2010. (d) Young male eastern fox squirrel's left ear showing severe chemical skin blisters in 2005. (e) Adult female dog with chemical blisters, summer 2013. (f) Adult female WTD with multiple skin growths in May 2010.

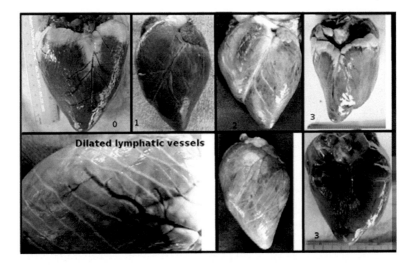

FIGURE 7.35 White-tailed deer heart conditions ranked from 0 to 3. 0. Normal heart. (1) Slightly enlarged right ventricle. (2) Moderately enlarged right ventricle. (3) Severely enlarged right ventricle. Dilated lymphatic vessels on heart surface of newborn fawn and close-up of dilated lymphatic vessels on newborn fawn. Corresponding numbers were used in the field to record the presence or severity of any abnormal heart condition observed.

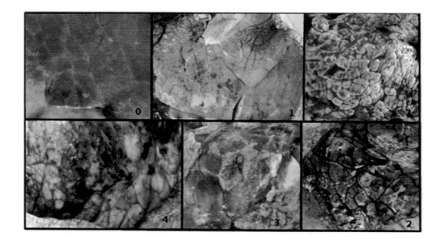

FIGURE 7.36 White-tailed deer lung conditions ranked 0–4. 0. Normal lungs. (1) Slightly bumpy on outer lobes. (2) Raised alveoli on much of lung area. (3) Raised alveoli and white areas in lungs. (4) Raised alveoli and bleeding lungs. Corresponding numbers were used in the field to record the presence or severity of any adverse lung conditions observed.

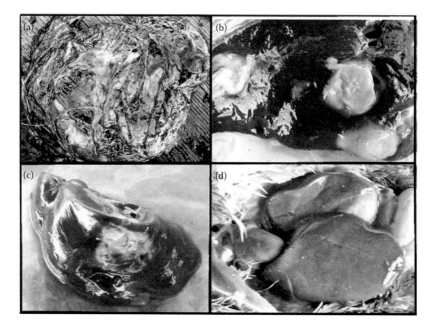

FIGURE 7.37 Liver conditions in wildlife. (a) Large tumor verified as cancer, 18 cm. (7 in.) in diameter, removed from the outside of the liver on a female gray wolf. (b) Tumorlike growths in the liver of an adult female domestic goat. (c) Tumorlike growths in the liver of a fledgling Rock Pigeon. (d) A black-billed magpie fledgling's enlarged, discolored liver.

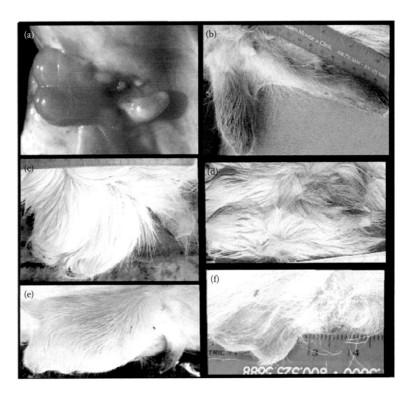

FIGURE 7.38 Normal and abnormal white-tailed deer male genitalia. (a) White-tailed deer fetus, normal genitalia. (b) One-year-old white-tailed deer, normal genitalia. (c) One and half-year-old white-tailed deer with misaligned hemiscrota and short penis sheath. (d) One and half-year-old white-tailed deer, no scrotum formed on external skin, testes ectopic under the skin (see bumps), short penis sheath. (e) Two-year-old white-tailed deer, horizontal misaligned hemiscrota, penis sheath normal. (f) Newborn white-tailed deer with misaligned hemiscrota and short penis sheath.

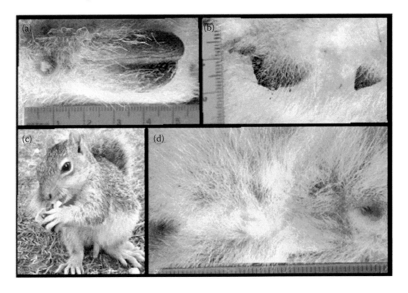

FIGURE 7.39 Normal and abnormal eastern fox squirrel male genitalia. (a) Normal scrotum, very short penis sheath. (b) Scrotum is misaligned with short empty skin flaps, penis sheath very short. (c) White spot where scrotum should be formed, penis sheath very short. (d) Live juvenile male with normal penis sheath for comparison.

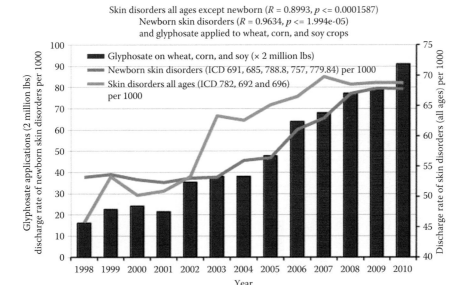

FIGURE 7.42 Hospital discharge rates for newborn skin disorders and skin disorders in the general population superimposed with glyphosate applications to wheat, corn, and soy crops. The newborn skin disorders are: atopic dermatitis (ICD 691); pilonidal cyst (ICD 685); erythema and urticaria (ICD 778.8); vascular hamartomas (ICD 757.32); pigment anomalies (ICD 757.33); unspecified deformities of hair, skin, and nails (ICD 757.9); and meconium staining (ICD779.84). The Pearson correlation coefficient is $R = 0.9634$. Skin disorders for the general population include rash, swelling, and changes in skin tone and texture (ICD 782); eczema (ICD 692); and psoriasis (ICD 696). The Pearson correlation coefficient is $R = 0.8993$.

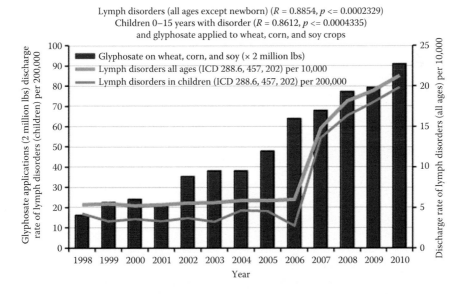

FIGURE 7.43 Hospital discharge rates for children with lymphatic disorder and lymphatic disorder in the general population superimposed with glyphosate applications to wheat, corn, and soy crops. The lymphatic disorders for children are: lymphedema (ICD 457); lymphocytosis (ICD 288.6); Castleman's disease (angiofollicular lymph node hyperplasia, ICD 202). The Pearson correlation coefficient is $R = 0.8612$. The lymphatic disorders for the general population are: lymphedema (ICD 457); lymphocytosis (ICD 288.6); Castleman's disease (angiofollicular lymph node hyperplasia, ICD 202). The Pearson correlation coefficient is $R = 0.8854$.

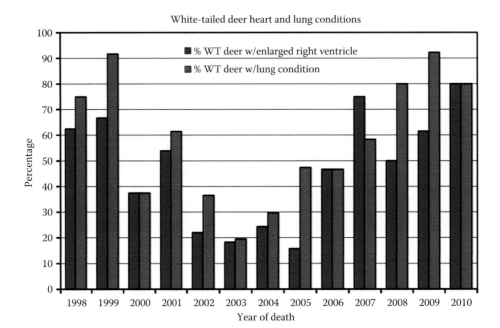

FIGURE 7.44   Percentage of white-tailed deer with heart and lung conditions, 1998–2010.

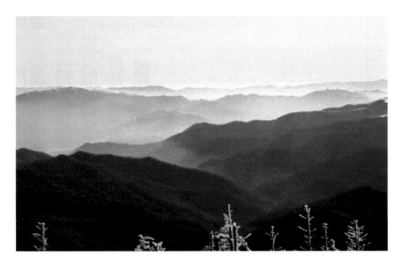

FIGURE 8.1   Picture of terpene haze. (From https://earthdata.nasa.gov/user-resources/sensing-our-planet/volatile-trees.

contraction, thrombogenesis and fibrinogenesis, and platelet activation and inhibition. Previous studies have demonstrated that mercury decreases the production of nitric oxide (NO) and alters the expression of NOS.[487] $HgCI_2$ at concentrations of 0.5–10 µM produces vasoconstriction, reduces the endothelial vasodilator response, and stimulates a COX-derived vasoconstrictor.[488] In addition, several studies have shown that mercury induces oxidative stress with subsequent oxidative damage to several organs or systems.[483] GSH depletion by mercury may be a trigger for the production of ROS that induce lipid, protein, and DNA oxidation.[483] Vascular endothelium is highly sensitive to oxidative stress and this is the main cause of endothelial dysfunction observed in cardiovascular diseases such as hypertension and atherosclerosis.[482,489] Most mercury toxicity studies are performed with high (micromolar) concentrations of mercury and under acute exposure. Then, given the idea that relatively high blood levels are more frequently used to indicate mercury as an environmental risk factor for cardiovascular diseases, Vassallo et al.[490] recently developed a methodology involving controlled chronic mercury administration that attains a concentration of 8 ng/mL (~29 nM) in blood[485] to better understand the endothelial modulation of vascular responses.

Although the TLV for mercury is 0.05 mg/m^3,[491] this standard may be falsely high, and it does not take into account individual susceptibility. The fact is mercury and its compounds are toxic to man. Individuals may be exposed to various sources of mercury such as mercury vapor, inorganic mercury salts, organic mercury compounds, alkyl mercury compounds, and seafood contaminated with mercury. Acute exposure to high levels of mercury compounds causes a variety of gastrointestinal symptoms and severe anuria with uremia, as well as precipitating chemical sensitivity. The clinical symptoms for chronic mercurialism involve the CNS, with tremor and various neuropsychiatric disturbances. They also involve the female reproductive system. For example, the first indicators of fetal toxicity were shown to occur when abortions were observed in women undergoing mercury treatment for syphilis.

A relaxation equal to or greater than 90% indicates functional integrity of the endothelium. Smooth muscle viability is tested using sodium nitroprusside (SNP, 0.1 mg/mL) in rings previously contracted with phenylephrine. After 30 minutes, cumulative concentration–response curves for phenylephrine (0.1 nM–300 µM) are generated.

The incubation of segments with mercury $HgCI_2$ for 60 minute promotes an increase in the reactivity to phenylephrine both at high (0.5–10 µM) and low (6 nM) concentrations.[492,493] This increased reactivity appears as an increase R_{max} and sensitivity. Gadolinium (3 µM as $GdCl_3$) promotes similar responses[494] but lead increases vascular reactivity when administered only at high concentration (100 µM). At lower lead concentration (5 nM), reactivity to phenylephrine decreases.

When controlled chronic mercury treatments are performed using exposure to low doses for 30 days, with a blood concentration of 8 ng/mL (~29 nM) being reached, vascular reactivity to phenylephrine increases in Hg-treated rats.[485,486] Mercury treatment also increases 5-HT-induced vasoconstriction in coronary arteries.[487] A similar increase of vascular reactivity was obtained with lead treatments for 30 days or more.[491] However, exposure of rats to low lead concentrations for 7 days decreased the contractile that the effects of lead are concentration and time dependent.[321] Regarding gadolinium, there are no reports about chronic treatments with low concentrations.

Other detrimental effects of mercury have been reported. Between 1953 and 1971, 134 cases of mercury poisoning were reported, including 78 adults and 56 children. During this period, 25 infants were born with brain damage, a result of *in utero* exposure to mercury. Six percent of these infants had cerebral palsy. Similar poisonings occurred in Nigata, Japan with 46 cases of mercurial poisonings being reported as a result of ingestion of mercury-contaminated fish. Also, in Iraq in 1971, barley and wheat grain treated with MeHg were distributed to farmers. The grain was used to make bread containing about 4 mg of mercury per loaf. Ingestion of this bread resulted in 6530 hospitalized cases of mercurial poison, including 459 deaths, for a mortality rate of 7%.

According to Ni et al.,[495] "the neurotoxicity of MeHg is well documented in both humans and animals. MeHg causes acute and chronic damage to multiple organs, most profoundly the CNS." Microglial cells are derived from macrophage cell linage, making up ~12% of cells in the CNS,

MeHg has adverse effect on microglial viability triggers ROS generation alters GSH level, redox homeostasis, and Nrf2 protein expression.[495]

Experimental studies have shown time-dependent increase in ROS generation, accompanied by a statistically significant decrease in the ratio of GSH and its oxidized form glutathione disulfide (GSSG) (GSH/GSSG ratio). MeHg increased the cytosolic Nrf2 protein level within 1 minute of exposure, followed by its nuclear translocation after 10 minute of treatment. Consistent with the nuclear translocation of Nrf2, this knockdown of Nrf2 greatly reduced the upregulation of the Ho-1, Ngo1, and xCT genes and increased microglial death upon Nrf2 knockdown by the shRNA approach. Thus, this study has demonstrated that microglial cells are exquisitely sensitive to MeHg and respond rapidly to MeHg by upregulating the Nrf2-mediated antioxidant response.[495]

Mercury is a potent neurotoxin that directly impairs many areas and functions of the neuron, including calcium channels,[496–498] protein synthesis,[499] mitochondria,[499] and neurite outgrowth.[500]

Both the aforementioned neurotoxicity and a human disease response to mercury exposure have been shown to be dependent on reaching a critical threshold concentration.[501] Therefore, in cases of acute mercury poisoning, the direct neurotoxic effect of mercury in the brain may surpass this threshold and elicit a disease response. However, in cases of chronic mercury exposure, mercury concentrations in the brain may remain beneath the critical threshold concentration and therefore a direct relationship between chronic mercury exposure and neurotoxicity is not evident, prima facie. In toxicological studies of chronic mercury exposure in primates, organic mercury has been shown to demethylate and form inorganic mercury deposits which persist in the brain for years.[495]

In both primates and humans, inorganic mercury deposits preferentially target the pituitary where they accumulate.[502,503]

The accumulation of inorganic mercury deposits in the body is reasoned to be detectable by changes of inorganic mercury level(s) in the blood.[504] In a recent human population dependent on fish, inorganic mercury accumulation in the blood has been shown to be associated with chronic mercury exposure.[505] In another recent study, Carvalho et al. used inorganic mercury exposure as the bioindicator of chronic mercury exposure within the U.S. population[506] and discovered a significant, inverse relationship between chronic mercury exposure and luteinizing hormone (LH).

Role of LH

LH is not only a high-affinity target for mercury, located in the prime area of mercury deposition and accumulation, but also regulates diverse systems whose impairment is symptomatic of mercury-associated disease. LH is secreted by the anterior pituitary and mediates androgen stimulation, mitogenesis, and immune regulation.[507–510]

Specific neuronal tracts have been shown to produce luteinizing hormone-releasing hormone (LHRH) within the adult brain to modulate glial formation and the complex neuronal-microglia networks that are crucial to brain development, plasticity, function, and the neuroimmune inflammatory response.[509] LHRH is also found on human peripheral lymphocytes, indicating a role for LH in mediating both the central and peripheral immune systems.[511] As a mitogen, LH is not only involved as a gonadotroph but also in the birth of neurons. Recently, LH was demonstrated in both mice[512] and sheep[513] to directly induce neurogenesis in the adult hippocampus, the area of the brain associated with learning and memory.

LH is directly involved in regulating all of the systems that are symptomatic of mercury-associated disease: impaired immune response, inflammation, disruption of glia-neuronal networks, and impaired neurogenesis. Therefore, it is reasonable to assume that the biological association between chronic mercury exposure and LH represents a causal mechanism to delineate the pathology from chronic mercury exposure and deposition to an impaired endocrine system and the defining characteristics of mercury-associated disease. In Mercury, LH, and associated disease, there are certainly strong and persistent associations.

The HPA is programmed during neonatal development, and early exposure to toxins can disrupt the delicate endocrine system to program an imbalanced immune system that is predisposed toward an inflammatory response.[508] Experts agree that any disturbance of the HPA system leads to an increased risk of infection, inflammation, and autoimmune disease.[514,515] Inflammatory response and an impaired immune system are characteristics of mercury neurotoxicity[516–519] and both neurodevelopmental[520,521] and neurodegenerative[522] diseases that are associated with mercury exposure. LH plays a key role in neuroprotection and inflammatory response within the CNS.[523]

The endocrine system has been implicated for a central role in the pathogenesis of autism.[524–526] LH is a gonadotroph and is primarily known for its role in the induction of androgens. Strikingly, autism is characterized by an imbalance in androgen levels.[527,528] While some medical professionals have hypothesized a direct interaction between mercury exposure and androgen receptors,[529] this perspective postulates that the effect of mercury is primarily upstream of those receptors, and, an alternative hypothesis is presented, that focal targeting of LH by mercury exposure and deposition in the pituitary is responsible for the apparent aberrant androgen levels in mercury-associated neurodevelopmental disease such as autism.

Mounting evidence indicates that inflammation impairs neurogenesis, the required migration of neuronal precursors, and the proper incorporation of new neurons into the cytoarchitecture.[530–532] The pituitary secretes hormones which regulate thyroid hormones. Mercury exposure has been demonstrated to impair thyroid hormone function.[533,534] Impaired thyroid hormone function has been linked to impaired migration of neuronal precursors and disruption of the delicate incorporation of neurons into the developing cytoarchitecture.[535] Inorganic mercury deposits are associated with neurotoxic and immune pathways associated with neurodegeneration and LH provides a compelling candidate to explain a causal relationship.[536]

As mentioned previously, mercury exposure has been associated with age-related neurodegenerative disease.[537–540] "Endocrine abnormalities of the HPA system in patients with Alzheimer's (AD) and Parkinson's disease (PD) have been described repeatedly."[541] AD pathology is marked by elevated serum and neuronal levels of LH.[542] Brain regions mostly affected by AD pathology show elevated expression of LH,[507] and moreover, in cell culture, LH accelerates the formation of amyloid plaques, a defining pathological characteristic of AD.

Trends of Chronic Mercury Exposure

From analysis of data on the human population from 1999 to 2000, it was estimated that 300,000–500,000 children may be born during those years with elevated risks of neurodevelopmental disease based on their exposure to mercury.[542] However, these risks of disease response to mercury exposure may be rising over time due to rising levels of chronic mercury exposure.[543] In fact, atmospheric mercury deposition is rising over time,[544] mercury levels are rising in the oceans,[545] and global mercury emissions are projected to continue rising in the future.[546] Therefore, while a causal mechanism between chronic mercury exposure and associated disease is not clearly understood, this time trend of rising exposure levels makes it a public health and medical imperative to investigate the mechanisms underlying mercury-associated disease in order to prevent, diagnose, and treat this serious, emergent health threat.

Conclusion

Certainly, it is well understood, in multiple human and animal models, that mercury exposure targets the endocrine system.[547] However, the relationship between endocrine impairment and mercury-associated disease is poorly understood. This perspective posits that LH represents a promising and viable candidate to provide a causal mechanism for mercury association.

During the past few years, three instances of mercury poisoning have been reported in Minimata, Japan, Iraq, and the Russia Minimata's disease occurred after 27 tons of MeHg chloride was dumped into Minimata Bay. Fish harvested from this bay were eaten and caused severe neurological problems.[535] The results of the incidents in Iraq and the Russia are unclear. Also, three recent case reports from Lund, Sweden, King County, Washington, and Alamogordo, New Mexico showed pregnant women whose fetuses had mercury toxicity.

Detectable levels of mercury in the bloodstream of humans have been attributed to silver amalgam fillings. James et al.[542] described a case of lichen planus due to mercury amalgam fillings. Finne et al.[544] described a series of 29 patients with lichen planus due to mercury amalgam fillings. Nylander[545] has shown deposits of mercury in the brain of people whose teeth have silver fillings. They have advocated removal of these fillings in order to reduce the complications of mercury, which is known to destroy the GSH replenishing systems and produce cytotoxic Type II immunological reactions. Exposure to pesticides containing mercury has been seen to exacerbate some chemically sensitive patients. Mercury is used in some pharmaceuticals.

Cracking the Mercury Methylation Code

Mercury (Hg) is a global pollutant that is transported over long distances. Although it occurs naturally, its concentration in the biosphere has increased dramatically over the past 200 years as a result of industrial activities. Mercury enters the environment in its inorganic form, but its bioaccumulation in organisms, biomagnification in food webs, and toxicity to humans depend on microbial MeHg synthesis.

The use of stable isotopes of mercury has improved the ability to trace and measure mercury in the environment,[548,549] but methods to predict MeHg synthesis in the environment remain scarce. Parks et al.[550] identify two genes required for mercury methylation. This discovery will be helpful for developing tools to study the synthesis and accumulation of MeHg and to improve the management of contaminated environments.

The crippling and deadly effects of MeHg have been recognized globally since the severe mercury poisoning event in Minamata, Japan in 1956, after the release of mercury from a nearby industry. Since then, studies have shown that mercury is methylated under anoxic conditions[551] by sulfate- and iron-reducing bacteria.[552,553] Biochemical studies suggested the possible involvement of corrinoid proteins in the methylation pathway.[554,555] However, no specific mercury methylation genes were identified, limiting understanding of the methylation pathway and hence the ability to track MeHg production.

Parks et al.[550] used comparative genomics and structural biology tools to identify candidate genes. They performed targeted gene deletion and complementation experiments to show that two genes, hgcA (which encodes a putative corrinoid protein) and hgcB (which encodes a 2[Fe-4S] ferredoxin), are required for mercury methylation.

On the basis of these findings, the authors propose a mechanistic model where a methyl group is transferred from the methylated HgcA protein to inorganic Hg(II) and the HgcB protein is required for HgcA turnover. This proposed pathway raises questions about the biophysical and biochemical mechanisms by which mercury is methylated. Most intriguing is the authors' prediction that the C-terminus of HgcA may be membrane embedded, possibly coupling methylation to the transport of Hg(II) and/or MeHg across the cell wall (Figure 4.19).

The authors' identified homologs of hgcA and hgcB in genomes of 52 bacteria and methanogenic archaea. Although most have not been tested for their ability to methylate mercury in pure culture, field studies have implicated methanogens in mercury methylation.[556] The distribution of methylation ability is sporadic, with methylating and nonmethylating strains occurring in the same species.[557] These observations raise the questions how methylation evolved and what its purpose might be. Methylation may be a detoxification mechanism,[558,559] possibly an ancient pathway used to deal with toxic inorganic mercury. Further experiments and analyses of the genomes in which hgcA and hgcB are found will help establish the evolutionary path of mercury methylation.[560]

Mercury is methylated in anoxic environments by microorganisms, one of which is illustrated in the inset. Parks et al.[550] show that the methylation reaction requires two genes, hgcA (encoding a putative methyltransferase [MeTr] corrinoid protein) and hgcB (encoding a putative [4Fe-4S] ferredoxin). Different colors for the HgcA protein indicate different redox states of the corrinoid HgcA enzyme. The toxic MeHg accumulates in aquatic species (bioaccumulation) and its concentrations

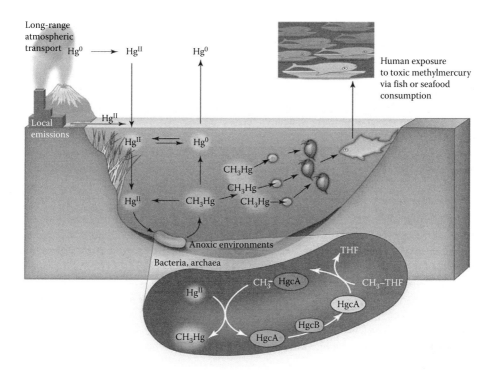

FIGURE 4.19 **(See color insert.)** Mercury geochemical cycle.[973] (From Poulain, A. J., T. Barkay. 2013. Cracking the mercury methylation code. *Science* 339(6125)1280–1281. With Permission from AAAS.)

increase with each trophic level (biomagnification), causing a threat to humans whose diets rely on fish. Tetrahydrofolate (THF) is also involved.

The Genetic Basis for Bacterial Mercury Methylation

MeHg is a potent neurotoxin produced in natural environments from inorganic mercury by anaerobic bacteria. However, until now, the genes and proteins involved have remained unidentified. Parks et al.[550] report a two-gene cluster, hgcA and hgcB, required for mercury methylation by *Desulfovibrio desulfuricans* ND132 and *Geobacter sulfurreducens* PCA. In either bacterium, deletion of hgcA, hgcB, or both genes abolishes mercury methylation. The genes encode a putative corrinoid protein, HgcA, and a 2 (4Fe-4S) ferredoxin, HgcB, consistent with roles as a methyl carrier and an electron donor required for corrinoid cofactor reduction, respectively. Among bacteria and archaea with sequenced genomes, gene orthologs are present in confirmed methylators but absent in nonmethylators, suggesting a common mercury methylation pathway in all methylating bacteria and archaea sequenced to date.

Mercury (Hg) is a pervasive global pollutant; in the form of MeHg (CH_3Hg^+), it bioaccumulates in the food web and is highly toxic to humans and other organisms.[561] Unlike inorganic forms of Hg which originate from atmospheric deposition and point discharges, MeHg is generated in the environment predominantly by anaerobic microorganisms.[562] Sulfate-reducing bacteria are the main producers of CH_3Hg^+,[563,564] although iron-reducing bacteria[565–567] and methanogens[568,569] can also be involved.

Production of CH_3Hg^+ by the model methylating bacteria *D. desulfuricans* ND 132 and *G. sulfurreducens* PCA involves cellular uptake of Hg(II) by active transport, methylation of Hg(II) in the cytosol, and export of CH_3Hg^+ from the cell.[559] Hg methylation is an enzyme-catalyzed process proposed to be associated with the reductive acetyl-coenzyme A (CoA) pathway (also called the Wood–Ljungdahl pathway[554]) and potentially linked to corrinoid proteins involved in this pathway.[568] However, no direct evidence firmly connects the acetyl-CoA pathway and the ability of bacteria to methylate Hg. Furthermore, phylogenetic analyses have not revealed any distinctive trends or clustering of methylating versus nonmethylating microorganisms.[557,567,570]

To understand the genetic and biochemical basis of microbial Hg methylation, Parks et al. analyzed the genomes of methylating and nonmethylating bacteria in the context of biochemical pathways involved in single-carbon metabolism. The well-characterized corrinoid iron–sulfur protein (CFeSP) is known to transfer methyl groups to a NiFeS cluster in acetyl-CoA synthase.[571] Therefore, recognizing that a corrinoid protein associated with the acetyl-CoA pathway could be required for Hg methylation. They reasoned that a protein similar to CFeSP might transfer a methyl group to a Hg substrate to yield CH_3Hg^+, and that genes encoding such a protein should be recognizable in the genome sequences of Hg-methylating bacteria. Complete genome sequences are available for six methylating and eight closely related nonmethylating bacterial species (Tables 4.23 and 4.24). Furthermore, molecular structures and functions have been determined for various enzymes of the reductive acetyl-CoA pathway, including CFeSP from *Moorella thermoacetica*[572] and *Carboxdothermus hydrogenoformans*.[573,574] Accordingly, they performed a BLASTP search with the sequence of the large subunit of CFeSP (CfsA, locus tag CHY_1223 from *C. hydrogenoformans* Z-2901 against the translated genome sequence of *D. desulfuricans* ND 132).[575] Sequence similarity was found between the C-terminal corrinoid-binding domain of DfsA and the N-terminus of DND132_1056, although DND132_1056 attacks both the TIM barrel domain and the C-terminal (4Fe-4S)-binding motif of CfsA. The C-terminal region showed no detectable similarity to any proteins of known structure, but exhibited features characteristic of a transmembrane domain.

They also performed comparative genomic analyses of known Hg methylators and nonmethylators on the basis of Pfam classifications,[576] with an emphasis on enzyme families known to be involved in methyl transfer reactions. The distribution of Pfam domains in the genomes is heterogeneous and, for the most part, does not coincide with the mercury methylation phenotype. However,

TABLE 4.23

Confirmed Mercury Methylating Bacteria with Completely Sequenced Genomes

Organism name	Goldstamp ID1	Culture collections	Reference
Desulfovibrio desulfuricans ND132	Gi03061	–	*(15)*
Desulfovibrio aespoeensis	Gc01651	DSM 10631	*(67)*
Desulfovibrio africanus Walvis Bay	Gi03062	ATCC 19997, NCIB 8397	*(22)*
Desulfobulbus propionicus 1pr3	Gc01599	DSM 2032, ATCC 33891	*(68)*
Geobacter sulfurreducens PCA	Gc00166	DSM 12127, ATCC 51573	*(6)*
Geobacter metallireducens GS-15	Gc00314	DSM 7210, ATCC 53774	*(6)*

TABLE 4.24

Confirmed Non-Methylating Bacteria with Completely Sequenced Genomes

Organism name	Goldstamp ID*	Culture collections	Reference
Desulfovibrio desulfuricans MB	Gc00931	DSM 6949, ATCC 27774	*(14); (15)*
Desulfovibrio vulgaris Hildenborough	Gc00184	DSM 644, ATCC 29579	*(14); (15)*
Desulfovibrio alaskensis G20	Gc00315	DSM 16109,	*(15)*
Desulfovibrio salexigens	Gc01109	DSM 2638, ATCC 14822	*(15)*
Desulfotomaculum acetoxidans	Gc01106	DSM 771, ATCC 49208	*(46)*
Desulfotomaculum nigrificans	Gi03933	DSM 574, ATCC 19998	*(46)*
Syntrophobacter fumaroxidans MPOB	Gc00453	DSM 10017	*(14)*
Desulfovibrio piger	Gi01734	ATCC 29098, DSM 749	*(67)*

the distribution of proteins of the CdhD family (PF03599, annotated as CO dehydrogenase/acetyl-CoA synthase delta subunit) encoded in the genomes correlates with the ability or inability of those organisms to methylate mercury. DND132_1056 is annotated as encoding a CdhD member, as are its close relatives in all five other confirmed methylators.

Analysis of the genomic context in the confirmed Hg methylators revealed genes similar to both the putative corrinoid protein-encoding gene and an additional, ferredoxin-like gene located downstream, which suggests that these two genes might be coexpressed and functionally related. In *D. desulfuricans* ND 132, the annotated coding sequences of the two genes (DND132_1056 and DND132_1057) are on the same strand and are separated by only 14 base pairs. Similar gene pairs were found in the genomes of 52 organisms with sequence translations available in public databases. The two genes are present in all sequenced, confirmed methylators and absent in the sequenced, confirmed nonmethylators. The other 46 organisms in which the genes are present have not been tested for Hg methylation.

They hypothesized that these two genes are key components of the bacterial Hg methylation pathway, with the putative corrinoid protein facilitating methyl transfer and the ferredoxin carrying out corrinoid reduction. Therefore, they deleted these genes individually, and also together, from *D. desulfuricans* ND132 (supplementary text). Additionally, they deleted the orthologs GSU1440 and GSU1441 together, and GSU1440 individually, from *G. sulfurreducens* PCA. In both of these organisms, CH_3Hg^+ production decreased in the deletion mutants by >99% relative to the parental strains. Complementation of the two-gene deletions by reincorporation of the genes into the chromosomes restored 26% and 87% of the wild-type methylation activity in *D. desulfuricans* ND132 and *G. sulfurreducens* PCA, respectively, as measured by inductively coupled plasma mass spectrometry (ICP-MS). Deletion of DND132_1057 alone yielded <0.2% of wild-type methylation activity, and subsequent complementation showed 97% methylation activity. Complementation of either gene alone into the double-deletion mutant did not restore detectable methylation activity (Figure 4.20). Restoration of ΔDND132_1056 was not performed. Although the relative location of the two genes is consistent with cotranscription, reverse transcription polymerase chain reaction confirmed the transcription of DND132_1056 in the ΔDND132_1057 strain and DND132_1057 in the ΔDND132_1056 mutant.

The above findings are consistent with both genes being required for Hg methylation activity, although other unidentified genes are also likely to be involved. Hereafter, they refer to the DND132_1056 gene and its inferred orthologs as hgcA, encoding putative corrinoid proteins required for CH_3Hg^+ production and DND132_1057 and its inferred orthologs as hgcB encoding putative corrinoid protein-associated 2(F3-4S) ferredoxins. To determine whether gene loss impairs metabolism on a more general scale, comparative growth curves were obtained. The deletion mutants showed no impairment in rate or extent of growth. Thus, under the conditions tested, the construction of the deletions did not cause major growth aberrations that might interfere with the detection of methylation activity. The native functions of hgcA and hgcB remain unknown, but these genes are not essential for cell survival or proliferation.

The above findings merit some mechanistic considerations. The requirement for HgcA and HgcB in methylation is largely consistent with a previously proposed Hg methylation pathway by Bartha and coworkers,[554] which are revised. The methyl group in CH_3Hg^+ originates from $CH_3–H_4$-folate in *D. desulfuricans* LS[554] and is likely first transferred (as CH_3^+) to cob(I)alamin-HgcA to form CH_3-cob(III)alamin-HgcA. This step may be catalyzed by a folate-binding MeTr similar to the $CH_3–H_4$-folate: CFeSP MeTr from the reductive acetyl-CoA pathway,[577,578] or by an unknown enzyme. The high affinity of thiolate ligands for Hg^{2+} (formation constants for $Hg(SR)_2$, log K = 40–43)[579] suggests that a possible substrate for HgcA could be a Hg(II) bis(thiolate) complex involving either free cellular thiols or cysteine residues from a protein. Methyl transfer from CH_3-cob(III)alamin-HgcA to a Hg substrated likely involves either CH_3^+ or CH_3^-. Although transfer of a carbon from methylcobalamin to Hg(II) nonenzymatically is known to occur,[580,581] enzymatic transfer of CH_3^- by a corrinoid protein has never been observed.

Further sequence analysis of the 52 HgcA orthologs revealed a highly conserved motif, Asn-(Val/Ile)-Trp-Cys-Ala-(Ala/Gly)-Gly-Lys, in the region of highest similarity to the CfsA subunit

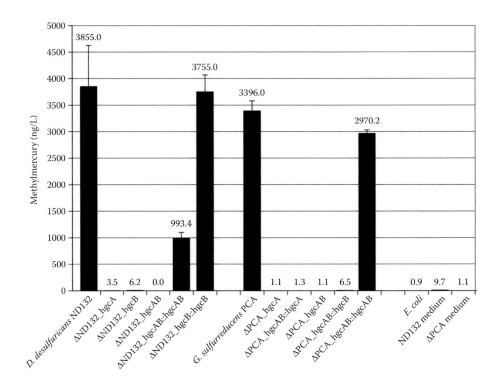

FIGURE 4.20 Production of methylmercury by *D. desulfuricans* ND132 and *G. sulfurreducens* PCA, by deletions of hgcA, hgcB, and hgcAB, and by complements in both bacteria. CH_3Hg^+ concentrations (ng/L) were determined after overnight incubations and measured by ICP-MS. The prefix Δ indicates a gene deletion; the symbol :: indicates complementation by chromosomal insertion. Values plotted are the average CH_3Hg^+ concentrations detected per strain from triplicate assays; error bars denote SD. Note that ΔPCA_hgcAB complemented with PCA_hgcA^+ or PCA_hgcB^+ is still deleted for PCA_hgcB or PCA_hgcA, respectively. (From Parks, J. M. et al. 2013. The genetic basis for bacterial mercury methylation. *Science* 339(6125):1332–1335. With Permission from AAAS.)

of CFeSP. This region corresponds to the cap helix of CFeSP, which is located near the lower axial face of the corrin ring.[573] In all HgcA sequences, a strictly conserved cysteine (Cys[93] in *D. desulfuricans* ND132) occupies the position corresponding to Thr[374] in CFeSP from *C. hydrogenoformans* Z-2901. Although Thr[374] is not considered a ligand for Co,[572,573] a cysteine might co-ordinate to Co, depending on its location relative to the cofactor and the Co oxidation state. Homology modeling and ultraviolet–visible spectra of the cocobalamin-binding domain of HgcaA suggest that Co–S co-ordination may be present in HgcA. Lower axial co-ordination of alkyl-cob(III) alamin by a biological thiolate has been proposed previously[582] but has never been observed for a corrinoid protein. The likely role of the ferredoxin-like protein HgcB is to accomplish the thermodynamically difficult reduction of Co(II) to Co(I) required for turnover, consistent with a previously suggested need for a ferredoxin as a reductant in Hg methylation.[554] The mechanistic details of methyl transfer, the integration of these two-gene products into carbon and energy metabolism, and their functioning with other potential as yet unidentified proteins remain to be determined.

In the absence of genome sequences for all Hg-methylating organisms, the generality of the present findings cannot yet be ascertained. However, their interpretation is in agreement with all currently available sequence information for methylating bacteria and archaea. The presence of the hgcAB cluster in the genomes of several sequenced, but so far untested, microorganisms leads them to hypothesize that these organisms are also capable of methylating mercury. The gene cluster appears to be quite sporadically distributed across two phyla of bacteria (Proteobacteria and

Firmicutes) and one phylum of archaea (Euryarchaeota). Organisms possessing the two-gene cluster include 24 strains of Deltaproteobacteria, 16 Clostridia, 1 Negativicutes, and 11 Methanomicrobia. Interestingly, they also found these genes in a psychrophile,[583] in a thermophile,[584] and in a human commensal methanogen.[585] The sporadic distribution of these genes and the lack of an obvious selective advantage related to mercury toxicity raise important questions regarding their physiological roles. Identification of these genes is a critical step linking specific microorganisms and environmental factors that influence microbial Hg methylation in aquatic ecosystems.

Gadolinium

Gadolinium is a trivalent lanthanide cation currently used as a magnetic resonance contrast medium, the gadobenate dimeglumine (Gd-bopta),[586] which blocks calcium channel stretch at high concentrations (10 μM).[587] However, concerns about contrast-induced nephropathy have been reported.[588]

In addition to acting as a calcium channel blocker, gadolinium, at low concentration, can interact with the signaling involved in intracellular and extracellular ATP hydrolysis.[589] Escalada et al.[590] reported that 3 μM gadolinium, a concentration that does not block calcium channels, has a potent inhibitory action on ectonucleoside triphosphate diphosphohydrolase (E-NTPDase) activity from the electric organ of *Torpedo marmorata*. Extracellular nucleotides are important molecules involved in the regulation of different biological processes, including vascular tone. When released as a neurotransmitter from the sympathetic terminals, ATP binds to P2X receptors of vascular smooth muscle cells, producing vasoconstriction. When binding to endothelial P2Y receptors, ATP leads to vasodilatation.[589,591] ATP exerts other effects on the vascular beds, such as control of smooth muscle and endothelial cell proliferation.[589,591] The action of extracellular nucleotides is terminated by the E-NTPDase family. NTPDase 1 is the major ectonucleotidase expressed in the vasculature[589,591] and its action limits platelet activation by ATP hydrolysis.[589,591] NTPDase 2 is another ectonucleotidase associated with the vasculature that preferentially converts ATP to ADP.[592] Following the action of E-NTPDases, ecto-5′-nucleotidase is responsible for the end of nucleotide signaling by converting AMP to adenosine.[593]

Gadolinium also affects ACE activity as a chelate by a transmetallation effect with zinc. This enzyme is a metallopeptidase containing zinc and therefore the possibility of a transmetallation effect is likely. *Angiotensin II* resulting from the action of ACE is the major effectors of the rennin–angiotensin system (RAS).[594] It activates the AT_1 receptor, has vasoconstriction and pressor effects, and also causes thrombosis, inflammation, and vascular and myocardial hypertrophy.[594]

Interestingly, despite these actions, gadolinium has not been defined as a toxic agent. There is no toxicological information and recommended exposure limits have not been defined.

Arsenic

Arsenic is a class I human carcinogen[595] to which ~150 million people worldwide, including 35 million in Bangladesh alone,[596] are chronically exposed through contaminated drinking water as is in more than 70 countries, including the United States, Mexico, Taiwan, Chili, Argentina, and India. In a previous survey of water As concentrations of all tube wells within their study region in Araihazar, Bangladesh,[597] 72% of the wells exceeded both the U.S. EPA[598] and the WHO[599] limits of 10 μg/L and 52% exceeded the Bangladesh standard of 50 μg/L. Chronic exposure to As has been associated with increased risk of several cancers, including lung, bladder, liver, and skin,[600] and deficits in intelligence in children.[601]

The TLV for arsenic and its compounds is 0.5 mg/m³.[64] Arsenic in higher doses has been known for centuries to cause death.

The primary health effects from the inhalation of the dust of arsenic trioxide and other inorganic arsenic compounds are irritation of the skin and injury to the mucous membranes. However, accumulation can occur with exposure to arsenical pesticides, the most common sources of arsenic today. It can also originate from chickens fed arsenic as a growth stimulator, wells, and treated wood. Also, ulcers and perforation of the nasal septum are not uncommon among arsenic workers. Arsenic has an affinity for keratin. Therefore, fingernails, hair, and skin will be affected by arsenic exposure. Arsenic in a water supply of a Mexican village was shown to cause arthritis and malaise in a large portion of the population. High levels of arsenic have been found in shellfish.

Arsenic being a class 1 human carcinogen causes hypertension associated with a variety of adverse health outcomes.[602–604] Chronic exposure to arsenic causes various types of skin lesions, including raindrop pigmentation, hyperpigmentation, hyperkeratosis, squamous cell carcinoma, basal cell carcinoma, and Bowen's disease.[602,605] Such dermal effects are hallmarks of the early stages of arsenic poisoning and are thought to be precursors of the arsenic-induced cancers.[606] Signs and symptoms are also found on other tissues of the body, including the tongue, gingival, and buccal mucosa.[607]

Toxic metals have profound effects on oral health. Melanocytes present in the basal cell layer of the oral mucosa are similar to those found in the skin.[608] Oral cancer is the sixth most common cancer worldwide after oral cavity lesions and continues to be a growing health concern.[609] The annual estimated incidence is around 275,000 for oral cancers, two-thirds of which occur in developing countries.[610] In particular, high levels of nickel and chromium were associated with oral cancer within the population in Taiwan,[611] thus competing with as a severe problem.

Similarly to these metals, arsenic can cause oral health problems. For example, arsenic is toxic to vital pulp, which can cause severe damage and osteomyelitis of the jaw.[612] In a recent study in Bangladesh, 75.5% of participants showed swelled vallate papillae as an indication of aresenicosis.[613] Exposure to arsenic may also manifest buccal mucous membrane melanosis.[614] Nevertheless, information about arsenic exposure and oral cavity lesions is very limited. To the best of our knowledge, no study to date has measured the relationship between arsenic exposure and oral cavity arsenical lesions and their associated factors, particularly of the gums, lips, and tongue, in Bangladesh or elsewhere at the population level. In this context, the Health Effects of Arsenic Longitudinal Study (HEALS) data represent a valuable opportunity for investigating the association between arsenic exposure and oral cavity arsenical lesions.

Therefore, in this study, Syed et al.[615] aimed to explore the relationship between arsenic exposure and oral cavity lesions among arsenic exposed people in Bangladesh. The information uncovered through this objective might be useful in developing appropriate strategies to support those affected in Bangladesh.

Out of 12,050 eligible participants, 11,746 were included in the HEALS baseline cohort. The response rate was 97.5%. Among 11,746 participants, 42.9% ($n = 5042$) were male and 57.5 ($n = 6704$) were female. The mean age of male participants was 41.6 (SD = 9.9) years and of female participants was 33.6 (SD = 8.8) years. The difference was statistically significant ($p < 0.001$). Table 4.1 shows the distribution of sociodemographic characteristics in relation to oral cavity lesions of the participants. The presence of arsenical lesions of the gums, lips, and tongue increased with age and was more common in men.

Findings from this study suggest that a higher level of uAs concentration is associated with a higher risk of arsenical lesions of the gums and tongue. To the best of our knowledge, this population-based study is the first study to examine the relationship between levels of uAs and oral cavity lesions. This result is supported by prior claims that high levels of toxic metals (nickel and chromium) have a detrimental impact on oral health.[611] In this study, Syed et al.[615] provided further direct evidence that arsenic concentration in urine has a stronger association with arsenicosis symptoms of the gums and tongue. These findings imply that contamination of drinking water with arsenic might also be a risk factor for arsenicosis of the gums and tongue.

A lesion related to arsenic exposure is an early signal of the subsequent development of cancers.[616] Moreover, several studies have highlighted that arsenic in drinking water is associated with cancers.[616–620] Exposure to toxic elements was implicated as a factor in the rapidly increasing rates of oral cancer in the population of Taiwan.[621] Thus, ecological studies have illustrated that high levels of nickel and chromium (toxic metals) in the soils are correlated with oral cancer incidence in Taiwan.[622,623] Thus, arsenic-exposed populations may develop oral cancers of the gums and tongue.

This study suggests that safe drinking water programs might have positive impacts on decreasing the rates of arsenical lesions of the gums and tongue.

In this study, women were less likely to develop arsenical lesions of the gums. This might be attributable to the higher arsenic methylation capabilities of women than men, which reduced their risk of developing arsenical lesions of the gums. This result is supported by several studies.[624,625] In addition, one previous study showed that women of child-bearing age had significantly higher arsenic methylation capacity compared with men.[626] They also found that manual workers (daily labor, farmer, factory workers, and other paid jobs) had fewer chances to develop arsenical lesions of the gums compared with those unemployed or homemakers. Most manual workers were men and about 94.0% (n = 6325) of female participants were homemakers. This result is supported by a previous study that showed men had higher prevalent rate of arsenicosis than women.[627] In this study, they observed that men tended to drink less water (mean 2875 mL) than women (mean 3095 mL). Men's lower tendency to drink water might be a contributing factor in their lower susceptibility to develop oral cavity lesions of the gums. A recent study reported that lifestyle characteristics of women are the most prevalent health concerns, as they were unknowingly harming their health through increased exposure to arsenic.[628] Therefore, further studies should incorporate health education sessions targeting those unemployed or homemakers and covering the health effects of arsenic exposure highlighted in their occupation in affected communities.

Consistent with a previous study,[627] Syed et al.[615] results found that age is associated with developing arsenical lesions of the tongue. It may be because older participants have lived in an arsenic-endemic area for a longer period of time. Nevertheless, with regard to health effects caused by arsenic poisoning, younger people may have a higher tolerant ability for arsenic exposure than older people.[627] This study suggests the benefits of a community-based awareness program for the age-specific arsenic-exposed population in Bangladesh.

In this study, Syed et al.[615] observed that smokers have greater chances to develop other pathologies of the gums, lips, and tongue. *Smoking* is one of the major lifestyle factors influencing human health and is also associated with poorer arsenic methylation capacity. It is also possible that some chemicals in cigarettes may play a significant role in the future development of oral cancer among arsenic-exposed populations. A recent hospital-based case–control study and a prospective follow-up study in Taiwan showed that smoking was associated with higher methylarsenic acid (MMA^V) percentage and lower dimethylarsenic acid (DMA^V) percentage in the noncancerous control participants.[629,630] One previous study also observed that cigarettes have a large number of chemical carcinogens, including arsenic, which can result in tissue-damaging effects in lips.[631] Since about one-third (29.0%) of male participants were smokers in this study, community-based health education might be a fruitful approach to the management of common human cancers within arsenic-exposed populations in Bangladesh.

Although a relationship has been studied between quid chewing and increased risk of arsenic-induced skin lesions,[632,633] this study showed no such association between betel leaf chewing and lesions of the gums, lips, and tongue. Recently, other studies also have found no association between betel leaf chewing and oral or oropharyngeal cancers.[634] This might be attributed to the reduced levels of carcinogenic substances added to certain products by tobacco manufacturing companies.[634] On the contrary, some people might not use lime or zarda, which might account for much of the associated risk for development of lesions of the oral cavity.

This study had three limitations. First, this study was limited by its cross-sectional analysis, which means that causality cannot be attributed. Nevertheless, the HEALS is a large-scale, methodologically rigorous epidemiological cohort study in a developing country setting where 60.0% of the participants were exposed to arsenic concentrations of 1–100 µg/L. This provides a unique opportunity to assess different ranges of arsenic exposure and the associated health effects. Second, this study only assessed arsenic concentration levels in the urine and oral cavity lesions of the participants. It is possible that some participants had other environmental exposures, which might affect the arsenical lesions of oral cavity. A previous study indicated that arsenic and nickel concentrations in farm soils are associated with oral cancer.[622] Third, there might have been possible errors during the diagnosis of arsenical lesions of oral cavity between the teams. Nevertheless, to minimize possible diagnostic errors, participants were diagnosed by trained study physicians for the presence of premalignant lesions following the same protocol.

Despite these limitations, this study had several strengths. First, it used data from a large population-based prospective study. The large sample size enabled adjustment for a large number of potential confounders and for a fully adjusted multivariate model. Second, although some participants were exposed to high levels of arsenic, most of the participants were exposed to relatively low levels of arsenic, making their results generalizable to a wide range of exposures. In addition, the measurement of total arsenic in urine was available for all participants. Therefore, findings of this study will add important information for the protection of arsenic-exposed people worldwide. Finally, the sociodemographic characteristics of Araihazar are similar to other rural areas of Bangladesh, which implies that inferences from these results may be extended to other regions of Bangladesh, where elevated arsenic concentrations in well water are a common phenomenon.

In conclusion, higher levels of arsenic exposure were positively associated with an increased risk of arsenical lesions of the gums and tongue.

Impact of Smoking and Chewing Tobacco on Arsenic-Induced Skin Lesions

Even moderately elevated concentrations of inorganic arsenic (InAs) in drinking water are of major public health concern worldwide.[635] In Bangladesh alone, more than 50 million inhabitants are drinking water that contains arsenic above the WHO guideline value of 10 μg/L.[636,637] In addition, there is increasing concern about arsenic exposure from food, especially rice products.[638] Chronic arsenic exposure is associated with an increased risk of cancer of the skin, lungs, bladder, liver, and possibly kidneys,[639] as well as a number of noncarcinogenic effects.[635,640,641] The earliest signs of toxicity from chronic exposure to InAs in humans are pigmentation changes and hyperkeratosis, which may proceed to skin cancer.[642] Unlike the arsenic-related cancers, which may appear first after two to three decades of exposure, these skin lesions may appear within a few years of exposure.[643,644]

A wide variation appears to exist in susceptibility to arsenic-induced toxicity. The best-documented risk-modifying factor for arsenic-related health effects is the metabolism of arsenic. InAs is methylated via one-carbon metabolism using arsenic (III) MeTr (AS34MT). The main metabolites excreted in urine are methylarsenic acid (MA) and dimethylarsenic acid (DMA), besides some unmethylated InAs, but major differences exist between individuals and population groups.[645] Numerous studies have demonstrated positive associations between the percentage of MA in urine and various cancers, chromosome aberrations, and oxidative stress.[646–658] Two recent studies[659,660] also reported increased risk for pigmentation changes and hyperkeratosis.

Another known risk-modifying factor is cigarette smoking. For quite some time, researchers have known that concurrent exposure to arsenic and smoking synergistically increases the risk of lung cancer,[661,662] and experimental studies showed that arsenic and cigarette smoke at environmentally relevant levels act synergistically to cause DNA damage.[663] Similarly, bladder cancer seemed to be significantly associated with arsenic exposure among smokers only.[664,665] Recently, an interaction between elevated arsenic exposure via drinking water and tobacco smoking was indicated also for the induction of skin lesions.[643]

It was recently reported that the well-documented less efficient methylation of arsenic in men, compared with women,[666] is the main reason for the observed higher prevalence of skin lesions in men.[660] Since smoking has been associated with less efficient arsenic methylation,[667,668] they evaluated potential interactions between smoking and arsenic metabolism for the risk of developing skin lesions.

This population-based case-referent study in Bangladesh is the first to evaluate the combined effects of arsenic exposure, arsenic metabolism, and use of tobacco for the risk of arsenic-related skin effects. All forms of tobacco use were associated with less efficient methylation of arsenic. Among men, there appeared to be an additive effect of poor arsenic methylation (high InAs and high %MA) and smoking for the development of arsenic-induced skin lesions, although a high %MA increased the risk more than smoking did. Since very few women smoked cigarettes or bidis, an interaction between arsenic methylation and smoking in women could not be evaluated. Another new finding in the present study was that tobacco chewing, which is much more common among Bangladeshi women than smoking, was also a risk factor for developing arsenic-related skin lesions in women. The high ORs for skin lesions among the women who chewed tobacco in the highest tertiles of %InAs or %MA (7.5 and 7.3, respectively) compared with nontobacco-using women with efficient arsenic methylation, suggest an interaction, although the RERI values were not quite significant. For men, an association between chewing tobacco and skin lesions was observed in the crude analysis only, but the sample size was small and the CIs wide. Further studies on larger cohorts are warranted for firm conclusions concerning the biologic interactions between various tobacco use, arsenic exposure, and arsenic metabolism. In any case, the use of various forms of tobacco should be considered in the risk assessment of arsenic and in the comparison of arsenic-related health risks among populations.

Arsenic Forecast for China

According to Michael, in China, pollution is pervasive and anthropogenic groundwater contamination has attracted attention.[669] Naturally occurring arsenic is perhaps less widespread, yet equally dangerous to those exposed. Though the problem has been known for decades[670] and mitigation is ongoing,[671] estimates of the exposed population differ widely.[672,673] Rodriguez-Lado et al.[674] assess the probability of the occurrence of unsafe arsenic levels in China's groundwater and identify at-risk areas where data are sparse. They suggest that more than 19 million Chinese may be drinking water above the WHO guideline of 10 µg/L. Such predictive models could guide action toward minimizing the impact of this widespread threat to human health.

More than two decades of research on groundwater arsenic that occurs naturally in aquifers has laid the foundation for predicting conditions in which arsenic concentrations are likely to be high. Two hydrogeologic settings that promote release of arsenic from sediments to the dissolved forms that contaminate and move with groundwater are shown to occur. In reducing environments under anoxic conditions, organic carbon drives chemical reactions that dissolve iron minerals on which arsenic is bound. This reductive dissolution often occurs in wet, flat regions and is the main mechanism producing high arsenic concentrations in the large river basins of South and Southeast Asia.[675,676] Arsenic release also occurs in toxic, high-pH water that promote desorption of arsenic from mineral oxides. This generally occurs in arid regions, for example, in Argentina, Spain, and the Southwest United States.[677] High arsenic concentrations resulting from both conditions occur in localized areas of China.[678,679]

Can arsenic-releasing environments be identified in areas where no testing has been done? Easily measurable characteristics of land surface that indicate conditions favoring release and buildup of high arsenic concentrations would be ideal predictors. However, identification of such proxies is challenging, because arsenic release is affected by complex, three-dimensional processes in the subsurface. Rodriguez-Lado et al.[674] meet this challenge by first identifying land surface characteristics that can indicate arsenic release and then using statistical analysis to determine which proxies have predictive power for aquifers in China. A combination of eight factors explains much of the variability in known arsenic concentrations and could therefore be used as a reliable set of indicators to predict the probability of arsenic occurrence in areas without data.

To estimate health risk, the authors combine the probability maps with population data. Although the estimated population affected may be high owing to mitigation efforts or model false positives, such estimates can be valuable tools for prioritizing action. In Bangladesh, where arsenic poisoning is perhaps most acute, a random survey to establish nationwide trends in arsenic concentration, completed in 2000,[675] provided a foundation for impact estimates and more targeted studies. China is 67 times the size of Bangladesh, with 9 times the population, but arsenic occurrence is likely much less pervasive. Nationwide monitoring activities are under way,[669,673] but risk maps could guide more targeted screening. Risk maps may also prompt private well-testing initiatives[680] or public pressure mitigation in affected areas.

Recognition of the extent of the problem is, however, only the first step toward relief of health impacts. Arsenic concentrations can vary widely on the scale of tens of meters. These small-scale patterns cannot be predicted from surface features that vary on the scale of kilometers. This variability is the result of a complex set of hydrological, geological, and biogeochemical factors that affect release of arsenic from sediments and the movement of dissolved arsenic through aquifers. Understanding this complexity, along with social and economic factors is critical for identifying appropriate mitigation options. In Bangladesh, despite decades of hydrogenochemical investigations and screening of about half of the existing wells,[681] tens of millions of people continue to be exposed,[682] illustrating the challenges in moving from identification to mitigation.

Many arsenic-affected basins, deltas, and floodplains are among the most populated in the world; humans have fundamentally changed these landscapes and altered their hydrology. Understanding the anthropogenic factors that affect natural hydrological and biogeochemical processes will be critical in predicting where arsenic and other problems exist, determining how they will evolve in the future, and implementing effective mitigation strategies to improve the health and livelihood of millions of people worldwide.

Arsenic Exposure and Hypertension: A Systematic Review

In this systematic review, Abhyankar et al.[683] identified an association between arsenic and the prevalence of hypertension. Interpreting a causal effect of environmental arsenic on hypertension is limited by the small number of studies, the presence of influential studies, and the absence of prospective evidence.[683]

Hypertension is a major risk factor for mortality and morbidity worldwide.[684–687] Risk factors for hypertension include high salt intake, increased body mass index (BMI), genetic predisposition, and exposure to psychosocial stress.[686,687] Additional evidence, however, suggests that environmental factors play a role in hypertension development.[686,688–693] The identification and mitigation of environmental exposures related to hypertension could contribute to reducing the worldwide burden of hypertension-related disease.

According to Abhyankar et al.,[683] among environmental exposures, epidemiologic and experimental evidence supports the possibility that arsenic plays a role in hypertension and other cardiometabolic diseases.[694–700] Arsenic-contaminated drinking water represents a major public health problem internationally.[701–706] The WHO and U.S. EPA standard for arsenic levels in drinking water is 10 μg/L.[687,698] In the United States alone, millions of persons are exposed to arsenic concentrations >10 μg/L (as shown in Chapter 3, Volume 5), whereas persons in Bangladesh, China, India, Cambodia, Ghana, Argentina, Mexico, and other countries around the world are exposed to arsenic levels in drinking water that are well beyond 10 μg/L.[696,698] Epidemiologic studies conducted in arsenic-endemic areas in Taiwan and Bangladesh have found a positive relationship between inorganic arsenic exposure from drinking water and hypertension.[702,706] Experimental studies have indicated that arsenic exposure may be involved in the development of hypertension through the promotion of inflammation, oxidative stress, and endothelial dysfunction.[697,698,707–709]

To evaluate the potential relationship between arsenic and hypertension, Abhyankar et al.[683] conducted a systematic review of epidemiologic studies that have investigated the association between inorganic arsenic exposure (using environmental measures or biomarkers) and hypertension outcomes (using hypertension status and systolic and diastolic blood pressure [SBP and DBP, respectively]). A total of 138 studies were not in English. Chen et al.[710] and Jones et al.[711] were the only studies including both hypertension and BP level end points.

Epidemiologic studies with data on arsenic exposure and hypertension outcomes were included. They excluded nonoriginal reports, experimental studies, case reports and case series, and studies without measures of arsenic exposure or hypertension end points. They also excluded one study that used hypertension mortality as the only end point[712] and two reports[713,714] that used the same study population as another included study.[702]

Study characteristics: Eleven studies, published between 1995 and 2011, were identified. All studies meeting the inclusion criteria were cross-sectional and published in English. Combined, the studies covered arsenic exposure and hypertension outcomes for >20,000 individuals. Eight studies were conducted at moderate to high levels of exposure (average levels in drinking water ≥50 µg/L or occupational studies),[702,706,710,715–719] and three studies were conducted at low levels of exposure (average levels in drinking water <50 µg/L).[699,711,720] Ten studies were conducted in general populations (two from Taiwan, two from Bangladesh, two from Inner Mongolia, two from the United States, one from Turkey, and one from Iran).[699,702,706,710,711,715,716,718–720] One study was conducted in an occupational setting in Denmark.[717] Five studies measured arsenic concentrations in drinking water,[702,706,710,718,720] three compared areas of high and low arsenic concentrations in drinking water,[715,716,719] two studies used biomarkers (hair, Wang et al.[699]; urine, Jones et al.[711]), and one study assigned arsenic exposure based on job title.[717] Eight studies assessed hypertension as the end point of interest,[699,702,706,710,711,716,719,720] five studies reported differences in mean SBP,[710,711,715,717,718] and four studies reported differences in mean DBP.[710,711,715,718]

Epidemiological Studies of Arsenic Exposure and Blood Pressure End Points

Five studies measure arsenic in drinking water at the individual level[699,710,711,718,719]; three of these studies measured individual arsenic exposure based on measured well water concentrations,[710,718,719] and two studies used a biomarker of exposure.[699,711] Five studies defined hypertension based on established cutoffs for SBP and DBP levels measured with a standardized protocol and self-reported physician diagnosis or antihypertensive treatment.[699,702,706,710,711] Five of the 11 studies did not adjust for potential confounders.[699,715–717,719] Other studies adjusted at least for age, sex, and BMI.

Criteria for Evaluation of Design and Data Analysis of Epidemiological Studies on Arsenic and Hypertension

ORs estimates for hypertension: For the association of hypertension with arsenic exposure, five of the eight studies found a positive association.[699,702,706,716,720] Among the studies that assessed hypertension at moderate to high levels of exposure, the OR estimates comparing highest with lowest arsenic exposure groups ranged from 0.71 (95% CI: 0.18, 2.63) in a small study in Turkey[719] to 16.5 (95% CI: 2.8, 668.5) in a study in Inner Mongolia.[716] Two studies from Bangladesh provided inconsistent results: an OR of 3.0 (95% CI: 1.5, 5.8) in the study by Rahman et al.[706] and OR of 1.02 (95% CI: 0.84, 1.23) in the study by Chen et al.[710] Among the studies that assessed hypertension at low levels of exposure, the OR estimates comparing highest with lowest arsenic exposure groups ranged from 1.17 (95% CI: 0.75, 1.83) in a study in the general U.S. population[711] to 2.00 (95% CI: 1.21, 3.31) in a study in central Taiwan.[699]

ORs of hypertension by arsenic exposure levels: The area of each square is proportional to the inverse of the variance of the estimated log OR. Horizontal lines represent 95% CIs. In the Chen et al.[710] study, arsenic concentrations ($\sum C_i T_i / \sum T_i$, where "C_i and T_i denote the well arsenic concentration and drinking duration for the well").

The pooled OR of hypertension comparing the highest and lowest arsenic exposure categories in eight studies with available information on hypertension was 1.27 (95% CI: 1.09, 1.47; *p*-value for heterogeneity = 0.001; I^2 = 70.2%). The corresponding pooled OR in five studies with moderate to high arsenic exposure was 1.15 (95% CI: 0.96, 1.37; *p*-value for heterogeneity = 0.002; I^2 = 46.6%). The pooled OR comparing the highest and lowest arsenic exposure categories in the three studies with low arsenic exposure was 1.56 (95% CI 1.21, 2.01; *p*-value for heterogeneity = 0.27; I^2 = 24.6%). They also restricted the overall pooled analysis to studies with multivariable adjust ORs (pooled OR = 1.22; 95% CI: 1.04, 1.42),[702,706,710,711,720] studies with a standard hypertension definition (pooled OR = 1.21; 95% CI: 1.03, 1.42),[702,706,710,711] and studies with individual assessment of arsenic exposure (pooled OR = 1.19; 95% CI: 1.02, 1.38).[699,710,711,720] Funnel plots did not suggest the presence of publication or related biases (data not shown).

They evaluated the dose response or six studies with ORs reported for three or more categories.[699,702,706,710,711,720] Among them, the Chen et al.[710] study in Bangladesh showed no dose–response relationship. Compared with the baseline category, the other study from Bangladesh[706] and the study from Taiwan[702] showed increased prevalence of hypertension for most of the arsenic exposure categories. Studies conducted at low levels of exposure in drinking water[699,711,720] showed an increased prevalence of hypertension throughout the range of arsenic exposure levels, although the association was not statistically significant for the intermediate arsenic categories.

This systematic review identified an association between arsenic exposure and the prevalence of hypertension. The association was present both in studies conducted in areas with moderate-to-high arsenic exposure levels and in studies conducted in areas with low exposure levels. A clear dose response was observed in several studies, and experimental evidence supports the hypertensive effects of arsenic. The interpretation of this association regarding the causal effect of arsenic on hypertension, however, is limited by the small number of studies, the heterogeneity across studies, and the absence of prospective evidence. In addition, some studies were affected by additional methodological limitations, such as the lack of standard hypertension definitions, individual assessment of arsenic exposure, or appropriate adjustment for relevant confounders. The evidence is particularly scarce for low levels of exposure and for evaluating the association with SBP and DBP levels as continuous outcomes. Overall, the evidence is suggestive but insufficient to infer a causal relationship between environmental arsenic exposure and hypertension.

Two studies from areas with high arsenic levels in drinking water in Southwestern Taiwan[702] and Bangladesh[706] and two studies conducted in areas with low levels of arsenic in drinking water in Wisconsin[720] and Central Taiwan[699] showed consistent associations of arsenic exposure with the prevalence of hypertension with increasing arsenic exposure.

Discrepancies in the association between arsenic and the prevalence of hypertension were observed in four studies.[710,715,716,719] The study with the strongest association (OR = 16.54[716]) and the study with inverse association (OR = 0.71[719]) had small numbers of cases, provided no definition of hypertension, and incorporated no adjustment for relevant confounders. Both studies were highly imprecise with large CIs. The two null studies were large high-quality studies conducted in Bangladesh and the United States.[710,711] The study in Bangladesh found no dose–response relationship, despite assessing arsenic at the individual level and defining hypertension based on BP measures.[710] However, this study did find an association between arsenic levels in drinking water with systolic hypertension and pulse pressure levels among participants with low folate and vitamin intake levels,[710] whereas subgroup analyses by folate and vitamin B concentrations were conducted in the study in the general U.S. population, with no differences.[711] In the study conducted among the general U.S. population, the association between arsenic exposure and hypertension was not statistically significant, and it was consistent with no association.[711] However, the magnitude of the association was compatible with a small increased prevalence of hypertension and consistent with the dose–response trend observed in other studies conducted at low-to-moderate exposure levels in Wisconsin and Central Taiwan.[699,711,720]

The potential association between exposure to inorganic arsenic and the development of hypertension is supported by experimental and mechanistic evidence, especially at high exposure levels. Arsenic promotes inflammation activity, oxidative stress, and endothelial dysfunction through several mechanisms including the activation of stress response transcription factors such as activator protein-1 and nuclear factor-κB.[710,721–724] *In vitro*, arsenite altered vascular tone in blood vessels by suppressing vasorelaxation[709] and increased the expression of COX-2 in endothelial cells.[721,725] In animal models, arsenite increased superoxide accumulation and impaired nitric oxide formation in endothelial cells.[726–728] Finally, the hypertensive effects of arsenic could be related to the possible chronic kidney effects of arsenic.[694,729] Additional experimental studies using arsenic exposure levels relevant to human populations are needed to characterize the etiopathogenesis of potential hypertensive effects of arsenic.

This is the first systematic review and meta-analysis evaluating the relationship between arsenic exposure and hypertension end points. Abhyankar et al.[683] identified a positive association between elevated arsenic exposure and the prevalence of hypertension, but the implications of this association from a causal perspective are unclear because of the limited number of studies as well as the studies' cross-sectional design, and methodological limitations. Prospective cohort studies in populations exposed to a wide range of arsenic exposure levels, from low through moderate-to-high levels of exposure, are needed to better characterize the relationship between arsenic and hypertension. Because of the widespread exposure to arsenic worldwide and the high burden of disease caused by hypertension, it is important that high-quality prospective studies are conducted with individual-level assessment of arsenic exposure and standardized measurements of BP. The studies should evaluate the shape of the dose response and whether the magnitude of the association is different in susceptible populations, including populations with nutritional deficiencies. If the hypertensive effects of arsenic are confirmed, they could partly explain the association between arsenic and cardiovascular disease.[695–700,730] Given the widespread arsenic exposure through drinking water and food, even a modest effect of arsenic on hypertension could have a substantial impact on morbidity and mortality.[718,731]

Relationship of Creatinine and Nutrition with Arsenic Metabolism

Basi et al.[732] reported the associations of both dietary and blood nutrient measures, as well as urinary creatinine (uCr), with arsenic (As) methylation capacity, as assessed by the proportions of urinary inorganic, monomethyl, and dimethyl As metabolites. One finding was that uCr was the strongest predictor of As methylation; participants with higher uCr concentrations had a higher percentage of total urinary As as dimethylarsenic acid (DMA) compared with those with lower uCR. This is consistent with what we have previously reported in Bangladeshi adults and children,[659,733,734] and is an interesting and potentially very important observation. Approximately 40% of S-adenosylmethionine (SAM)-derived methyl groups are devoted to the biosynthesis of creatine, the precursor of creatinine.[735,736] At high levels of As exposure (500–1000 µg/L), based on one-carbon kinetics,[737] Gamble and Hall[737] estimated that methylation of 80% of a daily dose of inorganic As (InAs) to DMA would require ~50 µmol SAM, thus consuming ca. 2%–4% of the SAM normally turning over in a well-nourished adult per day. Low dietary creatine intake associated with low-protein or vegetarian diets places an increased demand for SAM for creatine biosynthesis.[735] This could potentially reduce the availability of SAM for As methylation, providing a plausible mechanism underlying this highly reproducible observation. This assumes that uCr reflects, to some extent, dietary creatine intake, as we have observed (Gamble,[737] unpublished data). Conversely, dietary creatine intake and/or creatine supplementation downregulates endogenous creatine biosynthesis, potentially sparing SAM for methylation of other substrates such as As. Gamble and Hall[737] are currently testing this hypothesis in a randomized controlled trial of creatine supplementation. In addition, as Basu et al.[732] noted, and as they have previously reported,[738] one implication of the observed association between uCr and As methylation capacity is that urinary As should not be expressed per gram creatine to correct for urine concentration. Rather, uCr should be included as a covariate in regression models.

One concerning aspect of the study by Basu et al.[732] is the handling of blood samples used for nutrient measurements. As noted by Basu et al.[732] and in a previous publication on these same participants,[739] the blood samples were stored in an ice chest in the field for up to 24 hours before processing. This 24-hour delay can be problematic for some nutrients, especially folate, which is extremely sensitive to oxidative degradation.[740] Basu et al.[732] reported that in univariate analyses, they observed higher urinary percentages of InAs in individuals with higher serum folate concentrations. This finding is contrary to our previous findings that folate facilitates As methylation.[733,734,741–743] This discrepancy might be explained by differences in sample processing.

Basu et al.[732] also reported associations between dietary intake of several nutrients (assessed using a modified 24-hour recall) and As methylation capacity. One of the most critical and widely discussed issues in nutritional epidemiology is the method used to adjust for total energy intake (TEI).[744] The main reasons to adjust for TEI are to (1) adjust for potential confounding by TEI, (2) remove extraneous variation in nutrient intakes that is due only to their correlation with TEI, and (3) simulate a dietary intervention. What is often most relevant is diet composition or nutrient intake in relation to

TEI.[744] Several methods are available to adjust for TEI, and the best approach can vary depending on the nutrient and question of interest. Basu et al.[732] adjusted for TEI by dividing each nutrient intake by TEI (nutrient density method). While this approach is appealing because of its simplicity, in reality, it can create a complex variable.[745] For example, when TEI is related to the outcome of interest, the use of nutrient densities can actually induce confounding in the opposite direction. Although we cannot determine from Basu et al.'s[732] article whether TEI measured by the 24-hour recall was associated with As methylation, in theory, an association seems plausible. Also, because their statistical analysis tested for associations between multiple nutrients and urinary As metabolizes, it is best to acknowledge that some of the statistically significant associations might be due to chance alone.

Relationship of Creatinine and Nutrition with Arsenic Metabolism: Smith et al. Respond

In their article,[732] they cited their earlier results concerning urinary dimethylarsenic acid (DMA) and creatinine concentrations, noting that in 2005, they reported a strong correlation between uCr and the percentage of DMA (DMA%).[733] Smith et al.[746] noted rather similar findings from another group working in Bangladesh,[747] so together with their findings in India, there are three separate studies that have reported this association.[732,733,747] Their results highlight the strength of the relationship between uCr and urinary DMA% which was stronger than the relationship between DMA% and any of the 19 dietary factors and 16 blood micronutrients that we investigated.

Creatinine, Diet, Micronutrients, and Arsenic Methylation in West Bengal, India

Ingested inorganic arsenic (InAs) is methylated to monomethylated (MMA) and dimethylated metabolites (DMA). Methylation may have an important role in arsenic toxicity, because the monomethylated trivalent metabolite (MMA[III]) is highly toxic.

Basu et al.[732] assessed the relationship of creatinine and nutrition-using dietary intake and blood concentrations of micronutrients with arsenic metabolism, as reflected in the proportions of InAS, MMA, and DMA in urine, in the first study that incorporated both dietary and micronutrient data.

They studied methylation patterns and nutritional factors in 405 persons who were selected from a cross-sectional survey of 7638 people in an arsenic-exposed population in West Bengal, India. They assessed associations of urine creatinine and nutritional factors (19 dietary intake variables and 16 blood micronutrients) with arsenic metabolites in urine (Tables 4.25 and 4.26).

uCr had the strongest relationship with overall arsenic methylation to DMA. Those with the highest uCr concentrations had 7.2% more arsenic as DMA compared with those with low creatinine ($p < 0.001$). Animal fat intake had the strongest relationship with MMA% (highest tertile animal fat intake had 2.3% more arsenic as MA, $p < 0.001$). Low serum selenium and low folage were also associated with increased MMA%.

Urine creatinine concentration was the strongest biological marker of arsenic methylation efficiency, and therefore should not be used to adjust for urine concentration in arsenic studies. The new finding that animal fat intake has a positive relationship with MMA% warrants further assessment in other studies. Increased MMA% was also associated, to a lesser extent, with low serum selenium and folate.

Diet and arsenic methylation, and blood micronutrients and arsenic methylation, have previously been assessed separately.[734,748–751] This is the first comprehensive study of arsenic methylation including both dietary and micronutrient variables, along with uCr, considered together in the same analysis. New findings to emerge from this work include the fact that uCr was the strongest predictor of DMA% with a high uCr being associated with more InAs being fully methylated to DMA. Once uCr was taken into account, no nutritional factor was a significant predictor of DMA%. A high uCr was associated in the opposite direction with InAs%, which had a lower percentage in urine when creatinine was high. This association for InAs% decreased when lycopene and riboflavin were included in the model, with lycopene becoming the strongest predictor variable in that a high lycopene concentration was associated with a low InAs%. One previous study suggested that low plasma lycopene was associated with reduced arsenic methylation capacity.[729] However, we find that full methylation to DMA was more strongly related to uCr than to lycopene.

TABLE 4.25

Results of Toxin Removal Prototype (Values Expressed in μg/g of Creatinine)

	Arsenic	Cadmium	Lead	Mercury
		Subject A		
Baseline	5.8	0	0.8	0
Day 42	6.	0.3	2.5	0
Day 57	4.3	0.2	2.4	2.2
Day 64	5.2	0.3	0.5	1
Day 69	26	0.7	1.3	0.8
Day 77	12	0.2	0	1.1
Day 82	7.1	0	0	0.8
Day 110	7.1	0	0	0.8
Day 118	5.7	0	0	2.4
		Subject B		
Baseline	9.9	0.5	1.8	0
Day 20	17	0.7	0	13
Day 42	74	0.4	1.6	0
Day 57	14	0.7	1.4	1
Day 64	30	0.8	1.2	1.1
Day 69	13	0.6	1.4	0.9
Day 82	15	0.5	0	2.5
Day 110	48	0.4	3.1	0
Day 118	35	0.4	0	0.9
		Subject C		
Baseline	11	0	1.3	0.4
Day 42	5.2	0	2.8	1.7
Day 57	6.9	0.6	0	1.4
Day 64	9.1	0	1.8	1.8
Day 77	130	0.2	2	0
Day 82	11	0.3	0	0.4
Day 110	37	0	2.4	0
Day 118	17	0.2	0	0

The relationship between creatinine and arsenic methylation has been reported previously as an aside, without noting that it is the most important predictor nor being able to compare it with multiple nutritional factors as they have done here. In the past, uCr has usually been used to normalize for urine concentration, to compensate for variation in diuresis. However, problems with doing so have been identified,[752] in particular for studies of arsenic.[747,753] Gamble et al. reported a strong correlation between uCr and DMA% ($p < 0.001$),[733] and Nermell et al.[747] noted that uCr was correlated mainly with DMA. One recent study found that low uCr was associated with arsenic-induced skin lesions.[633] It is noteworthy that the formation of creatinine from methylation of guanidinoacetate accounts for ~75% of all folate-dependent transmethylation reaction.[736,752]

Another new finding was that animal fat in the diet was by far the strongest predictor of MMA%, with a high intake of animal fat being associated with a high MMA%. Some investigators have thought that a high MMA% would be due to an increase in the first step of methylation from InAs to MMA. However, because 85% of InAs, on average, is methylated, at least to MMA, and the large majority ends up as DMA, increases in MMA% are more likely due to a reduction in the second step of methylation from MMA to DMA. They do not know why a high intake of animal fat would reduce the second step of methylation from MMA to DMA. One possibility is

TABLE 4.26
Results of DMSA Challenge (Values Expressed in μg/g of Creatinine)

	Arsenic	Cadmium	Lead	Mercury
Subject A	8.1	<dL	9.3	1.6
Subject B	14	0.5	20	2.1
Subject C	11	<dL	8.8	4.7

that animal fat intake is related to some unknown confounding factor. The only published study that could find that mentioned fat intake and methylation was a study of 66 adults who were kept on a fixed diet.[753] The investigators reported that during the experimental period of the study, when dietary fat intake was higher than during the usual diet, blood SAM levels were inversely correlated with fat intake. The positive association between dietary animal fat and MMA% is a new finding not reported elsewhere. In a study on dietary intake and arsenic methylation based on a U.S. population ($n = 30$), Steinmaus et al.[751] did not find any relationship between fat intake and MMA% in urine. A possible reason why these findings were different from the U.S. study could be attributed to the different levels and patterns of nutrition between a U.S. population and this rural Indian population.

The inverse association between serum folate and selenium and MMA% is supported by findings from other epidemiological studies. Using data from a cross-sectional survey in a comparable Bangladeshi population ($n = 300$), Gamble et al.[733] reported that serum folate was inversely associated with InAs% (Spearman $r = -0.12$; $p < 0.05$) and MMA% ($r = -0.12$; $p = 0.04$) and was positively associated with serum homocysteine ($r = 0.21$; $p < 0.05$) and urinary DMA% ($r = 0.21$; $p < 0.001$).[733] Gamble and colleagues reported univariate correlation estimates of associations and did not report results of multivariate associations after adjustment of possible confounding variables. On the same population, Gamble et al.[733] conducted a follow-up double-blind randomized controlled trial ($n = 200$) that compared 12-week administrations of folate versus placebo and found that after 12 weeks of folic acid supplementation, the increase in the proportion of total uAs excreted as DMA in the folate group (72% at baseline and 79% after supplementation; $p < 0.0001$) was greater than that in the placebo group, as was the reduction in the proportions of total uAs excreted as MMA (13% and 10% respectively; $p < 0.0001$) and as InAs (15% and 11% respectively; $p < 0.001$). However, in this study, the intervention group and the placebo group were exposed to arsenic during the time of the trial.[741] Since this study was conducted among individuals concomitantly exposed to high concentrations of InAs, it cannot be inferred that folate supplementation would benefit individuals who were not longer exposed to arsenic in drinking water.

Studies have consistently reported higher MMA% in males than in females.[606] In the univariate comparison, the difference in MMA% between men and women was 1.9. This difference was not much less than for animal fat. The difference between males and females may be explained in part by differences in animal fat intake and by differences in uCr.

Associations that might have been expected but were largely absent include homocysteine, vitamin B_{12} (cobalamin), and methionine. Homocysteine was strongly related to MMA% in univariate analysis, but the association became weaker in multivariate modeling when folate was added. Heck et al.[748] reported a relationship between cobalamin and increased MMA to InAs ratio, but the authors found no evidence of it in this study (MMA% for the lowest tertile of vitamin $B_{12} = 8.0$ and for the highest tertile MMA% = 8.1; $p = 0.75$).

Data for this study came from a cross-sectional survey. Information on the dietary variables was collected at the same time as blood was sampled for estimation of serum micronutrients, and urine was collected for estimation of urinary InAs%, MMA%, and DMA%. This provides a snapshot of interrelationships between diet, micronutrients, and arsenic methylation variables.

Usually, the main limitation of cross-sectional studies pertains to inferring long-term outcomes from data obtained at 1 pint in time. However, this limitation does not apply here, because it is reasonable to believe that arsenic methylation patterns would relate to current nutritional factors. In addition, it has been found that arsenic methylation efficiency in individuals is relatively stable over time.[754] Another limitation is that because we did not have measures of urinary specific gravity, it was not possible to adjust for urine concentration. The authors' findings and those of others indicate that one should not use uCr to adjust for urine concentration in studies of arsenic, especially those involving speciation. However, it should be noted that the parameters of interest in this study were InAs%, MMA%, and DMA%. The proportion of arsenic in these various forms is unlikely to be related to urine concentration, even though the concentrations in absolute terms would be similar.

This study revealed that uCr in the highest versus lowest tertile had a stronger association with arsenic methylation to DMA than did similar contrasts for any of the dietary or micronutrient factors assessed. This finding provides further evidence that uCr should not be used to adjust urine concentrations for diuresis effects. Further studies are needed to investigate the determinants of urine creatinine concentrations in arsenic-exposed populations, because such factors are also likely to influence arsenic methylation. The new findings that plasma lycopene had an inverse relationship with InAs% and that animal fat intake had a positive relationship with MMA% are new and warrant further assessment in other studies.

Folate, Cobalamin, Cysteine, Homocysteine, and Arsenic Metabolism among Children in Bangladesh

According to Hall et al.,[734] $\sim$35 million people in Bangladesh are chronically exposed to inorganic arsenic (InAs) in drinking water. Methylation of InAs to monomethylarsenic (MMA) and dimethylarsenic acids (DMA) relies on folate-dependent one-carbon metabolism and facilitates uAs elimination.

They examined the relationships between folate, cobalamin, cysteine, total homocysteine (tHcys), and uAs metabolites in a sample of 6-year-old Bangladeshi children ($n = 165$).

Children provided blood sample for measurement of tHcys, folate, cobalamin, and cysteine, and urine specimens for the measurement of total uAs and As metabolites.

Consistent with their studies in adults, mean tHcys concentrations (7.9 μmol/L) were higher than those reported among children of similar ages in other populations. Nineteen percent of the children has plasma folate concentrations <9.0 nmol/L. The proportion of total uAs excreted as InAs was inversely correlated with folate ($r = -0.20$, $p = 0.01$) and cysteine ($r = -0.23$, $p = 0.003$), whereas the correlations between %DMA and both folate ($r = 0.12$, $p = 0.14$) and cysteine ($r = 0.11$, $p = 0.15$) were positive. Homocysteine was inversely correlated ($r = -0.27$, $p = 0.009$) with % MMA in males, and the correlation with %DMA was positive ($r = 0.13$, $p = 0.10$).

These findings suggest that similar to adults, folate and cysteine facilitate As methylation in children. However, the inverse correlation between tHcys and %MMA and positive correlation with %DMA are both opposite to our previous findings in adults. They propose that upregulation of one-carbon metabolism, presumably necessary to meet the considerable demands for DNA and protein biosynthesis during periods of rapid growth, results in both increased tHcys biosynthesis and increased As methylation.

As is metabolized in humans via reduction and methylation reactions with SAM serving as the methyl donor.[755] Methylation of inorganic As (InAs) to monomethylarsenic (MMA) and dimethylarsenic acids (DMA) occurs enzymatically via one-carbon metabolism and facilitates uAs elimination.[756] Methylation of As has generally been considered a detoxification pathway; studies show that a higher proportion of DMA in urine is associated with decreased risk of skin lesions,[659] skin,[646] and bladder cancers,[652,757] and peripheral vascular disease.[758] There is, however, accumulating evidence that the trivalent methylated As intermediate, MMA[III], may be the most toxic As species.[699,759]

Individuals show substantial variation in As methylation capacity, which may be partly attributable to availability of vitamins required for one-carbon metabolism (folate, vitamin B_{12} [cobalamin], and vitamin B_6) as well as intake of nutrients that are not required per se but contribute to the availability of methyl groups, such as protein, betaine, and choline. In animal models, folate deficiency decreases uAs excretion,[760] and dietary methyl donor deficiency increases As retention in tissues.[756] In Bangladeshi adults, plasma folate was inversely associated with %MMA and positively associated with %DMA in urine.[733] Further, in our randomized controlled trial, folic acid supplementation to folate-deficient adults was associated with increased %DMA in urine[741] and a statistically significant 14% reduction in total blood As,[742] primarily due to a decline in blood MMA. These findings emphasize the importance of adequate folate for the synthesis and relatively rapid elimination of As as DMA.

Hall et al.[734] have also previously observed that uCr—an analyte traditionally used to adjust for hydration status (and a catabolite of creating)—is a strong predictor of As methylation[659,733,738,741,743] and that participants with lower uCr are at increased risk for As-induced skin lesions.[633] uCr is influenced by dietary intake of creatine (derived from meat), which downregulates endogenous creatine biosynthesis. Because creatine biosynthesis is the major consumer of methyl groups,[736,762] downregulation by dietary sources may lower total homocysteine (tHcys)[763–765] and thereby increase the pool of methyl groups for methylation of As and other substrates.

Few studies have examined As methylation in children. Concha et al.[766] reported higher %InAs and lower %DMA in urine among children in Northern Argentina compared with women suggesting that children may have reduced capacity to methylate As. However, Chowdhury et al.[767] reported that children in Bangladesh had lower %InAs and %MMA and higher %DMA than adults. Both work in Bangladeshi children[601] and the results of a recent study conducted in China are not supportive of the finding by Concha et al.[766] For example, Sun and colleagues[268] reported that children had lower %MMA and higher %DMA in urine than adults when exposed to the same concentration of As in drinking water. Meza et al.[768] reported that three single-nucleotide polymorphisms in the AS3MT gene were associated with increased As methylation in children but not in adults.[768] Together, these studies suggest that children have a greater capacity to methylate As than adults.

To the best of our knowledge, there are no published reports pertaining to nutritional influences on As metabolism in children. Given that childhood may represent a critical period for exposure to As with regard to risk for long-term adverse health outcomes,[769–771] it is important to identify potentially modifiable risk factors that may favorably influence As metabolism and elimination. In this study, they examined the prevalence of folate deficiency and hyperhomocysteinemia and the relationships between folate, cobalamin, cysteine, tHcys, and As metabolism in 6-year-old Bangladeshi children.

Overview

This work is part of the Nutritional Influences on Arsenic Toxicity (NIAT) study[733,741,761] in collaboration with a larger, multidisciplinary program (The Columbia University Superfund Basic Research Program [CU-SBRP]). The main health project within the CU-SBRP is the HEALS,[772] a prospective cohort study of >12,000 married men and women living in Araihazar, Bangladesh, who are followed up at 2-year intervals. The study region and recruitment of HEALS participants have been previously described.[772] Araihazar was chosen because it has a wide range of As concentrations in drinking water and is within a reasonable commuting distance from Dhaka.

Study Participants and Procedure

Hall et al.[734] identified a sample of 6-year-old children of HEALS participants who were available at the time of a preliminary home visit and were willing to provide biological samples. The current study sample is a subset of 165 of 301 children selected at random for their previous study of water As exposure and intellectual function who were willing to provide both blood and urine samples.[770] This subset of 165 children did not differ from the 136 who gave only a urine sample with regard to total uAs or %uAs metabolites. However, the 136 children who did not give blood samples weighed

0.5 kg less, were 1.5 cm shorter, had head circumferences that were 0.3 cm smaller, and had higher water As (131 vs. 111 µg/L, respectively) than those who did donate blood.

Measurements of Plasma Nutrients

They analyzed plasma folate and cobalamin by radioimmunoassay (Quantaphase II; Bio-Rad Laboratories, Richmond, California) as previously described.[733,773] The within-day coefficient of variation (CV) was 3% for folate and 4% for cobalamin. The between-day CV was 5% for folate and 11% for cobalamin. They used high-performance liquid chromatography (HPLC) with fluorescence detection[774] to measure plasma tHcys and cysteine concentrations as described previously.[733] The within-day and between-day CVs were 3% and 6% for tHcys and 5% and 8% for cysteine, respectively.

Well Water As

Hall et al.[734] analyzed well water samples for total As by graphite furnace atomic absorption (GFAA) with a detection limit of 5 µg/L. Samples found to have a concentration <5 µg/L were reanalyzed by inductively coupled plasma mass spectrometry (ICP-MS) for which the detection limit is 0.1 µg/L.[775]

Total uAs and Creatinine

Total uAs was measured in the Columbia University Trace Metals Core Laboratory. Intraclass correlation coefficients between the laboratory's values and samples calibrated at the Quebec Laboratory were 0.99. uCr concentrations were analyzed using a method based on the Jaffe reaction.[776]

uAs metabolites

As metabolites were speciated using HPLC separation of arsenobetaine (AsB), arsenocholine (AsC), arsenate ($InAs^V$), arsenite ($InAs^{III}$), MMA, and DMA followed by detection using ICP-MS. After subtracting AsC and AsB from the total, we calculated the percentages of InAs ($InAs^{III} + InAs^V$), MMA ($MMA^{III} + MMA^V$), and DMA^V.

Results

The general characteristics of the study sample was by sex. As expected, males were taller and heavier than females and also had a larger head circumference. Based on age-specific growth charts from the Centers for Disease Control (CDC),[777] 52% of females and 49% of males had a BMI below the fifth percentile. Using WHO growth standards,[778] these percentages were 38.4% for females and 33.7% for males. Almost all of the children had albumin levels <3.8 g/dL. Using NHANES III data for 6–11-year-old U.S. children,[784] males had a higher prevalence of high homocysteine (78% >95th percentile, i.e., >7.0 µmol tHcys/L) than did females (64% >7.0 µmol/L). In the absence of published reference values for children, they used published adult reference values for marginal plasma folate (<9 nmol/L),[779] 18% of females and 21% of males were classified as having marginal folate nutritional status. Using the CDC adult cutoff of 6.8 nmol/L,[773] 4.1% of females and 3.3% of males were classified as having folate deficiency. Similarly, using adult reference values for cobalamin,[779] 7% of females and 5% of males had plasma levels <151 pmol/L, indicative of deficiency.

As expected, both plasma folate and cobalamin were inversely correlated with tHcys ($r = -0.21$, $p = 0.008$ and $r = -0.14$, $p = 0.07$, respectively). After adjustment for age and sex, plasma folate explained only 3.5% and cobalamin explained 2.3% of the variation in plasma tHcys. tHcys and cysteine were positively correlated ($r = 0.43$, $p < 0.0001$); this association was stronger among females ($r = 0.64$, $p < 0.0001$) than males ($r = 0.23$, $p = 0.03$) and the sex difference was statistically significant ($p < 0.01$).

Water As concentrations ranged from 0.1 to 864 g/L; 56% of the wells that served as the primary source of drinking water for these children had water As concentrations above the Bangladesh standard of 50 µg/L, whereas 79% were above the WHO standard of 10 µg/L. uCr concentrations were similar for males and females; both total uAs and total UAs per gram creatinine were significantly higher among males.

Consistent with their previous findings in adults, plasma folate was inversely associated with both total uAs ($r = -0.22$, $p = 0.004$) and uAs per gram creatinine ($r = -0.31$, $p < 0.0001$). Plasma levels of cobalamin, tHcys, and cysteine were not significantly associated with either total uAs or total uAs per gram creatinine. Overall, there were no statistically significant correlations between the plasma measures and uCr (data not shown). However, there was a positive association between plasma folate and uCr among females ($r = 0.22$, $p = 0.06$).

In this cross-sectional study of 6-year-old Bangladeshi children ($n = 165$), the associations between plasma folate and As metabolites observed were similar to those in Gamble et al.'s study of adults[741]; folate was inversely correlated with %InAs and positively correlated with %DMA, although the latter did not achieve statistical significance. These findings suggests that folate is required for both the first and second As methylation steps and are in line with the well-known role of folate as a methyl donor involved in the generation of SAM. Hall et al.[734] did not observe an association between folate and %MMA in children, whereas in adults there was a statistically significant inverse association. Consistent with previous results,[741] they did not find associations between plasma cobalamin and any of the uAs metabolites, although the ability to detect an association in the previous study was limited by the exclusion of cobalamin-deficient participants. The relatively small sample size and the small number of children with cobalamin deficiency may have constrained their ability to detect an association in this study.

Plasma cysteine showed a statistically significant inverse association with %InAs and was positively associated with %MMA and %DMA, suggesting that cysteine may be involved in As reduction, thus facilitating both the first and second As methylation steps. Cysteine is an amino acid that can be produced from the catabolism of Hcys and is an intermediate in the synthesis of GSH. Cysteine is involved in redox cycling[780] and can reduce As^{V} to As^{III} *in vitro*,[781] a necessary step before methylation. Although their findings suggest that the reported ability of cysteine to reduce As *in vitro* may also be relevant in humans, it is equally possible that the association is secondary to the role of cysteine in GSH biosynthesis; GSH is known to be capable of providing reducing equivalents for this reaction.

Plasma tHcys was significantly inversely associated with %MMA in males, and its estimated correlation with %DMA was positive, although not statistically significant among both males and females. These associations are opposite of those in adults. Although additional studies will be required to clarify the mechanism underlying these observations, the findings raise the question of whether there may be differences in the fundamental regulation of one-carbon metabolism between children and adults. Theoretically, one would expect overall upregulation of one-carbon metabolism during periods of rapid growth to meet the high demands for protein and DNA synthesis. In rats and rabbits, glycine-*N*-methyltransferase (GNMT) activity levels are very low at birth and increase continuously with age.[782] Since GNMT, which catalyzes the nonessential methylation of glycine to sarcosine, competes for SAM and generates SAH, lower activity during periods of rapid growth may be one mechanism whereby increased requirements for SAM during growth and development are achieved. Whether similar developmental changes occur in humans is unknown.

The mean plasma tHcys concentrations (7.9 μmol/L) in this study are generally higher than those reported among children of similar ages in other populations.[783–785] In 6–11-year-old participants in NHANES III (1988–1994, prefolate fortification), mean plasma tHcys concentrations were 5.2 μmol/L among boys and 5.3 μmol/L among girls.[784] Geometric mean plasma tHcys concentrations were somewhat higher in 6–9-year-old Greek children (6.5 μmol/L).[785] Differences in folate status may partially explain the higher tHcys concentrations in this population; in 4–11-year-old participants in NHANES III, mean plasma folate levels measured were 19.9 nmol/L,[786] substantially higher than the mean concentrations observed in this study (12.8 nmol/L). However, it is likely that other factors—for example, genetics—may contribute to these considerable population differences in tHcys concentrations, given that plasma folate explained only a small fraction of the variability in tHcys concentrations.

In Hall et al.[734] previous study of Bangladeshi adults,[733] they observed a pronounced sex difference in the prevalence of hyperhomocysteinemia (males > females); among children, the sex difference was of borderline statistical significance. Must et al.[784] also reported a sex divergence in tHcys concentrations that began at ~10 years of age and continued through adolescence. This sex difference is often attributed to steroid hormones, an explanation that is not relevant for this sample of young children not yet approaching puberty.

As expected, average tHcys concentrations were lower among children compared with the study by Halls et al. of adults (adults:females, 9.5 μmol/L and males, 15.3 μmol/L; children:females, 7.7 μmol/L and males, 8.0 μmol/L). However, using NHANES III cutoff values for each age category, it was observed an overall higher prevalence of high homocysteine (78% and 64% >7 μmol/L for males and females, respectively) than in this study of adults, in which the prevalence was 26% among females (>10.4 μmol/L) and 63% among males (>11.4 μmol/L).[733] Although a high prevalence of hyperhomocysteinemia among Asian adults has been previously reported,[787,788] this finding in children is somewhat surprising, given that the children have a lower prevalence of folate and cobalamin deficiencies. The correlations between plasma folate and tHcys, as well as between cobalamin and tHcys were also weaker in this study than in the adults,[733] and plasma folate accounted for a smaller portion of the variability of tHcys (3.5% vs. 15% for children and adults, respectively). Perhaps in children, homocysteine biosynthesis makes a relatively greater contribution to tHcys concentrations than its effective removal via remethylation compared with adults.

The current findings suggest that children have a lower mean urinary %InAs and %MMA and higher mean %DMA than adults, independent of water As and plasma folate levels, suggesting an overall higher As methylation capacity. This is in agreement with most other studies comparing adults and children and is consistent with the conjecture that one-carbon metabolism may be generally upregulated during periods of growth. Behaviors prevalent in Bangladeshi adults that are known to be associated with reduced As methylation, such as cigarette smoking and betel nut use, may also partially explain this finding.

The expression of uAs metabolites as percentages limits the interpretation of these findings, because the relative level of each metabolite is influenced by that of the others. Likewise, the lack of data on blood As metabolites is limited, because the relative distribution of As metabolites in urine does not closely reflect those in blood; MMA makes up a substantially greater proportion of total blood As than urine As both in adults[742] and in children.[743] However, urine As metabolites are still useful for indicating overall patterns of association.

In conclusion, the results of this cross-sectional study suggest that folate and cysteine facilitate As methylation in children; these findings are similar to those of adults. However, the observed negative association between tHcys and %MMA and the positive association with %DMA are opposite those of adults. Additional studies will be required to clarify the mechanism underlying these observations. The unusually high prevalence of high homocysteine concentrations among 6-year-old Bangladeshi children, despite a lower prevalence of folate deficiency than among adults from the same geographic area, was likewise unanticipated. Determinants of tHcys and the potential long-term health implications of high tHcys in children are not well characterized and warrant further study. Finally, these results suggest an overall high As methylation capacity in children compared with adults.

Arsenic competes with selenium, and selenium is known to reduce arsenic toxicity. Arsenicals were used as medicine, and arsenic acid and nitrophenol forms of arsenic are used as growth enhancers and for feed efficiency of pigs and poultry.[789–791] Arsenic is excreted, mainly through the urine, in its inorganic form and methylated derivatives. Because hair, nail, and liver show high levels of arsenic, they are considered excretory routes. Chronic toxicity is characterized by weakness, prostration, aching muscles, gastrointestinal upset, peripheral neuropathy (increased nerve conduction), and changes in pigmentation of the nails and skin. Arsenic antagonizes thyroid function with resultant goiter. It is a carcinogen or cocarcinogen.[791] Certainly, excessive arsenic exposure will exacerbate chemical sensitivity.

Cadmium

Cadmium is an element that occurs naturally in the earth's crust. Pure cadmium is a soft, silver-white metal; however, cadmium is not usually found in the environment as a metal. It is usually found as a mineral combined with other elements such as oxygen (cadmium oxide), chlorine (cadmium chloride), or sulfur (cadmium sulfate, cadmium sulfide). These compounds are solids that may dissolve in water but do not evaporate or disappear from the environment. All soils and rocks, including coal and mineral fertilizers, have some cadmium in them. Cadmium is often found as part of small particles present in air. You cannot tell by smell or taste that cadmium is present in air or water, because it does not have any definite odor or taste.

According to Eck,[792] cadmium can enter the environment in several ways. It can enter the air from the burning of coal and household waste, and metal mining and refining processes. It can enter water from disposal of wastewater from households or industries. Fertilizers often have some cadmium in them and fertilizer use causes cadmium to enter the soil. Spills and leaks from hazardous waste sites can also cause cadmium to enter soil or water. Cadmium attached to small particles may get into the air and travel a long way before coming down in the environment but can change into different forms. Most cadmium stays where it enters the environment for a long time. Some of the cadmium that enters water will bind to soil but some will remain in the water. Cadmium in soil can enter water or be taken up by plants. Fish, plants, and animals take up cadmium from the environment.

Most cadmium used in this country is extracted during the production of other metals such as zinc, lead, or copper. Cadmium has several uses in industry and consumer products, mainly batteries, pigments, metal coatings, and plastics.

Sources are air pollution, art supplies, and bone meal. In most cases, cadmium in the environment comes from cadmium-copper industrial plants and battery plants. It is used for plating steel. The TLV for cadmium fumes is 0.05 mg/m^3. For cadmium dust, it is 0.05 mg/m^3.[793]

The primary health effect from the inhalation of cadmium fumes is pulmonary edema. Fatal cases have been reported for exposures at 50 and 40 mg/m^3 for 1 hour. Proteinuria, emphysema, and other complaints have been reported in workers with exposures of 20 years to concentrations between 3 and 15 mg/m^3 of the dusts of cadmium and its oxide. Cadmium will also cause growth retardation, impaired reproduction, hypertension, teratogenesis, and carcinoma. It affects the GSH replenishing system, preventing the conversion of oxidant GSH to reduced GSH. It can stop the GSH replenishing mechanism similar to lead and mercury, exacerbating chemical sensitivity.

According to Eck and Wilson,[792] cadmium is an extremely toxic metal which has no known necessary function in the body. Cadmium toxicity contributes to a large number of health conditions, including the major killer diseases such as heart disease, cancer, and diabetes.

Cadmium displaces zinc in many metalloenzymes and many of the symptoms of cadmium toxicity can be traced to a cadmium-induced zinc deficiency.

Cadmium concentrates in the kidney, liver, and various other organs and is considered more toxic than either lead or mercury. It is toxic at levels one-tenth that of lead, mercury, aluminum, or nickel.

Cadmium toxicity is increasing in incidence today for several reasons. One of the primary reasons is a zinc deficiency in many commonly eaten foods. Zinc, which is protective against cadmium, is becoming increasingly deficient in the soil and consequently in foods. Food processing and eating of refined foods further reduces zinc intake.

Exposure to cadmium is also increasing due to its use as a coating for iron, steel, and copper. It is also used in copper alloys, stabilizers in rubber and plastics, cigarette papers, fungicides, and in many other products. Often these industries then pollute water, air, and food with this metal.

Sources of Cadmium

According to Eck,[792] the most common sources of cadmium toxicity are foods such as rice and wheat which are grown in soil contaminated by sewage sludge, superphosphate fertilizers, and irrigation water.

Large ocean fish such as tuna, codish, and haddock concentrate within their tissues relatively large amounts of cadmium. Oysters although containing large amounts of cadmium also contain large amounts of zinc which serves to protect against cadmium toxicity.

Besides contaminated produce and organ meats such as liver and kidneys, a significant source of cadmium toxicity is a diet high in refined foods. Zinc, which normally protects against the toxic effects of cadmium, is largely removed during the milling process, leaving cadmium behind.

For the average American, low levels of cadmium exposure occur through diet. Currently, these background exposures through diet are not believed to cause adverse health effects.

However, there are groups within the United States who suffer higher than average exposures to cadmium because of occupation, hobby, or personal habits such as smoking.

Additionally, there are certain regions of the globe, such as Japan, which are contaminated with high levels of cadmium in the environment. Since local food crops, such as rice, pick up high levels of cadmium, local people are exposed to cadmium through their diet.

Many processed foods have had the protective elements zinc and calcium removed in the refining process. Cadmium, however, remains and is readily absorbed since the zinc and calcium are not available to compete for absorption.

Cadmium may also be used as plating material in food-processing plants, thereby finding its way into processed food products. Processed meats, refined grains, instant coffee, and cola drinks are among the most common sources of cadmium toxicity.

Widespread use of white flour and white rice, along with causing various vitamin and mineral deficiencies, contribute to cadmium toxicity by their high cadmium/zinc ratio. An excessive carbohydrate intake also serves to reduce tissue zinc levels, further aggravating a cadmium toxicity problem.

Solder used to seal cans is a common source of cadmium. Cadmium used in industry finds its way into many water supplies. Soft water is more dangerous since the calcium in hard water has a protective effect. Old galvanized pipes and new plastic (PVC) pipes are sources of cadmium in drinking water.

Cadmium is used in numerous industries: in battery electrodes, semiconductors, etc. Workers in these industries are at risk of exposure. Dental amalgams and appliances may also contain cadmium.

One package of cigarettes deposits between 2 and 4 µg of cadmium into the smoker's lungs. Cigarettes are especially dangerous because cadmium is efficiently absorbed when inhaled.

Motor oil, exhaust and incineration of rubber goods, tires, plastics, and paints are also the sources of cadmium.

Cadmium levels are highest in urban areas where incineration takes place and where vehicle exhaust levels are higher.

Cadmium was passed to the fetal rat brain when a pregnant mother was given a subcutaneous cadmium injection. We commonly observe high concentrations of cadmium in babies and young children, with no other possible source except from the mother.

Congenital cadmium toxicity is becoming increasingly common and probably helps account for the increase in birth defects, hyperkinesis, learning disorders, minimal brain dysfunction, and the failure to thrive syndrome.

In the United States in the 1990s, ~297,000 workers were estimated to be at greatest risk of cadmium exposure.[794] There are no more recent estimates. The types of workers potentially exposed to direct occupational exposure include alloy makers, aluminum solder makers, ammunition maker, auto mechanics, battery makers, bearing makers, braziers and solderers, cable and trolley wire makers, cadmium alloy and cadmium-plate welders, cadmium platers, cadmium vapor lamp makers, ceramic and pottery makers, copper–cadmium alloy makers, dental amalgam makers, electric instrument makers, electrical condenser makers, electroplaters, engravers, glass makers, incandescent lamp makers, jewelers, lithographers, lithophane makers, metal sculptors, mining and refinery workers, municipal solid waste recover workers, paint makers, paint sprayers, pesticide makers, pharmaceutical workers, photoelectric cell makers, pigment makers, plastic products makers, smelterers, sold makers, and textile printers.

"Itai-Itai" Disease

"Itai-itai" or ouch-ouch disease was first described in postmenopausal Japanese women exposed to excessive levels of cadmium over their lifetimes. The women were exposed through their diet because the region of Japan in which they resided was contaminated with cadmium.[795,796]

Developmental Effects

In animals, cadmium crosses the placenta, and large parenteral doses during early gestation cause birth defects. During later pregnancy, doses greater than 2.5 mg/kg cause severe placental damage and fetal death.

Cadmium has not been reported to include birth defects in infants of women occupationally exposed to cadmium. However, there are reports that women in Japan with higher urinary cadmium levels have increased rates of preterm delivery than mothers with lower levels. These mothers also had infants with birth weights that were lower levels. These mothers also had infants with birth weights that were lower than those of newborns of unexposed women but this difference was felt to be due to the increased incidence of early deliveries.[797] However, other studies have not shown cadmium to cause preterm labor.[798] At this time, the evidence of cadmium's effects on pregnancy is inconsistent and requires further investigation.

Detection of Cadmium

Blood Tests

Even when high dietary cadmium is fed, the blood level of cadmium remains extremely low. Even intravenously injected cadmium rapidly disappears from the blood. Consequently, cadmium data from blood have little diagnostic value.

Challenge Tests

Chelating agents may be given and a 24-hour urine sample collected to detect cadmium in arteries and blood. However, cadmium which is stored in the liver, bones, joint, and other tissues will not be detected using challenge tests.

Hair Analysis

- Cadmium levels in the hair show statistically significant correlations with cadmium levels in the kidneys.
- However, excessive tissue cadmium is often not revealed on the first mineral test. As with the other toxic metals, cadmium can be so tightly bound that it may require months or even several years on a nutritional program before cadmium is released from storage and is revealed on a hair analysis.

Metabolism of Cadmium

Absorption

Absorption of cadmium is highest through inhalation. Women are more prone to cadmium toxicity than men. This may be due to the fact that females in general tend to have a lower metabolic rate than males.

Dietary absorption of cadmium is favored by a deficiency of calcium, zinc, copper, iron, and protein in the diet.

Retention

According to Eck,[792] about 50% of ingested or inhaled cadmium is stored in the liver and kidneys. High concentrations of cadmium are also deposited in the pancreas and salivary glands. Other storage sites may also include the joints, arteries, periosteum or covering of the bones, and virtually all body tissues.

In the blood, cadmium moves from the plasma to the red blood cells, where it binds mainly to metallothionein and hemoglobin.

Cadmium ingestion stimulates production of metallothionein, a zinc- and cadmium-binding protein.

The cadmium content of the body increases with age in industrialized societies, from <1 mcg in the newborn to 15–20 mg in adults.

Excretion

According to Eck,[792] metallothionein plays an important role in the excretion of cadmium, inasmuch as it acts as a chelating agent. Excretion of cadmium occurs through the kidneys and liver, but the excretion rate is normally very low. The biological half-life of cadmium is probably between 10 and 30 years.

Metabolic Effects of Cadmium

Effects on Energy Production

Cadmium is a well-known inhibitor of cellular respiration. It forms strong covalent bonds with many biomolecules and so its potential targets for damage are numerous. Some of the most vulnerable enzymes are GSH reductase and the enzymes of the Krebs energy cycle—pyruvate and α-ketoglutarate dehydrogenase.

Displacement of Zinc

Many of the toxic effects of cadmium, including kidney disease, neurological damage, arteriosclerosis, and birth defects, stem from the replacement of zinc in sensitive enzyme-binding sites.

Metallothionein binds zinc and copper as well as cadmium. Cadmium binds more tightly to metallothionein, and as a result, less copper and zinc are bound which results in a copper and zinc deficiency. Since binding to metallothionein is necessary for utilization of zinc and copper, cadmium poisoning can lead to a zinc and copper deficiency.

An interesting aspect of cadmium poisoning is that by replacing zinc in critical enzyme systems, cadmium can perform a homeostatic function. That is, many zinc-dependent enzymes can continue to function to a certain extent with cadmium instead of zinc. However, enzymatic activity is reduced and problems eventually occur as a result of impairment of the zinc-dependent enzymes.

Many of the toxic effects of cadmium stem from its accumulation in the kidneys. Renal dysfunction affects calcium, vitamin D, phosphorus, and sodium levels, resulting in proteinuria, glycosuria, renal hypertension, and other metabolic disorders.

Cadmium has been suggested as an etiologic factor in certain human cancers. Birth defects, probably due to zinc deficiency, have been observed in mice, rats, and hamsters.

It is difficult to describe metabolic dysfunctions to cadmium toxicity alone; inasmuch as many metabolic dysfunctions are the result of displacement of zinc or a zinc deficiency. However, the major categories of metabolic dysfunctions associated with cadmium toxicity include:

Neurotransmitters: Cadmium inhibits the release of acetylcholine, probably by interfering with calcium metabolism. Cadmium also activates the enzyme cholinesterase, while zinc inhibits cholinesterase activity. Cooper and Steinberg concluded that cadmium at any dose was a more potent blocking agent of cholinesterase activity than lead.

Adenylate cyclase and MAO activity is inhibited by cadmium. Uptake at synapses of choline, catecholamines, GABA, and glutamic acid is inhibited.

Cadmium also inhibits the methylation of phospholipids, interfering with cellular membrane functions.

Other damage: Cadmium causes hemorrhages in the autonomic ganglia with secondary nerve cell necrosis. Direct damage is also reported to nerve cells, particularly nerve fibers.

Peripheral neuropathy is also a result.

Alterations in calcium and phosphorus metabolism can result in osteoporosis, osteomalacia, and arthritic conditions. Interference with zinc metabolism can result in neuromuscular dysfunctions associated with a zinc deficiency.

Cadmium replaces zinc in the arterial walls, leading to reduced flexibility and strength of the arteries. The body then will coat the arteries to prevent aneurysms, resulting in atherosclerotic plaque, narrowing of arteries and hypertension.

Interference with zinc-dependent enzymes, such as carboxypeptidase, can result in *impaired digestion*. Cadmium may contribute to prostate difficulties and impotence by interfering with zinc enzymes and by interference with cellular energy production. Growth impairment and the failure to thrive syndrome are often associated with cadmium toxicity. Zinc is essential for normal growth. The major storage sites of cadmium are the kidneys. It is not known whether the cadmium itself or the cadmium bound to metallothionein is responsible for tubular damage, which can result in high blood pressure and other renal disease. Alterations in calcium and vitamin D metabolism can result in dental caries and tooth deformities. Cadmium is associated with hyperactivity and learning disability, most likely due to a cadmium-induced zinc deficiency. Inhibition of acetylcholine release may also result in hyperkinetic behavior.

Metabolic Dysfunctions Associated with Cadmium Toxicity

According to Eck,[792] *alcoholism* is frequently associated with zinc deficiency and with hypoglycemia. Cadmium may be implicated in alcoholism, principally due to its effect upon zinc metabolism. *Alopecia* is commonly associated with a cadmium-induced zinc deficiency. *Anemia* is an early sign of cadmium toxicity. Zinc is necessary for the optimal metabolism of fats. By interfering with zinc levels, cadmium toxicity can contribute to atherosclerosis. Zinc is required to maintain the normal elasticity of arteries. By displacing zinc, cadmium causes the arteries to become less elastic and therefore more vulnerable to rupture. The body may then deposit calcium plaques to help strengthen the arterial walls. Displacement of zinc by cadmium results in impaired protein synthesis. Inadequate protein synthesis interferes with regeneration of joint surfaces, which leads to pain and inflammation of the joints. Zinc is required for bone repair. Cadmium can also displace calcium in bone structures. Cadmium toxicity is intimately associated with various malignancies. A high percentage of cancer patients on tissue mineral analysis programs, at one time or another, revealed cadmium toxicity. Interference with zinc-dependent enzymes may be the link to malignancy.

Cardiovascular Disease

Tipton[799] noted that victims of cardiovascular disease, particularly stroke victims, had high levels of cadmium in their body tissues. Weakness and hardening of cerebral arteries, due to cadmium toxicity, result in an increased tendency for cerebral hemorrhage. Zinc deficiency due to cadmium impairs detoxification of alcohol in the liver, which may explain the connection between cadmium toxicity and liver cirrhosis. Zinc is required for the production, release, and transport of insulin. By interfering with zinc metabolism, cadmium can initiate or aggravate a diabetic condition. Cadmium from cigarettes acts as a lung irritant. Cadmium also replaces zinc in collagen causing brittleness and breakage of the fragile alveoli in the lungs.

An enlarged heart is often secondary to narrowed arteries and high blood pressure. Cadmium toxicity is a common contributor to these cardiovascular conditions.

Zinc is critical for male fertility. Sexual potency is decreased due to a cadmium-induced zinc deficiency.

This disorder involves deposition of excessive iron in the tissues. Hemochromatosis may be due to inadequate ability of the liver to detoxify iron. Cadmium toxicity may impair the ability of the liver to detoxify iron. A deficiency of zinc and copper due to cadmium toxicity may also be involved in this disorder.

By causing a zinc deficiency, excess cadmium can cause a rise in cholesterol levels. Levels of other fats may be adversely affected if liver function is impaired by cadmium toxicity.

High levels of cadmium are considered to be an important causative factor in hypertension. Cadmium, by impairing kidney function and causing hardening of the arteries, can result in high blood pressure.

A zinc deficiency, secondary to cadmium toxicity, is a frequent cause of hypoglycemia.

Cadmium causes increased retention of sodium by way of its action on the kidney. This aldosterone-like effect is capable of inducing an inflammatory process. Also, zinc has an anti-inflammatory effect. Zinc deficiency due to cadmium toxicity can increase inflammation.

By interfering with zinc metabolism, cadmium can cause impotency or decrease libido.

Lung Disease

Cadmium can adversely affect the elasticity of lung tissue. By interfering with zinc metabolism, cadmium toxicity may allow tissue copper buildup to occur, resulting eventually in the causation of migraine headaches.

Osteoporosis

High levels of cadmium can cause demineralization of the bones and total inhibition of bone repair mechanisms. Zinc is essential for bone mineralization. Cadmium concentrates in the kidneys, thus contributing to renal arteriosclerosis. Cadmium has a unique tendency to concentrate in the human kidney. There it can cause renal hypertension and proteinuria. Cadmium acts directly on the kidney to enhance sodium and water retention. No other substance, save aldosterone, is known to enhance resorption of sodium. Cadmium-induced schizophrenia is most likely due to displacement of zinc. Zinc is a CNS stabilizer and is now considered a neurotransmitter substance. A low zinc level may result in mood alterations and can allow copper to accumulate in excess in the brain. Copper toxicity is linked to a specific type of schizophrenia. When cadmium replaces zinc in the cerebral arteries, vascular elasticity is diminished. Frequently, the body coats the weakened arteries with fatty or calcium plaques to protect against rupture of the artery. If a bit of plaque or cholesterol breaks free, it can lodge in a cerebral artery, causing a stroke.

According to Eck,[792] their effects on other minerals as described above, cadmium can replace zinc in many metalloenzyme-binding sites.

Cadmium deposited in the kidneys disturbs the calcium and phosphorus balance, probably by altering vitamin D metabolism. A disturbance in the calcium/phosphorus ratio can result in osteoporosis, osteomalacia, and pseudofractures.

Cadmium has a potent inhibitory effect upon calcium incorporation, even when dietary calcium intake is adequate. This may be due to inhibition of 1,25-dihydroxycalciferol by the renal tubules.

By damaging the filtering capacity of the renal tubules, cadmium causes sodium retention which can contribute to a wide array of disorders ranging from hypertension to hyperactivity.

Cadmium reduces copper levels in the liver. Cadmium binds more tightly to metallothionein than does copper. Because copper is not adequately bound, it becomes biounavailable. Hepatic and renal manganese are apparently increased by cadmium. Adequate dietary iron protects against cadmium absorption. Induction of testicular tumors and sarcomas by cadmium is inhibited by selenium. Large amounts of vitamin C have been found to prevent signs of cadmium poisoning in quail.

Different sources of protein are more effective in protecting against cadmium toxicity than others. Egg white had a more protective effect than casein, soy, or gelatin, probably due to the high amounts of selenium in egg white. A low protein intake can contribute to increased cadmium toxicity. Pyridoxine (vitamin B6) appears to increase the toxic effects of cadmium, probably by enhancing its absorption.

Although the medical literature states that cadmium toxicity is largely irreversible, we have had excellent success in reversing cadmium-induced pathology using the mineral balancing approach. The nutritional method involves several aspects, all of which must be combined for greatest effectiveness.

The most important principle for correcting cadmium toxicity is increasing biochemical energy production, which frees more energy for all normal metabolic activities. This is accomplished by precisely balancing the tissue electrolyte levels and ratios as revealed in an unwashed hair sample.

Dietary cadmium absorption can be reduced by administration of iron, zinc, and copper. Zinc and calcium are cellular antagonists to cadmium. Selenium appears to reverse certain effects of cadmium toxicity.

Vitamin C can bind cadmium and facilitate its removal. Sulfur compounds may also be helpful. EDTA therapy is used by some doctors to remove cadmium from the kidneys.

Any therapy which improves the activity of the kidneys will assist detoxification of cadmium. Kidney glandular substance, combined with synergistic factors, to support kidney activity has proven to be effective.

Diet plays an important role not only in avoiding sources of cadmium, including refined and contaminated foods, but also to help balance the oxidation rate and provide adequate protein, mineral, and vitamins.

Reduce Exposure

Occupational cadmium exposure, cigarette smoking, and ingestion of cadmium-contaminated foods should be discontinued.

Combined Therapy

While these methods seem simple enough, their application at times is complex because cadmium may perform an adaptive function by raising sodium levels. In order to reduce cadmium levels, the need for this adaptation must be removed.

Over the past 12 years, Eck and Wilson[792] have researched many aspects of cadmium detoxification in over 10,000 cases and have identified those nutrients which are most effective.

The dosage of manganese, iron, calcium, zinc, inositol, choline, methionine, vitamin C, selenium, and other nutrients should be adjusted for each individual. A hair mineral retest should be performed every 3 months to maintain optimal mineral ratios and levels to assure optimal results.

Protection against a "Cadmium Crisis"

The active removal of cadmium from tissue storage occasionally results in a cadmium crisis which causes disagreeable symptoms. These symptoms may include fatigue, metallic taste in the mouth, low back pain, stomach distress, poor appetite, skin eruption, and/or headache.

These symptoms are temporary, but can be reduced or eliminated by increasing the intake of vitamin C and calcium. The dosage of vitamin C and calcium during a crisis period can be increased to 3000 mg for vitamin C and 1600 mg for calcium. The dosage can be reduced as symptoms subside.

Environmental Cadmium and Lead Exposures and Hearing Loss in U.S. Adults: The NHANES, 1999–2004

Background: Although cadmium and lead are known risk factors for hearing loss in animal—models, few epidemiologic studies have been conducted on their associations with hearing ability in the general population.

Objectives: Choi et al.[800] investigated the associations between blood cadmium and lead exposure and hearing loss in the U.S. general population while controlling for noise and other major risk factors contributing to hearing loss.

Methods: Choi et al.[800] analyzed data from 3698 U.S. adults 20–69 years of age who had been randomly assigned to the NHANES 1999–2004 Audiometry Examination Component. Pure-tone averages (PTAs) of hearing thresholds at frequencies of 0.5, 1, 2, and 4 kHz were computed, and hearing loss was defined as a PTA >25 dB in either ear.

Results: The weighted geometric means of blood cadmium and lead were 0.40 (95% CI: 0.39, 0.42) µg/dL and 1.54 (95% CI: 1.49, 1.60) µg/dL, respectively. After adjusting for sociodemographic and clinical risk factors and exposure to occupational and nonoccupational noise, the highest (vs. lowest) quintiles of cadmium and lead were associated with 13.8% (95% CI: 4.6%, 23.8%) and 18.6% (95% CI: 7.4%, 31.1%) increases in PTA, respectively (trends <0.05).

Conclusions: The results suggest that low-level exposure to cadmium and lead found in the general U.S. population may be important risk factors for hearing loss. The findings support efforts to reduce environmental cadmium and lead exposures.

Cerebral Atrophy and CFS

Ruggiero[801] has just published a novel technique to determine cerebral brain blood flow and the presence or absence of temporal lobe atrophy using an inexpensive, modified ultrasound methodology using a linear probe placed over the temporal area of CFS patients. He can see the structure of the temporal lobe cerebral cortex down to 200–300 µm and sufficient to accurately measure the cerebral cortical thickness and infer the volume of the temporal lobe as well as blood flow within the temporal lobe.

In his article, he suggests that heavy metals, especially cadmium with its ability to inhibit angiogenesis, may be a root cause of this although the angiogenesis inhibition of cadmium is itself linked to oxidative stress and therefore the issues may be broader than cadmium. He notes that magnesium and zinc are clinically indicated for cadmium poisoning and, of course, magnesium is very helpful to CFS cases in my experience, but magnesium is also a significant positive modulator or redox status by ETM as well and seen in seconds on the ETM. Magnesium couples ATP to ADP without directly increasing oxygen consumption, though ADP is positively correlated with oxygen throughput at the cell level according to Guyton.

Since ME/CFS is considered as a neurological disorder, several attempts have been made to detect alterations in the brains of ME/CFS patients. A recent study using a fully automated, observer-independent procedure to study morphological alterations of the CNS demonstrated that ME/CFS patients had an average decrease of the volume of the gray matter of about 8% compared with matched healthy controls.[803] The gray matter volume reduction was significantly associated with objective reduction of physical activity in ME/CFS patients.[803] Gray matter volume reduction was not localized in any particular area of the brain and it was not associated with a concomitant reduction in white matter, thus indicating that the phenomenon was specific to neurons. Gray matter volume reduction could then be held accountable for most of the symptoms of ME/CFS. It is therefore interesting to notice that it was recently demonstrated that cadmium-induced neuronal death in cortical neurons through a combined mechanism of apoptosis and necrosis involving ROS generation and lipid peroxidation.[804]

Since reduction of cerebral blood flow in ME/CFS patients occurs across nearly every region assessed by functional magnetic resonance imaging[805] or by xenon-computed tomography,[806] the temporal lobe could represent an easily accessible region of the human brain to be studied by transcranial sonography.

Note that the Japanese showed reversal of temporal lobe cortical atrophy (previously posted) in their CFS mouse model created by successive antigenic stimulation and then used resveratrol, a potent polyphenol found also in dark chocolate and the highly polyphenol-enriched humic acids (black water) which both test positive on the redox-sensitive ETM in CFS and seem helpful clinically as well.

BERYLLIUM

The source of beryllium is usually the fluorescent lamp industry. Beryllium was not thought to be a toxic element until it was commercially produced. Then workers engaged in extracting it from its ores began to suffer from a number of ailments such as dermatitis, tracheobronchitis, and pneumonitis. A study[807] showed that chronic lung disease developed among workers in fluorescent lamp plants, where fluorescent powder containing finely divided beryllium,[808] can cause chemical sensitivity. The particle size of beryllium oxide dust is a critical factor in exposure that leads to lung injury.[809] Although the TLV for beryllium is 0.992 mg/m^3, it may be too high for the chemically sensitive to tolerate.

IRON OXIDE

Iron is used in the steel industry and for making hard, durable pans and for medical supplementation. Exposure to iron oxide fumes has caused discreet densities in the chest x-rays of electric arc welders, carbon arc, and acetylene welders, silver polishers using rouge (a finely divided iron oxide), workers engages in the manufacture of electrolytic iron oxide, iron, and steel grinders in foundries, and boiler scalers. In the case of the hematite miners, iron and steel grinders in foundries, and the boiler scalers, the oxide fume exposure was associated with exposure to silica, and a number of workers developed a disabling pneumoconiosis. We have seen chemical sensitivity develop in iron workers that resulted in recurrent bronchitis for a description of iron excess and its metabolic changes.

The TLV for iron oxide fumes is 10 mg/m^3.[810] This level may, however, be too high for the general population. It is definitely excessive for the chemically sensitive.

ZINC

Zinc oxide fume fever may result from the inhalation of these fumes. The source is usually a fire in the metal industry or in the electric power generators. Zinc is found in galvanized pans and pipes. The symptoms of zinc excess include fever, chills, muscular pain, nausea, and vomiting, but complete recover occurs in 24–48 hour after exposure. The TLV for zinc oxide fumes is 5 mg/m^3.[811] Zinc oxide is used in some dental fillings. Excess zinc disturbs the zinc/copper ratio, yielding pathogenesis in the chemically sensitive. For zinc deficiency, see section Cadmium.

COPPER

The major industrial sources of copper are fumes occurring in copper and brass plants and in the welding of copper-containing metals. Lower levels of exposure can occur from water conduits, copper cooking pans, radiators, and intrauterine birth control coils.

Health effects consist of irritation of the upper respiratory tract, metallic or sweet tastes, nausea, metal fume fever, and in some cases, discoloration of the skin and hair. Inhalation of dusts and mists of copper salts can result in congestion of nasal mucous membranes, sometimes of the pharynx, and ulceration of the nasal septum. Larger concentrations reaching the gastrointestinal tract can produce salivation, nausea, vomiting, gastric pain, hemorrhagic gastritis, and diarrhea. Chronic exposure may result in anemia. On the skin, copper salts can produce itching and eczema, while on the eye, conjunctivitis or ulceration and turbidity of the cornea can occur.

The TLV for copper fumes is 0.11 mg/m^3 and for copper dust and mist 1.0 mg/m^3.[812] Our observations at the EHC-Dallas suggest that this level is too high for the chemically sensitive. Probably, it is excessive for the general population as well.

Obviously, the spreading phenomenon occurred in this patient developing sensitivity to other chemicals. The copper-to-zinc ratio is very important to body function. Excess copper can disturb zinc metabolism. In our experience, abnormal copper may result in hyperactivity in children and some adults. Disturbance in the ceruloplasmin (copper transportation) results in liver dysfunction. Histidine and threonine are amino acids that also transport copper. Other problems of chemical sensitivity may develop from excess copper as illustrated in this case report.

Case study: A 50-year-old woman was admitted to the environmental unit with complaints of headache, nausea, fatigue, diarrhea, dizziness, forgetfulness, chest pains, and myalgia. She had found that her symptoms were aggravated substantially at her workplace, an aircraft factory, where she was exposed to a variety of chemicals and solvents. She had a specific history of feeling sick when she was near exhaust fumes, gasoline, and other chemicals. Close proximity to pesticide spraying also made her very ill.

As with many environmentally sensitive patients, her erythrocyte sedimentation rate (ESR) was elevated. It was over 50, with a depressed white blood cell (WBC) count of 3500, with 54% lymphocytes and 43% polymorphonucleocytes. Her absolute T cells were low at 556 (normal >1000/mm^3), and her absolute B cells were similarly depressed at 253 (normal >500/mm^3). A chlorinated pesticide screen revealed the presence of detectable levels of beta-BHC, DDE, dieldrin, heptachlor epoxide, and hexachlorobenzene.

She was placed in a porcelain room and fed chemically less contaminated food and water. Oral and intradermal food challenges revealed reactions to a variety of foods, including beef, eggs, chicken, lamb, peas, corn, shrimp, oranges, wheat, potatoes, and others.

She was double-blind tested for inhaled chemicals in a steel and glass challenge booth, and she showed reactions to formaldehyde, pesticide, phenol, alcohol, and natural gas (Table 4.27).

On serum mineral testing, she was found to have a high serum copper at 220 ppm (normal, 80–120 ppm). This level was confirmed on several tests in the absence of any liver impairment or Wilson's disease. Liver function tests were normal.

Before development of her chemical sensitivities, she had installed in her home a solar water heating unit that was constructed largely of copper. This unit appeared to be the cause of her high copper levels.

She was treated with rotation diet, environmental control, and nutritional support, along with intravenous and oral vitamin C and antioxidant supplementation, and elimination of all copper-generating sources. Her copper levels fell afterwards to 126, and she showed considerable improvement in her overall health. Finally, these levels returned to normal, and the patient became asymptomatic.

TABLE 4.27

Double-Blind-Inhaled Challenge 50-Year-Old White Female with Copper Excess after 4 Days of Deadaptation in the ECU with Total Load Reduced

	Dose ppm	Reaction Signs and Symptoms Reproduced
Formaldehyde	<0.20	+
Phenol	<0.0020	+
Ethanol (petroleum derived)	<0.50	+
Pesticide (2,4-DNP)	<0.0034	+
Chlorine	<0.33	−
Saline	Placebo	−
Saline	Placebo	−
Saline	Placebo	

Source: Rea, W.J. 1994. *Chemical Sensitivity, Volume II*, Page 739, Table 5. With permission.

Copper excess has been associated with nausea, vomiting, diarrhea, abdominal pain, anemia, and myalgia. This case illustrates that environmentally sensitive people, who often have adverse reactions to foods and chemicals, may have other complicating factors, such as mineral imbalances, that can alter their total health picture.

In addition to inhaling nanoaluminum, such spraying will saturate the ground, water, and vegetation with high levels of aluminum. Normally, aluminum is poorly absorbed from the GI tract, but nanoaluminum is absorbed in much higher amounts. This absorbed aluminum has been shown to be distributed to a number of organs and tissues, including the brain and spinal cord. Inhaling this environmentally suspended nanoaluminum will also produce tremendous inflammatory reaction within the lungs, which will pose a significant hazard to children and adults with asthma and pulmonary diseases. We often see aluminum in hair samples of chemically sensitive patients.

Once the soil, plants, and water sources are heavily contaminated, there will be no way to reverse the damage that has been done.

Steps need to be taken now to prevent an impending health disaster of enormous proportions if this project is not stopped immediately. Otherwise, we will see an explosive increase in neurodegenerative diseases occurring in adults and the elderly in unprecedented rates as well as neurodevelopmental disorders in our children. We are already seeing a dramatic increase in these neurological disorders and it is occurring in younger people than ever before.

Tin

Tin is important as an ideal material for coating steel sheets because it is resistant to corrosion. About one-half of the world production of tin is used in the tin-plate industry for making cans for food. Tin alloys are used for soldering, especially in the electrical industry and in making bronzes. Some chemically sensitive patients do become sensitive to tin. Some chemically sensitive patients have high tin levels in their hair.

Phosphorus

Phosphorus does not occur in nature as an element since it is very reactive. It occurs as rock phosphate (Figure 4.21). Phosphorus compounds are necessary for plant and animal metabolism. Therefore, they are used in many fertilizers. Phosphorus is used in the manufacture of matches and detergents. It is also used in the preparation of fungicides, pesticides, and insecticides in the form of phosphorus pentasulfide. Phosphorus is also used in toothpastes, flame retardants in textiles, acidifying agents for beverages (soft drinks), and dyeing agents for gases (as a base for making dyes). It is used as an intermediate in preparing phosphate esters used as plasticizers and additives for motor fuels, and it is a catalyst for surface treatment of metals. We have seen excess phosphorus compounds exacerbate chemical sensitivity. This type exposure is particularly devastating when they are organophosphate insecticides that can induce chemical sensitivity. Phosphorus will become trapped in the phosphorus pool of the body causing the formation of more toxic substances. It must be emphasized that intercellular phosphorylation of Ca^{2+} entering the nerve and vascular cell can combine with protein kinase A and C and cause hypersensitivity up to 1000 times. This hypersensitivity is extremely important in cellular response to numerous actions, including NMDA and TRPV1, TRPA, TRPM8 reactions.

Nickel

Workers employed in nickel refineries have a greater-than-normal incidence of nasal, sinus, and lung cancer.[813] The specific carcinogenic agent is not well defined and is the subject of continuing research. A condition common among nickel platers is dermatitis, or "nickel itch."[814] This symptom appears to have two components: a simple dermatitis localized to the area of contact and chronic

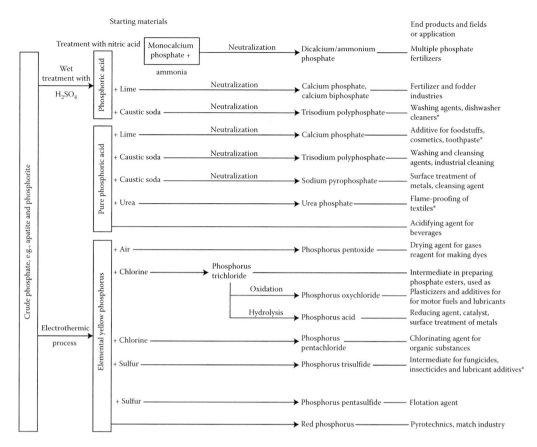

FIGURE 4.21 Products derived from phosphorus and phosphoric acids. Some of these will affect the chemically sensitive adversely. *Some may be trapped in the phosphorus pool of the chemically sensitive, causing protein binding of the cytochrome P-450 and antibody formation with subsequent malfunction. (From Hopp, V., I. Hennig. 1983. *Handbook of Applied Chemistry: Facts for Engineers, Scientists, Technicians, and Technical Managers*, Vol. II, pp. 6–14. Washington, DC: Hemisphere Publishing. With permission; Rea, W.J. 1994. *Chemical Sensitivity, Volume II*, Page 752, Figure 8. With permission.)

eczema or neurodermatitis without apparent connection to such contact, for example, systemic in origin. Nickel-containing bracelets can also cause dermatitis, and reports are appearing of people being sensitive to nickel in prostheses such as artificial hips and heart valves.[815] Titanium alloy used in many hip and spine implants long have contained nickel. These may have to be neutralized intradermally, in order to leave them in, if the patient reacts. Chronic nickel excess can result in heart muscle, brain, lung, liver, and kidney degeneration.[789,790] Nickel-containing heart valves have developed clots apparently due to sensitivity.

The TLV for nickel is 0.1 mg/m^3.[816] The effects of nickel at this level are unknown for both the general population and the chemically sensitive. Nickel appears to be one of the most highly sensitizing metals. Nickel concentrations in particulate matter PM$_{10}$ was measured at Midwestern sites, two urban sites with a large industrial component and one rural site, in samples collected from September 1985 to June 1988.[817] Nickel concentrations in the fine PM$_{10}$ particles (<1–2.5 μm) taken from collection sites in East St. Louis and Southeast Chicago averaged 2.1 ± 1.4 (1 SD and 2.7 ± 2.6 ng/m^3, respectively, and were similar to those measured in the coarser PM$_{10}$ particles (2.5–10 μm) of 1.8 ± 1.5 and 2.1 ± 1.0 ng/m^3, respectively. The concentrations of nickel measured in both the fine and coarse particles collected at the East St. Louis and Southeast Chicago sites were higher than the average concentration of nickel of 0.5 ± 0.3 and 0.7 ± 0.5 ng/m^3 measured in fine and coarse particles, respectively, collected from a rural site (Bondville, Illinois). The higher concentrations of nickel in the East St. Louis and Southeast Chicago sites are attributed to emissions from zinc smelters and steel mills/oil combustion, respectively.

Nickel concentrations in indoor air are generally <10 ng/m^3. In a study of 10 homes in the Southeast Chicago area, indoor and outdoor air samples were regularly sampled between June 1994 and April 1995.[818] Of the 48 samples taken, 35 had nickel concentrations above the detection limit of the assay with a mean (±1 SD) concentration of 0.002 ± 0.002 μg/m^3 and a maximum value of 0.008 μg/m^3. The median indoor nickel concentration of 0.003 μg/m^3 was similar to the median outdoor nickel concentration of 0.0034 μg/m^3. Indoor air samples taken from 394 homes in Suffolk and Onondaga Counties of New York State contained nickel concentrations that were similar to those found in the Chicago study.[819] A mean indoor nickel concentration of 2 ng/m^3 (0.002 μg/m^3) was derived from a sampling of 28 homes.

The New York study also examined nickel concentrations in indoor air as a function of combustion sources within the home (e.g., resident smoker, wood-burning stove, kerosene heater) and found no difference in the mean nickel concentrations between homes containing these combustion sources and homes without. Graney et al.[820] measured nickel levels in indoor air as part of a 1998 study of metal exposures for residents of a retirement home in Towson, Maryland. The study participants had a mean age of 84, were all nonsmokers, and did not typically cook their own meals. Median nickel concentrations of 1.02 and 1.71 ng/m^3 in air were reported in particulate matter (PM$_{2.5}$) samples collected from indoor air and personal exposure samplers, respectively.

In a study of 46 high school students in New York City conducted in the winter and summer of 1999, the concentrations of nickel in collected particulates (PM$_{2.5}$) to which these students were exposed was assessed using personal monitoring devices and stationary measurements of airborne nickel both within and outside the home.[821] The mean (±1 SD) air concentrations of nickel obtained from the outdoor, indoor, and personal monitors measured during the winter survey period were similar (32.3 ± 22.4, 31.6 ± 54.5, and 49.6 ± 114 ng/m^3, respectively). Likewise, the mean nickel concentrations obtained from all three monitors during the summer survey period were also found to be similar (11.7 ± 6.3, 12.6 ± 8.4, and 17.3 ± 24.7 ng/m^3, respectively), although somewhat lower than the winter concentrations. These results suggest that ambient concentrations of nickel are the dominating force in determining both indoor and personal exposures to nickel.

Because of the large number of nickel-releasing sources, the nickel concentration in ambient air may show considerable variation. In a remote area (Canadian Arctic), levels of 0.38–0.62 ng/m^3 were recorded,[822] as compared with 124 ng/m^3 in the vicinity of a nickel smelter.[823] In Northern Norway, a level of about 1 ng/m^3 was recorded in an unpolluted area as compared with about 5 ng/m^3 some 5 km distant from a nickel smelter (average values 1990–1991). The highest value recorded was 64 ng/m^3.[824,825] Concentrations of 18–42 ng/m^3 were recorded in eight U.S. cities.[826] These values correspond to the average value of 37 ng/m^3 for 30 U.S. Urban Air National Surveillance Network Stations for the period 1957–1968. This average decreased from 47 ng/m^3 for 1957–1960 to 26 ng/m^3 for 1965–1968. The mean (arithmetic) value for 1970–1974 was 13 ng/m^3.[827] Ranges of 10–50 and 9–60 ng/m^3 have been reported in European cities. Higher values (110–180 ng/m^3) have been reported from heavily industrialized areas.[828]

The mass medium diameter (MMD) of nickel in urban air is 0.83–1.67 μm and <1 μm in 28 55% of particles.[829] An MMD of 0.98 μm has also been reported.[830] The highest concentration of nickel was found in the smallest particles emitted from a coal-fired plant.[831] Particles with an MMD of 0.65–1.1 μm contained nickel at a concentration of 1600 mg/kg, while particles of 4.7–11 μm contained 400 mg/kg. Nickel-containing particles released from oil combustion (California, urban area) are in the fine size fraction, with MMDs of <1 μm.[832] Nickel carbonyl has never been demonstrated in ambient air.

Assuming a daily respiratory rate of 20 m^3, the amount of airborne nickel entering the respiratory tract is in the range 0.1–0.8 μg/day when concentrations are 5–40 ng/m^3 in ambient air. Owing to the variation in particle size and solubility between nickel compounds, no general statements can be made on the retention or absorption of nickel in the respiratory tract.[833] A total deposition of about 50% of the inhaled dose was estimated for particles with an MMD of 2.0 μm, while deposition was about 10% for those of 0.5 μm. For larger particles, >50% of the deposited dose was in the nasopharyngeal part of the respiratory tract as against <10% for the smaller particles.

In a single experiment, 95% of the nickel in a respirable aerosol of nickel-enriched fly ash was retained in the lung 1 month after the exposure.[834] Following intratracheal administration of nickel chloride, only 0.1% was retained in the lungs of rats at day 21.[835]

About 0.04–0.58 μg of nickel is released with the mainstream smoke of one cigarette.[836] Smoking 40 cigarettes per day may thus lead to inhalation of 2–23 μg of nickel. The possibility that nickel occurs in mainstream smoke in part as nickel carbonyl has never been substantiated.

Estimated releases of 404,413 lbs (~183 metric tons) of nickel and 942,117 lbs (~427 metric tons) of nickel compounds to the atmosphere from 2279 and 1286 domestic manufacturing and processing facilities in 2002, respectively, accounted for about 6.0% and 2.5% of the estimated total environmental releases, respectively, from facilities required to report to the TRI (TRI02 2004).

Nickel and its compounds are naturally present in the earth's crust, and releases to the atmosphere occur from natural processes such as windblown dust and volcanic eruption, as well as from anthropogenic activities. These latter releases are mainly in the form of aerosols. It is important to consider the background levels that are due to natural sources and distinguish them from levels that may result from anthropogenic activities. It is estimated that 8.5 million kg of nickel are emitted into the atmosphere from natural sources each year.[837,838] Based on this value, sources of nickel have been estimated as follows: windblown dust, 56%; volcanoes, 29%; vegetation, 9%; forest fires, 2%; and meteoric dust, 2%. A more recent and higher estimate of 30 million kg/year has been given for emission of nickel into the atmosphere from natural sources.[839,840] Anthropogenic sources of atmospheric nickel include nickel mining, smelting, refining, and production of steel and other nickel-containing alloys, fossil fuel combustion, and waste incineration.

Deposition of metals around large smelter complexes is a significant local problem. For example, at the Copper Cliff smelter in Sudbury, Ontario, it is estimated that 42% of nickel particulates emitted from the 381-m stack are deposited within a 60-km radius of the smelter.[841] The Copper Cliff smelter, one of three large nickel sources in the Sudbury area, emits 592 lbs (269 kg) of nickel per day.

A typical modern, coal-fired power plant emits ≈25 μg nickel per megajoule (MJ) of power produced compared with 420 μg/MJ for an oil-fired plant.[842]

It is estimated that in 1999, 570,000 tons of nickel were released from the combustion of fossil fuels worldwide.[843] Of this, 326 tons were released from electric utilities.[844]

From a public health point of view, the concentration of nickel associated with small particles that can be inhaled into the lungs is of greatest concern. The nickel content of aerosols from power plant emissions is not strongly correlated with particle size.[845] In one coal plant, 53% and 32% of nickel emissions were associated with particles of diameter <3 and <1.5 μm, respectively.[846] Other studies found that only 17%–22% of nickel emissions from coal-fired power plants were associated with particles of >2 μm, and that the MMD of nickel-containing particles from a plant with pollution control devices was 5.4 μm.[847,848] In one study, 40% of the nickel in coal fly ash was absorbed on the surface of the particles rather than being embedded in the aluminosilicate matrix.[845] Surface-absorbed nickel would be more available than embedded nickel.

Nickel emissions from municipal incinerators depend on the nickel content of the refuse and the design and operation of the incinerator. By comparing the nickel content of particles emitted from two municipal incinerators in Washington, DC, with that of atmospheric particulate matter, Greenberg et al.[849] concluded that refuse incineration is not a major source of nickel in the Washington area.

Nickel and nickel compounds have been identified in air samples collected from 20 of the 872 NPL hazardous waste sites where nickel or nickel compounds have been detected in environmental media.[850] Nickel or nickel compounds have been detected in air off-site of NPL sites at concentrations ranging from 0.4912 to 4000 ng/m^3.

Wastewater

Estimated releases of 151,725 lbs (~69 metric tons) of nickel and 516,804 lbs of nickel compounds (~234 metric tons) to surface water from 2279 and 1286 domestic manufacturing and processing facilities in 2002, respectively, accounted for about 2.2% and 1.4% of the estimated total environmental releases, respectively, from facilities required to report to the TRI (TR102 2004).

Emission factors have been estimated for the release of trace metals to water from various source categories and these have been used to estimate inputs of these metals into the aquatic ecosystem. The global anthropogenic input of nickel into the aquatic ecosystem for 1983 is estimated to be between 33 and 194 million kg/year with a median value of 113 million kg/year.[851] For 2014, it was ~193 million kg/year and an estimated projection for 195 million kg/year in 2015.

A survey of raw and treated wastewater from 20 industrial categories indicated that nickel is commonly found in some wastewaters. Those industries with mean effluent levels of >1000 μg/L in raw wastewater were inorganic chemicals manufacturing (20,000 μg/L), iron and steel manufacturing (1700 μg/L), battery manufacturing (6700 μg/L), coil coating (1400 μg/L), metal finishing (26,000 μg/L), porcelain enameling (19,000 μg/L), nonferrous metal manufacturing (<91,000 μg/L), and steam electric power plants (95,000 μg/L). Those industries with mean effluent levels >1000 μg/L in treated wastewater were porcelain enameling (14,000 μg/L) and nonferrous metal manufacturing (14,000 μg/L). The maximum levels in treated discharges from these industries were 67,000 and 310,000 μg/L, respectively. In addition, four other industrial categories had maximum concentrations in treated discharges >1000 μg/L.

In natural waters, nickel primarily exists as the hexahydrate. While nickel forms strong, soluble complexes with OH^-, SO_4^{2-}, and HCO_3^-, these species are minor compared with hydrated Ni^{2+} in surface water and groundwater with pH < 9.[852] Under anaerobic conditions, such as may exist in deep groundwater, nickel sulfide would reduce free aqueous nickel concentrations to low levels.

Drinking Water

Nickel concentrations in drinking water in European countries of 2–13 μg/L have been reported.[853] An average value of 9 μg/L and a maximum of 34 μg/L were recorded in Germany.[854] Nickel may, however, be leached from nickel-containing plumbing fittings, and levels of up to 500 μg/L have been recorded in water left overnight in such fittings.[855] In areas with nickel mining, levels of up to 200 μg/L have been recorded in drinking water. The average level of nickel in drinking water in public water supply systems in the United States was 4.8 μg/L in 1969.

Assuming a concentration of 5–10 μg/L, a daily consumption of 2 L of drinking water would result in a daily nickel intake of 10–20 μg (Table 4.28).

TABLE 4.28

Levels of Daily Nickel Intake (μg) by Humans from Different Types/Routes of Exposure

Type/Route of Exposure	Daily Nickel Intake	Absorption
Food	<300	45 (<15%)
Drinking water	<20	3 (<15%)
Ambient air (urban dweller)	<0.8	0.4 (50%)
Ambient air (smoker)	<23	12 (50%)

Food

In most food products, the nickel content is <0.5 mg/kg fresh weight. Cacao products and nuts may, however, contain as much as 10 and 3 mg/kg, respectively.[856] Total diet studies indicate a total average oral intake of 200–300 μg/day[857] (Table 4.28). Recovery studies indicate an absorption rate of <15% from the gastrointestinal tract.[858]

Relative Significance of Different Routes of Exposure

Percutaneous absorption of nickel is quantitatively minor, but is the most significant for cutaneous manifestations of nickel hypersensitivity.[859] Iatrogenic exposure to nickel may occur as a result of dialysis treatment, prostheses and implants, and medication. Such exposure is of minor importance for practical purposes.[860] Ear piercing, however, increases the probability of nickel sensitization.[861] However, there is a group of patients who have implant sensitivity. Intradermal neutralization is necessary when these patients are symptomatic. When this does not work, the implant will have to be removed which has occurred on numerous chemically sensitive patients. Often the nickel has been used as plates and screws and once bone fusion has occurred, they can be removed.

Both the gastrointestinal and respiratory uptake rates have been estimated on the basis of very limited experimental evidence.

Gastrointestinal uptake is of limited interest for effects other than nickel hypersensitivity. Moreover, even though a low-nickel diet has been reported to improve clinical symptoms in some hypersensitive individuals, other factors seem to be more important.

As the respiratory tract is a major target organ as well as an uptake organ for nickel, inhalation is the most significant route of exposure with regard to respiratory tract effects. Retention in the respiratory tract is more important than uptake into the general circulation because respiratory cancer is the critical effect. Given the particle distribution in ambient air, an ~50% retention figure seems reasonable for risk estimation. Effects in the lung resulting from oral intake cannot be excluded. Inhibition of 5′-nucleotidase activity and enhanced lipid peroxidation in pulmonary alveolar macrophages has been demonstrated in the respiratory tract following parenteral injection of nickel chloride in rats.[862] The relative importance for tumor development of respiratory tract exposure from the general circulation is not known.

Population Groups at High Probability of Exposure

Industrial activity accounts for most of the variability of nickel deposition on the earth's surface, but deposits from meteorites and volcanic eruptions may exceed releases from anthropogenic sources.[863] Point source emission increases nickel exposure, but an impact on health from such emissions has not been convincingly documented.[864,865]

An increased chance risk has been repeatedly demonstrated in the refining industry, but not for secondary users of nickel. Workroom air levels of nickel in secondary and end users of nickel are generally much lower than in the refining industry, often by a factor of 10–100.

At least 50% of a single-inhaled dose of nickel carbonyl is absorbed, the agent passing the alveolar wall intact.[866]

Domestic wastewater is the major anthropogenic source of nickel in waterways.[851] Another 31% of the nickel in influent streams is added at the wastewater treatment plant through the addition of water treatment chemicals. Storm water accounts for between 1% and 5% of the nickel in influent streams.

Soil

Estimated releases of 5.58 million lbs (~5530 metric tons) of nickel and 32.7 million lbs (~14,800 metric tons) of nickel compounds to soils from 2279 and 1286 domestic manufacturing and processing facilities in 2002, respectively, accounted for about 82% and 87% of the estimated total environmental releases, respectively, from facilities required to report to the TRI (TRI02 2004). An additional 55,185 lbs (~25 metric tons) of nickel and 634,432 lbs (~288 metric tons) of nickel compounds, constituting about 0.8% and 1.7% of the total environmental emissions, respectively, were released via underground injection (TRI02 2004).

Epigenetic Mechanisms of Nickel Carcinogenesis

The mechanism of nickel carcinogenesis, focusing primarily on the epigenetic changes associated with exposure of cells to carcinogenic nickel compounds, is described. A large percentage of nickel in sewage sludges exists in a form that is easily released from the solid matter.[867] Although the availability of nickel to plants grown in sludge-amended soil is correlated with soil-solution nickel, it is only significantly correlated with DTPA-extractable nickel.[868]

Distribution in the Body

The main carrier protein of nickel in serum is albumin, but nickel is also bound to α-2-macroglobulin and histidine.[869]

The body burden of nickel in adult humans averages about 0.5 mg per 70 kg. The highest concentrations of nickel are found in the lung and in the thyroid and adrenal glands (about 20–25 µg/kg wet weight). Most other organs (e.g., kidney, liver, brain) contain about 8–10 µg/kg wet weight.[870] Following parenteral administration to experimental animals, the kidney invariably showed the highest concentrations of nickel followed by either the lung or the pituitary glands.[871]

Values for serum/plasma are in the range 0.14–0.65 µg/L; values of around 0.2 µg/L seem to be the most reliable.[869,872] The corresponding values for urine are 0.9–4.1 µg/L, with values of 1–2 µg/L being the most reliable. For whole blood, values of 0.34–1.4 µg/L are given. These values are substantially lower than those reported prior to 1980 because of better analytical methods and improved control of contamination. The metal concentrations in the different samples were not influenced by *age or sex*. Various diseases (MI, acute stroke, thermal burns, hepatic cirrhosis) influence the kinetics of nickel metabolism.

Hypersensitivity Effects

Severe lung damage has been recorded following acute inhalation exposure to nickel carbonyl. Reversible renal effects (in workers), allergic dermatitis (most prevalent in women), and mucosal irritation and asthma (in workers) have been reported following exposure to inorganic nickel compounds.[873] Renal effects and dermatitis presumably relate both to nickel uptake by both inhalation and ingestion, in addition to cutaneous contact for dermatitis.

Allergic skin reactions to nickel (dermatitis) have been documented both in nickel worker and in the general population. However, the significance of nickel as a cause of occupationally induced skin reaction is decreasing. In contrast, there is evidence that nickel is increasingly a major allergen in the general population, especially in women. About 2% of males and 11% of females show a positive skin reaction to patch testing with nickel sulfate. Ear piercing considerablly increases the risk of nickel sensitization.[859]

The respiratory tract is also a target organ for allergic manifestations of nickel exposure. Allergic asthma has been reported among workers in the plating industry following exposure to nickel sulfate.

In nonsmokers, about 99% of the estimated daily nickel absorption stems from food and water; for smokers, the figure is about 75%. Nickel levels in the ambient air are in the range 1–10 ng/m^3 in urban areas, although much higher levels (110–180 ng/m^3) have been recorded in heavily industrialized areas and larger cities. There is, however, limited information on the species of nickel in ambient air.

Consumer products made from nickel alloys and nickel-plated items lead to cutaneous contact exposure.

Exposure to nickel levels of 10–100 mg/m^3 have been recorded from occupational groups with documented increased cancer risk. Exposure levels in the refining industry are currently usually <1–2 mg/m^3. Experimental and epidemiological data indicate that the nickel species in question are important for risk estimation. Nickel compounds are human carcinogens by inhalation exposure.

The present data are derived from studies in occupationally exposed human populations. Assuming a linear dose response, no safe level for nickel compounds can be recommended.

On the basis of the most recent information of exposure and risk estimated in industrial population, an incremental risk of 3.8×10^{-4} can be given for a concentration of nickel in air of $1\ \mu g/m^3$. The concentrations corresponding to an excess lifetime risk of 1:10,000, 1:100,000, and 1:1,000,000 are about 250, 25, and 2.5 ng/m^3, respectively (Figures 4.22 through 4.25).

SILICA

The dust of fused silica (SiO_2) or fused quartz is less active than unfused silica or quartz dust. It actually contains microcrystals of quartz and, therefore, is still fibrogenic but to a lesser extent than quartz dust. The crystalline variant of silica or quartz can produce silicosis in coal and metal miners; pegmatite, foundry, and pottery workers: and in practically anybody who is exposed to a chronic or acute exposure of silica (quartz sand, glass fiber) dust.

The TLV values for crystalline silica are different based on the method used for measuring its concentration in the air. The three methods for measuring it are as follows:

1. $\dfrac{300}{\%\ quartz + 10}$ million particles per cubic foot, using the particle count method

2. $\dfrac{10}{\%\ respirable\ quartz + 2}$ mg/m^3, using the respirable dust mass measurement method

3. $\dfrac{30}{\%\ quartz + 3}$ mg/m^3, using the total dust measurement method[874]

These particles may exacerbate chemical sensitivity.

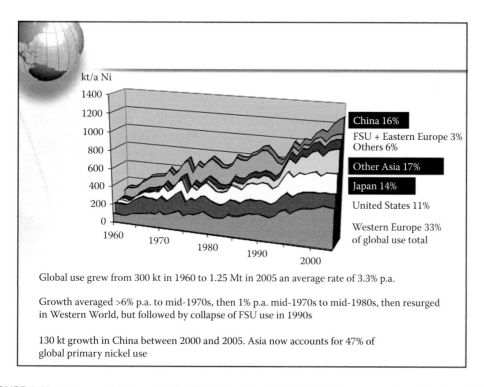

FIGURE 4.22 Primary nickel use 1960–2005. (Peter Cranfield, nickel industry consultant, October 2006.)

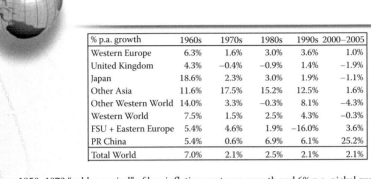

% p.a. growth	1960s	1970s	1980s	1990s	2000–2005
Western Europe	6.3%	1.6%	3.0%	3.6%	1.0%
United Kingdom	4.3%	−0.4%	−0.9%	1.4%	−1.9%
Japan	18.6%	2.3%	3.0%	1.9%	−1.1%
Other Asia	11.6%	17.5%	15.2%	12.5%	1.6%
Other Western World	14.0%	3.3%	−0.3%	8.1%	−4.3%
Western World	7.5%	1.5%	2.5%	4.3%	−0.3%
FSU + Eastern Europe	5.4%	4.6%	1.9%	−16.0%	3.6%
PR China	5.4%	0.6%	6.9%	6.1%	25.2%
Total World	7.0%	2.1%	2.5%	2.1%	2.1%

1950–1973 "golden period" of low inflation post-war growth and 6% p.a. nickel growth

First energy crisis (November 1973) marked the start of high inflation, low economic growth, and negative substitution, for example, loss of NiCr-plated steel bumpers, thin wall castings, near-net shape, better steel making replacing alloying elements

Stainless slab growth moved from Japan to Korea and Taiwan and European mills invested for export

Loss of 200 kt/a primary nickel use in FSU in the early 1990s

Since 2000, China has accounted for all net growth in global primary nickel use consumption growth constrained by supply/high price?

FIGURE 4.23   Primary nickel use growth rates. (Peter Cranfield, nickel industry consultant, October 2006.)

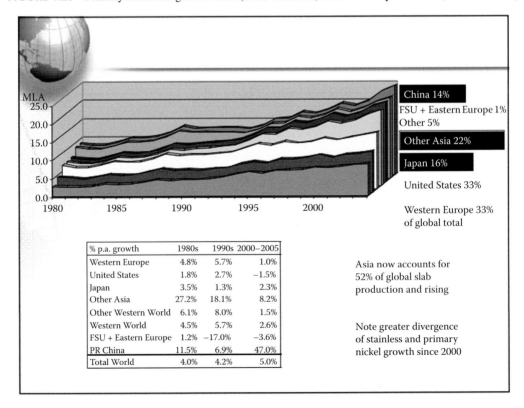

% p.a. growth	1980s	1990s	2000–2005
Western Europe	4.8%	5.7%	1.0%
United States	1.8%	2.7%	−1.5%
Japan	3.5%	1.3%	2.3%
Other Asia	27.2%	18.1%	8.2%
Other Western World	6.1%	8.0%	1.5%
Western World	4.5%	5.7%	2.6%
FSU + Eastern Europe	1.2%	−17.0%	−3.6%
PR China	11.5%	6.9%	47.0%
Total World	4.0%	4.2%	5.0%

Asia now accounts for 52% of global slab production and rising

Note greater divergence of stainless and primary nickel growth since 2000

FIGURE 4.24   Stainless slab production 1980–2005. (Peter Cranfield, nickel industry consultant, October 2006.)

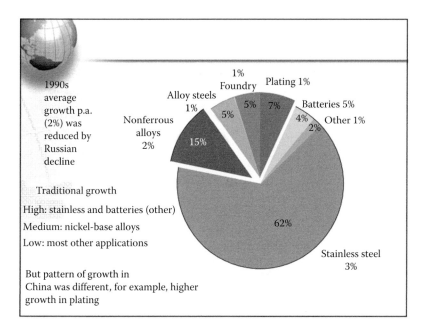

FIGURE 4.25 Global primary nickel by first use. (Peter Cranfield, nickel industry consultant, October 2006.)

ASBESTOS

Exposure to asbestos, one of the most pernicious indoor pollutants, has been linked to disease onset. For decades, scientific evidence of this relationship has been available.[875] Until recently, however, industry and government have, for the most part ignored, the warnings inherent in this evidence.

Tons of materials containing asbestos are used throughout our buildings. It is sprayed into walls, ceiling tiles, and conduits.[875] About 83,000 millions of asbestos water pipes are in use in the United States.[876]

As many as 30% of exposed workers in occupational settings succumb to asbestosis, mesothelioma, and other cancers of the lung, larynx, oral cavity, esophagus, colon, stomach, and kidney.[877] These diseases can result from a brief exposure and have latent periods of possibly 30 years before influencing cancer growth.[812] Studies by Kagen et al.[878] indicated that workers exhibiting either pleural thickening or parenchymal asbestos along with a definite history of occupational exposure to asbestos exhibited significantly reduced levels of IgA, IgG, IgM, and IgE as well as T-lymphocytes. This finding may indicate a possible role of asbestos in the induction of altered immune functioning and, in some cases, of chemical sensitivity.

People living in the area of asbestos and asbestos-using mining and manufacturing facilities, people using asbestos products, and people living in the homes of asbestos workers may suffer the same diseases as the workers. Brief exposures or very low cumulative exposures may produce asbestos-related diseases.[875] Selikoff et al.[880] found that ~15% of all deaths among asbestos workers are caused by mesotheliomas. This finding was reported for others who used these materials as well.

While the insurance industry virtually eliminated coverage for asbestos-related afflictions by 1918 and England regulated asbestos in the early 1930s, the United States waited until the 1970s to take steps toward significant control.[875] Unfortunately, the adopted standards appear inadequate. They currently allow a worker to inhale up to 1.6 billion fibers a day. Mounting evidence points toward synergistic effects of asbestos. One study states that asbestos workers who smoke cigarettes have 90 times more risk of contracting lung cancer than unexposed nonsmokers.[880] Selikoff et al.[880] reported that nonsmoking asbestos workers had few lung cancers, but those who smoked had significantly more lung cancers than would have been predicted had they not been asbestos workers.

TABLE 4.29

Age-Standardized Lung Cancer Death Rates for Cigarette Smoking and/or Occupational Exposure to Asbestos Dust Compared with No Smoking and No Occupational Exposure to Asbestos Dust

Group	Exposure to Asbestos	History Cigarette Smoking	Death Rate	Morality Difference	Mortality Ratio
Control	No	No	11.3	0.0	1.00
Asbestos workers	Yes	No	58.4	+47.1	5.17
Control	No	Yes	122.6	+111.3	10.85
Asbestos workers	Yes	Yes	601.6	+590.3	53.24

Source: Hammond, E. C. et al. 1979. Asbestos exposure, cigarette smoking and death rates. *Ann N. Y. Acad. Sci.* 330:473–490; Rea, W.J. 1994. *Chemical Sensitivity, Volume II*, Page 743, Table 6. With permission.

Note: Rate per 100,000 man-years standardized for age on the distribution of the man-years of all the asbestos workers. Number of lung deaths based on death certificate information.

In contrast to another finding, Selikoff et al.[880] showed that asbestos workers who smoked cigarettes have ~10 times more risk of developing lung cancer death rates as compared with nonsmoking asbestos workers (Table 4.29).

CHLORINE

In industry, chlorine comes from rock salt (NaCl). Chlorine is then used in drinking water and in a variety of industrial practices for the production of chlorinated solvents, for example, CCl_4, CCl_3, trichloroethane, plastics, and vinyl chlorides, etc. Mild mucous membrane irritation may occur at 0.2–16 ppm; eye irritation occurs at 7–8 ppm, throat irritation at 15 ppm, and cough at 30 ppm.[881] In several cases, prolonged symptoms following chlorine exposure may have been caused by aggravation of preexisting conditions, such as tuberculosis or heart disease.[882] Higher concentrations can cause severe poisoning in even shorter periods.[883] Chlorine dioxide also causes similar respiratory ailments.[883] Lower levels of chlorine concentrations can cause irritation of the lower respiratory passages, the eyes, the nose, and the throat. Excess chlorine may put a strain on the dehalogen oxidation and conjugation systems.

The TLV value for chlorine is 1 ppm, corresponding to about 3 mg/m^3,[884] which appears to be too high. In our studies at the EHC-Dallas, we found that some chemically sensitive patients who inhaled chlorine (<0.33 ppm) emanating from hot showers and baths were severely weakened. Also, we found that <0.33 ppm of chlorine triggers vascular phenomena[885] in the chemically sensitive. Further, ~37% of peripheral blood samples of our chemically sensitive patients contain chloroform, and most of these patients experience adverse reactions to chlorine challenge.[886] Since chlorine has a significant adverse impact on the lives of the chemically sensitive, they should avoid exposure to this chemical. They should stay away from chlorinated water used for drinking and bathing and soaps and degreasers.

When combined with organic materials, chlorine in the environment creates trihalomethanes which are very toxic to humans. When these trihalomethanes are subsequently ingested, they severely exacerbate chemical sensitivity.

HYDROGEN CHLORIDE

Hydrogen chloride (HCl) is a strong irritant of the throat and gastrointestinal system. In many cases of HCL poisoning, gastritis and chronic bronchitis have been observed. The TLV value for HCL in air is 5 ppm, corresponding to about 7 mg/m^3.[887] Again, this value is not valid in the susceptible individual. We have found HCl as the #1 sensitivity in the breath of a patient who lived in the middle of a gas field where HCl was used to frack shale to liberate natural gas.

BROMINE

Bromine comes from the mineral magnesium bromide ($CaBr_2$). Bromine is found in swimming pools, fumigants, and medications. Bromine is a respiratory irritant that can cause pulmonary edema. A detectable odor of bromine is produced when the concentration in the air reaches the 3–4 pm value. Excess bromine will put a strain on the detoxification systems involving oxidation and conjugation of halogens, and exposure will exacerbate chemical sensitivity. The TLV value for bromine (Br_2 is 0.1 ppm, which corresponds to about 0.7 mg/m^3).[888] Twenty percent of chemically sensitive patients seen at the EHC-Dallas have bromoforms in their blood.

FLUORINE AND FLUORIDE

Fluoride and fluorine come from fluorspar (CaF_2). Sodium fluoride, sodium fluorosilicates (Na_2SiF_2), and fluoroacetates (FCH_2COOH) are employed as insecticides, rodenticides, and delousing powders. Fluorine causes eye irritation and respiratory problems. Animal experiments have shown fluorine and fluoride only slightly damage pulmonary or renal tissues. The TLV value for fluorine is 1 ppm,[889] but again, this level is unacceptable for the chemically sensitive.

People and trees downwind from factories emanating high levels of fluoride have been found to be damaged. Fluoride placed in drinking water in order to stop dental cavities may be hazardous for some people. Some humans have developed chemical sensitivity from fluorine exposure.

Fluoride is an enzyme inhibitor and is commonly used as an anticoagulant and preservative in biologic specimens. It also increases the density of bones. Fluoride and fluorine cause irritation of the mucous membranes of the eyes, nose, and throat, then nausea, vomiting, respiratory distress, neurological abnormalities, gastrointestinal pain, and muscular fibrillation (tetany). Chronic excess fluoride, perhaps 10–80 mg over years, leads to crippling skeletal deformities characterized by excessive calcification of bone, stiffening of ligaments, and fusion of joints.[890–892]

Fluorocarbon comprises a group of synthetic halogen-substituted methane and ethane derivatives that are found extensively in aerosol propellants and refrigerants. Tons of fluorocarbon is found in the air of some cities. Some people who inhale these may experience environmentally triggered problems such as symptoms previously discussed. Fluorocarbon also destroys the ozone layer, allowing dangerous radiation into the atmosphere.

IODINE

Iodine comes from the mineral sodium iodate ($NaIO_3$) and seaweed. It is used for sterilization and treatment of thyroid problems. Iodine vapor (I_2) is a strong irritant and corrosive chemical, and is more dangerous than chlorine or bromine. In large concentrations in the air, iodine can cause pulmonary edema. Inhalation of iodine vapor causes epiphora, tightness in the chest, sore throat, and headache. Large doses result in pulmonary problems similar to the chlorine exposure. Excess iodine can suppress the thyroid gland. The TLV value of iodine is 0.1 ppm, corresponding to 0.1 mg/m^3.[893]

CYANIDES

Cyanides are compounds that are present in several organic and inorganic forms.

Cyanides are found naturally in apricot seeds, almonds, and walnuts. Cyanides are found in some foods, such as cassava, almonds, apricot pits, in vitamin B_{12}, and in sorghum. They can cause severe problems if the diet is not varied. Excess cyanide will paralyze the respiratory bursts of the cytochrome system and overload the sulfur conjugation detoxification system. Many chemically sensitive patients are sensitive to these cyanide compounds. In addition, damage to the detoxification systems may be so severe that some patients apparently cannot even tolerate vitamin B_{12} because of the cyanocobalamin complex in the B_{12} but they can tolerate hydroxyl or methylcobalamine.

Hydrogen cyanide (HCN) (hydrocyanic acid, prussic acid) is a highly poisonous liquid that smells like bitter almonds. It is manufactured on a large scale from ammonia and methane.

Cyanides are formed as follows: NH_3 and $CH_4 \rightarrow N - CN + 3H_2$. Their economic importance is large, with 450,000 tons produced worldwide in 1970 and 180,000 tons in the United.States in 1977. Production of cyanides has increased over the past 14 years. They are hazardous when used in industry and in agricultural fumigation. In addition to the original use of salt (cyanides) for the extraction of gold, cyanide is mainly used in the production of plastics and synthetic fibers. Cyanides are used in plating or metal hardening operations. Cyanides are used in forming urethanes, polymethacrylates, polyacrylonitrile, and polyamides. Cyanides in the form of alkali cyanide result in epistaxis and nasal ulceration at 5-mg/m³ concentrations. If alkali cyanides are mixed with hydrochloric acid, HCN may be formed. HCN is directly produced in some chemical industrial plants, and exposures at 20 ppm (or even less) may produce serious symptoms, particularly of a neurological nature. Concentrations of 100 ppm (or larger) may be fatal. Over 3000 people died at Bhopal, India, after the noted leak of methylisocyanate, and an estimated 300,000 or more were adversely affected, some of whom may have become chemically sensitive. The TLV value for alkali cyanides is 5 mg/m³.[894]

Toluene diisocynates are used as floor finishers and various other finishes. Diisocynates are very high sensitizers and account for asthma in some workers.

COBALT

Cobalt is used with nickel in manufacturing stainless steel. Pulmonary diseases have been reported with significant frequency in workers associated with the tungsten carbide industry and in workers who have been exposed to excess cobalt metal dust and fumes. In plasma, inorganic cobalt is distributed to albumin. Fourteen percent is deposited in bone, 43% in muscle, and smaller portions are distributed in other tissues, especially the kidney. Serious, and occasionally fatal, responses have occurred from exposures of the order of 1–2 mg/m³ of cobalt in the air. Severe pulmonary disease may occur among workers. The TLV value for cobalt is 0.1 mg/m³.[895] Large doses of cobalt salts enhance proliferation of erythropoietic cells and thyroid gland. Cobalt also has a cardiotoxic effect, and symptoms and signs of chemical sensitivity may be exacerbated by exposure to it.

CHROMIC ACID AND CHROMATES

Chrome-plating operations in different plants expose workers to chromic acid mist that can produce injury to the nasal tissues. Ulcers of the nasal septum; irritation of the mucous membranes of the larynx, pharynx, and conjunctiva; and asthmatic bronchitis have been reported among the workers. Chromium compounds are considered to cause cancer, and a significant increase in lung cancer cases has been observed in workers of chromate plants in England, Germany, and the United States in the 1950s.[896] The TLV value for chromic acid and chromates (as CrO_3) is 0.05 mg/m³.[897]

Chromate dyes are found in many carpets in the United States. These cause problems for the chemically sensitive.

ALUMINUM

Aluminum (Table 4.30) emanates from bauxite factories, antiperspirants, drinking water that has been treated by aluminum flocculation, aluminum cookware, aluminum radiators, and antacids.

TABLE 4.30
Nonprescription Drugs That Contain Aluminum[a]

Drug Class	Al Salts[b] Used	Al Dose (mg)	Possible Daily Al Dose (mg)
Antacids (1)	(a) Aluminum hydroxide	35–208	840–5000
	(b) Dihydroxyaluminum acetate	45–72	
	(c) Aluminum carbonate	NA[c]	
	(d) Aluminum oxide	41	
	(e) Bismuth aluminate	55	
	(f) Magaldrate	51–61	
	(g) Dihydroxyaluminum aminoacetate	100	
	(h) Dihydroxyaluminum sodium carbonate	63	
Internal analgesics	(a) Aluminum hydroxide	9–52	126–728
Buffered aspirins (2)	(b) Aluminum glycinate	10–15	
Antidiarrheals (3)	(a) Kaolin	120–1450	
	(b) Aluminum magnesium silicate	36	
	(c) Attapulgite	500–600	
Douches (4)	(a) Ammonium aluminum sulfate (5%–16%)	NA	
	(b) Potassium aluminum sulfate	NA	
	(c) "Alum"	NA	
Hemorrhoidal medications (5)	(a) Aluminum hydroxide	NA	

Source: Reprinted from Lione, A. 1983. The prophylactic reduction of alumina intake. *Food Chem. Toxicol.* 21(1):103–109. Copyright with kind permission from Pergamon Press, Ltd., Headington Hill Hall. Oxford OX3 OBW, U.K.; Rea, W.J. 1994. *Chemical Sensitivity, Volume II*, Page 748, Table 7. With permission.

[a] Penna, R. P. 1979. *Handbook of Nonprescription Drugs*, 6th ed., p. 205. Washington DC: American Pharmaceutical Association.

[b] Brand names (and manufacturer) for the aluminum salts used in each drug class (Penna, 1970): (1a) Albicon (Pfeiffer), AlternaGel (Stuart), Aludrox (Wyeth), Aluminum Hydroxide Gel (Philips Roxane), Alures (Rexall), Amphojel (Wyeth), A.M.T. (Wyeth), Antacid Powder (DeWitt), Banacid (Buffington), Rasellel Ex. Strength (Wyeth), Camalox (Rorer), Creamalin (Winthrop), Delcid (Merrell-National), Dialume (Armour), Di Gel (Plough), Estomul-M (Riker), Flacid (Amfre-Grant), Gelumina (Amer. Pharm.), Gelusil, M (Warner Chilcott), Geiusil II (Warner-Chilcott), Gelusi, (WEarner-Chilcott), Glycogel (Central Pharm.), Kessadrox (McKesson), Kolantyl (Merrill-National), Kudrox (Kremers-Urban), Liquid Antacide (McKesson), Maalox (Rorer), Maalox Plus (Rorer), Magna Gel (No. American), Magnatril (Lannet), Maxamag (Vitarine), Mylanta (Stuart), Mylanta II (Stuart), Nutrajel (Cenci), Pama (No. American), Silain-Gel (Robins), Syntrogel (Block), TGrimagel (Columbia Medical, TGrisogei (Lilly), WinGel (Winthrop); (1b) Aluscop (O'Neal); (1c) Basaljel (Wyeth) (1d) Magnesia and Alumina Oral (Philips Roxane) (1e) Noralae (No. American) (1f) Rioplan (Ayerst), Riopan Plus (Ayerst); (1 g) Robalate (Rocins); (1 h) Rolaids (Warner-Lambert); (2a) Arthritis Pain Formula (Whitehall), Ascriptin (Roer), Ascriptin A.D. (Rorer), B-a (O'Neal, Jones, and Feldman), Pabrin (Dorsey), Cama (Dorsey), Cope (Glenbrook), Vanquish Caplet (Gienbrook); (2b) Arthritis Strength Bufferin(Bristol-Myers), Bufferin (Bristol-Myers) (3a) Amogel (No. American), Bislad (Central), Diabismul (O'Neal, Jones & Feldman), Donngel-PG (Robins), Donnagel (Robins), Kaolin Pectin Suspension(Philips Roxane), Kaopectate (Upjohn), Kaopectate Concentrate (Upjohn), Parepectolin (Rorer), Pargel (Parke-Davis), Pektamalt (Warren-Teed); (3b) Pabisol with Paregoric (Rexall); (3c) Quintess (Lilly),k Rheaban (Pfizer) (4a) Massengil Douche Powder (Beecham Products), PMC Douche Powder (Thomas & Thompson); (4b) BoCarAl (Calgon), Summer's Eve (Personal Labs); (4c) V.A. (Norfcliff-Thayer).

[c] NA = not available.

Although aluminum is not thought to have any required essential metabolic function in man,[898–901] it is known to be absorbed by inhalation, transdermally, and gastrointestinally. Once absorbed, it can be stored in a variety of body tissues. The likelihood that it will be stored increases if kidney disease or other chronic illnesses are present.

Aluminum oxide, or alumina, appears mainly in the form of particulates in the air, and mainly china and pottery workers, bauxite mining workers, and aluminum refining workers are exposed to alumina fumes. Alumina particles of the size of 2 μm may be highly fibrogenic. The TLV value for aluminum oxide is 10 mg/m^3.[901] Other contaminations can come from heaters, cooking wares, antacids, public drinking water, and deodorants. There are also some food additives containing aluminum. These are sodium aluminum phosphates, aluminum sulfates, alums for pickling agents, and aluminum silicates used as anticaking agents and in chewing gums.

The aluminum ion (Al^{+3}) is one of the smallest ions known, with a very high electrical density, and biologic complexes tend to be very stable, once formed. Aluminum causes ion linkage between large molecules, a possible mechanism for carcinogenesis.[902,903] It is also toxic to enzyme hexokinase[904] and inhibits transaminations.[905] Gonadotoxic effects are similar to those of lead. Aluminum has been found to be teratogenic when administered to pregnant rats.[906] It has been noted to severely exacerbate chemical sensitivity.

Aluminum and Mineral Metabolism

Several reports now suggest that a high aluminum intake may have adverse effects on the metabolism of phosphorus, calcium, and fluoride in the human body and may induce or intensify skeletal abnormalities.[907] This fact may explain the altered calcium and phosphorus measured in some chemically sensitive patients.

The development of osteomalacia with pseudofractures as a result of the ingestion of aluminum hydroxide was first reported in 1960.[908] Lotz, Zisman, and Bartter[909] also described a phosphorus-depletion syndrome that was associated with chronic ingestion of large amounts of aluminum-containing antacids. The interaction of aluminum with dietary phosphorus can increase fecal excretion of phosphorus, decrease urinary phosphorus, and increase urinary calcium. These effects on mineral metabolism have been reported after relatively short periods of aluminum intake[910] and when small doses of aluminum-containing antacids have been administered.[911,912]

Recent studies have indicated that intestinal absorption of calcium is unchanged during the intake of aluminum-containing antacids,[913] suggesting that the elevation of urinary calcium caused by the aluminum-containing antacids may reflect increased bone resorption induced by phosphorus depletion.[909,911] Oarjubsib et al.,[914] reviewed the role of aluminum overload in the severe vitamin D-resistant osteomalacia ("Newcastle bone disease") that occurs in some patients with chronic renal failure.

Aluminum-containing antacids markedly decrease the absorption of fluoride in human subjects.[915,916] Fluoride may be important for the maintenance of normal bone structure, and several investigators described fluoride as an effective form of treatment for osteoporosis.[917–919] Other reports suggest that by interfering with the absorption of fluoride, the aluminum-containing antacids may contribute to the development of skeletal weakness and demineralization.[911,915,916]

Aluminum and the Parathyroid Glands

Mayor et al.[918] reported a significant positive correlation between the concentration of serum parathyroid hormone and aluminum in a group of 39 patients on renal dialysis. Some reports have suggested a role of parathyroid hormone in the uptake of aluminum from the gut.[918,920] Alfrey[921] critically reviewed these findings.

Conn et al.[922] analyzed the aluminum content of various human tissue and found that the parathyroid glands concentrate aluminum selectively. These investigators also found that the aluminum concentration in the parathyroid of patients who reported consuming aluminum-containing drugs was significantly higher than in a group of control subjects.

Aluminum Neurotoxicity

The encephalopathies that can be induced in cats and rabbits by toxic doses of aluminum have been characterized and studied extensively.[923–935] Some reports of aluminum-induced brain degeneration were initially criticized as physiologically irrelevant because the aluminum was administered intracranially. However, additional work has shown that extracranial administration of aluminum and intracranial aluminum produce forms of experimental brain degeneration that are indistinguishable from each other.[933]

The neurotoxicity of aluminum to patients with severe renal impairment was first reported by Alfrey et al.[936] These researchers demonstrated that uremic patients who died of dialysis-associated encephalopathy, "dialysis dementia," had significantly higher levels of aluminum in muscle, bone, and brain tissue than did control subjects or other dialysis patients.[937,938] Collaborative findings have also been reported[939–941] and have been reviewed in detail by Parkinson et al.[914]

Kaehny et al.[942] demonstrated the efficient transfer of dialysate aluminum into uremic patients during hemodialysis. The role of gastrointestinally absorbed aluminum in the encephalopathies developed by uremic patients has been described by several researchers who studied the incidence of degenerative brain disease in uremic patients who were not dialyzed.[943–946] These researchers reported that readministration of aluminum-containing drugs to two uremic patients was followed by recurrent encephalopathy, which was reversed only when oral aluminum intake was again restricted.

Craper and DeBoni[930] reviewed the existing evidence that implicates aluminum as a possible toxic agent in Alzheimer's disease. The characteristic pathology of this disease is the presence of degenerate brain cells that contain large cluster of tangle neurofilaments.[947] Peri and Brody[948] have recently shown that high concentrations of aluminum are bound to the nuclei of cells that display this distinctive neurofibrillary degeneration.

The nuclear binding of aluminum within the brain cells of patients with Alzheimer's disease[907] is consistent with earlier reports that showed elevated brain aluminum in patients with senile dementia of the Alzheimer's type[949,950] and histochemical association of brain aluminum with the nuclear chromatin in homogenized brain tissue from patients with Alzheimer's disease.[949] Some patients with chemical sensitivity react severely to aluminum exposure. Headaches and other vascular phenomena have been observed.

Nanoaluminum: Neurodegenerative and Neurodevelopmental Effects to Combat Global Warming

According to Blaylock,[951] there has been major concern that there is evidence that they are spraying tons of nanosized aluminum compounds. It has been demonstrated in the scientific and medical literature that nanosized particles are infinitely more reactive and induce intense inflammation in a number of tissues. Of special concern is the effect of these nanoparticles on the brain and spinal cord, as a growing list of neurodegenerative diseases, including Alzheimer's dementia, Parkinson's disease, and ALS disease, are strongly related to exposure to environmental aluminum.

Nanoparticles of aluminum are not only infinitely more inflammatory but also they easily penetrate the brain by a number of routes, including the blood and olfactory nerves. Studies have shown that these particles pass along the olfactory neural tracts, which connect directly to the area of the brain that is not only most effected by Alzheimer's disease, but also the earliest affected in the course of the disease. It also has the highest level of brain aluminum in Alzheimer's cases.

The intranasal route of exposure makes spraying of massive amounts of nanoaluminum into the skies especially hazardous, as it will be inhaled by people of all ages, including babies and small children for several hours. We know that older people have the greatest reaction to this airborne aluminum. Owing to the nanosizing of the aluminum particles being used, home filtering system will not remove the aluminum, thus prolonging exposure, even indoors.

Manganese

According to Kraft and Harry,[952] the vulnerability of the nigrostriatal dopaminergic pathway and the whole of this pathway in Parkinson's disease (PD) has been the focus of several studies examining the contribution of neuroinflammation to neuronal death. These efforts have focused on environmental agents that can produce similar clinical symptoms while sparing the nigral neurons[953] (e.g., manganese), or insults that lead to the loss of dopaminergic neurons (e.g., sepsis and rotenone).[954] A role of neuroinflammation and associated microglial or astrocyte responses has been suggested for a number of these exposure models. However, in the case of rotenone, although microglial activation and elevated neuroinflammatory factors are often observed, the reproducibility and robustness of nigral degeneration is widely variable.[955] However, this toxic has been observed to increase chemical sensitivity and chronic degenerative disease from breast implants.

Excessive occupational exposure to Mn as a component of welding fumes and mining has been associated with neuronal damage in the globus pallidus, with less severe damage in the striatum and minimal damage in other basal ganglia structures, such as the substantia nigra, that are routinely affected in PD.[956,957] In addition, Mn-exposed patients do not respond well to the classic PD levodopa therapy,[958–960] which may be related to both the lack of evidence of nigral neuron loss and damage to striatal or pallidal neurons possessing dopamine receptors capable of responding to the treatment. This lack of response can do with inability to decrease the levels or remove the Mn. Clinically, Mn-induced Parkinsonism is often associated with a high-frequency, postural, or kinetic tremor, but not the dyskinesia or resting tremor common in PD. Experimental models of primate exposure have confirmed a similar neuropathological profile with motor disturbances, neuronal loss, and gliosis in the globus pallidus, and a lack of responsiveness to levodopa treatment.[961] Recent work using positron emission tomography (PET) in nonhuman primates reported a marked decrease in dopamine release associated with elevated brain Mn levels.[962,963] Further work suggested a selective effect of Mn on the substantia nigra pars reticulate (SNr), as compared to the substantia nigra pars compacta (SNc). Interestingly, in young (5–6-year-old) nonhuman primates exposed to 5–6.7 mg Mn/kg body weight, 2 times/week/32–34 weeks, microglia within the SNc and SNr displayed retracted processes. In the SNr, microglia displayed morphology suggestive of a disintegration of distal processes.[964] The morphological pattern of dysmorphic microglia was similar to that observed in the aging brain and with neurodegenerative disorders,[965,966] suggesting that Mn exposure may have an adverse effect upon microglia and thus significantly influence the microenvironment of the dopaminergic neurons. Some chemically sensitive patients do have high red blood cells levels of Mn which could make them prone to Parkinson's or other neurological disorders.

Experimental rodent studies have attempted to model the human neurodegenerative effects of manganese; however, in several cases the rodent does not show sensitivity to manganese neurotoxicity and often fails to demonstrate the clinical signs relevant to the human and nonhuman primate. Recent work by Sriram et al.[967] suggested that direct pulmonary exposure of rats once a week for 7 weeks to complex mixtures of welding fumes containing either high or low levels of manganese, resulted in pulmonary inflammation, cytotoxicity, and, particularly with the high-Mn exposure, deposition of Mn within various brain regions, including the striatum and midbrain. Within 1 day post exposure, the midbrain showed a lower mRNA level for the dopamine D2 receptor and loss of TH protein with either exposure.

While this TH loss appeared to be transient and recovered in the low-Mn group, this effect persisted in animals exposed to high-Mn fumes beyond 105 days postexposure. In the midbrain, mRNA levels for the inflammatory factors, CXCL2, TNF-α, and IL-6 were unchanged in the high-Mn group and only TNF-α was increased in the low-Mn exposure group. This increase in TNF-α may have significant cause in the chemically sensitive group of patients.

In the striatum, however, mRNA levels for all three factors were elevated in both exposure groups. Interestingly, although the TH loss persisted, these inflammatory indicators were resolved by 105 days postexposure, mRNA levels for NOS2 were elevated in both exposure groups in both the striatum and the midbrain, but NOS1, NOS3, COX-2, and HO-1 mRNA levels remained unchanged. A microglial response, as determined by increased mRNA levels for Emr1 (f/80) and Itgam (OX42) in the midbrain, accompanied the TH loss in the striatum and midbrain of the high-Mn exposure group only.

However, these indicators of microglial activation recovered by 105 days postexposure, with the only change persisting alongside the midbrain TH loss being a decrease in GFAP levels for astrocytes. Of interest is the speculation that the changes observed, including cytotoxicity, were due to Mn exposure.

As previously stated, there is no clear evidence in human subjects or nonhuman primates that moderate levels of Mn initiate degeneration of dopaminergic pathways.[953] Thus, this data may reflect species differences or a synergy of Mn with other components of the complex mixtures of welding fumes. In any case, there series of experiments demonstrate the complex nature of examining markers of neuroinflammation, gliosis, and neuronal alterations *in vivo*, reiterating the need for multiple markers, regions, and times of examination in any interpretation of such effects.

Further studies examining the impact of inflammatory factors on manganese-induced dopaminergic neuron death have focused primarily on *in vitro* culture systems. Using an N9 microglial cell line, Chang and Liu[968] reported that manganese could exacerbate LPS-induced NO production. Such data raises the possibility that manganese exposure can alter the homeostatic balance of the brain, resulting in a system that is primed or preconditioned to respond differently upon classical activation of the immune system. Additional work suggested that the increased production of pro-inflammatory cytokines by LPS-activated microglia exposed to Mn was associated with increased and persistent activation of p38 kinase.[969]

Certainly, increased exposures to Mn resulting in the increased RBC Mn which occurs over years may continue to aggravate the CNS and eventually exceed its total Mn pollutant load and cause nerve damage. Also, the chemically sensitive may be exposed to other pollutants simultaneously which could cause a synergic reaction putting the individual over the threshold causing irreparable CNS damage.

Recent work using cocultured astrocytes/microglia and neurons suggested that $MnCl_2$ did not alter the number of TH-immunoreactive neurons until the concentrations reached 30 μM.[970] When cocultures were exposed to both $MnCl_2$ and LPS, a loss of TH[+] cells was observed at a lower dose. $MnCl_2$ exposure alone was not sufficient to elevate the protein levels, even at the 30 μM dose level for which TH[+] cell loss was observed. LPS, however, induced the production of TNF-α, IL-1β, and nitrite revealed that $MnCl_2$ exposure alone was not sufficient to elevate the protein levels, even at the 30 μM dose level for which TH[+] cell loss was observed. LPS, however, induced the production of TNF-α, IL-1β, and nitrite. The data at the high LPS dose level (2 ng/mL) suggested a synergistic effect of coexposure to $MnCl_2$ with a significant increase seen at $MnCl_2$ levels of 3 μM and above. Upon further examination, $MnCl_2$ was found to significantly potentiate LPS-induced release of TNF-1 an IL-1β in microglia, but not in astroglia. $MnCl_2$ and LPS were also more effective in inducing the formation of ROS and NO in microglia than in astroglia. Additionally, $MnCl_2$ and LPS-induced ROS and RNS generation, cytokine release, and dopamine neurotoxicity were significantly attenuated by pretreatment with the potential anti-inflammatory agents, minocycline and naloxone.[970]

Platinum

Platinum in the form of complex states (chloroplatinates, cis-platinum) may cause asthma and rhinitis when inhaled in 2–20 μg/m³ concentrations. The TLV value for soluble salts of platinum is 0.002 mg/m³.[971] Cis-platinum is a common anticancer drug.

CONCLUSION

The measures required for the control and elimination of inorganic air and oral pollutants depend on their chemical and physical characteristics. A general approach should be the elimination of their emissions into the air. If not possible, then improvement of ventilation and filtering of the circulated inside air is essential.

To control outdoor inorganic air pollutants, the Clean Air Act has set National Ambient Air Quality Standards for the criteria pollutants and national emission standards for hazardous air pollutants. These are not often met, and even when they are, they appear to be too high.[972] The objective should be to control these pollutants at the source by not allowing them into the air. It is clear that most, even in small doses, can bother the chemically sensitive who are exposed to them. However, understanding the total environmental pollutant load in relation to the total body pollutant load is paramount in helping the environmentally damaged, chemically sensitive, and EMS-sensitive patient.

REFERENCES

1. Suner, S., G. Jay. 2008. Carbon monoxide has direct toxicity on the myocardium distinct from effects of hypoxia in an *ex vivo* rat heart model. *Acad. Emerg. Med.* 15:59–65.
2. Rea, W. J. 1992. *Chemical Sensitivity*, Vol. 1, p. 47. Boca Raton, FL: Lewis Publishers.
3. Meyer, G., S. Tanguy, P. Obert, C. Reboul. 2011. Carbon monoxide urban air pollution: Cardiac effects. In *Advanced Topics in Environmental Health and Air Pollution Case Studies*, A. Moldoveanu, ed., pp. 171–173. New York: InTech.
4. Miranda, A. I., V. Martins, P. Cascão, J. H. Amorim, J. Valente, C. Borrego, A. J. Ferreira, C. R. Cordeiro, D. X. Viegas, R. Ottmar. 2012. Wildland smoke exposure values and exhaled breath indicators in firefighters. *J. Toxicol. Environ. Health A* 75:831–843.
5. Dallas, M. L. et al. 2012. Carbon monoxide induces cardiac arrhythmia via induction of the late Na$^+$ current. *Am. J. Respir. Crit. Care. Med.* 186:648–656.
6. Kerin E. J. et al. 2006. Mercury methylation by dissimilatory iron-reducing bacteria. *Appl. Environ. Microbiol.* 72:7919. doi:10.1128/AEM.01602-06 Medline.
7. Bauer, M. A., J. J. Utell, P. E. Morrow, D. M. Speers, F. R. Gibb. 1984. 0.30 ppm nitrogen dioxide inhalation potentiates exercise-induced bronchospasm in asthmatics. *Am. Rev. Respir. Dis.* 129:151.
8. Melia, J., C. Florey, Y. Sittampalam, C. Watkins. 1983. The relation between respiratory illness in infants and gas cooking in the U.K.: A preliminary report. In *Air Quality 6th World Congress: Proceeding International Union of Air Pollution Prevention Association*. Paris: SEPIC (APPA). pp. 263–269.
9. Melia, R. J. W., C. du Ve Florey, R. W. Morris, B. D. Goldstein, D. Clark, H. H. John. 1982. Childhood respiratory illness and the home environment. I. Relations between nitrogen dioxide, temperature, and relative humidity. *Int. J. Epidemiol.* 2:155–163.
10. Melia, R. J. W., C. du Ve Florey, R. W. Morris, B. D. Goldstein, D. Clark, H. H. John, I. B. Craighead, J. C. Mackinlay. 1982. Childhood respiratory illness and the home environment II. Association between respiratory illness and nitrogen dioxide, temperature and relative humidity. *Int. J. Epidemiol.* 2:164–169.
11. Ware, J. H., D. W. Dockery, A. Spiro III, F. E. Speizer, B. G. Ferris Jr. 1984. Passive smoking, gas cooking, and respiratory health of children living in six cities. *Am. Rev. Dis.* 129:366–374.
12. Kuraitis, K., A. Richters, R. P. Sherwin. 1981. Spleen changes in animals inhaling ambient levels of nitrogen dioxide. *J. Toxicol. Environ. Health* 7:851–859.
13. McGrath, J. J., F. J. Oyervides. 1982. Response of NO$_2$ exposed mice to Klebsiella challenge. In *Int. Symp. on the Biomedical Effects of Ozone and Related Photochemical Oxidants*, N. C. Pinehurst, S. D. Lee, M. G. Mustafa, M. A. Mehlman, eds., Princeton, NJ: Princeton Scientific Publications.
14. Ranchou-Peyruse, M. et al. 2009. Overview of mercury methylation capacities among anaerobic bacteria including representatives of the sulphate-reducers: Implications for environmental studies. *Geomicrobiol. J.* 26:1. doi:10.1080/01490450802599227.
15. Gilmour, C. C. et al. 2011. Sulfate-reducing bacterium *Desulfovibrio desulfuricans* ND132 as a model for understanding bacterial mercury methylation. *Appl. Environ. Microbiol.* 77:3938. doi:10.1128/AEM.02993-10 Medline.
16. Kleinman, M. R., R. M. Bailey, W. S. Linn, K. R. Anderson, J. D. Whynot, D. A. Shamoo, J. D. Hackney. 1983. Effects of 0.2 ppm nitrogen dioxide on pulmonary function and response to bronchoprovocation in asthmatics. *J. Toxicol. Environ. Health* 12:815–826.
17. Hazucha, M. J., J. F. Ginsberg, W. F. McDonnell, E. O. Haak Jr., R. L. Pimmel, S. A. Sallam, D. E. House, P. A. Bromberg. 1983. Effects of 0.1 ppm nitrogen dioxide on airways of normal and asthmatic subjects. *J. Appl. Physiol. Respir. Environ. Exer. Physiol.* 54:730–739.
18. Speizer, F. E., B. J. Ferris, Y. W. Bishop, J. Spengler. 1980. Respiratory disease rates and pulmonary function in children associated with NO$_2$ exposure. *Am. Respir. Dis.* 121(1):3–10.
19. Richters, A., V. Richters. 1983. A new relationship between air pollutant inhalation and cancer. *Arch. Environ. Health* 38:69–75.

20. Richters, A., K. Kuraitis. 1981. Inhalation of NO_2 and blood-borne cancer cell spread to the lungs. *Arch. Environ. Health* 36:36–39.

21. Lefkowitz, S. S., J. J. McGrath, D. L. Lefkowitz. 1982. Effects of NO_2 on interferon production in mice. In *Int. Symp. on the Biomedical Effects of Ozone and Related Photochemical Oxidants*, N. C. Pinehurst, S. D. Lee, M. G. Mustafa, M. A. Mehlman, eds., Princeton, NJ: Princeton Scientific Publications.

22. Brown, S. D. et al. 2011. Genome sequence of the mercury-methylating strain *Desulfovibrio desulfuricans* ND132. *J. Bacteriol.* 193:2078. doi:10.1128/JB.00170-11 Medline.

23. Trudel, J. R. 1985. Metabolism of nitrous oxide. In *Nitrous Oxide*, E. Eger II, ed., pp. 203–208. New York: Elsevier.

24. Brodsky, J. B. 1985. Toxicity of nitrous oxide. In *Nitrous Oxide*, E. Eger II, ed., p. 269. New York: Elsevier.

25. Snyder, S. H., D. S. Bredt. 1992. Biological roles of nitric oxide. *Sci. Am.* 266(5):68–77.

26. Hopp, V., I. Hennig. 1983. *Handbook of Applied Chemistry: Facts for Engineers, Scientists, Technicians, and Technical Managers*, Vol. II, pp. 3–16. Washington, DC: Hemisphere Publishing.

27. Miñana, M. D., V. Felipo, S. Grisolia. 1989. Assembly and disassembly of brain tubulin is affected by high ammonia levels. *Neurochem. Res.* 14(3):235–238.

28. American Conference of the Governmental Industrial Hygienists. 1976. *Ammonia. Documentation for the TLVs for Substances in Workroom Air*, 3rd ed., p. 289. Cincinnati: Signature Publications.

29. Baselt, R. C., ed. 1982. *Disposition of Toxic Drugs and Chemicals in Man*, 2nd ed., p. 120. Davis, CA: Biomedical Publications.

30. Delfino, R. J., H. Gong, W. S. Linn, Y. Hu, E. D. Pellizzari. 2003. Respiratory symptoms and peak expiratory flow in children with asthma in relation to volatile organic compounds in exhaled breath and ambient air. *J. Expo. Anal. Environ. Epidemiol.* 13(5):348–363.

31. Smargiassi, A., T. Kosatsky, J. Hicks, C. Plante, B. Armstrong, P. J. Villeneuve, S. Goudreau. 2009. Risk of asthmatic episodes in children exposed to sulphur dioxide stack emissions from a refinery point source in Montreal, Canada. *Environ. Health Perspect.* 117:653–659.

32. Segala, C., B. Fauroux, J. Just, L. Pascual, A. Grimfeld, F. Neukirch. 2002. Short-term health effects of particulate and photochemical air pollution in asthmatic children. *Eur. Resp. J.* 20(4):899–906.

33. Bascom, R., P. A. Bromberg, C. Hill. 1996. Health effects of outdoor air pollution (Part 1). *Am. J. Respir. Crit. Care. Med.* 153:3–50.

34. Schwartz, J. 1994. Air pollution and daily mortality: A review and meta-analysis. *Environ. Res.* 64:36–52.

35. Dockery, D. W., F. E. Speizer, D. O. Stram, J. H. Ware, J. D. Spengler, B. J. Ferris. 1989. Effects of inhalable particles on respiratory health of children. *Am. Rev. Respir. Dis.* 139:587–594.

36. Sandström, T. 1995. Respiratory effects of air pollutants: Experimental studies in humans. *Eur. Resp. J.* 8:976–995.

37. von Mutius, E., C. Fritzsch, S. K. Weiland, G. Röll, H. Magnussen. 1992. Prevalence of asthma and allergic disorders among children in united Germany: A descriptive comparison. *BMJ.* 305:1395–1399.

38. Braback, L., A. Breborowicz, S. Dreberg, A. Knutsson, H. Pieklik, B. Björkstein. 1994. Atopic sensitization and respiratory symptoms among Polish and Swedish school children. *Clin. Exp. Allergy* 24:826–835.

39. Forastière, F., G. M. Corbo, R. Pistelli, P. Michelozzi, N. Agabiti, G. Brancato, G. Ciappi, C. A. Perucci. 1994. Bronchial responsiveness in children in areas with different air pollution levels. *Arch. Environ. Health* 49:111–118.

40. Pönkä, A. 1991. Asthma and low level air pollution in Helsinki. *Arch. Environ. Health* 46:262–270.

41. Rossi, O. V. J., V. L. Kinnula, J. Tienari, E. Huhti. 1993. Association of severe asthma attacks with weather, pollen and air pollutants. *Thorax* 48:244–248.

42. Schwartz, J., D. Slater, T. V. Larson, W. E. Pierson, J. Q. Koenig. 1993. Particulate air pollution and hospital emergency room visits for asthma in Seattle. *Am. Rev. Respir. Dis.* 147:826–831.

43. Walters, S., R. K. Griffiths, J. G. Ayres. 1994. Temporal associations between hospital admissions for asthma in Birmingham and ambient levels of sulphur dioxide and smoke. *Thorax* 49:133–140.

44. Romieu, I., F. Meneses, J. Jose, J. J. Sienra-Monge, S. Huerta, S. Ruiz Velasco, M. C. White, R. A. Etzel, M. Hernandez-Avila. 1995. Effects of urban air pollutants on emergency visits for childhood asthma in Mexico City. *Am. J. Epidemiol.* 141:546–553.

45. Perry, G. B., H. Chai, W. Dickey, R. H. Jones, R. A. Kinsman, C. G. Morrill, S. L. Spector, P. C. Weiser. 1983. Effects of particulate air pollution on asthmatics. *Am. J. Public Health* 73:50–56.

46. Bridou, R., M. Monperrus, P. R. Gonzalez, R. Guyoneaud, D. Amouroux. 2011. Simultaneous determination of mercury methylation and demethylation capacities of various sulfate-reducing bacteria using species-specific isotopic tracers. *Environ. Toxicol. Chem.* 30:337. doi:10.1002/etc.395 Medline.

47. Moselholm, L., E. Taudorf, A. Frosig. 1993. Pulmonary function changes in asthmatics associated with low-level SO_2 and NO_2 air pollution, weather and medicine intake. *Allergy* 48:334–344.

48. Higgins, B. G., H. C. Francis, C. J. Yates, C. J. Warburton, A. M. Fletcher, J. A. Reid, C. A. Pickering, A. A. Woodcock. 1995. Effects of air pollution on symptoms and peak expiratory flow measurements in subjects with obstructive airways disease. *Thorax* 50:149–155.

49. Pope, C. A., D. W. Dockery, J. D. Spengler, M. E. Raizenne. 1991. Respiratory health and PM10 pollution. *Am. Rev. Respir. Dis.* 144:668–674.

50. Pope, C. A., D. W. Dockery. 1992. Acute health effects of PM10 pollution on symptomatic and asymptomatic children. *Am. Rev. Respir. Dis.* 145:1123–1128.

51. Roemer, W., G. Hoek, B. Brunekreef. 1993. Effects of ambient air pollution on respiratory health of children with chronic respiratory symptoms. *Am. Rev. Respir. Dis.* 147:118–124.

52. Ostro, B. D., M. J. Lipsett, J. K. Mann. 1995. Air pollution and asthma exacerbations among African-American children in Los Angeles. *Inhal. Toxicol.* 7:711–722.

53. Peters, A., D. W. Dockery, J. Heinrich, H. E. Wichmann. 1997. Short-term effects of particulate air pollution on respiratory morbidity in asthmatic children. *Eur. Respir. J.* 10:872–879.

54. Vedal, S., M. B. Schenker, A. Munoz, J. Samet, S. Batterman, F. E. Speizer. 1987. Daily air pollution effects on children's respiratory symptoms and peak expiratory flow. *Am. J. Public Health* 77:694–698.

55. Forsberg, B., N. Stjemberg, M. Falk, B. Lundbäck, S. Wall. 1993. Air pollution levels, meteorological conditions and asthma symptoms. *Eur. Respir. J.* 6:1109–1115.

56. Peters, A., I. F. Goldstein, U. Beyer, K. Franke, J. Heinrich, D. W. Dockery, J. D. Spengler, H. E. Wichmann. 1996. Acute effects of exposure to high levels of air pollution in Eastern Europe. *Am. J. Epidemiol.* 144:570–581.

57. Schwartz, J., D. Wypij, D. Dockery, J. Ware, S. Zeger, J. Spengler, B. Ferris Jr. 1991. Daily diaries of respiratory symptoms and air pollution: Methodological issues and results. *Environ. Health Perspect.* 90:181–187.

58. Braun-Fahdländer, C., U. Ackermann-Liebrich, J. Schwartz, H. P. Gnehm, M. Rutishauser, H. U. Wanner. 1992. Air pollution and respiratory symptoms in preschool children. *Am. Rev. Respir. Dis.* 145:42–47.

59. Rutishauser, M., U. Ackermann, C. Braun, H. P. Gnehm, H. U. Wanner. 1990. Significant associations between outdoor NO_2 and respiratory symptoms in preschool children. *Lung* 168(Suppl 1):347–352.

60. Mostardi, R. A., N. R. Woebkenberg, D. L. Ely, M. Conlon, G. Atwood. 1981. The University of Akron study on air pollution and human health effects II. Effects on acute respiratory illness. *Arch. Environ. Health* 36:250–255.

61. Bascom, R., P. A. Bromberg, D. L. Costa. 1996. Health effects of outdoor air pollution (Part 2). *Am. J. Respir. Crit. Care. Med.* 153:477–498.

62. von Mutius, E., D. L. Sherill, C. Fritzsch, F. D. Martinez, M. D. Lebowitz. 1995. Air pollution and upper respiratory symptoms in children from East Germany. *Eur. Respir. J.* 8:723–728.

63. Jaakkola, J. J. K., M. Paunio, M. Virtanen, O. P. Heinonen. 1991. Low-level air pollution and upper respiratory infections in children. *Am. J. Public Health* 81:1060–1063.

64. Beer, S. I., Y. I. Kannai, M. J. Waron. 1991. Acute exacerbation of bronchial asthma in children associated with afternoon weather changes. *Am. Rev. Respir. Dis.* 144:31–35.

65. Dales, R. E., I. Shweitzer, J. H. Toogood, M. Drouin, W. Yang, J. Dolovich, J. Boulet. 1996. Respiratory infections and the autumn increase in asthma morbidity. *Eur. Respir. J.* 9:72–77.

66. Zureik, M., R. Liard, C. Ségala, C. Henry, M. Korobaeff, F. Neukirch. 1995. Peak expiratory flow rate variability in population surveys: Does the number of assessment matter? *Chest* 107:418–423.

67. Graham, A. M., A. L. Bullock, A. C. Maizel, D. A. Elias, C. C. Gilmour. 2012. Detailed assessment of the kinetics of Hg-cell association, Hg methylation, and methylmercury degradation in several *Desulfovibrio* species. *Appl. Environ. Microbiol.* 78:7337. doi:10.1128/AEM.01792-12.

68. King, J. K., J. E. Kostka, M. E. Frischer, F. M. Saunders. 2000. Sulfate-reducing bacteria methylate mercury at variable rates in pure culture and in marine sediments. *Appl. Environ. Microbiol.* 66:2430. doi:10.1128/AEM.66.6.2430-2437.2000 Medline.

69. Quackenboss, J. J., M. D. Lebowitz, C. D. Crutchfield. 1989. Indoor-outdoor relationships for particulate matter: Exposure classifications and health effects. *Environ. Int.* 15:353–360.

70. Fontelle, J. P., N. Audoux, F. Moisson. 1992. *Inventaire des émissions SO2, NOx, poussières, COV, CH4 dans l'atmosphère d'Ile de France 1990*. Rapport CITEPA.

71. Société Française de Santé Publique. 1996. *La pollution atmosphérique d'origine automobile et la santé publique. Bilan de 15 ans de recherche internationale*. Collection Santé et Société No. 4, Paris.

72. Medina, S., W. Dab, P. Quénel, R. Ferry, B. Festy. 1996. La pollution atmosphérique urbaine pose toujours un problème de santé publique à Paris. *Forun Mondial de la Santé* 17:196–202.

73. Moseler, M., A. Hendel-Kramer, W. Karmaus, J. Forster, K. Weiss, R. Urbanek, J. Kuehr. 1994. Effect of moderate NO_2 air pollution on the lung function of children with asthmatic symptoms. *Environ. Res.* 67:109–124.

74. Samet, J. M., M. J. Utell. 1990. The risk of nitrogen dioxide: What we have learned from epidemiological and clinical studies? *Toxicol. Ind. Health* 6:247–262.

75. Dassen, W., B. Brunekreef, G. Hoek, P. Hofschreuder, B. Staatsen, H. de Groot, E. Schouten, K. Biersteker. 1986. Decline in children's pulmonary function during an air pollution episode. *J. Air Pollut. Control Assoc.* 36:1223–1227.

76. Brunekreef, B., P. L. Kinney, J. H. Ware, D. Dockery, F. E. Speizer, J. D. Spengler, B. G. Ferris Jr. 1991. Sensitive subgroups and normal variation in pulmonary function response to air pollution episodes. *Environ. Health Perspect.* 90:189–193.

77. Dockery, D. W., J. H. Ware, B. G. Ferris Jr., F. E. Speizer, N. R. Cook, S. M. Herman. 1982. Change in pulmonary function in children associated with air pollution episodes. *J. Air Pollut. Control Assoc.* 32:937–942.

78. Lunn, J. E., J. Knowelden, A. Handyside. 1967. Patterns of respiratory illness in Sheffield infant school children. *Br. J. Prev. Med.* 21(1):7–16.

79. Lunn, J. E., J. Knopwelden, J. A. Handyside. 1970. Patterns of respiratory illness in Sheffield infant school children. *Br. J. Prev. Med.* 24(4):223–228.

80. Pope, C. A., D. W. Dockery, J. D. Spengler, M. Raizenne. 1991. Respiratory health and PM10 pollution: A daily time series analysis. *Am. Rev. Respir. Dis.* 144(3 Pt 1):668–674.

81. Pope, C. A., D. W. Dockery. 1992. Acute health effects of PM10 pollution on symptomatic and asymptomatic children. *Am. Rev. Respir. Dis.* 145(5):1123–1128.

82. Roemer, W., G. Hoek, B. Brunekreef. 1993. Effects of ambient winter air pollution on respiratory health of children with chronic respiratory symptoms. *Am. Rev. Respir. Dis.* 147(1):118–124.

83. Ware, J. H., B. G. Ferris, D. W. Dockery, J. D. Spengler, D. O. Stram, F. Speizer. 1986. Effects of ambient sulfur oxides and suspended particles on respiratory health of preadolescent children. *Am. Rev. Respir. Dis.* 133(5):834–842.

84. Yang, C. Y., J. D. Wang, C. C. Chan, J. S. Hwang, P. C. Chen. 1997. Respiratory symptoms of primary school children living in a petrochemical polluted area in Taiwan. *Pediatr. Pulm.* 25(5):299–303.

85. Environmental Protection Administration, Republic of China. 1984–1992. *Annual Reports of Air pollution in Taiwan, 1983–1990.* Environmental Protection Administration, Taipei.

86. Randolph, T. G. 1962. *Human Ecology and Susceptibility to the Chemical Environment*, pp. 70–71. Springfield, IL: Charles C. Thomas.

87. American Conference of Governmental Industrial Hygienists. 1974. *Sulfur Dioxide. Documentation of the TLVs for Substances in Workroom Air*, 3rd ed., pp. 238–239. Cincinnati: Signature Publications.

88. Amdur, M. O. 1986. Air pollutants. In *Casarett and Doull's Toxicology: The Basic Science of Poisons*, 3rd ed., C. Klassen, M. O. Amdur, J. Doull, eds., p. 802. New York: Macmillan.

89. Dalgaad, J. N., F. Dencker, B. Fallentin, P. Hansen. 1972. Fatal poisoning and other health hazards connected with industrial fishing. *Br. J. Ind. Med.* 29:307–316.

90. Morse, D. L., M. A. Woodburg, K. Rentmeester, D. Farmser. 1981. Death cause by fermenting manure. *JAMA* 245(1):63–64.

91. Rea, W. J. 1992. *Chemical Sensitivity*, Vol. 1, p. 17. Boca Raton, FL: Lewis Publishers.

92. Balazs, T., J. P. Hanig, E. H. Herman. 1986. Toxic responses of the cardiovascular system. In *Casarett and Doull's Toxicology: The Basic Science of Poisons*, 3rd ed., C. Klassen, M. O. Amdur, J. Doull, eds., p. 802. New York: Macmillan.

93. Amdur, M. O. 1986. Air pollutants. In *Casarett and Doull's Toxicology: The Basic Science of Poisons*, 3rd ed., C. Klassen, M. O. Amdur, J. Doull, eds., pp. 813–405. New York: Macmillan.

94. Ehrlich, R. 1980. Interaction between environmental pollutants and respiratory infections. *Environ. Health Perspect.* 35:89–110.

95. Levine, S. A., P. M. Kidd. 1985. *Antioxidant Adaptation: Its Role in Free Radical Pathology*, p. 88. San Leandro, CA: Biocurrents Division, Allergy Research Group.

96. Hocking, W. G., D. W. Golde. 1979. The pulmonary-alveolar macrophage (Part 2). *N. Engl. J. Med.* 301:639–645.

97. Sarino, A., M. L. Peterson, D. House, A. G. Turner, H. E. Jeffries, R. Baker. 1978. The effect of ozone on human cellular and humoral immunity: Characterization of T and B lymphocytes by rosette formation. *Environ. Res.* 15(1):65–69.

98. Merz, T., M. A. Bender, H. D. Kerr, T. J. Kulie. 1975. Observations of aberrations in chromosomes of lymphocytes from human subjects exposed to ozone at a concentration of 0.5 ppm for 6 and 10 hours. *Mutat. Res.* 31(5):299–302.

99. Levine, S. A., P. M. Kidd. 1985. *Antioxidant Adaptation: Its Role in Free Radical Pathology*, p. 89. San Leandro, CA: Biocurrents Division, Allergy Research Group.

100. Kesner, L., R. J. Kindya, P. C. Chan. 1979. Inhibition of erythorocyte membrane ($Na^+ + K^+$)-activated. ATPase by ozone-treated phospholipids. *J. Biol. Chem.* 254(8):2705–2709.

101. Rage, E., V. Siroux, N. Kunzli, I. Pin, F. Kauffmann. 2009. Air pollution and asthma severity in adults. *Occup. Environ. Med.* 66(3):182–188.

102. Delfino, R. J., R. S. Zeiger, J. M. Seltzer, D. H. Street. 1998. Symptoms in pediatric asthmatics and air pollution: Differences in effects by symptom severity, anti-inflammatory medication use and particulate averaging time. *Environ. Health Perspect.* 106(11):751–761.

103. McDonnell, W. F., D. E. Abbey, N. Nishino, M. D. Lebowitz. 1999. Long-term ambient ozone concentration and the incidence of asthma in nonsmoking adults: The AHSMOG study. *Environ. Res.* 80(2):110–121.

104. Greer, J. R., D. E. Abbey, R. J. Burchette. 1993. Asthma related to occupational and ambient air pollutants in nonsmokers. *J. Occup. Environ. Med.* 4(5):909–915. http://journals.lww.com/joem/Abstract/1993/09000/Asthma_Related_to_Occupational_and_Ambient_Air.14.aspx.

105. Friedman, M. S., K. E. Powell, L. Hutwagner, L. M. Graham, W. G. Teague. 2001. Impact of changes in transportation and commuting behaviors during the 1996 Summer Olympic Games in Atlanta on air quality and childhood asthma. *J. Am. Med. Assoc.* 285(7):897–905.

106. Krzyzanowski M, W. Jeddychowski, M. Wysocki. 1986. Factors associated with change in ventilatory function and development of chronic obstructive pulmonary disease in a 13 year follow-up of the Cracow study: Risk of chronic obstructive pulmonary diseases. *Am. Rev. Respir. Dis.* 134:1011–1019.

107. Lebowitz, M, R. Knudson, B. Burrows. 1975. Tucson epidemiologic study of obstructive lung diseases. I. Methodology and prevalence of disease. *Am. J. Epidemiol.* 102:137–152.

108. Ferris, B. G., F. E. Speizer, J. D. Spengler, D. Dockery, Y. M. Bishop, M. Wolfson, C. Humble. 1979. Effects of sulfur oxides and respirable particles in human health: Methodology and demography of populations in study. *Am. Rev. Respir. Dis.* 120:767–779.

109. Korn, R. J., D. W. Dockery, F. E. Speizer, J. H. Ware, B. G. Ferris. 1987. Occupational exposures and chronic respiratory symptoms: A population based study. *Am. Rev. Respir. Dis.* 136:298–304.

110. Prediletto, R., G. Viegi, P. Paoletti, L. Carrozzi, F. Di Pede, M. Vellutini, C. Di Pede, C. Giuntini, M. D. Lebowitz. 1987. Effects of occupational exposure on respiratory symptoms and lung functions in a general population sample. *Am. Rev. Respir. Dis.* 143(3):135.

111. Lebowitz, M. 1977. Occupational exposures in relation to symtomatology and lung function in a community population. *Environ. Res.* 44:59–67.

112. Becklake, M. R. 1989. Occupational exposures: Evidence for casual association with chronic obstructive pulmonary disease. *Am. Rev. Respir. Dis.* 140(3 pt 2):S85–S91.

113. US Department of Health and Human Services. 1991. *Environmental Tobacco Smoke in the Workplace: Lung Cancer and Other Health Effects.* Cincinnati, OH: US Department of Health and Human Services, Public Health Service, Centers for Disease Control, National Institute for Occupational Safety and Health, DHHS (NIOSH) (pub no. 91-108).

114. Euler, G. L., D. E. Abbey, J. E. Hodgkin, A. R. Magie. 1987. Chronic obstructive pulmonary disease symptoms effects of long-term cumulative exposure to ambient levels of total suspended particulates and sulfur dioxide in California seventh-Day Adventists Residents. *Arch. Environ. Health.* 42:213–222.

115. Abbey, D. E., F. F. Peterson, P. K. Mills, W. L. Beeson. 1993. Long term ambient concentrations of total suspended particulates and ozone and incidence of respiratory symptoms in a nonsmoking population. *Arch Environ Health.* 94:43–50.

116. Abbey, D. E., P. K. Mills, F. F. Peterson, W. L. Beeson. 1991. Long-term ambient concentrations of total suspended particulates and oxidants as related to incidence of chronic disease in California Seventh-Day Adventists. *Arch. Environ. Health.* 94:43–50.

117. McWhorter, W. P., M. A. Polis, R. A. Kaslow. 1989. Occurrence, predictors, and consequences of adult asthma in NHANES I and follow-up survey. *Am. Rev. Respir. Dis.* 139:721–724.

118. Broder, I., M. W. Higgins, K. P. Matthews, J. B. Keller. 1962. Epidemiology of asthma and allergic rhinitis in a total community, Tecmuseh, Michigan. IV. Natural history. *J. Allergy Clin. Immunol.* 54:100–110.

119. Barbee, R. A., R. Dodge, M. L. Lebowitz. 1985. The epidemiology of asthma. *Chest* 83(suppl.):21–25.

120. Lebowitz, M. D., R. J. Knudson, B. Burrows. 1984. Risk factors for airways obstructive disease. *Chest* 85:11S–12S.

121. Burrows, B., R. A. Barbee, M. Cline, R. J. Knudson, M. D. Lebowitz. 1991. Characteristics of asthma among elderly adult in a sample of the general population. *Chest* 100:935–942.

122. Higgins, M. W.et al. 1984. Risk of chronic obstructive pulmonary disease. *Am. Rev. Respir. Dis.* 130:380–385.

123. Chan-Yeung, M., S. Lam. 1986. Occupational asthma: State of the art. *Am. Rev. Respir. Dis.* 133:686–703.

124. Brooks, S. M., A. R. Kalica. 1987. NHLBI workshop summary. Strategies for elucidating the relationship between occupational exposures and airflow obstruction. *Am. Rev. Respir. Dis.* 135:268–273.

125. Taylor, A. J. Newmann. 1980. Occupational asthma. *Thorax* 35:268–245.

126. Majedi, M. R., H. Kazemi, D. C. Johnson. 1990. The effects of passive smoking on the pulmonary function of adults. *Thorax* 45:27–31.

127. Fielding, J. E., K. J. Phenow. 1988. Health effects of involuntary smoking. *N. Engl. J. Med.* 319:1452–1460.

128. Kreit, J. W., K. B. Gross, T. B. Moore, T. J. Lorenzen, J. D'arcy, W. L. Eschembacher. 1989. Ozone-induced changes in pulmonary function and bronchial responsiveness in asthmatics. *J. Appl. Physiol.* 66:217–222.

129. Spektor, D. M., M. Lippmann, G. D. Thurston, P. J. Lioy, J. Stecko, G. O'Connor, E. Garshick, F. E. Speizer, C. Hayes. 1989. Effects of ambient ozone on respiratory function in healthy adults exercising outdoors. *Am. Rev. Respir. Dis.* 138:821–828.

130. Linn, W. S., E. L. Avol, D. A. Shamoo, R. C. Peng, L. M. Valencia, D. E. Little, J. D. Hackney. 1988. Repeated laboratory ozone exposures of volunteer Los Angeles residents: An apparent seasonal variation in response. *Toxicol. Ind. Health.* 4:505–520.

131. Krzyanowski, M., J. J. Quackenboss, M. D. Lebowitz. 1992. Relation of peak expiratory flow rates and symptoms to ambient ozone. *Arch. Environ. Health.* 47:107–115.

132. Bergofsky, E. H. 1991. The lung mucosa: A critical environmental battleground. *Am. J. Med.* 91(suppl. 4a):4S–10S.

133. Gelzleicher, T., H. Witschi, J. Last. 1992. Concentration-response of rat lungs to exposure to oxidant pollutants: A critical test of Harber's Law for ozone and nitrogen dioxide. *Toxicol. Appl. Pharamacol.* 112:73–80.

134. Yania, M., T. Ohuri, T. Aikawa, H. Okayama, K. Sekizawa, K. Maeyama, H. Sasaki, T. Takishima. 1990. Ozone increases susceptibility to antigen inhalation in allergic dogs. *J. Appl. Physiol.* 68:2267–2273.

135. Koening, J. Q., D. S. Covert, Q. S. Hanley, G. van Belle, W. E. Pierson. 1990. Prior exposure to ozone potentiates subsequent response to sulfur dioxide in adolescent asthmatic subjects. *Am. Rev. Respir. Dis.* 141:377–380.

136. Abbey, D. E., R. J. Burchette. 1996. Relative power of alternative ambient air pollution metrics for detecting chronic health effects in epidemiological studies. *Environmetrics* 7:453–470.

137. Biagini, R. E., W. J. Moorman, T. R. Lewis, I. L. Bernstein. 1986. Ozone enhancement of platinum asthma in a primate model. *Am. Rev. Respir. Dis.* 134:719–725.

138. Triosi, R. J., W. C. Willett, S. T. Weiss, D. Trichopoulos, B. Rosner, F. E. Speizer. 1995b. Menopause, postmenopausal estrogen preparations, and the risk of adult- onset asthma. *Am. J. Respir. Crit. Care Med.* 152:1183–1188.

139. Triosi, R. J., W. C. Willett, S. T. Weiss, D. Trichopoulos, B. Rosner, F. E. Speizer. 1995a. A prospective study of diet and adult-onset asthma. *Am. J. Respir. Crit. Care Med.* 151:1401–1408.

140. Devlin, R. B., W. F. McDonnell, R. Mann, S. Becker, D. E. House, D. Schreinemachers, H. S. Koren. 1991. Exposure of humans to ambient levels of ozone for 6.6 hours causes cellular and biochemical changes in the lung. *Am. J. Respir. Cell Mol. Biol.* 4:72–81.

141. Kehlr, H. R., L. M. Vincent, R. J. Kowalsky, D. H. Horstman, J. J. O'Neil, W. H. McCartney, P. A. Bromberg. 1987. Ozone exposure increases respiratory epithelial permeability in human. *Am. Rev. Respir. Dis.* 135:1124–1128.

142. Holtzman, M. J., J. H. Cunningham, J. R. Sheller, G. B. Irsigler, J. A. Nadel, H. A. Boushey. 1979. Effect of ozone on bronchial reactivity in atopic and nonatopic subjects. *Am. Rev. Respir. Dis.* 120:1059–1067.

143. Horstman, D. H., L. J. Folinsbee, P. J. Ives, S. Abdul-Salaam, W. F. McDonnell. 1990. Ozone concentration and pulmonary response relationships for 6.6-hour exposures with five hours of moderate exercise to 0.08, 0.10, 0.12 ppm. *Am. Rev. Respir. Dis.* 142:1158–1163.

144. Tyler, W. S., N. K. Tyler, J. A. Last, M. J. Gillespie, T. G. Barstow. 1988. Comparison of daily and seasonal exposures of young monkeys to ozone. *Toxicology* 50:131–144.

145. Sheppard, D., Y. Yokosaki. 1996. Roles of airway epithelial integrins in health and disease: The Parker B. Francis Lectureship. *Chest* 109(suppl.):29S–33S.

146. Huang, X. Z., J. F. Wu, D. Cass, D. J. Erie, D. Corry, S. G. Young, R. V. Farese, D. Sheppard. 1996. Inactivation of the integrin beta 6 subunit gene reveals a role of epithelial integrins in regulating inflammation in the lung and skin. *J. Cell Biol.* 133:921–928.

147. Biagini, R. E., W. J. Moorman, T. R. Lewis, I. L. Bernstein. 1986. Ozone enhancement of platinum asthma in a primate model. *Am. Rev. Respir. Dis.* 134:719–725.

148. Osebold, J. W., Y. C. Zee, L. J. Gershwin. 1988. Enhancement of allergic lung sensitization in mice by ozone inhalation. *Proc. Soc. Exp. Biol. Med.* 188:259–264.

149. Jorres, R., D. Nowak, H. Magnussen. 1996. The effect of ozone exposure on allergen responsiveness in subjects with asthma or rhinitis. *Am. J. Respir. Care Med.* 153:56–64.

150. Thurston, G. D., M. Lippmann, M. B. Scott, J. M. Fine. 1997. Summertime haze air pollution and children with asthma. *Am. J. Respir. Crit. Care Med.* 155:654–660.

151. Whittemore, A. S., E. L. Korn. 1980. Asthma and air pollution in the Los Angeles area. *Am. J. Public Health* 70:687–696.

152. Lebowitz, M. D., L. Collins, C. J. Holberg. 1987. Time series analyses of respiratory responses to indoor and outdoor environmental phenomena. *Environ. Res.* 43:332–341.

153. Weisel, C. P., R. P. Cody, P. J. Lioy. 1995. Relationship between summertime ambient ozone levels and emergency department visits for asthma in central New Jersey. *Environ. Health.* 103(suppl. 2):97–102.

154. White, M. C., R. A. Etzel, W. D. Wilcox, C. Lloyd. 1994. Exacerbations of childhood asthma and ozone pollution in Atlanta. *Environ. Res.* 65:56–68.

155. Abbey, D. E., B. L. Hwang, R. J. Burchette, M. A. Vancuren, P. K. Mills. 1995. Estimated long-term ambient concentrations of PM_{10} and development of respiratory symptoms in a nonsmoking population. *Arch. Envrion. Health.* 50:139–152.

156. Yunginger, J. W., C. E. Reed, E. J. O'Connell, L. J. Melton III, W. M. O'Fallon, M. D. Silverstein. 1992. A community based study of the epidemiology of asthma. *Am. Rev. Respir. Dis.* 146:888–894.

157. Erzen, D., K. C. Carriere, N. Dik, C. Mustard, L. L. Roos, J. Manfreda, N. R. Anthonsien. 1997. Income level and asthma prevalence and care patterns. *Am. Crit. Care Med.* 155:895–901.

158. Lebowitz, M. D., S. Spinaci. 1993. The epidemiology of asthma. *Eur. Repir. Rev.* 3:415–423.

159. Gilmour, M. I., P. Park, M. J. Selgrade. 1996. Increased immune and inflammatory responses to dust mite antigen in rats exposed to 5 ppm NO_2. *Fundam. Appl. Toxicol.* 31:65–70.

160. Brunekreef, B., S. T. Holgate. 2002. Air pollution and health. *Lancet,* 360:1233–1242.

161. Pope, C. A. 3rd, D. W. Dockery. 2006. Health effects of fine particulate air pollution: Lines that connect. *J. Air. Waste Manag. Assoc.* 56:709–742.

162. Künzli, N., I. B. Tager. 2005. Air pollution: From lung to heart. *Swiss Med. Wkly.* 135:697–702.

163. Boezen, H. M., J. M. Vonk, S. C. van der Zee. 2005. Susceptibility to air pollution in elderly males and females. *Eur. Respir. J.* 25:1018–1024.

164. Gent, J. F., E. W. Triche, T. R. Holford. 2003. Association of low-level ozone and fine particles with respiratory symptoms in children with asthma. *JAMA.* 290:1859–1867.

165. Desqueyroux, H., J. C. Pujet, M. Prosper. 2002. Short-term effect of low-level air pollution on respiratory health of adults suffering from moderate to severe asthma. *Environ. Res. (Section A).* 89:29–37.

166. Hiltermann, T. J. N., J. Stolk, S. C. van der Zee. 1998. Asthma severity and susceptibility to air pollution. *Eur. Respir. J.* 11:686–693.

167. Rage, E., V. Siroux, N. Kunzli, I. Pin, F. Kauffmann. 2009. Air Pollution and Asthma Severity in Adults. *Occup. Environ. Med.* 66(3):182–188.

168. Sunyer, J., C. Spix, P. Quénel. 1997. Urban air pollution and emergency admissions for asthma in four European cities: The APHEA project. *Thorax* 52:760–765.

169. Neuhaus-Steinmetz, U., F. Uffhausen, U. Herz, H. Renz. 2000. Priming of allergic immune responses by repeated ozone exposure in mice. *Am. J. Respir. Cell Mol. Biol.* 23:228–233.

170. Peden, D. B., B. Boehlecke, D. Horstman. 1997. Prolonged acute exposure to 0.16 ppm ozone induces eosinophilic airway inflammation in asthmatic subjects with allergies. *J. Allergy Clin. Immunol.* 100:802–808.

171. Oryszczyn, M. P., E. Bouzigon, J. Maccario. 2007. Interrelationships of quantitative asthma-related phenotypes in the EGEA study. *J. Allergy Clin. Immunol.* 119:57–63.

172. Romieu, I., M. Ramirez-Aguilar, J. J. Sienra-Monge. 2006. GSTM1 and GSTP1 and respiratory health in asthmatic children exposed to ozone. *Eur. Respir. J.* 28:953–959.

173. Frey, U., T. Bordbeck, A. Majumdar. 2005. Risk of severe asthma episodes predicted from fluctuation analysis of airway function. *Nature* 438:667–670.

174. Wenzel, S. E. 2006. Asthma: Defining of the persistent adult phenotypes. *Lancet* 368:804–813.

175. Global strategy for asthma management and prevention update 2006. Global Initiative for Asthma (GINA). [Accessed March 14, 2007].

176. Schildcrout, J. S., L. Sheppard, T. Lumley. 2006. Ambient air pollution and asthma exacerbations in children: An eight-city analysis. *Am. J. Epidemiol.* 164:505–517.

177. Schindler, C., N. Künzli, J. P. Bongard. 2001. Short-term variation in air pollution and in average lung function among never-smokers (SAPALDIA). *Am. J. Respir. Crit. Care Med.* 163:356–361.

178. U.S. EPA. 2006. *Air Quality Criteria for Ozone and Related Photochemical Oxidants (Final).* Washington, DC: U.S. Environmental Protection Agency.

179. Darby, A. E., J. P. Dimarco. 2012. Management of atrial fibrillation in patients with structural heart disease. *Circulation* 125(7):945–957. http://circ.ahajournals.org/content/125/7/945.short

180. Fuster, V. et al. 2006. ACC/AHA/ESC 2006 guidelines for the management of patients with atrial fibrillation: A report of the American College of Cardiology/American Heart Association Task Force on Practice Guidelines and the European Society of Cardiology Committee Practice Guidelines (Writing Committee to Revise the 2001 Guidelines for the Management of Patients With Atrial Fibrillation): Developed in collaboration with the European Heart Rhythm Association and the Heart Rhythm Society. *Circulation* 114:e257–e354.

181. Miyasaka, Y., M. E. Barnes, B. J. Gersh, S. S. Cha, K. R. Bailey, W. P. Abhayaratna, J. B. Seward, T. S. M. Tsang. 2006. Secular trends in incidence of atrial fibrillation in Olmsted County, Minnesota, 1980 to 2000 and implications on the projections for future prevalence. *Circulation* 114:119–125.

182. Steinberg, J. S. et al. and the AFFIRM Investigators. 2004. Analysis of cause specific mortality in the Atrial Fibrillation Follow-up Investigation of Rhythm Management (AFFIRM) Study. *Circulation* 109:1973–1980.

183. DiMarco, J. P. 2009. Atrial fibrillation and acute decompensated HF. *Circ. Heart Fail.* 2:72–73.

184. Miyasaka, Y., M. E. Barnes, K. R. Bailey, S. S. Cha, B. J. Gersh, J. B. Seward, T. S. M. Tsang. 2007. Mortality trends in patients diagnosed with first atrial fibrillation: A 21-year community based study. *J. Am. Coli. Cardiol.* 49:986–992.

185. Miyasaka, Y., M. E. Barnes, B. J. Gersh, S. S. Cha, K. R. Bailey, J. B. Seward, T. S. M. Tsang. 2008. Changing trends of hospital utilization in patients after their first episode of atrial fibrillation. *Am. J. Cardiol.* 102:568–572.

186. Gage, B. F., A. D. Waterman, W. Shannon, M. Boechler, M. W. Rich, M. J. Radford. 2001. Validation of clinical classification schemes for predicting stroke: Results from the National Registry of Atrial Fibrillation. *JAMA* 285:2863–2870.

187. Lip, G. Y. H., R. Nieuwlaat, R. Pisters, D. A. Lane, H. J. G. M. Crijins. 2010. Refining clinical risk stratification for predicting stroke and thromboembolism in atrial fibrillation using a novel risk factor-based approach: The Euro Heart Survey on Atrial Fibrillation. *Chest* 137:263–272.

188. Braunwald, E. 1997. Shattuck lecture: Cardiovascular medicine at the turn of the millennium: Triumphs, concerns, and opportunities. *N. Engl. J. Med.* 337:1360–1369.

189. Kannel, W. B., R. D. Abbott, D. D. Savage, P. M. McNamara. 1982. Epidemiologic features of chronic atrial fibrillation: The Framingham study. *N. Engl. J. Med.* 306:1018–1022.

190. Benjamin, E. J., D. Levy, S. M. Vaziri, R. B. D'Agostino, A. J. Belanger, P. A. Wolf. 1994. Independent risk factors for atrial fibrillation in a population-based cohort: The Framingham heart study. *JAMA* 271:840–844.

191. Maisel, W. H., L. W. Stevenson. 2003. Atrial fibrillation in heart failure: Epidemiology, pathophysiology, and rationale for therapy. *Am. J. Cardiol.* 91:2D–8D.

192. Ehrlich, J. R., S. Nattel, S. H. Hohnloser. 2002. Atrial fibrillation and congestive heart failure: Specific considerations at the intersection of two common and important cardiac disease sets. *J. Cardiovasc. Electrophysiol.* 13:399–405.

193. Seiler, J., W. G. Stevenson. 2010. Atrial fibrillation in congestive heart failure. *Cardiol. Rev.* 8:38–50.

194. Krum, H., R. E. Gilbert. 2003. Demographics and concomitant disorders in heart failure. *Lancet* 362:147–158.

195. Adams, K. F., G. C. Fonarow, C. L. Emerman, T. H. LeJemtel, M. R. Costanzo, W. T. Abraham, R. L. Berkowitz, M. Galvao, D. P. Horton. 2005. Characteristics and outcomes of patients hospitalized for heart failure in the United States: Rationale, design, and preliminary observations from the first 100,000 cases in the Acute Decompensated Heart Failure National Registry (ADHERE). *Am. Heart J.* 149:209–216.

196. Grogan, M., H. C. Smith, B. J. Gersh, D. L. Wood. 1992. Left ventricular dysfunction due to atrial fibrillation in patients initially believed to have idiopathic dilated cardiomyopathy. *Am. J. Cardial.* 69:1570–1573.

197. Camm, A. J. et al. 2010. Guidelines for the management of atrial fibrillation. *Europace* 12:1360–1420.

198. Wyse, D. O. et al. 2002 For the Atrial Fibrillation Follow-up Investigation of Rhythm Management (AFFIRM) Investigators. A comparison of rate control and rhythm control in patients with atrial fibrillation. *N. Engl. J. Med.* 347:1825–1833.

199. Van Gelder, I. C. et al.; for the Rate Control Versus Electrical Cardioversion for Persistent Atrial Fibrillation Study Group. 2002. A comparison of rate control and rhythm control in patients with recurrent persistent atrial fibrillation. *N. Engl. J. Med.* 347:1834–1840.

200. Mustafić, H. et al. 2012. Main Air Pollutants and Myocardial Infarction. *JAMA* 307(7):713.

201. Dickey, L. D. 1976. *Clinical Ecology.* Charles, C. ed., Springfield, IL: Thomas Publisher.

202. Ayres, J. G. Cardiovascular disease and air pollution: A report by the Committee on the Medical Effects of Air Pollutants. [Accessed December 13, 2011] http://www.advisorybodies.doh.gov.uk/comeap/statementsreports/CardioDisease.pdf

203. Bhaskaran, K., S. Hajat, A. Haines, E. Herrett, P. Wilkinson, L. Smeeth. 2009. Effects of air pollution on the incidence of myocardial infarction. *Heart* 95(21):1746–1759.

204. Peng, R. D., H. H. Chang, M. L. Bell, A. McDermott, S. L. Zeger, J. M. Samet, F. Dominici. 2008. Coarse particulate matter air pollution and hospital admissions for cardiovascular and respiratory diseases among Medicare patients. *JAMA* 299(18):2172–2179.

205. Dominici, F., R. D. Peng, M. L. Bell, L. Pham, A. McDermott, S. L. Zeger, J. M. Samet. 2006. Fine particulate air pollution and hospital admission for cardiovascular and respiratory diseases. *JAMA* 295(10):1127–1134.

206. Filleul, L. et al. 2001. Short-term relationships between urban atmospheric pollution and respiratory mortality: Time series studies [in French]. *Rev. Mal. Respir.* 18(4 pt 1):387–395.

207. Braga, A. L., A. Zanobetti, J. Schwartz. 2001. The lag structure between particulate air pollution and respiratory and cardiovascular deaths in 10 US cities. *J. Occup. Environ. Med.* 43(11):927–933.

208. Koken, P. J., W. T. Piver, F. Ye, A. Elixhauser, L. M. Olsen, C. J. Portier. 2003. Temperature, air pollution, and hospitalization for cardiovascular diseases among elderly people in Denver. *Environ. Health Perspect.* 111(10):1312–1317.

209. Barnett, A. G., G. M. Williams, J. Schwartz, T. L. Best, A. H. Neller, A. L. Petroeschevsky, R. W. Simpson. 2006. The effects of air pollution on hospitalizations for cardiovascular disease in elderly people in Australian and New Zealand cities. *Environ. Health Perspect.* 114(7):1018–1023.

210. Berglind, N., P. Ljungman, J. Möller, J. Hallqvist, F. Nyberg, M. Rosenqvist, G. Pershagen, T. Bellander. 2010. Air pollution exposure: A trigger for myocardial infarction? *Int. J. Environ. Res. Public Health.* 7(4):1486–1499.

211. Cendon, S., L. A. Pereira, A. L. Braga, G. M. S. ConceiçãoI, A. C. Junior, H. Romaldini, A. C. Lopes, P. H. N. Saldiva. 2006. Air pollution effects on myocardial infarction. *Rev. Saude Publica.* 40(3):414–419.

212. Linn, W. S., Y. Szlachcic, H. Gong Jr., P. L. Kinney, K. T. Berhane. 2000. Air pollution and daily hospital admissions in metropolitan Los Angeles. *Environ. Health Perspect.* 108(5):427–434.

213. Pope, C. A. III, M. L. Hansen, R. W. Long, K. R. Nielsen, N. L. Eatough, W. E. Wilson, D. J. Eatough. 2004. Ambient particulate air pollution, heart rate variability, and blood markers of inflammation in a panel of elderly subjects. *Environ. Health Perspect.* 112(3):339–345.

214. Bräuner, E. V., P. Møller, L. Barregard, L. O. Dragsted, M. Glasius, P. Wåhlin, P. Vinzents, O. Raaschou-Nielsen, S. Loft. 2008. Exposure to ambient concentrations of particulate air pollution does not influence vascular function or inflammatory pathways in young healthy individuals. *Part. Fibre Toxicol.* 5:13.

215. Peters, A., A. Döring, H. E. Wichmann, W. Koenig. 1997. Increased plasma viscosity during an air pollution episode: A link to mortality? *Lancet.* 349(9065):1582–1587.

216. Lucking, A. J. et al. 2008. Diesel exhaust inhalation increases thrombus formation in man. *Eur. Heart J.* 29(24):3043–3051.

217. Bouthillier, L., R. Vincent, P. Goegan, I. Y. Adamson, S. Bjarnason, J. Stewart, J. Guénette, M. Potvin, P. Kumarathasan. 1998. Acute effects of inhaled urban particles and ozone: Lung morphology, macrophage activity, and plasma endothelin-1. *Am. J. Pathol.* 153(6):1873–1884.

218. Zhang, Z. M., E. A. Whitsel, P. M. Quibrera, R. L. Smith, D. Liao, G. L. Anderson, R. J. Prineas. 2009. Ambient fine particulate matter exposure and myocardial ischemia in the Environmental Epidemiology of Arrhythmogenesis in the Women's Health Initiative (EEAWHI) study. *Environ. Health Perspect.* 117(5):751–756.

219. Liao, D., E. A. Whitsel, Y. Duan, H. M. Lin, P. M. Quibrera, R. Smith, D. J. Peuquet, R. J. Prineas, Z. M. Zhang, G. Anderson. 2009. Ambient particulate air pollution and ectopy: The environmental epidemiology of arrhythmogenesis in Women's Health Initiative study, 1999–2004. *J. Toxicol. Environ. Health A.* 72(1):30–38.

220. Chardon, B., S. Host, A. Lefranc, F. Millard, I. Gremy. 2007. What exposure indicator should be used to study the short-term respiratory health effect of photochemical air pollution? A case study in the Paris metropolitan area (2000–2003). *Environ. Risques. Santé.* 6(5):345–353.

221. Dilaveris, P., A. Synetos, G. Giannopoulos, E. Gialafos, A. Pantazis, C. Stefanadis. 2006. Climate impacts on myocardial infarction deaths in the Athens Territory: The CLIMATE study. *Heart* 92(12):1747–1751.

222. Yusuf, S. et al.; INTERHEART Study Investigators. 2004. Effect of potentially modifiable risk factors associated with myocardial infarction in 52 countries (the INTERHEART study): Case-control study. *Lancet* 364(9438):937–952.

223. Henrotin, J. B., M. Zeller, L. Lorgis, Y. Cottin, M. Giroud, Y. Béjot. 2010. Evidence of the role of short-term exposure to ozone on ischaemic cerebral and cardiac events: The Dijon Vascular Project (DIVA). *Heart* 96(24):1990–1996.

224. Nuvolone, D., D. Balzi, M. Chini, D. Scala, F. Giovannini, A. Barchielli. 2011. Short-term association between ambient air pollution and risk of hospitalization for acute myocardial infarction: Results of the cardiovascular risk and air pollution in Tuscany (RISCAT) study. *Am. J. Epidemiol.* 174(1):63–71.

225. Bhaskaran, K., S. Hajat, B. Armstrong. 2011. The effects of hourly differences in air pollution on the risk of myocardial infarction: Case crossover analysis of the MINAP database. *BMJ.* 343:d5531.

226. Medina, S., A. Le Tertre, P. Quénel, Y. Le Moullec, P. Lameloise, J. C. Guzzo, B. Festy, R. Ferry, W. Dab. 1997. Air pollution and doctors' house calls: Results from the ERPURS system for monitoring the effects of air pollution on public health in Greater Paris, France, 1991–1995: Evaluation des Risques de la Pollution Urbaine pour la Santé. *Environ Res.* 75(1):73–84.

227. Hoek, G., B. Brunekreef, A. Verhoeff, J. van Wijnen, P. Fischer. 2000. Daily mortality and air pollution in The Netherlands. *J. Air Waste Manag. Assoc.* 50(8):1380–1389.

228. Mann, J. K., I. B. Tager, F. Lurmann, M. Segal, C. P. Quesenberry Jr., M. M. Lugg, J. Shan, S. K. Van Den Eeden. 2002. Air pollution and hospital admissions for ischemic heart disease in persons with congestive heart failure or arrhythmia. *Environ. Health Perspect.* 110(12):1247–1252.

229. Ruidavets, J. B., M. Cournot, S. Cassadou, M. Giroux, M. Meybeck, J. Ferrières. 2005. Ozone air pollution is associated with acute myocardial infarction. *Circulation.* 111(5):563–569.

230. Eilstein, D., P. Quénel, G. Hédelin, J. Kleinpeter, D. Arveiler, P. Schaffer. 2001. Air pollution and myocardial infarction: Strasbourg France, 1984–1989 [in French]. *Rev. Epidemiol. Sante. Publique.* 49(1):13–25.

231. Henrotin, J. B., M. Zeller, L. Lorgis, Y. Cottin, M. Giroud, Y. Béjot. 2010. Evidence of the role of short-term exposure to ozone on ischaemic cerebral and cardiac events: The Dijon Vascular Project (DIVA). *Heart* 96(24):1990–1996.

232. Nabel, E. G., E. Braunwald. 2012. A tale of coronary artery disease and myocardial infarction. *N. Engl. J. Med.* 366:54.

233. Bloom, D. E., E. T. Cafiero, M. E. McGovern, K. Prettner, A. Stanciole, J. Weiss, S. Bakkila, L. Rosenberg. 2011. *The Global Economic Burden of Noncommunicable Diseases.* Geneva: World Economic Forum. pp. 5–45.

234. Swirski, F. K., M. Nahrendorf. 2013. Leukocyte behavior in atherosclerosis, myocardial infarction, and heart failure. *Science* 339(6116):161–166.

235. Tabas, I., K. J. Williams, J. Boren. 2007. Subendothelial lipoprotein retention as the initiating process in atherosclerosis: Update and therapeutic implications. *Circulation* 116:1832.

236. Stary, H. C. 1999. *Atlas of Atherosclerosis: Progression and Regression.* p. 131. New York: The Parthenon Publishing Group Inc.

237. Hansson, G. K., P. Libby. 2006. The immune response in atherosclerosis: A double-edged sword. *Nat. Rev. Immunol.* 6:508.

238. Gerrity, R. G. 1981. The role of the monocyte in atherogenesis: I. Transition of blood-borne monocytes into foam cells in fatty lesions. *Am. J. Pathol.* 103:181.

239. Gerrity, R. G. 1981. The role of the monocyte in atherogenesis: II. Migration of foam cells from atherosclerotic lesions. *Am. J. Pathol.* 103:191.

240. Moore, K. J., I. Tabas. 2011. Macrophages in the pathogenesis of atherosclerosis. *Cell.* 145:341.

241. Duewell, P. et al. 2010. NLRP3 inflammasomes are required for atherogenesis and activated by cholesterol crystals. *Nature* 464:1357.

242. Rajamaki, K., J. Lappalainen, K. Oörni, E. Välimäki, S. Matikainen, P. T. Kovanen, K. K. Eklund. 2010. Cholesterol crystals activate the NLRP3 inflammasome in human macrophages: A novel link between cholesterol metabolism and inflammation. *PLoS One* 5:e11765.

243. Manning-Tobin, J. J., K. J. Moore, T. A. Seimon, S. A. Bell, M. Sharuk, J. I. Alvarez-Leite, M. P. de Winther, I. Tabas, M. W. Freeman. 2009. Loss of SR-A and CD36 activity reduces atherosclerotic lesion complexity without abrogating foam cell formation in hyperlipidemic mice. *Arterioscler. Thromb. Vasc. Biol.* 29:19.

244. Menu, P., M. Pellegrin, J.-F. Aubert, K. Bouzourene, A. Tardivel, L. Mazzolai, J. Tschopp. 2011. Atherosclerosis in ApoE-deficient mice progresses independently of the NLRP3 inflammasome. *Cell. Death Dis.* 2:e137.

245. Spann, N. J. et al. 2012. Regulated accumulation of desmosterol integrates macrophage lipid metabolism and inflammatory responses. *Cell* 151:138.

246. Geissmann, F., M. G. Manz, S. Jung, M. H. Sieweke, M. Merad, K. Ley. 2010. Development of monocytes, macrophages, and dendritic cells. *Science* 327:656.

247. Yvan-Charvet, L. et al. 2010. ATP-binding cassette transporters and HDL suppress hematopoietic stem cell proliferation. *Science* 328:1689.

248. Murphy, A. J. et al. 2011. ApoE regulates hematopoietic stem cell proliferation, monocytosis, and monocyte accumulation in atherosclerotic lesions in mice. *J. Clin. Invest.* 121:4138.

249. Westerterp, M., S. Gourion-Arsiquaud, A. J. Murphy, A. Shih, S. Cremers, R. L. Levine, A. R. Tall, L. Yvan-Charvet. 2012. Regulation of hematopoietic stem and progenitor cell mobilization by cholesterol efflux pathways. *Cell Stem Cell* 11:195.

250. Robbins, C. S. et al. 2012. Extramedullary hematopoiesis generates Ly-6C(high) monocytes that infiltrate atherosclerotic lesions. *Circulation* 125:364.

251. Hilgendorf, I., F. K. Swirski. 2012. Making a difference: Monocyte heterogeneity in cardiovascular disease. *Curr. Atheroscler. Rep.* 14:450.

252. Tacke, F. et al. 2007. Monocyte subsets differentially employ CCR2, CCR5, and CX3CR1 to accumulate within atherosclerotic plaques. *J. Clin. Invest.* 117:185.

253. Combadiere, C., S. Potteaux, M. Rodero, T. Simon, A. Pezard, B. Esposito, R. Merval, A. Proudfoot, A. Tedgui, Z. Mallat. 2008. Combined inhibition of CCL2, CX3CR1, and CCR5 abrogates Ly6C(hi) and Ly6C(lo) monocytosis and almost abolishes atherosclerosis in hypercholesterolemic mice. *Circulation* 117:1649.

254. Saederup, N., L. Chan, S. A. Lira, I. F. Charo. 2008. Fractalkine deficiency markedly reduces macrophage accumulation and atherosclerotic lesion formation in CCR2$^{-/-}$ mice: Evidence for independent chemokine functions in atherogenesis. *Circulation* 117:1642.

255. van Gils, J. M. et al. 2012. The neuroimmune guidance cue netrin-1 promotes atherosclerosis by inhibiting the emigration of macrophages from plaques. *Nat. Immunol.* 13:136.

256. Nahrendorf, M., F. K. Swirski, E. Aikawa, L. Stangenberg, T. Wurdinger, J. L. Figueiredo, P. Libby, R. Weissleder, M. J. Pittet. 2007. The healing myocardium sequentially mobilizes two monocyte subsets with divergent and complementary functions. *J. Exp. Med.* 204:3037.

257. Zhu, S. N., M. Chen, J. Jongstra-Bilen, M. I. Cybulsky. 2009. GM-CSF regulates intimal cell proliferation in nascent atherosclerotic lesions. *J. Exp. Med.* 206:2141.

258. Choi, J. H., Y. Do, C. Cheong, H. Koh, S. B. Boscardin, Y. S. Oh, L. Bozzacco, C. Trumpfheller, C. G. Park, R. M. Steinman. 2009. Identification of antigen-presenting dendritic cells in mouse aorta and cardiac valves. *J. Exp. Med.* 206:497.

259. Choi, J. H. et al. 2011. Flt3 signaling-dependent dendritic cells protect against atherosclerosis. *Immunity* 35:819.

260. Koltsova, E. K. et al. 2012. Dynamic T cell-APC interactions sustain chronic inflammation in atherosclerosis. *J. Clin. Invest.*

261. Grabner, R. et al. 2009. Lymphotoxin beta receptor signaling promotes tertiary lymphoid organogenesis in the aorta adventitia of aged ApoE$^{-/-}$ mice. *J. Exp. Med.* 206:233.

262. Andersson, J., P. Libby, G. K. Hansson. 2010. Adaptive immunity and atherosclerosis. *Clin. Immunol.* 134:33.

263. Lahoute, C., O. Herbin, Z. Mallat, A. Tedgui. 2011. Adaptive immunity in atherosclerosis: Mechanisms and future therapeutic targets. *Nat. Rev. Cardiol.* 8:348.

264. Kyaw, T., P. Tipping, B. H. Toh, A. Bobik. 2011. Current understanding of the role of B cell subsets and intimal and adventitial B cells in atherosclerosis. *Curr. Opin. Lipidol.* 22:373.

265. Kyaw, T., P. Tipping, A. Bobik, B. H. Toh. 2012. Protective role of natural IgM-producing B1a cells in atherosclerosis. *Trends Cardiovasc. Med.* 22:48.

266. Stemme, S., B. Faber, J. Holm, O. Wiklund, J. L. Witztum, G. K. Hansson. 1995. T lymphocytes from human atherosclerotic plaques recognize oxidized low density lipoprotein. *Proc. Natl. Acad. Sci. U.S.A.* 92:3893–3897.

267. Yla-Herttuala, S., W. Palinski, S. W. Butler, S. Picard, D. Steinberg, J. L. Witztum. 1994. Rabbit and human atherosclerotic lesions contain IgG that recognizes epitopes of oxidized LDL. *Arterioscler. Thromb.* 14:32.

268. Sun, J., G. K. Sukhova, P. J. Wolters, M. Yang, S. Kitamoto, P. Libby, L. A. MacFarlane, J. Mallen-St Clair, G. P. Shi. 2007. Mast cells promote atherosclerosis by releasing proinflammatory cytokines. *Nat. Med.* 13:719.

269. Huo, Y., A. Schober, S. B. Forlow, D. F. Smith, M. C. Hyman, S. Jung, D. R. Littman, C. Weber, K. Ley. 2003. Circulating activated platelets exacerbate atherosclerosis in mice deficient in apolipoprotein E. *Nat Med.* 9:61.

270. Pinto, A. R., R. Paolicelli, E. Salimova, J. Gospocic, E. Slonimsky, D Bilbao-Cortes, J. W. Godwin, N. A. Rosenthal. 2012. An abundant tissue macrophage population in the adult murine heart with a distinct alternatively-activated macrophage profile. *PLoS One* 7:e36814.

271. Dewald, O., P. Zymek, K. Winkelmann, A. Koerting, G. Ren, T. Abou-Khamis, L. H. Michael, B. J. Rollins, M. L. Entman, N. G. Frangogiannis. 2005. CCL2/Monocyte Chemoattractant Protein-1 regulates inflammatory responses critical to healing myocardial infarcts. *Circ. Res.* 96:881.

272. Lee, W. W. et al. 2012. PET/MRI of inflammation in myocardial infarction. *J. Am. Coll. Cardiol.* 59:153.

273. Hofmann, U., N. Beyersdorf, J. Weirather, A. Podolskaya, J. Bauersachs, G. Ertl, T. Kerkau, S. Frantz. 2012. Activation of CD4+ T lymphocytes improves wound healing and survival after experimental myocardial infarction in mice. *Circulation* 125:1652.

274. Anzai, A. et al. 2012. Regulatory role of dendritic cells in postinfarction healing and left ventricular remodeling. *Circulation* 125:1234.

275. Leuschner, F. et al. 2012. Rapid monocyte kinetics in acute myocardial infarction are sustained by extramedullary monocytopoiesis. *J. Exp. Med.* 209:123.

276. Leuschner, F. et al. 2011. Therapeutic SiRNA Silencing in Inflammatory Monocytes in Mice. *Nat. Biotechnol.* 29(11):1005–1010.

277. Swirski, F. K. et al. 2009. Identification of splenic reservoir monocytes and their deployment to inflammatory sites. *Science* 325:612.

278. Dutta, P., G. Courties, Y. Wei, F. Leuschner, R. Gorbatov, C. S. Robbins, Y. Iwamoto. 2012. Myocardial infarction accelerates atherosclerosis. *Nature.* 487:325.

279. Wright, A. P., M. K. Öhman, H. Hayasaki, W. Luo, H. M. Russo, C. Guo, D. T. Eitzman. 2010. Atherosclerosis and leukocyte-endothelial adhesive interactions are increased following acute myocardial infarction in apolipoprotein E deficient mice. *Atherosclerosis* 212:414.

280. Oka, T. et al. 2012. Mitochondrial DNA that escapes from autophagy causes inflammation and heart failure. *Nature* 485:251.

281. Panizzi, P., F. K. Swirski, J. L. Figueiredo, P. Waterman, D. E. Sosnovik, E. Aikawa, P. Libby, M. Pittet, R. Weissleder, M. Nahrendorf. 2010. Impaired infarct healing in atherosclerotic mice with Ly-6C(hi) monocytosis. *J. Am. Coll. Cardiol.* 55:1629.

282. Engstrom, G., O. Melander, B. Hedblad. 2009. Leukocyte count and incidence of hospitalizations due to heart failure. *Circ. Heart Fail.* 2:217.

283. Tsujioka, H. et al. 2009. Impact of heterogeneity of human peripheral blood monocyte subsets on myocardial salvage in patients with primary acute myocardial infarction. *J. Am. Coll. Cardiol.* 54:130.

284. Assmus, B. et al. 2012. Acute myocardial infarction activates progenitor cells and increases Wnt signalling in the bone marrow. *Eur. Heart J.* 33:1911.

285. Massa, M. et al. 2005. Increased circulating hematopoietic and endothelial progenitor cells in the early phase of acute myocardial infarction. *Blood* 105:199.

286. Rea, W. J. 1992. *Chemical Sensitivity*, Vol. 1, p. 731. Boca Raton, FL: Lewis Publishers.

287. U.S. Environmental Protection Agency. 1981. *Air Quality Criteria for Oxides of Nitrogen.* Washington, DC: U.S. EPA. EPA-600/8-82-026F.

288. U.S. Environmental Protection Agency. 1984. *Revised Evaluation of Health Effects Associated with Carbon Monoxide Exposure: An Addendum to the 1979 EPA Air Quality Criteria Document for Carbon Monoxide.* Washington, DC: U.S. EPA. EPA-600/8-83-033F.

289. IFR Action. 2005. *Inhert Ingredient Tolerance Reassessment—Titanium Dioxide.* Washington DC: U.S. EPA. pp. 1–10.

290. EPA. 1998. U.S. Environmental Protection Agency. Titanium Dioxide; Exemption from the Requirement of a Tolerance. Final Rule. 63 FR 14360; [Accessed March 25, 1998] http://www.epa.gov/fedrg.str/EPA-PEST11998/March/Dav-25/u74.

291. Pflucker, F., V. Wendel, H. Hohenberg, E. Gartner, T. Will, S. Pfeiffer, R. Wepf, H. Gers-Barlag. 2001. The human stratum corneum layer: An effective barrier against dermal uptake of different forms of topically applied micronised titanium dioxide. *Skin Pharmacol. Appl. Skin Physiol.* 14(suppl. 1):92–97.

292. Lee, K. P., H. J. Trochimowicz, C. F. Reinhardt. 1985. Pulmonary response of rats exposed to titanium dioxide (TiO_2) by inhalation for two years. *Toxicol. Appl. Pharmacol.* 79(2):179–192.

293. Hext, P. M., J. A. Tomenson, P. Thompson. 2005. Titanium Dioxide: Inhalation Toxicology and Epidemiology. *Ann. Occup. Hyg.* 49(6):461–472.

294. Rossi, E. M., L. Pylkkänen, A. J. Koivisto, H. Nykäsenoja, H. Wolff, K. Savolainen, H. Alenius. 2010. Inhalation exposure to nanosized and fine TiO2 particles inhibits features of allergic asthma in a murine model. *Part. Fibre Toxicol.* 7(1):35.

295. Lötvall, J., A. Frew. 2006. *For the European Academy of Allergology and Clinical Immunology: Allergy: An Epidemic That Must Be Stopped.* Brussels: European Academy of Allergology and Clinical Immunology. [Accessed on August 17, 2017] http://www.eaaci.net/media/PDF/E/820.pdf.

296. Weinmayr, G. et al. 2007. Isaac Phase Two Study Group: Atopic sensitization and the international variation of asthma symptom prevalence in children. *Am. J. Respir. Crit. Care. Med.* 176:565–574.

297. Yazdanbakhsh, M., P. G. Kremsner, R. van Ree. 2002. Allergy, parasites, and the hygiene hypothesis. *Science* 296:490–494.

298. Gavett, S. H., H. S. Koren. 2001. The role of particulate matter in exacerbation of atopic asthma. *Int. Archives Allergy Immunol.* 124:109–112.

299. Nordenhall, C., J. Pourazar, M. C. Ledin, J. O. Levin, T. Sandstrom, E. Adelroth. 2001. Diesel exhaust enhances airway responsiveness in asthmatic subjects. *Eur. Respir. J.* 17:909–915.

300. Pandya, R. J., G. Solomon, A. Kinner, J. R. Balmes. 2002. Diesel exhaust and asthma: Hypotheses and molecular mechanisms of action. *Environ. Health Perspectives.* 110:103–112.

301. Baan, R., K. Straif, Y. Grosse, B. Secretan, F. El Ghissassi, V. Cogliano. 2006. Carcinogenicity of carbon black, titanium dioxide, and talc. *The Lancet Oncology.* 7:295–296.

302. Chen, X., S. S. Mao. 2007. Titanium dioxide nanomaterials: Synthesis, properties, modifications, and applications. *Chem. Rev.* 107:2891–2959.

303. Hamelmann, E., J. Schwarze, K. Tadeka, A. Oshiba, G. L. Larsen, C. G. Irvin, E. W. Gelfand. 1997. Noninvasive measurement of airway responsiveness in allergic mice using barometric plethysmography. *Am. J. Respir. Crit. Care Med.* 156:766–767.

304. Harkema, J., A. Mariassy, J. St. George, D. Hyde, C. Plopper. 1991. Epithelial cells of the conducting airways: A species comparison. In *The Airway Epithelium: Physiology, Pathophysiology and Pharmacology.* S. Farmer, D. Hay, eds., pp. 3–39. New York: Dekker.

305. Rossi, E. M. et al. 2010. Airway exposure to silica-coated TiO_2 nanoparticles induces pulmonary neutrophilia in mice. *Toxicol. Sci.* 113:422–433.

306. Lee, K. et al. 2009. Lung injury study by 15 days inhalation exposure of titanium dioxide nanoparticles in rats. *Toxicol. Lett.* 189:S186–S186.

307. Otani, N., S. Ishimatsu, T. Mochizuki. 2008. Acute group poisoning by titanium dioxide: Inhalation exposure may cause metal fume fever. *Am. J. Emerg. Med.* 26:608–611.

308. Garabrant, D., L. Fine, C. Oliver, L. Bernstein, J. Peters. 1987. Abnormalities of pulmonary function and pleural disease among titanium metal production workers. *Scand. J. Work Environ. Health* 13:47–51.

309. Last, J. A., R. Ward, L. Temple, K. E. Pinkerton, N. J. Kenyon. 2004. Ovalbumin-induced airway inflammation and fibrosis in mice also exposed to ultrafine particles. *Inhal. Toxicol.* 16:93–102.

310. Määttä, J., R. Haapakoski, M. Lehto, M. Leino, S. Tillander, K. HusgafvelPursiainen, H. Wolff, K. Savolainen, H. Alenius. 2007. Immunomodulatory effects of oak dust exposure in a murine model of allergic asthma. *Toxicol. Sci.* 99:260–266.

311. Thatcher, T. H., R. P. Benson, R. P. Phipps, P. J. Sime. 2008. High-dose but not low-dose mainstream cigarette smoke suppresses allergic airway inflammation by inhibiting T cell function. *Am. J. Physiol. Lung Cell Mol. Physiol.* 295:L412–L421.

312. Ryan, J. J., H. R. Bateman, A. Stover, G. Gomez, S. K. Norton, W. Zhao, L. B. Schwartz, R. Lenk, C. L. Kepley. 2007. Fullerene nanomaterials inhibit the allergic response. *J. Immunol.* 179:665–672.

313. Larsen, S. T., M. Roursgaard, K. A. Jensen, G. D. Nielsen. 2010. Nano titanium dioxide particles promote allergic sensitization and lung inflammation in mice. *Basic Clin. Pharmacol. Toxicol.* 106:114–117.

314. Leino, M. S., H. T. Alenius, N. Fyhrquist-Vanni, H. J. Wolff, K. E. Reijula, E.-L. Hintikka, M. S. Salkinoja-Salonen, T. Haahtela, M. J. Makela. 2006. Intranasal exposure to *stachybotrys chartarum* enhances airway inflammation in allergic mice. *Am. J. Respir. Crit. Care Med.* 173:512–518.

315. Mitchell, L. A., J. Gao, R. V. Wal, A. Gigliotti, S. W. Burchiel, J. D. McDonald. 2007. Pulmonary and systemic immune response to inhaled multiwalled carbon nanotubes. *Toxicol. Sci.* 100:203–214.

316. Fedulov, A. V., A. Leme, Z. Yang, M. Dahl, R. Lim, T. J. Mariani, L. Kobzik. 2008. Pulmonary exposure to particles during pregnancy causes increased neonatal asthma susceptibility. *Am. J. Respir. Cell Mol. Biol.* 38:57–67.

317. Goyer, R. A. 1986. Toxic effects of metals. In *Cassarett and Doull's Toxicology: The Basic Science of Poisons*, 3rd ed., C. D. Klassen, M. O. Amdur, J. P. Doull, eds., pp. 598–604. New York: Macmillan.
318. WHO (World Health Organization). 1989. *IPCS (International Program in Chemical Safety). Environmental Health Criteria-85-Lead Environmental Aspects.* Geneva: World Health Organization.
319. ATSDR (Agency for Toxic Substances and Disease Registry). 2005. Toxicological profile for lead (draft for public comment). Annual report. Atlanta: Department of Health and Human Services, Public Health Service.
320. Patrick, L. 2006. Lead toxicity Part II: The role of free radical damage and the use of antioxidants in the pathology and treatment of lead toxicity. *Altern. Med. Rev.* 11:114–127.
321. Carmignani, M., P. Boscolo, A. Poma, A. R. Volpe. 1999. Kininergic system and arterial hypertension following chronic exposure to inorganic lead. *Immunopharmacology* 44:105–110.
322. Navas-Acien, A., E. Guallar, E. K. Silbergeld, S. J. Rothenberg. 2007. Lead exposure and cardiovascular disease—A systematic review. *Environ. Health Perspect.* 115:472–482.
323. Lustberg, M., E. Silbergeld. 2002. Blood lead levels and mortality. *Arch. Intern. Med.* 162:2443–2449.
324. Vupputuri, S., J. He, P. Muntner, L. A. Bazzano, P. K. Whelton, V. Batuman. 2003. Blood lead level is associated with elevated blood pressure in blacks. *Hypertension* 41:463–468.
325. Den Hond, E., T. Nawrot, J. A. Staessen. 2002. The relationship between blood pressure and blood lead in NHANES III. National Health and Nutritional Examination Survey. *J. Hum. Hypertens.* 16:563–568.
326. Ehrlich, R. et al. 1998. Lead absorption and renal dysfunction in a South African battery factory. *Occup. Environ. Med.* 55:453–460.
327. Grizzo, L. T., S. Cordellini. 2008. Perinatal lead exposure affects nitric oxide and cyclooxygenase pathways in aorta of weaned rats. *Toxicol. Sci.* 103:207–214.
328. Farmand, F., A. Ehdaie, C. K. Roberts, R. K. Sindhu. 2005. Lead-induced dysregulation of superoxide dismutases, catalase, glutathione peroxidase, and guanylate cyclase. *Environ. Res.* 98:33–39.
329. Khalil-Manesh, F., H. C. Gonick, E. W. Weiler, B. Prins, M. A. Weber, R. E. Purdy. 1993. Lead-induced hypertension: Possible role of endothelial factors. *Am. J. Hypertens.* 6:723–729.
330. Carmignani, M., A. R. Volpe, P. Boscolo, N. Qiao, M. Di Gioacchino, A. Grilli, M. Felaco. 2000. Catecholami.ne and nitric oxide systems as targets of chronic lead exposure in inducing selective functional impairment. *Life Sci.* 68:401–415.
331. Vaziri, N. D., Y. Ding, Z. Ni. 2001. Compensatory up-regulation of nitric-oxide synthase isoforms in lead-induced hypertension; reversal by a superoxide dismutase-mimetic drug. *J. Pharmacol. Exp. Ther.* 298:679–685.
332. Kasperczyk, S., A. Kasperczyk, A. Ostalowska, M. Dziwisz, E. Birkner. 2004. Activity of glutathione peroxidase, glutathione reductase, and lipid peroxidation in erythrocytes in workers exposed to lead. *Biol. Trace Elem. Res.* 102:61–72.
333. Bakir, F. et al. 1973. Methylmercury poisoning in Iraq. *Science* 181:230–241.
334. Heydari, A., A. Norouzzadeh, A. Khoshbaten, A. Asgari, A. Ghasemi, S. Najafi, R. Badalzadeh. 2006. Effects of short-term and subchronic lead poisoning on nitric oxide metabolites and vascular responsiveness in rat. *Toxicol. Lett.* 166:88–94.
335. Zhang, L. F., S. Q. Peng, S. Wang. 2009. Decreased aortic contractile reaction to 5-hydroxytryptamine in rats with long-term hypertension induced by lead (Pb^{2+}) exposure. *Toxicol. Lett.* 186:78–83.
336. Pecanha, F. M., G. A. Wiggers, A. M. Briones, J. V. Perez-Giron, M. Miguel, A. B. Garcia-Redondo, D. V. Vassallo, M. J. Alonso, M. Salaices. 2010. The role of cyclooxygenase (COX)-2 derived prostanoids on vasoconstrictor responses to phenylephrine is increased by exposure to low mercury concentration. *J. Physiol. Pharmacol.* 61:29–36.
337. Zuo, M. 2013. Pollution from heavy metals devastates farmland. South China Morning Post. [Accessed April 26, 2016] http://www.scmp.com/news/china/article/1151311/pollution-heavy-metals-devastates-farmland
338. Underwood, E. J. 1977. *Trace Elements in Human and Animal Nutrition*, 4th ed., p. 417. New York: Academic Press.
339. Forbes, S. B., J. C. Regina. 1972. Effect of age on gastrointestinal absorption (Fe, Sn, Pb) in the rat. *J. Nutr.* 102:647.
340. Taylor, C. V., F. O. Thomas, M. G. Brown. 1933. Studies on protozoa. IV. Lethal effects of X-radiation on a sterile culture medium for Aulpidium Can phylum. *Physiol. Zool.* 6:467.
341. Schultz, J., N. J. Smith. 1958. A quantitative study for the absorption for food iron in infants and children. *Am. J. Dis. Child.* 95:109.
342. HMSO. 1983. Royal commission on environmental pollution (ninth report): Lead in the environment. p. 137. London: HMSO.

343. Calabrese, E. J. 1981. *Nutrition and Environmental Health: The Influence of Nutritional Status on Pollutant Toxicity and Carcinogenicity, Vol. 2, Minerals and Macronutrients*, p. 93. New York: John Wiley & Sons.

344. Kello, D., K. Kostial. 1974. The effect of milk diet on lead metabolism in rats. *Environ. Res.* 6:355.

345. Holtzman, R., F. H. Llcewicz. 1966. Lead-210 and polmium-210 in tissues of cigarette smokers. *Science* 153:1259–1260.

346. Gordon, G. F. 1986. *Lead Toxicity*. Vol. 20, issue 2. Sacramento, CA: American Academy of Medial Preventics.

347. Stansfield, K. H., J. R. Pilsner, Q. Lu, R. O. Wright, T. R. Guilarte. 2012. Dysregulation of BDNF-TrkB signaling in developing hippocampal neurons by Pb^{2+}: Implications for an environmental basis of neurodevelopmental disorders. *Toxicol. Sci.* 127(1):277–295.

348. Opler, M. G., A. S. Brown, J. Graziano, M. Desai, W. Zheng, C. Schaefer, P. Factor-Litvak, E. S. Susser. 2004. Prenatal lead exposure, deltaaminolevulinic acid, and schizophrenia. *Environ. Health Perspect.* 112:548–552.

349. Opler, M. G. et al. 2008. Prenatal exposure to lead, delta-aminolevulinic acid, and schizophrenia: Further evidence. *Environ. Health Perspect.* 116:1586–1590.

350. Mielke, H. W., C. R. Gonzales, P. W. Mielke Jr. 2011. The continuing impact of lead dust on children's blood lead: Comparison of public and private properties in New Orleans. *Environ. Res.* 111:1164–1172.

351. Nriagu, J., R. Senthamarai-Kannan, H. Jamil, M. Fakhori, S. Korponic. 2011. Lead poisoning among Arab American and African American children in the Detroit metropolitan area, Michigan. *Bull. Environ. Contam. Toxicol.* 87:238–244.

352. Toscano, C. D., T. R. Guilarte. 2005. Lead neurotoxicity: From exposure to molecular effects. *Brain Res. Brain Res. Rev.* 49:529–554.

353. Dooyema, C. A. et al. 2012. Outbreak of fatal childhood lead poisoning related to artisanal gold mining in Northwestern Nigeria, 2010. *Environ. Health Perspect.* 120:601–607.

354. Nichani, V., W. I. Li, M. A. Smith, G. Noonan, M. Kulkarni, M. Kodavor, L. P. Naeher. 2006. Blood lead levels in children after phase-out of leaded gasoline in Bombay, India. *Sci. Total Environ.* 363:95–106.

355. Stromberg, U., T. Lundh, S. Skerfving. 2008. Yearly measurements of blood lead in Swedish children since 1978: The declining trend continues in the petrol-lead-free period 1995–2007. *Environ. Res.* 107:332–335.

356. Zheng, L. et al. 2008. Blood lead and cadmium levels and relevant factors among children from an e-waste recycling town in China. *Environ. Res.* 108:15–20.

357. Jusko, T. A., C. R. Henderson, B. P. Lanphear, D. A. Cory-Slechta, P. J. Parsons, R. L. Canfield. 2008. Blood lead concentrations <10 microg/dL and child intelligence at 6 years of age. *Environ. Health Perspect.* 116:243–248.

358. Lanphear, B. P. 2005. Childhood lead poisoning prevention: Too little, too late. *J. Am. Med. Assoc.* 293:2274–2276.

359. Bellinger, D. C., K. M. Stiles, H. L. Needleman. 1992. Low-level lead exposure, intelligence and academic achievement: A long-term follow-up study. *Pediatrics* 90:855–861.

360. Conaway, M. R., C. Waternaux, E. Allred, D. Bellinger, A. Leviton. 1992. Pre-natal blood lead levels and learning difficulties in children: An analysis of non-randomly missing categorical data. *Stat. Med.* 11:799–811.

361. Canfield, R. L., C. R. Henderson Jr., D. A. Cory-Slechta, C. Cox, T. A. Jusko, B. P. Lanphear. 2003. Intellectual impairment in children with blood lead concentrations below 10 microg per deciliter. *N. Engl. J. Med.* 348:1517–1526.

362. Hu, H., M. M. Tellez-Rojo, D. Bellinger, D. Smith, A. S. Ettinger, H. Lamadrid-Figueroa, J. Schwartz, L. Schnaas, A. Mercado-Garcia, M. Hernandez-Avila. 2006. Fetal lead exposure at each stage of pregnancy as a predictor of infant mental development. *Environ. Health Perspect.* 114:1730–1735.

363. Neal, A. P., K. H. Stansfield, P. F. Worley, R. E. Thompson, T. R. Guilarte. 2010. Lead exposure during synaptogenesis alters vesicular proteins and impairs vesicular release: Potential role of NMDA receptor dependent BDNF signaling. *Toxicol. Sci.* 116:249–263.

364. Alkondon, M., A. C. Costa, V. Radhakrishnan, R. S. Aronstam, E. X. Albuquerque. 1990. Selective blockade of NMDA-activated channel currents may be implicated in learning deficits caused by lead. *FEBS Lett.* 261:124–130.

365. Guilarte, T. R., J. L. McGlothan. 1998. Hippocampal NMDA receptor mRNA undergoes subunit specific changes during developmental lead exposure. *Brain Res.* 790:98–107.

366. Omelchenko, I. A., C. S. Nelson, J. L. Marino, C. N. Allen. 1996. The sensitivity of N-methyl-D-aspartate receptors to lead inhibition is dependent on the receptor subunit composition. *J. Pharmacol. Exp. Ther.* 278:15–20.

367. Ujihara, H., E. X. Albuquerque. 1992. Developmental change of the inhibition by lead of NMDA-activated currents in cultured hippocampal neurons. *J. Pharmacol. Exp. Ther.* 263:868–875.

368. Guilarte, T. R., J. L. McGlothan. 1998. Hippocampal NMDA receptor mRNA undergoes subunit specific changes during developmental lead exposure. *Brain Res.* 790:98–107.

369. Nihei, M. K., N. L. Desmond, J. L. McGlothan, A. C. Kuhlmann, T. R. Guilarte. 2000. N-methyl-D-aspartate receptor subunit changes are associated with lead-induced deficits of long-term potentiation and spatial learning. *Neuroscience* 99:233–242.

370. Nihei, M. K., T. R. Guilarte. 1999. NMDAR-2A subunit protein expression is reduced in the hippocampus of rats exposed to Pb^{2+} during development. *Brain Res. Mol. Brain Res.* 66:42–49.

371. Toscano, C. D., J. L. McGlothan, T. R. Guilarte. 2003. Lead exposure alters cyclic-AMP response element binding protein phosphorylation and binding activity in the developing rat brain. *Brain Res. Dev. Brain Res.* 145:219–228.

372. Toscano, C. D., H. Hashemzadeh-Gargari, J. L. McGlothan, T. R. Guilarte. 2002. Developmental Pb^{2+} exposure alters NMDAR subtypes and reduces CREB phosphorylation in the rat brain. *Brain Res. Dev. Brain Res.* 139:217–226.

373. Greer, P. L., M. E. Greenberg. 2008. From synapse to nucleus: Calcium dependent gene transcription in the control of synapse development and function. *Neuron* 59:846–860.

374. Shieh, P. B., S. C. Hu, K. Bobb, T. Timmusk, A. Ghosh. 1998. Identification of a signaling pathway involved in calcium regulation of BDNF expression. *Neuron* 20:727–740.

375. Tabuchi, A., H. Sakaya, T. Kisukeda, H. Fushiki, M. Tsuda. 2002. Involvement of an upstream stimulatory factor as well as cAMP-responsive element-binding protein in the activation of brain-derived neurotrophic factor gene promoter I. *J. Biol. Chem.* 277:35920–35931.

376. Tao, X., S. Finkbeiner, D. B. Arnold, A. J. Shaywitz, M. E. Greenberg. 1998. Ca2þ influx regulates BDNF transcription by a CREB family transcription factor-dependent mechanism. *Neuron* 20:709–726.

377. Guilarte, T. R., C. D. Toscano, J. L. McGlothan S. A. Weaver. 2003. Environmental enrichment reverses cognitive and molecular deficits induced by developmental lead exposure. *Ann. Neurol.* 53:50–56.

378. Tao, X., A. E. West, W. G. Chen, G. Corfas, M. E. Greenberg. 2002. A calcium-responsive transcription factor, CaRF, that regulates neuronal activity-dependent expression of BDNF. *Neuron* 33:383–395.

379. Metsis, M., T. Timmusk, E. Arenas, H. Persson. 1993. Differential usage of multiple brain-derived neurotrophic factor promoters in the rat brain following neuronal activation. *Proc. Natl. Acad. Sci. U.S.A.* 90:8802–8806.

380. Andres, M. E., C. Burger, M. J. Peral-Rubio, E. Battaglioli, M. E. Anderson, J. Grimes, J. Dallman, N. Ballas, G. Mandel. 1999. CoREST: A functional corepressor required for regulation of neural-specific gene expression. *Proc. Natl. Acad. Sci. U.S.A.* 96:9873–9878.

381. Lewis, J. D., R. R. Meehan, W. J. Henzel, I. Maurer-Fogy, P. Jeppesen, F. Klein, A. Bird. 1992. Purification, sequence, and cellular localization of a novel chromosomal protein that binds to methylated DNA. *Cell* 69:905–914.

382. Chen, W. G., Q. Chang, Y. Lin, A. Meissner, A. E. West, E. C. Griffith, R. Jaenisch, M. E. Greenberg. 2003. Depression of BDNF transcription involves calcium-dependent phosphorylation of MeCP2. *Science* 302:885–889.

383. Martinowich, K., D. Hattori, H. Wu, S. Fouse, F. He, Y. Hu, G. Fan, Y. E. Sun. 2003. DNA methylation-related chromatin remodeling in activity-dependent BDNF gene regulation. *Science* 302:890–893.

384. Zhou, Z. et al. 2006. Brain-specific phosphorylation of MeCP2 regulates activity-dependent Bdnf transcription, dendritic growth, and spine maturation. *Neuron* 52:255–269.

385. Chiaruttini, C., M. Sonego, G. Baj, M. Simonato, E. Tongiorgi. 2008. BDNF mRNA splice variants display activity-dependent targeting to distinct hippocampal laminae. *Mol. Cell. Neurosci.* 37:11–19.

386. Hartmann, M., R. Heumann, V. Lessmann. 2001. Synaptic secretion of BDNF after high-frequency stimulation of glutamatergic synapses. *EMBO. J.* 20:5887–5897.

387. Lessmann, V., K. Gottmann, M. Malcangio. 2003. Neurotrophin secretion: Current facts and future prospects. *Prog. Neurobiol.* 69:341–374.

388. Tao, X., S. Finkbeiner, D. B. Arnold, A. J. Shaywitz, M. E. Greenberg. 1998. Ca2þ influx regulates BDNF transcription by a CREB family transcription factor-dependent mechanism. *Neuron* 20:709–726.

389. Tongiorgi, E., M. Righi, A. Cattaneo. 1997. Activity-dependent dendritic targeting of BDNF and TrkB mRNAs in hippocampal neurons. *J. Neurosci.* 17:9492–9505.

390. Colin, E., D. Zala, G. Liot, H. Rangone, M. Borrell-Pages, X. J. Li, F. Saudou, S. Humbert. 2008. Huntingtin phosphorylation acts as a molecular switch for anterograde/retrograde transport in neurons. *EMBO. J.* 27:2124–2134.

391. Zala, D., E. Colin, H. Rangone, G. Liot, S. Humbert, F. Saudou. 2008. Phosphorylation of mutant huntingtin at S421 restores anterograde and retrograde transport in neurons. *Hum. Mol. Genet.* 17:3837–3846.

392. Jovanovic, J. N., F. Benfenati, Y. L. Siow, T. S. Sihra, J. S. Sanghera, S. L. Pelech, P. Greengard, A. J. Czernik. 1996. Neurotrophins stimulate phosphorylation of synapsin I by MAP kinase and regulate synapsin I-actin interactions. *Proc. Natl. Acad. Sci. U.S.A.* 93:3679–3683.

393. Zuccato, C., E. Cattaneo. 2007. Role of brain-derived neurotrophic factor in Huntington's disease. *Prog. Neurobiol.* 81:294–330.

394. Gauthier, L. R. et al. 2004. Huntingtin controls neurotrophic support and survival of neurons by enhancing BDNF vesicular transport along microtubules. *Cell* 118:127–138.

395. Metzler, M., L. Gan, G. Mazarei, R. K. Graham, L. Liu, N. Bissada, G. Lu, B. R. Leavitt, M. R. Hayden. 2010. Phosphorylation of huntingtin at Ser421 in YAC128 neurons is associated with protection of YAC128 neurons from NMDA-mediated excitotoxicity and is modulated by PP1 and PP2A. *J. Neurosci.* 30:14318–14329.

396. Ciammola, A., J. Sassone, M. Cannella, S. Calza, B. Poletti, L. Frati, F. Squitieri, V. Silani. 2007. Low brain-derived neurotrophic factor (BDNF) levels in serum of Huntington's disease patients. *Am. J. Med. Genet. B Neuropsychiatr. Genet.* 144B:574–577.

397. Zuccato, C. et al. 2001. Loss of huntingtin-mediated BDNF gene transcription in Huntington's disease. *Science* 293:493–498.

398. Zuccato, C. et al. 2003. Huntingtin interacts with REST/NRSF to modulate the transcription of NRSE-controlled neuronal genes. *Nat. Genet.* 35:76–83.

399. Jiang, X., F. Tian, K. Mearow, P. Okagaki, R. H. Lipsky, A. M. Marini. 2005. The excitoprotective effect of N-methyl-D-aspartate receptors is mediated by a brain-derived neurotrophic factor autocrine loop in cultured hippocampal neurons. *J. Neurochem.* 94:713–722.

400. Neal, A. P., T. R. Guilarte. 2010. Molecular neurobiology of lead (Pb^{2+}): Effects on synaptic function. *Mol. Neurobiol.* 42:151–160.

401. Zafra, F., E. Castren, H. Thoenen, D. Lindholm. 1991. Interplay between glutamate and gamma-aminobutyric acid transmitter systems in the physiological regulation of brain-derived neurotrophic factor and nerve growth factor synthesis in hippocampal neurons. *Proc. Natl. Acad. Sci. U.S.A.* 88:10037–10041.

402. Omelchenko, I. A., C. S. Nelson, J. L. Marino, C. N. Allen. 1996. The sensitivity of N-methyl-D-aspartate receptors to lead inhibition is dependent on the receptor subunit composition. *J. Pharmacol. Exp. Ther.* 278:15–20.

403. Ujihara, H., E. X. Albuquerque. 1992. Developmental change of the inhibition by lead of NMDA-activated currents in cultured hippocampal neurons. *J. Pharmacol. Exp. Ther.* 263:868–875.

404. Greer, P. L., M. E. Greenberg. 2008. From synapse to nucleus: Calcium dependent gene transcription in the control of synapse development and function. *Neuron* 59:846–860.

405. Tao, J. et al. 2009. Phosphorylation of MeCP2 at Serine 80 regulates its chromatin association and neurological function. *Proc. Natl. Acad. Sci. U.S.A.* 106:4882–4887.

406. Bihaqi, S. W., H. Huang, J. Wu, N. H. Zawia. 2011. Infant exposure to lead (Pb) and epigenetic modifications in the aging primate brain: Implications for Alzheimer's disease. *J. Alzheimer's Dis.* 27:819–833.

407. Abuhatzira, L., K. Makedonski, Y. Kaufman, A. Razin, R. Shemer. 2007. MeCP2 deficiency in the brain decreases BDNF levels by REST/CoREST-mediated repression and increases TRKB production. *Epigenetics* 2:214–222.

408. Guy, J., B. Hendrich, M. Holmes, J. E. Martin, A. Bird. 2001. A mouse Mecp2-null mutation causes neurological symptoms that mimic Rett syndrome. *Nat. Genet.* 27:322–326.

409. Chang, Q., G. Khare, V. Dani, S. Nelson, R. Jaenisch. 2006. The disease progression of Mecp2 mutant mice is affected by the level of BDNF expression. *Neuron* 49:341–348.

410. Sun, Y. E., H. Wu. 2006. The ups and downs of BDNF in Rett syndrome. *Neuron* 49:321–323.

411. Huang, E. J., L. F. Reichardt. 2003. Trk receptors: Roles in neuronal signal transduction. *Annu. Rev. Biochem.* 72:609–642.

412. Fitzsimonds, R. M., M. M. Poo. 1998. Retrograde signaling in the development and modification of synapses. *Physiol. Rev.* 78:143–170.

413. Numakawa, T., T. Matsumoto, N. Adachi, D. Yokomaku, M. Kojima, N. Takei, H. Hatanaka. 2001. Brain-derived neurotrophic factor triggers a rapid glutamate release through increase of intracellular Ca(2+) and Na(+) in cultured cerebellar neurons. *J. Neurosci. Res.* 66:96–108.

414. Numakawa, T., S. Yamagishi, N. Adachi, T. Matsumoto, D. Yokomaku, M. Yamada, H. Hatanaka. 2002. Brain-derived neurotrophic factor induced potentiation of Ca(2+) oscillations in developing cortical neurons. *J. Biol. Chem.* 277:6520–6529.

415. Blum, R., A. Konnerth. 2005. Neurotrophin-mediated rapid signaling in the central nervous system: Mechanisms and functions. *Physiology (Bethesda)* 20:70–78.

416. Minichiello, L., A. M. Calella, D. L. Medina, T. Bonhoeffer, R. Klein, M. Korte. 2002. Mechanism of TrkB-mediated hippocampal long-term potentiation. *Neuron* 36:121–137.

417. Gruart, A., C. Sciarretta, M. Valenzuela-Harrington, J. M. Delgado-Garcia, L. Minichiello. 2007. Mutation at the TrkB PLC{gamma}-docking site affects hippocampal LTP and associative learning in conscious mice. *Learn. Mem.* 14:54–62.

418. Nihei, M. K., N. L. Desmond, J. L. McGlothan, A. C. Kuhlmann, T. R. Guilarte. 2000. N-methyl-D-aspartate receptor subunit changes are associated with lead-induced deficits of long-term potentiation and spatial learning. *Neuroscience* 99:233–242.

419. Jovanovic, J. N., A. J. Czernik, A. A. Fienberg, P. Greengard, T. S. Sihra. 2000. Synapsins as mediators of BDNF-enhanced neurotransmitter release. *Nat. Neurosci.* 3:323–329.

420. Sudhof, T. C. 2004. The synaptic vesicle cycle. *Annu. Rev. Neurosci.* 27:509–547.

421. Zagrebelsky, M., A. Holz, G. Dechant, Y. A. Barde, T. Bonhoeffer, M. Korte. 2005. The p75 neurotrophin receptor negatively modulates dendrite complexity and spine density in hippocampal neurons. *J. Neurosci.* 25:9989–9999.

422. Kiraly, E., D. G. Jones. 1982. Dendritic spine changes in rat hippocampal pyramidal cells after postnatal lead treatment: A Golgi study. *Exp. Neurol.* 77:236–239.

423. Koshimizu, H. et al. 2009. Multiple functions of precursor BDNF to CNS neurons: Negative regulation of neurite growth, spine formation and cell survival. *Mol. Brain* 2:27.

424. Wright, C. E., S. R. Kunz-Ebrecht, S. Iliffe, O. Foese, A. Steptoe. 2005. Physiological correlates of cognitive functioning in an elderly population. *Psychoneuroendocrinology* 30(9):826–838.

425. Fiedler, N., C. Weisel, R. Lynch, K. Kelly-McNeil, R. Wedeen, K. Jones, I. Udasin, P. Ohman-Strickland, M. Gochfeld. 2003. Cognitive effects of chronic exposure to lead and solvents. *Am. J. Ind. Med.* 44(4):413–423.

426. Schwartz, B. S. et al. 2001. Associations of blood lead, dimercaptosuccinic acid-chelatable lead, and tibia lead with neurobehavioral test scores in South Korean lead workers. *Am. J. Epidemiol.* 153(5):453–464.

427. Schwartz, B. S., B. K. Lee, K. Bandeen-Roche, W. Stewart, K. Bolla, J. Links, V. Weaver, A. Todd. 2005. Occupational lead exposure and longitudinal decline in neurobehavioral test scores. *Epidemiology* 16(1):106–113.

428. Stewart, W. F., B. S. Schwartz, D. Simon, K. I. Bolla, A. C. Todd, J. Links. 1999. Neurobehavioral function and tibial and chelatable lead levels in 543 former organolead workers. *Neurology* 52(8):1610–1617.

429. Winker, R., E. Ponocny-Seliger, H. W. Rüdiger, A. Barth. 2006. Lead exposure levels and duration of exposure absence predict neurobehavioral performance. *Int. Arch. Occup. Environ. Health* 79(2):123–127.

430. Balbus-Kornfeld, J. M., W. Stewart, K. I. Bolla, B. S. Schwartz. 1995. Cumulative exposure to inorganic lead and neurobehavioural test performance in adults: An epidemiological review. *Occup. Environ. Med.* 52(1):2–12.

431. Muldoon, S. B., J. A. Cauley, L. H. Kuller, L. Morrow, H. L. Needleman, J. Scott, F. J. Hooper. 1996. Effects of blood lead levels on cognitive function of older women. *Neuroepidemiology* 15(2):62–72.

432. Shih, R. A., H. Hu, M. G. Weisskopf, B. S. Schwartz. 2007. Cumulative lead dose and cognitive function in adults: A review of studies that measured both blood lead and bone lead. *Environ. Health Perspect.* 115:483–492.

433. Weuve, J., S. A. Korrick, M. A. Weisskopf, L. M. Ryan, J. Schwartz, H. Nie, F. Grodstein, H. Hu. 2009. Cumulative exposure to lead in relation to cognitive function in older women. *Environ. Health Perspect.* 117:574–580.

434. Levy, A., S. Dachir, I. Arbel, T. Kadar. 1994. Aging, stress, and cognitive function. *Ann. N. Y. Acad. Sci.* 717:79–88.

435. Mahoney, A. M., J. T. Dalby, M. C. King. 1998. Cognitive failures and stress. *Psychol. Rep.* 82(3 Pt 2):1432–1434.

436. Vitaliano, P. P., D. Echeverria, J. Yi, P. E. Phillips, H. Young, I. C. Siegler. 2005. Psychophysiological mediators of caregiver stress and differential cognitive decline. *Psychol. Aging* 20(3):402–411.

437. Cory-Slechta, D. A., M. B. Virgolini, A. Rossi-George, M. Thiruchelvam, R. Lisek, D. Weston. 2008. Lifetime consequences of combined maternal lead and stress. *Basic Clin. Pharmacol. Toxicol.* 102(2):218–227.

438. Zheng, G., X. Zhang, Y. Chen, Y. Zhang, W. Luo, J. Chen. 2007. Evidence for a role of GABAA receptor in the acute restraint stress-induced enhancement of spatial memory. *Brain Res.* 1181:61–73.

439. Cohen, S., T. Kamarck, R. Mermelstein. 1983. A global measure of perceived stress. *J. Health Soc. Behav.* 24(4):385–396.

440. Lazarus, R. S., S. Folkman. 1984. *Stress, Appraisal, and Coping.* New York: Springer. 456 p.

441. Lupien, S. J., F. Maheu, M. Tu, A. Fiocco, T. E. Schramek. 2007. The effects of stress and stress hormones on human cognition: Implications for the field of brain and cognition. *Brain Cogn.* 65(3):209–237.

442. McEwen, B. S. 2007. Physiology and neurobiology of stress and adaptation: Central role of the brain. *Physiol. Rev.* 87(3):873–904.

443. McEwen, B. S. 2008. Central effects of stress hormones in health and disease: Understanding the protective and damaging effects of stress and stress mediators. *Eur. J. Pharmacol.* 583(2–3):174–185.

444. Virgolini, M. B., K. Chen, D. D. Weston, M. R. Bauter, D. A. Cory-Slechta. 2005. Interactions of chronic lead exposure and intermittent stress: Consequences for brain catecholamine systems and associated behaviors and HPA axis function. *Toxicol. Sci.* 87(2):469–482.

445. Virgolini, M. B., A. Rossi-George, R. Lisek, D. D. Weston, M. Thiruchelvam, D. A. Cory-Slechta. 2008. CNS effects of developmental Pb exposure are enhanced by combined maternal and offspring stress. *Neurotoxicology* 29(5):812–827.

446. Agrawal, R., J. P. Chansouria. 1989. Adrenocortical response to stress in rats exposed to lead nitrate. *Res. Commun. Chem. Pathol. Pharmacol.* 65(2):257–260.

447. Kim, D., D. A. Lawrence. 2000. Immunotoxic effects of inorganic lead on host resistance of mice with different circling behavior preferences. *Brain Behav. Immun.* 14(4):305–317.

448. Glass, T. A., K. Bandeen-Roche, M. McAtee, K. Bolla, A. C. Todd, B. S. Schwartz. 2009. Neighborhood psychosocial hazards and the association of cumulative lead dose with cognitive function in older adults. *Am. J. Epidemiol.* 169(6):683–692.

449. Weisskopf, M. G., R. O. Wright, J. Schwartz, A. Spiro III, D. Sparrow, A. Aro, H. Hu. 2004. Cumulative lead exposure and prospective change in cognition among elderly men: The VA Normative Aging Study. *Am. J. Epidemiol.* 160(12):1184–1193.

450. Weisskopf, M. G., S. P. Proctor, R. O. Wright, J. Schwartz, A. Spiro III, D. Sparrow, H. Nie, H. Hu. 2007. Cumulative lead exposure and cognitive performance among elderly men. *Epidemiology* 18(1):59–66.

451. Wright, R. O., S. W. Tsaih, J. Schwartz, A. Spiro III, K. McDonald, S. T. Weiss, H. Hu. 2003. Lead exposure biomarkers and Mini-Mental Status Exam scores in older men. *Epidemiology* 14(6):713–718.

452. Rosner, B. 1983. Percentage points for a generalized ESD many-outlier procedure. *Technometrics* 25(2):165–172.

453. Sapolsky, R. M., L. C. Krey, B. S. McEwen. 1986. The neuroendocrinology of stress and aging: The glucocorticoid cascades hypothesis. *Endocr. Rev.* 7(3):284–301.

454. Pardon, M. C. 2007. Stress and ageing interactions: A paradox in the context of shared etiological and physiopathological processes. *Brain Res. Rev.* 54(2):251–273.

455. Lupien, S. J., A. Fiocco, N. Wan, F. Maheu, C. Lord, T. Schramek, M. T. Tu. 2005. Stress hormones and human memory function across the lifespan. *Psychoneuroendocrinology* 30(3):225–242.

456. Cohen, S, D. A. Tyrrell, A. P. Smith. 1993. Negative life events, perceived stress, negative affect, and susceptibility to the common cold. *J. Pers. Soc. Psychol.* 64(1):131–140.

457. Bushnell, P. J., S. E. Shelton, R. E. Bowman. 1979. Elevation of blood lead concentration by confinement in the rhesus monkey. *Bull. Environ. Contam. Toxicol.* 22(6):819–826.

458. Cetin, A., Y. Gökçe-Kutsal, R. Celiker. 2001. Predictors of bone mineral density in healthy males. *Rheumatol. Int.* 21(3):85–88.

459. Dennison, E., P. Hindmarsh, C. Fall, S. Kellingray, D. Barker, D. Phillips, C. Cooper. 1999. Profiles of endogenous circulating cortisol and bone mineral density in healthy elderly men. *J. Clin. Endocrinol. Metab.* 84(9):3058–3063.

460. Reynolds, R. M., E. M. Dennison, B. R. Walker, H. E. Syddall, P. J. Wood, R. Andrew, D. I. Phillips, C. Cooper. 2005. Cortisol secretion and rate of bone loss in a population-based cohort of elderly men and women. *Calcif. Tissue. Int.* 77(3):134–138.

461. Peters, J. L., L. Kubzansky, E. McNeely, J. Schwartz, A. Spiro III, D. Sparrow, R. O. Wright, H. Nie, H. Hu. 2007. Stress as a potential modifier of the impact of lead levels on blood pressure: The Normative Aging Study. *Environ. Health Perspect.* 115:1154–1159.

462. Chuang, H. Y., K. Y. Chao, S. Y. Tsai. 2005. Reversible neurobehavioral performance with reductions in blood lead levels—A prospective study on lead workers. *Neurotoxicol. Teratol.* 27(3):497–504.

463. Bremner, J. D., B. Elzinga, C. Schmahl, E. Vermetten. 2008. Structural and functional plasticity of the human brain in posttraumatic stress disorder. *Prog. Brain Res.* 167:171–186.

464. Wang, J., M. Korczykowski, H. Rao, Y. Fan, J. Pluta, R. C. Gur, B. S. McEwen, J. A. Detre. 2007. Gender difference in neural response to psychological stress. *Soc. Cogn. Affect Neurosci.* 2(3):227–239.

465. Chiamvimonvat, N., B. O' Rourke, T. J. Kamp, R. G. Kallen, F. Hofmann, V. Flockerzi, E. Marban. 1995. Functional consequences of sulfhydryl modification in the pore-forming subunits of cardiovascular Ca^{2+} and Na^+ channels. *Circ. Res.* 76:325–334.

466. Clarkson, T. W. 1972. The pharmacology of mercury compounds. *Annu. Rev. Pharmacol.* 12:375–406.

467. Abramson, J. J., G. Salama. 1989. Critical sulfhydryls regulate calcium release from sarcoplasmic reticulum. *J. Bioenerg. Biomembr.* 21:283–294.

468. Anner, B. M., M. Moosmayer, E. Imesch. 1992. Mercury blocks Na-KATPase by a ligand-dependent and reversible mechanism. *Am. J. Physiol.* 262:F830–F836.

469. Hechtenberg, S., D. Beyersmann. 1991. Inhibition of sarcoplasmic reticulum Ca(2+)-ATPase activity by cadmium, lead and mercury. *Enzyme* 45:109–115.

470. Stern, A. H. 2005. Balancing the risks and benefits of fish consumption. *Ann. Intern. Med.* 142:949.

471. McKelvey, W., R. C. Gwynn, N. Jeffery, D. Kass, L. E. Thorpe, R. K. Garg, C. D. Palmer, P. J. Parsons. 2007. A biomonitoring study of lead, cadmium, and mercury in the blood of New York City adults. *Environ. Health Perspect.* 115:1435–1441.

472. Chen, C. et al. 2005. Increased oxidative DNA damage, as assessed by urinary 8-hydroxy-2′-deoxyguanosine concentrations, and serum redox status in persons exposed to mercury. *Clin. Chem.* 51:759–767.

473. Klaassen, C. D. 1990. Heavy metals and the heavy metals antagonists. In *Goodman and Gilman's the Pharmacological Basis of Therapeutics*, 8th ed., A. G. Gilman, T. W. Rall, A. S. Nies, P. Taylor, eds., pp. 1592–1614. New York: Pergamon Press.

474. Bakir, F. et al. 1973. Methylmercury poisoning in Iraq. *Science* 181:230–241.

475. WHO (World Health Organization). 1990. *Environmental Health Criteria 101: Methylmercury.* Geneva: World Health Organization.

476. Nriagu, J. O., W. C. Pfeiffer, O. Malm, C. M. Magalhaes de Souza, G. Mierle. 1992. Mercury pollution in Brazil. *Nature* 356:389.

477. Clarkson, T. W., L. Magos, G. J. Myers. 2003. The toxicology of mercury-current exposures and clinical manifestations. *N. Engl. J. Med.* 349:1731–1737.

478. Halbach, S. 1995. Combined estimation of mercury species released from amalgam. *J. Dent. Res.* 74:1103–1109.

479. Bjorkman, L., G. Sandborgh-Englund, J. Ekstrand. 1997. Mercury in saliva and feces after removal of amalgam fillings. *Toxicol. Appl. Pharmacol.* 144:156–162.

480. Langworth, S., G. Sallsten, L. Barregard, I. Cynkier, M. L. Lind, E. Soderman. 1997. Exposure to mercury vapor and impact on health in the dental profession in Sweden. *J. Dent. Res.* 76:1397–1404.

481. Wakita, Y. 1987. Hypertension induced by methyl mercury in rats. *Toxicol. Appl. Pharmacol.* 89:144–147.

482. Salonen, J. T., K. Seppanen, T. A. Lakka, R. Salonen, G. A. Kaplan. 2000. Mercury accumulation and accelerated progression of carotid atherosclerosis: A population-based prospective 4-year follow-up study in men in eastern Finland. *Atherosclerosis* 148:265–273.

483. Houston, M. C. 2007. The role of mercury and cadmium heavy metals in vascular disease, hypertension, coronary heart disease, and myocardial infarction. *Altern. Ther. Health Med.* 13:S128–S133.

484. Vassallo, D. V., C. M. Moreira, E. M. Oliveira, D. M. Bertollo, T. C. Veloso. 1999. Effects of mercury on the isolated heart muscle are prevented by DTT and cysteine. *Toxicol. Appl. Pharmacol.* 156:113–118.

485. Wiggers, G. A., F. M. Pecanha, A. M. Briones, J. V. Perez-Giron, M. Miguel, D. V. Vassallo, V. Cachofeiro, M. J. Alonso, M. Salaices. 2008. Low mercury concentrations cause oxidative stress and endothelial dysfunction in conductance and resistance arteries. *Am. J. Physiol. Heart Circ. Physiol.* 295:H1033–H1043.

486. Pecanha, F. M., G. A. Wiggers, A. M. Briones, J. V. Perez-Giron, M. Miguel, A. B. Garcia-Redondo, D. V. Vassallo, M. J. Alonso, M. Salaices. 2010. The role of cyclooxygenase (COX)-2 derived prostanoids on vasoconstrictor responses to phenylephrine is increased by exposure to low mercury concentration. *J. Physiol. Pharmacol.* 61:29–36.

487. Furieri, L. B. et al. 2011. Endothelial dysfunction of rat coronary arteries after exposure to low concentrations of mercury is dependent on reactive oxygen species. *Br. J. Pharmacol.* 162:1819–1831.

488. da Cunha, V., L. V. Rossoni, P. A. Oliveira, S. Poton, S. C. Pretti, D. V. Vassallo, I. Stefanon. 2000. Cyclooxygenase inhibition reduces blood pressure elevation and vascular reactivity dysfunction caused by inhibition of nitric oxide synthase in rats. *Clin. Exp. Hypertens.* 22:203–215.

489. Touyz, R. M. 2004. Reactive oxygen species, vascular oxidative stress, and redox signaling in hypertension: What is the clinical significance? *Hypertension* 44:248–252.

490. Vassallo, D. V., M. R. Simões, L. B. Furieri, M. Fioresi, J. Fiorim, E. A. S. Almeida, J. K. Angeli, G. A. Wiggers, F. M. Peçanha, M. Salaices. 2011. Toxic effects of mercury, lead and gadolinium on vascular reactivity. *Braz. J. Med. Biol. Res.* 44(9):939–946.

491. Silveira, E. A., J. H. Lizardo, L. P. Souza, I. Stefanon, D. V. Vassallo. 2010. Acute lead-induced vaso-constriction in the vascular beds of isolated perfused rat tails is endothelium-dependent. *Braz. J. Med. Biol. Res.* 43:492–499.

492. Wiggers, G. A., I. Stefanon, A. S. Padilha, F. M. Pecanha, D. V. Vassallo, E. M. Oliveira. 2008. Low nanomolar concentration of mercury chloride increases vascular reactivity to phenylephrine and local angiotensin production in rats. *Comp. Biochem. Physiol. C Toxicol. Pharmacol.* 147:252–260.

493. da Cunha, V., H. P. Souza, L. V. Rossoni, A. S. Franca, D. V. Vassallo. 2000. Effects of mercury on the isolated perfused rat tail vascular bed are endothelium-dependent. *Arch. Environ. Contam. Toxicol.* 39:124–130.

494. Angeli, J. K., D. B. Ramos, E. A. Casali, D. O. Souza, J. J. Sarkis, I. Stefanon, D. V. Vassallo, C. R. Fürstenau. 2011. Gadolinium increases the vascular reactivity of rat aortic rings. *Braz. J. Med. Biol. Res.* 44:445–452.

495. Ni, M., X. Li, Z. Yin, H. Jiang, M. Sidoryk-Wegrzynowicz, D. Milatovic, J. Cai, M. Aschner. 2010. Methylmercury induces acute oxidative stress, altering Nrf2 protein level in primary microglial cells. *Toxicolo. Sci.* 116(2):590–603.

496. Szucs, A., C. Angiello, J. Salanki, D. O. Carpenter. 1997. Effects of inorganic mercury and methylmer-cury on the ionic currents of cultured rat hippocampal neurons. *Cell Mol. Neurobiol.* 17:273–288.

497. Shafer, T. J., C. A. Meacham, S. Barone Jr. 2002. Effects of prolonged exposure to nanomolar concentra-tions of methylmercury on voltage-sensitive sodium and calcium currents in PC12 cells. *Brain Res. Dev. Brain Res.* 136:151–164.

498. Tarabova, B., M. Kurejova, Z. Sulova, M. Drabova, L. Lacinova. 2006. Inorganic mercury and meth-ylmercury inhibit the Cav3.1 channel expressed in human embryonic kidney 293 cells by different mechanisms. *J. Pharmacol. Exp. Ther.* 317:418–427.

499. Yoshino, Y., T. Mozai, K. Nakao. 1966. Biochemical changes in the brain in rats poisoned with an alkymercury compound, with special reference to the inhibition of protein synthesis in brain cortex slices. *J. Neurochem.* 13:1223–1230.

500. Parran, D. K., S. Barone Jr., W. R. Mundy. 2003. Methylmercury decreases NGF-induced TrkA auto-phosphorylation and neurite outgrowth in PC12 cells. *Brain Res. Dev. Brain. Res.* 141:71–81.

501. Bakir, F. et al. 1973. Methylmercury poisoning in Iraq. *Science* 181:230–241.

502. Vahter, M. E., N. K. Mottet, L. T. Friberg, S. B. Lind, J. S. Charleston, T. M. Burbacher. 1995. Demethylation of methyl mercury in different brain sites of *Macaca fascicularis* monkeys during long-term subclinical methyl mercury exposure. *Toxicol. Appl. Pharmacol.* 134:273–284.

503. Cornett, C. R., W. D. Ehmann, D. R. Wekstein, W. R. Markesbery. 1998. Trace elements in Alzheimer's disease pituitary glands. *Biol. Trace. Elem. Res.* 62:107–114.

504. Sallsten, G., L. Barregard, A. Schutz. 1993. Decrease in mercury concentration in blood after long term exposure: A kinetic study of chloralkali workers. *Br. J. Ind. Med.* 50:814–821.

505. Passos, C. J., D. Mergler, M. Lemire, M. Fillion, J. R. Guimaraes. 2007. Fish consumption and bioindi-cators of inorganic mercury exposure. *Sci. Total Environ.* 373:68–76.

506. Carvalho, C. M., E. H. Chew, S. I. Hashemy, J. Lu, A. Holmgren. 2008. Inhibition of the human thiore-doxin system. A molecular mechanism of mercury toxicity. *J. Biol. Chem.* 283:11913–11923.

507. Casadesus, G., C. S. Atwood, X. Zhu, A. W. Hartzler, K. M. Webber, G. Perry, R. L. Bowen, M. A. Smith. 2005. Evidence for the role of gonadotropin hormones in the development of Alzheimer disease. *Cell. Mol. Life Sci.* 62:293–298.

508. Morale, M. C. et al. 2001. Neuroendocrine-immune (NEI) circuitry from neuron-glial interactions to function: Focus on gender and HPA-HPG interactions on early programming of the NEI system. *Immunol. Cell Biol.* 79:400–417.

509. Marchetti, B., F. Gallo, Z. Farinella, C. Tirolo, N. Testa, S. Caniglia, M. C. Morale. 2000. Gender, neuroendocrine-immune interactions and neuron-glial plasticity. Role of luteinizing hormone-releasing hormone (LHRH). *Ann. N Y Acad. Sci.* 917:678–709.

510. Marchetti, B., F. Gallo, Z. Farinella, C. Tirolo, N. Testa, C. Romeo, M. C. Morale. 1998. Luteinizing hormone-releasing hormone is a primary signaling molecule in the neuroimmune network. *Ann. N Y Acad. Sci.* 840:205–248.

511. Azad, N., N. La Paglia, K. A. Jurgens, L. Kirsteins, N. V. Emanuele, M. R. Kelley, A. M. Lawrence, N. Mohagheghpour. 1993. Immunoactivation enhances the concentration of luteinizing hormone-releasing hormone peptide and its gene expression in human peripheral T-lymphocytes. *Endocrinology* 133:215–223.

512. Mak, G. K., E. K. Enwere, C. Gregg, T. Pakarainen, M. Poutanen, I. Huhtaniemi, S. Weiss. 2007. Male pheromone-stimulated neurogenesis in the adult female brain: Possible role in mating behavior. *Nat. Neurosci.* 10:1003–1011.

513. Hawken, P. A., T. J. Jorre, J. Rodger, T. Esmaili, D. Blache, G. B. Martin. 2009. Rapid induction of cell proliferation in the adult female ungulate brain (Ovis aries) associated with activation of the reproductive axis by exposure to unfamiliar males. *Biol. Reprod.* 80:1146–1151.

514. Webster, J. I., L. Tonelli, E. M. Sternberg. 2002. Neuroendocrine regulation of immunity. *Annu. Rev. Immunol.* 20:125–163.

515. Chrousos, G. P. 1995. The hypothalamic–pituitary–adrenal axis and immune-mediated inflammation. *N. Engl. J. Med.* 1995332:1351–1362.

516. Abedi-Valugerdi, M., G. Moller. 2000. Contribution of H-2 and non-H-2 genes in the control of mercury-induced autoimmunity. *Int. Immunol.* 12:1425–1430.

517. Hultman, P., H. Hansson-Georgiadi. 1999. Methyl mercury-induced autoimmunity in mice. *Toxicol. Appl. Pharmacol.* 154:203–211.

518. Nielsen, J. B., P. Hultman. 2002. Mercury-induced autoimmunity in mice. *Environ. Health Perspect.* 110:877–881.

519. Havarinasab, S., E. Bjorn, J. Ekstrand, P. Hultman. 2007. Dose and Hg species determine the T-helper cell activation in murine autoimmunity. *Toxicology* 229:23–32.

520. Vargas, D. L., C. Nascimbene, C. Krishnan, A. W. Zimmerman, C. A. Pardo. 2005. Neuroglial activation and neuroinflammation in the brain of patients with autism. *Ann. Neurol.* 57:67–81.

521. Cohly, H. H., A. Panja. 2005. Immunological findings in autism. *Int. Rev. Neurobiol.* 71:317–341.

522. Shepherd, C. E., G. C. Gregory, J. C. Vickers, G. M. Halliday. 2005. Novel "inflammatory plaque' pathology in presenilin-1 Alzheimer's disease. *Neuropathol. Appl. Neurobiol.* 31:503–511.

523. Barron, A. M., S. J. Fuller, G. Verdile, R. N. Martins. 2006. Reproductive hormones modulate oxidative stress in Alzheimer's disease. *Antioxid. Redox Signal* 8:2047–2059.

524. Schulkin, J. 2007. Autism and the amygdala: An endocrine hypothesis. *Brain Cogn.* 65:87–99.

525. Colborn, T. 2004. Neurodevelopment and endocrine disruption. *Environ. Health Perspect.* 112:944–949.

526. Chen, C. Y., K. H. Chen, C. Y. Liu, S. L. Huang, K. M. Lin. 2008. Increased risks of congenital, neurologic, and endocrine disorders associated with autism in preschool children: Cognitive ability differences. *J. Pediatr.* 154(3):345–350.

527. Mills, J. L., M. L. Hediger, C. A. Molloy, G. P. Chrousos, P. Manning-Courtney, K. F. Yu, M. Brasington, L. J. England. 2007. Elevated levels of growth-related hormones in autism and autism spectrum disorder. *Clin. Endocrinol. (Oxf.).* 67:230–237.

528. Geier, D. A., M. R. Geier. 2007. A prospective assessment of androgen levels in patients with autistic spectrum disorders: Biochemical underpinnings and suggested therapies. *Neuro. Endocrinol. Lett.* 8:565–573.

529. Geier, D. A., M. R. Geier. 2006. A clinical trial of combined anti-androgen and anti-heavy metal therapy in autistic disorders. *Neuro. Endocrinol. Lett.* 27:833–838.

530. Ekdahl, C. T., J. H. Claasen, S. Bonde, Z. Kokaia, O. Lindvall. 2003. Inflammation is detrimental for neurogenesis in adult brain. *Proc. Natl. Acad. Sci. U.S.A.* 100:13632–13637.

531. Monje, M. L., H. Toda, T. D. Palmer. 2003. Inflammatory blockade restores adult hippocampal neurogenesis. *Science* 302:1760–1765.

532. Vallieres, L., I. L. Campbell, F. H. Gage, P. E. Sawchenko. 2002. Reduced hippocampal neurogenesis in adult transgenic mice with chronic astrocytic production of interleukin-6. *J. Neurosci.* 22:486–492.

533. Nishida, M., K. Muraoka, K. Nishikawa, T. Takagi, J. Kawada. 1989. Differential effects of methylmercuric chloride and mercuric chloride on the histochemistry of rat thyroid peroxidase and the thyroid peroxidase activity of isolated pig thyroid cells. *J. Histochem. Cytochem.* 37:723–727.

534. Kawada, J., M. Nishida, Y. Yoshimura, K. Mitani. 1980. Effects of organic and inorganic mercurials on thyroidal functions. *J. Pharmacobiodyn.* 3:149–159.

535. Soldin, O. P., D. M. O'Mara, M. Aschner. 2008. Thyroid hormones and methylmercury toxicity. *Biol. Trace Elem. Res.* 126:1–12.

536. Counter, S. A., L. H. Buchanan. 2004. Mercury exposure in children: A review. *Toxicol. Appl. Pharmacol.* 198:209–230.

537. Thompson, C. M., W. R. Markesbery, W. D. Ehmann, Y. X. Mao, D. E. Vance. 1988. Regional brain trace-element studies in Alzheimer's disease. *Neurotoxicology* 9:1–7.

538. Hock, C., G. Drasch, S. Golombowski, F. Muller-Spahn, B. Willershausen-Zonnchen, P. Schwarz, U. Hock, J. H. Growdon, R. M. Nitsch. 1998. Increased blood mercury levels in patients with Alzheimer's disease. *J. Neural. Transm.* 105:59–68.

539. Yu, W. H., W. J. Lukiw, C. Bergeron, H. B. Niznik, P. E. Fraser. 2001. Metallothionein III is reduced in Alzheimer's disease. *Brain Res.* 894:37–45.

540. Khan, A., A. E. Ashcroft, V. Higenell, O. V. Korchazhkina, C. Exley. 2005. Metals accelerate the formation and direct the structure of amyloid fibrils of NAC. *J. Inorg. Biochem.* 99:1920–1927.

541. Hartmann, A., J. D. Veldhuis, M. Deuschle, H. Standhardt, I. Heuser. 1997. Twenty-four hour cortisol release profiles in patients with Alzheimer's and Parkinson's disease compared to normal controls: Ultradion secretory pulsatility and diurnal variation. *Neurobiol. Aging* 18:285–289.

542. Mahaffey, K. R., R. P. Clickner, C. C. Bodurow. 2004. Blood organic mercury and dietary mercury intake: National Health and Nutrition Examination Survey, 1999 and 2000. *Environ. Health Perspect.* 112:562–570.

543. Laks, D. R. 2009. Assessment of chronic mercury exposure within the US population, National Health and Nutrition Examination Survey, 1999–2006. *Biometals.* 22(6):1103–1114.

544. N. A. listed. 2007. The Madison declaration on mercury pollution. *AMBIO: A Journal of the Human Environment.* 36(1):62–66.

545. Sunderland, M., D. Krabbenhoft, J. Moreau, S. Strode, W. Landing. 2009. Mercury sources, distribution, and bioavailability in the North Pacific Ocean: Insights from data and models. *Global Biogeochem. Cycles* 23:1–14.

546. Streets, D. G., Q. Zhang, Y. Wu. 2009. Projections of global mercury emissions in 2050. *Environ. Sci. Technol.* 43:2983–2988.

547. Tan, S. W., J. C. Meiller, K. R. Mahaffey. 2009. The endocrine effects of mercury in humans and wildlife. *Crit. Rev. Toxicol.* 39:228–269.

548. Hintelmann, H., K. Keppel-Jones, R. D. Evans. 2000. Constants of mercury methylation and demethylation rates in sediments and comparison of tracer and ambient mercury availability. *Environ. Toxicol. Chem.* 19:2204.

549. Bergquist, B. A., J. D. Blum. 2007. Mass-dependent and -independent fractionation of hg isotopes by photoreduction in aquatic systems. *Science* 318:417.

550. Parks, J. M. et al. 2013. The genetic basis for bacterial mercury methylation. *Science* 339(6125):1332–1335.

551. Jensen, S., A. Jernelöv. 1969. Biological methylation of mercury in aquatic organisms. *Nature* 223:753.

552. Compeau, G., R. Bartha. 1985. Sulfate-reducing bacteria: Principal methylators of mercury in anoxic estuarine sediment. *Appl. Environ. Microbiol.* 50:498.

553. Kerin, E. J., C. C. Gilmour, E. Roden, M. T. Suzuki, J. D. Coates, R. P. Mason. 2006. Mercury methylation by dissimilatory iron-reducing bacteria. *Appl. Environ. Microbiol.* 72:7919. doi:10.1128/AEM.01602-06 Medline.

554. Choi, S. C., T. Chase Jr., R. Bartha. 1994. Metabolic pathways leading to mercury methylation in *Desulfovibrio desulfuricans* LS. *Appl. Environ. Microbiol.* 60:4072.

555. Wood, J. M., F. S. Kennedy, C. G. Rosen. 1968. Synthesis of methyl-mercury compounds by extracts of a methanogenic bacterium. *Nature* 220:173.

556. Hamelin, S., M. Amyot, T. Barkay, Y. Wang, D. Planas. 2011. Methanogens: Principal methylators of mercury in lake periphyton. *Environ. Sci. Technol.* 45:7693.

557. Gilmour, C. C., D. A. Elias, A. M. Kucken, S. D. Brown, A. V. Palumbo, C. W. Schadt, J. D. Wall. 2011. Sulfate-reducing bacterium *Desulfovibrio desulfuricans* ND132 as a model for understanding bacterial mercury methylation. *Appl. Environ. Microbiol.* 77:3938.

558. Landner, L. 1971. Biochemical model for the biological methylation of mercury suggested from methylation studies *in vivo* with *Neurospora crassa*. *Nature* 230:452.

559. Schaefer, J. K., S. S. Rocks, W. Zheng, L. Liang, B. Gu, F. M. Morel. 2011. Active transport, substrate specificity, and methylation of Hg(II) in anaerobic bacteria. *Proc. Natl. Acad. Sci. U.S.A.* 108:8714.

560. Boto, L., I. Doadrio, R. Diogo. 2009. Prebiotic world, macroevolution, and Darwin's theory: A new insight. *Biol. Philos.* 24(1):119–128.

561. Wood, J. M. 1974. Biological cycles for toxic elements in the environment. *Science* 183:1049.

562. Hintelmann, H. 2010. Organomercurials. Their formation and pathways in the environment. *Met. Ions Life Sci.* 7:365.

563. Compeau, G. C., R. Bartha. 1985. Sulfate-reducing bacteria: Principal methylators of mercury in anoxic estuarine sediment. *Appl. Environ. Microbiol.* 50:498.

564. Gilmour, C. C., E. A. Henry, R. Mitchell. 1992. Sulfate stimulation of mercury methylation in freshwater sediments. *Environ. Sci. Technol.* 26:2281.

565. Fleming, E. J., E. E. Mack, P. G. Green, D. C. Melson. 2006. Mercury methylation from unexpected sources: Molybdate-inhibited freshwater sediments and an iron-reducing bacterium. *Appl. Environ. Microbiol.* 72:57.

566. Kerin, E. J., C. C. Gilmour, E. Roden, M. T. Suzuki, J. D. Coates, R. P. Mason. 2006. Mercury methylation by dissimilatory iron-reducing bacteria. *Appl. Environ. Microbiol.* 72:7919.

567. Yu, R. Q., J. R. Flanders, E. E. Mack, R. Turner, M. B. Mirza, T. Barkay. 2012. Contribution of coexisting sulfate and iron reducing bacteria to methylmercury production in freshwater river sediments. *Environ. Sci. Technol.* 46:2684.

568. Choi, S. C., T. Chase Jr., R. Bartha. 1994. Metabolic pathways leading to mercury methylation in *Desulfovibrio desulfuricans* LS. *Appl. Environ. Microbiol.* 60:1342.

569. Ekstrom, E. B., F. M. Morel, J. M. Benoit. 2003. Mercury methylation independent of the acetyl-coenzyme A pathway in sulfate-reducing bacteria. *Appl. Environ. Microbiol.* 69:5414.

570. Doukov, T. I., T. M. Iverson, J. Servalli, S. W. Ragsdale, C. L. Drennan. 2002. A Ni-Fe-Cu center in a bifunctional carbon monoxide dehydrogenase/acetyl-CoA synthase. *Science* 298:567.

571. Kung, Y., N. Ando, T. I. Doukov, L. C. Blasiak, G. Bender, J. Seravalli, S. W. Ragsdale, C. L. Drennan. 2012. Visualizing molecular juggling within a B12-dependent methyltransferase complex. *Nature* 484:265.

572. Ragsdale, S. W., P. A. Lindahl, E. Münck. 1987. Mössbauer, EPR, and optical studies of the corrinoid/iron-sulfur protein involved in the synthesis of acetyl coenzyme A by *Clostridium thermoaceticum*. *J. Biol. Chem.* 262:14289.

573. Svetlitchnaia, T., V. Svetlitchnyi, O. Meyer, H. Dobbek. 2006. Structural insights into methyltransfer reactions of a corrinoid iron-sulfur protein involved in acetyl-CoA synthesis. *Proc. Natl. Acad. Sci. U.S.A.* 103:14331.

574. Goetzl, S., J. H. Jeoung, S. E. Hennig, H. Dobbek. 2011. Structural basis for electron and methyl-group transfer in a methyltransferase system operating in the reductive acetyl-CoA pathway. *J. Mol. Biol.* 411:96.

575. Brown, S. D. et al. 2011. Genome sequence of the mercury-methylating strain *Desulfovibrio desulfuricans* ND132. *J. Bacteriol.* 193:2078.

576. Punta, M. et al. 2012. The Pfam protein families database. *Nucleic Acids Res.* 40(database issue):D290–301.

577. Drake, H. L., S. I. Hu, H. G. Wood. 1981. Purification of five components from *Clostridium thermoaceticum* which catalyze synthesis of acetate from pyruvate and methyltetrahydrofolate. Properties of phosphotransacetylase. *J. Biol. Chem.* 256:11137.

578. Doukov, T., J. Seravalli, J. J. Stezowski, S. W. Ragsdale. 2000. Crystal structure of a methyltetrahydrofolate- and corrinoid-dependent methyltransferase. *Structure* 8:817.

579. Cardiano, P., G. Falcone, C. Foti, S. Sammartano. 2011. Sequestration of Hg^{2+} by some biologically important thiols. *J. Chem. Eng. Data* 56:4741.

580. DeSimone, R. E., M. W. Penley, L. Charbonneau, S. G. Smith, J. M. Wood, H. A. Hill, J. M. Pratt, S. Ridsdale, R. J. Williams. 1973. The kinetics and mechanism of cobalamin-dependent methyl and ethyl transfer to mercuric ion. *Biochim. Biophys. Acta* 304:851.

581. Hill, H. A. O., J. M. Pratt, S. Ridsdale, F. R. Williams. 1970. Kinetics of substitution of co-ordinated carbanions in Colbalt (III) Corrinoids. *J. Chem. Soc. Chem. Commun.* 6:341–324.

582. Schrauzer, G. N., J. W. Sibert. 1970. Coenzyme B12 and coenzyme B12 model compounds in the catalysis of the dehydration of glycols. *J. Am. Chem. Soc.* 92:3509.

583. Zhang, G. S., N. Jiang, X. L. Liu, X. Z. Dong. 2008. Methanogenesis from methanol at low temperatures by a novel psychrophilic methanogen, *Methanolobus psychrophilus* sp. nov., prevalent in Zoige wetland of the Tibetan plateau. *Appl. Environ. Microbiol.* 74:6114–6120.

584. Slobodkina, G. B., A. L. Reysenbach, A. N. Panteleeva, N. A. Kostrikina, I. D. Wagner, E. A. Bonch-Osmolovskaya, A. I. Slobodkin. 2012. Deferrisoma camini gen. nov., sp. nov., a moderately thermophilic, dissimilatory iron(III)-reducing bacterium from a deep-sea hydrothermal vent that forms a distinct phylogenetic branch in the Deltaproteobacteria. *Int. J. Syst. Evol. Microbiol.* 62:2463.

585. Dridi, B., M. L. Fardeau, B. Ollivier, D. Raoult, M. Drancourt. 2012. Methanomassiliicoccus luminyensis gen. nov., sp. nov., a methanogenic archaeon isolated from human faeces. *Int. J. Syst. Evol. Microbiol.* 62:1902.

586. Klein, C., R. Gebker, T. Kokocinski, S. Dreysse, B. Schnackenburg, E. Fleck, E. Nagel. 2008. Combined magnetic resonance coronary artery imaging, myocardial perfusion and late gadolinium enhancement in patients with suspected coronary artery disease. *J. Cardiovasc. Magn. Reson.* 10:45.

587. Caldwell, R. A., H. F. Clemo, C. M. Baumgarten. 1998. Using gadolinium to identify stretch-activated channels: Technical considerations. *Am. J. Physiol.* 275:C619–C621.

588. Perazella, M. A. 2008. Gadolinium-contrast toxicity in patients with kidney disease: Nephrotoxicity and nephrogenic systemic fibrosis. *Curr. Drug Saf.* 3:67–75.

589. Burnstock, G. 2006. Pathophysiology and therapeutic potential of purinergic signaling. *Pharmacol. Rev.* 58:58–86.

590. Escalada, A., P. Navarro, E. Ros, J. Aleu, C. Solsona, M. Martin-Satue. 2004. Gadolinium inhibition of ecto-nucleoside triphosphate diphosphohydrolase activity in Torpedo electric organ. *Neurochem. Res.* 29:1711–1714.

591. Sevigny, J., C. Sundberg, N. Braun, O. Guckelberger, E. Csizmadia, I. Qawi, M. Imai, H. Zimmermann, S. C. Robson. 2002. Differential catalytic properties and vascular topography of murine nucleoside triphosphate diphosphohydrolase 1 (NTPDase1) and NTPDase2 have implications for thromboregulation. *Blood* 99:2801–2809.

592. Khalil-Manesh, F., H. C. Gonick, E. W. Weiler, B. Prins, M. A. Weber, R. E. Purdy. 1993. Lead-induced hypertension: Possible role of endothelial factors. *Am. J. Hypertens.* 6:723–729.

593. Frassetto, S. S., M. R. Schetinger, R. Schierholt, A. Webber, C. D. Bonan, A. T. Wyse, R. D. Dias, C. A. Netto, J. J. Sarkis. 2000. Brain ischemia alters platelet ATP diphosphohydrolase and 5′-nucleotidase activities in naive and preconditioned rats. *Braz. J. Med. Biol. Res.* 33:1369–1377.

594. Touyz, R. M., C. Berry. 2002. Recent advances in angiotensin II signaling. *Braz. J. Med. Biol. Res.* 35:1001–1015.

595. IARC (International Agency for Research on Cancer). 2004. Some drinking-water disinfectants and contaminants, including arsenic. *IARC Monogr. Eval. Carcinog. Risks Hum.* 84:241–267.

596. Kinniburgh, D. G., P. L. Smedley. 2001. *Arsenic Contamination of Groundwater in Bangladesh. Final Report.* BGS Technical Report. Keyworth, UK: British Geological Survey.

597. Van Geen, A. et al. 2002. Promotion of well-switching to mitigate the current arsenic crisis in Bangladesh. *Bull. WHO* 80(9):732–737.

598. U.S. EPA. 2001. National primary drinking water regulations: Arsenic and clarifications to compliance and new source contaminants monitoring. *Final Rule Fed. Reg.* 66(14):6975–7066.

599. WHO. 2004. *Recommendations. Guidelines for Drinking Water Quality.* 3rd ed. Geneva: World Health Organization.

600. California Environmental Protection Agency. 2004. *Public Health Goals for Arsenic in Drinking Water.* Sacramento: California Environmental Protection Agency, Office of Environmental Health Hazard Assessment.

601. Wasserman, G. A. et al. 2004. Water arsenic exposure and children's intellectual function in Araihazar, Bangladesh. *Environ. Health Perspect.* 112:1329–1333.

602. International Agency for Research on Cancer (IARC). 2004. Monographs on the evaluation of carcinogenic risk of chemicals to humans: Some drinking water disinfectants and contaminants, including arsenic. *IARC Monorg. Eval. Carcinog. Risks Hum.* 84:1–477.

603. European Chemicals Bureau. European chemical substances information system (ESIS). 2007. European Chemicals Bureau. [Accessed May 24, 2011] http://ecb.jrc.it/esis

604. Environmental Protection Agency. Integrated Risk Information system (IRIS). 2007. Environmental Protection Agency. [Accessed May 24, 2011] http://www.epa.gov./iris

605. Rahman, M. M. et al. 2003. Arsenic groundwater contamination and sufferings of people in North 24-Pargans, one of the nine arsenic affected districts of West Bengal, India. *J. Environ. Sci. Health A Tox. Hazard Subst. Environ. Eng.* 38:25–59.

606. National Research Council (NRC). 1999. *Arsenic in Drinking Water.* Washington, DC: National Academy Press.

607. Ahmad, S. A. 2000. *Water Contamination and Health Hazard*, p. 23. Rajshahi: Udayan Press.

608. Muller, S. 2010. Melanin-associated pigmented lesions of the oral mucosa: Presentation, differential diagnosis, and treatment. *Dermatol. Ther.* 23:220–229.

609. Khlifi, R., A. Hamza-Chaffai. 2010. Head and neck cancer due to heavy metal exposure via tobacco smoking and professional exposure: A review. *Toxicol. Appl. Pharmacol.* 248:71–88.

610. Ferlay, J., P. Pisani, D. M. Parkin. 2004. *Cancer Incidence, Mortality and Prevalence Worldwide. IARC Cancer Base (2002 Estimates).* Lyon: IARC Press. pp. 481–488.

611. Yuan, T. H., I. B. Lian, K. Y. Tsai, T. K. Chang, C. T. Chiang, C. C. Su, Y. H. Hwang. 2011. Possible association between nickel and chromium and oral cancer: A case-control study in central Taiwan. *Sci. Total Environ.* 409:1046–1052.

612. Wang, X., J. Zhang, M. Liu, F. C. Wei. 2008. Aseptic necrosis of the maxilla after devitalisation of the teeth with arsenic trioxide. *Br. J. Oral Maxillofac. Surg.* 46:79–82.

613. Sarwar, A. F. M., S. A. Ahmad, M. H. Kabir. 2010. Swelling of vallate papillae of the tongue following arsenic exposure. *Bangladesh Med. Res. Counc. Bull.* 36:1–3.

614. Rahman, M. M. et al. 2001. Chronic arsenic toxicity in Bangladesh and West Bengal, India—A review and commentary. *J. Toxicol. Clin. Toxicol.* 39:683–700.

615. Syed, E. H. et al. 2013. Arsenic exposure and oral cavity lesions in Bangladesh. *J. Occup. Environ. Med.* 55(1):59–66.

616. Yu, H. S., W. T. Liao, C. Y. Chai. 2006. Arsenic carcinogenesis in the skin. *J. Biomed. Sci.* 13:657–666.

617. Celik, I. et al. 2008. Arsenic in drinking water and lung cancer: A systematic review. *Environ. Res.* 108:48–55.

618. Mink, P. J., D. D. Alexander, L. M. Barraj, M. A. Kelsh, J. S. Tsuji. 2008. Low-level arsenic exposure in drinking water and bladder cancer: A review and meta-analysis. *Regul. Toxicol. Pharmacol.* 52:299–310.

619. Liu, J., M. P. Waalkes. 2008. Liver is a target of arsenic carcinogenesis. *Toxicol. Sci.* 105:24–32.

620. Yuan, Y., G. Marshall, A. H. Smith, C. Ferreccio, C. Steinmaus, J. Liaw, M. Bates. 2010. Kidney cancer mortality: Fifty-year latency patterns related to arsenic exposure. *Epidemiology* 21:103–108.

621. Su, C. C., K. Y. Tsai, Y. Y. Hsu, Y. Y. Lin, I. B. Lian. 2010. Chronic exposure to heavy metals and incidence of oral cancer in Taiwanese males. *Oral Oncol.* 46:586–590.

622. Su, C. C., Y. Y. Lin, T. K. Chang, C. T. Chiang, J. A. Chung, Y. Y. Hsu, I. B. Lian. 2010. Incidence of oral cancer in relation to nickel and arsenic concentrations in farm soils of patients' residential areas in Taiwan. *BMC Public Health* 10:67. doi: 10.1186/1471-2458-10-67.

623. Chiang, C. T., Y. H. Hwang, T. H. Yuan, C. C. Su, K. Y. Tsai, I. B. Lian, T. K. Chang. 2010. Elucidating the underlying causes of oral cancer through spatial clustering in high-risk areas of Taiwan with a distinct gender ratio of incidence. *Geospat. Health* 4:230–242.

624. Gao, J., J. Yu, L. Yang. 2011. Urinary arsenic metabolites of subjects exposed to elevated arsenic present in coal in Shaanxi Province, China. *Int. J. Environ. Res. Public Health* 8:1991–2008.

625. Lindberg, A. L., E. C. Ekstrom, B. Nermell, M. Rahman, B. Lönnerdal, L. A. Persson, M. Vahter. 2008. Gender and age differences in the metabolism of inorganic arsenic in a highly exposed population in Bangladesh. *Environ. Res.* 106:110–120.

626. Lindberg, A. L., R. Kumar, W. Goessler, R. Thirumaran, E. Gurzau, K. Koppova, P. Rudnai, G. Leonardi, T. Fletcher, M. Vahter. 2007. Metabolism of low dose inorganic arsenic in a Central European population-influence of gender and genetic polymorphism. *Environ. Health Perspect.* 115:1081–1086.

627. Wang, J. P., R. Maddalena, B. Zheng, C. Zai, F. Liu, J. C. Ng. 2009. Arsenicosis status and urinary malondialdehyde (MDA) in people exposed to arsenic contaminated-coal in China. *Environ. Int.* 35:502–506.

628. Al-Rmalli, A. W., R. O. Jenkins, P. I. Haris. 2011. Betel quid chewing elevates human exposure to arsenic, cadmium and lead. *J. Hazard. Mater.* 190:69–74.

629. Pu, Y. S., S. M. Yang, Y. K. Huang, C. J. Chung, S. K. Huang, A. W. Chiu, M. H. Yang, C. J. Chen, Y. M. Hsueh. 2007. Urinary arsenic profile affects the risk of urothelial carcinoma even at low arsenic exposure. *Toxicol. Appl. Pharmacol.* 218:99–106.

630. Huang, Y. K., Y. S. Pu, C. J. Chung, H. S. Shiue, M. H. Yang, C. J. Chen, Y. M. Hsueh. 2008. Plasma folate level, urinary arsenic methylation profiles, and urothelial carcinoma susceptibility. *Food Chem. Toxicol.* 46:929–938.

631. Arain, M. B., T. G. Kazi, J. A. Baig, M. K. Jamali, H. I. Afridi, N. Jalbani, R. A. Sarfraz, A. Q. Shah, G. A. Kandhro. 2009. Respiratory effects in people exposed to arsenic via the drinking water and tobacco smoking in southern part of Pakistan. *Sci. Total Environ.* 407:5524–5530.

632. McCarty, K. M., E. A. Houseman, Q. Quamruzzaman, M. Rahman, G. Mahiuddin, T. Smith, L. Ryan, D. C. Christiani. 2006. The impact of diet and betel nut use on skin lesions associated with drinking-water arsenic in Pabna, Bangladesh. *Environ. Health Perspect.* 114:334–340.

633. Pilsner, J. R., X. H. Liu, H. Ahsan, V. Ilievski, V. Slavkovich, D. Levy, P. Factor-Litvak, J. H. Graziano, M. V. Gamble. 2009. Folate deficiency, hyperhomocysteinemia, low urinary creatinine, and hypomethylation of leukocyte DNA are risk factors for arsenic-induced skin lesions. *Environ. Health Perspect.* 117:254–260.

634. Critchley, J. A., B. Unal. 2003. Health effects associated with smokeless tobacco: A systematic review. *Thorax* 58:435–443.

635. WHO (World Health Organization). 2001. Arsenic and Arsenic Compounds. *EHC 224.* Geneva: International Programme on Chemical Safety, WHO.

636. British Geological Survey (BGS) and Department of Public Health Engineering (DPHE). 2001. *Arsenic Contamination of Groundwater in Bangladesh. Vol. 3: Hydrochemical Atlas*, D. G. Kinniburgh, P. L. Smedley, eds., BGS Report WC/00/19. Keyworth, UK: British Geological Survey.

637. Chakraborti, D. et al. 2004. Groundwater arsenic contamination and its health effects in the Ganga-Meghna-Brahmaputra plain. *J. Environ. Monit.* 6(6):74N–83N.

638. Sun, G. X., P. N. Williams, A. M. Carey, Y. G. Zhu, C. Deacon, A. Raab, J. Feldmann, R. M. Islam, A. A. Meharg. 2008. Inorganic arsenic in rice bran and its products are an order of magnitude higher than in bulk grain. *Environ. Sci. Technol.* 42(19):7542–7546.

639. IARC (International Agency for Research on Cancer). 2004. Arsenic in drinking water. *IARC Monogr. Eval. Carcinog. Risks Hum.* 84:39–267.

640. Rahman, A., M. Vahter, E. C. Ekström, M. Rahman, A. H. Golam Mustafa, M. A. Wahed, M. Yunus, L. A. Persson. 2007. Association of arsenic exposure during pregnancy with fetal loss and infant death: A cohort study in Bangladesh. *Am. J. Epidemiol.* 165(12):1389–1396.

641. States, J. C., S. Srivastava, Y. Chen, A. Barchowsky. 2009. Arsenic and cardiovascular disease. *Toxicol. Sci.* 107(2):312–323.

642. Yu, H. S., W. T. Liao, C. Y. Chai. 2006. Arsenic carcinogenesis in the skin. *J. Biomed. Sci.* 13(5):657–666.

643. Chen, Y., J. H. Graziano, F. Parvez, I. Hussain, H. Momotaj, A. van Geen, G. R. Howe, H. Ahsan. 2006. Modification of risk of arsenic-induced skin lesions by sunlight exposure, smoking, and occupational exposures in Bangladesh. *Epidemiology* 17(4):459–467.

644. Saha, K. C. 2003. Diagnosis of arsenicosis. *J. Environ. Sci. Health A Tox. Hazard. Subst. Environ. Eng.* 38(1):255–272.

645. Vahter, M. 2002. Mechanisms of arsenic biotransformation. *Toxicology* 181–182:211–217.

646. Chen, Y. C., Y. L. Guo, H. J. Su, Y. M. Hsueh, T. J. Smith, L. M. Ryan, M. S. Lee, S. C. Chao, J. Y. Lee, D. C. Christiani. 2003. Arsenic methylation and skin cancer risk in southwestern Taiwan. *J. Occup. Environ. Med.* 45(3):241–248.

647. Chen, Y. C., H. J. Su, Y. L. Guo, E. A. Houseman, D. C. Christiani. 2005. Interaction between environmental tobacco smoke and arsenic methylation ability on the risk of bladder cancer. *Cancer Causes Control* 16(2):75–81.

648. Chen, C. J. et al. 2005. Biomarkers of exposure, effect, and susceptibility of arsenic-induced health hazards in Taiwan. *Toxicol. Appl. Pharmacol.* 206(2):198–206.

649. Chen, Y. C., H. J. Su, Y. L. Guo, E. A. Houseman, D. C. Christiani. 2005. Interaction between environmental tobacco smoke and arsenic methylation ability on the risk of bladder cancer. *Cancer Causes Control* 16(2):75–81.

650. Chung, C. J., C. J. Huang, Y. S. Pu, C. T. Su, Y. K. Huang, Y. T. Chen, Y. M. Hsueh. 2008. Urinary 8-hydroxydeoxyguanosine and urothelial carcinoma risk in low arsenic exposure area. *Toxicol. Appl. Pharmacol.* 226(1):14–21.

651. Hsueh, Y. M., H. Y. Chiou, Y. L. Huang, W. L. Wu, C. C. Huang, M. H. Yang, L. C. Lue, G. S. Chen, C. J. Chen. 1997. Serum beta-carotene level, arsenic methylation capability, and incidence of skin cancer. *Cancer Epidemiol. Biomarkers Prev.* 6(8):589–596.

652. Huang, Y. K., Y. L. Huang, Y. M. Hsueh, M. H. Yang, M. M. Wu, S. Y. Chen, L. I. Hsu, C. J. Chen. 2008. Arsenic exposure, urinary arsenic speciation, and the incidence of urothelial carcinoma: A twelve-year follow-up study. *Cancer Causes Control.* 19(8):829–839.

653. Li, X., J. Pi, B. Li, Y. Xu, Y. Jin, G. Sun. 2008. Urinary arsenic speciation and its correlation with 8-OHdG in Chinese residents exposed to arsenic through coal burning. *Bull. Environ. Contam. Toxicol.* 81(4):406–411.

654. Mäki-Paakkanen, J., P. Kurttio, A. Paldy, J. Pekkanen. 1998. Association between the clastogenic effect in peripheral lymphocytes and human exposure to arsenic through drinking water. *Environ. Mol. Mutagen.* 32:301–313.

655. Pu, Y. S., S. M. Yang, Y. K. Huang, C. J. Chung, S. K. Huang, A. W. Chiu, M. H. Yang, C. J. Chen, Y. M. Hsueh. 2007. Urinary arsenic profile affects the risk of urothelial carcinoma even at low arsenic exposure. *Toxicol. Appl. Pharmacol.* 218(2):99–106.

656. Steinmaus, C. et al. 2006. Arsenic methylation and bladder cancer risk in case-control studies in Argentina and the United States. *J. Occup. Environ. Med.* 48(5):478–488.

657. Xu, Y., Y. Wang, Q. Zheng, X. Li, B. Li, Y. Jin, X. Sun, G. Sun. 2008. Association of oxidative stress with arsenic methylation in chronic arsenic exposed children and adults. *Toxicol. Appl. Pharmacol.* 232(1):142–149.

658. Yu, R. C., K. H. Hsu, C. J. Chen, J. R. Froines. 2000. Arsenic methylation capacity and skin cancer. *Cancer Epidemiol. Biomarkers Prev.* 9(11):1259–1262.

659. Ahsan, H., Y. Chen, M. G. Kibriya, V. Slavkovich, F. Parvez, F. Jasmine, M. V. Gamble, J. H. Graziano. 2007. Arsenic metabolism, genetic susceptibility, and risk of premalignant skin lesions in Bangladesh. *Cancer Epidemiol. Biomarkers Prev.* 16(6):1270–1278.

660. Lindberg, A. L., M. Rahman, L. A. Persson, M. Vahter. 2008. The risk of arsenic induced skin lesions in Bangladeshi men and women is affected by arsenic metabolism and the age at first exposure. *Toxicol. Appl. Pharmacol.* 230(1):9–16.

661. Mostafa, M. G., J. C. McDonald, N. M. Cherry. 2008. Lung cancer and arsenic exposure in rural Bangladesh. *Occup. Environ. Med.* 65(11):765–768.

662. Pershagen, G., F. Bergman, J. Klominek, L. Damber, S. Wall. 1987. Histological types of lung cancer among smelter workers exposed to arsenic. *Br. J. Ind. Med.* 44(7):454–458.

663. Hays, A. M., D. Srinivasan, M. L. Witten, D. E. Carter, R. C. Lantz. 2006. Arsenic and cigarette smoke synergistically increase DNA oxidation in the lung. *Toxicol. Pathol.* 34(4):396–404.

664. Bates, M. N., O. A. Rey, M. L. Biggs, C. Hopenhayn, L. E. Moore, D. Kalman, C. Steinmaus, A. H. Smith. 2004. Case-control study of bladder cancer and exposure to arsenic in Argentina. *Am. J. Epidemiol.* 159(4):381–389.

665. Steinmaus, C., Y. Yuan, M. N. Bates, A. H. Smith. 2003. Case-control study of bladder cancer and drinking water arsenic in the western United States. *Am. J. Epidemiol.* 158(12):1193–1201.

666. Vahter, M., A. Akesson, C. Lidén, S. Ceccatelli, M. Berglund. 2007. Gender differences in the disposition and toxicity of metals. *Environ. Res.* 104(1):85–95.

667. Hopenhayn-Rich, C., M. L. Biggs, A. H. Smith, D. A. Kalman, L. E. Moore. 1996. Methylation study of a population environmentally exposed to arsenic in drinking water. *Environ. Health Perspect.* 104:620–628.

668. Lindberg, A. L., E. C. Ekström, B. Nermell, M. Rahman, B. Lönnerdal, L. A. Persson, M. Vahter. 2008. Gender and age differences in the metabolism of inorganic arsenic in a highly exposed population in Bangladesh. *Environ. Res.* 106(1):110–120.

669. Li, J. L., C. Y. Jiang, S. Li, S. W. Xu. 2013. Cadmium induced hepatotoxicity in chickens (*Gallus domesticus*) and ameliorative effect by selenium. *Nature* 499:14.

670. Wang, L., J. Huang, 1994. Arsenic in the environment, Part II. In *Human Health and Ecosystems Effects*, J. O. Nriagu, ed., pp. 159–172. New York: Wiley.

671. Sun, G., Y. Xu, Q. Zheng, S. Xi. 2011. Arsenicosis history and research progress in Mainland China. *Kaohsiung J. Med. Sci.* 27:377.

672. Sun, G., G. Yu, Q. Zheng. 2007. Health effects of exposure to natural arsenic in groundwater and coal in China: An overview of occurrence *Environ. Health Perspect.* 115:636.

673. Lan, Z., C. Changjie. 1997. *J. Hyg. Res.* 26:310.

674. Rodriguez-Lado, L., G. Sun, M. Berg, Q. Zhang, H. Xue, Q. Zheng, C. A. Johnson. 2013. Groundwater arsenic contamination throughout China. *Science* 341:866.

675. Kinniburgh, D. G., P. L. Smedley, eds. 2001. *Arsenic Contamination of Ground Water in Bangladesh.* BGS Technical Report WC/00/19, Keyworth, UK: British Geological Survey, Vol. 2.

676. Fendorf, S., H. A. Michael, A. van Geen. 2010. Spatial and temporal variations of groundwater arsenic in South and Southeast Asia. *Science* 328:1123.

677. Ravenscroft, P., H. Brammer, K. Richards. 2009. *Arsenic Pollution: A Global Synthesis*, Oxford: Blackwell-Wiley.

678. He, J., L. Charlet. 2013. A review of arsenic presence in China drinking water. *J. Hydrol.* 492(2013):79–88.

679. Currell, M. J., I. Cartwright, D. C. Bradley, D. M. Han. 2010. Recharge history and controls on groundwater quality in the Yuncheng Basin, north China. *J. Hydrol.* 385:216–229.

680. George, C. M., J. Inauen, S. M. Rahman, Y. Zheng. 2013. The effectiveness of educational interventions to enhance the adoption of fee-based arsenic testing in Bangladesh: A cluster randomized controlled trial. *Am. J. Trop. Med. Hyg.* 89:138.

681. Johnston, R. B., M. H. Sarker. 2007. Arsenic mitigation in Bangladesh: National screening data and case studies in three upazilas. *J. Environ. Sci. Health A.* 42:1889.

682. Flanagan, S. V., R. B. Johnston, Y. Zheng. 2012. Arsenic in tube well water in Bangladesh: Health and economic impacts and implications for arsenic mitigation. *Bull. World Health Organ.* 90:839.

683. Abhyankar, L. N., M. R. Jones, E. Guallar, A. Navas-Acien. 2011. Arsenic Exposure and Hypertension: A Systematic Review. *Environ. Health Perspect.* 120(4):494–500.

684. Lopez, A. D., C. D. Mathers, M. Ezzati, D. T. Jamison, C. J. Murray. 2006. Global and regional burden of disease and risk factors, 2001: Systematic analysis of population health data. *Lancet* 367:1747–1757.

685. Murray, C. J., A. D. Lopez. 1997. Mortality by cause for eight regions of the world: Global Burden of Disease Study. *Lancet* 349:1269–1276.

686. Oparil, S., M. A. Zaman, D. A. Calhoun. 2003. Pathogenesis of hypertension. *Ann Intern Med.* 139:761–776.

687. Whitworth, J. A. 2003. 2003 World Health Organization (WHO)/International Society of Hypertension (ISH) statement on management of hypertension. *J. Hypertens.* 21:1983–1992.

688. Houston, M. C. 2007. The role of mercury and cadmium heavy metals in vascular disease, hypertension, coronary heart disease, and myocardial infarction. *Altern. Ther. Health Med.* 13:S128–S133.

689. Klahr, S. 2001. The role of nitric oxide in hypertension and renal disease progression. *Nephrol. Dial. Transplant.* 16(suppl. 1):60–62.

690. Laclaustra, M., A. Navas-Acien, S. Stranges, J. M. Ordovas, E. Guallar. 2009. Serum selenium concentrations and hypertension in the US population. *Circ. Cardiovasc. Qual. Outcomes* 2:369–376.

691. Navas-Acien, A., E. Guallar, E. K. Silbergeld, S. J. Rothenberg. 2007. Lead exposure and cardiovascular disease—A systematic review. *Environ. Health Perspect.* 115:472–482.

692. Navas-Acien, A., B. S. Schwartz, S. J. Rothenberg, H. Hu, E. K. Silbergeld, E. Guallar. 2008. Bone lead levels and blood pressure endpoints: A meta-analysis. *Epidemiology* 19:496–504.

693. Vaziri, N. D. 2008. Mechanisms of lead-induced hypertension and cardiovascular disease. *Am. J. Physiol. Heart Circ. Physiol.* 295:H454–H465.

694. Chen, J. W., H. Y. Chen, W. F. Li, S. H. Liou, C. J. Chen, J. H. Wu, S. L. Wang. 2011. The association between total urinary arsenic concentration and renal dysfunction in a community-based population from central Taiwan. *Chemosphere* 84:17–24.

695. Medrano, M. A., R. Boix, R. Pastor-Barriuso, M. Palau, J. Damian, R. Ramis, J. L. Del Barrio, A. Navas-Acien. 2010. Arsenic in public water supplies and cardiovascular mortality in Spain. *Environ. Res.* 110:448–454.

696. Navas-Acien, A., A. R. Sharrett, E. K. Silbergeld, B. S. Schwartz, K. E. Nachman, T. A. Burke, E. Guallar. 2005. Arsenic exposure and cardiovascular disease: A systematic review of the epidemiologic evidence. *Am. J. Epidemiol.* 162:1037–1049.

697. Smedley, P. L., D. G. Kinniburgh. 2002. A review of the source, behaviour and distribution of arsenic in natural waters. *Appl. Geochem.* 17:517–568.

698. DHHS (Department of Health and Human Services). 2005. *Toxicological Profile for Arsenic.* Washington, DC: U.S. DHHS. p. 494.

699. Wang, S. L., F. H. Chang, S. H. Liou, H. J. Wang, W. F. Li, D. P. Hsieh. 2007. Inorganic arsenic exposure and its relation to metabolic syndrome in an industrial area of Taiwan. *Environ. Int.* 33:805–811.

700. Wu, M. M., T. L. Kuo, Y. H. Hwang, C. J. Chen. 1989. Dose–response relation between arsenic concentration in well water and mortality from cancers and vascular diseases. *Am. J. Epidemiol.* 130:1123–1132.

701. Chappell, W. R., C. O. Abernathy, R. L. Calderon, D. J. Thomas, eds. 2002. *Arsenic Exposure and Health Effects V: Proceedings of the Fifth International Conference on Arsenic Exposure and Health Effects.* Amsterdam: Elsevier. pp. 521–533.

702. Chen, C. J., Y. M. Hsueh, M. S. Lai, M. P. Shyu, S. Y. Chen, M. M. Wu, T. L. Kuo, T. Y. Tai. 1995. Increased prevalence of hypertension and long-term arsenic exposure. *Hypertension* 25:53–60.

703. Chilvers, D. C., P. J. Peterson. 1987. Global cycling of arsenic. In *Lead, Mercury, Cadmium and Arsenic in the Environment*, T. C. Huthchinson, K. M. Meema, eds., pp. 279–303. Chichester: John Wiley & Sons.

704. Hinkle, S. R., D. J. Polette. 1999. *Arsenic in Ground Water of the Willamette Basin, Oregon.* Portland, OR: U.S. Geological Survey, U.S. Department of the Interior. pp. 1–24.

705. Mukherjee, A., M. K. Sengupta, M. A. Hossain, S. Ahamed, B. Das, B. Nayak, D. Lodh, M. M. Rahman, D. Chakraborti. 2006. Arsenic contamination in groundwater: A global perspective with emphasis on the Asian scenario. *J. Health Popul. Nutr.* 24:142–163.

706. Rahman, M., M. Tondel, S. A. Ahmad, I. A. Chowdhury, M. H. Faruquee, O. Axelson. 1999. Hypertension and arsenic exposure in Bangladesh. *Hypertension* 33:74–78.

707. Aposhian, H. V., R. A. Zakharyan, M. D. Avram, M. J. Kopplin, M. L. Wollenberg. 2003. Oxidation and detoxification of trivalent arsenic species. *Toxicol. Appl. Pharmacol.* 193:1–8.

708. Balakumar, P., T. Kaur, M. Singh. 2008. Potential target sites to modulate vascular endothelial dysfunction: Current perspectives and future directions. *Toxicology* 245:49–64.

709. Lee, M. Y., B. I. Jung, S. M. Chung, O. N. Bae, J. Y. Lee, J. D. Park, J. S. Yang, H. Lee, J. H. Chung. 2003. Arsenic-induced dysfunction in relaxation of blood vessels. *Environ. Health Perspect.* 111:513–517.

710. Chen, Y., P. Factor-Litvak, G. R. Howe, J. H. Graziano, P. Brandt-Rauf, F. Parvez, A. van Geen, H. Ahsan. 2007. Arsenic exposure from drinking water, dietary intakes of B vitamins and folate, and risk of high blood pressure in Bangladesh: A population-based, cross-sectional study. *Am. J. Epidemiol.* 165:541–552.

711. Jones, M. R., M. Tellez-Plaza, A. R. Sharrett, E. Guallar, A. Navas-Acien. 2011. Urine arsenic and hypertension in US adults: The 2003–2008 National Health and Nutrition Examination Survey. *Epidemiology* 22:153–161.

712. Lewis, D. R., J. W. Southwick, R. Ouellet-Hellstrom, J. Rench, R. L. Calderon. 1999. Drinking water arsenic in Utah: A cohort mortality study. *Environ. Health Perspect.* 107:359–365.

713. Hsueh, Y. M., P. Lin, H. W. Chen, H. S. Shiue, C. J. Chung, C. T. Tsai, Y. K. Huang, H. Y. Chiou, C. J. Chen. 2005. Genetic polymorphisms of oxidative and antioxidant enzymes and arsenic-related hypertension. *J. Toxicol. Environ. Health A*. 68:1471–1484.

714. Huang, Y. K., C. H. Tseng, Y. L. Huang, M. H. Yang, C. J. Chen, Y. M. Hsueh. 2007. Arsenic methylation capability and hypertension risk in subjects living in arseniasis-hyperendemic areas in southwestern Taiwan. *Toxicol. Appl. Pharmacol*. 218:135–142.

715. Dastgiri, S., M. Mosaferi, M. A. Fizi, N. Olfati, S. Zolali, N. Pouladi, P. Azarfam. 2010. Arsenic exposure, dermatological lesions, hypertension, and chromosomal abnormalities among people in a rural community of northwest Iran. *J. Health Popul. Nutr*. 28:14–22.

716. Guo, J. X., L. Hu, P. Z. Yand, K. Tanabe, M. Miyatalre, Y. Chen. 2007. Chronic arsenic poisoning in drinking water in Inner Mongolia and its associated health effects. *J. Environ. Sci. Health A. Tox. Hazard Subst. Environ. Eng*. 42:1853–1858.

717. Jensen, G. E., M. L. Hansen. 1998. Occupational arsenic exposure and glycosylated haemoglobin. *Analyst* 123:77–80.

718. Kwok, R. K. et al. 2007. Drinking water arsenic exposure and blood pressure in healthy women of reproductive age in Inner Mongolia, China. *Toxicol. Appl. Pharmacol*. 222:337–343.

719. Yildiz, A., M. Karaca, S. Biceroglu, M. T. Nalbantcilar, U. Coskun, F. Arik, F. Aliyev, O. Yiginer, C. Turkoglu. 2008. Effect of chronic arsenic exposure from drinking waters on the QT interval and transmural dispersion of repolarization. *J. Int. Med. Res*. 36:471–478.

720. Zierold, K. M., L. Knobeloch, H. Anderson. 2004. Prevalence of chronic diseases in adults exposed to arsenic-contaminated drinking water. *Am. J. Public Health*. 94:1936–1937.

721. Bunderson, M., J. D. Coffin, H. D. Beall. 2002. Arsenic induces peroxynitrite generation and cyclooxygenase-2 protein expression in aortic endothelial cells: Possible role in atherosclerosis. *Toxicol. Appl. Pharmacol*. 184:11–18.

722. Carmignani, M., P. Boscolo, N. Castellino. 1985. Metabolic fate and cardiovascular effects of arsenic in rats and rabbits chronically exposed to trivalent and pentavalent arsenic. *Arch. Toxicol. Suppl*. 8:452–455.

723. Druwe, I. L., R. R. Vaillancourt. 2010. Influence of arsenate and arsenite on signal transduction pathways: An update. *Arch. Toxicol*. 84:585–596.

724. Pi, J. et al. 2000. Decreased serum concentrations of nitric oxide metabolites among Chinese in an endemic area of chronic arsenic poisoning in Inner Mongolia. *Free Radic. Biol. Med*. 28:1137–1142.

725. Tsai, S. H., Y. C. Liang, L. Chen, F. M. Ho, M. S. Hsieh, J. K. Lin. 2002. Arsenite stimulates cyclooxygenase-2 expression through activating IκB kinase and nuclear factor κB in primary and ECV304 endothelial cells. *J. Cell Biochem*. 84:750–758.

726. Barchowsky, A., E. J. Dudek, M. D. Treadwell, K. E. Wetterhahn. 1996. Arsenic induces oxidant stress and NF-κB activation in cultured aortic endothelial cells. *Free Radic. Biol. Med*. 21:783–790.

727. Barchowsky, A., R. R. Roussel, L. R. Klei, P. E. James, N. Ganju, K. R. Smith, E. J. Dudek. 1999. Low levels of arsenic trioxide stimulate proliferative signals in primary vascular cells without activating stress effector pathways. *Toxicol. Appl. Pharmacol*. 159:65–75.

728. Lee, P. C., I. C. Ho, T. C. Lee. 2005. Oxidative stress mediates sodium arsenite-induced expression of heme oxygenase-1, monocyte chemoattractant protein-1, and interleukin-6 in vascular smooth muscle cells. *Toxicol. Sci*. 85:541–550.

729. Hsueh, Y. M., C. J. Chung, H. S. Shiue, J. B. Chen, S. S. Chiang, M. H. Yang, C. W. Tai, C. T. Su. 2009. Urinary arsenic species and CKD in a Taiwanese population: A case-control study. *Am. J. Kidney Dis*. 54:859–870.

730. Chen, Y. et al. 2011. Arsenic exposure from drinking water and mortality from cardiovascular disease in Bangladesh: Prospective cohort study. *BMJ*. 342:d2431; doi: 10.1136/bmj.d2431 [Online May 5, 2011]

731. Manson, J. E., H. Tosteson, P. M. Ridker, S. Satterfield, P Hebert, G. T. O'Connor, J. E. Buring, C. H. Hennekens. 1992. The primary prevention of myocardial infarction. *N. Engl. J. Med*. 326:1406–1416.

732. Basu, A., S. Mitra, J. Chung, D. N. Guha Mazumder, N. Ghose, D. A. Kalman, O. S. von Ehrenstein, C. Steinmaus, J. Liaw, A. H. Smith. 2011. Creatinine, diet, micronutrients, and arsenic methylation in West Bengal, India. *Environ. Health Perspect*. 119:1308–1313.

733. Gamble, M. V., X. Liu, H. Ahsan, R. Pilsner, V. Ilievski, V. Slavkovich, F. Parvez, D. Levy, P. Factor-Litvak, J. H. Graziano. 2005. Folate, homocysteine, and arsenic metabolism in arsenic-exposed individuals in Bangladesh. *Environ. Health Perspect*. 113:1683–1688.

734. Hall, M. N., X. Liu, V. Slavkovich, V. Ilievski, J. R. Pilsner, S. Alam, P. Factor-Litvak, J. H. Graziano, M. V. Gamble. 2009. Folate, cobalamin, cysteine, homocysteine, and arsenic metabolism among children in Bangladesh. *Environ. Health Perspect*. 117:825–831.

735. Brosnan, J. T., R. P. da Silva, M. E. Brosnan. 2011. The metabolic burden of creatine synthesis. *Amino Acids* 40(5):1325–1331.

736. Mudd, S. H., J. R. Poole. 1975. Labile methyl balances for normal humans on various dietary regimens. *Metabolism* 24(6):721–735.

737. Gamble, M. V., M. N. Hall. 2012. Relationship of creatinine and nutrition with arsenic metabolism. *Environ. Health Perspect.* 120(4): A145–146.

738. Gamble, M. V., X. Liu. 2005. Urinary creatinine and arsenic metabolism [Letter]. *Environ. Health Perspect.* 113:A442.

739. Chung, J. S. et al. 2006. Blood concentrations of methionine, selenium, beta-carotene, and other micro-nutrients in a case-control study of arsenic-induced skin lesions in West Bengal, India. *Environ. Res.* 101(2):230–237.

740. Drammeh, B. S., R. L. Schleicher, C. M. Pfeiffer, R. B. Jain, M. Zhang, P. H. Nguyen. 2008. Effects of delayed sample processing and freezing on serum concentrations of selected nutritional indicators. *Clin. Chem.* 54(11):1883–1891.

741. Gamble, M. V. et al. 2006. Folate and arsenic metabolism: A double-blind, placebo-controlled folic acid-supplementation trial in Bangladesh. *Am. J. Clin. Nutr.* 84(5):1093–1101.

742. Gamble, M. V. et al. 2007. Folic acid supplementation lowers blood arsenic. *Am. J. Clin. Nutr.* 86(4):1202–1209.

743. Hall, M. et al. 2007. Determinants of arsenic metabolism: Blood arsenic metabolites, plasma folate, cobalamin, and homocysteine concentrations in maternal–newborn pairs. *Environ. Health Perspect.* 115:1503–1509.

744. Willett, W. C., G. R. Howe, L. H. Kushi. 1997. Adjustment for total energy intake in epidemiologic studies. *Am. J. Clin. Nutr.* 65(suppl. 4):1220S–1228S.

745. Willett, W., M. Stampfer. 1998. Implications of total energy intake for epidemiologic analysis. In *Nutritional Epidemiology*, 2nd ed., W. Willett, ed., pp. 273–301. New York: Oxford University Press.

746. Smith, A. H., J. Liaw, C. Steinmaus. 2012. Relationship of creatinine and nutrition with arsenic metabolism: Smith et al. *Respond. Environ. Health Perspect.* 120(4):a16–a17.

747. Nermell, B., A. L. Lindberg, M. Rahman, M. Berglund, L. A. Persson, S. El Arifeen, M. Vahter. 2008. Urinary arsenic concentration adjustment factors and malnutrition. *Environ. Res.* 106(2):212–218.

748. Heck, J. E., M. V. Gamble, Y. Chen, J. H. Graziano, V. Slavkovich, F. Parvez, J. A. Baron, G. R. Howe, H. Ahsan. 2007. Consumption of folate-related nutrients and metabolism of arsenic in Bangladesh. *Am. J. Clin. Nutr.* 85(5):1367–1374.

749. Heck, J. E., J. W. Nieves, Y. Chen, F. Parvez, P. W. Brandt-Rauf, J. H. Graziano, V. Slavkovich, G. R. Howe, H. Ahsan. 2009. Dietary intake of methionine, cysteine, and protein and urinary arsenic excretion in Bangladesh. *Environ. Health Perspect.* 117:99–104.

750. Huang, Y. L., Y. M. Hsueh, Y. K. Huang, P. K. Yip, M. H. Yang, C. J. Chen. 2009. Urinary arsenic methylation capability and carotid atherosclerosis risk in subjects living in arsenicosis-hyperendemic areas in southwestern Taiwan. *Sci. Total Environ.* 407(8):2608–2614.

751. Steinmaus, C., K. Carrigan, D. Kalman, R. Atallah, Y. Yuan, A. H. Smith. 2005. Dietary intake and arsenic methylation in a U.S. population. *Environ. Health Perspect.* 113:1153–1159.

752. Barr, D. B., L. C. Wilder, S. P. Caudill, A. J. Gonzalez, L. L. Needham, J. L. Pirkle. 2005. Urinary creatinine concentrations in the U.S. population: Implications for urinary biologic monitoring measurements. *Environ. Health Perspect.* 113:192–200.

753. Poirier, L. A., C. K. Wise, R. R. Delongchamp, R. Sinha. 2001. Blood determinations of S-adenosylmethionine, S-adenosylhomocysteine, and homocysteine: Correlations with diet. *Cancer Epidemiol. Biomarkers Prev.* 10(6):649–655.

754. Concha, G., G. Vogler, B. Nermell, M. Vahter. 2002. Intra-individual variation in the metabolism of inorganic arsenic. *Int. Arch. Occup. Environ. Health* 75(8):576–580.

755. Marafante, E., M. Vahter. 1984. The effect of methyltransferase inhibition on the metabolism of [74As] arsenite in mice and rabbits. *Chem. Biol. Interact.* 50(1):49–57.

756. Vahter, M., E. Marafante. 1987. Effects of low dietary intake of methionine, choline or proteins on the biotransformation of arsenite in the rabbit. *Toxicol. Lett.* 37(1):41–46.

757. Chen, Y. C., H. J. Su, Y. L. Guo, Y. M. Hsueh, T. J. Smith, L. M. Ryan, M. S. Lee, D. C. Christiani. 2003. Arsenic methylation and bladder cancer risk in Taiwan. *Cancer Causes Control* 14(4):303–310.

758. Tseng, C. H., Y. K. Huang, Y. L. Huang, C. J. Chung, M. H. Yang, C. J. Chen, Y. M. Hsueh. 2005. Arsenic exposure, urinary arsenic speciation, and peripheral vascular disease in blackfoot disease-hyperendemic villages in Taiwan. *Toxicol. Appl. Pharmacol.* 206(3):299–308.

759. Styblo, M., Z. Drobna, I. Jaspers, S. Lin, D. J. Thomas. 2002. The role of biomethylation in toxicity and carcinogenicity of arsenic: A research update. *Environ. Health Perspect.* 110(suppl. 5):767–771.

760. Spiegelstein, O., X. Lu, X. C. Le, A. Troen, J. Selhub, S. Melnyk, S. J. James, R. H. Finnell. 2003. Effects of dietary folate intake and folate binding protein-1 (Folbp1) on urinary speciation of sodium arsenate in mice. *Toxicol. Lett.* 145(2):167–174.

761. Gamble, M. V., X. Liu, H. Ahsan, R. Pilsner, V. Ilievski, V. Slavkovich, F. Parvez, D. Levy, P. Factor-Litvak, J. H. Graziano. 2005. Folate, homocysteine, and arsenic metabolism in arsenic-exposed individuals in Bangladesh. *Environ. Health Perspect.* 113:1683–1688.

762. Stead, L. M., J. T. Brosnan, M. E. Brosnan, D. E. Vance, R. L. Jacobs. 2006. Is it time to reevaluate methyl balance in humans? *Am. J. Clin. Nutr.* 83(1):5–10.

763. Korzun, W. J. 2004. Oral creatine supplements lower plasma homocysteine concentrations in humans. *Clin. Lab. Sci.* 17(2):102–106.

764. Stead, L. M., K. P. Au, R. L. Jacobs, M. E. Brosnan, J. T. Brosnan. 2001. Methylation demand and homocysteine metabolism: Effects of dietary provision of creatine and guanidinoacetate. *Am. J. Physiol. Endocrinol. Metab.* 281(5):E1095–E1100.

765. Taes, Y. E., J. R. Delanghe, A. S. De Vriese, R. Rombaut, J. Van Camp, N. H. Lameire. 2003. Creatine supplementation decreases homocysteine in an animal model of uremia. *Kidney Int.* 64(4):1331–1337.

766. Concha, G., B. Nermell, M. V. Vahter. 1998. Metabolism of inorganic arsenic in children with chronic high arsenic exposure in northern Argentina. *Environ. Health Perspect.* 106:355–359.

767. Chowdhury, U. K., M. M. Rahman, M. K. Sengupta, D. Lodh, C. R. Chanda, S. Roy, Q. Quamruzzaman, H. Tokunaga, M. Ando, D. Chakraborti. 2003. Pattern of excretion of arsenic compounds [arsenite, arsenate, MMA(V), DMA(V)] in urine of children compared to adults from an arsenic exposed area in Bangladesh. *J. Environ. Sci. Health A Tox. Hazard Subst. Environ. Eng.* 38(1):87–113.

768. Meza, M. M., L. Yu, Y. Y. Rodriguez, M. Guild, D. Thompson, A. J. Gandolfi, W. T. Klimecki. 2005. Developmentally restricted genetic determinants of human arsenic metabolism: Association between urinary methylated arsenic and CYT19 polymorphisms in children. *Environ. Health Perspect.* 113:775–781.

769. Smith, A. H., G. Marshall, Y. Yuan, C. Ferreccio, J. Liaw, O. von Ehrenstein, C. Steinmaus, M. N. Bates, S. Selvin. 2006. Increased mortality from lung cancer and bronchiectasis in young adults after exposure to arsenic in utero and in early childhood. *Environ. Health Perspect.* 114:1293–1296.

770. Wasserman, G. A. et al. 2007. Water arsenic exposure and intellectual function in 6-year-old children in Araihazar, Bangladesh. *Environ. Health Perspect.* 115:285–289.

771. Yuan, Y., G. Marshall, C. Ferreccio, C. Steinmaus, S. Selvin, J. Liaw, M. N. Bates, A. H. Smith. 2007. Acute myocardial infarction mortality in comparison with lung and bladder cancer mortality in arsenic-exposed region II of Chile from 1950 to 2000. *Am. J. Epidemiol.* 166(12):1381–1391.

772. Ahsan, H., Y. Chen, F. Parvez, M. Argos, A. I. Hussain, H. Momotaj, D. Levy, A. van Geen, G. Howe, J. Graziano. 2006. Health Effects of Arsenic Longitudinal Study (HEALS): Description of a multidisciplinary epidemiologic investigation. *J. Expo. Sci. Environ. Epidemiol.* 16(2):191–205.

773. Pfeiffer, C. M., S. P. Caudill, E. W. Gunter, J. Osterloh, E. J. Sampson. 2005. Biochemical indicators of B vitamin status in the US population after folic acid fortification: Results from the National Health and Nutrition Examination Survey 1999–2000. *Am. J. Clin. Nutr.* 82(2):442–450.

774. Pfeiffer, C. M., D. L. Huff, E. W. Gunter. 1999. Rapid and accurate HPLC assay for plasma total homocysteine and cysteine in a clinical laboratory setting. *Clin. Chem.* 45(2):290–292.

775. Cheng, Z., Y. Zheng, R. Mortlock, A. Van Geen. 2004. Rapid multielement analysis of groundwater by high-resolution inductively coupled plasma mass spectrometry. *Anal. Bioanal. Chem.* 379(3):512–518.

776. Slot, C. 1965. Plasma creatinine determination. A new and specific Jaffe reaction method. *Scand. J. Clin. Lab. Invest.* 17(4):381–387.

777. Kuczmarski, R. J., C. L. Ogden, S. S. Guo, L. M. Grummer-Strawn, K. M. Flegal, Z. Mei, R. Wei, L. R. Curtin, A. F. Roche, C. L. Johnson. 2002. 2000 CDC growth charts for the United States: Methods and development. *Vital Health Stat.* 11(246):1–190.

778. de Onis, M., A. W. Onyango, E. Borghi, A. Siyam, C. Nishida, J. Siekmann. 2007. Development of a WHO growth reference for school-aged children and adolescents. *Bull.* 85(9):660–667.

779. Christenson, R. H., G. A. Dent, A. Tuszynski. 1985. Two radioassays for serum vitamin B12 and folate determination compared in a reference interval study. *Clin. Chem.* 31(8):1358–1360.

780. Jones, D. P., Y. M. Go, C. L. Anderson, T. R. Ziegler, J. M. Kinkade Jr., W. G. Kirlin. 2004. Cysteine/cystine couple is a newly recognized node in the circuitry for biologic redox signaling and control. *FASEB J.* 18(11):1246–1248.

781. Celkova, A., J. Kubova, V. Stresko. 1996. Determination of arsenic in geological samples by HG AAS. *Anal. Bioanal. Chem.* 355(2):150–153.

782. Heady, J. E., S. J. Kerr. 1975. Alteration of glycine N-methyltransferase activity in fetal, adult, and tumor tissues. *Cancer Res.* 35:640–643.

783. Bates, C. J., M. A. Mansoor, J. Gregory, K. Pentiev, A. Prentice. 2002. Correlates of plasma homocysteine, cysteine and cysteinyl-glycine in respondents in the British National Diet and Nutrition Survey of young people aged 4–18 years, and a comparison with the survey of people aged 65 years and over. *Br. J. Nutr.* 87(1):71–79.

784. Must, A., P. F. Jacques, G. Rogers, I. H. Rosenberg, J. Selhub. 2003. Serum total homocysteine concentrations in children and adolescents: Results from the third National Health and Nutrition Examination Survey (NHANES III). *J. Nutr.* 133(8):2643–2649.

785. Papandreou, D., I. Mavromichalis, A. Makedou, I. Rousso, M. Arvanitidou. 2006. Reference range of total serum homocysteine level and dietary indexes in healthy Greek schoolchildren aged 6–15 years. *Br. J. Nutr.* 96(4):719–724.

786. Pfeiffer, C. M., C. L. Johnson, R. B. Jain, E. A. Yetley, M. F. Picciano, J. I. Rader, K. D. Fisher, J. Mulinare, J. D. Osterloh. 2007. Trends in blood folate and vitamin B-12 concentrations in the United States, 1988–2004. *Am. J. Clin. Nutr.* 86(3):718–727.

787. Carmel, R., P. V. Mallidi, S. Vinarskiy, S. Brar, Z. Frouhar. 2002. Hyperhomocysteinemia and cobalamin deficiency in young Asian Indians in the United States. *Am. J. Hematol.* 70(2):107–114.

788. Chambers, J. C., O. A. Obeid, H. Refsum, P. Ueland, D. Hackett, J. Hooper, R. M. Turner, S. G. Thompson, J. S. Kooner. 2000. Plasma homocysteine concentrations and risk of coronary heart disease in UK Indian Asian and European men. *Lancet* 355(9203):523–527.

789. Venugopal, B., T. D. Luckey, eds. 1978. *Metal Toxicity in Mammals*, Vol. 2. New York: Plenum Press. 409 p.

790. Underwood, E. J. 1977. *Trace Elements in Human and Animal Nutrition*, 4th ed. New York: Academic Press.

791. Linder, M. C. 1985. Nutrition and metabolism of the trace elements. In *Nutritional Biochemistry and Metabolism with Clinical Applications*, M. C. Linder, ed., pp. 191–192. New York: Elsevier.

792. Eck, P. C., L. Wilson. 1989. *Toxic Metals in Human Health and Disease.* Eck Institute of Applied Nutrition and Bioenergetics, Ltd.

793. American Conference of Governmental Industrial Hygienists. 1976. *Cadium Fume-As Cd. Documentation of the TLVs for Substances in Workroom Air*, 3rd ed., p. 292. Cincinnati: Signature Publications.

794. National Institute of Occupational Safety and Health. 1990. *Testimony on Occupational Exposure to Cadmium*, J. D. Millar, September 18, 1990.

795. Ikeda, M., Z. W. Zhang, S. Shimbo, T. Watanabe, H. Nakatsuka, C. S. Moon, N. Matsuda-Inoguchi, K. Higashikawa. 2000. Urban population exposure to lead and cadmium in east and south-east Asia. *Sci. Total Environ.* 249(1–3):373–384.

796. Watanabe, T., Z. W. Zhang, C. S. Moon, S. Shimbo, H. Nakatsuka, N. Matsuda-Inoguchi, K. Higashikawa, M. Ikeda. 2000. Cadmium exposure of women in general populations in Japan during 1991–1997 compared with 1977–1981. *Int. Arch. Occup. Environ. Health.* 73(1):26–34.

797. Nishijo, M., H. Nakagawa, R. Honda, K. Tanebe, S. Saito, H. Teranishi, K. Tawara. 2002. Effects of maternal exposure to cadmium on pregnancy outcome and breast milk. *Occup. Environ. Med.* 59:394–397.

798. Zhang, Y. L. et al. 2004. Effect of environmental exposure to cadmium on pregnancy outcome and fetal growth: A study on healthy pregnant women in China. *J. Environ. Sci. Health A.* 39(9):2507–2715.

799. Tipton, I. H., M. J. Cook, R. L. Steiner, C. A. Boye, H. M. Perry Jr., H. A. Schroeder. 1963. Trace Elements in Human Tissue. Part I. Methods. *Health Phys.* 9:89.

800. Choi, Y. H., H. Hu, B. Mukherjee, J. Miller, S. K. Park. 2012. Environmental cadmium and lead exposures and hearing loss in U.S. adults: The National Health and Nutrition Examination Survey, 1999 to 2004. *Environ. Health Perspect.* 120(11):1544–1550.

801. Ruggiero, M., S. Peter, M. G. Flower, B. Chiarelli, G. Morucci, J. J. V. Branca, M. Gulisano, S. Pacini. 2013. Transcranial sonography: A technique for the study of the temporal lobes of the human and non-human primate brain. *Ital. J. Anat. Embryol.* pp. 241–255.

802. Guyton, A. C., J. E. Hall. 2006. Transport of oxygen and carbon dioxide in blood and tissue fluids. In *Textbook of Medical Physiology*, 11th ed., A. C. Guyton, J. E. Hall, eds., p. 508. Philadelphia: Elsevier/Saunder, Figure 40-10.

803. de Lange, F. P., J. S. Kalkman, G. Bleijenberg, P. Hagoort, J. W. M. Van Der Meer, I. Toni. 2005. Gray matter volume reduction in the chronic fatigue syndrome. *Neuro. Image* 26(3):777–781.

804. Lopez, E., C. Arce, M. J. Oset-Gasque, S. Cánadas, M. P. Gõnzalez. 2006. Cadmium induces reactive oxygen species generation and lipid peroxidation in cortical neurons in culture. *Free Radic. Biol. Med.* 40(6):940–951.

805. Fischler, B., H. D'Haene, R. Cluydts, V. Michils, K. Demets, A. Bossuyt, L. Kauffman, K. DeMierlier. 1996. Comparison of [99M]TC HMPAO SPECT scan between chronic fatigue syndrome, major depression and healthy controls: An exploratory study of clinical correlates of regional cerebral blood flow.

806. Yoshiuchi, K., J. Farkas, B. H. Natelson. 2006. Patients with chronic fatigue syndrome have reduced absolute critical blood flow. *Clin. Physiol. Funct. Imaging.* 26:83–86.

807. Hardy, H. L., I. R. Tabershaw. 1946. Delayed chemical pneumonitis occurring in workers exposed to beryllium compounds. *J. Ind. Hyg. Tox.* 28:197.

808. Swanborg, R. H. 1984. Immune response in toxicology. In *Toxicology: Principles and Practice*, Vol. 2, F. Sperling, ed., p. 117. New York: John Wiley & Sons.

809. Anon. 1964. Hygenic Guide Series: Beryllium and its compounds. *Am. Ind. Hyg. Assoc. J.* 25:614.

810. American Conference of Governmental Industrial Hygienists. 1976. *Iron Oxide Fume. Documentation of the LVs for Substances in Workroom Air*, 3rd ed., pp. 325–326. Cincinnati: Signature Publications.

811. Rea, W. J. 1992. *Chemical Sensitivity*, Vol. 1, p. 58. Boca Raton, FL: Lewis Publishers.

812. American Conference of Governmental Industrial Hygienists. 1976. *Copper as Cu. Documentation of the LVs for Substances in Workroom Air*, 3rd ed., pp. 305–306. Cincinnati: Signature Publications.

813. National Institute for Occupational Safety and Health. 1977. *Criteria for a Recommended Standard.* Occupational Exposure to Inorganic Nickel. (NIOSH) 77-164, pp. 205–221. Washington, DC: U.S. Department of Health, Education, and Welfare.

814. Browning, E. 1969. *Toxicity of Industrial Metals*, 2nd ed., pp. 249–260. London: Butterworth.

815. Norseth, T. 1984. Clinical effects of nickel. In *Nickel in the Human Environment: Proceedings Joint Symposium. Held at IARC*, Lyon, France, March 8–11, 1983, F. W. Sunderman Jr. et al., eds., p. 395. London: Oxford University Press.

816. American Conference of Governmental Industrial Hygienists. 1976. *Nickel, Soluble Inorganic Salts. Documentation of the LVs for Substances in Workroom Air*, 3rd ed., p. 388. Cincinnati.

817. Sweet, C. W., S. J. Vermette, S. Landsberger. 1993. Sources of toxic trace elements in urban air in Illinois. *Environ. Sci. Technol.* 27:2502–2510.

818. van Winkle, M. R., P. A. Scheff. 2001. Volatile organic compounds, polycyclic aromatic hydrocarbons and elements in the air of ten urban homes. *Indoor Air.* 11:49–64.

819. Koutrakis, P., S. L. K. Briggs, B. P. Leaderer. 1992. Source apportionment of indoor aerosols in Suffolk and Onondaga Counties, New York. *Environ. Sci. Technol.* 26:521–527.

820. Graney, J. R., M. S. Landis, G. A. Norris. 2004. Concentrations and solubility of metals from indoor and personal exposure PM2.5 samples. *Atmos. Environ.* 38(2):237–247.

821. Kinney, P. L., S. N. Chillrud, S. Ramstrom, J. Ross, J. D. Spengler. 2002. Exposure to multiple air toxics in New York City. *Environ. Health Perspect.* 110(suppl. 4):539–546.

822. Hoff, R. M., L. A. Barrie. 1986. Air chemistry observations in the Canadian artic. *Water Sci. Technol.* 18:97–107.

823. Chan, W. H., M. A. Lusis. 1986. Smelting Operations and Trace Metals in Air and Precipitation in the Sudbury Basin. *Adv. Environ. Sci. Technol.* 17:113–143.

824. Norseth, T. 1994. Environmental Pollution around Nickel Smelters in the Kola Peninsula (Russia). *Sci. Total Environ.* 148:103–108.

825. Sivertsen, B. 1991. *Air Pollution in the Border Areas of Norway/Soviet Union January 1990-March 1991.* Lillestrøm: Norwegian Institute for Air Research (NILU OR: 69/91; Ref:0-8976). Analytik, Institut fur Anorganische und Angewandte Chemie, Universitat Hamburg, Germany.

826. Saltzman, B. E., J. Cholak, L. J. Schafer. 1985. Concentrations of Six Metals in the Air of Eight Cities. *Environ. Sci. Technol.* 19:328–333.

827. Schmidt, J. A., A. W. Andren. 1990. The atmospheric chemistry of nickel. In *Nickel in the Environment*, Vol. 1999, J. O. Nriagu, ed., pp. 93–137. New York: Wiley.

828. Bennett, B. J. 1994. Environmental nickel pathways to man. In *Nickel in the Human Environment*, F. W. Sunderman Jr., ed., pp. 487–495. Lyon: Lyon International Agency for Research on Cancer.

829. Lee, R. E., D. J. Von Lehmden. 1973. Trace metal pollution in the environment. *J. Air Pollut. Control Assoc.* 23:853–857.

830. Milford, J. B., C. I. Davidson. 1985. The sizes of particulate trace elements in the atmosphere—A review. *J. Air Pollut. Control Assoc.* 35:1249–1260.

831. Natusch, D. F. S., J. R. Wallace, C. A. Evans Jr. 1974. Toxic trace elements: Preferential concentration in respirable particles. *Science* 183:202–204.

832. Cass, G. R., G. J. Mcrae. 1983. Source receptor reconciliation of routine air monitoring data for trace metals: An emission inventory-assisted approach. *Environ. Sci. Technol.* 17:129–139.

833. Oberdörster, G. 1992. Lung dosimetry: Extrapolation modeling from animals to man. In *Nickel and Human Health: Current Perspectives*, E. Nieboer, J. O. Nriagu, eds., pp. 421–436. New York: Wiley.

834. Wehner, A. P., G. E. Dagle, E. M. Milliman. 1981. Chronic inhalation exposure of hamsters to nickel-enriched fly ash. *Environ. res.* 26:195–216.

835. Carvalho, S. M., P. L. Ziemer. 1982. Distribution and clearance of [63]Ni administered as [63]NiCl2 in the rat: Intratracheal study. *Archives of Environ. Contam. Toxicol.* 11:245–248.

836. Nickel. Geneva, World Health Organization, 1991 (Environmental Health Criteria, No. 108).

837. Bennett, B. G. 1984. Environmental nickel pathways in man. In *Nickel in Human Environment*. Sunderman, F. W. Jr., ed., *Proceedings of a Joint Symposium IARC*. Scientific Publication No. 53. Lyon, France: International Agency for Research on Cancer, pp. 489–495.

838. Schmidt, A. W., J. A. Andren. 1980. The atmospheric chemistry of nickel. In *Nickel in the Environment*, J. O. Nriagu, ed., pp. 93–135. New York: John Wiley and Sons.

839. Duce, R. A. et al. 1991. The atmospheric input of trace species to the world ocean. *J. Global Biogeochem. Cycles* 5(3):193–259.

840. Giusti, L., Y. L. Yang, C. N. Hewitt, J. Hamilton-Taylor, W. Davison. 1991. The solubility and partition-ing of atmospherically derived trace metals in artificial and natural waters: A review. *Atmos. Environ.* 27A:1567–1578.

841. Taylor, Gregory J., A. A. Crowder. 1983. Accumulation of atmospherically deposited metals in Wetland soils of Sudbury, Ontario. *Water, Air, Soil Pollut.* 19(1):29–42.

842. Hasanen, E., V. Pohjola, M. Hahkala, R. Zilliacus, K. Wickstrom. 1986. Emissions from power plants fueled by peat coal, natural gas and oil. *Sci. Total Environ.* 54:29–51.

843. Zilliacus Rydh, C. J., B. Svärd. 2003. Impact on global metal flows arising from the use of portable rechargeable batteries. *Sci. Total Environ.* 302:167–184.

844. Leikauf, G. D. 2002. Hazardous air pollutants and asthma. *Environ. Health Perspect.* 110(suppl. 4):505–526.

845. Hansen, L. D., J. L. Fisher. 1980. Elemental distribution in coal fly ash particles. *Environ. Sci. Technol.* 14:1111–1117.

846. Sabbioni, E., L. Goetz, G. Bignoli. 1984. Health and environmental implications of trace metals released from coal-fired power plants: An assessment study of the situation in the European community. *Sci. Total Environ.* 40:141–154.

847. Gladney, E. S., S. E. Gordon, W. H. Zoller. 1978. Coal combustion: Source of elements in urban air. *J. Environ. Sci. Health A* 13:481–491.

848. Lee, R. E. Jr. et al. 1975. Concentration and size of trace metal emissions from a power plant, a store plant and a cotton gin. *Environ. Sci. Technol.* 9:643–647.

849. Greenberg, R. R., W. H. Zoller, S. E. Gordon. 1978. Composition and size distribution of particles released in refuse incinerators. *Environ. Sci. Technol.* 12:566–573.

850. HazDat. 2005. Atlanta, GA: Agency for Toxic Substances and Disease Registry (ATSDR).

851. Nriagu, J. O., J. M. Pacyna. 1988. Quantitative assessment of worldwide contamination of air, water and soils by trace metals. *Nature* 333:134–139.

852. Rai, D., J. M. Zachara. 1984. *Chemical Attenuation Rates, Coefficients, and Constants in Leachate Migration. Volume 1: A Critical Review*. Palo Alto, CA: Electric Power Research Institute.

853. Amavis, R., W. J. Hunter, J. G. P. M. Smeets. 1976. Hardness of drinking water and public health. *Proceedings of the European Scientific Colloquium*, Luxembourg, May 1975 (EUR 5447). Oxford: Pergamon Press. 553 p.

854. Scheller, R. et al. 1988. Chemical and technological aspects of food for a diet poor in nickel for endog-enous nickel contact eczema. *Hautarzt* 39:491–497.

855. Andersen, K. E. et al. 1983. Nickel in tap water. *Contact Dermatitis.* 9:140–143.

856. International Agency for Research on Cancer (IARC). 1990. Nickel and nickel compounds. In *IARC Monographs on the Evaluation of Carcinogenic Risks to Humans: Chromium, Nickel and Welding*, Vol. 49, pp. 257–445.

857. WHO—World Health Organization. 1991. *Nickel.* Geneva: Environmental Health Criteria, No. 108.

858. Sunderman, F. W. Jr., S. M. Hopfer, K. R. Sweeney, A. H. Marcus, B. M. Most, J. Creason. 1989. Nickel absorption and kinetics in human volunteers. *Proc. Soc. Exp. Biol. Med.* 191:5–11.

859. Theler, B., C. Bucher, L. E. French, B. Ballmer Weber, G. F. L. Hofbauer. 2009. Clinical expres-sion of nickel contact dermatitis primed by diagnostic patch test. *Dermatology* 219:73–76. doi: 10.1159/000212119.

860. Prognostic markers in resectable non-small cell lung cancer a multivariable analysis.

861. Nielsen, N. H., T. Menne. 1992. Allergic contact sensitization in an unselected Danish population. The Glostrup Allergy Study, Denmark. *Acta Derm. Venereol. Suppl. (Stockh.)* 72:456–460.

862. Sunderman, F. W., S. M. Hopfer, S. M. Lin, M. C. Plowman, T. Stanjovic, S. H. Y. Wong, O. Sharia, L. Ziebka. 1989. Toxicity to alveolar macrophages in rats following parenteral injection of nickel chloride. *Toxicology and Applies Pharmacology.* 100(1):107–118.

863. Brimblecombe, P. 1994. Long-term changes in elemental deposition at the earth's surface. *Environ. Pollut.* 83:81–85.

864. Chan, W. H., M. A. Lusis. 1986. Smelting operations and trace metals in air and precipitation in the Sudbury Basin. *Adv. Environ. Sci. Technol.* 17:113–143.

865. Norseth, T. 1994. Environmental pollution around nickel smelters in the Kola Peninsula (Russia). *Sci. Total Environ.* 148:103–108.

866. Sadig, M., C. G. Enfield. 1984a. Solid Phase formation and solution chemistry of nickel in soils. *I. Theor. Soil Sci.* 138:262–270.

867. Rudd, T., D. L. Lake, I. Mehorta, R. M. Sterritt, P. W. W. Kirk, J. A. Campbell, J. N. Lester. 1988. Characterization of metal forms in sewage sludge by chemical extraction and progressive acidification. *Sci. Total Environ.* 74:149–175.

868. Adams, J. F., D. E. Kissel. 1989. Zinc, copper and nickel availabilities as determined by soil solution and DTPA extraction of a sludge-amended soil. *Commun. Soil Sci. Plant Anal.* 20:139–158.

869. Sunderman, F. W. 1993. *Scand. J. Work Environ. Health.* 19:34.

870. Rezuke, W. N., J. A. Knight, F. W. Sunderman. 1987. *Ann. J. Ind. Med.* 11:419.

871. Mushak, P. 1980. Metabolism and systemic toxicity of nickel. In *Nickel in the Environment*, J. O. Nriagu, ed., pp. 499–524. New York: Wiley.

872. Templeton, D. M., F. W. Sunderman, R. F. M. Herber Jr. 1994. *Sci. Total Environ.* 148:243.

873. National Geographic Society. *How Megafires Are Remaking American Forests.* 1996–2015 National Geographic.

874. American Conference of Governmental Industrial Hygienists. 1971. Documentation of the threshold limit values.

875. Selikoff, I. J., W. J. Nicholson, A. M. Langer. 1972. Asbestos air pollution. *Arch. Environ. Health.* 25:1.

876. U.S. Environmental Protection Agency. 1982. *Corrosion in Potable Water Systems.* Washington, DC: U.S. Environmental Protection Agency.

877. Hathaway, G. J., N. H. Proctor, J. P. Hughes, M. L. Fischman. 1991. *Proctor and Hughes' Chemical Hazards of the Workplace*, 3rd ed., p. 97. New York: Van Nostrand Reinhold.

878. Kagen, E., A. Solomon, J. C. Cochrane, P. Kuba, P. H. Rocks, I. Webster. 1977. Immunological studies of patients with asbestosis. II. Studies of circulating lymphoid cell numbers and humoral immunity. *Clin. Exp. Immunol.* 28:268–275.

879. Selikoff, I. J., J. Churg, E. C. Hammond. 1965. Relation between exposure to asbestos and mesothelioma. *N. Engl. J. Med.* 272(11):560–565.

880. Selikoff, I. J., J. Churg, E. C. Hammond. 1968. Asbestos exposure, smoking and neoplasia. *JAMA* 204:106–112.

881. National Research Council Committee on Medical and Biological Effects of Environmental Pollutants. 1976. *Chlorine and Hydrogen Chloride*, pp. 116–123. Washington, DC: National Academy of Sciences.

882. National Institute for Occupational Safety and Health. 1976. *Criteria for a Recommended Standard. Occupational Exposure to Chlorine.* (NIOSH) 76–100, pp. 29, 36, 56. Washington, DC: National Academy of Sciences.

883. Anon. 1958. Hygienic guide series: Beryllium and its compounds. *Am. Ind. Hyg. Assoc. J.* 19:261.

884. American Conference of Governmental Industrial Hygienists. 1976. *Chlorine.. Documentation of the LVs for Substances in Workroom Air*, 3rd ed., p. 46. Cincinnati.

885. Rea, W. J. 1980. Review of cardiovascular disease in allergy. In *Biannual Review of Allergy*, C. A. Frazier, ed., pp. 282–347. Springfield, IL: Charles C. Thomas.

886. Rea, W. J., Y. Pan, J. L. Laseter, A. R. Johnson, E. J. Fenyves. 1987. Toxic volatile organic hydrocarbons in chemically sensitive patients. *J. Clin. Ecol.* 5(2):70–74.

887. American Conference of Governmental Industrial Hygienists. 1976. *Hydrogen Chloride. Documentation of the LVs for Substances in Workroom Air*, 3rd ed., p. 129. Cincinnati: Signature Publications.

888. American Conference of Governmental Industrial Hygienists. 1976. *Bromine. Documentation of the LVs for Substances in Workroom Air*, 3rd ed., p. 27. Cincinnati: Signature Publications.

889. American Conference of Governmental Industrial Hygienists. 1976. *Fluorine (F2). Documentation of the LVs for Substances in Workroom Air*, 3rd ed., pp. 321–322. Cincinnati: Signature Publications.

890. Hodge, H. C., F. A. Smith. 1977. Occupational fluoride exposure. *J. Occup. Med.* 19:12–39.

891. Waldbot, G. L. 1979. Preskeletal fluorosis near an Ohio enamel factory: A preliminary report. *Vet. Hum. Tox.* 21:4–8.
892. Baselt, R. C., ed. 1982. *Disposition of the Toxic Drugs and Chemical in Man*, 2nd ed., p. 331. Davis, CA: Biomedical Publications.
893. American Conference of Governmental Industrial Hygienists. 1976. *Iodine. Documentation of the LVs for Substances in Workroom Air*, 3rd ed., p. 135. Cincinnati: Signature Publications.
894. American Conference of Governmental Industrial Hygienists. 1976. *Cyanides (as CN). Documentation of the LVs for Substances in Workroom Air*, 3rd ed., p. 64. Cincinatti: Signature Publications.
895. American Conference of Governmental Industrial Hygienists. 1976. *Cobalt (Metal Dust and Fume). Documentation of the LVs for Substances in Workroom Air*, 3rd ed., pp. 364–365. Cincinnati: Signature Publications.
896. Goyer, R. A. 1986. Toxic effects of metal. In *Casarett and Doull's Toxicology: The Basic Science of Poisons*, 3rd ed., C. D. Klaassen, M. O. Amdur, J. Doull, eds., p. 597. New York: Macmillan.
897. American Conference of Governmental Industrial Hygienists. 1976. *Chromic Acid and Chromates. Documentation of the LVs for Substances in Workroom Air*, 3rd ed., pp. 55–56. Cincinnati: Signature Publications.
898. Greger, J. L., H. W. Lane. 1987. The toxicology of dietary tin, aluminum and selenium. In *Nutritional Toxicology*, Vol. II, Hathcock, ed., p. 228. Orlando: Academic Press.
899. Underwood, E. J. 1977. *Trace Elements in Human and Animal Nutrition*, 4th ed., New York: Academic Press.
900. Elsenhans, B., K. Schümann, W. Forth. 1991. Toxic metals: Interactions with essential metals. In *Nutrition, Toxicity and Cancer*, I. R. Rowland, ed., p. 243. Boca Raton, FL: CRC Press.
901. Hathaway, G. J., N. H. Proctor, J. P. Hughes, M. L. Fischman. 1991. *Proctor and Hughes' Chemical Hazards of the Workplace*, 3rd ed., New York: Van Nostrand Reinhold.
902. Bischoff, F., G. Bryson. 1964. Carcinogenesis through solid state surfaces. *Proc. Exp. Tumor Res.* 5:85–133.
903. Léonard, A., G. B. Gerber. 1988. Mutagenicity, carcinogenicity, and teratogenicity of aluminum. *Mutat. Res.* 196(3):247–257.
904. Viola, R. E., J. F. Morrison, W. W. Cleland. 1980. Interaction of metal (III)-adenosine 5′-triphosphate complexes with yeast hexokinase. *Biochemistry* 19:3131–3137.
905. Buys, S. S., J. P. Kushner. 1989. Hemotologic effects of aluminum toxicity. In *Aluminum and Health. A Critical Review*, H. J. Gitelman, ed., p. 251. New York: Marcel Dekker.
906. Paternain, J. L., J. L. Domingo, J. M. Llobet, J. Corbella. 1988. Embryotoxic and teratogenic effects of aluminum nitrate in rats upon oral administration. *Teratology* 38(3):253–257.
907. Lione, A. 1983. The prophylactic reduction of aluminum intake. *Food Chem. Toxicol.* 21(1):103–109.
908. Bloom, W. L., D. Flinchum. 1960. Osteomalacia with pseudoiractures caused by the ingestion of aluminum hydroxide. *J. Am. Med. Assoc.* 174:1327.
909. Lotz, M., E. Zisman, F. C. Bartter. 1968. Evidence for a phosphorus-depiction syndrome in man. *N. Engl. J. Med.* 278:409.
910. Shields, H. M. 1978. Rapid fail of serum phosphorus secondary to antacid therapy. *Gastrointerology* 75:1137.
911. Spencer, H., M. Lender. 1979. Adverse effects of aluminum-containing antacids on mineral metabolism. *Gastroenterology* 76:603.
912. Spencer, H., C. Norris, J. Coffey, E. Wiatrowski. 1975. Effect of small amounts of antacids on calcium, phosphorus and fluoride metabolism in man. *Gastroenterology* 68:990.
913. Spencer, H., L. Kramer, C. Norris, D. Osis, E. Wiatrowski. 1980. Effect of aluminum on fluoride and calcium metabolism in man. In *Trace Substances in Environmental Health*, Vol. 14, D. D. Hemphill, ed., p. 94. Columbia: University of Missouri.
914. Parkinson, I. S., M. K. Ward, D. N. S. Kerr. 1981. Dialysis encephalopathy, bone disease and anaemia: The aluminum intoxication syndrome during regular haemodialysis. *J. Clin. Pathol.* 34:1285.
915. Spencer, H. L., L. Kramer, C. Norris, E. Wiatrowski. 1980. Effect of aluminum hydroxide on fluoride metabolism. *Clin. Pharmocol. Ther.* 28:529.
916. Spencer, H. L., L. Kramer, C. Norris, E. Wiatrowski. 1981. Effect of aluminum hydroxide on plasma fluoride excretion during high fluoride intake in man. *Toxic Appl. Pharmacol.* 58:140.
917. Jowsey, J., B. L. Riggs, P. J. Kelly, D. L. Hoffman. 1972. Effect of combined therapy with sodium fluoride, vitamin D, and calcium in osteoporosis. *Am. J. Med.* 53:43.
918. Mayor, G. H., J. A. Keiser, D. Makdani, P. K. Ku. 1977. Aluminum absorption and distribution: Effect of parathyroid hormone. *Science* 197:1187–1189.

919. Spencer, H. L., D. Lewin, D. Osis, J. Samachson. 1970. Studies of fluoride and calcium metabolism in patients with osteoporosis. *Am. J. Med.* 49:814.

920. Mayor, G. H., R. F. Remedi, S. M. Sprague, K. L. Lovell. 1980. Central nervous system manifestations of oral aluminum effect of parathyroid hormone. In *Aluminum Neurotoxicity*, L. Liss, ed., p. 33. Park Forest South, IL: Pathotox Publishers.

921. Alfery, A. C. 1980. Aluminum metabolism in uremia. In *Aluminum Neurotoxicity*, L. Liss, ed., p. 43. Park Forest South, IL: Pathotox Publishers.

922. Cann, C. E., S. G. Prussin, G. S. Gordan. 1979. Aluminum uptake by the parathyroid glands. *J. Clin. Endocrinol. Metab.* 49(4):543–545.

923. Crapper, D. R. 1974. Dementia: Recent observations on Alzheimer's disease and experimental aluminum encephalopathy. In *Frontiers of Neurology and Neuroscience Research*, P. H. Seeman, G. M. Brown, eds., p. 97. Toronto: University of Toronto Press.

924. Crapper, D. R. 1976. Functional consequences of neurofibrillary degeneration. In *Neurobiology of Aging*, R. Terry, S. Gershon, eds., p. 405. New York: Raven Press.

925. Crapper, D. R., A. J. Dalton. 1973. Alteration in short-term retention, conditioned avoidance response acquisition and motivation following aluminum induced neurofibrillary degeneration. *Physiol. Behav.* 10:925.

926. Crapper, D. R., U. DeBoni. 1977. Aluminum and the genetic apparatus in Alzheimer's disease. In *The Aging Brain and Senile Dementia*, K. Nandy, L. Sherwin, eds., p. 229. New York: Plenum Press.

927. Crapper, D. R., S. Karlik, U. DeBoni. 1978. Aluminum and other metals in senile (Alzheimer's) dementia. In *Alzheimer's Disease: Senile Dementia and Related Disorders*, Katzman, R. D. Terry, K. L. Bick, eds., p. 271. New York: Raven Press.

928. Crapper, D. R., S. S. Krishman, A. J. Dalton. 1973. Brain aluminum distribution in Alzheimer's disease and experimental neurofibrillary degeneration. *Science* 180:511.

929. Crapper, D. R., G. J. Tomko. 1975. Neuronal correlates of an encephalopathy associated with aluminum neurofibrillary degeneration. *Brain Res.* 97:253.

930. Crapper, D. R., U. DeBoni. 1980. Aluminum in human brain disease—and overview. In *Aluminum Neurotoxicity*, L. Liss, ed., p. 3. Park Forest South, IL: Pathotox Publishers.

931. DeBoni, U., D. R. Crapper. 1978. Paired helical filaments of the Alzheimer type in cultured neurons. *Nature* 271:566.

932. DeBoni, U., J. W. Scott, D. R. Crapper. 1974. Intracellular aluminum binding: A histochemical study. *Histochemistry* 40:31.

933. DeBoni, U., A. Otvos, J. W. Scott, D. R. Crapper. 1976. Neurofibrillary degeneration induced by systemic aluminum. *Acta Neuropathol.* 35:285.

934. Klatzo, I., H. Wisniewski, E. Strerener. 1965. Experimental production of neurofibrillary degeneration. I. Light microscopic observations. *J. Neuropathol. Exp. Neurol.* 24:187.

935. Terry, R. D., C. Pena. 1965. Experimental production of neurofibrillary degeneration. II. Electron microscope observations. *J. Neuropathol. Exp. Neurol.* 24:200.

936. Alfrey, A. C., G. R. LeGendre, W. D. Kaehny. 1976. The dialysis encephalopathy syndrome: Possible aluminum intoxication. *N. Engl. J. Med.* 294:184–188.

937. Mahurkar, S. C., S. K. Dhar, R. Salta, L. Meyers Jr., E. C. Smith, G. Dunea. 1973. Dialysis dementia. *Lancet* 1:1412.

938. Rozas, V., F. K. Port. 1979. Progressive dialysis encephalopathy [letter]. *Ann. Neurol.* 6:88.

939. Alfrey, A. C., A. Hegg, P. Craswell. 1980. Metabolism and toxicity of aluminum in renal failure. *Am. J. Clin. Nutr.* 33:1509.

940. Arieff, A. L., J. D. Cooper, D. Armstrong, V. C. Lazarowitz. 1979. Dementia renal failure and brain aluminum. *Ann. Intern. Med.* 90:741.

941. McDermott, J. R., A. L. Smith, M. K. Ward, I. S. Parkinson, D. N. S. Kerr. 1978. Brain-aluminum concentration in dialysis encephalopathy. *Lancet* 1:901.

942. Kaehny, W. D., A. P. Hegg, A. C. Alfrey. 1977. Gastrointestinal absorption of aluminum from aluminum-containing antacids. *N. Engl. J. Med.* 296:1389.

943. Balyarte, H. J., A. B. Gruskin, L. D. Hiner, C. M. Foley, W. D. Grover. 1977. Encephalopathy in children with chronic renal failure. *Proc. Clin. Dial. Transpl. Forum.* 7:95.

944. Masselot, J. P., J. P. Adhemar, M. C. Jaudon, D. Kleinknecht, A. Galli. 1978. Reversible dialysis encephalopathy: Role for aluminum-containing gels. *Lancet* 2:1386.

945. Nathan, E., S. E. Pedersen. 1980. Dialysis encephalopathy in a non-dialysed uraemic boy treated with aluminum hydroxide orally. *Acta Paediat. Scand.* 69:793.

946. Poisson, M., R. Mashaly, B. Lattorgue. 1979. Progressive dialysis encephalopathy: Role of aluminum toxicity [letter]. *Ann. Neurol.* 6:88.

947. Gilroy, J., M. J. Sterling. 1979. *Medical Neurology*, 3rd ed., p. 177. New York: Macmillan.

948. Peri, D. P., A. R. Brody. 1980. Alzheimer's disease: X-ray spectrometric evidence of aluminum in neurofibrillary tangle-beating neuron. *Science* 208:297.

949. Crapper, D. R., S. S. Krishnan, S. Quittkat. 1976. Aluminum neurofibrillary degeneration and Alzheimer's disease. *Brain* 99:67.

950. Trapp, G. A., G. D. Miner, R. L. Zimmerman, A. R. Mastri, L. L. Heston. 1978. Aluminum levels in brain in Alzheimer's disease. *Biol. Psychiat.* 13:709.

951. Blaylock, R. L. 2012. Aluminum induced immunoexcitotoxicity in neurodevelopmental and neurodegenerative disorders. *Curr. Inorg. Chem.* 2:46–53.

952. Kraft, A. D., G. J. Harry. 2011. Features of microglia and neuroinflammation relevant to environmental exposure and neurotoxicity. *Int. J. Environ. Res. Public Health* 8:2980–3018.

953. Guilarte, T. R. 2010. Manganese and Parkinson's disease: A critical review and new findings. *Environ. Health Perspect.* 118:1071–1080.

954. Greenamyre, J. T., J. R. Cannon, R. Drolet, P. G. Mastroberardino. 2010. Lessons from the rotenone model of Parkinson's disease. *Trends Pharmacol. Sci.* 31, 141–142; author reply 142–143.

955. Schmidt, W. J., M. Alam. 2006. Controversies on new animal models of Parkinson's disease pro and con: The rotenone model of Parkinson's disease (PD). *J. Neural. Transm. Suppl.* 70:272–276.

956. Aschner, M., T. R. Guilarte, J. S. Schneider, W. Zheng. 2007. Manganese: Recent advances in understanding its transport and neurotoxicity. *Toxicol. Appl. Pharmacol.* 221:131–147.

957. Perl, D. P., C. W. Olanow. 2007. The neuropathology of manganese-induced Parkinsonism. *J. Neuropathol. Exp. Neurol.* 66:675–682.

958. Calne, D. B., N. S. Chu, C. C. Huang, C. S. Lu, W. Olanow. 1994. Manganism and idiopathic Parkinsonism: Similarities and differences. *Neurology* 44:1583–1586.

959. Cersosimo, M. G., W. C. Koller. 2006. The diagnosis of manganese-induced Parkinsonism. *Neurotoxicology* 27:340–346.

960. Pal, P. K., A. Samii, D. B. Calne. 1999. Manganese neurotoxicity: A review of clinical features, imaging and pathology. *Neurotoxicology* 20:227–238.

961. Olanow, C. W., P. F. Good, H. Shinotoh, K. A. Hewitt, F. Vingerhoets, B. J. Snow, M. F. Beal, D. B. Calne, D. P. Perl. 1996. Manganese intoxication in the rhesus monkey: A clinical, imaging, pathologic, and biochemical study. *Neurology* 46:492–498.

962. Guilarte, T. R. et al. 2008. Impairment of nigrostriatal dopamine neurotransmission by manganese is mediated by pre-synaptic mechanism(s): Implications to manganese-induced Parkinsonism. *J. Neurochem.* 107:1236–1247.

963. Guilarte, T. R. et al. 2006. Nigrostriatal dopamine system dysfunction and subtle motor deficits in manganese-exposed non-human primates. *Exp. Neurol.* 202:381–390.

964. Verina, T., S. F. Kiihl, J. S. Schneider, T. R. Guilarte. 2011. Manganese exposure induces microglia activation and dystrophy in the substantia nigra of non-human primates. *Neurotoxicology* 32:215–226.

965. Streit, W. J., N. W. Sammons, A. J. Kuhns, D. L. Sparks. 2004. Dystrophic microglia in the aging human brain. *Glia* 45:208–212.

966. Lopes, K. O., D. L. Sparks, W. J. Streit. 2008. Microglial dystrophy in the aged and Alzheimer's disease brain is associated with ferritin immunoreactivity. *Glia* 56:1048–1060.

967. Sriram, K., G. X. Lin, A. M. Jefferson, J. R. Roberts, R. S. Chapman, B. T. Chen, J. M. Soukup, A. J. Ghio, J. M. Antonini. 2010. Dopaminergic neurotoxicity following pulmonary exposure to manganese-containing welding fumes. *Arch. Toxicol.* 84:521–540.

968. Chang, J. Y., L. Z. Liu. 1999. Manganese potentiates nitric oxide production by microglia. *Brain Res. Mol. Brain Res.* 68:22–28.

969. Crittenden, P. L., N. M. Filipov. 2008. Manganese-induced potentiation of *in vitro* proinflammatory cytokine production by activated microglial cells is associated with persistent activation of p38 MAPK. *Toxicol. In Vitro* 22:18–27.

970. Zhang, P., K. M. Lokuta, D. E. Turner, B. Liu. 2010. Synergistic dopaminergic neurotoxicity of manganese and lipopolysaccharide: Differential involvement of microglia and astroglia. *J. Neurochem.* 112:434–443.

971. American Conference of Governmental Industrial Hygientists. 1976. *Platinum (Soluble Salts as Pt). Documentation of the TLVs for Substances in Workroom Air*, 3rd ed., pp. 213–214. Cincinnati: Signature Publications.

972. Godish, T. 1985. *Air Quality*, p. 217. Chelsea, MI: Lewis Publishers.

973. Poulain, A. J., T. Barkay. 2013. Cracking the mercury methylation code. *Science*, 339(6125) 1280–1281.

5 Organic Chemicals

INTRODUCTION

Organic contaminants are chemical compounds that contain carbon–hydrogen bonds in their basic molecular structures, where most of them are mixtures. These are often combined with a large variety of other atoms. Their source can be either natural products or synthetics, especially those derived from oil, gas, and coal. The number of organic compounds already known is more than 2 million.[1] About 100,000 synthetic organic compounds are commercially available at present, and more than 2000 new organic compounds are produced annually by the chemical industry.[2] These facts are at times overwhelming to the clinician who has to sift through different groups of organic compounds that are aggravating or triggering the individual patient. Often, the clinician will have to settle for a group of chemicals that make up the total body pollutant load and eliminate these for successful prescription for health.

According to the findings of the studies of Randolph[3] and Dickey,[4] diverse chemicals cause chemical sensitivity. This has been established and confirmed by many physicians and scientists over the last 40 years such as Rea,[5] Meggs,[6] Morgan (Morgan, H. 1994. Personal communication), and Ross.[7] These chemicals can be organic and/or inorganic. This chapter deals primarily with organic chemicals, although some inorganic chemicals are mentioned for completeness. Basic scientific studies have been developed by Szallasi,[8] Nicolson,[9] Pall,[10] Calderon-Garciduenas,[11] Meggs,[12] and many others who elaborate the basic mechanisms of chemical sensitivity. Pall[10] has shown that a diverse number of chemicals, at least in part, act as toxicants via the excessive N-methyl-D-aspartic acid (NMDA) activity, which initiate chronic disease, including chemical sensitivity and many chronic degenerative diseases. Szallasi[8] has elaborated this by defining some mechanisms altered by calcium, it meters the nerve when triggered by the pollutant's entry and injury. The transient receptor potential, TRPV1, TRPA, TRPM8, etc., response can trigger the vascular endothelin inside the nerve cell membrane. The Ca^{2+}-triggered TRPV1 activates protein kinases A and C to phosphorylate, thus increasing the sensitivity of the sensory nerve, receptors, and nonimmune system by as much as 1000 times.[12] This increase in sensitivity would at least partially account for chemical sensitivity. Also, with K^+ leaving the cell when the neurovascular membrane leaks, weakness and fatigue result, again causing another basic physiological phenomenon. The oxidative stress and NMDA receptors of the sensory nerves, blood vessels, and immune system appear to be the main triggering mechanisms for most of these chemicals, resulting in chemical sensitivity and chronic degenerative diseases. However, hormone mimics, cancer, and arteriosclerosis can also be produced by toxic chemicals. Each category will be discussed in this chapter.

Diverse Chemicals That Act as Toxicants via Excessive Oxidative Stress, NMDA Activity for the Initiating of Chemical Sensitivity, and Chronic Degenerative Disease

Mechanisms

Organic contaminants may exist in the form of gas (vapor), liquid, or solid particles in the atmosphere, food, and/or water. Having relatively high vapor pressure, some organic compounds will be in the particles in the air, or they can occur in gas or vapor form at normal temperatures. These can cause vascular spasms resulting in hypoxia, thus creating oxidative stress.

Volatile organic chemicals generally have vapor pressures $>10^{-2}$–10^{-8} Kpare-10^{-2} Kpa, that is, methane, ethane, propane, butane. Compounds with vapor pressures between 10^{-2}–10^{-8} Kpare-10^{-2} Kpa are described as semivolatile organic compounds (SVOCs). This class of compounds includes pesticides, herbicides, polychlorinated biphenyl (PCB), polychlorinated benzodioxins, and polyaromatic hydrocarbons (PAHs) (Wallace IC-33 15p-1 McGrun hX 14 16 200). For instance, volatiles such as methane, the simplest organic compound in the air, outgas continuously from the earth, which leads to a background level of 1.5 ppm across the world.[13] Methane levels in fracking areas can be in the thousands of parts per billion.

Terpenes and terpenoids also outgas from plants, yielding another one-third of the chemicals present along with methane (Table 5.1).

Most of them affect the chemically sensitive immediately, while many take years before chronic degenerative disease develops. The classification of organics varies but we will focus on the natural. This can be somewhat arbitrary; however, the intermediates and the final products will be classified as synthetic substances where the naturals would be classified as natural sources. Coal, gas, and oil are naturals from the earth as are the odors, coal products, and terpenes. Any of these can affect the chemically sensitive and cause chronic degenerative disease and make the chemically sensitive very ill or be very helpful. There are separate chapters on the terpenes and pesticides, formaldehyde and natural gas. Table 5.2 shows the volatile organics. Table 5.3 shows terpenes exceeding the prescribed limit in a house (Table 5.4).

Breath Analysis

Breath analysis[14] has also become the tool for evaluating chemical detoxification and exposure along with the outdoor and indoor air analytical laboratory (Table 5.5).[15]

TABLE 5.1

Outdoor Air Analysis of Some Original Chemicals That Are Concentrated to Intermediate Products and Then Final Products Made from Crude Oil, Gas, and Coal

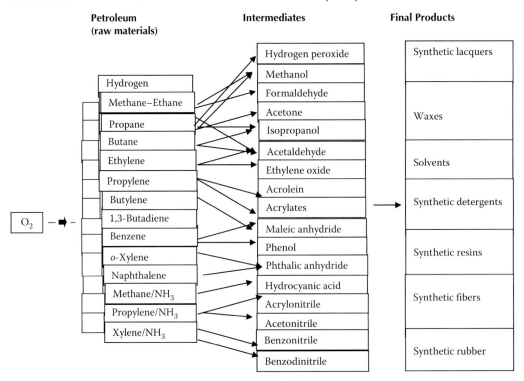

Source: Hopp, V., I. Henning, eds. 1983. *Handbook of Applied Chemistry: Facts for Engineers, Scientists, Technicians, and Technical Manager*, pp. IV/3–IV18. Washington, DC: Hemisphere Publishing. With permission.

TABLE 5.2
Volatile Organic Compounds: Indoor Air Analysis

Compound	4582-1 Family Room		4582-2 Sauna		4582-3 Attic		Recommended Maximum Chronic Concentration	Typical Sources
	μg/m³	ppbv	μg/m³	ppbv	μg/m³	ppbv	μg/m³	
n-Butane	<0.1	<0.1	<0.1	<0.1	1.2	0.5	1900	Gasoline, natural gas, and
Isopentane	1.5	0.5	2.2	0.8	<0.1	<0.1	350	aerosol propellants
Ethyl alcohol	47.3	25.2	1.8	1.0	123	65.4	1880	Cleaners, personal care products, and beverages
Isopropyl alcohol	<0.1	<0.1	<0/1	<0.1	11.9	4.9	785	Personal care products and cleaners, adhesives, solvents, and nail polish remover
Benzene	2.8	0.9	<0.1	<0.1	<0.1	<0.1	4.5	Gasoline and solvents
Toluene	10.7	2.9	5.3	1.4	23.3	6.2	1200	
o-, m-, and p-Xylenes	9.3	2.1	5.5	1.3	3.9	0.9	208	
Nonane	3.4	2.7	<0.1	<0.1	<0.1	<0.1	1050	
Decane	1.7	1.2	<0.1	<0.1	2.0	1.4	1000	
Dodecane	1.9	0.3	<0.1	<0.1	3.7	0.5	350	
Acetone	38.3	16.2	11.1	4.7	32.7	13.8	590	Personal care products, cleaners, adhesives, solvents, nail polish remover, and human emissions
Methyl ethyl ketone	<0.1	<0.1	<0.1	<0.1	2.1	0.7	390	Paints, solvents, nail polish, nail polish removers
Ethyl acetate	<0.1	<0.1	<0.1	<0.1	4.1	1.1	1440	Solvents, fragrances, and nail
N-Butyl acetate	2.9	0.6	6.4	1.4	3.4	0.7	36	polish removers
Acetic acid	24.6	10.0	233	95.1	129	52.7	25	Food products, silicone caulks/ sealants, and glass cleaners
Methyl amyl ketone	5.2	1.1	1.3	0.3	7.4	1.6	840	Fragrances
d-Limonene	40.3	7.2	8.4	1.5	33.5	6.0	100	Cleaners, disinfectants,
α-Pinene	79.7	14/.3	18.2	3.3	68.8	12.4	6	fragrances, perfumes, wood
β-Pinene	23.3	4.2	4.3	0.8	22.3	4.0	6	products
d-Carene	20.7	3.7	24.0	4.3	33.0	5.9	100	
Eucalyptol	10.9	1.7	<0.1	<0.1	13.7	2.2	nl	
β-Phellandrene	13.2	2.4	28.9	5.2	23.7	4.3	200	
Mycrene	4.1	0.7	2.1	0.4	6.9	1.2	100	
Camphene	3.0	0.5	2.0	0.4	3.8	0.7	2	
Styrene	<0.1	<0.1	<0.1	<0.1	2.8	0.7		Plastics, resins, and coatings
2-Ethyl furan	<0.1	<0.1	3.0	0.8	<0.1	0.7	nl	
Propionic acid	<0.1	<0.1	4.3	1.4	<0.1	<0.1	10	
Cyclohexanone	<0.1	<0.1	0.9	0.2	1.0	0.2	48	
Hexanoic acid	<0.1	<0.1	3.9	0.08	5.4	1.1	3	
Naphthalene	<0.1	<0.1	<0.1	<0.1	1.8	0.3	44	Diesel fuel and gasoline
3-Methylcyclopentanol	<0.1	<0.1	<0.1	<0.1	1.5	0.4	nl	
Isopropyltoluene	<0.1	<0.1	<0.1	<0.1	5.7	1.0	nl	
Total other VOCs as toluene[1/]	81.2	98.4	129.4	125.1	165.4	90.8		
Total	426	120	496	160	737	235	200	

Source: Environmental Health Center-Dallas.

Note: Primarily all gasoline and petroleum distillate hydrocarbons. nl, normal limits.

TABLE 5.3

Aldehydes

Sampling Method: Collection on DNPH Silica Gel
Analytical Method: HPLC–UV

Compound	μg/m³	ppbv	Recommended Maximum Chronic Concentration		Typical Sources
			μg/m³	Agency	
Formaldehyde	7	6	3.3/20	1/12.2/	Paint, particle board, plywood, adhesives, and fiberglass insulation
Acetaldehyde	4	2	9	1/	Food products, perfumes, tobacco smoke, auto exhaust, and paints
Propionaldehyde	<1	<1	2	1/	Food products and paints
Crotonaldehyde	<1	<1	0.9	1/	
Butyraldehyde	<1	<1	1.4	1/	Food products, degradation of fats and oils
Benzaldehyde	<1	<1	2.2	1/	Oil alkyd paints, coatings, and
Tolualdehyde, *o*-, *m*-, and *p*-	<1	<1	2.2	1/	adhesives
Valeraldeyde	<1	<1	10	1/	
Hexaldehyde	<1	<1	8 (odor)	1/	
Heptaldehyde	<1	<1	nl	1/	
Total	60	41			

Source: Environmental Health Center-Dallas.
Note: nl, normal limits.

The most common chemicals found in the breath air analysis (Menssana Research, Inc.) of 500 chemically sensitive patients seen at the EHC-Dallas are shown in Table 5.6:

1. 1,3-Butadiene-2-methyl is the most common chemical found in breath analysis. This is an isoprene (terpene) chemical (isoprene) that is a building block for cholesterol. However, it can come in extraneously from various sources, including natural rubber and many synthetics.

2. Cyclopropane, ethylidine is found in 68% of the patients. It is a component of pyrethroid pesticide, which is ubiquitous in commercial buildings and homes due to pesticide use. It is extremely dangerous to the chemically sensitive and chronic degenerative diseased patients, obviously putting a strain on the detoxification systems. Organic phosphate pesticide is also found commonly and is tied with natural gas as the most common chemical found indoors.

3. Acetone, found in 38% of chemically sensitive patients, comes from car exhaust, refineries, varnishes, sealants, and a variety of synthetic compounds. These chemicals can challenge the detoxification systems, putting a strain on them.

4. Limonenes, found in 23% of the patients, come from various terpenes in pine, cedar, and other conifer woods. These will add to the burden of detoxification.

5. Butane, found in 18% of the patients, comes from natural gas. This contaminate is commonly found in patients from heating the building, which puts a strain on various detoxification systems.

6. Various other chemicals come from petroleum-derived products or the breakdown of a few natural chemicals. Clearly, all these have an effect on the detoxification systems, which they can easily overload. In fact, the attempts by the body to detoxify may be seen since many chemicals have groups attached to them as they come out through the breath.

TABLE 5.4

Semivolatile Organic Compounds: Indoor Air Continued

Sampling Method: Collection on PUF Filters
Analytical Method: GC/MS

Analyte	Dining Room		Recommended Maximum Chronic Concentration		Typical Sources
Polycyclic Aromatic Hydrocarbons	$\mu g/m^3$	ppbv	$\mu g/m^3$	Agency	
Acenaphthene	<0.1	<0.1	0.1	1/	Tobacco smoke, combustion processes
Acenaphthylene	<0.1	<0.1	0.1	1/	(fireplaces, diesel engine exhaust,
Anthracene	<0.1	<0.1	0.05	1/	chimneys, and candles), paints and
1,2-Benzanthracene	<0.1	<0.1	nl	1/	adhesives containing tar oil or bitumen,
Benzo(b)fluoranthene	<0.1	<0.1	0.5	1/	wood protection agents and fungicides
Benzo(k)fluoranthene	<0.1	<0.1	0.5	1/	
1,12-Benzoperylene	<0.1	<0.1	nl	1/	
Benzo(a)pyrene	<0.1	<0.1	0.003	1/	
2-Chloronaphthalene	<0.1	<0.1	2	1/	
Chrysene	<0.1	<0.1	0.5	1/	
1,2:5,6-Dibenzanthracene	<0.1	<0.1	nl	1/	
Fluoranthene	<0.1	<0.1	nl	1/	
Fluorene	<0.1	<0.1	nl	1/	
Indeno (1, 2, 3-C, D) pyrene	<0.1	<0.1	0.05	1/	
Naphthalene	<0./1	<0.1	44	1/	
Phenanthrene	<0.1	<0.1	0.05	1/	
Pyrene	<0.1	<0.1	0.05	1/	
Phthalates	$\mu g/m^3$	Ppbv	$\mu g/m^3$	Agency	
Bis(2-ethylhexyl)phthalate	<0.1	<0.1	5	1/	Plasticizer in vinyl cellulosic and
Butyl benzyl phthalate	<0.1	<0.1	5	1/	acrylate plastics and synthetic rubber
Di-n-butyl phthalate	<0.1	<0.1	5	1/	
Diethyl phthalate	<0.1	<0.1	5	1/	
Dimethyl phthalate	<0.1	<0.1	5	1/	
Di-n-octyl-phthalate	<0.1	<0.1	5	1/	
Other semivolatile organic compounds					

Source: Environmental Health Center-Dallas.
Note: nl, normal limits.

Table 5.2 shows the substances we have found by analytical air analysis in the homes of patients with chemical sensitivity and chronic degenerative disease. We see the fumes of natural gas, pesticides, formaldehydes, solvents, terpenes, SVOC, and particulate matter (PM). Probably many more could be found had the laboratory not been limited to those found. However, when you compare the environmental chemicals to those seen in the breath analysis, they are generally the same. Thus, indoor pollution has a profound effect on the individual's detoxification systems. The methyl groups present on these chemicals may well be for detoxification of phase II methylation but most likely the alkyl and aromatics are the original methyl groups from the air.

TABLE 5.5

High Propensity of Chemicals in Breath Air Analysis in 150 Chemically Sensitive Patients That Found 840 Chemicals

Name	%
1,3-Butadiene, 3-methyl	85
Cyclopropane, ethylidene, pyrethroid, ONP insecticides	69
Acetone	38
d-Limonene	23
Benzene ethanol,*a,a*-dimethyl-	18
Butane, natural gas, methane, ethane, propane	17
Cyclohexene, 1-methyl-4-(1-methyl ethyl)-	11
Hexane	11
Heptane, 5-ethyl-2,2,2-trimethyl-	10
Pentane	9
Pentane, 2,2,4,4-tetramethyl-	9
Pentane, 2,2,4-trimethyl-	9
Pentane, 2-methyl-	9
Octane, 2,3,3-trimethyl-isoctane	9
1,3-Pentadiene,(*E*)-	9
Toluene	9

Source: Breath analysis of 150 chemically sensitive patients with 840 chemicals randomly selected from the analysis. Performed in less chemically polluted environment controlled room to exclude extraneous chemicals. EHC-Dallas, 2010–2012—Messana Corp. With permission.

The less polluted air has a very significant effect on the detoxification systems, which showed that the avoidance resulting in the reduction in total air pollutant load of a minimum of five times less as compared to the normal toxic outdoor and indoor air has a marked effect in the increase in detoxification. The patient would develop more energy and be able to handle specific and general toxic environments for longer times without developing impaired brain, cardiac, or other bodily functions. The chemically sensitive patient could right themselves and outperform a normal individual without chemical sensitivity.

Table 5.7 shows the breath analysis of an individual who was initially extremely chemically sensitive and unable to function but after living and working in a less polluted and controlled environment for years had only minor propensity of pollutants on breath analysis. Obviously, the strain on the detoxification systems was decreased, allowing for more efficient detoxification. When the patient went on a trip to the Amazon from the United States, the pollutant load from the air trip and commercial accommodations showed high levels of cyclopropane and butane. The data in Table 5.8 obviously showed an overload of the detoxification systems from overexposures in different airplanes and hotels.

It is clear from clinical improvements and analytical data that a decrease in total body pollutant load will enhance the detoxification systems, allowing for an individual to normalize.

Solvent profiles of 134 patients are shown in Table 5.9. As time went by, these patients' symptoms abated and the profiles went to normal. Again, this shows how relieving the strain on the detoxification systems by environmental control is efficacious. By using the ECU to study the chemically sensitive and chronically degenerative diseased patients, we have observed that less polluted environments have resulted in increased detoxification and pushed the patients toward health.

Table 5.10 shows the signs and symptoms of chemically sensitive patients under environmentally controlled conditions. This study is for the various types of pesticides. However, the findings could

---

TABLE 5.6

Most Common Inhalants Causing Symptoms Indoors in Chemically Sensitive Patients

Formaldehydes	Terpenes
Acetaldehyde	α-β-Pinene
Acrolein	d-Limonene
Other aldehydes	d-Carene
Solvents	Semivolatile organics
Benzene	Polycyclic
Toluene	Aromatic hydrocarbons
Styrene	Anthrocene
Hexane	Benzopyrene
Isooctane	Pyrene
2,+3-Methylpentane	Phthalates
Volatile organic hydrocarbons	Particulates—dust
Isobutane	Mold spores
Ethyl alcohol	Pollen
Isopropyl	Natural fibers
Acetone	Glass fibers
Acetic acid	Synthetic fibers
	Quartz
	Clay
	Iron oxide
	Calcium sulfate (gypsum)
	Calcium carbonate (limestone)
Fumes of natural gas, propanes, octane, methane, ethanes	Pesticides

Source: Matrix Analytical Laboratories Portable Collection Kits, Environmental Health Center-Dallas, 2012.

---

be substantiated for most chemically sensitive and chronic degenerative diseased patients no matter their exposure.

Methane is the main component of natural gas, which can also contain ethane, propane, butane, pentane, hexane, heptanes, octane, etc. VOCs are ubiquitous. Even in a rural outdoor environment, air samples will contain some 50–100 VOCs at levels on the order of 0.01–1 part per billion by volume (ppbv).[16] Organic compounds are extremely important in initiating and propagating chemical sensitivity because they are often volatile or semivolatile and can be easily absorbed, and by sheer volume can overload the detoxification systems.

NMDA

They create NMDA (aspartate), further damaging and allowing penetration and entry of the other toxics and nontoxics, resulting in the absorption of greater quantities of hydrophiles than would be absorbed if toxics were not present. The toxics can make holes by peroxynitrate–superoxide, in lipid cell membranes, allowing Ca^{2+} to enter, thus triggering the TRPV1, TRPA, and TRPM8 mechanisms, resulting in fatigue and weakness when this compound disturbs the mitochondrial membrane, resulting in a leak with an ATP decrease causing weakness and fatigue. Once these cellular membranes are penetrated, a series of enzymes like endolipase, proteases, nitro oxide synthetase, endonucleases, protein kinase, etc., are triggered, resulting in deranged physiology. The combination of Ca^{2+} + protein kinases A and C is phosphorylated. This deranged physiology, when phosphorylated, can increase sensitivity in nerve cells and vascular endothelial cells up to 1000 times, which will result in chemical sensitivity.[8]

TABLE 5.7

Patient before Trip to the Amazon

Patient Id	Compound	Air Gradient	Breath Gradient	Alveolar Gradient
317550	Pentane, 2,2,4-trimethyl-	0	1.402095	1.402095
317550	Undecane, 3,7-dimethyl-	0.093076	1.076027	0.982951
317550	Dodecane, 2,7,10-trimethyl-	0	0.952417	0.952417
317550	Undecane, t,7-dimethyl-	0	0.917727	0.917727
317550	1,3-Hexadien-5-yne	0	0.717116	0.717116
317550	Isotridecanol-	0	0.672264	0.672246
317550	Pentadecane	0	0.5775	0.5775
317550	Octane, 2,3,6-trimethyl-	0	0.564772	0.564772
317550	Decane, 2,4-dimethyl-	0	0.550534	0.550534
317550	Undecane, 4,6-dimethyl-	0	0.549181	0.549181
317550	Dodecane, 4,6-dimethyl-	0	0.401954	0.401954
317550	Octane, 2,3,7-trimethyl-	0.190102	0.564772	0.37467
317550	Nonane, 4-methyl-t-propyl-	0	0.341242	0.341242
317550	Undecane, 4-ethyl-	0	0.336442	0.336442
317550	Undecane, 2-dimethyl-	0.245707	0.549181	0.303474
317550	Decane, 2-cyclohexyl-	0	0.281293	0.281293
317550	Undecane, 4,8-dimetyl-	0	0.252724	0.252724
317550	Pentadecane, 2-methyl-	0	0.239795	0.239795
317550	Dodecane, 4-methyl-	0	0.217909	0.217909
317550	Decane, 4-methyl-	0.135536	0.341242	0.205706

Source: Environmental Health Center-Dallas.

TABLE 5.8

Patient after Trip to the Amazon

Patient Id	Compound	Air Gradient	Breath Gradient	Alveolar Gradient
x317550	Cyclopropane, ethylidene-	8.58835	126.811	118.2226
x317550	Butane	0	49.8668	49.8668
x317550	Pentane, 3-ethyl-2,2-dimethyl-	0	2.141433	2.141433
x317550	Heptane, 3,4-dimethyl-	0	1.875919	1.875919
x317550	Ethylbenzene	0.638953	1.874642	1.235688
x317550	1,3-Hexadien-5-yne	0	1.053669	1.053669
x317550	Isotridecanol	0	0.835682	0.835682
x317550	2,4-Dimethyl-1-heptene	0.128923	0.819384	0.69091
x317550	Tetradecane	0	0.677717	0.677717
x317550	Undecane, 3,7-dimethyl-	0	0.672187	0.672187
x317550	Undecane, 3,8-dimethyl-	0	0.640294	0.640294
x317550	Undecane, 2,6-dimethyl-	0.292789	0.887335	0.594547
x317550	Dodecane, 4,6-dimethyl	0	0.545848	0.545848
x317550	Octane	0.249534	0.781883	0.532348
x317550	Decane, 2,9-dimethyl-	0	0.512026	0.512026
x317550	Pent-2-ynal	0	0.466736	0.466736
x317550	Undecane, 4,8-dimethyl-	0	0.464866	0.464866
x317550	Undecane, 4-ethyl-	0	0.431727	0.431727
x317550	Dodecane, 4-methyl-	0	0.4144534	0.411534
x317550	Furan, 3-methyl-	0.092706	0.466736	0.37403

Source: Environmental Health Center-Dallas.

TABLE 5.9

Toxic Volatile Organic Chemicals Found in 134 Chemically Sensitive Patients Blood Compared with Overall Patient Population Blood Studied by the Laboratory

Compound	No. of Patients below Detection Limits 0.1–0.3 ppb (All Volatiles Negative) 1987	No. and Percent (%) of 134 Patients Detectable TVOC Levels (0.3–36.2 ppb) EHC-Dallas 1987	Percent of Patient Population (>500 Persons) Tested Accu-Chem
Volatile Aromatic Hydrocarbons			
Benzene	20	16 (11%)	23.4
Toluene	20	55 (44.0%)	63.2
Ethylbenzene	20	22 (16.4%)	39.2
Xylenes	20	51 (38.1%)	59.7
Styrene	20	7 (5.2%)	22.0
Trimethylbenzene	20	10 (7.5%)	3.2
Volatile Chlorinated Hydrocarbons			
Chloroform	20	13 (9.7%)	36.9
Dichloromethane	20	21 (15.7%)	49.7
1,1,1-Trichloroethane	20	42 (31.3%)	50.5
Trichloroethylene	20	14 (10.4%)	8.6
Tetrachloroethylene	20	72 (53.7%)	83.1
Dichlorobenzene	20	17 (12.7%)	10.5

Compound	No. and Percent (%) of 134 Patients Detectable TVOC Levels (0.3–36.2 ppb) EHC-Dallas 2010–2014	No. of Patients below Detection Limits 0.1–0.3 ppb (All Volatiles Negative) 2010–2014
Volatile Aromatic Hydrocarbons		
Benzene	45 (45%)	20
Toluene	50 (50%)	20
Ethylbenzene	30 (30%)	20
Xylenes	45 (45%)	20
Styrene	20 (20%)	20
Trimethylbenzenes	15 (15%)	20
Volatile Chlorinated Hydrocarbons		
Chloroform	20 (20%)	20
Dichloromethane	25 (15%)	20
1,1,1-Trichloroethane	45 (45%)	20
Trichloroethylene	20 (20%)	20
Tetrachloroethylene	60 (60%)	20
Dichlorobenzene	30 (30%)	20

Source: Rea, W. J. et al. 1987. Toxic volatile organic hydrocarbons in chemically sensitive patients. *Clin. Ecol.* 5(2):70–74. With permission.

TABLE 5.10

Signs and Symptoms of Chemically Sensitive Patients

1. Odor sensitivity
2. Chronic weakness and fatigue
3. Disturbed sleep and/or insomnia
4. Fibromyalgia and arthritis
5. Gas, bloating, GI upset, constipation, diarrhea
6. Spontaneous bruising, petechiae, acneform lesions, edema
7. Cold sensitivity, inability to seat
8. Rhinosinusitis, postnasal drip, ears ringing, popping, headache
9. Cough, wheezing
10. Bladder frequency, burning, vaginal discharge, premenstrual tension

Source: Environmental Health Center-Dallas.

NMDA Receptor

The NMDA (aspartate), a glutamate receptor, is the predominant molecular device for controlling synaptic plasticity and memory function[17] due to chemical and EMF exposure.

The NMDA is a specific type of ionotropic glutamate receptor. NMDA is methyl-D-aspartate— the name of a selective agonist that binds to NMDA receptors but not to other glutamate receptors. The activation of NMDA receptors results in the opening of an ion channel that is nonselective to captions with an equilibrium potential near 0 mV. A property of the NMDA receptor is its voltage-dependent activation, which opens the nerve or vascular intracellular channel which has occurred as a result of an ion channel block by extracellular Mg^{2+} ions. This opening allows the flow of Na^+ and small amounts of Ca^{2+} ions into the cell and K^+ to go out of the cell to be voltage dependent.[18–21] This can soon cause weakness and fatigue due to K^+ loss and hypersensitivity due to the combination of Ca^{2+} with protein kinases A and C when being phosphorylated.

Calcium flux through the NMDA receptor and cell membrane is thought to be critical in synaptic plasticity, a cellular mechanism for learning and memory deficiency is observed in many cases of chemical sensitivity. The NMDA receptor is distinct in two ways: first, it is both ligand gated and voltage dependent; second, it requires coactivation by two ligands: glutamate and either D-serine or glycine[22] transcripts and differential expression of the NR2 subunits.

Each receptor subunit has modular design and each structural module also represents a functional unit.

Ligands

The activation of NMDA receptors requires binding of glutamate or aspartate (aspartate does not simulate the receptors as strongly).[23] In addition, NMDAs also require the binding of the coagonist glycine for the efficient opening of the ion channel, which is a part of this receptor.

D-Serine has also been found to coagonize the NMDA receptor with even greater potency than glycine.[24] D-Serine is produced by serine racemase, and is enriched in the same areas as NMDA receptors. Removal of D-serine can block NMDA-mediated excitatory neurotransmission in many areas. Recently, it has been shown that D-serine can be released by neurons and astrocytes to regulate NMDA receptors.

In addition, a third requirement is membrane depolarization. A positive change in transmembrane potential will make it more likely that the ion channel in the NMDA receptor will open by expelling the Mg^{2+} ion that blocks the channel from the outside. This function allows leaks in the membrane, allowing the K^+ efflux and the Na^+ and Ca^{2+} into the cell. This property is fundamental to the role of the NMDA receptor in memory and learning, and it has been suggested that this channel is a biochemical substrate of Hebbian learning, where it can act as a coincidence detector for membrane depolarization and synaptic transmission.

The known NMDA receptor agonists include aminocyclopropanecarboxylic acid, D-cycloserine, *cis*-2,3-piperidinedicarboxylic acid, L-aspartate, quinolinate, homocysterate, D-serine, ACPL, L-alanine, and GLYX-13. The partial agonists are NMDA and 3,5-dibromo-L-phenylalanine.[25]

Antagonists of the NMDA receptor are used as anesthetics for animals and sometimes humans, and are often used as recreational drugs due to their hallucinogenic properties, in addition to their unique effects at elevated dosages such as dissociation. When NMDA receptor antagonists are given to rodents in large doses, they can cause a form of brain damage called Olney's lesions. So far, the published research on Olney's lesions is inconclusive in its occurrence on human or monkey brain tissues with respect to an increase in the presence of NMDA receptor antagonists.[26]

Common NMDA receptor antagonists include amantadine,[27] ketamine, methoxetamine, phencyclidine (PCP), nitrous oxide, dextromethorphan and dextrorphan, memantine, ethanol, riluzole (used in ALS),[28] xenon, HU-211 (also a cannabinoid), lead (Pb^{2+}),[29] conantokins, and huperzine A. Dual opioid and NMDA receptor antagonists include ketobemidone, methadone, dextropropoxyphene, tramadol, kratom alkaloids, and ibogaines.

The NMDA receptor is modulated by a number of endogenous and exogenous compounds.[30]

For example, Mg^{2+} not only blocks the NMDA channel in a voltage-dependent manner but also potentiates NMDA-induced responses at positive membrane potentials. Treatment with forms of magnesium glycinate and magnesium taurinate has been used to produce rapid recovery from depression[31] and agitation modalities in the chemically sensitive and at EHC-Dallas.

Na^+, K^+, and Ca^{2+} not only pass through the NMDA receptor channel but also modulate the activity of NMDA receptors.

Zn^{2+} and Cu^{2+} generally block NMDA current activity in a noncompetitive and a voltage-independent manner. However, zinc may potentiate or inhibit the current depending on the neural activity.

Pb^{2+} (lead) is a potent NMDA antagonist. Presynaptic deficits resulting from Pb^{2+} exposure during synaptogenesis are mediated by disruption of NMDA-dependent BDNF signaling. Similar type of reaction occurs with other heavy metals such as cadmium, mercury, etc. to which the chemically sensitive patient is exposed.

It has been demonstrated that polyamines do not directly activate NMDA receptors, instead they act to potentiate or inhibit glutamate-mediated responses.

Aminoglycosides have been shown to have a similar effect to polyamines, and this may explain their neurotoxic effect. The activity of NMDA receptors is also strikingly sensitive to the changes in H^+ concentration, and is partially inhibited by the ambient concentration of H^+ under physiological conditions.[32] The level of inhibition by H^+ is greatly reduced in receptors containing the NR1, a subtype, which contains the positively charged insert Exon 5. The effect of this insert may be mimicked by positively charged polyamines and aminoglycosides, explaining their mode of action. The counteraction of this H^+ effect in the treatment of the chemically sensitive patient with bicarbonates is highly significant. Often, the response to a hypersensitive reaction is acidosis. When sodium bicarbonates, potassium bicarbonates, and calcium carbonates are used, the reaction rapidly terminates.

NMDA receptor function is also strongly regulated by chemical reduction and oxidation, via the "redox modulatory site."[33] Through this site, reductants dramatically enhance NMDA channel activity, whereas oxidants either reverse the effects of reductants or depress native responses. It is generally believed that NMDA receptors are modulated by endogenous redox agents such as glutathione, lipoic acid, and the essential nutrient pyrroloquinoline quinone. Src kinase enhances NMDA receptor currents.[34] Reelin modulates NMDA function through Src family kinases and DAB1,[35] significantly enhancing LTP in the hippocampus. CDK5 regulates the amount of NR2B-containing NMDA receptors on the synaptic membrane, thus affecting synaptic plasticity.[36,37]

Proteins of the major histocompatibility complex class 1 are endogenous negative regulators of NMDA-mediated currents in the adult hippocampus,[38] and modify NMDA-induced changes in AMPAR trafficking[38] and NMDA-dependent synaptic plasticity.

According to Pall, pollutants therefore result in a release of arachidonic acid, which triggers inflammation. Toxics lead to an increase in the sensitivity to NMDA receptors. Toxics also increase membrane partial depolarization, which gives lowered energy metabolism with mitochondria dysfunction which yields an ATP decrease, NO/OONO cycle is a sensory irritant mechanism TRPB1, TRPA, TRPM, giving increases in intracellular glutamate.

According to Pall,[39] antioxidants include MPTP, rotomone, carbon monoxide, hypoxia, fluoroquin, aminoglycoside, β-lactam, isoniazid, salicylate (inner ear), domic acid, brevetoxins, ciguartoxin, Hg, Hg-Murcurals, A-1, and mangamen.

According to Pall,[39] oxidants include NO/OONO cycle superoxide and peroxynitrite nitric oxide/ and $OO \rightarrow OONO$, ↑ transcription factor NF-κB, OONO → with $CO_3 \rightarrow HO$, CO_3, NO_2—free radicals, ONOO oxidant produces oxidative stress→imbalance between oxidants and antioxidants. ↑ NF-κB, NF-κB→↑ transcription of inducible INOS synthase. NF-κB→↑ inflammatory cytokines—1L, 1B, IL-6, IL-8, TNF-α, IFN-γ. Each cytokine, →↑ NO INOS→↑ NO > ONOO inactivates Ca-ATPase→intracellular Ca^{2+} Other oxidants→↑ or ↓ Ca^{2+} ATPase. ↑ Ca^{2+}–intracellular–↑ OO(superoxide) in mitochondria→ATPase. Viscous cycle ↓ ATP→↓ATP→↑ intracellular Ca^{2+}, intracellular Ca^{2+}→↑nNOS and eNOS form of N.O. synthase-Ca^{2+} dependent, ↑ nNOS and eNOS→↑ NO synthesis OONO oxidizes BH_4→↓, BH_4↓→ partial uncoupling of 3 NO synthases →OO instead of N.O.

Nicking of nuclear DNA by hydroxyl and carbonate radicals can produce a massive stimulation of poly-ADP-ribosylation of chromosomal proteins, leading, in turn, to a massive depletion of NAD/ NADH pools because NAD is the substrate for such poly-ADP-ribosylation. NADH depletion lowers, in turn, ATP production in the mitochondrion decreases.

Other changes causing ATP depletion come from a cascade of events occurring within the mitochondrion. The cascade starts with NO, possibly produced by mitochondrial NO synthase (mtNOS which is thought to be largely a form of nNOS), with NO binding to cytochrome oxidase, competitively inhibiting the ability of molecular oxygen to bind. This inhibits the ability of cytochrome oxidase to serve as the terminal oxidase of the mitochondrial electron transport chain.

The action of NO by nicking DNA increases massive depletion of NADH, which decreases DNA production above produces increase superoxide production by the electron transport chain.

Peroxynitrite, produced from the combination of nicking nuclear DNA and mitochondrial changes resulting in ATP ↓ above, also acts to produce increased superoxide from the electron transport chain.

Peroxynitrite, superoxide, and their products lead to lipid peroxidation of the cardiolipin in the inner membrane of the mitochondrion. Cardiolipin is highly susceptible to such peroxidation because most of the fatty acids that make up its structure in mammals are polyunsaturated fatty acids, which are much more susceptible to peroxidation than are other fatty acids.

Cardiolipin peroxidation leads to lowered activity of some of the enzymes in the electron transport chain, leading to further lowering of ATP synthesis. Cardiolipin peroxidation also leads to increased superoxide generation from the electron transport chain in the mitochondrion.

Peroxynitrite produces inactivation of the mitochondrial superoxide dismutase (mn-SOD), leading in turn to increased superoxide levels in the mitochondrion.

Peroxynitrite, superoxide, and nitric oxide inactivate or inhibit the aconitase enzyme, lowering citric acid cycle activity and subsequent ATP synthesis.

Oxidative stress leads to oxidation of cysteine residues in the enzyme xanthine reductase, converting it into xanthine oxidase, which produces superoxide as a product, thus increasing superoxide generation.

Increased activity of the enzyme NADPH, which produces superoxide as a product, is an important part of the inflammatory cascade, and contributes, therefore, to the cascade by producing increased superoxide.

The activity of the NMDA receptors allows calcium influx into the cell, raising intracellular calcium levels.

The activity of transfer receptor potential (TROP) receptors also allows calcium influx into the cell, again raising intracellular calcium levels, presumably leading to increased nitric oxide production.

The main physiological agonist of the NMDA receptors is glutamate whose extracellular concentration is lowered after release, by energy-dependent transport. It follows that ATP depletion produces increased NMDA stimulation by lowering glutamate transport.

The activity of the NMDA receptors is also greatly increased by ATP depletion within the cells containing the NMDA receptors. The mechanism here is that the ATP depletion lowers the electrical potential across the plasma membrane which produces, in turn, increased susceptibility of the NMDA receptors to stimulation.

Three of the TRP groups of receptors have been shown to be stimulated by increased superoxide and/or oxidative stress of their downstream consequences, these being the TRPV1, TRPA1, and TRPM2 receptors, with the increased TRPV1 and TRPA1 activity being produced in part through the oxidation of cysteine residue side chains. Several TRP receptors are also activated by nitric-oxide-mediated nitrosylation.

In TRPV1, TRPA1, and probably several other TRP group receptors, stimulation has each been repeatedly shown to lead to increased NMDA activity, with neurons containing these TRP family of receptors acting in part by releasing glutamate, a major physiological NMDA agonist.

SOURCES OF ORGANICS

There are literally thousands of organic chemicals in the urban atmosphere, homes, food, and water.[3–5,11,16,40] Some of these chemicals, with relatively low boiling points, are used primarily as gasoline additives, solvents, and components of plastic production. Parts and all of these entering sources can enter the body and has to be dealt with either by detoxification or by surrounding it and parking in the muscle, connective tissue, or fat.

The primary source of organic chemicals is the petroleum industry. They are also present in automobile emissions. Their annual production in the United.States is calculated to be millions of tons per year. A large fraction of these chemicals volatilizes directly into the atmosphere. As a consequence, the ratio of man-made to natural volatile organics in large urban centers is usually greater than one, thus doubling the amount of pollutants to which man would normally be exposed to and accounting for a large increase in total pollutant body load. For example, if a person stands by a busy road, his pollutant count doubles. If he runs along the road, the pollutant load increases eight times.[41] Natural organics, which are discussed in areas individually, are composed of about 70% methane and 29% terpenes. (For further discussion of terpenes, see Chapter 8).

Comparison of the types of volatile organics found in various large urban areas reveals that their qualitative composition is very similar and constant.[42] The data collected from three urban sites in New Jersey exemplify this relative frequency of selected volatile organics. Studies at the EHC-Dallas have shown that many volatile organics are in the blood, tissue, and breath of the chemically sensitive, no matter where they are from, and upon subsequent exposure to them, these patients react (Tables 5.1 through 5.3). According to Calderon-Garciduenas, Mexico City has the worst air pollution.[11]

The occurrence of specific volatile organic chemicals in the urban environment depends on several factors, including the amount and variability of emissions from environmental sources, such as car and diesel emissions, factories, etc., the chemical reactivity of the volatile organic chemicals, weather conditions, and location on the earth (hills, valleys, plains). Common manufacturing processes that use various basic synthetic processes produce many volatile organic chemicals. Thus, many complex chemical substances can easily be released into the environment.

Concerns about VOCs in the atmosphere, indoor air, food, and water are threefold. First, they promote photochemical reactions that produce ozone in the lower atmosphere. Second, they significantly increase indoor air pollution. Finally, they threaten individual health in which they cause and propagate chemical sensitivity and chronic degenerative disease (arthritis, autoimmune disease, cancer, arteriosclerosis, etc.).

CLASSIFICATION OF ORGANIC CHEMICALS

In order for these clinicians to evaluate systematically the effects of different organic chemicals on the chemically sensitive and chronic degenerative diseased patient, classification of these chemicals is essential. However, since it is impossible, within the confines of this text, to present all of the thousands of different types of volatile organics that are produced in and pollute urban environments, we present a simple classification of a few of the more common organic chemicals that are known to affect the chemically sensitive adversely (see outline in the beginning of this chapter). These include components of gas, oil, and coal, which are original sources, followed by intermediates and final products and their substituted forms, such as chlorinated products, fluorinated products, etc. These final products can be aliphatic or aromatic, single or multiple with elemental substitutes like cyanide, sulfur, and nitrogen in many. The classification of organics can be done by many ways but we will use the natural and synthetic ones. This can be somewhat arbitrary; however, through the intermediates, the final products, that is, Table 5.1, will be classified as synthetic, while the naturals would be classified as the sources. Coal, gas, and oil are natural substances from the Earth as are the odor and colors and plant produces the terpenes. Any of these can disturb the chemically sensitive and chronic degenerative diseased and make them very ill or at times can be very helpful. Separate chapters are devoted to terpenes, pesticides, formaldehyde, and other substances. Table 5.11 shows terpenes exceeding the theoretical limit in a house (Tables 5.12 and 5.13).

Petrochemistry is an important subdivision of the chemical industry. Various industrial processes and methods of chemical synthesis specific to this industry use hydrocarbons as their starting material. The primary sources of these hydrocarbons are crude oil, natural gas, and coal. The primary products produced from these raw materials are hydrogen, methane, ethane, ethylene, propane, 1-butane, 1,5-butane, 1,3-butadiene, acetylene, propylene, benzene, toluene, and *o*- and *p*-xylene. All of these have been shown to trigger the chemically sensitive and chronic degenerative diseased patient. They are frequently found in breath and indoor and outdoor air analyses (Table 5.14).

Subsequent to their production, primary petrochemical materials are used to derive synthetically intermediate and end products. The intermediate products produced from petroleum include many substances, such as phenols, acetone, and acrylonitrile. The end products produced from crude oil and sometimes natural gas are solvents, synthetic lacquers, detergents, resins, fibers, waxes, and rubbers (Table 5.1).

TABLE 5.11
Terpenes with 29% of Outdoor Air

α-Pinene

β-Pinene

Limonene

Isoprene—1,3-butadiene 2-methyl

Eucalyptol

Phellandrene

Camphene

Turpentine

Source: Environmental Health Center-Dallas, 2012.

TABLE 5.12

Relative Frequency for Detection of Selected Volatile Organics in Urban Sites in the United States

Ubiquitous (>75%)	Occasional (20%–75%)	Rare (<20%)
Vinylidene chloride	Carbon tetrachloride	Vinylchloride
Methylene chloride	1,1,2-Trichloroethene	Ethylene dichloride
Chloroform	1,4-Dioxane	Ethylene dibromide
Trichloroethylene	*o,p*-Chlorotoluene	1,1,2,2-Tetrachloroethane
Tetrachloroethylene	Insecticides–fungicides	
Chlorobenzene	Phenols	
o,p-Dichlorobenzene	Acetone	
Benzene	Acrylonitrile	
Toluene	Acetic acid	
o,m,p-Xylene	Pentane	
Styrene	Hexane	
Ethylbenzene	Cyclopropane	
Nitrobenzene	Octane	
Formaldehyde	Halogenated hydrocarbons	
Urethane		
Polyvinyl		
Natural gas (methane, ethane, propane, butane)		
Organophosphate pesticide		
Pyrethroid pesticide		

Source: Wallace, L. A. 1987. *The Total Exposure Assessment Methodology (TEAM) Study: Summary and Analysis*, Vol. 1. EPA/600/6-87/002A, Washington, DC: U.S. Environmental Protection Agency; Modified from Rea, W. J. 2010–2012. Breath analysis of 500 chemical sensitive patients. Environmental Halth Center-Dallas. Rea, W.J. 1994. *Chemical Sensitivity, Volume II*, page 767, table 1. With permission.

What is important about these primary, intermediate, and end products is that they all have the potential to compromise the health of the chemically sensitive and chronic degenerative diseased. While some are generally quite toxic and sensitizing to humans, many have been found in the blood and breath of the chemically sensitive and chronic degenerative diseased patients at the

TABLE 5.13

Relative Reactivity of Various Classes of Hydrocarbons

Internally bonded alkenes (olefins)

Terminally bonded alkenes (olefins)

Dialkyl and trialkyl benzenes (aromatics)

Diolefins

Ethylene

Toluene and other monoalkyl benzenes

C_6 + alkanes (paraffins)

C_1—C_5 alkanes (paraffins); acetylene and benzene

Source: Environmental Health Center, 2012. Rea, W.J. 1994. *Chemical Sensitivity, Volume II*, page 772, table 2. With permission.

TABLE 5.14

Indoor Air Analysis—Aldehyde Problem

VOCs and Aldehydes	Test Results ($\mu g/m^3$)	Reference Levels ($\mu g/m^3$)	Comparison to Reference Levels (%)
Volatile Organic Compounds and Aldehydes—Bedroom Old Bldg., Antwerp, Belgium 55-Year-Old Housewife			
Benzene	7	4.5	155.6
Acetaldehyde	44	45	97.8
Camphene	4	5	80.0
Formaldehyde	18	20	90.0
Benzaldehyde	2	9	22.2
Tolualdehyde, *o*, *m*, and *p*	2	9	22.2
Acetic acid	4	25	16.0
d-Carene	13	112	11.6
2,2,4-Trimethylpentane	4	75	5.3
Hexaldehyde	4	80	5.0
Propionaldehyde	2	46	4.3
Acetone	24	590	4.1
Limonene	4	110	3.6
o, *m*, and *p*-Xylenes	7	180	3.9
1-Methyl(1-methylethenyl)-benzene	7	245	2.9
n-Pentane	7	350	2.0
Valeraldehyde	2	180	1.1
Toluene	9	1200	0.8
Isopentane	2	350	0.6
n-Octane	2	350	0.6
Nonane	2	1050	0.6
Ethyl benzene	2	1250	0.2
Hexamethylcyclotrisiloxane	4	n/l	0.2
Total other VOCs as toluene	40		
Total VOCs and aldehydes	216	<200	

Source: Environmental Health Center-Dallas, 2006.

EHC-Dallas. They have been proven extremely harmful to them upon challenge, often reproducing their sensitivity signs and exacerbating their diseases. All have been shown, in some instances, to affect the chemically sensitive adversely.

The main component of natural gas is methane. Since it is a much lighter molecule than the larger, relatively more inert hydrocarbon molecules that occur in petroleum, it is a gas at room temperature. There is much conjecture as to whether this substance is harmful to humans. Evidence from the EHC-Dallas suggests that it is harmful to the chemically sensitive and chronic degenerative diseased, usually triggering their symptoms of their illness. Depression and fatigue and other neurological as well as vascular dysfunction such as spasm, spontaneous bruising, petechiae, acne-like lesions, peripheral edema, etc. are some of their predominant symptoms. Methane has been shown to be bubbling from the Earth, where the polar ice cap has melted.[43]

In petrochemistry, reactive molecules are produced from these relatively nonreactive hydrocarbons by either splitting off the hydrogen, which leads to C=C or aromatic hydrocarbons (benzene), or by substitution, for example, replacing its atoms by reactive atoms or groups of atoms (Cl, Fl, Br, CN, CH, etc.). At the EHC-Dallas, we have shown that these more reactive molecules are, in many instances, definitely harmful to humans, especially to the chemically sensitive and chronic degenerative diseased patients. Halogenated organics seem to be some of the most damaging.

Oil and gas have become more important than coal as a source of raw material for the $-CH_2-$ group because ethylene groups are present in chain forms, whereas in coal they have to be inefficiently produced with steam. Therefore, it is cheaper initially to use oil and gas and their raw, natural products in industry for the production of final products. The hydrogen content of the hydrocarbons in oil and gas constitute the real value for manufacturing final products. We see many ethylene molecules in the breath analysis and also propane and butane compounds.

Methyl alcohol can cause blindness. Many methane products can cause distress in the chemically sensitive and methyl alcohol and its products are often seen in the breath analyses of chemically sensitive and chronic degenerative diseased patients. In calculating the cost of oil and gas products, little consideration is given to the hidden costs of environmental pollution and subsequent medical care for individuals affected by exposure to these pollutants, all of which can cause problems in the chemically sensitive and chronic degenerative diseased. These hidden costs, however, should be calculated, along with production expenses, in order to assess accurately the total cost of using refining and marketing of oil and gas products but of course they are not.

Hundreds of different compounds can be detected in crude oil. These range from very small volatile components to large molecules that remain in tar when crude oil is distilled. Irrespective of the site where it is formed, crude oil consists almost entirely of hydrocarbons. In addition, it contains various forms of oxygen, sulfur, and nitrogen. Sulfur-containing compounds must be removed before the oils can be commercially used. Removing the sulfur-containing compounds adds to the cost of the refining process; therefore, sulfur oil is more expensive initially. When the costs of damage to the environment and chemically sensitive and chronic degenerative diseased individuals are factored into its total costs, the cost of crude oil rises.

Paraffins, naphthenic crude oils that contain primarily alicyclic hydrocarbons (in particular, derivatives of cyclopentane and cyclohexane) and aromatic hydrocarbons (United States, Venezuela, and Romania), and crude oils of mixed composition (these usually come from the Middle East and Africa) are the three types of crude oils. The type or intensity of chemical sensitivity and chronic degenerative diseased that might result from exposure to these oils could vary due to the qualities unique to the oils produced in various parts of the world. These different compositions can have different effects on the chemically sensitive and chronic degenerative diseased patients.

Crude oils are extracted from bore holes sunk in porous sandstone or limestone rocks, and not from subterranean lakes. Capillary action brings them to the surface. Over 700,000 bore holes are used for extracting oil in the world, 625,000 of which are in the United States. One can see how these numbers of underground disturbances, if near the local water tables, might affect underground ecology in the area. Many chemically sensitive patients have reported problems with contaminated water in these areas containing bore holes.

The composition of natural gas varies depending on its origin. It usually contains methane, and it can contain ethane. In addition, it contains propane, butane, hydrogen, nitrogen, carbon dioxide, hydrogen sulfide, and helium. The H_2 must be removed from natural gas before it can be used for heating or a raw material in manufacturing primary products. Natural gas occurs frequently as gas bubbles near oil fields, or it is dissolved in crude oil or surrounding coal fields, as a product of subsequent carbonization. It also comes from the fracking of shale. These with chronic degenerative disease may not initially perceive the contamination and are exposed for years before chemical sensitivity or the fatal cancer or arteriosclerosis occurs. When they are tapped, these gas and oil fields emanate odors that pollute the air and adversely affect the chemically sensitive and chronic degenerative diseased in the area. Natural gas from shale is the latest problem in the United States as many people living in the area have become ill by the fumes and thus pollutants; this phenomenon shows chemical sensitivity or chronic degenerative disease often occurs as does hormone deregulation, cancer, or arteriosclerosis.

Distillation is the most important process employed in refining crude oil and is the reason for the development of the large commercial distiller, the refinery. Refineries are constructed in the open with their furnace, reactors, columns, and pipes outdoors in order to allow gases to leak. While this ventilation reduces the immediate explosive potential of the refinery, it also contributes greatly to local atmosphere contamination. (See the Texas City and local refinery air pollution section in Chapter 4.) On days of weather inversion, especially, pollutants released into the air via this type of ventilation produce high air pollution levels. Higher winds push polluted air to areas remote from the refinery, causing pollutants to be dumped on other people. As we have seen in many areas, many chemically sensitive people develop symptoms when exposed to fumes from these sources.

During the refining process, moving from gas to solid form, the fractions to which crude oil is separated are gas consisting of hydrocarbons with a chain length of C_2–C_4 (ethane, propane, butane) and naphtha, heavy naphtha, kerosene, diesel and fuel oil, lubricating oil, and bitumen. These separate at different boiling endpoints. The fractions used as gasoline must have a precise mixture of 100 octanes to n-heptanes to prevent engine knocking. Parts of these different fractions of gasoline have been identified in the blood and breath of the chemically sensitive and chronic degenerative diseased, and have been shown to adversely affect their function. Isooctane is often found in the chemically sensitive breath and blood solvent profile (Table 5.6).

Diesel fuel and gasoline produce straight-chain paraffins (aliphatics—alkanes C–C). Subtle differences in the composition and end combustion products that occur as crude oil are fractioned and may explain why some chemically sensitive and chronic degenerative diseased patients seem to have more visible problems from diesel fuel than from gasoline. However, these patients usually experience problems from exposure to both; the problems caused by one are often simply more severe than those from the other. For example, the chemically sensitive individual who fills his car gas tank may get a runny nose. When exposed to diesel exhaust, however, he may become dysfunctional. Also, when chronically exposed to gas fumes, this same person, over time, may become nonfunctional by developing neurodegenerative disease, arteriosclerosis, or cancer.

As thousands of different types of volatile organics are produced in, and pollute, urban environments, it is impossible, within the confines of this text, to talk about all of them. A few of the known, significant hydrocarbons that cause problems in the chemically sensitive and chronic degenerative diseased breath analysis are generally classified as short-chained compounds, such as ketones, alcohols, and aldehydes, aliphatic hydrocarbons (C–C) and aromatic cyclic compounds with one or more benzene rings.

Major components of primary straight-chain hydrocarbon pollution in urban areas are aldehyde (RCHO) (e.g., formaldehyde, acetaldehyde, acrolein); ketones (RCHOR) (e.g., acetone); alkanes (paraffins) (C–C) (e.g., methane, isoethane, propane, n-butane, isopentane); cycloalkanes (e.g., cyclohexane, methylcyclopentane); olefins (alkenes) C=C (e.g., ethylene, propylene, butene); cycloolefins (e.g., cyclohexene); alkynes (C≡C) (e.g., acetylene), as well as other halogenated derivates. The closed-ring group (toluene, xylene) and their halogenated (e.g., hexachlorobenzene), nitrogenated, and sulfated derivatives make up the aromatic compounds. The complex multiple benzene ring compounds form a separate class. These include benzapyrenes, anthracenes, etc. Some components can create brain dysfunction as shown in the following case reported by Stein et al.[44]

Exposure and Susceptibility: Schizophrenia in a Young Man Following Prolonged High Exposures to Organic Solvents

There is an abundant literature on the deleterious effects of solvents on the neurobehavioral performance, higher brain functions, and chronic solvent-induced encephalopathy.[44] However, literature establishing a cause–effect relationship between solvent exposure and schizophrenia is sparse, consisting mostly of case reports, case series reports, and cross-sectional comparisons.

Schizophrenia is defined as any of several psychotic disorders characterized by distortions of reality, impairments of thought and language, and withdrawal from social contact.[45] The disease is traditionally considered to be triggered by unknown factors intrinsic to the patient. Few studies have focused on occupational exposures as possible causes of schizophrenia. As with other diseases, the pathogenesis and clinical expression of schizophrenia may involve gene–environment interactions and genetic susceptibility.[46,47] Here is a report on a patient with schizophrenia, first diagnosed with acute psychosis which was precipitated by a sustained period of exposures to neurotoxic solvents in an occupational setting.

Case Report

The patient was a 30-year-old man, the 9th of 10 siblings, son of a 43-year-old father and 35-year-old mother at the time of his birth. His family immigrated to Israel from Tajikistan. The patient was hospitalized in November 1997 at the age of 24 for an acute attack of what was diagnosed as severe psychosis, subsequently requiring several months of hospitalization. He presented in the Emergency Room with acute delirium, disorganized and violent behavior, and was agitated, restless, and unable to restrain himself, with fits of shouting and crying, suicidal thoughts, unsteady gait, muscle pain, and insomnia. On neurological examination, he was found to have horizontal nystagmus, which later disappeared. During the period before hospitalization, his family, including his mother, noted that he behaved as though he were drunk, even though he was a teetotaler. His family denied abuse of hashish or alcohol, including vodka, to which he said he was allergic. His family, at that time, was unaware of occupational exposures to potentially toxic compounds.

The behavioral change was gradual. In the weeks and months prior to hospitalization, he experienced irritation of skin and airways. The conjunctivae in his eyes were noted to be red; his skin color was described as yellow. He suffered from headache, dizziness, nausea, fatigue, irritability, forgetfulness, and loss of appetite. He felt depressed and agitated. His speech was slurred and its content was incoherent, as though drunk. His urine was dark in color.

Serum transaminase levels were elevated and mild thrombocytopenia was detected on his first hospitalizations.

Occupational History

The patient's psychotic attack occurred following 6 months of work in a paint factory, beginning in May 1997, where he was exposed for up to 17 hours a day to paints and many organic solvents, in a closed small caravan 12 m^3 in volume. He worked as a painter of computer with metal components, in a small room containing a stove, a waterfall device for absorbing droplets of paint, and two chimneys. Among the agents were toluene, xylene, n-butyl acetate, ethylene glycol, monomethyl ether acetate, methoxy propranolol, trimethylbenzene, isobutanol, as well as organic and inorganic pigments, strontium chromate, lead, and acetone. There were several dermal and respiratory exposures at extremely high levels, under extremely poor working conditions. There were neither windows nor ventilation systems in his working environment. His work consisted of spraying the paints onto the electronic components and cleaning the equipment by immersing it in acetone by his bare hands. He had no gloves to use. He used a nonprotective cotton face mask which he received from his employer. He ate alone in the caravan and had not been informed on the exposures and possible health risks. No surveys or environmental measurements had been performed at the workplace.

Prior to employment, he had been healthy, strong, and alert. He completed high school, where he was popular and excelled in sports. Given his high military medical profile, he served full compulsory service in the Israeli Defense Forces (IDF) as a combat solider in an infantry unit from which he was honorably discharged.

A twin sister had died soon after birth, in Tajikistan. A 20-year-old brother was found dead after disappearing, 1 year after immigrating to Israel, without a known prior psychiatric history. A mental health diagnosis of the patient's brother had not been performed.

It was a tightly knit family. His sister, especially, was extremely supportive. We had no information on any problems with crime, drugs, or violence in the family.

The patient's first discharge diagnosis was acute psychotic stress, either from toxic (organic) of functional (nonorganic) cause. In the following years, although he was no longer exposed to solvents or other toxic substances, the patient was repeatedly hospitalized due to severe psychotic attacks, in which he became violent and required restraint. Between psychotic episodes, he did not resume his former high level of function but was mostly idle, secluded, and withdrawn. At some point, there was also a failed marriage. In February 2000, he was hospitalized again and the diagnosis of schizophrenia was first established.

When examined in 2003, at the age of 30, the patient was spending much of his time in bed. He was found to suffer from concentration difficulties, especially when reading, and was described by his psychiatrists as lacking motivation (Apulia), suffering from chronic fatigue, and depressed. On physical examination, he appeared apathetic; there were no disturbances in organization of thoughts, concepts, judgment, and perception; and there was no disorientation in relation to time, place, or self. He required sedatives, antidepressants, and tranquilizers.

The patient underwent a comprehensive neurocognitive assessment in 2003. Memory was evaluated using the Wechsler Memory Scale.[44] His learning capacity skills were tested using the Rey Auditory Verbal Learning Test. This patient showed impairment, particularly in immediate working memory. His scores were two standard deviations below the norm and his learning curve I–V was very flat: trial I = 3, II = 5, III = 8, IV = 8, and V = 8. Such low scores probably reflect, at least partly, the effort invested in performing the tests rather than true cognitive abilities. Lack of volition is regarded as a "negative sign" of schizophrenia and frontal subdominant organic brain damage, as well as a clinical feature of depression. His physicians and close family members have reported a slight improvement in his memory since then.

Repeated electroencephalographies (EEGs) and magnetic resonance imaging (MRI) brain scans showed unremarkable findings, but these tests were performed 3 years after his acute exposures, by the time the acute effects on electrophysiological parameters of brain function, would not necessarily have persisted. The absence of findings on imaging is consistent with experience that imaging procedures cannot be relied upon as gold standard tests of brain disease from toxic exposures.[44] However, triple-camera SPECT brain scans were not performed or even considered which most likely would have shown toxic changes as performed at the EHC-Dallas. Didriksen toxic brain functions profiles could have shown abnormalities had the patient been able to perform them. Furthermore, EEG reflects first and foremost the electrical cortical activity, while functional solvent-induced impairment is mainly in the subcortical long tracts and associative neural pathways.

These are relevant to the case report because (1) they have richness in individual detail lacking in larger analytic studies, (2) they enable us to relate our findings to those from prior knowledge, and (3) they also generate hypotheses for testing interesting associations, relevant to our hypothesis regarding exposure and susceptibility.

Wada et al.[48] compared a group of solvent-exposed patients and a group of schizophrenic patients. Overlap in signs and symptoms between patients diagnosed as having solvent-induced psychosis and patients with schizophrenia is described; these include delusion, hallucination, anxiety, emotional instability, and loss of motivation. It is interesting to note that the symptom of loss of motivation, characteristic of patients suffering from solvent-induced psychosis, is very similar to the negative signs typical to schizophrenia.

Other cases of brain dysfunction have been described such as the one by Stein et al.[44] There is an abundant literature on the adverse effects of solvents on the neurobehavioral performance, higher brain functions, and chronic solvent-induced encephalopathy.[44] However, the occurrence of solvent-related schizophrenia is rare, with few reports on the link between solvent exposure and schizophrenia. Here, Stein[44] reports on a patient with schizophrenia, presenting after a sustained period of 6 months of everyday exposure to high levels of toxics in a contained area to neurotoxic solvents in an unprotected occupational setting in Haifa, Israel.

In light of the similarity of symptoms of schizophrenia and chronic solvent encephalopathy (CSE), they call for further epidemiologic studies to examine the potential contribution of solvent exposure to the etiology and evolution of schizophrenia in selected cases. This case study and review of relevant literature underscores the importance of obtaining detailed histories on occupational exposures to search for agents which can trigger psychotic episodes. In the meantime, policies to prevent such exposures at the source can be expected to contribute to the prevention of a nontrivial proportion of neurotoxic diseases, including, possibly, schizophrenia in worker populations.

Case reports are interesting in which they suggest, but analogous, the possibility that exposures that lead to syndromes somewhat similar to schizophrenia, can also lead to schizophrenia.

Case-referent studies face the difficulty of selecting comparisons. Daniels and Latcham[49] presented 29 male and 5 female schizophrenic patients, from an island in which self-induced exposure to solvents is common (petrol sniffing). Compared to matched referents, the schizophrenic patients had a much higher probability of past exposure to solvents—an association which suggests the possibility of a cause–effect relationship.

Cohort Studies

Cohort-type studies are presented. Schizophrenia is difficult to capture in prospective cohort studies because of the relatively low prevalence of the condition—1%[45]; yet, large population-based cohorts have managed to extract suggestions of increased risks for schizophrenia with prior exposures to solvents and other agents[50] twin status,[51] and older age of the father[52]—all of which are relevant to this patient. Two large birth cohorts were followed, a registry of 12,094 births between 1959 and 1966 from Oakland, California[50]; and a registry of 88,829 births between 1964 and 1976 from Jerusalem.[53,54]

Mikkelsen[55] reviewed epidemiologic studies of occupational mixed solvent exposure for evidence of exposure-related neuropsychiatric disorders, mental symptoms, and impaired neurobehavioral performance. Although the reviewed psychiatric morbidity studies did not find a clear relation between occupational solvent exposure and admission to a hospital for psychiatric illness, the author concluded that the cumulative findings strongly suggest that occupational solvent exposure may be the cause of mental and cognitive impairment, which may become chronic and disabling.

Several studies have described patients presenting with signs and symptoms which were also seen in this patient following exposure to solvents, that is, depressed mood, anxiety, irritability, and aggressive behavior. The patients were later diagnosed as CSE.[56–59] These studies do not present patients with psychotic signs and symptoms, and do not address a possible outcome of schizophrenia.

Bolla et al.[60] observed the neuropsychiatric symptoms in paint manufacturers. The paper examined all 187 participants with the Present State Exam, structured psychiatric interview. Exposure data were thorough and complete, and statistical analyses focused on cumulative dose–response relationships. An outcome of depression was found to be significantly related to solvent exposure, and there were other nontrivial associations. The Q16 and exposure data in the paper suggest that even in the highest of four exposure groups, exposures were much lower than those in this patient. These higher exposures in the patient may account for the greater spectrum and severity of his signs and symptoms.

Van Valen et al.[61] reviewed the epidemiologic literature to provide an overview of the course and prognostic factors of CSEs following exposure to solvents, but did not reach any definite conclusions and did not address the outcome of schizophrenia.

In summary, case reports, case series, and case–case reports, despite many limitations, suggest some overlap between symptoms and signs of CSE and "negative signs" of schizophrenia (regarding memory loss and cognitive decline). The presence of psychotic symptoms (positive signs) of schizophrenia, such as delusions, hallucinations, and thought disturbances, distinguishes between these conditions.

Cohort-type studies suggest that exposures below regulatory thresholds may increase risks for subsequent neurotoxic and neurobehavioral impairment.

The patient presented with nonspecific neurotoxic signs and symptoms, hospitalized and diagnosed first as suffering from acute psychosis; when it became clear that his condition was chronic, his diagnosis was established as schizophrenia. The case of causality between the patient's exposures and schizophrenia was based on the "weight of the evidence" approach to his history. The fact that the patient's acute symptoms appeared following his sustained and massive exposure to organic solvents suggested that the exposure triggered schizophrenia. His symptoms were known to be produced by solvent exposure. The transient elevation of transaminases is the clinical evidence that his liver functions had been affected by exposure to solvents. The absence of findings on imaging is consistent with experience that imaging procedures cannot be relied upon as gold standard tests of brain disease from toxic exposures.[62] The fact that only 30% of the patients with schizophrenia have neuroradiologic abnormalities means that 70% do not. This is when MRIs and pet scans are used. However, when triple-camera SPECT scans are used, one can show neurotoxicity, but blood and breath levels of solvents were not performed. In our experience, when performed, they would most likely be positive.

The obscure circumstances in which the patient's brother disappeared and died could possibly represent a familial factor which eventually caused him to be more susceptible to his occupational exposure to solvent, in such obviously appalling working conditions and in prolonged solitude. One should also note that his father was 43 years old when the patient was born, which is a borderline age in regard to the excess risk of schizophrenia, found over paternal age of 45.[52] These factors may have interacted with his exposures and added to his susceptibility.

This sequence of an intense, symptomatic exposure, directly followed by nonspecific neurotoxic symptoms accompanied by an acute psychotic state with signs and symptoms typical to schizophrenia, restates and strengthens the case for a cause–effect relationship.

In the light of the foregoing, there appears to be a two-stage model in which the patient's exposures led to organic psychosis and his organic psychosis then was later diagnosed, by all doctors who examined him, as schizophrenia. This two-stage model states the case for a model of genetic risk for schizophrenia being modified or triggered by a high exposure to neurotoxic agents, without which there either would have been no clinical expression, less severe expression, or onset later on in life, perhaps also triggered by extrinsic factors. It is suggested that this model takes into account current paradigms or exposure–susceptibility.

They suggest the need to take into account the possibility that extreme external exposure can trigger disease—even in relatively uncommon disease such as schizophrenia, which has not been proven to be associated with this exposure—in persons in whom there is preexisting susceptibility.

Current psychiatric terminology shows a distinction between schizophrenia without any known organic or environmental trigger, and clinically identical syndromes associated with the exposure as the trigger.[63]

We cannot confidently rule out the possibility that this patient's occupational exposure and the symptoms, which led to the diagnosis of schizophrenia were a mere coincidence. However, this is not the first report of such a coincidence. The reproducibility of the association and the severity of the exposures in this patient make chance an unlikely explanation.

This patient's case history reinforces the case of taking careful occupational histories of past exposures in patients with schizophrenia and other psychoses—a routine that is not always followed. More case–control studies are needed to explore the contributory role of neurotoxic exposures in triggering expression of organic mental syndromes in individuals with prior indications of susceptibility.

The pertinent questions are: If the exposures in this case were missed, in how many other patients diagnosed with schizophrenia were they not looked for? If the associations in this case were not reported, how many others have not been reported? How many patients diagnosed as having schizophrenia, have in fact developed the disease as a consequence of prior exposures, possibly following primary nonspecific neurotoxic signs and symptoms? If the associations in this case were not reported, how many others have not been reported? How many patients diagnosed as having schizophrenia, have in fact developed the disease as a consequence of prior exposures, possibly following primary nonspecific neurotoxic signs and symptoms? Did the label—schizophrenia—disable the diagnostician? Does making the diagnosis divert attention from possible triggers? We suggest that the current pathogenetic models of schizophrenia may not adequately take into account the role of high exposure at the level of the individual patient. One also has to recognize that at the global level, the absence of evidence on the proportional contribution of solvent exposures to schizophrenia, and for that matter, all so-called organic psychoses and neurobehavioral impairments should not be equated with the absence of the evidence. In the interim, there remains an ethical import to delay, and the case for action remains to prevent exposures at the source to solvents and other neurotoxic agents, by substitution and enclosure.

EDR and OB provided expert medical opinions in support of the case for a cause–effect relationship between patient's exposures and medical status, as part of their work in Hebrew University–Hadassah Medical Center.

According to the EHC-Dallas and Didriksen,[64] there are neurocognitive and personality/behavioral concomitants of neurotoxic exposure.

Neuropsychological assessment is an important component of a comprehensive evaluation of patients who have been exposed to neurotoxic substances. Test results provide information regarding the degree of cognitive and behavioral impairment for the referring physician for treatment planning purposes and extends documentation for litigation worker's compensation, and disability issues (private and social security) and most important—the patient's health.

The Environmental Protection Agency (EPA) in 1998 defined neurotoxicity as "an adverse change in the structure or function of the central and/or peripheral nervous system following exposure to a chemical, physical, or biological agent." The classes of neurotoxic substances include gases (carbon monoxide, cyanide, hydrogen sulfide), metals (mercury, lead, manganese), monomers used for chemical synthesis in the production of polymers, resins, and plastics, (acrylamide, styrene), organic solvents (toluene, xylene, white spirit), pesticides (organophosphates, organochlorines, carbamates), and others (hydrazine, pyridine, arsine, and tetrodotoxin).[65,66] Although the neurotoxicity of toxigenic molds and EMF remains somewhat controversial, data collection in this clinic strongly suggests their neurotoxic properties.

The majority of patients who are referred for neuropsychological assessment have been exposed to a neurotoxic agent in the workplace, primarily via inhalation of absorption. However, many patients have also been exposed in their homes, for example, misapplication of pesticides, water intrusion resulting in exposure to toxigenic molds, hobbies requiring the use of solvents, extra-small electrical apparatus, smart meter, cellular phones, TV, etc. A few patients have become ill after drinking contaminated water or from intentional exposure from mosquito abatement or an inadvertent exposure from crop dusting.

Regardless of the neurotoxin, the effects observed on neuropsychological assessment are quite similar. The damage to the central nervous system (CNS) is diffuse, rather than localized as in tumor or stroke, and in this regard is very similar to the deficits observed in patients following mild traumatic head injury as well as similar to deficits found in patients with diseases involving infectious processes, for example, chronic fatigue syndrome or Lyme disease.

The majority of patients seeking evaluation and treatment for neurotoxic exposures in the past were primarily solvent-exposed individuals. The majority of patients assessed at this time are reporting exposures to toxigenic molds. Fewer pesticide-exposed patients are seen at this time, as well.

The effects of solvent exposure were classified at a meeting of the WHO in Copenhagen in 1985. These classifications may also be appropriately applied to patients exposed to other neurotoxic agents as they present with similar symptoms. The classifications include:

1. *Affective syndrome*: Neuropsychiatric symptoms reported, no objective findings, considered reversible
2. *Mild chronic toxic encephalopathy*: Neuropsychiatric symptoms impairments
3. *Severe chronic toxic encephalopathy*: Severe neuropsychiatric symptoms

Illness may be a result of chronic low-level exposure over a period of months to years or due to an acute exposure lasting only minutes, but of a very high concentration of the neurotoxic substance. Damage to central and peripheral neurons may occur due to anoxia, changes in the nerve cell membrane, impairment of oxidative metabolism, interference with neurotransmitters, and structural damage to the neuron. Many neurotoxic substances may cross the blood–brain barrier. Other organs in the body may be damaged, resulting in indirect impairment of the nervous system, for example, lung damage.[66]

Three symptom checklists have been developed and constantly revised over more than 20 years from the reported physical, psychological, and neurocognitive symptoms of neurotoxically exposed individuals. These symptoms are consistent with those reported in the literature following neurotoxic exposure with some variation from patient to patient depending on various factors, including prior exposures, infectious processes, excessive use of prescription drugs, illicit drugs, or alcohol, metabolic conditions, diseases indirectly affecting the brain (e.g., sleep apnea), prior head injury, frequency, intensity, and duration of exposure, and others.

Primary physical symptoms reported in the Physical Symptom Checklist include fatigue, low energy, weakness, sleep disturbances, headaches, balance and coordination problems, tremor, decreased libido, and inability to tolerate excessive environmental or sensory stimuli. Primary symptoms reported in the Psychological Symptom Checklist include present performance inferior to prior performance or level of functioning, difficulty in getting started in the morning, decreased coping ability, worrying about bodily dysfunction, difficulty in setting and reaching goals, diminished self-confidence and self-esteem, anxiety, depression, and irritability. Primary neurocognitive symptoms include decreased attention, concentration, memory, comprehension, and executive functions, expressive speech difficulties, confusion, and slowed thinking and information processing, resulting in an inability to complete tasks in a timely manner.

Adverse effects of neurotoxic exposure reported in the literature include decreased attention, concentration, memory, intelligence, and executive functions, mental slowing, as well as sensory, motor, and visuospatial impairments. Personality and behavioral changes reported include anxiety, tension, depression, fatigue, irritability, decreased coping ability, anger, psychosis, and social isolation and withdrawal.

The Halstead-Reitan Neuropsychological Test Battery, a fixed battery, is primarily utilized to assess neurocognitive functioning in toxically exposed patients who are involved in litigation or who are applying for disability benefits with private companies. It is the most widely used instrument for the assessment of brain–behavior relationships in the United States and Canada and is sensitive to cerebral damage. It is able to compare the subject's level of functioning to others, and to compare performances on the same tasks on two sides of the body to permit inferences regarding the status of each hemisphere. The HRB meets the Daubert criteria for admissibility of expert testimony in federal courts.

The HRB includes general tests that are sensitive to all areas of the cerebral cortex as well as specific neuropsychological tests which reflect the functional status or regionally or specifically localized areas. Results from the Weschler Adult Intelligence Scale are also utilized to compute the General Neuropsychological Deficit Scale score, the overall score which indicates the degree of impairment. Several tests of the HRB are used to compute the Impairment Index, which indicates the consistency of impairment over cognitive domains.

The majority of patients who have been evaluated in Didriksen' office following neurotoxic exposure score in a mildly impaired range, overall, on the Halstead-Reitan Battery. Greatest impairment is typically observed on two measures of higher cortical functions, the Halstead Category Test and Tactual Performance Test. The majority of patients score within normal limits on two measures of visual tracking and scanning (Trail Making Tests A and B) with greater impairment typically observed on Trails B, which requires divided attention and the ability to alternate between two sets of stimuli (mental flexibility).

The majority of patients score within normal limits on the Speech Sounds Perception Test, a measure of sustained attention and concentration for slowly presented, verbal auditory stimuli.

Greater impairment is observed in the Seashore Rhythm Test, a measure of sustained attention and concentration for more rapidly presented, nonverbal auditory stimuli.

Some impairment is observed on measures of specific neuropsychological abilities, including sensory and motor functions. Weakness and motor slowing are typical findings. The majority of patients score within normal limits on measures of sensory–tactile functioning as well as on measures of bilateral, simultaneous stimulation in the auditory, visual, and tactile modalities. The most frequently observed pathognomonic signs in the Reitan-Indiana Aphasia Screening Test include constructional dyspraxia and dyscalculia. The majority of patients do not show a significant difference between right and left hemisphere scores due to the diffuse nature of neurotoxic effects.

The majority of neurotoxically exposed individuals score in the average to high-average ranges on one of the Weschler Adult Intelligence Scales. Verbal comprehension appears less affected than perceptual organization, working memory, and information processing speed. The greatest impairment is typically observed on measures of information processing speed which may reduce the Performance IQ score as many of the tests are timed. Verbal IQ scores are typically less affected than Performance IQ scores (acquired verbal knowledge and reasoning vs. nonverbal fluid reasoning).

Memory functioning, as measured by the Weschler Memory Scale-III is typically slightly below the population mean (50th percentile) for auditory and visual, immediate and delayed memory. Scores are also typically below average on measures of attention and concentration.

Scores of the Benton Visual Retention Test with known sensitivity for neurotoxic effect deviate to some degree from the expected scores for a patient's age and intellectual level, but generally fall within normal limits unless a patient is assessed shortly after exposure. This measure is included in the WHO core battery of tests with known sensitivity for neurotoxic effects.

The Clinical Analysis Questionnaire (CAQ), a 272-item, self-report questionnaire developed by Cattell et al.[67] had been utilized for many years. The CAQ, unlike the Minnesota Multiphasic Personality Inventory (MMPI), measures normal personality traits in addition to 12 clinical factors, which include 7 depression scales. The PsychEval Questionnaire, the current revision of the CAQ, is now being used. It is a factor-analytically derived measure of normal personality traits as well as clinically relevant traits, yielding normal personality scales and pathology-oriented scales. Each part of the test augments the information available from the other, in contrast to established clinical instrument such as the MMPI, primarily oriented to measuring psychopathological traits.[67]

A study examining the CAQ data of mold-exposed individuals indicated that the results were quite similar to a population of normal adults used for the standardization sample and no scores measuring the 16 normal personality traits differed significantly from the sample. Scores for the exposed individuals suggested a tendency toward greater detachment from others, decreased coping ability, greater conformity, conscientiousness, persistence, social awareness, and conservatism, as well as greater pessimism and caution. Scores for the exposed males compared with females indicated a somewhat higher degree of tension, frustration, and impatience, as well as greater restraint, caution, and social awareness, and diminished coping ability.

Scores of the clinical factors for both males and females indicated a significantly greater number of somatic complaints as would be expected, as well as depression associated with low energy and fatigue compared with the normative group. A trend was also observed toward a greater degree of confusion and diminished self-confidence and self-esteem. Both groups had a tendency toward greater difficulty formulating ideas into verbal expression, less of a tendency toward uninhibited behavior, and greater compassion for others. No significant differences were noted between scores of the present study and those of a prior study which examined the CAQ scores of patients exposed to a variety of neurotoxins and/or who were chemically/environmentally sensitive, and referred for neuropsychological assessment.

Neuropsychological assessment of individuals exposed to neurotoxic substances is complex, particularly when attempting to establish a cause–effect relationship between the observed neurocognitive deficits and the reported toxic exposure for litigation issues. There should be evidence of the exposure by test reports, material safety data sheets, medical examination, etc. Many potentially confounding variables must be considered. These include age, educational level, frequency, intensity and duration of exposure, prior neurotoxic exposures, head trauma, other neurological conditions, metabolic disorders (e.g., hypothyroidism) infections, past or current drug and alcohol use/abuse, medication effects, length of time from cessation of exposure to evaluation, and malingering/secondary gain. The majority of patients tested, probably >95%, have not shown insufficient effort on specific tests of effort and motivation or on embedded measures of poor effort. Correlation between neuropsychological test results and medical evidence, as well as consistency among scores of similar measures are also considered in addition to any transient condition which may have affected performance at the time of the evaluation, including anxiety, fatigue, chronic or acute pain, inadvertent exposures, and medication effects.

The majority of patients who have been evaluated in Didriksen's office have educational levels beyond high school, including advanced degrees. Many show impairment on several measures, including measures of higher cortical functions. However, even when test scores fall within normal limits, statistically, they may not represent preexposure levels of functioning for the individual. Evidence of prior levels of functioning may be obtained from academic transcripts, work reviews, promotion, leadership positions, and/or awards or special recognition, aiding in the interpretation of test results.

An unfortunate and relatively frequent consequence of neurotoxic exposure is an inability to maintain gainful employment. Many patients have attempted to continue working, despite illness and despite exposures to toxic substances in the workplace due to the obvious necessity of earning a living and maintaining benefits, including health insurance, retirement plans, etc., until they are no longer able to do so. Neuropsychological evaluation extends documentation of the disabled condition.

Many patients have positions which require higher cortical functions, including abstract reasoning, new learning, problem-solving, decision-making, etc. as well as adequate attention, concentration, and memory. Employment failure is often the result of impairment in many of these areas in addition to an inability to attend to detail, often resulting in frequent errors, as well as slowed information processing, resulting in an inability to maintain pace and persistence. Changes in personality and behavioral functioning such as increased anxiety, depression, and irritability and decreased coping ability may also contribute to employment failure.

The long-term sequelae of neurotoxic exposures are also important considerations. Some patients may not improve, despite treatment interventions, which may be due to a lack of compliance with the prescribed treatment program, for example, an inability to afford continuing treatment and an inability to avoid exposures, for example, unable to obtain safe living conditions. The neurocognitive condition of some patients may decline over time. An increased risk for neurodegenerative diseases, including Parkinson's disease (PD) and Alzheimer's disease is indicated in the literature.

Cognitive decline may be prevented or slowed to some degree by medical, cognitive (pollutant avoidance, nutrition, oxygen therapy, immune modulation), and behavioral interventions. Primary interventions which may improve cognitive functioning and prevent or slow decline in individuals exposed to neurotoxic substances include avoidance of neurotoxins, full participation in the prescribed treatment program, active learning in the form of reading, computer skills, formal/informal classes, etc., stress management and relaxation techniques, particularly meditation, greater social interaction, exercise, and online neurocognitive rehabilitation programs. Compensatory techniques for memory problems (lists, schedules, reminders, etc.), particularly when reacting to environmental incitants, should be utilized as well. Repeated neuropsychological evaluation will determine whether an individual's cognitive and personality/behavioral status has improved, regressed, or remained stable.

ENVIRONMENTAL EFFECTS OF ORGANIC POLLUTANTS

The relative reactivity of various classes of volatile organics varies (Table 5.13). As a group, orchos olefins (alkenes) (cycloolefins) are the most reactive hydrocarbons, followed by aromatic compounds with two or more alkyl groups. Aromatics with only one alkyl group are only slightly reactive in the environment. The least reactive hydrocarbons are C_1-C_5 (alkanes/paraffins) and acetylene. Regardless of the level of reactivity of these hydrocarbons, they contribute to outdoor and indoor pollution. Reactive hydrocarbons play an important role in the city environment, where a series of complex reactions between NO_2 and ambient oxygen, which produce ozone on sunny days, occurs. It should be emphasized that the degree of reactivity in the outdoor environment is aggravated by other chemicals in the air. This reactivity is not necessarily carried into an individual who has been contaminated by multiple chemicals. This observation is emphasized by the fact that we have seen many patients react to the exposure of propane and butane (relatively low environmental reactors) gas heat and cooking stoves just as severely as to other more reactive products in the environment. Chronic long-term exposure to natural gas is the number 1 offender along with pesticides in a home for the development of chemical sensitivity and chronic degenerative diseased with chronic fatigue. This reaction is often subtle at first, showing weakness, fatigue, and brain fog. Also, even though it is thought to be a low-level air reactant, benzene is known to trigger some forms of leukemia. Benzene is found in the breath analysis as well as the indoor and outdoor air analysis of chemically sensitive and chronic degenerative diseased patients in many forms. It adversely affects the chemically sensitive and chronic degenerative diseased patients and its removal causes them to function much more easily. The same principle applies to paraffins, which, when implanted in humans, can cause scleroderma-like syndromes and other connective tissue neurovascular reactions.

A large number of the volatile organics found in urban atmospheres and able to have a negative impact on human health are those defined as bacterial and viral mutagens and suspect carcinogens (e.g., vinyl chloride, acrylonitrile, 1,2-dichloroethane, and 1,2-dibromoethane).[68] Also, at concentrations much higher than those found in ambient air, many volatile organics are known to have toxic effects.[42] Synthetic halogenated hydrocarbons appear to be the most devastating to the chemically sensitive and chronic degenerative diseased. Most came into major use after 1950, and since then their production has increased with a doubling time of 6 years. Along with exposure to toxic chemicals in food, water, and the workplace environment, continuous exposure to "low levels" of volatile organics in ambient air may enhance the frequency of cancer occurring in the urban population. Increases in cancer have been seen in chemical dump areas of New Jersey[42] and also in high-herbicide areas in Iowa.[69] Also, these levels are clearly associated with chemical sensitivity and chronic degenerative disease. It has now been shown that petrochemicals are responsible for obesity and diabetes.

In 1961, Randolph[3] pointed out that the indoor environment is more highly contaminated by chemical pollutants than the outdoor environment. A wide variety of organic chemicals is found indoors (Chapter 2). An analysis by Molhave et al.[70] of new Danish homes in 1978 to the present showed higher levels of VOCs compared to outdoor ambient air. Later works by Wallace et al.,[71] Lebret et al.,[72] Jarke,[73] Seifert,[74] DeBartoli et al.,[75] and Mage and Gammage[76] in the United States, Italy, and Germany confirmed Randolph and Molhave's work. Measurements of the total amounts of VOCs in new homes have indicated levels as high as 19 mg/m³. A reduction of as much as 1000 times has been seen in homes over 3 years old, and even higher reduction in environmentally safe housing is common (Chapter 3). Pathways through which these chemicals enter the human body and go to the specific organs they affect are discussed in Chapter 2 and Volume II of this work, the clinical chapters.

Combining the aldehyde levels far exceeds what a control population can handle.

An example is seen in the indoor air analysis of a 55-year-old housewife from Antwerp, Belgium. Her home is in the center of the town where there is a lot of traffic. One can see that the prime product in the air is benzene which was caused by influx of traffic fumes in an old leaky home. She also had many aldehydes in her indoor air analysis, which was caused by her recent remodeling. This indoor air was part of the problems that was making her ill. She would go to a less polluted area of the earth and her sensitivities would go away. She had been ill for 15 years. Now, with a clean house and being in less polluted air, she lives a vigorous medication-free life.

Toxic Brain Syndrome

Many patients have toxic brain syndrome as shown in Tables 5.15 through 5.26. Of the patients who had toxic brain syndrome and evaluation by neuropsychological consultation, there were a total of 64 patients: female = 35, male = 29; age = 30–72 years, average age = 47.4 years.

Triple-camera SPECT scans were performed on 17 chemically sensitive patients. The rest had neuropsychological profiles. Seventeen of the brain scans were positive for toxicity as others had neuropsychological profiles.

Thermography was performed on 39 patients (Table 5.17). Head points were rigid in 39 of 39 patients. All patients could not stand on their toes or walk a straight line with their eyes open or closed. Therefore, accomplished posturography examination was performed (balance test—Table 5.19). Heart rate variability was also performed as another autonomic NS test. Table 5.20 shows the changes. $N = 52$. All patients had neuropsychological consultation. Twelve patients underwent inhaled challenges after depollution in a less polluted environment. Chemical inhalant challenge and intradermal chemical skin test provoking the patient's symptoms and signs. Testing was performed in a controlled less polluted environment and the patients were residing in a less polluted environment. $N = 46$.

Chemical Sensitivity: Sources of Total Body Pollutant Load

The sources of total body pollutant load include indoor, outdoor, air, food, and water pollutants.

TABLE 5.15
Associated Diagnosis

By Systems Were not Shown	No.	%
Headache, neurotoxicity, vertigo, memory loss, dizziness	33	51.6
M.S. (fibromyalgia, arthralgia, fatigue, back pain)	55	85.9
Respiratory (ARS, bronchospasm, chest tightness, SOB cough, reactive airway)	48	75.0
GI (IBS, vomiting, bloating, constipation, nausea)	21	32.8
CV (angioedema, chest pain, arrhythmia, hypertension, vasculitis)	16	25.0
Endocrine	4	6.3
Breast implant	1	1.6
Skin	1	1.6

Source: Environmental Health Center-Dallas.
Note: 55 Year Old White Female from Belgium—Fatigue, Fibromyalgia, Vasculitis.

TABLE 5.16
Associated Diagnosis

By Composed hx and Rx	No.	%
Inhalant sensitivity	41	64.1
Food sensitivity	36	56.3
EMF sensitivity	1	1.6

Source: Environmental Health Center-Dallas.

TABLE 5.17
Thirty-Nine Chemically Sensitive Patients—100%
Positive—Thermography EHC-Dallas in ECU
(Age: 22–80 Years, Male: 19, Female: 20)

Point	No.	%
RN (radis nasi)	1	2.6
FS1 (frontal sinus right)	8	20.5
FS2 (frontal sinus left)	14	35,9
T1 (temple right)	16	41.0
T2 (temple left)	15	38.5
CP1 (commissural palpebrarum medialis right)	14	35.9
CP2 (commissural palpebrasum medialis left)	17	43.6
M1 (mastoid right)	15	38.5
M2 (mastoid left)	13	33.3
OSE1 (os ethmoidale right)	9	23.1
OSE2 (os ethmoidale left)	7	17.9
MS1 (maxillary sinus right)	3	7.7
MS2 (maxillary sinus left)	3	7.7

Source: Environmental Health Center-Dallas.

TABLE 5.18
(Pupillography $N = 57$)—Chemically Sensitive
Patients—EHC-Dallas in Less Polluted ECU
(Age: 22–80 Years, Male: 28, Female: 29)

Pupillography $N = 57$	No.	%
Cholinergic	2	3.5
Sympatholytic	2	3.5
Cholinergic and sympatholytic	2	3.5
Abnormal		
Cholinolytic	9	15.8
Sympathomimetic	12	21.1
Cholinologic and sympathomimetic	1	1.8
Nonspecific change	25	43.9
Normal	4	7.0

Source: Environmental Health Center-Dallas.

Aldehydes, ketones, and alcohols are derived from solvents and are major sources of free radical species in photochemical smog, usually from car and truck exhaust, factory emissions, insecticide spraying, electromagnetics, etc. Both formaldehyde and acetaldehyde are highly reactive and will readily absorb sunlight to dissociate into free radicals. Excess aldehyde, ketone, and alcohol intake can overload the oxidative metabolic breakdown systems in the body, causing metabolic dysfunction with secondary food and chemical sensitivity. Combinations of the chemical are particularly involved in triggering chemical sensitivity and chronic degenerative disease. One of many can trigger the disease, while single or combinations can propagate the problem. (For further discussion of

TABLE 5.19

Posturography—EHC-Dallas on Chemically Sensitive Patients in Less Polluted ECU (Age: 22–80 Years, Male: 14, Female: 15)

$N = 29$	No.	%
Normal	4	13.8
Abnormal	25	86.2
Sensory Organization Test	23	92
Motor Organization Test	17	68

Source: Environmental Health Center-Dallas.

TABLE 5.20

Abnormal = 52, 100% Abnormal—Heart Rate Variability EHC-Dallas on Chemically Sensitive Patients in Less Polluted ECU (Age: 22–80 Years, Male: 26 Female: 26)

	No.	%
Parasympathetic system decreased and sympathetic increased	31	59.6
Parasympathetic system decreased and sympathetic even	9	17.3
Influence of sympathetic system	7	13.5
Parasympathetic increased and sympathetic increased	1	1.9
Parasympathetic decreased and sympathetic decreased	1	1.9
Autonomic balance on average	2	3.8

Source: Environmental Health Center-Dallas.

TABLE 5.21

$N = 64$—EHC-Dallas—Chemically Sensitive in Less Polluted ECU (Age: 22–80 Years, Male: 32, Female: 32)

	Diagnosis	No.	%
ICD-9	Toxic encephotopathy	43	67.1
	Psychological factors associated with physical condition classified elsewhere	38	59.3
DSM-IV	Axis I cognitive disorder not otherwise specified	23	34.3
	Dysthymic disorder	2	0.28
		19	29.6
	Axis II no diagnosis	22	32.8
	Axis III Chemical/environmental sensitivity	22	32.8
	Axis IV Illness, disability	22	32.8
	Axis V 35–40	1	0.15
	GAF 40	1	0.15
	40–50	1	0.15
	45	1	0.15
	45–50	6	0.93
	50	6	0.93
	55–60	1	0.15

Source: Environmental Health Center-Dallas.

TABLE 5.22
Reproducing the Chemical-Sensitive Patient's Symptoms,
$N = 12$ **(Double Blind with Saline Placebos—EHC-Dallas in the**
Less Polluted ECU; Age: 22–80 Years, Male: 6, Female: 6)

Chemical	Positive No.	Positive %	Negative No.	Negative %
Ethanol	7	87.5	1	12.5
Formaldehyde	5	62.5	3	37.5
Toluene	5	100	0	0
Xylene	2	100	0	0
Hexane	1	100	0	0
Benzene	1	100	0	0
Chlorine	0	0	2	100
Phenol	3	75.0	1	25.0
Placebo	2	15.4	11	84.6

Source: Environmental Health Center-Dallas.

TABLE 5.23
Toxic Chemical in Blood Analysis, $N = 35$—**Chemically Sensitive**
Patients—EHC-Dallas (Age: 22–80 Years, Male: 17, Female: 18)

Chemical	No.	%
2-Methylpentane	3	8.6
3-Methylpentane	23	65.7
n-Hexane	15	42.9
n-Heptane	2	5.7
Toluene	1	2.9
Chloroform	2	5.7
Dichloromethane	1	2.9
Dichlorobenzene	2	5.7
HCB	3	8.6
Heptachlor	1	2.9
Endosulfan II	1	2.9
DDE	6	17.1
DDT	2	5.7
Creatinine	6	17.1
Diethylphosphate	3	8.6
Diethyl phosphorothioate	1	2.9
Dimethyl phosphorothioate	1	2.9
Hippuric acid	1	2.9
Phenol urine	1	2.9

Source: Environmental Health Center-Dallas.

TABLE 5.24
Intradermal Challenge of the Biological Inhalant Skin Test for Chemically Sensitive Patients in Less Polluted ECU at EHC-Dallas (Age: 22–80 Years, Male: 21, Female: 21)

Components making up part of the total body pollutant load $N = 42$

Pollutant	No.	%
Mold	37	88.1
Algae	25	59.5
Dust	23	54.8
Mite	23	54.8
Danders	11	26.2
Terpenes	15	35.7
Smuts	11	26.2
Cotton	8	19.0
TOE	15	35.7
Candida	18	42.9
Trees	25	59.5
Grass	24	57.1
Weeds	23	54.8

Source: Environmental Health Center-Dallas.

TABLE 5.25
Intradermal Provocation Test in the Less Polluted ECU at EHC-Dallas (Age: 22–80 Years, Male: 23, Female: 23)

Pollutant	No.	%
Natural gas—methane	11	23.9
Propane gas	11	23.9
Cigarette smoke	28	60.9
Chlorine—SL	17	37.0
Ethanol	21	45.7
Formaldehyde	31	67.4
Ladies cologne	13	28.3
Men's cologne	15	32.6
Orris root	25	54.3
News material	9	19.6
Phenol	11	23.9
Unl/Diesel	14	30.4
Fireplace smoke	5	10.9
Jet fuel	2	4.3
Xylene	2	4.3
Toluene	4	8.7
Hexane	2	4.3
Benzene	1	2.2

Source: Environmental Health Center-Dallas.

TABLE 5.26
Intradermal Metals Test under a Less Polluted Controlled
Environments at EHC-Dallas (N = 16, Age: 22–80 Years, Male: 8,
Female: 8)

Metal	No.	%
Aluminum	5	31.3
Copper	2	12.5
Gold	3	18.8
Lead	4	25.0
Nickel sulfate	13	81.3
Silver	5	31.3
Tin	4	25.0
Titanium	3	18.8
Zinc sulfate	13	81.3
Stainless steel	1	6.3
Porcelain	1	6.3

Source: Environmental Health Center-Dallas Intradermal Food Test in 36 patients showed
positive range: 1–35 kinds of foods; mean = 10 kinds of foods.

sources and metabolism of aldehydes, ketones, and alcohol, see Chapter 2.) In addition to entering the body, many of these substances are made in the course of normal metabolism of foods, as well as being breakdown products in the metabolism of foreign chemicals that have entered the body. It appears that the chemically sensitive individual who is already overloaded reacts when additionally exposed to these substances.

A 53-year-old white female developed severe anxiety and fatigue, immune deregulation, and vasculitis, and before she came to the EHC-Dallas, she was incapacitated for 1 year. The air analysis in her house showed high levels of formaldehyde and other aldehydes. When the sources were removed, she recovered her health (Table 5.27).

If ingested, abdominal pain, nausea, vomiting, and chemical pneumonias can occur. With change in her environment and eliminating most of the aldehyde sources, her symptoms and signs were relieved and she became well. Intradermal and inhaled provocation reproduced all her symptoms, leading to the fact that her total body formaldehyde load was in excess and also apparently caused her illness.

Another case involved a 6-year-old (Table 5.28) Indian boy. He was born in Canada and had difficulty with learning and behavior. As one can see, the indoor air analysis was full of aldehydes. A number 5 dilution (3000) intradermal injection provocation with formaldehyde reproduced all his symptoms acutely. After some time, using less polluted water and diet, he also moved out of this house. He has performed extremely well and has become a superior student (Table 5.29).

Nonchlorinated Aliphatic Hydrocarbons (Paraffins)

Nonchlorinated aliphatic hydrocarbons include alkanes (C–C), cycloalkanes, alkenes (C=C), cycloalkenes, and alkynes (C≡C). The straight-chain (four of them) and branch-chain aliphatics are discussed.

Alkanes (C–C)

Alkanes with up to four carbons (methane, ethane, propane, and butane) are gases and are present in natural gas. Methane and ethane are simple asphyxiants and in the past have not usually been

TABLE 5.27

Volatile Organic Compounds and Aldehydes: Indoor Air—53-Year-Old White Female

VOCs and Aldehydes	Test Results (µg/m³)	Reference Levels (µg/m³)	Comparison to Reference Levels (%)
Formaldehyde	24	20	100+
Acetic acid	14	25	56.0
Furfuraldehyde	2	8	25.0
Butyraldehyde	14	74	18.9
Naphthalene	4	50	8.0
Acetaldehyde	3	45	6.7
Hexaldehyde*	3	80	3.8
Limonene	3	110	3.7
Methyl ethyl ketone	14	590	2.4
o-, m-, and p-Xylenes	3	180	1.7
Isopropyl alcohol	8	492	1.6
3-Methylpentane	5	350	1.4
Cyclohexane	2	140	1.4
Isopentane	3	350	0.9
1,2,4-Trimethylbenzene	1	125	0.8
1,2,4,5-Tetramethylbenzene	1	125	0.8
Styrene	1	140	0.7
Methylpentane	2	350	0.6
α-Pinene	2	350	0.6
n-Pentane	2	350	0.6
n-Hexane	1	200	0.5
Acetone	2	590	0.3
Toluene	4	1200	0.3
Tridecane	1	350	0.3
Decane	1	1000	0.1
2,4-Dimethylpentane	2	n/l	
Total other VOCs as toluene	57		
Total VOCs and aldehydes	157	<200	

Source: Matrix Laboratory and Environmental Health Center-Dallas, Texas.

thought to produce nonlocalized effects. However, there is a suggestion that chemically sensitive patients react to them specifically (brain dysfunction, fatigue, weakness) but certainly the daughter products like methanol and ethanol also cause problems. Many chemically sensitive patients react to marsh gas and to the fumes of natural gas. Whether this reaction is due to methane or other components is not 100% certain. Intradermal skin tests and inhaled challenge produce signs of the offender in the home that causes reaction and upon scientific inhalation studies at the EHC-Dallas. Clearly, we have seen many people in the thousands who have become ill by methane, ethane, propane, and butane fumes in homes heated by these substances. We have seen few moderately severe chemically sensitive patients who improved while remaining in a natural gas home environment. Natural gas is the number 1 offender for pollutant injury along with pesticides in the home. For health reason, they need to be removed.

The higher-molecular-weight alkanes are liquids, and their vapors produce CNS effects that may result in depression, dizziness, and loss of coordination. Nonspeech central neuropathy, PD, and Alzheimer's disease can be the ultimate result.

TABLE 5.28

Volatile Organic Compounds (VOCs) and Aldehydes: 6-Year-Old Male

VOCs and Aldehydes	Test Results ($\mu g/m^3$)	Reference Levels TCEQ—Long-Term ESL ($\mu g/m^3$)
Formaldehyde	31.0	3.3
Butyraldehyde	4.0	1.4
Propionaldehyde	4.0	2
α-Pinene	7.1	6
p-Dichlorobenzene	1.6	2
Isoamyl alcohol	1.1	1.4
Benzaldehyde	1.0	2.2
Acetaldehyde	60.0	9
Hexaldehyde	3.0	8
Hexanedioic acid	0.9	6
4-Isopropyl toluene	1.1	8
β-Pinene	0.8	6
Valeraldehyde	1.0	10
o-, m-, and p-Xylenes	6.0	208
Tetradecane acid	0.9	350
Isopentane	4.6	5
Acetic acid	19.6	25
Ethyl alcohol	28.4	100
Naphthalene	1.9	44
Mycrene	15.0	350
Acetone	5.7	590
Isopropyl alcohol	6.2	785
d-Limonene	0.6	100
β-Phellandrene	2.0	485
Dodecane	1.1	350
Toluene	2.8	1200
n-Pentane	2.7	1900
n-Butane	1.5	1880
Glycol Ether EB	1.3	1880
2-Methylpentane	0.7	1050
Nonane	0.6	1050
Linalool	14.3	nl
Toluene	2.8	1200
n-Pentane	2.7	1900
n-Butane	1.5	1880
2-Methylpentane	0.7	1050
Nonane	0.6	1050
Linalool	14.3	nl
Total volatile organic compounds	142.0	200

Source: Matrix Laboratory and Environmental Health Center-Dallas, Texas, 2005.

Note: A 6-year-old Indian boy's home air analysis. High levels of aldehydes triggered his problems of difficulty in learning and abnormal behavior, and when eliminated, he got well. nl, normal limits.

TABLE 5.29
Volatile Organic Compounds: 6-Year-Old Boy

Sampling Method: Thermal Desorption Tube

Analytical Method: GC/MS

	Test Results		
Compound	**μg/m³**	**ppbv**	**Typical Sources**
n-Butane	1.5	0.6	Gasoline, natural gas, and aerosol products
Isopentane	4.6	1.6	
Ethyl alcohol	28.4	15.1	Cleaners, personal care products, and beverages
Isopropyl alcohol	6.2	2.5	Personal care products and cleaners, adhesives, solvents, nail polish removers
Acetone	5.7	2.4	Personal care products and cleaners, adhesives, solvents, nail polish removers and human emissions
Acetic acid	19.6	8.0	Food products, silicone caulks and sealants and glass cleaners
Glycol ether EB	1.3	0.3	Cleaners and degreasers
α-Pinene	7.1	1.3	Cleaners, disinfectants, fragrances, perfumes, and wood products
β-Pinene	0.8	0.1	
Linalool	14.3	2.3	
β-Phellandrene	2.0	0.4	
Myrcene	15.0	2.7	
d-Limonene	0.6	0.1	
Naphthalene	1.9	0.4	Diesel fuels and gasoline
n-Pentane	2.7	0.9	Gasoline and solvents
2-Methyl pentane	0.7	0.2	
Nonane	0.6	0.5	
Dodecane	1.1	0.2	
Toluene	2.8	0.7	
o-, m- and p-Xylenes	6.0	1.4	
Isoamyl alcohol	1.1	0.3	Medicinals, solvents, and flavorings
p-Dichlorobenzene	1.6	0.3	Moth repellant
Tetradecane acid	0.9	0.1	
4-Isopropyl toluene	1.1	0.2	
Hexanedioic acid	0.9	0.2	
Total other VOCs as toluene[a]	13.5	42.3	
Total	14.2	45.9	

Source: Matrix Laboratory and EHC-Dallas, Texas.

[a] Primarily gasoline range hydrocarbons.

Extremely high levels of C_5-C_8 hydrocarbon vapor (pentane, hexane, heptane, octane) levels, usually derived from gasoline products, result in the death of experimental animals and disrupt human functions. At lower levels, alkanes trigger a myriad of symptoms in the chemically sensitive, and they are often found in their blood and breath. Hexane and 2- and 3-methylpentane are found in the intravenous (IV) solutions from plastic bags but not from glass bottles.

2,2-Dimethylbutane (2,2-bimethylbutane) is a common environmental pollutant because of its presence in gasoline (0.68%). It threatens the health of the chemically sensitive and chronic degenerative diseased who tend to react negatively to it upon exposure.

n-Pentane

n-Pentane (Table 5.30) is the most important isomer of pentane and is found in volatile petroleum fractions (gasoline contains up to 13.05% *n*-pentane, some of which is used as a solvent for fuel and chemical synthesis). The pure compound is employed in the manufacturing of ice and low-temperature thermometers and as a blowing agent for plastics in solvent extraction processes.[77] Pentane is used as a blowing (foaming) agent in fracking operations. Some *n*-pentane is generated in the body by the action of free radicals (produced by other toxic chemicals) on lipids, especially in lipid membranes. Wispe et al.[78] reported that peroxidation of the unsaturated fatty acid constituents of tissue is one proposed mechanism of *in vivo* oxidant damage. In addition to pentane, the volatile hydrocarbon ethane is a product of unsaturated fatty acid peroxidation. These two hydrocarbons are eliminated in expired air and may be used as measurements to reflect *in vivo* lipid peroxidations.[78] One sees both in breath analysis of some chemically sensitive patients (Table 5.31).

The chief effects of inhalation of the *n*-pentane vapor are narcosis and irritation of the respiratory passages.[79,80] We have seen this narcosis in several patients who will go to sleep after eating or other exposure. This response is often accompanied by bloating and other vagus nerve symptoms. Following exposure to *n*-pentane vapor, many of our chemically sensitive patients reported sleepiness and brain fog, eye, ear, nose, throat, and skin irritation, and cough. This reaction could reflect the effects of this chemical either alone or in combination with others already in their system or inhaled mixtures of toxic chemicals.

Sore throat, headache, shortness of breath, dizziness, loss of coordination, and arrhythmia occur due to the breakdown products of gasoline (Table 5.30). These have been found in the blood and breath of some chemically sensitive patients, who may have inhaled and absorbed these substances by filling their gas tanks or perhaps by being in traffic.

If patients are living near commercial or military airports, they will breathe hydrocarbons that contaminate their air when raw fuel is dumped for safety before landings or perhaps when they are exposed directly to jet exhausts. We have seen several patients who had chemical sensitivity and were chronically exposed to jet fuel. One patient, a 43-year-old white female, was totally incapacitated for a period of time when her blood levels showed extremely high levels of the products of jet fuel. Intradermal jet fuel provocation under environmentally controlled conditions resulted in a reproduction of her systems and signs. Her extreme weakness and fatigue disappeared as her blood levels of these substances decreased.

TABLE 5.30

Analysis of the 0–145°F Gasoline Distillation[a]

Compound	Weight % in Gasoline[a]	% of Chemically Sensitive Patients with These Substances in Their Blood[b]
n-Pentane	13.05	40.3
2,2-Dimethylbutane	0.68	9.7
Cyclopentane	0.94	22.2
2-Methylpentane	9.19	68.1
3-Methylpentane	4.27	62.5
n-Hexane	1.5	61.1
n-Heptane	0.01	18.1
Ethanol	10.0	70.0
Total	29.64	

Source: Environmental Health Center-Dallas, 2012.

TABLE 5.31

Symptoms and Signs of Sensitivity to Pentane Exposure

1. Mild sleepiness due to narcosis
2. Respiratory irritation—shortness of breath
3. Brain fog
4. Eye, ear, nose, and throat irritation, cough
5. Headache
6. Dizziness
7. Loss of coordination
8. Arrhythmia

Source: Environmental Health Center-Dallas.

2-Methylpentane: Gasoline contains up to 9.19% 2-methylpentane. 2-Methylpentane has been found in the blood of a subset (68%) of the chemically sensitive individuals. Table 5.32 shows that its decrease in the blood parallels improvement in these patients.

3-Methylpentane: Gasoline contains 4.27% of 3-methylpentane. This substance is found in a large subset (62.5%) of chemically sensitive patients who may have inhaled it from ambient air or absorbed it from direct contact with gas fumes at the pump or in traffic (Table 5.30). Improvement in the chemically sensitive patient contaminated with 3-methylpentane parallels a decrease of this chemical in their blood.

Perbellini et al.[81] reported tissue/air partition coefficients for nine aliphatic hydrocarbons: *n*-pentane, 2,2-dimethylbutane, 2-methylpentane, 3-methylpentane, methylcyclopentane, *n*-hexane, cyclohexane, 2-methylhexane, and *n*-heptane. Their mean solubility in different tissues was higher than the solubility in the blood by the following factors: lung 1.4, heart 3.9, liver 5.6, kidney 5.2, brain 6.5, muscle 7.6, and fat 205 (Table 5.32). Because of the tissue differences, a much higher end-organ load that produces an increased total body burden occurs. This increased load, in turn, will exacerbate the chemically sensitive for longer periods of time, resulting in chronic illness until the toxic compounds are cleared.

Forty percent of pentane is excreted from the lungs. Most of these as well as other chemicals will have some removal via this route. If the lungs are damaged or functioning ineffectively, clearing is

TABLE 5.32

Main Tissue/Air Partition Coefficient (from Blood to Other Organs): *n*-Pentane; 2,2-Dimethyl Butane; 2-Methylpentane; 3-Methylpentane; Methyl Cyclopentane; *n*-Hexane; 2-Methylhexane; and *n*-Heptane

Organ	Coefficient
Lung	1.4
Heart	3.9
Liver	5.6
Kidney	5.2
Brain	6.5
Muscle	7.6
Fat	205.0

Source: Perbellini. L. et al. 1985. Partition coefficients of some industrial aliphatic hydrocarbons (C5-C7) in blood and human tissues. *Br. J. Ind. Med.* 42:162–167.

impeded, resulting in increased chemical sensitivity. This route of excretion through the lungs supports our observation of adverse reactions between patients who are close together in heat depuration and environmental control units and who are made ill from each other's outgasing.

n-Hexane

n-Hexane is widely used as a solvent in numerous industries. Technical grades contain about 40% *n*-hexane, together with various amounts of isomers and related compounds such as 2-methylpentane, 3-methylpentane, 2,2-dimethylbutane, 2,3-dimethylbutane, and cyclohexane. These are used in solvents and in quick-drying rubber cements and inks. Hexane is found in intravenous plastic saline bags as compared to none in glass bottles. Hexane and 2-hexane (methyl butyl ketone) are produced during the refining and distillation of crude oil. These are used in glues, paints, and varnishes and as a dilutant in the production of plastics and rubber. Hexane is also used for extracting oil from seeds.[82,83] Thus, it may be found in cooking oils available in the commercial market. Also, gasoline contains up to 1.5% hexane.[84] Exposure to hexane via these products or other similarly tainted may explain the chemically sensitive patient's intolerance to it.

An estimated 2.5 million workers are exposed to *n*-hexane.[85–87] 2-Hexanone, a derivative, is used as a paint thinner, in cleaning agents, as a solvent for dye printing, and in the lacquer industry. Acute exposure to *n*-hexane causes CNS depression. Chronic exposure to an average air concentration of 450–650 ppm for as little as 2 months may result in peripheral neuropathy. This neuropathy is characterized by muscular weakness, loss of sensation, and impaired gait.[88,89] We do not know the consequences of lower-level exposures, but many of our chemically sensitive patients with hexane in their blood or breath do show signs of early neuropathy, which can be accentuated by inhaled challenge.

The first cases of *n*-hexane polyneuropathy were reported in 1964 in workers who were involved in laminating polyethylene products. In 1969, a major outbreak of disease was reported in a cottage industry in Japan that involved the use of glue containing *n*-hexane to assemble sandals.[87,90,91] The neuropathy is sensory motor, with numbness and paraesthesia.[87,88,92] If the injury goes untreated long enough, axonal swelling on the proximal side of the node of Ranvier, demyelination, and nerve fiber degeneration, resembling "dying back" neuropathy result. Such syndromes have been seen in the chemically sensitive at the EHC-Dallas.

Hexane, like other aliphatics, is usually oxidized and excreted in the urine.[93] Disruption of this process can cause or exacerbate chemical sensitivity.

A 48-year-old white female developed chronic fatigue, fibromyalgia for several years. She became incapacitated and was found to have hexane compounds as well as 1,2-butadiene, acetone, and ethylene in her breath analysis. Intradermal provocation under environmentally controlled conditions studies of dilute hexane (1–5, 1–25, 1–625) reproduced her sensitivities. These toxics were apparently causing her symptoms because when they were eliminated, she became well and vigorous.

n-Heptane

n-Heptane is a standard for octane-rating measurements. Triptane, one of nine isomers of heptane, is used in aviation fuel. All isomers are employed in organic synthesis and are ingredients of gasoline and rubber solvent naphtha and other petroleum solvents that are used as fuels and solvents.[94] Gasoline contains up to 0.01% *n*-heptane.[84]

The signs and symptoms of CNS involvement in *n*-heptane occurred in the absence of noticeable mucous membrane irritation and were first observed by the patient upon entering a contaminated atmosphere. Brief exposures (4 minutes) to high levels (5000 ppm) produced complaints of nausea, loss of appetite, and a gasoline taste that persisted for several hours. Fatal concentrations were 16,000 ppm.[95]

Patty and Yant[80] reported that *n*-heptane at 1000 ppm caused slight dizziness after a 6-minute exposure. Higher concentrations for shorter periods resulted in marked vertigo, incardination, and hilarity.

n-Octane

Octane is a hydrocarbon and alkane with the chemical formula of C_8H_{18}. Octane has many structural isomers that differ in the amount and location of branching in the carbon chain. One of the standard isomers is 2,2,4-trimethylpentane, which is isooctane used as one of the standard values in the octane rating scale. Octane is very flammable. Isooctane is used to reduce engine knock.

Cycloalkanes (Cyclopentane)

Cyclopentane is used chiefly as a reagent in the laboratory. It is found in petroleum ether and other commercial solvents that are used as a fuel in fat and wax extraction, in paints, and in the shoe industry.[94] It is a CNS depressant.[96] Symptoms of acute exposure to high concentrations are excitement, loss of equilibrium, stupor, coma, and, rarely, respiratory failure. Studies at the EHC-Dallas, which revealed cyclopentane in the blood of 22% of chemically sensitive patients (Tables 5.33 and 5.34), suggest that symptoms due to long-term, low-level exposures are similar to those due to acute exposures (Chapter 3).

Alkenes (=C, Olefins)

Alkenes include ethylene, propylene, butene, etc. Alkenes such as the dienes and trienes are hydrocarbons containing two or more double bonds. These include (1,2), (1,3), or 2-methyl-1,3-butadiene and 1,3,5-hexatriene.

Ethylene (oxirane, methyl): Ethylene is one of the most common substances in breath analysis. Ethylene can be formed directly from crude oil (Figure 5.1). Ethylene oxide is used as a sterilizing solution for a number of types of medical equipment. Numerous adverse effects, including death, resulting from ethylene oxide exposure have been reported in the literature.[97,98] One episode of contamination with resultant fatalities occurred during the sterilization of the heart lung machines used for babies. Ethylene gas is used to ripen bananas and other fruits artificially. Many chemically sensitive cannot tolerate fruit ripened artificially but have no problem with naturally ripened fruit. Ethylene at times has been used as a fungicide. Ethylene is also used as a dispersant in coating composition for silicone crucibles and also as a blending fuel for enhancement of cold start performance of gasoline and ethanol.

TABLE 5.33
Common Exposure Sources of Volatile Organic Chemicals[a]

Volatile Organic (GVST™)	Fuel and Exhaust	Paint Thinners and Building Products	Plastic	Product of Disinfection of Drinking Water
Chloroform				X
Dichloromethane				X
Trichloroethane		X		X
Trichloroethylene	X	X		
Tetrachloroethylene				X
Dichlorobenzenes[b]				X
Xylene	X	X		
Benzene	X	X		
Toluene	X	X		
Ethylbenzene	X	X		
Trimethylbenzene	X	X		
Styrene			X	

[a] Any or all of these are common groundwater and atmospheric contaminants in association with industrial activity and chemical waste sites.

[b] The para-isomer of dichlorobenzene is used in mothballs and similar insecticide preparations.

TABLE 5.34

Common Exposure Sources of Volatile Organic Chemicals[a]

Volatile Organic (GVST™)	Soil, Grain Building Fumigant	Industrial Degreaser and Solvent	Refrigerant Impurity	Laundry and Dry Cleaning
Chloroform	X	X	X	
Dichloromethane	X	X	X	
Trichloroethane	X	X		
Trichloroethylene		X		X
Tetrachloroethylene	X	X		
Dichlorobenzenes[b]	X			
Xylene		X		
Benzene		X		
Toluene		X		
Ethylbenzene		X		
Trimethylbenzene				
Styrene				

[a] Any or all of these are common groundwater and atmospheric contaminants in association with industrial activity and chemical waste sites.

[b] The para-isomer of dichlorobenzene is used in mothballs and similar insecticide preparations.

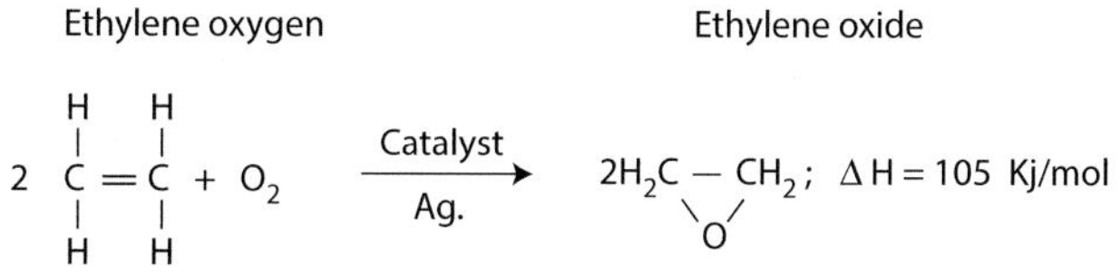

FIGURE 5.1 Process by which ethylene is formed. Ethylene is oxidized directly to ethylene oxide over a silver catalyst by means of oxygen. (Rea, W.J. 1994. *Chemical Sensitivity, Volume II*, page 779, figure 2. With permission.)

Polyethylene is the most important large-tonnage plastic, taking precedence over polyvinyl chloride (PVC), which is second, and polystyrene, which is third. In 1979, the production of polyethylene amounted to 5628 million tons in the United States and to 4 million tons in Japan and Europe. In 2014, it amounted to 108.1 billion tons in the United States. Ethylene is obtained from oil products by dehydrogenation by thermal cracking.

Polyethylene occurs when energy (heat or light) acts upon an ethylene molecule (2NC=C)
to yield an ethylene radical (2N + C−C−). Threadlike molecules are formed (C−C−C−C−C−C),
yielding polyethylene materials. Synthetic fiber materials of this type include PVC, polypropylene, polyacrylnitrile, etc. All of this poses problems for the chemically sensitive.

Polyester is usually polyethylene glyco tetraphthalate. It is made from *p*-xylene and nitric acid. The macromolecule of the polyester formed from tetraphthalic acid and glycol is linked between the two. Approximately 100–150 units are linked together in a polymer. After solidification, the polycondensate is converted to polyester chips, becoming the raw material for polyester fibers.[99] The chemically sensitive cannot tolerate materials made of these. Ethylene (oxirane) can also be used as a fumigate and can cause severe reactions in the chemically sensitive and also trigger vasculitis, immune deregulation, chronic fatigue, itching, and severe pain. The case report of A.F. is an example where he had a high propensity of ethylene in addition to 1,3-pentadienes. Some of the functions of ethylene (oxirane, methyl) include fungicide, coatings of integrated circuitry and silicon crucibles, and a blending fuel often enhances the cold-start performance of gasoline and ethanol. Both ethylene and 1,3-pentadiene are often found in the breath analysis of the chemically sensitive.

Cycloalkenes

Cyclical olefins are cyclohexene and cyclohexadene. These are some of the chemical sources for a wide range of synthetics that may adversely affect the chemically sensitive. 1,3-Butadiene and 1,2-butadiene-3-methyl are some of the most common chemicals along with 1,3-pentadiene, found in the human breath. It can come from the body as well as external sources. When originally from the body, it supplies isoprene units which act as a reflection of cholesterol function for normal body function. When coming from external sources, it can be quite toxic to the body.

Alkynes (C≡C)

Alkynes are unsaturated hydrocarbons containing triple bonds. These include ethyne (acetylene), propyne (methylacetylene), and 1-butyne (ethylacetylene).

In contrast to the saturated hydrocarbons, the unsaturated hydrocarbons constitute only a small part of natural gas and petroleum. The large quantities that are required for some industries are obtained by the chemical modification of the raw materials in oil refineries. Unsaturated hydrocarbons are reactive compounds. Due to marked tendency to react, they constitute readily convertible raw materials for many kinds of synthesis carried out industrially on a large scale. The C·C and C^C bonds are reactive sites that undergo important reactions, especially additions, including polymerization. Molecules that add on readily include hydrogen, halogens, hydrogen halides, water, and oxygen. Polymerization is a special kind of addition. Unsaturated molecules are not only able to add on molecules of a different kind but can also add on to one another. An example is polyethylene (previously shown).

Each of the aforementioned group of solvents and natural gas products can trigger the NMDA receptor, TRPV1, TRPA1, TRPM, and other sensory nerves and receptors. These cycles can be quite devastating to the chemically sensitive and chronic degenerative diseased patient causing a vicious cycle of illness.

CHLORINATED ALIPHATIC HYDROCARBONS

Chlorinated aliphatic hydrocarbons are generally more toxic than nonchlorinated aliphatic hydrocarbons. Halomethanes are commonly the result of chlorination of drinking water and are some of the most toxic substances known to humans. They can trigger symptoms in chemically sensitive individuals. Due to the special adverse effects of halogenated compounds, these compounds will be discussed individually.

Carbon Tetrachloride (CCl₄)

Carbon tetrachloride is used in the manufacturing of fluorocarbon propellants. It is used as a solvent for oils, fats, lacquers, varnishes, rubber, waxes, and resins. It is also used as a degreasing and cleaning agent and as a fumigant.[100] It is found in worm killers, fire extinguishers, shampoos, and bathroom cleaners.[101,102] CCl_4 is a toxic substance that can enter the body by several routes, including the skin, lungs, and gastrointestinal tract. It is highly toxic to the liver and kidney.[103] Large acute exposures result in liver necrosis. Exposures can result in mucous membrane irritation, CNS depression, and changes in blood cells and metabolism.[103] Both acute and chronic exposures can be hazardous to health,[104] resulting in the frequently noted symptoms of upset stomach, nausea, vomiting, drowsiness, headache, and dizziness.[101] Alcohol potentiates the CCl_4 intoxication.[105–107] While fatalities have occurred following accidental or medicinal ingestion of CCl_4, most deaths have resulted from inhalation of its vapors. Elkins[101] reported a serious illness following "a few days exposure" to CCl_4 levels of 130 ppm. Other reports detail illness occurring upon chronic exposure to concentrations of CCl_4 between 25 and 100 ppm.[108–112] Liver damage was seen in laboratory animals following daily exposures of 10 ppm, and questionable damage was observed in the guinea pig at 5 ppm.[71]

Chloroform (CHCl₃)

Chloroform is used in the preparation of pharmaceuticals, artificial silks, insecticides, floor polishes, lacquers, and cleaning solvents. It is a known general anesthetic, although its use in surgery has ceased since many complications of chloroform have been recognized. Though it is a common by-product of water chlorination, average air in New Jersey homes was found to contain 10 mg/m.[113] Chloroform compounds affect the CNS and liver; acute exposure to higher levels will cause acute liver necrosis and/or death by CNS suppression, while long-term, low-level exposure chronically assaults the liver. Halocarbon fumigants affect cardiac irritability, giving arrhythmias. Liver damage without increased SGOT, LDH, SGPT, etc. may occur. Thirty-seven percent of 500 chemically sensitive patients surveyed at the EHC-Dallas had chloroform in their blood. The presence of chloroform in these patients appeared to account for several symptoms, including mental cloudiness. They were apparently partially anesthetized.

Trichloroethylene (Cl₂C=CHCl)

Trichloroethylene (TCE) is found in paint thinners, drinking water disinfectants, industrial detergents and solvents, anesthetics, and dry cleaning fluids. TCE influences the metabolism of riboflavin. Thiamine deficiency enhances this pollutant's toxicity, and this pollutant enhances thiamine deficiency. Of 500 chemically sensitive patients seen at the EHC-Dallas, 8.6% had TCE in their blood. Some patients actually had their symptoms reproduced by "low-level" inhaled challenge of this substance (Figure 5.2) as was the case with a 36-year-old white female who was a secretary in a building adjacent to a plant that made TCE. She developed spontaneous bruising and fatigue that became so severe that she was unable to work. After some time in the ECU, these symptoms cleared. They were then reproduced by inhaled challenge.

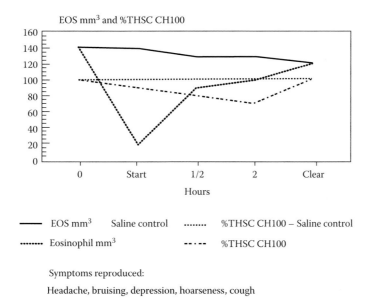

FIGURE 5.2 36-year-old white female. Double-blind challenge of trichlor-ethylene (15-sec exposure) in the ECU after 4 days deadaptation with total load decreased. (Rea, W.J. 1994. *Chemical Sensitivity, Volume II*, page 782, figure 3. With permission.)

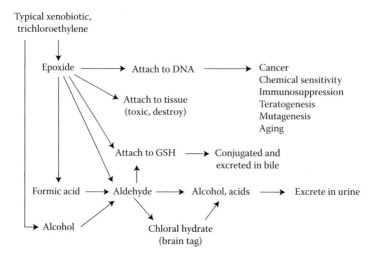

FIGURE 5.3 Degradation of trichlorethylene causing toxic intermediates that harm the chemically sensitive. (*Source*: Rogers, S. 1988. Personal communication.) (Rea, W.J. 1994. *Chemical Sensitivity, Volume II*, page 782, figure 4. With permission.)

Some of the degradation pathways for TCE are presented in Figure 5.3. TCE overload can result in a range of effects, from chemical sensitivity to malignancy. CNS suppression is also a problem in these patients with TCE in their blood. They also appear to be anesthetized.

Solvent Exposures and PD Risk in Twins

Several case reports have linked solvent exposure to PD, but few studies have assessed associations with specific agents using an analytic epidemiologic design. Goldman et al.[114] tested the hypothesis that exposure to specific solvents is associated with PD risk using a discordant twin pair design.

Ninety-nine twin pairs discordant for PD ascertained from the National Academy of Sciences/National Research Council World War II Veteran Twins Cohort were interviewed regarding lifetime occupations and hobbies using detailed job task-specific questionnaires. Exposures to six specific solvents selected *a priori* were estimated by expert raters unaware of case status.

Every exposure to TCE was associated with significantly increased risk of PD (odds ratio [OR]: 6.1, 95% CI 1.2–33, $p = 0.034$), and exposure to perchloroethylene (PERC) and carbon tetrachloride (CCl_4) tended toward significance (OR: 10.5, 95% CI: 0.97–113, $p = 0.053$; OR: 2.3, 95% CI: 0.9–6.1, $p = 0.088$, respectively). Results were similar for estimates of exposure duration and cumulative lifetime exposure.

Exposure to specific solvents may increase the risk of PD. TCE is the most common organic contaminant in groundwater; and PERC and CCl_4 are also ubiquitous in the environment. Their findings require replication in other populations with well-characterized exposures, but the potential public health implications are substantial.

To the best of our knowledge, this is the first confirmation of a significant association between TCE exposure and PD risk in a population-based study. Two other chlorinated solvents, PERC and CCl_4, tended toward significantly increased risk. Results were similar in analyses considering no exposure, exposure duration, or lifetime cumulative exposure. Their findings are consistent with prior case reports[115–117] and a rodent model of TCE-induced parkinsonism that recapitulates key pathological and neurochemical features of PD.[118] In this model, TCE caused selective dose-dependent loss of dopaminergic neurons in the substantia nigra pars compacta (SNpc), and selective accumulation of α-synuclein protein in the dorsal motor nucleus of the vagus nerve and SNpc, a pattern consistent with human pathological staging of PD.[119] TCE also reduced mitochondrial complex 1 activity, similar to the neurotoxin 1-methyl-4-phenylpridinium (Mpp+), the insecticide rotenone, and the mitochondrial deficiency seen in typical PD.[120,121] Like TCE, PERC[122,123] and CCl$_4$[124–126] have also been shown to increase markers of oxidative and nitrative stress, activate microglia, and disrupt mitochondrial function.[127–131] Due to their lipophilic nature, each of these compounds readily distributes in body tissues and particularly the brain.[132–134]

TCE, PERC, and CCl$_4$ have been used extensively worldwide for decades.[132,135] TCE has been used as a dry cleaning and degreasing agent, and as an additive in many common household products, including typewriter correction fluid, adhesives, paints, and carpet cleaners, and spot removers. In 1977, the U.S. Food and Drug Administration banned its use as a general anesthetic, skin disinfectant, grain fumigant, and coffee decaffeinating agent.[132] Today, it is primarily used as a degreasing agent in metal parts fabrication. Approximately 50 million pounds of TCE are still released annually into the environment in the United States. It is detected in air, soil, food, and human breast milk, and is the most frequently reported organic contaminant in groundwater, found in up to 30% of the U.S. drinking water supplies.[132–134]

Applications of PERC are similar to those of TCE.[132] PERC has been the leading dry cleaning solvent since the 1950s.[136] It is also used in textiles manufacturing and as a degreasing agent, and is found in many common household products. PERC persists in air and groundwater for several months or longer and is ubiquitous in human tissues. CCl$_4$ was the first chlorinated solvent used in dry cleaning, predominating from 1930 until the early 1950s. The major use of CCl$_4$ has historically been for the production of chlorofluorocarbon, which is used as a refrigerant. CCl$_4$ has also been used as an anesthetic and antihelminth, and in common household products. Until recently, it was used as a fumigant to kill insects in grain. Due to its toxicity, consumer and fumigant uses were phased out by 2000, but industrial uses remain. CCl$_4$ is a stable chemical that is degraded very slowly, so it has gradually accumulated in the environment, mainly the atmosphere.[135]

TCE and PERC are primarily metabolized by CYP2E1 and glutathione transferase.[123,137] A proposed proximate toxic species is 1-trichloromethyl-1,2,3,4-tetrahydro-β-darboline, a potent mitochondrial complex 1 inhibitor, dopaminergic toxin, and structural analog of MPP+ that forms in the presence of tryptamine after CYP2E1-mediated oxidation.[138–140] Consistent with this hypothesis, pooled exposure to either TCE or PERC was associated with markedly increased PD risk in a study.

Although ORs were greater than unity for the other solvents studied, their magnitude of association with PD was modest, and none approached significance. Similarly, risk associated with exposure to any solvent or with job categories was modest, and nonsignificant. This is consistent with the modest associations reported by two prior mortality studies,[141,142] and the lack of association reported by others,[143–145] when broadly defined occupational solvent exposure categories were used.

The term "solvent" encompasses a wide range of compounds, whose only common characteristics are their ability to dissolve other substances. Although **most solvents are oxidative stressors**,[146–148] there is little reason to assume these disparate molecular compounds share a common neuronal toxicity.[149] As most prior studies of occupational solvents and PD explored exposures in a nonspecific manner, relationships with any particular etiologic agent may have been obscured.

This study has several strengths. Because twins share both genes and environment, the discordant twin pair design is more resistant to confounding by unrecognized genetic and environmental factors than standard case–control designs, reducing the likelihood of spurious results.[150] They used validated exposure assessment methods to minimize reporting bias. The traditional method to obtain retrospective exposure information is to directly query subjects about the use of specific compounds, but this method is prone to recall bias—the predilection of case subjects to report exposures due to heightened awareness or concern—and workers are often unaware of the specific chemicals they are exposed to.[151–154]

Although the present work focused on occupational exposures, solvents are ubiquitous in the environment, and this is particularly true for those implicated in this study—TCE, PERC, and CCl$_4$. Their findings require replication in other populations with well-characterized exposures, but the potential public health implications are considerable. One remarkable observation made in all the reports linking TCE exposure with PD is the very long time lag (10–40 years) between exposure and clinical disease. These observations suggest that exposure may trigger a degenerative cascade dependent on the passage of time, providing a critical window of opportunity to arrest the disease process before clinical symptoms are manifested.

Vinyl Chloride ($H_2C=CC1H$) (Chloroethylene)

Vinyl chloride is an intermediate in the synthesis of several major chemicals, including PVC (see "Biopolymers" section), and has been used as an aerosol propellant. Polyvinyl can contaminate air, food, and water. Soft and hard plastics containing vinyl are known to leach into the substances with which they come in contact. This leaching is especially true of the softer containers, such as wrappings for foods and intravenous containers as well as drinking water containers.[154] Vinyl chloride can cause CNS damage, depression, dizziness, light-headedness, nausea, dulling of the senses, and headache. Other significant chronic effects include vascular malformations with aneurysms of the small vessels,[154] vasculitis, thrombocytopenia,[154] splenomegaly,[154] hepatomegly,[154] and hepatofibrosis.[155] PVC is a carcinogen producing angiosarcoma of the liver and also malignancy of the brain.[156] Most chemically sensitive individuals react to PVCs.

The IV bags have been shown to leach off toxic hydrocarbons. About 10 ppb of the hydrocarbon re: n-pentane 4 ppb, n-hexane 2 ppb, 2-methylpentane 5 ppb, 2,2,4-trimethylpentane 2 ppb, 2,20-trimethyl octane 1 ppb, leach into the solution. Therefore, most people in the United States who need IV solution get a transient infusion of at least 10 ppb of hydrocarbon with each saline administration.

1,1,1-Trichloroethane (CH_3CCl_3) (Methylchloroform)

1,1,1-Trichloroethane is commonly used in the manufacturing of computer chips and electrical components. It is a degreaser for metals and a dry cleaning agent also found in lacquers, printing inks, paints, and refrigerants and is an extracting agent in the decaffeination of coffee. Half of 500 chemically sensitive patients seen at the EHC-Dallas had this substance in their blood. Due to its lipophilicity and chemical formulation, this compound is one of the most difficult to remove once it enters the body. After using hospitalized environmental control or outpatient treatment using heat chamber depuration, only 48% of our patients had cleared this compound from their blood. Treatment takes a much longer time than other chlorinated or aliphatic compounds.

Dichloromethane (CH_2Cl_2) (Methylene Chloride)

Dichloromethane is a major component of paint strippers and degreasers. It is also used as a solvent for oils, fats, and waxes. At the EHC-Dallas, 15.7% of chemically sensitive patients studied had this substance identified in their blood. After using environmental control or outpatient treatment using heat depuration, 66% of these patients had cleared this substance from their blood.

Tetrachloroethylene ($Cl_2C=CCl_2$) (Perchloroethylene)

Tetrachloroethylene is a dry cleaning agent. It is used for manufacturing pharmaceuticals, metal degreasing, and grain fumigation. Of the 500 chemically sensitive patients surveyed at the EHC-Dallas, 83% had tetrachloroethylene in their blood. This chemical because of its lipophilicity and chemical configuration is difficult to be eliminated from the body. A single exposure can stay in the body for months, even though, theoretically, it should be eliminated within 45 days. In addition, liver damage can occur from contamination with tetrachloroethylene, as shown by the changes in this patient, and liver damage may account for the body's inability to eliminate this pollutant.

Solvent-Exposed Workers

Workers chronically exposed to solvent mixtures frequently exhibit significantly compromised attention, processing speed, and working memory relative to demographically similar unexposed controls.[55,157,158] Anatomical studies using MRI and computed tomography (CT) have detected structural changes, which are typically seen only in subjects with severe solvent exposures such as workers diagnosed with chronic toxic encephalopathy[159,160] or organic solvent abusers.[161–164] Moreover, many of these studies suffered from poor characterization of exposure, confounding, inability to determine dose–response, and biased subject selection.[165] Other studies involving workers with varying levels and durations of exposure have also reported no cognitive correlations.[166,167]

In the absence of a clear neurobiological basis for compromised cognitive performance, several investigators have questioned the validity of solvent-induced cognitive impairment.[167] However, cognitive changes observed in solvent-exposed subjects may be due to neurochemical alterations that can be detected with functional imaging. For example, position emission tomography (PET) scans revealed that subjects diagnosed with CSE ($N = 6$) did not use typical areas of anterior activation and showed less anterior activity than controls ($N = 6$) without solvent exposure but with comparable behavioral performance on the experimental task, dorsolateral prefrontal cortex (DLPFC).[168] The Haut study, however, included a small number of subjects ($N = 6$) diagnosed with cognitive dysfunction based on a previous comprehensive neuropsychological evaluation and therefore, may not reflect the larger group of workers chronically exposed to solvents. Simon and Hickey working at the EHC-Dallas showed SPECT scans (triple camera) changed in solvent exposure in 1000 chemically sensitive patients (Simon, T. D. Hickey. 1993. Metabolic imaging. Personal communication).

Thus, the purpose of the study by Tang et al.[169] was to evaluate neural activation patterns with functional MRI (fMRI) during performance of working memory tasks among construction workers with and without chronic exposure to solvents and without a diagnosed cognitive impairment.

There were 133 solvent-exposed subjects (industrial painters) and 78 controls (drywall/tapers, glazers, carpenters) recruited for the study that included a screening medical evaluation; a structured psychiatric interview Composite International Diagnostic Interview (CIDI) for DSM-IV[170]; cognitive and sensory testing; assessment of lifetime use of alcohol, marijuana, and cocaine; and lifetime solvent exposure history. A subgroup of these subjects volunteered to participate in the fMRI study by study ($N = 46$ solvent-exposed, $N = 39$ controls). There were no females among the participants. Solvent-exposed workers had at least 10 years employment in their respective trades. Control subjects who reported solvent exposure were excluded ($N = 4$). After screening for psychiatric conditions, current medication use, MRI compatibility, incidental findings, ability to perform the N-Back task, and excessive motion during the scans, 19 workers exposed to solvents and 12 controls were eliminated from further analysis. For the depression assessment, they used the Beck Depression Inventory-II Questionnaire, a widely used depression scale with excellent reliability.[171]

Exposure assessment: A cumulative lifetime exposure index was calculated for each subject who reported ever working with solvent-based paints. The work duration and time spent performing specific job tasks (spray, roller, brush, rag/sponge, and cleaning equipment) was determined based on the completion of a computerized questionnaire administered by a trained technician. Subjects reported painting activities in 5-year intervals, estimating the percent of time spent in each activity and the protective equipment worn during those activities for their working lifetime. Subjects reported in the questionnaire that they uniformly wore clothing that covered their skin during bridge and other industrial painting tasks, so no estimate of dermal exposure from solvents was included in the final exposure calculation.

To assess representative air concentrations of solvents during current painting activities, field samples were collected in a series of weeklong sampling programs during different seasons at New Jersey Department of Transportation (NJDOT) and New York City Bridge Maintenance work sites.[172] Historic estimates of exposure to solvents were estimated from the changes in paint composition determined by the U.S. EPA regulations, to reduce ozone, research literature reports from the past 25 years (e.g., PubMed, TOXLINE), regulatory documents (e.g., Health Hazard Evaluation, EPA, Material Safety Data Sheets), and commercial sources (e.g., National Paints and Coatings Association, Journal of Protective Coatings and Linings). This approach was followed since only limited data exist documenting historical air concentrations of organic solvents during construction painting.

Working memory task: They applied the N-Back task during the fMRI acquisition for activation of the working memory circuitry. The N-Back task[173,174] is a continuous performance task that is commonly used in functional imaging for the study of cognition where memory loads can be adjusted using the parameter N.

Results: Among the painters, 19 subjects were excluded from the analysis due to current psychiatric disorder ($N = 3$), current use of medication ($N = 3$), no solvent exposure ($N = 5$), and incomplete data ($N = 8$). Among the controls, 12 were excluded as follows: exposure to solvents ($N = 4$), current psychiatric disorder ($N = 1$), medication use ($N = 2$), anatomical finding ($N = 1$), and incomplete data ($N = 4$). Solvent-exposed subjects were similar to controls in age, education, number of years worked, lifetime alcohol, marijuana, and cocaine use, and Beck depression scores. Although from similar occupational groups, the solvent-exposed subjects had significantly lower reading test scores (North American Adult Reading Test [NAART] and significantly higher blood lead concentrations than controls. Controls were more likely to be Caucasian than solvent-exposed workers.

The performance scores of the N-Back task showed that solvent-exposed subjects scored significantly fewer correct hits ($p = 0.005$) and more false hits ($p = 0.016$) than controls, consistent with previous neurobehavioral studies.[175–179] For the 0-Back condition (press button when target appears) used to estimate reaction time, solvent-exposed subjects were slower than controls ($p = 0.034$).

The statistical parametric mapping (SPM) group maps show areas of activation consistent with other fMRI studies using working memory paradigms in normal controls. Significant activated clusters were detected in the anterior cingulated cortex (ACC), DLPFC, parietal cortex (PC), and insular cortices (ICs). Due to the imbalance in race (no African-Americans in the control group), the between group comparisons were performed on Caucasians only. After correcting for VIQ and lead exposure, SPM maps showed that relative to controls, solvent-exposed subjects had reduced activation in areas in the ACC and bilateral DLPFC. Accounting for task performance differences, the ANCOVA showed that the solvent-exposed subjects had significantly reduced activation in the left DLPFC and increased activation in the left parietal regions compared with controls. Among solvent-exposed subjects, lifetime solvent exposure was significantly and negatively correlated with activation detected in the ACC, DLPFC, and PC after control for confounders Z. Percent activation values that were extracted from the ROIs also showed significant correlations with lifetime solvent exposure.

This is one of the few human fMRI studies to evaluate activation patterns among individuals with chronic occupational exposure to solvent mixtures and control of potential confounders. As hypothesized, this study showed a negative correlation between solvent exposure and activation in the ACC, DLPFC, and PC among the solvent-exposed group, suggesting defects in the brain circuitry underlying performance of attention and working memory tasks. Moreover, solvent-exposed subjects exhibited significantly lower activation of the ACC and DLPFC and significantly worse performance on the N-back task than controls. Their findings of lower activity in the ACC and DLPFC of solvent-exposed painters compared with controls is consistent with studies performed using nuclear tracer techniques such as SPECT or PET, where reduced blood flow was found in these areas.[168,180,181]

The behavioral performances between the two groups were significantly different, and one might argue that the resulting activation differences are the result of performance. They ran a voxel-by-voxel ANCOVA to take into account the behavioral performance differences between the groups. This result showed that the left DLPFC had reduced activation in the solvent-exposed subjects but regions in their left PC showed increased activity relative to the controls. Evidence of compensatory increases in the function of regions in the PC was also reported in a PET study by Haut et al.[168] Although in that study a much smaller number of subjects were imaged (six exposed to organic solvents vs. six controls) using a different working memory task, they also reported reduced activation in the left DLPFC. One explanation of this left-sided significance is that our working memory task involved letters and thus was likely to be verbally mediated.[182,183] It has been widely accepted that working memory is supported by a tightly integrated network of the frontal and parietal regions.[184–186] A dysfunctional prefrontal cortex may cause aberrant activation patterns in the posterior aspects of the brain. Their finding of increased activity in the parietal lobe in solvent-exposed subjects compared with controls supports this idea. In some fMRI studies, one finds that a population sample has hyperactivity in the target brain region as an indicator of dysfunction. This hyperactivity is assumed to be an indicator of local compensatory function; the less "efficient" brain region has to work harder (showing increased blood flow) in order to perform the same task as has been shown in studies of normal cognition and intelligence.[187,188] In other fMRI studies, a different pattern of activation is detected in the population sample and is taken as an indicator of brain plasticity, where other brain regions have taken over the function of the target brain region, which is allegedly defective. This has been reported in alcohol studies[189] as well as solvent exposure studies.[168] The observed hypoactivity is similar to studies that found reduced activation in areas affected by traumatic brain injury[190,191] or Alzheimer's disease.[192] This reduced activity in the DLPFC was shown to be more specific in the left DLPFC after they accounted for the task performance. The reduced activation in the **affected brain areas is consistent with altered neuronal pathology**, which might be altered blood supply mechanism or neuronal death or toxicity due to solvent exposure rather than due to performance.

As part of the study, Nin Tang had also acquired proton density and T2-weighted images for the purpose of screening for incidental pathologies. Patients with white matter abnormalities, as determined by hyperintensities in the T2-weighted images, were excluded from the analysis. This suggests that the loci that differed between the solvent-exposed subjects and the controls involved gray matter regions, although one cannot rule out the possibility that white matter played a role as well. A study using other imaging techniques such as diffusion tensor imaging[193] might elucidate the role of white matter. Nin Tang's correlation results also show an inverse relationship between activation and lifetime solvent exposure among the solvent-exposed subjects, supporting a direct relationship between exposure and blood flow in brain regions that subserve working memory as proposed to indirect compensatory or other cognitive effects.

The prefrontal cortex together with the parietal cingulated cortex and ACC form the neural substrate for working memory and attention.[184,194,195] The prefrontal cortex is the last brain region to develop in the human brain and may be the most vulnerable to physical or chemical insults. The prefrontal cortex is most vulnerable in neurodegenerative disorders and atrophy of the prefrontal cortex is also one of the morphological changes in aging as well.[196–198] The chemically sensitive often has a different pathway of entry from the olfactory tract to the normal pathway. In the normal pathway, odorants enter through the nasal tract going directly to the limbic system then the prefrontal area. The patient's chemical sensitivity impulses go to the prefrontal area and then go to the limbic system.

A few studies have looked into solvent effects on neurotransmitters such as dopamine, acetylcholine, and gamma-amino butyric acid (GABA) with limited consistent results. Brain dopamine concentrations with solvent exposure have been studied in rodent models and both increases as well as decreases[199] have been reported albeit using different methodologies. The dopamine relationship is certainly relevant considering that it is an important neurotransmitter involved in DLPFC signaling.[200] Increases in striatal acetylcholine with exposure levels have also been reported.[201–203] Changes in GABA binding have also been detected in rats' frontal cortex that depended on the chronic or subchronic exposure levels.[204,205] GABA might be reasonable target considering the addictive effects in the recreational use of certain solvents. A large number of additional studies on the effects of solvents on other neurotransmitters actions such as GABA, glycine, NMDA, nicotine, and 5HT$_3$ have been performed.[206] Studies at the EHC-Dallas using intradermal provocation (under less polluted environmentally controlled conditions) with different mini doses of dopamine, norepinephrine, capsaicin, histamine, serotonin, metcholine, and acetylcholine have shown that there are changes in subtle brain function with short-term memory loss. Intradermal neutralization of the precise dose can often restore function if the physiology and not the anatomy is disturbed (Table 5.26). These include dopamine, epinephrine, norepinephrine, methcholine, capsaicin, and serotonin.

Anatomical studies of solvent exposure in humans have shown diffuse atrophy in the cerebellar regions, brainstem as well as frontal cortex and PC.[160,207,208] This condition was observed clinically at the EHC-Dallas by having the patient standing on his toes and walking a straight line with the eyes opened and closed. It was then documented by computerized posturography (Table 5.19). Most of these anatomical findings were nonspecific and some included the frontal and parietal regions postsolvent exposure where we found evidence of functional deficits. The results of their functional imaging study in the frontal and parietal regions are also consistent with the diminished cognitive function observed among solvent-exposed subjects.

The solvent-exposed subjects in Tang et al.'s[169] study have worked with solvent mixtures for an average of 22 years. Unfortunately, they do not have actual historical measurements of solvent exposure for their subjects, and therefore cannot determine a specific dose–response analysis for the imaging results in this study. Nevertheless, the highly significant relationship between their lifetime solvent exposure metric and activation patterns validates the neural basis for alterations in cognitive function so often observed among these workers. Future studies are needed to better understand what exposure concentrations over a working lifetime are associated with neurological effects among workers.

The current OSHA permissible exposure limits (PELs) for toluene is 200 ppm, the same value as for general industry. The (NIOSH) PEL is 100 ppm, whereas the threshold limit value (TLV) for toluene as recommended by American Conference of Governmental Industrial Hygienists (ACGIH) is 50 ppm. Unfortunately, without actual historical exposure measurements for subjects, one cannot be certain of the exact solvent concentrations to which subjects were exposed. Although many manufacturing sites follow current and historical ACGIH recommendations, worksites for construction painters are often less well controlled and industrial hygiene measurements are not routinely collected.[172] Therefore, excursions from recommended solvent exposure limits may have occurred. In addition, it is not unreasonable to believe that the sample of solvent-exposed subjects was exposed to higher concentrations historically than those recommended currently by ACGIH based on their average (i.e., 22 years) and minimum length (10 years) of time spent working with solvent-based paints. Under these estimated exposure conditions, their results show changes in the biological substrates that are consistent with the neurobehavioral observations documented in an extensive literature of workers who continue to be exposed to solvent mixtures during their working lifetime. It is clear from studies at the EHC-Dallas that once an individual develops chemical sensitivity and chronic degenerative disease, extremely small doses in the parts per billion can trigger sensitivity, including memory loss and brain fatigue, confusion, and other subtle brain dysfunctions.

Phosgene (COCl$_2$)

Phosgene is a severely toxic nerve gas. It is important because it is an intermediate product in the development of 150 cyanates. It reacts readily with amines containing H$_2$N groups and with alcohol-containing HO groups. Phosgene was used as a nerve gas in World War I, damaging respiratory function in those who were contaminated by it. Today, it has been found to emanate from electrostatic precipitators, causing severe reactions in the chemically sensitive.

1,2-Dichloropropane (CH$_3$CHClCH$_2$Cl) and 1,2-Dibromo-3-Chloropropane (CH$_2$BrCHBrCH$_2$Cl)

1,2-Dibromochloropropane and 1,2-dibromo-3-chloropropane have reportedly caused sterility in plant workers in the manufacturing industry and reduced sperm counts in highly exposed applicators.

Among the halogenated hydrocarbons are several other industrially important agents used as solvents, chemical intermediates, and consumer products. Many are powerful liver and kidney toxic compounds. Some are carcinogens. Limited space prevents a detailed discussion of these here (Table 5.6). Most textbooks on chemistry, however, provide ample information about halogenated hydrocarbons.

Trimethyl propane phosphate need data for pilots and cabin air—tricresyl phosphate brief—most should be indoor air (Chapter 2).

Aliphatic Amines

Aliphatic amines make up a separate category of altered aliphatic hydrocarbons (Table 5.35). Selected ones can be extremely toxic as well as damaging to the chemically sensitive.

A variant of the alkanes is ethanolamine (NH_2CH_2CHOH). The TLV is 3 ppm over a short period of time, not over a 24-hour period.

Ethanolamine is produced by the chemical industry. At very high (lethal) doses, the symptoms of ethanolamine poisoning relate to CNS depression. At low doses, ethanolamine stimulates the CNS. However, inhalation of ethanolamine over an extended time may result in depression. Ethanolamine is also an irritant. It has a necrotic effect on skin. Toxicity studies carried out on rats, mice, rabbits, guinea pigs, and dogs have shown similar effects. Phosphoethanol amine occurs naturally as a breakdown product in the body and is often seen to be elevated when measuring amino acids in a subset of chemically sensitive patients.

TABLE 5.35
Aliphatic Amines (Toxic)

Name	Source	TLV (Air)[a] (8-Hour Work Day)
Hydrazine	Industrial plants	1 ppm
	Rocket industry	
Methylamine	Animal waste	10 ppm
	Fish processing	
	Tobacco smoke	
	Industrial plants	
Dimethylamine	Animal waste	10 ppm
	Fish processing	
	Tobacco smoke	
Dimethylformamide	Industrial solvent	10 ppm
Dimethylhydrazine	Industrial plants	0.5 ppm
N-Nitrosodimethylamine	Amine manufacturing	Extremely toxic
	Tobacco smoke	
Ethylamine	Animal waste	10 ppm
	Sewage treatment	
	Tobacco smoke	
Ethanolamine	Industrial gas production	3 ppm
	Natural gas production	
Diethylamine	Fish processing	25 ppm
	Chemical solvent	
	Tobacco smoke	
Triethylamine	Animal waste	25 ppm
	Sewage treatment	
	Chemical solvent	
Isopropylmine	Animal waste	5 ppm
	Fertilizer manufacturing	
	Fish processing	
	Sewage treatment	

Source: Rea, W. J. 1994. *Chemical Sensitivity: Sources of Total Body Load.* Vol. 2., page 786, table 7. Boca Raton: Lewis Publishers. With permission.

[a] No safe values for optimum health have been found.

Aromatic Hydrocarbons

There are two major categories of aromatic hydrocarbons. These include the monocyclic and polycyclic aromatic hydrocarbons (PAHs). The monocyclic can be nonchlorinated or chlorinated. These are some of the most common activators and exacerbators of chemical sensitivity.

Nonchlorinated Monocyclic Aromatic Hydrocarbons

Nonchlorinated monocyclic aromatic hydrocarbons contain many toxic compounds. Of these, the chemicals most commonly found in the chemically sensitive are benzene, ethylbenzene, trimethylbenzenes, toluene, xylene, styrene, and phenols. Therefore, we will discuss these in detail. Nicotine,[209] salicylate derivatives, tartrazine, and toluene diisothiocyanate, which may be significant triggers of chemical sensitivity, are discussed independently in various chapters.

Benzene

Benzene is found in gasoline, petroleum products, processed foods, and cigarette smoke. It is used in the manufacturing of detergents, polymers, pesticides, pharmaceuticals, and paint products. Benzene intoxication enhances urinary excretion of B vitamins. It is known to seriously affect the hematopoietic system, inducing blood dyscrasias such as aplastic anemia and hemolytic anemia. Low concentrations can cause CNS effects such as drowsiness, dizziness, tachycardia, headaches, fever, nose bleeds, fatigue, tremor, and confusion.

Indoor Air Quality Handbook (2000)[210] has reported that in volatile benzene exposure to 200 trip study of commuters carried out in both the summer and winter seasons. They found an average benzene exposure of 13 pbb for commuters during the rush hours, which showed an order of five times that of a fixed ratio of 5.1:1:1.[210] A North Carolina study showed five to eight times background.[210] Although controversial, a causal relationship appears to exist between benzene exposure and the onset of leukemia. Iron-deficient patients may be particularly susceptible to developing benzene-induced anemia. Twelve percent of the chemically sensitive patients seen at the EHC-Dallas have benzene in their blood, and upon challenge, benzene appears to be one of the triggers of their chemical sensitivity.[211] Benzene breakdown as alkyl benzenes is usually through the glucuronic conjugation pathway, which, when overloaded, can malfunction in the chemically sensitive

Ethylbenzene is used as a chemical intermediate for paint, lacquer thinners, and styrene production. It also serves as an antiknock agent for gasoline. The blood of 16% of the chemically sensitive seen at the EHC-Dallas contains ethylbenzene, which when present composes a significant part of their total body load (burden). It can cause liver and kidney damage, nervous system and blood changes, and birth defects.

Trimethylbenzenes are used as chemical intermediates for paint thinners, perfumes, dyes, and fuel additives. Seven-and-a-half percent of the chemically sensitive studied at the EHC-Dallas had trimethylbenzene in their blood, suggesting that, for some reason, these carcinogens and others may bioaccumulate in susceptible patients and thereby play a role in the induction and/or propagation of chemical hypersensitivity. Low levels can cause headache, fatigue, drowsiness, irritation of the skin, and chemical pneumatics.

Toluene

One estimate of the domestic production of both isolated and nonisolated toluene in 1978 was 31×10^6 kg.[212] It is used predominantly as a component of gasoline and as a solvent for gums, fats, adhesives, petroleum products, marker pens, and paint products. Gasoline is about 15% by weight of 6% by volume.[213] The U.S. EPA conducted a survey in 1988 and found toluene in groundwater, surface water, or soil, that was 29% of the toluene at hazardous waste sites surveyed. The average amounts of toluene at hazardous waste sites were 21 ppb in groundwater and 7.5 ppb in surface water. The amount in soil was 77 ppb.[214] It can also be found in urban air, usually in the low parts per billion range. CNS depression is a primary result of exposure, and this solvent is frequently abused for its narcotic-like effect. Long-term abuse and exposure is known to cause permanent brain damage with behavioral change; it can also induce chemical bronchitis, hepatomegaly, paresthesia, and renal damage along with drowsiness, ataxia, lack of coordinating balance and weaving gait, limb and eye movement, nystagmus tremors, and cerebral atrophy.

Ototoxicity: Analysis of Human Studies

The data on toluene's effects on human hearing originate mainly from case reports of acute toluene poisoning. In the studies that focused on the voluntary inhalation of toluene, severe hearing loss in the central auditory pathways was reported.[215,216] One study on workers with normal hearing ability (evaluated by pure-tone audiometry) and exposed to 97 ppm of toluene for 12–14 years showed a change in auditory brainstem-evoked responses. This test demonstrated auditory nervous system modification before the appearance of clinical signs due to chronic toluene exposure.[217] A change in auditory brainstem-evoked responses was also observed in another study carried out on workers, but data on noise exposure were not reported (Table 5.36).[218,219]

Ototoxicity: Analysis of Animal Studies

Thirty-five studies on rats were identified. In 31 studies, the rats were exposed to toluene by inhalation; in two studies, the exposure was orally, and in one study, the rats received toluene intravenously. The inhaled concentrations were 600 ppm[220] or more, and the exposure duration varied between 30 minutes[221] and 23 weeks.[222] Hearing losses were measured by behavioral methods and confirmed by electrophysiological tests. Most often, permanent high-frequency hearing loss was reported. Factors such as concentrations and duration of exposure seem to affect the loss of hearing sensitivity in rats. The daily concentration is far more significant than the total duration of the exposure.[223] Also, toluene, rather than its metabolites, seems to be responsible for the ototoxic effects.[224,225] However, toluene's ototoxicity was also observed in a quiet environment during a study on rats orally exposed to toluene, which excludes noise caused by the inhalation system as a possible causal factor for the ototoxic effect.[226] The LOAEL for the ototoxicity of toluene in rats is between 700 and 1500 ppm.

In rats, the evidence suggests that toluene exposure causes permanent damage to the outer hair cells (OHCs) of the cochlea. In several rat studies, no changes in the latencies of the auditory brainstem responses was noted,[224–229] suggesting that damage is localized in the cochlea and not in the central auditory pathways.[230] The effect on OHCs has been confirmed by morphological examinations of the cochlea, showing a loss of OHCs, mainly in the third row.[226,231,232] The examinations show that cochlear toxicity is in the frequencies from 16 to 29 kHz and from 4 to 5 kHz. Inner hair cells seem to be preserved.[233] Hair cell loss seems to be progressive and continues even after exposure ends.[231] Also, the results from the intravenous study suggest that toluene exposure might change the response of protective acoustic reflexes.[234]

TABLE 5.36

Toluene Quebec Permissible Exposure Values: TWAEV: 188 mg/m³ (50 ppm)

Conclusion about ototoxicity	Strength of evidence
Ototoxic substance	Human studies: medium
	Animal studies: strong
	Overall: strong
Conclusion about interaction with noise	Strength of evidence
Evidence of interaction	Human studies: strong
	Animal studies: medium
	Overall: strong

Source: Environmental Health Center-Dallas.

Three inhalation studies on guinea pigs were identified. In two studies, toluene concentrations of 600 and 1000 ppm induced no effect[220,235] while in the third study, an ototoxic effect was observed with a LOAEL of 250 ppm. One inhalation study on chinchillas exposed to 1000 ppm showed no toluene-related ototoxicity.

Interaction with Noise: Analysis of Human Studies

Four studies on workers were identified, two of which used the data from the same experiment.[236,237] In a well-conducted study on plant workers,[238] simultaneous exposure to toluene (100–365 ppm) and noise (88–98 dB[A]) significantly increased the predicted probability of developing hearing loss compared to a group of workers exposed to comparable noise levels. The acoustic reflex measurements suggested that the hearing losses found in the group exposed to the two agents might be due to lesions in the central auditory system.

Another well-conducted study identified hearing impairment from simultaneous exposure to toluene (33–165 ppm) and 85 dB noise in workers.[239] However, no hearing impairment was observed in the study in which workers were simultaneously exposed to up to 45 ppm toluene and 82 dB noise, indicating that the threshold for developing hearing loss due to toluene exposure could be above 50 ppm.[236,237]

Interaction with Noise: Analysis of Animal Studies

Six rat studies were identified. Toluene interaction with noise, producing additive or synergic cochlear damage, was suggested in five studies. The reduction in hearing sensitivity of rats exposed to toluene followed by noise was greater than the sum of the effects of toluene and noise alone (synergic effect).[240,241] When exposures were in the reverse order (namely, noise followed by toluene exposure), the loss in sensitivity was greater than the individual loss caused by toluene or noise, but did not exceed the sum of the two losses.[242] Also, one study showed a greater effect of impact noise than wideband noise during simultaneous coexposure to 500–1500 ppm to toluene.[243] However, the value of the results of these studies is limited with respect to occupational exposure, because the daily exposures were long (10–16 hours/day), the exposure durations were short (2–4 weeks), and the noise and toluene exposure was not simultaneous in three of the studies.[227,240,242] The results of the single study in which the daily exposures as well as the exposure durations were more representative (6 hours/day, 90 days for rats exposed to 100–500 ppm toluene) were negative and the authors found a hearing protective effect for exposures to low concentrations of toluene.[243] One study on guinea pigs[235] and one study on chinchillas were negative.

Discussion

While certain ototoxic effects have been reported for workers, other human studies are necessary to arrive at a final conclusion. However, a series of animal studies clearly revealed ototoxic effects in relation to high toluene concentrations. In rats, toluene affects auditory function mainly in the mid-frequency range of the cochlea. There is convincing evidence of an ototoxic interaction after combined exposure to toluene and noise in workers and rats. Taking into account the results of the human studies and the evidence provided by the animal studies, we recommend that toluene be considered an ototoxic agent that can also interact synergically with noise to cause more severe hearing loss.

Because toluene is very widely used in modern society, it is difficult to avoid entirely. Even casual contact can affect the susceptible individual. Sixty-three percent of 500 chemically sensitive patients surveyed at the EHC-Dallas had toluene in their blood. In the chemically sensitive, this chemical can produce widespread long-term effects. The following case is illustrative of the devastating effects of acute and chronic toluene exposure.

Case Study

A 45-year-old white chairwoman of the Department of Physiology at a university medical school in the United States was admitted to the EHC-Dallas with the chief complaints of brain dysfunction, malaise, fatigue, edema, hormonal dysfunction, odor sensitivity, cyanosis, gastrointestinal upset, and obesity. Her illness started years previously, coinciding with a toluene leak discovered in the area of the Department of Physiology.

This patient had worked continually in a medical school environment for 23 years prior to collapse, when she had been healthy and highly productive. A few months before she collapsed, her family physician of many years detected elevated blood pressure, gastritis, and extreme fatigue. These conditions were followed by metrorrhagia of 3 weeks' duration. Her fatigue worsened until viral-like symptoms began early in January 1986. Many other individuals in her immediate work environment complained of similar symptoms and reported a heavy odor of toluene in the hallways. Her office was located above a passageway for automobile traffic. In addition, the PET building, immediately adjacent to her building, was being repaired, and heavy black smoke was released from the lines into the air.

Because of her history of exposure to toluene, the presence of toluene in her blood (1.4 ng/mL; control: <1.0 ng/mL), and the known cerebral and endocrinological effects of toluene exposure, she underwent double-blind inhalation challenge testing in a chemically free booth to assess sensitivity to toluene. She was tested with two controls and toluene. No reaction to the controls was observed. On exposure to toluene, she experienced head flushing, a dizzy sensation, and flushed feelings in her arms. She appeared very distant and foggy in her thinking. Independent neurological assessment by a psychologist before and after each inhalation challenge test showed significant worsening on neurological screening and on visuoperceptual motor functioning with exposure to toluene. She was also perceived by the objective tester to be affected adversely by toluene exposure, with clumsiness, tremulousness, and unsteady movement of hands and legs. These responses confirmed sensitivity to toluene. These effects were not seen on the control challenges. Nine months later, upon reexposure to toluene (1989), she deteriorated rapidly and again went on the amino acid liquid diet (70 g/day). After 3 weeks on this program, the patient showed improvement; toluene in her blood was 0.8 ng/ mL. She is currently working on developing an uncontaminated, preservative- and additive-free diet plan for the future maintenance of her health.

Xylene

In 1980, the annual production of xylene in the United States was 11.1×10^9 pounds.[244] This production has steadily increased over the last 32 years. Xylenes are used for industrial cleaning, degreasing, processing, extracting, and thinning solvents.[245] Mixed xylenes are used a diluents in the paint industry, in agricultural sprays for insecticides and in gasoline blends, synthetic resins, rubbers, and inks. Gasoline is about 9% xylenes by weight.[246] Like toluene, xylenes causes CNS depression and can cause erythema, defatting dermatitis, conjunctivitis, renal damage, and paresthesia of the extremities. Xylene is metabolized by oxidation. It is then conjugated to methylhippuric acid and excreted in the urine. It has half-life of 20–30 hours, except in the chemically sensitive, where it may linger for weeks. Only about 5% of xylene is exhaled unchanged.

We saw one 35-year-old female who had sustained three nonfatal cerebral infarcts after using xylene to strip a room. She wore no protective clothing, gloves, or mask, since the product she used was commercially available. She realized during the stripping process that she felt ill and needed fresh air, and each time she left the room to get fresh air from outside, her symptoms cleared. Nonetheless, she persisted in finishing the stripping of the room. Afterward, she developed incapacity and was hospitalized. Her brain scans revealed three areas of acute infarction. She recovered with mild residual effects, but she remains severely chemically sensitive. Inhaled, double-blind challenge reproduced her symptoms.

Sixty percent of 500 chemically sensitive patients seen at the EHC-Dallas were found to have xylene in their blood. Xylene remains one of the more difficult aromatics to remove from the chemically sensitive (Table 5.8).

Styrene is used as a solvent for synthetic rubber resins and is an intermediate in the chemical synthesis and manufacture of polymerized synthetic materials. Along with irritation of mucosal membranes and dermatitis it is also associated with chromosomal damage. It can cause abnormal CNS function. Twenty-two percent of 500 chemically sensitive patients surveyed at the EHC-Dallas had styrene in their blood. It is the easiest chemical to be removed from the blood. In our series, we were able to remove 100% styrene out of our patients.[247] However, others have speculated that styrene may not be removed. It may, instead, convert to another toxic substance and subsequently remain undetected in the body. Although this scenario is possible, it seems unlikely since patients continue to improve after analytical evidence of clearing occurs (Tables 5.37 and 5.38).

General volatile blood screening tests can be performed on patients suspected of being chemically sensitive. Often, these tests will reveal multiple substances in the parts per billion (Table 5.38). Stronger proof of a causal relationship between the chemically sensitive and the presence of toxic substances is the reduction of symptoms as the levels of toxic chemicals decrease over a period of

TABLE 5.37
Clearing of Toxic Hydrocarbons in the Chemically Sensitive after Heat Depuration Physical Therapy and Avoidance

Chemical	Percent[a]	Chemical	Percent[b]
Styrene	100.0	Toluene	54.1
Dichlorobenzenes	90.0	1,1,1-Trichloroethane	47.3
Trimethylbenzenes	88.9	Cyclopentane	71.4
Chloroform	83.3	n-Hexane	46.7
Trichloroethylene	76.2	n-Pentane	44.8
Dichloromethane	65.7	3-Methylpentane	43.4
Ethylbenzene	61.5	2,2-Dimethylbutane	41.7
Xylenes	60.3	2-Methylpentane	40
Benzene	60.0		
Tetrachloroethylene	59.0		

Source: [a] Rea, W. J., Y. Pan, A. R. Johnson. 1987/88. Clearing of toxic volatile hydrocarbons from human. *Clin. Ecol.* 5(4):166–170; [b]Rea, W. J. 1989. The effect of sauna physical therapy on clearing aliphatic hydrocarbon solvents from the body. Presented in American Academy of Environmental Medicine, Twenty-Third Scientific Session and Twenty-Fourth Ann. Meet. Hyatt Regency Kavinia at Atlanta Perimeter, Atlanta, GA, October 28–31, 1989.

TABLE 5.38
General Volatile Screening Test (GVST)

Sources of Chemicals	Chemicals Found in Blood	
Household products	Benzene	Chloroform
Chlorination of potable water	Toluene	Dichloromethane
Paint and paint thinners	Xylene	1,1,1-Trichloroethane
Degreasers	Ethylbenzene	Trichloroethylene
Dry cleaning operations	Styrene	Tetrachloroethylene
Petroleum products	Trimethylbenzene	Dichlorobenzene
Natural gas	Pentane	Cyclopentane
Plastics	2,3-Methylpentane	
Fugitive emissions from	Hexane	
Chemical manufacturing	Heptane	
operations		

Source: Rea, W.J. 1994. *Chemical Sensitivity, Volume II*, page 792, table 9. With permission.

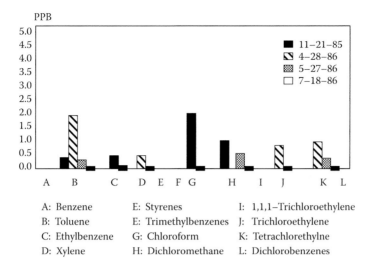

A: Benzene   E: Styrenes   I: 1,1,1–Trichloroethylene

B: Toluene   E: Trimethylbenzenes   J: Trichloroethylene

C: Ethylbenzene   G: Chloroform   K: Tetrachlorethylne

D: Xylene   H: Dichloromethane   L: Dichlorobenzenes

FIGURE 5.4 40-year-old white female nurse — ECU study (time in ECU). (Rea, W.J. 1994. *Chemical Sensitivity, Volume II*, page 793, figure 7. With permission.)

time in the controlled environment (Figures 5.4 and 5.5). Of course, the best proof of this causal relationship between the chemically sensitive and the presence of toxic substances is an individual, inhaled challenge, which we have used thousands of times at the EHC-Dallas to demonstrate sensitivity in our chemically sensitive patients (see Chapters 2 and 6 on clinical effects).

Phenols are benzene compounds with hydroxyl groups attached to them. If a single OH group is present in benzene, it is a monocyclic phenol. This substance is also known as carbolic acid and was the antiseptic that Lister used for his antiseptic surgical techniques. It is still used today in most hospitals throughout the world. It is very toxic to tissues and will kill most microorganisms as well as human tissue. Chemically sensitive patients can react to the extremely small amounts used as preservatives in many allergy medications and antigens. Basically, it is degraded through sulfur and glucuronic conjugation systems. These systems are often impaired in the chemically sensitive, thus compromising their health. Thus, the chemically sensitive will exacerbate.

Resorcinol is a benzene ring with two hydroxyl groups stuck out. Gaitan[248] has shown that resorcinol triggers thyroiditis (see the section "Endocrine"). Various plastics are made from phenols.

Phenolic resins are polymers resulting from the combination of formaldehyde with phenol or, less commonly, with other phenolic compounds, such as *p-tert*-butylphenol, resorcinol, or cashew nut oil (pentadecacatechol).

The manufacturing conditions for products derived from phenol (e.g., ratio of starting reactants, pH) are determined by the intended application of the final material.[249,250] For example, there are two types of phenol formaldehyde resins: resols and novolacs. Resols are prepared with an alkaline catalyst, using a molar excess of formaldehyde to phenol. At the first stage, a brittle resin, the resol, is produced; this alcohol-soluble compound mainly contains methylol and methylene-ether bridges. The resol can be used in molding powders and laminates. With further heating, the resin passes through a partially soluble stage before conversion to the fully polymerized, insoluble, infusible form (resite). In contrast, novolac resins are prepared using an acid catalyst and less formaldehyde than phenol. The novolacs, containing methylene linkages, are thermoplastic and require a curing agent for polymerization; this may be hexamethylene tetramines.

Because of bond stability, phenol formaldehyde polymers rarely emit formaldehyde except when heated during curing. However, the chemically sensitive still have problems when exposed to plywood that has been treated by this process. Some phenolic resins, such as PTPB-formaldehyde, have been implicated as sensitizers, possibly due to intermediates or degradation products other than

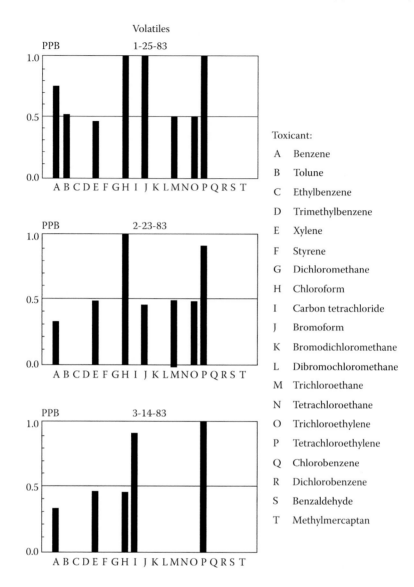

FIGURE 5.5   Time in a less-polluted environment. (Rea, W.J. 1994. *Chemical Sensitivity, Volume II*, page 794, figure 8. With permission.)

formaldehyde. Over 10,000 chemically sensitive patients have had their symptoms triggered by the inhalation or injection of phenol under controlled conditions at the EHC-Dallas and many of these react to phenol formaldehyde. Formaldehyde is the third most common substance after natural gas and pesticide, which triggers chemical sensitivity.

Bisphenol A

According to Melzer et al.,[251] bisphenol A (BPA) is one of the world's highest produced volume chemicals,[252] used in polycarbonate plastics in many consumer products and epoxy resins lining food and beverage containers. BPA is an endocrine-disrupting chemical first synthesized with a novel estrogenic molecular structure in the 1930s.[253] The American Endocrine Society[254] has called for further research on endocrine-disrupting chemicals, including BPA, citing a strong basis for concern about possible links between endocrine-disrupting chemicals, obesity, and related disorders.

The global population is subject to repeated exposure to BPA, primarily through packaged food, drinking water, dental sealants, dermal exposure, and inhalation of household dusts,[255] with detectable concentrations of metabolites in the urine of >90% of the population worldwide.[256,257] In the first major epidemiological analysis of adult health effects associated with BPA, Melzer et al.[251] found that higher BPA concentrations were associated with cardiovascular diagnoses (OR per 1-SD increase in BPA concentrations = 1.39: 95% CI, 1.18–1.63; $p = 0.001$ with full adjustment; the survey-weighted SD of uBPA was SD = 6.68 ng/mL, and geometric mean = 2.47 ng/mL; data from authors). With the release of new (independent) data from NHANES 2005–2006 ($n = 1493$), they replicated the association of higher uBPA concentrations with coronary heart disease (OR per Z-score increase in BPA = 1.33; 95% CI = 1.01–1.75; $p = 0.043$), despite a significant decrease in NHANES sample uBPA concentrations since the 2003–2004 survey (NHANES 2005–2006 geometric mean = 1.79 ng/mL; 95% CI = 1.64–1.96). Initially reported associations with diabetes mellitus and some liver enzyme changes did not reach significance in the 2005–2006 data but remained significant in pooled data.[258]

These analyses were cross-sectional, and it is theoretically possible, for example, that participants with coronary artery disease (CAD) change their exposures to BPA (perhaps through change of diet) after diagnosis. Longitudinal data demonstrating temporality (i.e., higher BPA concentrations predicting subsequent first diagnoses of disease) would greatly strengthen the evidence for BPA playing a causal role.[259,260] Their aim was to estimate the prospective association between uBPA and incident CAD. Data were available on 861 controls and 758 cases of incident CAD (total $n = 1619$). The mean $\pm$SD age of cases was 64.1 $\pm$ 7.5 years and controls was 63.8 $\pm$ 7.3 years. There were marginally fewer men in the case group (62% vs. 66.1% in controls), and fewer had never smoked. As expected, CAD risk markers were associated with case status. uBPA concentrations were relatively low. The median uBPA concentration in controls was 1.24 ng/mL and in cases was 1.35 ng/mL (geometric means, 1.23 and 1.39 ng/mL, respectively; 1.304 ng/mL combined). The distributions were strongly skewed with, for example, 12.5% (108/861) of the controls having uBPA concentrations ≥4 ng/mL were compared with 16.6% (126/758) of the cases. Among controls, those with higher uBPA concentrations (top 50% >1.243 ng/mL vs. bottom 50%) tended to be less likely from professional or managerial occupational backgrounds, but there were no other differences on demographic or CAD risks (Tables 5.39 and 5.40).

In NHANES 2003–2004[261] and again in NHANES 2005–2006, higher uBPA concentrations were associated with heart disease (pooled $p < 0.001$).[258] A major limitation of the NHANES analyses is their cross-sectional nature, making it theoretically possible, for example, that CAD patients might have changed their behaviors and incidentally increased their BPA exposure. To strengthen the evidence for causal inference, Melzer et al.[251] conducted the longitudinal study presented here, which provides the first report of similar trends in associations between higher BPA exposure (evidenced as higher uBPA metabolite concentrations) and incident CAD. The prospective design adopted shows that such reverse causation cannot account for BPA–CAD associations.

The concentrations of uBPA seen in this sample are relatively low. The overall median value was 1.3 ng/mL when compared with 7 ng/mL (interquartile range, 1.0–5.4 ng/mL) in the US NHANES 2003–2004 study in which the uBPA association with cardiovascular disease was first identified.[262] The relative paucity of more highly exposed study subjects clearly reduces our power to detect true associations, which makes our results more noteworthy. This reduced power may explain the marginal loss of two-sided significance for the fully adjusted unmatched linear model. In our NHANES 2003–2004 analysis, the SD of uBPA was 6.68 ng/mL, and produced a (per-SD) OR of 1.39 (95% CI: 1.18–1.63; $p = 0.001$) for cardiovascular diagnoses in fully adjusted models. To compare this estimate with the present EPIC-Norfolk results (SD = 4.56 ng/mL; per-SD OR = 1.11; 95% CI: 1.00–1.23), we can rescale by raising the EPIC OR to the power of the result by dividing the NHANES SD by the EPIC SD. With this approach, the EPIC per 6.68 ng/mL uBPA OR is 1.17 (95% CI: 1.00–1.35; $p = 0.058$) for incident CAD. Thus, associations between higher uBPA concentrations and incident CAD in EPIC-Norfolk showed similar although somewhat smaller trends compared with the cross-sectional results in NHANES 2003–2004.

TABLE 5.39

Sociodemographic and Risk Factor Characteristics of Cases (With Incident Coronary Artery Disease) and Controls

	Controls	SD	Cases	SD	P
No.	861		758		
Age, years	63.8	7.3	64.1	7.5	0.412
Male sex, %	62.0		86.1		0.088
Educational attainment, %[a]					9.4×10^{-4}
No qualification (<15 years of schooling)	38.6		44.0		
"0" level or equivalent (15 years)	8.1		7.7		
"A" level or equivalent (17 years)	40.2		41.0		
Oistc = school or postdegree qualification	13.1		7.3		
Occupational social class, %					0.010
Professional	8.1		5.2		
Managerial	36.2		34.6		
Skilled nonmanual	16.6		15.9		
Skilled manual	23.4		22.6		
Semiskilled	11.9		15.3		
Nonskilled	3.3		5.7		
Uncoded	0.5		0.7		
Smoking status, %					2.3×10^{-8}
Current		9.6		17.1	
Past	46.4		51.5		
Never	43.9		31.5		
Physical activity, %					0.0029
Inactive	31.2		39.5		
Moderately inactive	27.9		25.7		
Moderately active	22.4		21.8		
Active	18.5		14.1		
Body mass index, kg/m²	26.2	3.4	27.2	3.8	2.5×10^9
LDL-C, mmol/L (n = 1532)	4.1	1.0	4.3	1.0	5.1×10^{-6}
HDL-C, mmol/L (n = 1532)	1.4	0.4	1.3	0.4	1.5×10^{-9}
Total cholesterol, mmol/L (n = 1595)	6.33	1.19	6.56	6.47	5.5×10^{-5}
Triglycerides, mmol/L (n = 1594)	1.91	1.32	2.18	1.13	6.0×10^{-6}
Systolic blood pressure, mmHg (n = 1615)	137.5	17.8	143	18.7	2.6×10^{-10}
Urinary Bisphenol A Concentration, ng/mL (n = 1619)					
Median (25th to 75th percentile)	1.24		1.35		0.042[b]
	(0.59–2.52)		(0.67–2.70)		
Geometric mean	1.23	2.95	1.39	3.02	0.027

Source: Melzer, D. et al. 2012. Urinary bisphenol a concentration and risk of future coronary artery disease in apparently healthy men and women. *Circulation* 125 (12):1482–1490. Used by permission from Wolters Kluwer.

Note: Data are presented as arithmetic mean (SD) or percentage. Means and percentages may be based on marginally fewer observations than the indicated number of subjects. LDL-C, low-density lipoprotein cholesterol; HDL-C, high-density lipoprotein cholesterol.

[a] One case had unknown educational status.

[b] Mann–Whitney rank sum test (Melzer, D. et al., 2012.)

The BPA measures in EPIC-Norfolk (as in NHANES) are from single-spot urine specimens. Ingested BPA in humans is excreted rapidly, and hence urine is used in biomonitoring.[256] They used urine samples taken at the same time of day for each respondent to minimize interindividual variation. In regard to the use of single-spot samples as measures of longer-term exposure, a study of temporal variability found that a single-spot sample had moderate sensitivity for predicting and

TABLE 5.40

Sociodemographic and Coronary Artery Disease Risk Factor Status by Lower and Higher Urinary Bisphenol A Concentration (Dichotomized at uBPA = 1.243 ng/mL) in Controls

	Lower uBPA Concentration ≤1.243 ng/mL	SD	Higher uBPA Concentration >1.243 ng/mL	SD	Unadjusted p^{a}
N	842		842		
Age, years	63.8	(7.19)	63.8	(7.38)	0.91
Male sex %	62.9		62.8		0.99
Smoking status, %					0.42
Never		8.1	10.5		
Past		48.5	45.9		
Current		43.5	33.8		
Education, %		0.072			
No qualification (<15 years of schooling)		36.9	42.0		
"0" level or equivalent (15 years)	6.7	9.6			
"A" level or equivalent (17 years)	41.9	37.0			
Postschool or postdegree Qualification	15.6	11.5			
Occupational social class, %		0.034			
Professional	8.3	7.8			
Managerial	40.3			32.1	
Skilled nonmanual	15.0	17.8			
Skilled manual	21.6		25.2		
Semiskilled	10.0	14.0			
Nonskilled	4.6	2.5			
Uncoded	0.2	0.7			
Physical activity, %			0.49		
Inactive	30.5	34.6			
Moderately inactive	29.2		26.3		
Moderately active		23.0		20.9	
Active	17.4	18.3			
Body mass index categories, kg/m²	0.21				
<18.4	0.43%	0.0%			
18.4–24.9	38.2%	33.7%			
25.0–29.9	47.0%	52.8%			
30.0–34.9	12.9%	11.3%			
>35	1.5%	2.2%			
LDL-C, mmol/L	4.06	(1.04)	4.11	(0.97)	0.45
HDL-C, mmol/L	1.36	(0.39)	1.36	(0.41)	0.93
Total cholesterol, mmol/L	6.31	(1.30)6.28	(1.08)	0.78	
Triglycerides, mmol/L	2.03	(1.68) 1.87		(1.02)	0.097
Systolic blood pressure, mmHg	138.4	(16.6)	137.8	(17.6)	0.59

Source: Melzer, D. et al. 2012. Urinary bisphenol A concentration and risk of future coronary artery disease in apparently healthy men and women. *Circulation* 125(12):1482–1490. Used by permission from Wolters Kluwer.

Note: Data are presented as arithmetic mean (SD) or percentage; uBPA indicates urinary bisphenol A; LDL-C, low-density lipoprotein cholesterol; and HDL-C, high-density lipoprotein cholesterol.

[a] Unadjusted ξ^{2} or test estimate.

individual's tertiary BPA categorization.[263] Nepomnaschy et al.[264] measured the stability of BPA over 2-week intervals in first-voided urine samples from 60 women and found a Spearman correlation of 0.5, indicating that within-individual BPA exposures were generally stable over periods of weeks. Ye et al.[265] similarly reported changes between spot measures during each day and across 7 days but concluded that spot samples may adequately reflect population average exposures.

Although humans can rapidly eliminate BPA when it is provided as a single bolus,[266] continuous external BPA exposure through diet appears to lead to sustained concentrations that are detectable in serum or plasma. A recent study in which denuded BPA was used found that the half-life of BPA was six times longer for diet-fed mice than for those who received a bolus, a phenomenon consistent with an inhibitory effect of food on first-pass metabolism.[267] Stahlhut et al.[268] reported the half-life population of BPA to be considerably >6 hours on the basis of NHANES data on fasting time. The supposition is that BPA, which is lipophilic, is redistributed to lipid-rich tissues, from which slow release may occur. However, there is an absence of human pharmacokinetic data for BPA to fully explain these findings, and extrapolations from animal studies have been hindered by species-specific differences in the metabolism and toxicity of BPA,[269] the multiple potential routes by which humans may be exposed, including dermal exposure,[270] and inhalation of dusts, which would avoid first-pass metabolism. Once ingested, BPA is metabolized in the intestines and liver,[271] with the major metabolite BPA-monoglucuronide eliminated in humans via urine but in rats via bile. Glucuronidation and enterohepatic recirculation also show differences between rodents, primates, and humans although the effect of this on pharmacokinetics is not yet clear.[272]

Any misclassification of longer-term BPA body burden is likely to have resulted in a smaller (diluted) estimate of the strength of association between BPA and CAD; the true association is likely to be stronger. Some[273] have suggested that BPA disease associations are driven by higher dietary intakes, which would result in obesity-related risks and incidental higher BPA excretions. However, our sensitivity analyses show that exclusion of those with obesity and adjustment for blood lipid concentrations and levels of physical activity have little effect on the association, making such an explanation unlikely. Similarly, the lack of effect of adjustment for vitamin C makes diets poor in fruits and vegetables an unlikely explanation.[274] Liver and kidney function changes, resulting in altered BPA metabolism or excretion, are also possible confounding factors, but excluding those with high blood creatinine concentrations or adjusting for live enzymes sensitive to cell damage show these as unlikely explanations. In any observational study, it is impossible to exclude the possibility that some unmeasured confounder is present. It is clear, however, that any such confounder must be independent of classic CAD risk factors.

There are several potential mechanisms by which BPA could plausibly raise CAD incidence rates. BPA and metabolites have well-documented estrogenic, antiandrogenic,[275] and additional receptor-mediated modes of toxicity.[275] Given the known receptor-mediated effects of estrogen on cardiovascular tissues, it is biologically plausible that BPA might exert estrogenic effects or antagonize and endogenous estrogens in cardiovascular tissues by binding to soluble or membrane-bound estrogen receptors.[276]

The mean uBPA concentration in our study was 3.65 ng/mL with an assumption of an average 24-hour urine volume for adults of 1600 mL, a 100% excretion rate, and a total blood volume of 6 L, which would give an estimated BPA blood concentration in the nanograms per milliliter range. BPA shows relatively weak estrogenic agonist activities against both human estrogen receptor-α and receptor-β subtypes (ERα, ERβ) that control many estrogen-mediated activities. The half-maximal inhibitory concentration for receptor binding of BPA to human ERα and ERβ is in the low micromolar range when calculated *in vitro* and, if extrapolated directly to the *in vivo* situation (without considering competitive binding to serum-binding proteins, for instance), this would imply low ER occupancy rates in blood and potential target tissues. However, BPA binds to other estrogen-related receptors with high affinity, including the estrogen-related receptor-γ (ERRγ), for which optimal receptor binding is in the nanomolar range.[277] A recent study has reported positive associations between increased BPS exposure and *in vivo* estrogenic gene expression in adults, including ERβ and the estrogen-related receptor α (ERRα).[278] ERRα is an orphan nuclear receptor involved in estrogenic signaling and energy homeostatis that is coordinately regulated with ERRγ. It is relevant to note that expression of ERRα is highest in tissues that preferentially use fatty acids as energy sources, including adipose tissue, skeletal muscle, and heart.

In addition to its estrogenic mode of action, BPA has been shown to possess antiandrogenic activity,[279] and uBPA levels have been associated with higher blood testosterone concentrations in Italian men.[280] Lee et al.[279] showed BPA to affect multiple steps in the activation and function of the androgen receptor. Conversely, the enzyme responsible for BPA conjugation in the intestine and liver, uridine diphosphate-glucuronosyltransferase (UGT), is itself down regulated by androgens,[280] which could result in an increase in serum BPA concentration under hyperandrogenic conditions. It is unlikely that such metabolic change could alter 24-hour urinary BPA excretion in the context of repeated ingestion of BPA at the population level, although it has been suggested that a combination of hyperandrogenemia and insulin resistance may further enhance BPA levels in younger populations, especially in women with syndromes associated with increased cardiovascular disease markers and cardiovascular disease.[281] The relationship between androgen homeostasis and cardiovascular risk remains to be comprehensively established, although an increased risk of cardiovascular adverse events was recently reported in a trial of testosterone supplementation in older men.[282]

Because the pharmacokinetic behavior of BPA in humans is not comprehensively documented for practical and ethical reasons, it is not possible to rule out the conversion of BPA to metabolites that shows enhanced estrogenic activity. The major metabolite of BPA, BPA-monoglucuronide, has no estrogenic activity, but oxidative cleavage of BPA to form the estrogenically active metabolite 4-methyl-2,4-bis(4-hydroxyphenyl)pent-1-ene (MBP) has been shown in rat liver; MBP was 500-fold more potent as an inducer of dose-dependent changes of estrogen receptor genes *in vivo* compared with BPA itself.[283] The extent to which MBP may be present in humans is not known, but the oxidation product BPA-catechol, which also shows estrogenic activity, is reported to be a minor ($\approx 10\%$) metabolite in both human and rat microsomal models. Given these potential contributory factors, a comprehensive documentation of BPA phase 1 metabolism is clearly merited.

Other potential mechanisms of BPA toxicity may be relevant to the results presented here. Maxi-K channels and the β1 subunit in particular[284] play key roles in regulating smooth muscle excitability and are estrogen sensitive. BPA in the micromolar range activates Maxi-K (kcal.1) ion channels in human coronary smooth muscle cells in culture to a degree sufficient to hyperpolarize the membrane potential.[285] Laboratory exposure studies have shown that BPA can induce liver and oxidative cellular damage,[286] disrupt pancreatic β-cell function,[287] and have obesity-promoting effects,[288] all of which could plausibly contribute toward CAD risk. Certain BPA derivatives, including bisphenol A diglycidyl ether (BADGE), are peroxisome proliferator-activated receptor-γ agonists, which may activate or inhibit ion channel activity in vessel walls directly,[289] providing an alternative mechanism worthy of further investigation.

Much remains unknown about the mechanisms involved in the BPA–CAD association in humans. Future scientific work in humans is, of course, constrained by ethical limits and the practicality of repeated BPA exposure measures in long-term and large follow-up studies. Without these constraints, controlled trials would be needed to prove causation in humans, but such evidence is almost certainly beyond reach.

Associations between higher BPA exposure (reflected in higher urinary concentrations) and incident CAD during >10 years of follow-up in the EPIC-Norfolk study showed trends similar to previously reported cross-section findings in the more highly exposed NHANES 2003–2004 and 2005–2006 study respondents. More work is needed to accurately estimate the shape of the dose–response relationship. Work is also needed to identify the mechanism underlying the association between higher BPA exposure and incident.

Cresol ($CH^3C^6H^4OH$) is a mixture of the three isomeric cresols: *ortho-*, *meta-*, and *para*-cresol. It is colorless, yellowish, brownish yellow, or pinkish liquid with a phenolic odor. Cresols are soluble in alcohol, glycol, and dilute alkalis. Also, they may be combustible. Synonyms for cresol include cresylic acids, cresylol, hydroxytoluene, methyl phenol, oxytoluene, and tricresol.

Cresol is used as a disinfectant, as an ore flotation agent, as a preservative in railroad ties, and as an intermediate in the manufacturing of chemicals, dyes, plastics, and antioxidants. Tricresol phosphate is used as a jet engine fuel. A mixture of isomers is generally used; the concentrations of the components are determined by the source of the cresol. o-Cresol is also a metabolite of toluene in the urine of humans.

According to federal standards, the PELs of cresol is 5 ppm for odor (22 mg/m^3 for skin).[290]

Cresol enters the body through inhalation or percutaneous absorption of liquid or vapor. On humans, its harmful effects are both local and systemic. Locally, cresol is very corrosive to all tissues. It may cause burns if it is not removed completely from contaminated areas of the body very quickly, which may result in death. When it comes in contact with skin, cresol may not produce any immediate sensation. After a few moments, however, prickling and intense burning occur. This reaction is followed by loss of feeling. The affected skin shows wrinkling with discoloration and softening. Later, gangrene may occur. If the chemical comes in contact with the eyes, it may cause extensive damage and blindness. A skin rash may result from repeated or prolonged exposure of the skin to low concentrations of cresol. Discoloration of the skin may also occur from this type of exposure.

Cresol may cause systemic poisoning when it is absorbed into the body via the lungs, skin, mucous membranes, or by swallowing. The signs and symptoms of systemic poisoning may develop in 30–40 minutes. These toxic effects include weakness of the muscles, headache, dizziness, dimness of vision, ringing of the ears, rapid breathing, mental confusion, loss of consciousness, and sometimes death.

Prolonged or repeated absorption of low concentrations of cresol through the skin, mucous membranes, or respiratory tract may cause chronic systemic poisoning. Symptoms and signs of chronic poisoning include vomiting, difficulty in swallowing, salivation, diarrhea, loss of appetite, headache, fainting, dizziness, mental disturbances, and skin rash. Death may result if there has been severe damage to the liver and kidneys.[291]

Some chemically sensitive people do become sensitive to cresol. Those living in the desert experience problems with the odor from the creosote bush; others have problems near telephone poles and railroad ties treated with creosote, while others develop symptoms from exposure to other emitters such as airplane cabin air. We have seen one chemically sensitive patient who was a brittle diabetic living near a cresol plant. She became sensitized to cresol and developed several swings in her blood sugar. It was found that cresol was used in the insulin compounding, so that each time she took her insulin shot, her condition worsened. She moved to an area where she was not exposed to cresol in the air and was neutralized to the cresol by the intradermal method. She has done well since.

The most devastating exposure of tricresyl phosphate is in jet fuel. We have seen four pilots, one in the U.S. Air Force and the others from Australia who were severely damaged. Of course, mixtures of these with other substances may cause even more devastating effects.

Tricresyl phosphate—see airplane cabin air in Chapter 2.

Chlorinated Monocyclic Aromatic Hydrocarbons

Aromatic chemicals used in industry can be significantly contaminated with toxic chlorinated derivatives created during the production process. Included in this group are chlorinated hydrocarbons, benzenes, phenols, nicotine, salicylate derivatives, and toluene types.

Chlorinated phenol derivatives are widely used because of their antimicrobial, antifungal, herbicidal, and molluscacidal properties. A brief discussion is given here.

The chlorinated aromatics are substances such as the chlorinated napthalenes, PCB, polybrominated biphenyl (PBB), chlordane, dieldrin, and dioxins. In this chapter, we discuss chlorinated benzenes, dichlorobenzene, pentachlorophenol, hexachlorophene, PCBs, and polybrominated biphenyl.

Dichlorobenzene

Dichlorobenzenes are 1,2; 1,3; and 1,4 forms and 20:1 ratio of indoor to outdoor pollutant. Dichlorobenzene is used as an intermediate in deodorants, disinfectants, insecticides, fumigants, metal polishes, moth proofing, lacquers, and paint products. Lower concentrations will cause mucous membrane irritation, while higher levels produce nausea, anemia, jaundice, and headaches. Long-term exposure is associated with hepatic necrosis and cirrhosis. Ten percent of 500 chemically sensitive patients surveyed at the EHC-Dallas had this substance in their blood. It composed a significant part of their total body load (burden).

Pentachlorophenol

Pentachlorophenol is widely used as a wood preservative and a fungicide in leather, especially for shoes. Chlorinated phenols are produced in quantities of more than 50 million lb/year, and they are commonly found in human tissues. Chloracne dermatitis, a severe skin disorder that often results from human exposure to PCP, may actually be due to the presence of chlorinated aromatic hydrocarbons, such as dioxins, predioxins, and dibenzofurans, in the PCP. Dioxin is a common contaminant in PCP and other aromatic hydrocarbons. PCP has been isolated from the blood of chemically sensitive patients. The mean range of 12 ppm of PCP was seen in a series of 30 chemically sensitive patients at the EHC-Dallas (Table 5.41).

Hexachlorophene (2,2'-Methylene-Bis-3,4,6-Trichlorophenol)(Hexachlorophene, pHisoHex)

Hexachlorophene is an antibacterial agent that is used in commercial hygiene soaps. It is extensively used in hospitals, especially for scrubs in surgery and nurseries. It may also be found in mouthwash (0.5%) and soaps and antiseptic solutions. Baseline blood levels of hexachlorophene in "normal" adults averaged 0.028 mg/L (range: 0–0.089).[292] Adults using mouthwash containing the 0.5% hexachlorophene for 3 weeks averaged 0.06 mg/L. Those who did whole-body washing with soaps containing hexachlorophene averaged 0.24 mg/L (range: 0.10–0.38).[293]

Repeated exposure of newborns to hexachlorophenols was associated with vascular encephalopathy of the brainstem and reticular formation and spongy degeneration of myelin in the spinal cord.[294] An increased incidence of congenital malformations has been observed in neonates born to mothers who use soaps containing hexachlorophene.[295] Increased levels were seen in adult burn patients with diplopia, irritability, vomiting, and seizures.[296] Surgeons scrubbing with hexachlorophene soaps were found to have higher levels in their blood.[297] Contact dermatitis was another common finding in nurses who used soaps containing hexachlorophene.

Polychlorinated Biphenyls

PCBs are found in coolants and insulating oils used for electric utility transformers, heat transfer fluids, hydraulic fluids, plasticizers, carbonless paper, flame retardants for wood products, pump

---

TABLE 5.41

Means and Standard Deviation of Pentachlorophenol in 30 Patients

Variety Name	Size	Mean	Sample Std. Dev.	Sample Std. Err.	
Penta	30	12.06667	6.75142	1.23263	
Volume Size	**Size**	**Median**	**Minimum**	**Maximum**	**Range**
Penta	30	9	6	28	22

Source: Environmental Health Center-Dallas. Rea, W.J. 1994. *Chemical Sensitivity, Volume II*, page 798, table 10. With permission.

oils, plasticizers for plastics and coatings, caulking compounds, adhesives, and printing products. In 1970, the North American environment was bombarded with an estimated 1 to 2×10^3 tons by evaporation, 4 to 5×10^3 tons by leaks and disposal, and 22×10^3 tons from incineration and burial.[298]

High levels of PCBs are found in freshwater fish, especially in Lake Michigan. In one study, blood levels were observed to increase 50% in two volunteers within hours after they ingested fish meal containing 128–181 μg of PCB.[299] PCB residues were found in 43% of plasma specimens from residents of the Southeastern United States in concentrations up to 29 μg/L.[300]

All PCB isomers are lipid soluble and tend to accumulate in adipose tissue with repeated exposure.[301] The more highly chlorinated compounds are extremely long lived in mammals.[302] Of 37 specimens of adipose tissue obtained from members of the U.S. population, 69% contained less than 1 mg/kg of PCB. Twenty-six percent contained from 1 to 2 mg/kg, and 5% more than 2 mg/kg.[303] In 30 Japanese citizens, levels averaged 1 mg/kg and ranged 0.4–2.5 mg/kg.[304] In six other Japanese citizens, liver concentrations of PCB averaged 0.09 mg/kg and ranged from 0.03 to 0.32 mg/kg.[305] Persistent organic pollutants (POPs) especially PCBV have been associated with arteriosclerosis (preceding pages).

PCBs cause chloracne and nervous system and liver dysfunction, as seen in many chemically sensitive people. Mass poisoning with PCB-contaminated rice oil occurred in Japan, affecting 2000 individuals.

In one U.S. survey, almost all mothers nursing had PCB in their breast milk, with 30% having more than 0.05 ppm. Fifty percent of Michigan mothers had more than 1.35 ppm in their milk.[306] Neurological and developmental impairments in children have been linked to exposure to PCBs through ingestion of mother's milk. Rats, rabbits, and guinea pigs exposed to PCBs showed liver damage with fatty infiltrates, central lobe atrophy, and necrosis.[307] PCBs interfere with liver metabolism, with three major biochemical effects being the indicator of a mixed-function oxidase system. PCBs have major contaminants dibenzofuran and dibenzodioxine, both of which are potent mixed-function oxidase inducers. PCBs are potent immune suppressants and carcinogens.[307] Following human exposure to PCBs, the neurological signs have included headache, fatigue, nervousness, dizziness, and decreased sensory nerve conduction.[308] PCBs can cause lymphoid atrophy in rabbits, chickens, and guinea pigs. A splenic and/or thymic atrophy can occur in monkeys. PCBs affect vitamin A absorption; they inhibit the synthesis of retinal binding protein.[309] Exposure to PCBs may cause selenium and/or vitamin E deficiency in chickens.[310] PCBs are inducers of hepatic microsomal mixed-function oxidases and can affect selenium-induced growth functions of depleted rats by affecting their utilization.[311] They are strong inducers of liver microsomal enzyme and possibly may affect selenium depletion. Hepatic biopsy in Yusho patients who have been accidentally exposed to PCBs in oil showed hypertrophy of the smooth endoplasmic reticulum, indicative of microsomal enzyme induction.[312] Seven years after the accident, very high levels were still found in several Yusho patients, with 92.0 and 230 ppb being reported in two patients.[312] Exposure to PCBs results in enlargement of the thyroid gland in rats.[313] Clinical short-term responses of humans and monkeys to PCBs are summarized in Table 5.42.[314]

PCB levels according to sex showed higher values in males.[312] In animal studies, PCBs have been shown to cause a host of metabolic effects like porphyria, altered steroid metabolism, decreased hormone production, and others.[314] Pregnant rhesus monkeys fed PCBs showed resorption or abortion of fetuses, or their offspring had low birth weights, shortened long bones, and decreased skull circumference.

Polybrominated Biphenyl (PBB)

PBB is used as a flame retardant on carpets, mattresses, furniture, clothing, construction products, and plastics. 2,2′,4,4′,5,5′-Hexabromobiphenyl is commonly used.

In Michigan 1973, FireMaster PB-6, a commercially prepared fire retardant composed primarily of a mixture of polybrominated biphenyls (PBBs), was accidentally substituted for Nutrimaster, an

---

TABLE 5.42

Short-Term Clinical Responses of Humans and Monkeys to PCBs

Response	Man	Monkey
Susceptibility	High	High
Acne	Yes	Yes
Hyperpigmentation of skin	Yes	Only infants
Hyperactive meibomian eye glands	Yes	Yes
Conjunctivitis	Yes	Yes
Edema of eyelids	Yes	Yes
Subcutaneous edema	Yes	Yes
Keratin cysts in hair follicles	Yes	Yes
Hyperplasia of hair follicle epithelium	Yes	Yes
Gastric hyperplasia	NAb	Yes
Hepatic hypertrophy	Yes	Yes
Liver enzyme change	NAb	Yes
Decreased number of red blood cells	Yes	Yes
Decreased hemoglobin	Yes	Yes
Serum hyperlipidemia	Yes	Hypo
Leukocytosis	Yes	Yes

Source: Letz, G. 1982. The toxicology of PCB's. An overview with emphasis on human health effects and occupational exposure. Health hazard and information service. State of California, Department of Health Services.

---

animal feed supplement. This food substitution subsequently contaminated cows, pigs, chickens, and ultimately humans via the food chain.

In 1976–1977, a group of unexposed farmers had nearly uniformly undetectable serum PBB concentrations, while Michigan farmers and consumers showed concentrations ranging from undetectable to 100 µg/L, with most in the 1–5 µg/L range.[315] Serum levels ranged from 1 to 15,340 µg/L in 14 workers at a PBB production plant.[316]

Concentrations of PBBs in the adipose tissue of most members of the general population are below detectable levels, but in 1975, they averaged 226 µg/kg in urban residents of Michigan, 516 µg/kg in nonquarantined farmers, and 1965 µg/kg in quarantined farmers. After 1974, fat levels of PBBs were found to decline by an average of 39% (range: 11–12) in 16 acutely exposed persons over a 6-month period. No consistent relationship was found between concentrations of PBBs in fat and serum. The ratio of PBBs in fat to that in breast milk averaged about 2.[317,318]

Symptoms of PBB contamination include fatigue, joint pain and stiffness, headache, muscle pain, dizziness, sleepiness, and skin rash. Liver damage was seen in the Michigan farmers. Chemical sensitivity has resulted in the survivors.

In 1978%, 97% of individuals residing in Michigan had measurable levels of PBBs in their adipose tissue.[319] In the ensuing years, animal studies have suggested that PBBs may be hepatotoxic, neurotoxic, immunotoxic, and carcinogenic.[320–323] Halogenated aromatic hydrocarbons, such as PCBs and PBBs administered to experimental animals have been shown to cause wasting syndromes, immunotoxicity, skin disorders, endocrine and reproductive deficits, porphyria and hepatotoxic, neurotoxic, and genotoxic effects.[324] Similar effects have been recorded in humans for these compounds, as seen in both a subset of chemically sensitive and complaints by individuals exposed to PBBs that included headache, joint pain, loss of memory, nervousness, etc.[324]

Residents of contaminated Michigan in whom PBBs persist will probably bear this xenobiotic burden throughout their lives.[315,316,325–327] Certainly, every chemically sensitive patient from Michigan that we have seen at the EHC-Dallas in 2012–2014 bears these effects. PBBs are transmitted transplacentally to human fetuses and into maternal breast milk.[318,328,329] These observations have also been made for PCBs in humans[330–333] and for both compounds in animals.[327,334,335] More recently, Miceli and Marks[327] demonstrated the persistence of PBBs in human postmortem tissue and its distribution into 15 different tissues 10 years following exposure. If these lipophilic substances were sequestered only in lipid deposits (evidence indicates this sequestering is not the case[336]) and did not mobilize from such tissues, the threat to human health presumably would be low. However, mobilization of lipids within the body occurs throughout the day, can be induced by several mechanisms, and involves both the active and inactive fraction of the adipose tissue. The active fraction constitutes only 5% of total adipose tissue and does not appear to contain many of the xenobiotics found in the inactive fraction.[337] Apparently, autotransfusions occur as chemicals are mobilized from stress, exercise, etc.

PHTHALATES (PHTHALIC ACID ESTERS)

The greatest amount of data has been accumulated for the PVC plasticizers, the phthalic acid esters. These have been seen to affect the chemically sensitive adversely and therefore are discussed in detail. They have recently been banned from the use of liquid containers.

The production of phthalates is ~400 million lb/year. Phthalates are plasticizers and are added to plastic products in significant quantities, usually to keep the plastics soft. As much as half the mass of a PVC container can be phthalates.[338] Another large part of plastic is organophosphates similar to these found in organophosphate pesticide. Plastic containers are widely used in industry and consumer products, and phthalates can leach from the PVC walls of containers and contaminate the fluid contents. Studies by Kalin and Brooks[339] and our work at the EHC-Dallas have shown that the chemically sensitive may be made ill by this leaching. Specific phthalic esters with short alkyl groups, such as dimethyl and di-n-butyl phthalate (DBP), are appreciably soluble in water. Most other dialkyl phthalates, including di-(2-ethylhexyl) phthalate (DEHP), are selectively soluble in aqueous medium because of their lipophilic structures. Volatiles are said to be generally of low standard temperature and pressure for the long-chain and branched compounds such as DEHP. Many edible oils are stored in these containers and will absorb the phthalates.

Phthalate esters, principally DEHP, can be introduced directly into the circulatory system by use of plasticized PVC medical equipment, (e.g., syringes and tubing) or infusions from plasticized PVC blood and intravenous solutions. For other than occupationally or medically exposed populations, the most common mode of human contact with phthalate esters is by ingestion of foods or liquids. Laseter (Laseter, J. L. 1987, personal communication) showed decreased amounts of synthetics in water stored in glass versus those stored in plastic (see Chapter 3, Volume 5 on Water). In addition, many studies have shown that solutions stored in plastic intravenous bottles will retain synthetic molecules from the plastic itself.

This problem is not seen with glass containers. Phthalates, which are fat soluble, can be absorbed through the skin. They have a broad range of toxic effects and can be teratogenic and mutagenic.[340] In mammals, the main target organs are the liver and testes.[341] The chemically sensitive react to fluids stored in plastic containers. Oils stored in plastics are the worst for leaching phthalates because of their lipophilicity.

Over 90% of food stored in plastic contains phthalates, which when absorbed usually go to the urine. Some absorption studies show that phthalates are absorbed and lost mostly in the urine. Virtually, all DEHP in blood is protein bound, ~80% to lipoproteins, and the rest to albumin. DEHP and DBP are rapidly cleared from the body within 24 hours to 3–5 days in a normal individual. There is little or no evidence of tissue accumulation. This rapid excretion may not be true in the chemically sensitive individual, the genetically deficient individual, or any individual who is old or diseased. Fat, absorptive organs (especially the gastrointestinal tract), and excretory organs (liver, kidney, gastrointestinal tract) are the major initial repositories of the dialkyl esters. The excretory organs probably accumulate the phthalate esters as a mechanism of excretion. DEHP was reported to be retained for several months in the livers of rhesus monkeys infused with small doses.

Phthalates can also significantly modify the functioning and inducibility of liver enzymes. Humans exposed to tetrachlorophthalic anhydride (TCPA) in the production of epoxy resins developed recurrent respiratory symptoms and physiologic abnormalities. Inhalation challenge with TCPA reproduced symptoms and demonstrated both immediate and delayed (4–6 hours) physiological responses.[342] Phthalates can be metabolized by both the MFO and mitochondrial systems. Phthalates can significantly modify the functioning and inducibility of liver mixed-function oxidase enzymes.[343] Metabolites of phthalates can alter MFO induction that has been stimulated by pentobarbital, carbon tetrachloride, or ethanol. They stimulate some MFO enzymes to increase activity and inhibit the activities of others. A recent report suggests that DEHP is hepatocarcinogenic.[344]

Phthalate esters are hydrolyzed and conjugated with glucuronic acid in the liver. Overload of this conjugation system will initiate and exacerbate chemical sensitivity. Phthalates are now being taken off the market due to their toxicity (Tables 5.43 and 5.44).

Bicyclic Aromatic Hydrocarbons

Aromatic bicyclic hydrocarbons are benzene and naphthalene derivatives found in diesel exhaust, tobacco smoke, plastic, the polymer industry, and coal–tar manufacturing. They are also known to overload oxidative and conjugation systems and damage cytochrome oxidase systems, thus exacerbating chemical sensitivity.

Polyaromatic Hydrocarbons

PAHs with two or more fused benzene rings are potent carcinogens and inducers of chemical sensitivity and are ubiquitous. Usually, PAHs are benzopyrenes and anthracenes. They occur in fossil fuels and are liberated with solvent fermentation (charcoal production) and oil refining. Incomplete burning of organic matter, such as found in car exhaust, will liberate these polycyclic aromatic hydrocarbons. One finds the benzopyrenes high in charcoal-broiled and charcoal-soaked foods, vegetable fats and oils, the incineration of plastics, and polluted air (especially cigarette smoke).

The PAHs occur in a variety of environmental products such as soot, coal, tar, tobacco smoke, petroleum, and cutting oils. The input of petroleum hydrocarbons into the marine environment has been substantial. These then go into sea life and back to man. It is difficult to differentiate PAHs synthesized from plants, bacteria, fungi, marine seeps, and forest and grass fires from anthropogenic sources.

TABLE 5.43

Unopened Injectable Saline Solution Packaged in Plastic Bag Container (Standard Intravenous Bags for Infusions)

Analysis of Volatile Organic Compounds
Reference Method: Purge and Trap: GC/MS

Compounds Detected	Concentration μg/L (ppb)
n-Pentane	4
n-Hexane	2
2-Methylpentane	5
2,2,4-Trimethylpentane	2
2,2,6-Trimethyloctane	1
Other VOCs	Not detected <1

Source: Matrix Laboratory, Dallas, Texas.

TABLE 5.44

Analysis of Semivolatile Organic Compounds: Glass Bottle

Reference Method: GC/MS

Compounds Detected	Concentration µg/L (ppb)
None detected	0

Source: Matrix Laboratory, Dallas, Texas.

Studies show the bulk of PAHs are in harbors and near the seashores. Gasgosian et al.[345] were unable to detect individual PAHs in uncontaminated air at Enewetak Atoll, Marshall Islands, in the Pacific Ocean. Concentrations of 2,3-benzopyrenes have been found in mollusks, oysters, soft-shell clams, crabs, shrimp, sea urchins, starfish, sea cucumbers, mullet, sole, cod, eels, menhaden, and sardines off the coast of Europe, North America, and Greenland.[346]

The facts concerning PAHs resulting from petroleum spills; leaching from dumps, oil wells, and coal beds; surface water runoffs; sewage effluents; and industrial processes are hard. Also, PAHs may occur from evaporation and photochemical oxidation, microbial degradation, and sedimentation. Neoplasias in fish have been observed in lakes and rivers of the United States. These fish include bullhead catfish, white sucker, Atlantic tomcod, sauger and wall eye, winter flounder, sole, staghorn sculpin and drum, and are thought to be due to the PAHs.[347]

Substitution of methyl groups of benzopyrenes enhances carcinogenicity. Thus, 7,12-dimethyl-benz[*a*]anthracene (DMBA) is one of the most powerful carcinogens known.[348] Biotransformation of PAHs occurs by oxidation to an eventual formation of dihydrodiol epoxide. These are then conjugated and detoxified and go out of the body. Inhibition of the carcinogenicity of this class of compounds by xenobiotics depends on increasing the level of detoxification reactions.[349] PAHs have been observed to make the chemically sensitive extremely ill. They often trigger recurrent respiratory and sinus infections, among other conditions (Tables 5.45).

PAHs are oxidatively metabolized in the liver by the aryl hydrocarbon hydroxylase system, which is roughly equivalent to the mixed-function oxidase (MFO) system, but incorporates other cytochromes in addition to, or in place of, the P-450 forms. Therefore, overload of these systems will cause local accumulation and exacerbation of chemical sensitivity.

While the common PAHs are discussed at the beginning of this section, there are many other polycyclic aromatic compounds that contain atoms such as nitrogen, sulfur, and oxygen and are frequently referred to at PAHs. Though closely related, they are not true PAHs because they are substituted for carbon. Nonetheless, we work within convention when choosing to treat these as if they were the same type of poly aromatic hydrocarbon.

ORGANICS OF OUTDOOR AIR

DIESEL EXHAUST PARTICLES—MANY SUBSTANCES SUCH AS POLY AROMATIC HYDROCARBON ARE FOUND IN DIESEL FUEL

According to Kraft and Harry,[350] microglia-mediated neuroinflammation has been implicated in the pathology induced by exposure to PM present in polluted air of which diesel exhaust particles (DEPs) are a major component. The chemically sensitive in some cases are extremely prone to exposure to diesel exhausts. This substance can cause a myriad of reactions, including sudden weakness, brain fog, neuropathy, vascular spasm, confusion, arrhythmias, bloating, gas, urinary urgency, etc.

Diesel exhaust contains greater than 40 toxic air pollutants, including known neuromodulatory contaminants such as nitric oxide, carbon monoxide, benzene, lead, and zinc. These substances often show in the blood and breath analysis of the chemically sensitive. It should be noted that this

TABLE 5.45

Aromatic Bicyclic Hydrocarbons Benzene and Naphthalene Derivatives

Name	Source
Methylindane	Diesel exhaust, tobacco smoke
Dimethylindane	Diesel exhaust
Trimethylindane	Diesel exhaust
Indene	Tobacco smoke, polymer manufacturing
Ethylindene	Tobacco smoke
Benzeindene	Tobacco smoke, coal combustion
Azulene	Tobacco smoke
Biphenyl	Diesel exhaust, tobacco smoke, plasticsindustry
4-Methylbiphenyl	Tobacco smoke
Ethylmethylbiphenyl	Tobacco smoke
Trinaphthene benzene	Car emission
Naphthalene	Diesel exhaust, polymer industry, tobacco smoke, brewing
1,2,3,4-Tetrahydronaphthalene	Diesel exhaust, tobacco smoke
1-Methylnaphthalene	Car emission, brewing, diesel exhaust, coal tar manufacturing, tobacco smoke
2-Methylnaphthalene	Landfill, tobacco smoke
Dimethylnaphthalene	Coal tar manufacturing, tobacco smoke
Trimethylnaphthalene	Diesel exhaust, tobacco smoke

Source: Rea, W. J. 1994. *Chemical Sensitivity: Sources of Total Body Load.* Vol. 2., page 805, table 12. Boca Raton: Lewis Publishers. With permission.

pollution consists of not only PM but also significant amounts of other possible confounders such as ozone, LPS, tobacco smoke, and gasoline exhaust.[351]

The work by Hartz et al.[352] suggested that exposure of isolated brain capillaries in culture to DEP produced an upregulation of the efflux transporter, P-glycoprotein via oxidative stress and TNFα-dependent mechanisms. Direct exposure to DEPs (50 μg/mL), specifically, has been reported to decrease dopamine uptake and mesencephalic midbrain neuronal cultures 8–9 days posttreatment *in vitro*. This selective effect upon cultured dopaminergic neurons was reported to be dependent upon activation of microglia to elaborate superoxide via NOX in response to phagocytosis of DEP.[353]

As would be expected with cells of the monocyte lineage, the phagocytic function of the cells was observed with the addition of DEP to the culture media. A shift in the morphological phenotype of the microglia was observed within 6 hours of DEP exposure, consistent in timing with other literature examining the phagocytic uptake of fluorescent beads by cultured microglia.

Phagocytes like microglia can physically stimulate and will be activated to engulf any foreign material within the media. This can result in a cascade of microglial activation responses, including elaboration of proinflammatory cytokines which can punch holes in the neurocell membrane triggering aspartate (NMDA) and glutamate nerves and receptors triggering the TRPV1, TRPA, TRPM mechanism. Even if maintained in the presence of other CNS cells and in the absence of known stimulatory factors, cultured microglia display a quasi-activated phenotype.[354–356]

This activation probably occurs in the chemically sensitive who are exposed to DEPs. They have a lot of dopaminergic reactions some of which can be neutralized by intradermal antigen techniques. A similar pattern of susceptibility of dopaminergic neurons in culture dependent upon activation of microglia-like BV2 cells has been reported for nanosize titanium dioxide[357] which many chemically sensitive patients react to when challenged intradermally (EHC-Dallas) or have as implants.

In the absence of a filtered DEPs solution, the contribution of other contaminants in the media and the responses of other glia or neurons in these culture system remains a concern. Since DEPs can absorb organic chemicals and metals from the surrounding environment, it is unknown how this property affects the integrity of *in vitro* systems, particularly as regards DE uptake and microglial activation.

In addition, the treatment of cells with DEPs after shaking to remove microglia from the astrocyte monolayer produces a population of microglia in a significantly more activated state than would be found *in vivo*. Such a shift in the activation state is also observed with the use of the BV2 microglia cell line. Thus, further examination along these lines of investigation will bolster the ability to translate the effects observed *in vitro* to those that would occur *in vivo*. Identification of the underlying mechanisms will require a significant level of attention to detail and control to determine specificity of the response. Support for similar effects occurring *in vivo* is provided by a limited number of studies.

Campbell et al.[358] exposed mice (4 hours, 5 days/week for 2 weeks) to concentrated airborne particulates at a site near heavily trafficked highways in Los Angeles, California. All animals were treated with intranasal instillation of ovalbumin to induce lung sensitization. Of course, this sensitization can usually happen to both areas and sensitivity to other chemicals and is seen particularly to other foods. In the chemically sensitive, this condition gives them a particularly unique setup for more diesel pollutants entry causing or exacerbating the chemically sensitive and chronic degenerative diseased. It often results in addition to food sensitivity and sensitivity to molds and more chemicals. This state creates a generalized hypersensitivity condition to both the sensory nerves and the immune system. Under these conditions, exposure to either ultrafine or combined ultrafine and fine particles increased NF-κB activation in isolated brain nuclear fractions. In the cytoplasmic fraction, IL-1a protein was increased under both exposure conditions, while TNFα elevation was increased only with the combined particle exposure.

However, caution should be applied when interpreting these results as indicative of particle-mediated activation of microglial inflammatory processes. For example, when air treated with PM collected from sites at varying proximity from traffic sources, immortalized macrophages displayed no traffic density-dependent elaboration of TNFα or IL-6; rather, these responses appeared to be depended more on the quantity and composition of endotoxin and transition metals contaminating these particles.[359]

If this condition occurs in the chemically sensitive by either or both mechanisms, it would not only explain the chemically sensitive reacting to DEPs but also other environmental substances. Of course, most chemically sensitive react to food, acting like or in fact the ovalbumin, setting up the target tissue for the endotoxin and/or metal sensitivity. Food and mold sensitivity reactions may play a more important role than scientists have appreciated in diesel damage which can propagate many aberrant physiological functions, creating chronic disease. Gerlofs-Nijland et al.[360] exposed rats to 0.4 ppm ozone for 12 hours in a whole-body inhalation chamber 24 hours prior to initiating nose-only exposure to diesel engine exhaust (DEE) for 6 hours/day; 5 days/week for 4 weeks. DEE exposure in the absence of preozone exposure was not conducted. In these studies, TNFα and IL-1a proteins levels were selectively elevated in the striatum. mRNA levels for TNFα and TNFp55 receptor (TNFR1) were not altered by DEE exposure in any of the brain regions examined.

This finding would be compatible with that in the chemically sensitive, who is sensitive to DEPs. They suffer great reactions that clear after the exposure terminates. In contrast with the earlier study by Campbell et al.,[358] NF-κB activation was also not altered in any of the brain regions examined.

In a study using Indian ink as a PM donor, it was shown that a direct injection in the perivascular space led to scavenging of particles solely by MHCII+ perivascular cells, with no ingestion by pericytes, microglia, or other macrophages,[361] suggesting a localized phagocytic response and the lack of penetration of the particles into the brain parenchyma or blood vessels.

This fact appears to be consistent for DEPs based on similar deposition across most, but not all, brain regions after exposure. Interestingly, in rats, XO (4000 ppm) inhalation exposure for 15 minutes produced no evidence of neuronal pathology or astrogliosis with 1-hour postexposure; however, evidence for reactive microglia was observed,[362] suggesting a rapid response to exposure in the absence of cell death. This sequence of events could occur in the chemically sensitive who are exposed to DEPs or DEE in that they clear their brain dysfunction after the exposure terminates. We frequently see this in the chemically sensitive patients after cessation of the diesel exposure. The clearing may take minutes to hours depending on how damaged the detoxification mechanisms are and on how overloaded they are with toxins. Chronic exposure for years has shown the Mexico City population to develop Alzhiemer's disease, multiple sclerosis, PD, and other neuron vascular responses.[350]

Air pollution may be associated with CNS inflammation and disrupted neural transmission,[363,364] which one sees in the chemically sensitive as evidenced by the Triple-Camera Brain SPECT scan correlating with clinical signs of confusion and inability to walk a straight line or stand on their toes with eyes open or closed or have concentrated brain function. According to Kraft and Harry, exposure to diesel exhaust, which makes up a significant portion of the air pollution present in a number of the Mexican cities from which animal and human cohorts have been examined, is associated with gliosis and brain damage in rats, dogs, and humans.[365,366] In an earlier study, Calderon-Garciduenas et al.[11] examined cortical brain tissue of feral dogs of mixed breed, from less than 1 year to 12 years of age, with uncontrolled diet and genetic background, living in a highly polluted region (Southwest Metropolitan Mexico City, SWMMC), as compared with dogs from a less polluted region (Tlaxcala, Mexico). From these random cohorts, the authors interpreted the data of elevated NF-κB activation, iNOS levels, and astrogliosis to 1 PM in the brain.

In further examination of neuroinflammation in association with high air pollution, Calderon-Garciduenas et al.[367] examined the brains following autopsy of human patients (between 2 and 45 years; average ~25 years of age) who died suddenly. Subjects were from low-exposure housing environments in Tlaxcala and Veracruz, Mexico ($n = 12$) or high-exposure housing environments in Mexico City, Mexico ($n = 35$). In this cohort, the high exposure group displayed evidence of BBB disruption and increased GFAP, COX-2, IL-1B, and CD14 (an LPS receptor) levels in the olfactory bulb and in secondary sites, including the frontal cortex and the substantia nigra. No changes were observed in the hippocampus.

Histopathology showed a prominent increase in perivascular mononuclear cells and other indicators of vascular damage in multiple brain regions. PM appeared to penetrate the CNS and was observed within olfactory bulb neurons (in 4/35 subjects from the 2008 Calderon-Garciduenas cohort); however, in other regions, its presence appeared to be restricted to the capillary and perivascular space, at least partly within or in contact with abundant mononuclear cells or mononuclear cell-ingested red blood cells (RBCs).[367,368]

Similarly, dogs in high pollution areas exhibit enlarged cortical, perivascular space, and accompanying hypertrophy of surrounding astroglia, presumably activated to maintain barrier integrity.[369] Based upon MRI, prefrontal white matter lesions, which were presumed to be neuroinflammatory in nature, were more frequent (56.5% vs. 7.6%) in MRIs of children from the cities representing high-pollutant versus low-pollutant areas ($n = 23$ and 13, respectively).[370] Further examination of the brainstem from nine children from these localities indicated evidence of inflammation and pathology in the auditory nuclei and, in live subjects, a delay in brainstem auditory evoked potentials in relation to exposure.[363] We would expect these to be the case in some chemically sensitive brains due to previous SPECT scan findings although their changes reflect glutathione deficiencies.

Complicating the connection between exposure and effects on the nervous system are the known, non-CNS changes induced by diesel exhaust. These include cardiovascular and respiratory effects which appear to involve elevated systemic inflammatory responses, at least for responses to levels well above ambient concentrations.[371] These include exacerbation of asthma and bronchitis with chronic cough in some chemically sensitive or the development of arrhythmias and even heart failure in times of high or even subnormal environmental exposure, once they are sensitized.

Vascular function is influenced by air pollution, including vasoconstriction effects that are enacted even in the absence of the particles themselves and may involve reduced NO.[372–374] Restricted blood flow to the brain can cause hypoxia and associated neurological events, including activation of resident microglia and elaboration of cytokines or reactive oxygen species, which may be incorrectly attributed to responses associated with CNS-penetrating DEP. Additionally, *in vitro* systems incorporating lung epithelial cells reveal that DEPs can alter lung barrier properties, including reductions in the tight junction protein occluding[375]; induction of MMP-1, NOX, and ROS[376] and elaboration of IL-8, GM-CSF, and ICAM-1, the latter even after removal of the particles and independent of particle size.[377] At the BBB, these changes particularly increased endothelial cell expression of occludins and ICAM-1, which indicate barrier dysfunction and could result in secondary activation of brain microglia. The neurons can also be activated when the NMDA and glutamate receptors become hypersensitive enlarging holes in the membranes. These holes allow currents of K^+ to go out and Na^+ and Ca^{2+} to enter the neuron. The Ca^{2+} then combines with the protein kinases A and C which when phosphorylated increases sensitivity 1000 times.

In studies such as this, preexisting vascular pathology, as may exist due to atherosclerosis or CAD, should be considered as influencing susceptibility. We do see patients with coronary disease and other areas of atherosclerosis who have brain dysfunction if they are also chemically sensitive. This underlying pathology can influence the influx of infiltrating monocytes and lymphocytes, the activation state (increased hypertrophy and cellular density) of parenchymal cells, and sensitivity of specific neuronal populations, such as those in the substantia nigra.[378–380]

Fine PM such as that isolated from diesel exhaust has been reported to elicit the production of 8-hydroxy-2′-deoxyguanosine and hydroxyl radicals in isolated, *in vitro* systems and, in an immortalized microglia cell line, can reduce ATP and GSH, cause mitochondrial membrane depolarization, and induce TNFα and IL-6 mRNA expression, as well as alter genes associated with "oxidative stress" and innate immunity.[381,382] Most chemically sensitive and chronic degenerative diseased patients have a reduction of both of these ATP and GSH. The reduction in ATP is ordered by the fact that these patients have external weakness and fatigue, and it is relieved by avoidance of DEPs and the energy augmented by ATP administration. The GSH deficiency is observed by the SPECT brain scan where the dye is dependent upon glutathione physiology. Areas with no dye uptake in the brain are glutathione dependent. Intravenous glutathione helps these chemically sensitive patients with brain dysfunction to correct the deficiency and allows the patient to function better.

In this study, the PMs with the most robust effects separated (based on induction of NF-κB in respiratory epithelial cells) were identified as having higher concentrations of nickel and vanadium. It is possible that the transport of these metals to neurons or glia near to PM deposits after exposure may disrupt function and/or induce excavation. Almost all chemically sensitive and chronic fatigued patients have depleted energy, and it would not be surprising that they had not only microglia dysfunction in the brain but also phagocytic and active cardiac and skeletal muscle cellular dysfunction which would explain their weakness when exposed to diesel particulates. While interesting, the existing literature is insufficient to characterize the neuroinflammatory properties of brain resident cells as causative of neuronal pathology that may be related to diesel exhaust exposure; however, the data warrant consideration for future *in vivo* animal experiments and carefully designed epidemiological studies (Table 5.46).

Aromatic and Heterocyclic Amines

Aromatic and heterocyclic amines are chemicals composed of single- and multiple-ring systems with an exocytic amino group. They do not occur in nature except for complex heterocyclines that are generated during pyrolysis. They are synthetics used in dye and drug manufacturing and as antioxidants.[383] The typical monoarylamines and polyarylamines with carcinogenic potential include aniline and *o*-toluidine (sarcoma), *o*-anisidine and *p*-cresidine (bladder cancer), and phenacetin[384] (Table 5.48). At high doses, anilines are carcinogenic, and through its metabolite phenylhydroxylamine, aniline is a powerful hematopoietic poison producing methemoglobinemia. *o*-Toluidine and 2,6-dimethylaniline are released from the local anesthetics prilocaine and lidocaine.[385] High-level chronic abuse, but not ordinary intermittent drug use, of phenacetin has led

TABLE 5.46
Aromatic Polycyclic Hydrocarbons

Name	Source
Fluorene	Car emission, coal combustion, tobacco smoke
Methylfluorene	Coal combustion, refuse combustion, tobacco smoke
Dimethylfluorene	Diesel exhaust
Trimethylfluorene	Diesel exhaust
Phenanthrene	Aluminum manufacturing, car exhaust, petroleum manufacturing, refuse combustion, coal combustion, tobacco smoke
Methylphenanthrene	Coal combustion, coal tar manufacturing, tobacco smoke
Anthracene	Petroleum manufacturing, aluminum manufacturing, asphalt manufacturing, auto exhaust, coal combustion, refuse combustion, tobacco smoke
Methylanthracene	Aluminum manufacturing, auto emission, coal combustion, diesel exhaust, tobacco smoke
Benz[a]anthracene	Aluminum manufacturing, auto emission, coal combustion, diesel exhaust, tobacco smoke
Methylbenz-anthracene	Tobacco smoke, auto emission, coal combustion
Fluoranthene	Petroleum manufacturing, aluminum manufacturing, asphalt manufacturing, auto emission, diesel exhaust, refuse combustion, coal combustion, tobacco smoke
Methylfluoranthene	Tobacco smoke, aluminum manufacturing
Acephenanthrylene	Tobacco smoke
Pyrene	Petroleum manufacturing, aluminum manufacturing, asphalt manufacturing, auto emission, coal combustion, refuse combustion, tobacco smoke
Methylpyrene	Aluminum manufacturing, coal combustion, tobacco smoke
Chrysene	Aluminum manufacturing, auto emission, diesel exhaust, refuse combustion, tobacco smoke
Naphthacene	Auto emission
Perylene	Auto emission, coal combustion, petroleum manufacturing, refuse combustion, tobacco smoke
Pentacene	Asphalt manufacturing
Coronene	Auto emission, coal combustion, petroleum industry, refuse combustion, tobacco smoke

Source: Rea, W. J. 1994. *Chemical Sensitivity: Sources of Total Body Load*. Vol. 2., page 806, table 13. Boca Raton: Lewis Publishers. With permission.

to human bladder cancer.[386] These aforementioned aromatic amines have been observed to trigger chemical sensitivity.

Typical dicyclic and polycyclic arylamines include 2-naphthylamine, 1-naphthylamine, 4-aminobiphenyl, benzidine, 2-furylfuramine, 2-anthramine, 2-phenanthrylamine, 6-amino-chrysene, and 4-aminostilbene. Many are carcinogenic, but some are both genotoxic and mutagenic. The metabolism of aromatic or heterocyclic amines can lead to ring epoxy derivatives that, in turn, can be reduced to dihydrodiols or rearranged to phenols. Ring epoxidation may be important in some. Humans have the ability to *n*-hydroxylate arylamines, but there are quantitative differences between individuals. Again, this difference in the ability to break down toxic substances may partially explain the susceptibility of the chemically sensitive to these potentially toxic chemicals (Figures 5.6 and 5.7).

Aromatic Amines Other than Naphthalamines, Phenylamine, and Tyrosine

Other existing aromatic amines include 4-aminodiphenyl, 2,3,4-aminopyridines, quinolines, azaarenes, and nitroso compounds. These can be quite toxic and have adverse effects on the chemically sensitive. Each will be discussed separately.

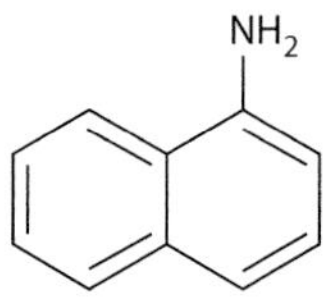

FIGURE 5.6 1-Naphthylamine.

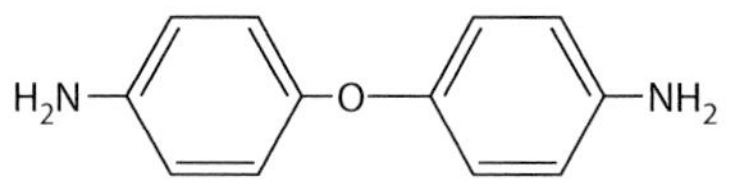

FIGURE 5.7 4-Aminodiphenyl.

4-Aminodiphenyl has produced carcinogenicity both in animals and humans, and therefore is dangerous to the chemically sensitive. It is considered one of the most potent bladder carcinogens. Development of bladder tumors in 11% of 171 workers in a chemical plant manufacturing 4-aminodiphenyl has been shown. The tumors appeared 5–19 years after initial exposure, which lasted for 1.5–19 years (Tables 5.47 and 5.48).[387]

1,2-Dichloropropane ($NH_2C_5H_4N$)

2-Aminpyridine has a TLV of 0.5 ppm (2 mg/m³). Its major sources are chemical plants. Acute poisoning symptoms are headache, nausea, and increased blood pressure. One fatal accident was reported[388] in a chemical plant manufacturing 2-aminopyridine. 2-Aminopyridine can trigger symptoms in the chemically sensitive (Figures 5.8 and 5.9).

3-Aminopyridine and 4-Aminopyridine

These are more toxic than 2-aminopyridine and thus may cause greater problems for the chemically sensitive (Figure 5.10).

Simple azo compounds consist of two aromatic rings joined by an azo-N=N–length. The azo acts as a chromophore and hence as dyes (see section on Pigments and Dyes). Azos are known to induce liver and bladder cancer in some laboratory animals. Only heavy occupational contact with arylamines has been linked to bladder cancer in humans.[389]

This major class of chemical carcinogens is characterized by chemicals derived from secondary amines or amides by nitrosamides that are synthetic as well as naturally occurring substances. Nitrosoamine compounds are hepatotoxic and known to exacerbate chemical sensitivity (Figures 5.11 and 5.12).

Quinolines and Azaarenes

Quinolines and azaarenes are aromatic homocyclic compounds that represent many important structures upon which drugs are based. Quinoline itself is carcinogenic, leading to hepatocellular cancer and hemangioendotheliomas in rats and mice. Among the chemicals obtained from the action of frying or boiling meats under realistic home cooking conditions were several compounds based on an imidazoquinoline or quinzoline ring system. These chemicals were among the most mutagenic compounds found. They may be the agents associated with cancer of the colon, and certainly they exacerbate chemical sensitivity. When 4-nitroquinolone-*N*-oxide is combined with a carcinogenic growth promoter, croton oil, and painted on the skin of rats, it causes papillomas and carcinomas. Some of the other quinolines include benzo(*g*)quinoline, benzo(*f*)quinoline, 2-amino-3-methylimidazo(4,5-*f*)quinoline, 4-nitro-2-formamido-4-(5-nitro-2-furyl)thiazole.

TABLE 5.47

Concentrations of 3,4-Benzopyrene in Tissues of Aquatic Organisms

Organism	Location	BP (μs/kg dry wt.)
Mollusks		
Mussels (*Mytilus edulis*)	Seine Estuary, France	ND-380a
	Tillamook Bay, Oregon	<0.4–67.4
	Yaquina Bay, Oregon	0.48–120.8
	St. Efflam, France	5.0
	Vancouver, Canada	
	Outer Harbor	8 + 1
	Wharf Marina, and	
	Dock areas	72 + 20
	False Creek	168 + 24
Oyster (*Crassostrea virginica*)	Norfolk Harbor, Virginia	20–60
Soft-shell clam (*Mya arenaria*)	Tillamook Bay, Oregon	1.2
	Coos Bay, Oregon	1.32–26.64
Cockle (*Cardium edule*)	Seine Estuary, France	220–780
Crustaceans		
Crabs		
(*Callinectes sapidus*)	Chesapeake Bay, Virginia	<2.0
(*Maia squinado*)	Brest, France	3.5
Shrimp (*Penaeus aztecus*)	Palacios, Texas	<4
Isopods (*Ligia* sp.)	Clipperton Lagoon,	
	Equatorial Pacific	536
Echinoderms		
Sea urchin (UNID)a	St. Efflam, France	ND
Starfish (UNID)	North Sea coast, France	ND-126
Sea cucumber (UNID)	West coast of Greenland	ND
Annelids		
Freshwater oligochaetes	Freshwater pool, Italy	50
(*Fublifex* sp.)		
Fish		
Mullet (*Mugil chelo*)	Bay of St. Malo, France	17.3 (flesh)
		155 (viscera)
		22 (scales)
Sole (*Solea solea*)	Bay of St. Malo, France	10.0
Cod (*Gadus* sp.)	Holsteinborg, Greenland	15
	Atlantic, 40 km off Toms	<10
	River, New Jersey	
Eel (*Anguilla* sp.)	Dunkerque, France	30
Menhaden	Raritan Bay, New Jersey	6.0
Sardine	Bay of Naples, Italy	65.4

Source: Rea, W. J. 1994. *Chemical Sensitivity: Sources of Total Body Load.* Vol. 2., pp. 808–809, table 14, Boca Raton: Lewis Publishers. With permission.

[a] ND = not detectable; UNID = unidentified; wet weight values were converted to dry weights using a factor of 4.

N-NITROSO COMPOUNDS

Nitroso compounds are used extensively as industrial intermediates and have been found in diesel exhausts (Figure 5.13). Nitroso compounds can be reduced readily to hydroxylamine derivatives and then to amines. Many pathways of nitrocompounds are derived from the combination of nitric acids with petroleum products.

TABLE 5.48
Aromatic Amines (Toxic)

Name	Source	TLV (Air)[a] (8-Hour Period)
Aniline	Chemical industry, plastics combustion, tobacco smoke	5 ppm
Toluidine	Chemical industry, plastics combustion, tobacco smoke	5 ppm
Xylidine	Chemical industry	5 ppm
Dimethylaniline	Chemical industry	5 ppm
Diphenylamine	Chemical industry	10 mg/m^3
Naphthylamine	Chemical industry	Very toxic
Carbaryl	Pesticide	5 mg/m^3

Source: Rea, W. J. 1994. *Chemical Sensitivity: Sources of Total Body Load.* Vol. 2., page 810, table
        15, Boca Raton: Lewis Publishers. With permission.
[a] No safe values for optimum health have been found.

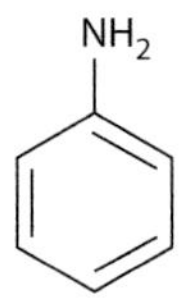

FIGURE 5.8   Aniline.

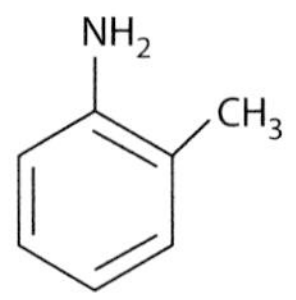

FIGURE 5.9   Toluidine.

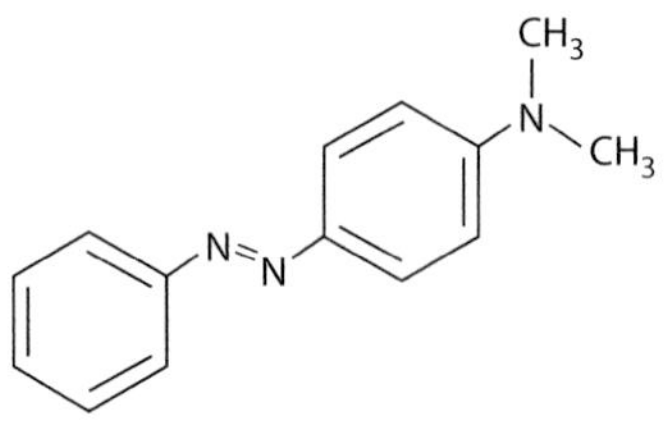

FIGURE 5.10   Azo compounds (dimethylaminoazobenzene) 4-dimethylaminoazobenzene.

Besides synthetics, sulfur organic compounds are used in medicinal products, dye stuffs, preservatives, chemotherapeutic agents, sweeteners (saccharin), disinfectants, and antidiabetic drugs.
Most of the nitro and sulfur compounds combined with petroleum products seem to have adverse
effects on the chemically sensitive.

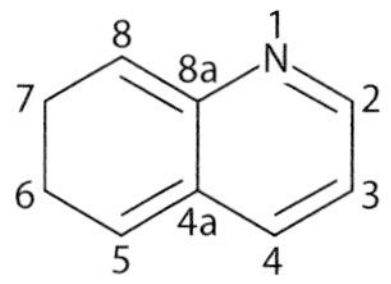

FIGURE 5.11 Quinolines and azaarenes.

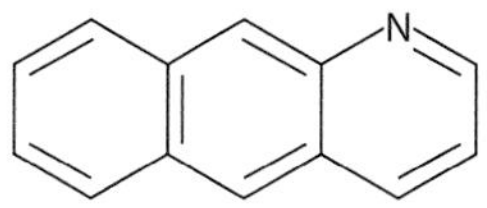

FIGURE 5.12 Benzoquinoline.

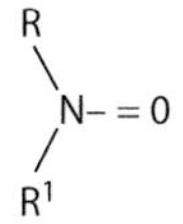

FIGURE 5.13 *N*-nitroso compounds.

Carcinogenic Substances Able to Exacerbate Chemical Sensitivity

Many chemical substances have been shown to be carcinogens. These chemicals are divided, according to Casarett and Doull,[390] into DNA reactive, epigenetic, and unclassified categories. All of these almost always exacerbate the chemically sensitive (Figure 5.14).

Nitrofurans and nitroheterocyclics are drugs and potent carcinogens. Many nitrofurans have been synthesized for drugs with antibacterial activity. These are not only used particularly in veterinary practice but also in humans.

Nitrofuran FAN FT 2 Formamido-4-(5 Nitro-2 Furyl) Thiazole

AF-2 or furylfuramide was used as a food additive in Japan until it was found to be mutagenic and carcinogenic (Figure 5.15). In animals, bladder and mammary cancer have been induced by some nitrofurans.

Azaserine

Serine diazoacetate, which is produced by streptomyces, is thought to be an antifumer agent. It inhibits purine biosynthesis through the inhibition of the enzyme 2-formamide-*N*-ribosyl acetamide

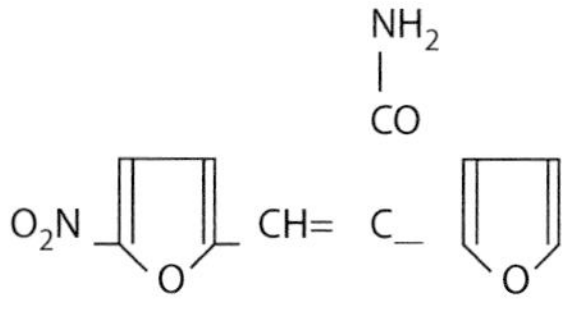

[e.g., 2-(2-fury1)-3-(5-nitro 2-fury1) acrylamide (AF-2)]

FIGURE 5.14 Nitrofurans and nitroheterocyclics.

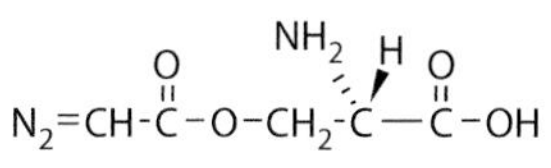

FIGURE 5.15 2-(2-Furyl)3-(5-nitro-2-furyl) acrylamide (AF-2).

5-phosphate: L-glutamine amido-ligase. Azaserine has been shown to produce primarily pancreas and kidney cancer in rats.

As with cancer, there is no single mode of action to the production of chemical sensitivity. Carcinogens enhance neoplastic conversion, while promoters enhance neoplastic development. The same principle may hold for the chemically sensitive. The neoplastic state is heritable at the cellular level (e.g., the progeny of the neoplastic cells inherit the neoplastic potential). Carcinogens, therefore, interact with DNA or RNA to alter genetic and epigenetic mechanisms. Carcinogens that interact with and alter DNA are called "genitotoxic" mechanisms. They are also mutagenic (Table 5.49).

Carcinogens for which no evidence of DNA change exists have "epigenetic" mechanisms involving cytotoxicity, chronic tissue injury, intracellular generation of reactive tissues, and hormonal imbalance, immunologic effects, or promotional activity. These same activities have been observed in most chemicals that trigger chemical sensitivity. Some carcinogenic agents could indirectly cause genetic alterations and neoplastic conversion by means of production of inaccurate DNA synthesis, reactive oxygen free radicals, aberrant methylation, and chromosomal abnormalities. Alternatively, some carcinogens could produce neoplastic conversion by epigenetic effects on gene expression. Many of these carcinogens probably do not produce neoplastic conversion at all, but rather act in the sequence of neoplastic development to facilitate tumor development by cells that are already genetically altered or have been independently altered by genetic carcinogens. Benzopyrenes can apparently act in any of the aforementioned ways, as can many of the other toxic hydrocarbons (Table 5.16). The development of disease from any of these substances may take a similar pathway to a point and then deviate, causing sensitivity rather than cancer.

Direct carcinogens are alkyl imine (ethylene imino-), alkylene epoxides (1,2,3,4-butadiene epoxide), small-ring lactenes (β-propiolactone), propane sultone, sulfate esters (dimethyl sulfate, methyl methanesulfonate, 1,4-butacaine dimethanesulfonate [Myleran]), mustards (bis[2-chloroethyl] sulfide mustard gas, Yperite), bis(2-chloroethyl)amine (nor-nitrogen mustard R−H, nitrogen mustard R−CH$_3$), cyclophosphamide (cytoxin), 2-naphthylamine mustard (chlornaphazine), triethylenemelamine chloride, methyl iodide, dimethylcarbamyl chloride, PAHs (anthracene, benzopyrene), aromatic amines (aniline, toluidine, *o*-anisidine, *p*-cresidine, phenacetin). Quinolones and aza are nitranologues of carcinogenic aromatic urethane, ethionine, formaldehyde, hexamethyl phosphoramide, carbamates, and halogenated hydrocarbons. Inorganics include uranium, polonium,

---

TABLE 5.49
Classification of Carcinogenic Chemicals

Category	Class Example
1. DNA—reactive (genotoxic)	Carcinogens
a. Activation independent	Alkylatory agent
b. Activation dependent	Polycyclic aromatic hydrocarbon
2. Epigenetic carcinogens	Nitrosamine
a. Promoter	Organochlorine pesticides, saccharins
b. Cytotoxic	Nitrol acetic acid
c. Hormone modifying	Estrogen, amitrole
d. Immunosuppressor	Purine analog
e. Solid state	Plastics
3. Unclassified	
a. Peroxisome proliferators	Clofibrate, phthalate esters
b. Miscellaneous	Dioxanes

Source: Rea, W. J. 1994. *Chemical Sensitivity: Sources of Total Body Load.* Vol. 2., page 813, table 16, Boca Raton: Lewis Publishers. With permission.

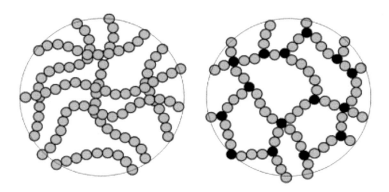

FIGURE 5.16 Section of the amorphous three-dimensional network of a cured thermosetting material. Since the cross-linking takes place in all directions of the space, an enormous number of close-meshed networks are formed, linked to one another, and coiled. In the ideal case, an article made from a thermosetting plastic consists of a single, gigantic, spatially cross-linked molecule.

radium, radon gas, titanium, nickel chromium under special conditions, cobalt, lead, manganese, beryllium, selenium, and arsenic.

There are also carcinogens produced in nature, either by microorganisms or by plants. Those originating from the microorganisms are aflatoxins, sterigmatocystin, luteoskyrin, islanditoxin, griseofulvin, actinomycins, mitomycin C, adriamycin, daunomycin, elaiomycin, ethionine, azaserine, nitrosonornicotine, and streptozotocin, some of which have been observed to trigger chemical sensitivity. Carcinogens produced by plants are tobacco, betel nut, cycavin, pyrrolizidine (senecio), coltsfoot, bracken fern, mushroom toxins, safrole, β-asarone (calamus oil), thiourea, goitrogens (resorcinol), and phorbol esters. Most of these substances can also trigger chemical sensitivity.

BIOPOLYMERS

Biopolymers are used as a basis for all kinds of synthetic materials to which the chemically sensitive react. These include plastics, synthetic fabrics, pigments, dyes, and detergents.

Plastics

Thermosetting materials are curable plastics consisting of phenols (cresol or resorcinol), formaldehydes, urea, and melamines. Synthetic resins are materials used in the production of plastics (in an unshaped state as powders or liquids) and their precursors. During fabrication, chemical reactions take place under the influence of initiators (curing agents) or by application of heat, and these reactions produce huge spatially cross-linked molecules through interlinking (Figure 5.6).

Plastics may be soft or hard. The soft plastics consist of fabrics, adhesives, binders, and paint lacquers. The hard plastics are moldings and laminates. Cured thermosetting materials are glassy, hard, and infusible (Figure 5.17). The cured articles made from these materials are no longer plastic but can only be shaped by machinery. Thermosetting materials that are to be shaped by machine are available commercially in a dissolved form or in powders, emulsions, dispersions, pastes, casting resins, compression molding materials, or adhesives. Bending materials by means of adhesion has become a process of great industrial importance. The following survey summarizes important groups of synthetic resins from which corresponding thermosetting plastics are manufactured. Some of these resins affect the chemically sensitive more than others do, depending on their volatility.

Phenoplastics come from phenol (cresol or resorcinol) formaldehyde. Amino plastics come from urea and melamine formaldehyde resins. Reactive resins come from unsaturated polyesters in styrene and epoxide resins. Silicones come from silicone resins. Many of the soft substances cause stray outgasing and make the chemically sensitive individual very ill.

A. Polyolefins	Basic chemical unit
Polyethylene, PE	$-CH_2-CH_2-$
Polypropylene, PP	$-CH_2-CH-$ $\qquad\quad CH_3$

B. Polymers containing halogens	
Polyvinyl chloride, PVC	$-CH_2-CH-$ $\qquad\quad Cl$
Polytetrafluoroethylene, PTFE	$-CF_2-CF_2-$

C. Styrene polymers	
Polystyrene, PS	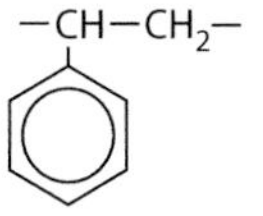 $-CH-CH_2-$ (phenyl ring)
ABS copolymers, ABS	Copolymers and blends of the components acrylonitrile/butadiene/styrene
MBS copolymers, MBS	Copolymers formed from methyl methacrylate/styrene/butadiene
ASA copolymers, ASA	Copolymers formed from acrylonitrile/styrene/acrylates

D. Other homopolymers containing a	$-C-C-$chain
Polyvinyl acetate, PVA	$-CH_2-CH-$ $\qquad\quad O-COCH_3$
Polymethyl methacrylate, PMMA	$\qquad\quad CH_3$ $-CH_2-C-$ $\qquad\quad COOCH_3$

E. Polymers containing heteroatoms (O and N) in their chains, so-called heteropolymers

Polyacetals, for example, polyoxymethylene, POM	$-CH_2-O-$
Polyamides, PA, for example, polyamides 6, PA 6	$\qquad\qquad\qquad O$ $\qquad\qquad\qquad \|\|$ $-NH-(CH_2)_5-C-$
Polyester, for example, polycarbonates, PC	$\qquad\quad O$ $\qquad\quad \|\|$ $-R-O-C-O-$
And polyethylene glycol terephthalate, PETP	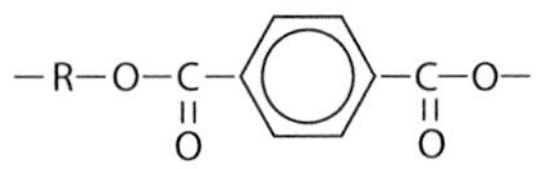 $-R-O-C-\bigcirc-C-O-$ $\qquad\quad \|\| \qquad\qquad\quad \|\|$ $\qquad\quad O \qquad\qquad\qquad O$
Cellulose esters, for example, cellulose acetate, CA cellulose propionate, CP cellulose acetobutyrate, CAB	

FIGURE 5.17   Important thermoplastics able to cause problems in the chemically sensitive. (Hopp, V., and I Hennig, Eds., 1983. *Handbook of Applied Chemistry: Facts for Engineers, Scientists, Technicians, and Technical Managers*, pp. IV/3-18. Washtington, D.C.: Hemisphere Publishing. With permission; Rea, W.J. 1994. *Chemical Sensitivity, Volume II*, page 816, figure 11. With permission.)

The thermosetting materials can have some outgasing problems if their sources are (such as phenol, formaldehyde, resorcinol, or melamine) outgas or if their filler (such as ground minerals, pine acid flour, short-fiber asbestos, cellulose flocks, chopped paper or textiles, or glass fiber) chips off. Most of these latter solid materials are less problematic for the chemically sensitive than are the volatiles. However, asbestos, pine, and fiber glass have been seen to create a problem in the chemically sensitive.

Elastomers are plastics with a wide-meshed three-dimensional cross-linked network. They are rubber elastic or rigid elastic, in contrast to the thermosetting materials which are rigid. The degrees of cross-linking are much less than that of the thermosetting plastics. Therefore, elasticity occurs. Sulfur is used to vulcanize and harden. Natural rubber is C15-1,4-polyisoprene (see Chapter 8).

Synthetic rubber can be any of many different cross-linked elastomers, such as styrene–butadiene copolymer, acrylonitrile–butadiene copolymer, C15-1,4-polybutadiene, isobutylene–isoprene copolymer (butyl rubber), poly-2-chloro-butadiene (chloroprene rubber), ethylene/vinyl acetate copolymer, ethylene–propylene copolymer, polyester polyurethane, PVC partially cross-linked plasticizers, and silicone rubber.

The behavior of different plastics with heat is important to the chemically sensitive. Thermoplastic noncross-linked threadlike molecules and lightly cross-linked elastomers soften with heat and decompose, thus causing toxic outgasing. The hard, strongly cross-linked thermosetting materials have much less outgasing and are much less troublesome to the chemically sensitive.

SYNTHETIC FIBERS

The synthetic fibers are polyamides, esters, ethylenes, vinyls, acrylonitriles, urethanes, and elastomers. Most synthetic fabrics (Figure 5.18) have toxic chemicals such as phosgene and/or cyanide compounds, ammonia, or xylene as their intermediates, initiates, or side products. Therefore, it

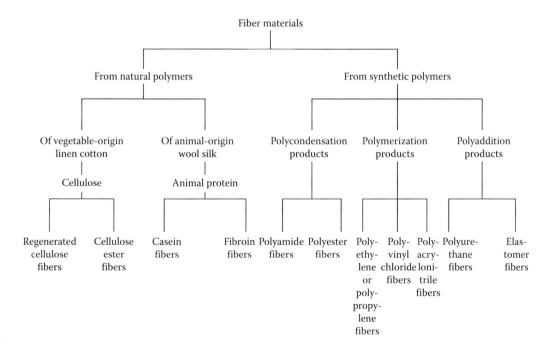

FIGURE 5.18 Family tree of fibers—Classification of synthetic fibers. (From Hopp V., I. Hennig, eds. 1983. *Handbook of Applied Chemistry: Facts for Engineers, Scientists, Technicians, and Technical Managers,* p. IV/3–IV18. Washington, DC: Hemisphere Publishing. With permission; Rea, W.J. 1994. *Chemical Sensitivity, Volume II,* page 818, figure 12. With permission.)

is possible that residuals will be on fibers, thereby enhancing their toxicity potential. Certainly, the people who make these fibers can be dangerously exposed to these chemicals, and some may develop chemical sensitivity. In addition, in the spinning process, organic solvents such as dimethylformamide are used after spun synthetic products are treated to give strength and elasticity to the thread. This after treatment is usually a water-soluble emulsion of fats and oils.

This emulsion not only makes the filaments more pliable and easy to process but also protects the fibers from picking up a static charge. All steps in the creation of synthetic fabrics may add contamination to the fabric. These are some of the reasons the chemically sensitive have problems with synthetic fibers.[391]

The demand for textiles in the last four decades of the twentieth century grew faster than the production of natural fiber. Therefore, more use of synthetics came into being.

The production of synthetic fibers grew faster than the production of cotton and wool. At the turn of the twentieth century, the world production of wool was 730,000 tons for a world population of 1.6 billion people. Since then, the population has increased to 6.2 billion people; the production of wool rose to 1.6 million tons. Thus, the per capita production of wool has remained constant over 70 years. The world production of synthetic fibers increased to 14 million tons in 1980 and has now exceeded 50% of the world fiber market. Before 1950, there was a miniscule use of synthetic fibers.[392] The massive increase in the use of synthetic fibers has created a severe problem for the chemically sensitive since many materials used in public buildings, cars, and homes are made of synthetics which increase their total pollutant body load and cause patients to be more prone to reactions and chemical sensitivity.

The United States is the world leader in the production of synthetics (Figure 5.19). The leading consumer is also the United States. This increase in manufacture and consumption of synthetics greatly increases the total environmental and societal load. This large volume often is hazardous to the chemically sensitive patient who is trying to survive in today's society.

The various properties of synthetic versus natural fibers are outlined in Table 5.17. Clearly, distinct differences between some naturals and synthetics exist. What is not presented in this table is the increase in noxious outgasing potentials, the opposite charge in the synthetics, or the content of toxic chemicals, all of which adversely affect the chemically sensitive individual.

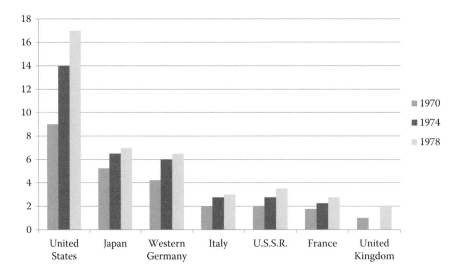

FIGURE 5.19 Manufacture of plastics in leading countries (in million tons). (From Hopp, V., I. Hennig, eds. 1983. *Handbook of Applied Chemistry: Facts for Engineers, Scientists, Technicians, and Technical Managers*, pp. IV/3–IV18. Washington, DC: Hemisphere Publishing. With permission.)

Urethanes

Urethanes are hydrocarbons that are combined with cyanide compounds. Some of these are quite detrimental to the chemically sensitive. Others, such as the one used as varnish, are less damaging.

The reactions of amines and phosgene give isocyanates and carbamate esters. Isocyanates are of great importance for making polyurethanes. Polyurethanes are polyaddition products formed from diisocyanates and dehydric alcohols or diamines. Polyurethane is a textile raw material for elastomers, for example, rubber-elastic continuous-filament yarns, and starting materials for foam plastics.

The properties of polyurethanes (ethylcarbamates) can range from adhesives, to extremely hard and abrasion-resistant lacquers, to gear wheels. They will even be used as foam plastics. Urethanes are carcinogenic in animals and definitely are known to exacerbate chemical sensitivity in humans.

Some chemically sensitive individuals can sometimes tolerate urethane finishes on hard wood after much curing, but many others cannot tolerate them. Therefore, cautious use of these products on woods in the homes of the chemically sensitive is recommended. Figure 5.20 contains the results of a double-blind challenge of a polyurethane-sensitive patient. This individual became nonfunctional after a single exposure. After the patient's symptoms were cleared in the ECU, inhaled, double-blind challenges reproduced the symptoms. A program of avoidance allowed the patient to regain his health (Table 5.50).

Hydrogen cyanide (HCN) and its salts poison by inactivating the cytochrome oxidase of cells in critical tissues, primarily the heart and brain. (See Chapter 4, Sulfur Compounds.[393]) Acrylonitrile degrades slowly to HCN in the body and, therefore, acts primarily by the same mechanism, although the slow release of free cyanide renders it somewhat less toxic than HCN itself. Both HCN and acrylonitrile (found in wallboard) are sufficiently absorbable across the skin to cause poisoning in the absence of inhalation exposure. Manifestations of poisoning are mainly due to intracellular anoxia of brain tissue (leading to respiratory failure) and the circulatory insufficiency that results from myocardial weakness. The liver has substantial capacity for converting cyanide to the less toxic thiocyanate, a metabolic conversion that is accelerated by therapeutically administered thiosulfate. Cyanide is much more difficult for the chemically sensitive to detoxify and will exacerbate chemical sensitivity.

Polycarbonates

Carbonate esters are important as solvents and the starting materials in making polycarbonates.[394]

Polycarbonates are used in containers for many liquids as well as in oxygenators for heart–lung machines and other extracorporeal medical devices. Polycarbonates leach off synthetics, which causes problems in the chemically sensitive; however, polycarbonates are not as toxic as most plastics.

Propylene

Propylene is used to manufacture the monomer acrylonitrile. It is converted by a catalytic reaction involving ammonia and oxygen. Sixty percent is converted into synthetic fibers. Twelve percent is used as a constituent of copolymers (e.g., acrolein) for synthetic rubber and a further 12% is used for acrylonitryl, butadiene, styrene (ABS) polymers. Acrylonitrile has been found in sheetrock paper and is suspected of being carcinogenic.[392,395–397] The most chemically sensitive patient does not tolerate clothes made of these materials or newly hung drywall.

$$[C-N-(CH_2)_6-N-C-O-CH_2)_4-O]_n$$
$$\underset{O \ H}{\| \ |} \qquad \underset{H \ O}{| \ \|}$$

FIGURE 5.20 Polyurethane (ethylcarbamate).

TABLE 5.50
Properties of Natural and Synthetic Fibers

Properties Type of Fiber	Strength (cN) (tex)	Elongation %	Moisture Content (%)	Water Absorption (%)	Density (g/cm^3)	Melting Point (Range °C)	Resistance to Acids/ Alkalis
Cotton	15–35 (50)[a]	7–10	7–8	35–75	1.53	Carbonizes	Nonresistant/good
Wool	10–16	25/48	15	28–42	1.30	Carbonizes	Good/nonresistant
Silk	30–45	18–24	11	54	1.25	Carbonizes	Good/nonresistant
Staple viscose (rayon)	20–30 (40)[a]	15–20 (30)	13	80–125	1.52	Carbonizes	Nonresistant/good
Acetate	13–17	16–31	6.5	50	1.31	Carbonizes	Nonresistant/good
Polyamide	35–55 (75)[a]	15–31	4	10–14	1.15	Nylon 225 Perlon 215	Moderate/very good
Polyester	40–60 (68)[a]	10–25	0.5	1–2	1.38	255–256	Good–very good/good
Polyacrylonitrile	20–30 (50)[a]	15–18	1	2.5–3	1.18	Softens and decomposes 200–250	Very good/moderate
Structural steel (comparison) Special types[a]		27	8				

Source: Hopp, V., J. Hennig, eds. 1983. *Handbook of Applied Chemistry: Facts for Engineers, Scientists, Technicians, and Technical Managers,* pp. IV/3–IV18. Washington, DC: Hemisphere Publishing. With permission; Rea, W.J. 1994. *Chemical Sensitivity, Volume II,* page 821, table 17. With permission.

[a] Length.

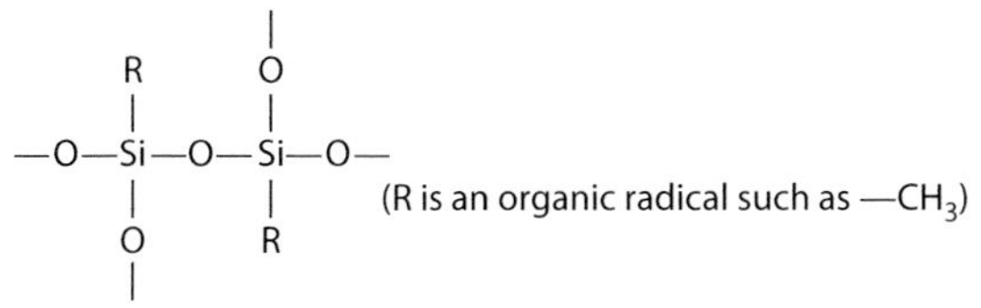

(R is an organic radical such as —CH$_3$)

FIGURE 5.21 Silicone rubber.

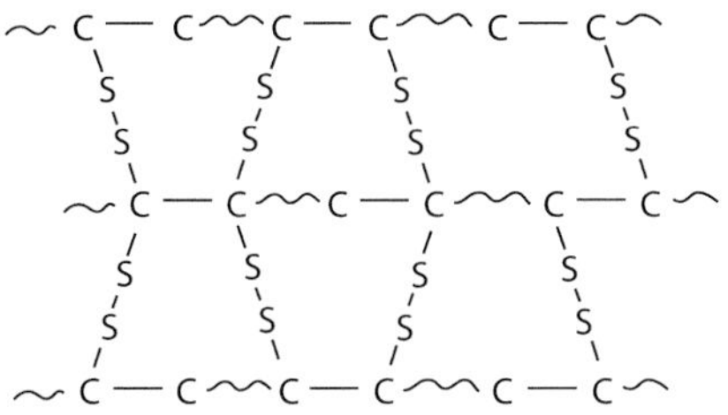

FIGURE 5.22 Vulcanized rubber. Elastomers are plastics with a wide-meshed three-dimensional cross-linked network. They are rubber-elastic to rigid-elastic.

Silicone rubber is a macromolecule with an inorganic base. The outstanding properties of silicone rubbers are their heat and weathering stability. Pure silicone rubber is acceptable for sealants in the houses of the chemically sensitive if it is used sparingly. Also, there appears to be less triggering of the clotting mechanism and vessel wall irritation in catheters made of pure silicone rubber. Arthritic and myalgic symptoms have occurred in chemically sensitive patients with silicone implants. Silicone breast implants and other silicone implants have been shown to be toxic to many individuals. They have been shown to create and exacerbate chemical sensitivity and chronic degenerative disease.[41] However, some patients have been shown to tolerate cataract eye implants (Figure 5.21).[41]

Vulcanized Rubber

The vulcanization of caoutchouc (rubber) with sulfur produces a material with wide meshed cross-linking rubber (Figure 5.22). In hard-rubber vulcanite, there are more sulfur bridges. This presence of the sulfur appears to cause problems in the chemically sensitive since there is some outgasing. The harder the substance, the less offensive it is.

PIGMENTS AND DYES

A pigment is an organic or inorganic, colored or colorless colorant that is virtually insoluble in solvents and/or vehicles. A dyestuff is an organic colorant that is soluble in solvents and/or vehicles.

Organic pigments are natural, synthetic, or combinations. The natural colorants come from fish and vegetables. Examples of the different categories of dyestuffs are mauveine and fuchsin, indigo, azo dyestuffs, indanthrene, phthalocyaines, and the reactive dyestuffs. The starting materials for organic colorants must contain inter alia, double bonds, or aromatic compounds. The basic aromatic compounds used as the bases of dyes are benzene, phenol, naphthalene, and diphenyl, all of which cause considerable problems for the chemically sensitive. Classification of organic colorants is as follows: azo, anthraquinone, indigoid, triarylmethane, sulfur, phthalocyanine, acridine, quinacridone, and perylene colorants.

Inorganic pigments include natural earth pigments (chalk, manganese ore, iron-containing aluminum, silicates), synthetic inorganic mineral pigments (bronzes), and carbon pigments (carbon black). These substances tend not to bother the chemically sensitive as much as organics.

Many of these dyes have been found to bother the chemically sensitive. The aniline dyes were known to cause bladder cancer in workers in the 1920s,[398] while the chromates are highly sensitizing. Many chemically sensitive individuals have severe adverse reactions to material dyed with aniline and chromate. Manganese toxicity has been seen to occur and the manganese is often found in chemically sensitive patients who have titanium alloy implants which cause problems with chemical sensitivity.

DETERGENTS

Detergents are substances that allow the penetration of water into lipid areas that are non-water-soluble. Hydrocarbons such as petrol and mineral oils are completely insoluble in water while acids such as acetic or sulfuric acids are miscible with water. This solubility is connected with the fact that both are polar compounds. Decomposition of fats and oils occurs naturally by means of alkalis, yielding the alkali metal salts of fatty acids, the soaps, or artificially by synthetic aliphatic hydrocarbons attaching to acids. The attaching of acids makes them polar and more hydrophilic. There are anionic, cationic, and nonionic substances. The anions, especially the natural ones, are the least toxic and often tolerated by most of the chemically sensitive. Natural soaps are sodium salts of stearic and palmitic acid while soft soaps consist of potassium salts of these acids. The most important synthetic anionic soaps include sodium alkylbenzene sulfonate, sodium alkyl sulfonate, and sodium alkyl sulfate. These, in themselves, may cause less environmental damage with degradation occurring in 10 days versus other synthetic detergents.[399] However, these synthetics may be troublesome to the chemically sensitive individual. Cationic detergents (positively charged), for example, quaternary ammonium salts, are poisonous to microorganisms and can be used for disinfection. These substances are generally not very harmful to humans, but we have seen some chemically sensitive individuals react to them. At the EHC-Dallas, we use benzalkoniums as disinfectants because of their lesser reactivity in the chemically sensitive.

Substances such as polyethylene glycols do not form ions in aqueous solutions. These solutions do not foam, so they are used in washing machines. They were thought to be physiologically inert and, therefore, are used as emulsifiers in medicines and cosmetics. However, reactions have now been found to substances like the glycols, and these detergents present a problem with many of the chemically sensitive patients. They can overload the alcohol oxidative reduction systems during detoxification.

Surface-active substances order and layer the lipophilic and hydrophilic part of substances. The droplets of oil or dirt particles become electrically charged. As they have a similar charge, the individual particles have a mutual repulsion for one another. This repulsion makes agglomeration more difficult but promotes further dispersion. The lipophilic part is lined up to the air and the hydrophilic part is in the water. Thus, it is washed away. The addition of surface-active substances makes it easier for water to penetrate cavities in textiles and to wet water-repellant substances such as fat, dirt, and oil.

The synthetic sulfonates are superior to soaps because they form soluble salts with the Ca and Mg of hardwater. Since Ca and Mg have hardly any detergent action, polyphosphates are added to bond them. Besides their use as detergents, surface-active substances are used as firefighting foam and dust suppressors, in the production of emulsions of plastics and bitumen in the building industry, and for boring and cutting oils. All of these substances can cause problems in humans by decreasing the surface activity of the skin and lungs.

TEFLON TOXICOSIS

This entity can occur in 2–5 minutes on a conventional stovetop. Cookware coated with Teflon and other nonstick surfaces can exceed temperatures at which the coating breaks apart and emits toxic particles and gases linked to hundreds, perhaps thousands, of pet bird deaths and an unknown number of human illnesses each year, according to tests commissioned by Environmental Working Group (EWG).

A generic nonstick frying pan preheated on a conventional, electric stovetop burner reached 736°F in 3 minutes and 20 seconds, with temperatures still rising when the tests were terminated. A Teflon pan reached 721°F in just 5 minutes under the same test conditions, as measured by a commercially available infrared thermometer. DuPont studies show that the Teflon offgases toxic particulates at 464°F. At 680°F, Teflon pans release at least six toxic gases, including two carcinogens, two global pollutants, and MFA, a chemical lethal to humans at low doses. At temperatures that DuPont scientists claim are reached on stovetop drip pans (1000°F), nonstick coatings break down to a chemical warfare agent PFIB, and a chemical analog of the WWII nerve gas phosgene.

For the past 50 years, DuPont has claimed that their Teflon coatings do not emit hazardous chemicals through normal use. DuPont wrote that "significant decomposition of the coating will occur only when temperatures exceed about 660°F (340°C). These temperatures alone are well above the normal cooking range."

These new tests show that cookware exceeds these temperatures and turns toxic through the common act of preheating a pan, on a burner set on high.

In cases of "Teflon toxicosis," as the bird poisonings are called, the lungs of exposed birds hemorrhage and fill with fluid, leading to suffocation. DuPont acknowledges that the fumes can also sicken people, a condition called "polymer fume fever." DuPont has never studied the incidence of the fever among users of the billions of nonstick pots and pans sold around the world. Neither has the company studied the long-term effects from the sickness, or the extent to which Teflon exposures lead to human illnesses often believed erroneously to be the common flu.[400]

The government has not assessed the safety of nonstick cookware. According to a Food and Drug Administration (FDA) food safety scientist, "You won't find a regulation anywhere on the books that specifically addresses cookwares," although the FDA approved Teflon for contact with food in 1960 based on a food frying study that found higher levels of Teflon chemicals in hamburger cooked on heat-aged and old pans. At the time, FDA judged these levels to be of little health significance.

Of the 6.9 million bird-owning households in the United States that claim an estimated 19 million pet birds, many do not know that Teflon poses an acute hazard to birds. Most nonstick cookware carries no warning label. DuPont publicly acknowledges that Teflon can kill birds, but the company-produced public service brochure on bird safety discusses the hazards of ceiling fans, mirrors, toilets, and cats before mentioning the dangers of Teflon fumes.

As a result of the new data showing that nonstick surfaces reach toxic temperatures in a matter of minutes, EWG has petitioned the Consumer Product Safety Commission (CPSC) to require that cookware and heated appliances bearing nonstick coatings must carry a label warning of the acute hazard the coating poses to pet birds. Additionally, they recommend that bird owners completely avoid cookware and heated appliances with nonstick coatings. Alternative cookware includes stainless steel, cast iron, and glass, none of which offgases persistent pollutants that kill birds.

Bird deaths have been documented during or immediately after the following normal cooking scenarios: New Teflon-lined Amana oven was used to bake biscuits at 325°F; all the owner's baby parrots died (Stewart, Bob. 2002. Personal communication with Dr. Jennifer Klein, Environmental Working Group. May 9, 2002; Stewart, Bob. 2002. Personal email communication with Anne Morgan, Environmental Working Group). Four stovetop burners, underlined with Teflon-coated drip pans, were preheated in preparation for Thanksgiving dinner; 14 birds died within 15 minutes.[401,402] Nonstick cookie sheet was placed under oven broiler to catch the drippings; 107 chicks died. Self-cleaning feature on the oven was used; a $2000 bird died.[402] Set of Teflon pans, including egg poaching pan, were attributed to seven bird deaths over 7 years.[403] Water burned off a hot pan; more than 55 birds died.[404] Electric skillet at 300°F and space heater were used simultaneously; pet bird died.[405] Toaster oven with a nonstick coating was used to prepare food at a normal temperature; bird survived but suffered respiratory distress.[406] Water being heated for hot cocoa boiled off completely; pet bird died (Anonymous 2003. Email correspondence to Environmental Working Group.

TABLE 5.51
Presence of Aldehydes in Buildings

Compound Aldehydes	4555-1 Bedroom μg/m³	4555-1 Bedroom ppbv	4555-2 Kitchen μg/m³	4555-2 Kitchen ppbv	4555-3 Living Room μg/m³	4555-3 Living Room ppbv	Typical Sources
Formaldehyde	45	37	35	29	45	37	Paint, particle board, plywood, and adhesives
Acetaldehyde	18	10	14	8	21	12	Food products, perfumes, tobacco smoke, auto exhaust, and paints
Acrylaldehyde	<1	<1	<1	<1	<1	<1	Cooking oils
Propionaldehyde	<1	<1	<1	<1	<1	<1	Food products and paints
Crotonaldehyde	<1	<1	<1	<1	<1	<1	
Butyraldehyde	3	1	2	1	3	1	Food products, degradation of fats, and oils
Benzaldehyde	1	<1	<1	<1	<1	<1	Oil alkyd paints, coatings, and adhesives
Tolualdehyde, *o*, *m*, and *p*	<1	<1	<1	<1	<1	<1	
Valeraldehyde	4	1	3	1	7	2	
Hexaldehyde	32	8	14	3	29	6	
Heptaldehyde	<1	<1	<1	<1	<1	<1	
Total	103	57	68	42	105	58	

Source: Environmental Health Center-Dallas.

April 2003).[407] Grill plate on gas stove used to prepare food at normal temperatures; two birds died on two separate occasions[408] (Anonymous 2003. Email correspondence to Environmental Working Group. April 2003).

DuPont claims that its coating remains intact indefinitely at 500°F.[409] Experiences of consumers whose birds have died from fumes generated at lower temperatures show that this is not the case. In one case, researchers at the University of Missouri documented the deaths of about 1000 broiler chicks exposed to offgas products from coated heat lamps at 396°F.[410]

DuPont also claims that human illness will be produced only in cases that involved gross over-heating or burning of the food to an inedible state.[409] Yet DuPont's own scientists have concluded that polymer fume fever in humans is possible at 662°F, a temperature easily exceeded when a pan is preheated on a burner or placed beneath a broiler, or in a self-cleaning oven.[411]

The relationship of organic chemicals to chemical sensitivity is legion. We have only scratched the surface in this chapter. The student of chemical sensitivity will have to study chemistry texts to learn the effects of specific chemicals and apply this knowledge to particular cases (Table 5.51).

ENDOCRINE DISRUPTORS OBESITY

PLEIOTROIC ACTIONS OF INSULIN RESISTANCE AND INFLAMMATION IN METABOLIC HOMEOSTASIS

Metabolism and immunity are inextricably linked both to each other and organism-wide function, allowing mammals to adapt to changes in their internal and external environments. In the modern context of obesogenic diets and lifestyles, however, these adaptive responses can have deleterious consequences. In this review, Odegaard and Chawla[412] discussed the pleiotropic actions of inflammation and insulin resistance in metabolic homeostasis and disease.[412] This information is coupled with our inputs of other aspects of the environmental pollution and obesity. An appreciation of the adaptive context in which these responses arose is useful for understanding their pathogenic actions in disease.[412]

According to Odegaard and Chawla,[412] humans have evolutionarily confronted three primary killers: starvation, infection, and predation. Through modern agriculture, hygiene, and our relatively recent elevation to top predator status, we have made remarkable progress in mitigating these, only to find new, evolutionary novel threats taking their place, principally, cardiovascular disease, diabetes, and cancer. Unmasked by our successes against more ancient challenges, these modern diseases represent a rapidly increasing share of human morbidity and mortality in both relative and absolute terms and threaten the gains in life expectancy already achieved. In recent years, obesity has emerged as the driving force behind these disturbing trends.

From 1980 to 2008 alone, the number of overweight individuals worldwide doubled to more than half a billion people, eclipsing the number of underweight individuals for the first time in history and driving the obesity attributable death rate to 3 million per year.[413] More poignantly, even a spare handful of extra pounds in midlife is associated with a (20–59) 40% increase in all-cause mortality, obesity with an ~100% increase, and morbid obesity with an ~300% increase.[414] Despite such chilling numbers, the true effect of obesity is still likely to be understated.

Notwithstanding its catastrophic consequences, obesity's importance went long unappreciated because it acts less by overt effect than by promoting/exacerbating cardiovascular disease, diabetes, and cancer among other diseases. Indeed, the mechanistic links between obesity and better established pathologies have been highly investigated over the past two decades. Odegaard and Chawla[412] primarily explore the cellular and molecular connections between chronic low-grade inflammation, insulin resistance, and obesity-induced metabolic disease. They begin by summarizing the current mechanistic understanding of obesity-induced insulin resistance and then discuss the importance of the histologic and evolutionary context within which it arises. Specifically, the argument presented that key mediators of obesity-induced metabolic disease, such as insulin resistance and inflammation, are evolutionarily conserved adaptive traits with maladaptive effects in the modern obesogenic environment. Clearly, organic chemicals play a large part of the problem. Total body and individual specific pollutant load in the form of organic and inorganic chemicals, as well as particulate, must be considered.

Obesity-Induced Insulin Resistance

The fundamental characteristic of obesity is chronic imbalance between caloric intake and energy expenditure, resulting in the storage of excess nutrients in which white adipose tissue (WAT)[415] is the prime result. In lean individuals, metabolic tissues such as WAT, liver, and skeletal muscle readily buffer excess nutrients by storing them as triglycerides and glycogen. Along with these nutrients is the storage of toxic chemicals and responses to EMF which enters in excess from the environment. With chronic over nutrition, however, the storage capacity of metabolic tissues is eventually exceeded. According to Odegaard and Chawla,[412] this causes intracellular buffering mechanisms within dedicated nutrient-storing cells to break down with excess nutrients overflowing into physiologic compartments that are ill equipped for substrate handling. This breakdown releases toxic chemicals as well as nutrients. Consequently, both professional metabolic and bystander tissues are exposed to super-physiologic levels of metabolic substrates, as well as toxic chemicals, resulting in cell-intrinsic and cell-extrinsic dysfunction.[416,417] This dysfunction is aided by the release of toxic chemicals back into the local and at times into the general bloodstream, often causing localized or generalized metabolic dysfunction. The primary cell-intrinsic dysfunctions include lipid deregulation (e.g., accumulation of intracellular diacylglycerols saturated fatty acids, and ceramides), abnormal intracellular protein modification, mitochrondrial dysfunction, oxidative stress, and endoplasmic reticulum/membrane stress. Ectopic lipid deposition, abnormal extracellular protein modification (such as hemoglobin A1c and advanced glycation end-products), and adipokine deregulation represent the major cell-extrinsic pathways. With persistent imbalance between energy intake and expenditure, these processes escalate and eventually lead to adipocyte death as is observed in obese WAT.[418]

Obesity-induced cellular dysfunction activates a diverse range of stress-responsive and counter-regulatory signaling pathways, including kinases (JNK), inhibitor of nuclear factor $_k$B (I_kB) kinase β (IKKβ), endoplasmic reticulum-to-nucleus signaling 1 (IRE-1), to mammalian target of rapamycin (mTOR), extracellular signal-regulated kinases (ERKs), protein kinase Cθ(PKCθ), suppressor of cytokine signaling (SOCS) proteins, and RNA-activated protein kinase (PKR)[416,417,419–423] Although a detailed discussion is beyond the scope of this review, these pathways collaborate to produce two metabolically important effects. According to Odegaard and Chawla,[412] first, each pathway converges on and inhibits insulin signaling pathways, primarily through serine phosphorylation of insulin receptor substrate (IRS) proteins, which blunts insulin action in stressed target tissues and stems the influx of nutrients into already overwhelmed cells. Second, these signals converge on two main inflammatory signaling pathways, JNK and IKKβ, to initiate, support, and augment an inflammatory response within metabolic tissues. In parallel with these actions, deregulated nutrient intake can also bypass cellular stress responses entirely and trigger inflammatory activation through a variety of mechanisms, including triggering of innate immune receptors (e.g., saturated fatty acids-fetuin A ligation of Toll-like receptor 4),[424] increased gut-derived lipopolysaccharide (LPS) translocation, and intestinal dysbiosis.[425] In selected patients and perhaps most or all obese, develop an entry of Ca^{2+} into the cell and then combine with protein kinases A and C which when phosphorylated increases the sensitivity to pollutant entry and injury up to 1000 times.

Despite using similar pathways and mediators, the inflammatory response in obesity differs substantially in duration and intensity from that observed in the more familiar setting of infection. For instance, infectious inflammation involves short-lived, high-amplitude responses, whereas metabolic inflammation, like other chronic inflammatory conditions, smolders at low levels for years to decades. Although the underlying mechanisms contributing to these differences are not entirely clear, it seems likely that hormonal or epigenetic programming may permanently reassign certain systemic and tissue-specific parameters, such as body weight and leukocyte activation, in obesity.[426] Once the hypersensitivity to environmental pollutants occurs, the total body pollutant load accelerates the body to many abnormal responses increasing the dysmetabolism response hormones like insulin.

According to Odegaard and Chawla,[412] inflammatory activation within metabolic tissues potentiates insulin resistance and metabolic disease by three principal means.[427] First, inflammatory signaling pathways, such as cellular stress-induced and counter-regulatory cascades, inhibit insulin signaling through direct inhibitory serine phosphorylation of IRS proteins by JNK and IKKβ.[421] Second, secreted inflammatory mediators (such as the chemokine [C–C Motif] ligand 2 [CcL2], Ccl5, and Ccl8 which are produced by lipid-engorged adipocytes) recruit circulating leukocytes (such as Ll7C^{Hi} monocytes) to stressed tissue to augment the inflammatory signaling and tissue remodeling capacity of tissue-resident cells.[427] Third, secreted inflammatory mediators communicate insulin resistance systemically as well as locally to recruited leukocytes, biasing them toward an inflammatory phenotype.[423,427] Although the first effect involves professional nutrient handling cells, such as adipocytes, hepatocytes, and skeletal myocytes, the latter two establish a stable, feed-forward signaling loop in which tissue-resident and recruited leukocytes sustain and augment both local and systemic inflammation and insulin resistance.

According to Odegaard and Chawla,[412] as might be expected, activation of this inflammatory circuit is accompanied by shifts in leukocyte populations and activation status that have profound effects on systemic metabolic parameters. In obesity, for example, macrophages increase from ~10% of all adipose tissue cells to over 50%, shift from an even to a clustered topographic distribution (primarily because of the appearance of necrotic adipocytes), and swap an immunoregulatory M2 phenotype (CD206$^+$, Arg1$^+$, and CD301$^+$) for a proinflammatory M1 bias (CD11c$^+$, nitric oxide synthase 2$^+$ [NOS2$^+$], and tumor necrosis factor-α$^+$(TNFα$^+$).[428–431] Adipose-tissue-associated lymphocytes undergo a similar reorganization with the small T helper 2(T_H2)/regulatory T cell

(T_{reg}cell)-dominated repertoire associated with lean individuals giving way to a much larger and more inflammatory T_H1/CD8-dominated population in the obese.[432–434] Furthermore, interleukin-4 (IL-4)-expressing eosinophils resident in lean WAT are displaced by waves of ingressing neutrophils, mast cells, and B cells in obese individuals.[435–437]

According to Odegaard and Chawla,[412] the marked shift in leukocyte population represents a key mechanistic link in the progression from overfeeding-related cellular stress to metabolic deregulation to frank disease.[438] In lean mice, alternative M2 macrophages, T_{re} cells, eosinophils, and invariant natural killer T cells collaborate to maintain an insulin-sensitive, tolerogenic immune environment.[429,432,435,439–443] Functional depletion of any of these leukocyte lineages disrupts this collaborative effort, destabilizing the anti-inflammatory environment, negatively affecting adipocyte insulin signaling, and exacerbating the deleterious effects of high-fat diets. Supplementation of any one of these cellular constituents has the opposite effect. Through the mechanisms discussed above, obesity reorganized the leukocyte landscape into an insulin-resistant, proinflammatory milieu in which the tolerogenic leukocyte network is disrupted and replaced with inflammatory (M1 macrophages, CD8+ T cells, and T_H1 cells). Functional depletion of any one of these lineages weakens this inflammatory influence, lessening the effects of obesogenic diets, whereas their supplementation exacerbates inflammation and disease.[433,434,444] Furthermore, even interventions that prevent or augment recruitment of new leukocytes to WAT without influencing the existing leukocyte populations (e.g., abrogation or amplification of the Ccl2–Ccr2 chemotactic axis) can dramatically modulate obesity-associated insulin resistance.[445,446]

According to Odegaard and Chawla,[412] although WAT, the most structurally dynamic nutrient-storing tissue, demonstrates dramatic alterations in obesity, similar leukocyte shifts take place in other metabolically important organs as well. For example, obesity precedes restructuring of pancreas- and liver-associated leukocyte populations (although the latter occurs without substantial change in macrophage number),[440,447,448] whereas brain and skeletal muscle acquire inflammatory microenvironments without substantial numeric alterations in leukocyte complements.[449,450] Coincident with this shift, the major tissue targets of insulin action begin to advertise the hallmarks of insulin resistance: increased triglyceride lipolysis in WAT; increased insulin production in pancreatic islets; elevated gluconeogenesis, glycogenolysis, and lipogenesis in the liver; decreased insulin-stimulated glucose disposal in skeletal muscle; and decreased satiety signaling in the brain. Shifts in the leukocyte populations occurring in these organs have systemic importance similar in scope to those occurring in adipose tissue. For example, liver-selective abrogation of alternative M2 macrophage activation results in increased obesity and systemic metabolic disease in response to high-fat diet,[439,440] a phenotype similar to that seen in whole-animal abrogation of the alternative M2 program.[429,441,442,451] These data support an integral role for resident leukocytes in local, tissue-specific manifestations of metabolic disease, and indicate that leukocyte deregulatiaon in even one tissue bed increases systemic susceptibility to metabolic disease.

According to Odegaard and Chawla,[412] although obesity-induced metabolic disease promotes and exacerbates pathology through numerous disease-specific mechanisms, most pathology ultimately arises from obesity's characteristic milieu of chronic low-grade inflammation and insulin resistance; the most important fact being what stimulates and triggers this low-grade inflammation and what can be done to eliminate it. For example, obesity has been recognized for decades as an important risk factor for cardiovascular disease; however, only recently that risk has been mechanistically understood as a result of obesity's accompanying inflammation and insulin resistance.[452] Similarly, hyperlipidemia, another well-described contributor to cardiovascular disease, arises as a consequence of inflammatory insulin resistance through increased adipose tissue lipolysis and hepatic lipogenesis. Even the biomechanical dynamics of cardiovascular disease, arterosclerotic plaque formation, remodeling, and rupture, are influenced by the inflammatory milieu.[452] It is necessary for long-run reduction of the total environmental and total body pollutant load in order to reduce the biodynamics of not only cardiovascular disease but also of inflammation and obesity. Indeed, the efficacy of some antihyperlipidemic therapies correlates with their immunomodulatory potency as much as with their lipid-lowering capacity (such as statins and salicylates).[453] Given the shared pathophysiology, it is not surprising that individuals with one cardiovascular disease risk factor often have multiple others and observation that forms the basis for metabolic syndrome.

Insulin Resistance as an Adaptive Trait

Because inflammatory insulin resistance underpins much of the overt pathology associated with obesity and excess caloric intake, there is an adopted biased view of this physiology as a maladaptive response to overfeeding. Although the clinical consequences of obesity are undoubtedly grim, three lines of evidence call into question the current view of insulin resistance as an injurious response to mounting adiposity. First, numerous examples exist in which obesity and insulin resistance are divorced, including both lean, insulin-resistant (such as lipodystrophy and mice in which caveolin-1 has been knocked out[454] and obese, insulin-sensitive states such as mice in which Fabp4 has been knocked out[455]) and cold-adapted mammals.[456] Indeed, the relationship between insulin resistance and obesity in humans is similarly disjointed,[457] with many obese individuals exhibiting better insulin sensitivity than expected for their adiposity.[458] Moreover, many of the most widely used insulin-sensitizing pharmaceuticals are associated with an increase in adiposity rather than a decrease (e.g., thiazolidinedione treatment).[459] This is why proper diet and a less polluted environment are so necessary for some people.

Second, insulin resistance develops as an evolutionarily conserved adaptive response in specific physiologic contexts unassociated with obesity. For example, both infection and pregnancy require organisms to reserve priority nutrient access for an emerging metabolic requirement-immune system activation and fetal development, respectively, in this instance. According to Odegaard and Chawla,[412] organisms meet these requirements by decreasing systemic insulin sensitivity (developing insulin resistance), decreasing nutrient uptake by nonpriority tissues, and reserving glucose for priority cells. Indeed, the resulting adaptive physiology in both situations closely resembles that which develops in the context of obesity.[426,460]

According to Odegaard and Chawla,[412] lastly, extreme diet-induced obesity, complete with systemic insulin resistance, hyperinsulinemia, and hyperlipidemia is observed as an evolutionarily conserved, adaptive, and entirely pathology-free response in mammalian hibernators.[456] These animals circannually engage in postreproduction periods of overfeeding and rapidly eat themselves into what in humans would be morbid obesity; some *Zapus* species, for example, enter hibernation with fat comprising more than 80% of their body weight (for comparison, the threshold for human obesity is ~25% in males and ~32% in females).[461] For most hibernators, autumnal obesity is accompanied by physiologic hallmarks of type 2 diabetes and metabolic syndrome, including decreased insulin sensitivity in primary target tissues and substantial elevations in LDL cholesterol levels.[456,462] Although its exact role is unclear, insulin resistance may function in this context as both a sensor of nutrient stores and as an instructive signal for tissues to switch from glucose to fatty acid metabolism in preparation for hibernation.

Despite meeting clinical criteria for type 2 diabetes and metabolic syndrome, hibernators demonstrate no pathologic consequences of their brief bout with obesity; after shedding their extra fat during the winter fast, animals are able to immediately enter into the reproductive cycle. Nor are the ill effects of circannual obesity transient; in one Swedish study, atherosclerotic lesions were entirely absent from the major vessels of obese, insulin-resistant hibernators despite marked hyperlipidemia.[462] Similarly, obese hibernators fail to develop the smoldering inflammation that characterizes human obesity despite similar metabolic parameters.[456,463] The absence of pathology despite remarkably similar metabolic states suggests that transient obesity and insulin resistance are not necessarily pathologic and may in fact be part of an adaptive, evolutionarily conserved response to excess nutrient storage. The fact that may be missing is the understudy of the effects of the testing in this scenario may be the key for not developing inflammation and insulin resistance. We have used testing, avoidance, and intradermal treatment as a therapeutic tool in the hypersensitive neurovascular patient for 40 years very successfully. Often, the hypersensitivity is eliminated and metabolism restored in these environmentally sensitive patients. Weight loss and inflammation often subside.

According to Odegaard and Chawla,[412] pregnancy, sepsis, and hibernation-associated insulin resistance demonstrate that transient inhibition of insulin signaling can be advantageous in certain adaptations between organisms as diverse as flies and humans, demonstrating that the capacity for insulin resistance is sufficiently advantageous to be conserved through millions of years of evolutionary divergence. This observation, however, is hardly surprising given the evolutionary primacy of infection, starvation, predation, and, above all, reproduction. Indeed, insulin resistance confers evolutionary advantages and enhances organism fitness in each of these categories: fueling immune function to combat infection, switching hibernator metabolic substrate preference from glucose to lipids to avoid starvation, and reserving metabolic resources for fetal development to optimize reproduction. Insulin resistance is even likely advantageous in predation-driven selection because the "fight-or-flight" response involves antagonism of insulin signaling by the stress-responsive hormones, catecholamines, and glucocorticoids.[464] In this context, acute inhibition of insulin's anabolic actions mobilizes stored nutrients to fuel a heightened state of arousal and combat the threat of predation. The pleiotropy and evolutionary importance of variable insulin sensitivity may then explain the diversity of metabolic, inflammatory, hormonal, dietary, and behavioral pathways that influence insulin signaling.

Many of these conserved and evolutionarily important pathways are active in obesity-induced metabolic disease, and although much of the resulting physiology appears pathologic, insulin resistance's full effect remains unclear. For example, one of the consequences of insulin resistance in obesity is to limit further nutrient uptake by overloaded cells. Certainly, nutrient toxicity is consequences worth avoiding, which include necrosis of engorged adipocytes found in obese adipose tissue.[418] Without insulin resistance to limit further nutrient uptake, this fate may well extend to other adipocytes, decreasing the storage pool available for excess nutrients and establishing a vicious cycle in which fewer and fewer cells are available to shoulder already overwhelming metabolic burdens. After the adipose tissue depots collapse, skeletal myocyte and hepatocyte depots would similarly fail, followed closely by nonprofessional nutrient-storage tissues. Organisms would be able to quite literally eat themselves to death.

Appreciation of this possibility has led some to reconsider the therapeutic potential of insulin-sensitizing treatments as a core approach to obesity-associated metabolic disease.[465] Targeting a potentially adaptive response to overfeeding, although moderately, is effective in reducing its unfortunate long-term consequences, which is unlikely to effectively treat the underlying physiologic defect. Rather, effective therapies are more likely to target the fundamental energetic imbalance that underpins the entire state.[466] These modalities include 1000 caloric intake of less chemically contaminated food and less pollutant containing air and water.

Also, a less toxic and hypoallergenic diet of iron stops the food craving allowing for massive weight loss. Certainly, fasting the individual for periods of time helps the obesity-induced metabolism to clear and change the body to physiologic state.

ADAPTIVE METABOLIC LEUKOCYTE ACTIVATION

Careful study of diet-induced obesity has identified chronic leukocyte-mediated low-grade inflammation within professional metabolic tissues as the characteristic pathophysiology of metabolic syndrome.[423,427] This focus on obesity, however, has limited our understanding of leukocyte activation to the role in promoting metabolic disease. Nonetheless, leukocytes are normally present in metabolic tissues, where they perform nonredundant, supportive functions.[438] In lean WAT, for example, eosinophil-derived IL-4 drives the production of IL-10 and other mediators by macrophages. This phenotype is critical for the maintenance of both adipocyte insulin sensitivity (IL-10 directly potentiates insulin signaling in adipocytes[428]) and the general anti-inflammatory timbre of the WAT microenvironment (both directly and through support of adipose tissue resident T_{reg} cells).[427] Congruent with these observations, disruption of IL-4 production or signaling in adipose tissue macrophages results in adipocyte dysfunction, insulin resistance, and metabolic disease.[429,435,439–441] In contrast, augmentation of IL-4 signaling blunts the deleterious effects of high-fat-diet challenge.[435,467]

Alternatively, activated M2 macrophages are also an indispensable component of the nonshivering thermogenic response of brown adipose tissue (BAT), the sole dedicated thermogenic tissue in mammals.[468] Cold exposure elicits this response via hypothalamic stimulation of BAT-innervating efferents of the sympathetic nervous system that, in turn, activates brown adipocytes by releasing catecholamines. Once activated, brown adipocytes oxidize fatty acids and dissipate the resulting mitochondrial proton gradient via uncoupling protein-1, liberating heat.[468] Alternative MS macrophages form an indispensable component of this adrenergic synapse, accounting for ~50% of the total catecholamine content of cold-stimulated brown and WATs.[468] In response to cold exposure, alternative M2 macrophages produce catecholamines, which together with sympathetic efferents induce the thermogenic program in brown adipocytes while simultaneously inducing lipolysis in adipocytes.[468] Disinterage animals lacking alternative M2 macrophages are thus unable to mount an effective thermogenic response or mobilize the fatty acids necessary to support it.

Even within the context of obesity-induced metabolic disease, leukocyte activation can be adaptive. For example, WAT infiltration by inflammatory (M1) macrophages is a well-known, necessary component of metabolic disease; however, augmentation of this leukocyte population might be necessary for certain adaptive roles as well. Infiltration of Ly6c^{Hi} monocytes/M1-biased macrophages in early obesity seems to be driven by the necrosis/apoptosis of hypertrophic adipocytes.[418] Although surrounding parenchymal cells can clear apoptotic debris in most organs, adipocyte death yields large lipid droplets whose uncontrolled lipolysis can be toxic to neighboring cells. This toxicity may be due to the liberation of toxic fat and also stored chemicals. Thus, in obese WAT, newly recruited M1 macrophages would encapsulate and sequester the lipid droplet and eventually eliminate it.[418] Without professional phagocyte intervention, these adipocyte corpses would presumably persist, releasing necrotic cellular debris and free lipids as well as toxic chemicals to the detriment of surrounding tissue.

Although their intervention is undoubtedly necessary, these phagocytic macrophages demonstrate a M1 bias presumably in response to necrotic debris and are thought to be a major source of inflammatory cytokines in obese adipose tissue.[428] Disposal of apoptotic cell corpses, however, is not necessarily associated with an inflammatory phenotype.[469] Indeed, clearance of apoptotic cells potently suppresses macrophage activation and is strongly associated with a regulatory phenotype not entirely dissimilar from that of lean adipose-tissue-associated macrophages. Therapeutic manipulation of the manner in which macrophages dispose off, dying adipocytes may thus remove a major proinflammatory influence without compromising necessary function.

INTEGRATING TISSUE ARCHITECTURE WITH FUNCTION

According to Odegaard and Chawla,[412] the work in obesity, adipose tissue homeostasis, and thermogenesis suggests a close, functional integration of adipocytes, and tissue-resident leukocytes in both BAT and WAT. Indeed, the numeric and spatial distribution of these cells within the tissue suggests that this would be the case.[470] At baseline, adipose-tissue-resident leukocyte number and distribution vary little between individuals and are maintained even across species, whereas their depletion results in rapid and precise restoration of the original leukocyte complement without changes in representation/distribution or encroachment by other populations.[438] Some adipose-tissue-resident leukocytes even display distinct, tissue-specific features that distinguish them from cells of similar lineage present elsewhere in the body. For example, WAT-resident T_{reg} cells demonstrate a different transcriptional profile characterized by the expression of genes more characteristically associated with neighboring adipocytes, including peroxisome proliferator activated receptor γ (PPARγ), the "master regulator" of adipogenesis.[471] These data suggest that resident leukocytes may acquire specific features in support of functional roles particular to the tissue in which they reside.

Despite our focus on it thus far, adipose tissue is not singular in its incorporation of leukocytes. Most tissues, in fact, demonstrate orderly components of resident leukocytes, suggesting that perhaps tissue-resident leukocytes play integrated roles elsewhere as well. Indeed, like adipose-tissue-associated macrophages, Kupffer cells of the liver, sinusoidal macrophages of the spleen, microglia of the brain, and alveolar macrophages of the lung are all phenotypically distinct populations with characteristic gene expression patterns and spatial distributions.[472] Although there are well-described functional specializations underlying these phenotypic differences in many tissues (e.g., senescent red blood cell clearance by splenic red pulp macrophages[472]) and neural synapse pruning by microglia,[473] the roles of resident leukocytes remain unexplored in others.

According to Odegaard and Chawla,[412] the recognition of obesity as a primary source of human disease has engendered fierce interesting metabolic dysfunction and identified inflammatory insulin resistance as its central pathophysiology. The focus in this matter, however, largely has been on the study of artificial metabolic extremes such as high-fat-diet challenge, lipid infusion, and monogenic models, total and specific environmental toxic lead exposure in air, food, and water. These approaches and the simplifications they circumscribe yield valuable insight into human disease; however, they are limited in their ability to describe the complex, nonextreme forms of obesity-induced metabolic disease that dominate the clinical landscape. For example, a genetically defined caged rodent fed mounds of sugared milk fat and lard over a few months, the basic experimental model of diet-induced obesity approximates, but will never faithfully recapitulate, an obese human. Our challenge then is to place experimental observations in a more nuanced, relevant context.

First, observations from reductionist disease models such as high-fat feeding must be compared with the disease itself with clinical observation and intervention. For example, identification of leptin as a potent regulator of feeding behavior by using the ob/ob mouse was popularly hailed as an "obesity cure" and was only placed in proper context by subsequent clinical characterization of obesity-related leptin resistance.[465] This argument implies that the current popularity of genetic intervention (e.g., gene knockouts, floxed alleles, and gain- or loss-of-function mutants) must be tempered by careful search for similar aberrations in human cohorts, as exemplified by the recent studies on Gpr120.[474] Moreover, this comparison can also be exploited in the reverse direction. Due to the "trial and error" approach of several clinical research, both therapeutic success and failures are often instructive, as demonstrated by both the relative success of surgical approaches and failure of pharmaceuticals in the treatment of obesity.[475] The contamination of food, water, and air and theory combined with EMF exposure chemical sensitivity must be taken into account as to the etiology of obesity.

Second, disease models and clinical observations must be compared with similar models and clinical observations of health. For example, leukocyte activation is a central pathophysiology in diet-induced obesity; however, the proactive effects of WAT- and liver-associated macrophages and WAT-associated T cells in lean, healthy rodent clearly demonstrate that leukocyte activation is context-dependent and explains the otherwise paradoxical exacerbation of metabolic pathology that accompanies complete loss of these lineages. Indeed, these observations have suggested novel therapeutic avenues, including pharmacologic skewing of macrophages and lymphocytes toward regulatory phenotypes. In addition, a number of inflammatory pathways that regulate energy expenditure and insulin resistance as IKKe, PKR, and Gpr120 might be suitable for therapeutic targeting of obesity-associated metabolic disease.[422,474,476,477]

Last, disease models and clinical observations must be compared with physiologically similar but pathologically distinct situations. The negative effects of insulin resistance, for instance, are much less clear in the context of pregnancy and infection, whereas the pathology-free "metabolic syndrome" of obese hibernators suggests that our current understanding of causality in human diet-induced obesity is incomplete. Although studies focusing on this particular context are rare, Odegaard and Chawla[412] have already discussed three biological scenarios, pregnancy, infection, and hibernation, in which aspects of obesity-induced metabolic disease manifest and regress. Careful study of how organisms reestablish metabolic normality after these events may provide insights into how we might reestablish the same in obesity-induced metabolic disease. Of course, the fasting of the animal in hibernation has been overlooked as an essential tool in the prevention and treatment of the metabolic syndrome in obesity. We at the EHC-Dallas have used fasting as a tool for 30 years in the chemically sensitive obese individual successfully as shown throughout the text.

Our current knowledge of metabolic biology and the basic mechanisms of obesity-induced metabolic disease are impressive. The remarkable progress in this field, however, has largely failed to translate into meaningful therapeutic advances in our struggle with obesity and metabolic disease, in part, because of a failure to place empiric studies in the proper clinical, physiological, and biological context. Especially, the environmental science and the total environmental and total body pollutant load are poorly and rarely considered. More attention has to be paid to this avenue of science and thinking. The challenge going forward, then, is to provide that context for the wealth of information available in order to identify root pathophysiologies and to appropriately target emerging therapeutics.

REFERENCES

1. Schnare, D. W., M. Ben, M. G. Shields. 1984. Body burden reductions of PCBs, PBBs, and chlorinated pesticides in human subjects. *Ambio* 13:378–380.
2. Schnare, D. W., G. Denk, M. Shields, S. Brunton. 1982. Evaluation of detoxification regimen for fat stored xenobiotics. *Med. Hypotheses* 9:265–282.
3. Randolph, T. H. 1962. *Human Ecology and Susceptibility to the Chemical Environment*. Springfield, IL: Charles C. Thomas.
4. Dickey, L. D., ed. 1976. *Clinical Ecology*. Springfield, IL: Charles C. Thomas.
5. Rea, W. J., M. J. Mitchell. 1982. Chemical sensitivity and the environment. *Immun. Allerg. Prac.* Sept/Oct:21–31.
6. Meggs, W. J. 1999. Mechanisms of allergy and chemical sensitivity. *Toxicol. Ind. Health* 15:331–338.
7. Ross, G. H. 1992. History and clinical presentation of the chemically sensitive patient. *Toxicol. Ind. Health* 8 (4):21–28.
8. Szallasi, A. 2001. Vanilloid receptor ligands: Hopes and realities for the future. *Drugs Aging* 18 (8): 561–573.
9. Nicolson, G. L., N. L. Nicolson. 1998. Gulf War illnesses: Complex medical, scientific and paradox. *Med. Confl. Surviv.* 14:156–165.
10. Pall, M. L. 2002. NMDA sensitization and stimulation by peroxynitrite, nitric oxide, and organic solvents as the mechanism of chemical sensitivity in multiple chemical sensitivity. *FASEB J.* 16 (11): 1407–1417.
11. Calderon-Garciduenas, L., B. Azzarelli, H. Acuna, R. Garcia, T. M. Gambling, N. Osnaya, S. Monroy, M. R. DEL Tizapantzi, J. L. Carson, A. Villarreal-Calderon, B. Rewcastle. Air pollution and brain damage. *Toxicol. Pathol.* 30:373–389.
12. Hennies, K., H.-P. Neitzke, H. Voigt. 2000. Mobile Telecommunications and Health.
13. Godish, T., ed. 1985. *Air Quality*, pp. 2, 12. Chelsea, MI: Lewis Publishers.
14. Rea, W. J. 2010–2012. Breath analysis of 500 chemical sensitive patients. EHC-Dallas.
15. Menssana Research Inc., Breathtaking Technology. Retrieved February 24, 2016.
16. Wallace, L. A. 2000. Assessing human exposure to volatile organic compounds. In *Indoor Air Quality Handbook*, J. D. Spengler, J. M. Samet, J. F. McCarthy, eds. pp. 33.1–33.35. New York City: McGraw-Hill.
17. Li, F., J. Z. Tsien. 2009. Memory and the NMDA receptors. *N. Engl. J. Med.* 361 (3):302–303.
18. Dingledine, R., K. Borges, D. Bowie, S. F. Traynelis. 1999. The glutamate receptor ion channels. *Pharmacol. Rev.* 51 (1): 7–61.
19. Liu, Y., J. Zhang. 2000. Recent development in NMDA receptors. *Chin. Med. J. (Engl.)* 113 (10):948–956.
20. Cull-Candy, S., S. Brickley, M. Farrant. 2001. NMDA receptor subunits: Diversity, development and disease. *Curr. Opin. Neurobiol.* 11 (3):327–335.
21. Paoletti, P., J. Neyton. 2007. NMDA receptor subunits: Function and pharmacology. *Curr. Opin. Pharmacol.* 7 (1):39–47.
22. Kleckner, N. W., R. Dingledine. 1988. Requirement for glycine in activation of NMDA-receptors expressed in *Xenopus* oocytes. *Science* 241 (4867):835–837.

23. Chen, P. E., M. T. Geballe, P. J. Stansfeld, A. R. Johnston, H. Yuan, A. L. Jacob, J. P. Snyder, S. F. Traynelis, D. J. Wyllie. 2005. Structural features of the glutamate binding site in recombinant NR1/NR2A N-methyl-D-aspartate receptors determined by site-directed mutagenesis and molecular modeling. *Mol. Pharmacol.* 67 (5):1470–1484.

24. Wolosker, H. 2006. D-Serine regulation of NMDA receptor activity. *Sci. STKE* 2006 (356): p. 41.

25. Zhang, L., T. Xu, S. Wang, L. Yu, D. Liu, R. Zhan, S. Y. Yu. 2013. NMDA GluN2B receptors involved in the antidepressant effects of curcumin in the forced swim test. *Prog. Neuropsychopharmacol. Biol. Psychiatry* 40:12–17.

26. Matteucci, A., R. Cammarota, S. Paradisi, M. Varano, M. Balduzzi, L. Leo, G. C. Bellenchi, C. De Nuccio, G. Carnovale-Scalzo. 2011. Curcumin protects against NMDA-induced toxicity: A possible role for NR2A subunit. *Invest. Ophthalmol. Vis. Sci.* 52 (2):1070–1077.

27. Yarotskyy, V., A. V. Glushakov, C. Sumners, N. Gravenstein, D. M. Dennis, C. N. Seubert, A. E. Martynyuk. 2005. Differential modulation of glutamatergic transmission by 3,5-dibromo-L-phenylalanine. *Mol. Pharmacol.* 67 (5):1648–1654.

28. Moskal, J., D. Leander, R. Burch. 2010. Unlocking the therapeutic potential of the NMDA receptor. *Drug Discovery and Development News.* Retrieved February 17, 2016.

29. Anderson, C. 2003. The Bad News Isn't In: A Look at Dissociative-Induced Brain Damage and Cognitive Impairment. Erowid DXM Vaults: Health. Retrieved February 17, 2016.

30. Flight, M. H. 2013. Trial watch: Phase II boost for glutamate-targeted antidepressants. *Nat. Rev. Drug Discov.* 12 (12):897.

31. Vécsei, L., L. Szalárdy, F. Fülöp, J. Toldi. 2012. Kynurenines in the CNS: Recent advances and new questions. *Nat. Rev. Drug Discov.* 12 (1):64–82.

32. Traynelis, S., S. Cull-Candy. 1990. Proton inhibition of N-methyl-D-aspartate receptors in cerebellar neurons. *Nature* 345 (6273):347–350.

33. Aizenman, E., S. A. Lipton, R. H. Loring. 1989. Selective modulation of NMDA responses by reduction and oxidation. *Neuron* 2 (3):1257–1263.

34. Yu, X. M., R. Askalan, G. J. Keil, M. W. Salter. 1997. NMDA channel regulation by channel-associated protein tyrosine kinase Src. *Science* 275 (5300):674–678. doi: 10.1126/science.275.5300.674.

35. Chen, Y., U. Beffert, M. Ertunc, T. S. Tang, E. T. Kavalali, I. Bezprozvanny, J. Herz. 2005. Reelin modulates NMDA receptor activity in cortical neurons. *J. Neurosci.* 25 (36):8209–8216.

36. Hawasli, A. H., D. R. Benavides, C. Nguyen, J. W. Kansy, K. Hayashi, P. Chambon, P. Greengard, C. M. Powell, D. C. Cooper, J. A. Bibb. 2007. Cyclin-dependent kinase 5 governs learning and synaptic plasticity via control of NMDAR degradation. *Nat. Neurosci.* 10 (7):880–886.

37. Zhang, S., L. Edelmann, J. Liu, J. E. Crandall, M. A. Morabito. 2008. Cdk5 regulates the phosphorylation of tyrosine 1472 NR2B and the surface expression of NMDA receptors. *J. Neurosci.* 28 (2):415–424.

38. Fourgeaud, L., C. M. Davenport, C. M. Tyler, T. T. Cheng, M. B. Spencer, L. M. Boulanger. 2010. MHC class I modulates NMDA receptor function and AMPA receptor trafficking. *Proc. Natl. Acad. Sci. U S A.* 107 (51):22278–22283.

39. Pall, M. 2013. The NO/ONOO-cycle as the central cause of heart failure. *Int. J. Mol. Sci.* 14 (11):22274–22330.

40. Spengler, J., K. Sexton. 1983. Indoor air pollution: A public health perspective. *Science* 221 (4605):9–17.

41. Rea, W. J. 1994. *Chemical Sensitivity: Sources of Total Body Load.* Vol. 2. Boca Raton: Lewis Publishers.

42. Wallace, L. A. 1987. *The Total Exposure Assessment Methodology (TEAM) Study: Summary and Analysis*, Vol. 1. EPA/600/6-87/002A, Washington, DC: U.S. Environmental Protection Agency.

43. Mason, I. December 19, 2008. Methane bubbling up from undersea permafrost? *National Geographic News.* Retrieved May 14, 2009.

44. Stein, Y., Y. Finkelstein, O. Levy-Nativ, O. Bonne, M. Aschner, E. D. Richter. 2010. Exposure and susceptibility: Schizophrenia in a young man following prolonged high exposures to organic solvents. *NeuroToxicology* 31 (5):603–607.

45. Mueser, K. T., S. R. McGurk. 2004. Schizophrenia. *Lancet* 363 (9426):2063–2072.

46. Tsuang, M. T., J. L. Bar, W. S. Stone, S. V. Faraone. 2004. Gene-environment interactions in mental disorders. *World Psychiatry* 3 (2):73–83.

47. Caspi, A., T. E. Moffitt. 2006. Gene-environment interactions in psychiatry: Joining forces with neuroscience. *Nat. Rev. Neurosci.* 7:583–590.

48. Wada, K., K. Nakayama, H. Koishikawa, M. Katayama, S. Hirai, T. Yabana, T. Aoki, S. Iwashita. 2005. Symptomatological structure of volatile solvent-induced psychosis: Is "solvent psychosis" a discernible syndrome? *Nihon Arukoru Yakubutsu Igakkai Zasshi* 40 (5):471–484.

49. Daniels, A. M., R. W. Latcham. 1984. Petrol sniffing and schizophrenia in a Pacific Island paradise. *Lancet* 1 (8373):389.

50. Opler, M. G., A. S. Brown, J. Graziano, M. Desai, W. Zheng, C. Schaefer, P. Factor-Litvak, E. S. Susser. 2004. Prenatal lead exposure, delta-aminolevulinic acid, and schizophrenia. *Environ. Health Perspect.* 112:548–552.

51. Kleinhaus, K., S. Harlap, M. C. Perrin, O. Manor, R. Calderon-Margalit, Y. Friedlander, D. Malaspina. 2008. Twin pregnancy and the risk of schizophrenia. *Schizophr. Res.* 105 (1–3):197–200.

52. Malaspina, D., S. Harlap, S. Fennig, D. Heiman, D. Nahon, D. Feldman, E. S. Susser. 2001. Advancing paternal age and the risk of schizophrenia. *Arch. Gen. Psychiatry* 58 (4):361–367.

53. Harlap, S Et al. 2007. The Jerusalem Perinatal Study cohort, 1964–2005: Methods and a review of the main results. *Paediatr. Perinat. Epidemiol.* 21 (3):256–273.

54. Perrin, M. C., M. G. Opler, S. Harlap, J. Harkavy-Friedman, K. Kleinhaus, D. Nahon, S. Fennig, E. S. Fennig, D. Malaspina. 2007. Tetrachloroethylene exposure and risk of schizophrenia: Offspring of dry cleaners in a population birth cohort, preliminary findings. *Schizophr. Res.* 90 (1–3):251–254.

55. Mikkelsen, S. 1997. Epidemiological update on solvent neurotoxicity. *Environ. Res.* 73 (1–2):101–112.

56. Bast-Pettersen, R. 2009. The neuropsychological diagnosis of chronic solvent induced encephalopathy (CSE)—a reanalysis of neuropsychological test results in a group of CSE patients diagnosed 20 years ago, based on comparisons with matched controls. *NeuroToxicology* 30:1195–1201.

57. Juntunen, J. 1993. Neurotoxic syndromes and occupational exposure to solvents. *Environ. Res.* 60 (1):98–111.

58. Keski-Säntti, P., A. Kaukiainen, H. K. Hyvärinen, M. Sainio. 2010. Occupational chronic solvent encephalopathy in Finland 1995–2007: Incidence and exposure. *Int. Arch. Occup. Environ. Health* 83 (6):703–712.

59. Saddik, B., A. Williamson, D. Black, I. Nuwayhid. 2009. Neurobehavioral impairment in children occupationally exposed to mixed organic solvents. *NeuroToxicology* 30:1166–1171.

60. Bolla, K. I., B. S. Schwartz, J. Agnew, P. D. Ford, M. L. Bleecker. 1990. Subclinical neuropsychiatric effects of chronic low-level solvent exposure in US paint manufacturers. *J. Occup. Med.* 32 (8):671–677.

61. van Valen, E., E. Wekking, G. van der Laan, M. Sprangers, F. van Dijk. 2009. The course of chronic solvent induced encephalopathy: A systematic review. *NeuroToxicology* 30:1172–1186.

62. Lubman, D. I., D. Velakoulis, P. D. McGorry, D. J. Smith, W. Brewer, G. Stuart, P. Desmond, B. Tress, C. Pantelis. 2002. Incidental radiological findings on brain magnetic resonance imaging in first-episode psychosis and chronic schizophrenia. *Acta Psychiatr. Scand.* 106:331–336.

63. DSM-IV-TR. Diagnostic and Statistical Manual of Mental Disorders fourth edition (Text Revision). *Diagnostic Criteria for Schizophrenia and Associated Disorders.* The American Psychiatric Association; 2000.

64. Didreksen, N. A. 2010. Assessment of Environmentally Ill-Patients for Disability. Retrieved February 24, 2016.

65. Arlien-Soborg, P., L. Simonsen. 1998. *Chemical Neurotoxic Agents. Encyclopaedia of Occupational Health and Safety,* 4th ed., Geneva: International Labour Office.

66. Valciukas, J. A. 1991. *Foundations of Environmental and Occupational Neurotoxicology.* New York: Van Nostrand Reinhold. 635 p.

67. Cattell R. B., A. K. Cattell, H. E. P. Cattell, M. T. Russell, S. Bedwell. PsychEval Personality Questionnaire. PsycTESTS Dataset.

68. Williams, G. M., J. H. Weisburger. 1986. Chemical carcinogens. In *Cassarett and Doull's Toxicology: The Basic Science of Poisons,* 3rd ed., C.D. Klaassen, M. O. Amdur, J. Doull, eds., p. 125. New York: Macmillan.

69. Isacson, P., J. A. Bean, R. Splinter, D. B. Olson, J. Kohler. 1985. Drinking water and cancer incidence in Iowa. *Am. J. Epidemiol.* 121 (6):856–869.

70. Mølhave L., J. Maller, I. Anderson. 1979. The content of gases, vapours, and dust in new houses. *Ugeskr. Laeger* 141:956–961.

71. Wallace, L. A., E. Prllizzari, T. Hartwell. 1984. Analysis of exhaled breath of 355 urban residents for volatile organic compounds. *Proceedings of International Conference on Indoor Air Quality and Climate (Stockholm)* 4:15–20.

72. Lebret, E., H. J. Varde Weil, H. T. Bos, D. Noij, J. S. M. Boleij. 1984. Volatile hydrocarbons in Dutch homes. *Proceedings of International Conference on Indoor Air Quality and Climate* 4:169–174.

73. Jarke, F. H. *Organic Contaminants in Indoor air Contaminants.* ASHRAE Report No. 183, IITRI project no C8276. Chicago: Illinois Institute of Technology Research Institute.

74. Seifert, B. 1985. *Results of the 1984 Saltzjaobaden WHO Meeting on Indoor Air Pollution. Report on the Third Annual International Symposium on Man and His Environment in Health and Disease,* Dallas, TX.

75. DeBartoli, M., H. Knoppel, E. Pecchio, A. Peil, L. Rogora, H. Schanenburg, H. Schlitt, H. Vissero. 1984. Integrating real life measurements of organic pollution in indoor and outdoor air of homes in northern Italy. *Proceedings of International Conference on Indoor Air Quality and Climate (Stockholm)* 4:21–26.

76. Mage, D. T., R. B. Gammage. 1985. Evaluation of changes in indoor air quality occurring over the past several decades. In *Indoor Air and Human Health*. R. B. Gammage, S. V. Kaye, V. A. Jacobs, eds., Chelsea, MI: Lewis Publishers.

77. American Conference of Governmental Industrial Hygienists. 1986. *Documentation of the Threshold Limit Values and Biological Exposure Indices*, 5th ed., p. 463. Cincinnati.

78. Wispe, J. R., E. F. Bell, R. J. Roberts 1985. Assessment of lipid peroxidation in newborn infants and rabbits by measurements of expired ethane and pentane: Influence of parenteral lipid infusion. *Pediatr. Res.* 19 (4):374–379.

79. Fühner, H. 1921. Die narkotisch Wirkung des Benszins und Seiner Bestand-teile (Pentan, Hexan, Heptan, Octan). *Biochem. Zeitschrift* 115:235–261.

80. Patty, F. A., W. P. Yant. 1929. *Odor Intensity and Symptoms Produced by Commercial Propane, Butane, Pentane, Hexane, and Heptane Vapor.* U.S. Bureau of Mines, Report of Investigations, No. 2979.

81. Perbellini, L., F. Brugnone, D. Caretta, G. Maranelli. 1985. Partition coefficients of some industrial aliphatic hydrocarbons (C5-C7) in blood and human tissues. *Br. J. Ind. Med.* 42:162–167.

82. Baselt, R. C., ed. 1982. *Disposition of Toxic Drugs and Chemicals in Man*, 2nd ed., p. 475. Davis, CA: Biomedical Publications.

83. Proctor, N. H., J. P. Hughes, eds. 1978. *Chemical Hazards of the Workplace*, p. 282. Philadelphia: Lippincott.

84. Aranyi, C., W. J. O'Shea, C. A. Halder, C. E. Holdsworth, B. Y. Cockrell. 1986. Absence of hydrocarbon-induced nephropathy in rats exposed subchronically to volatile hydrocarbon mixtures pertinent to gasoline. *Toxicol. Ind. Health* 2 (1):85–98.

85. Gonzales, E. G., J. A. Downey. 1972. Polyneuropathy due to n-hexane. *Arch. Phys. Med.* 53:333–337.

86. Paulson, G. W., G. W. Waylonis. 1976. Polyneuropathy due to n-hexane. *Arch. Physiol. Med.* 136 (8):880–882.

87. Yamamura, Y. 1969. n-Hexane polyneuropathy. *Folia. Psychiatr. Neurol. Jpn.* 23:45–57.

88. Herkowitz, A., N. Ishii, H. Schaumburg. 1971. N-Hexane neuropathy. A syndrome occurring as a result of industrial exposure. *N. Engl. J. Med.* 285:82–85.

89. Ruff, R. L., C. K. Petito, L. S. Acheson. 1981. Neuropathy associated with chronic low level exposure to n-hexane. *Clin. Toxicol.* 18:515–519.

90. Yamada, S. 1964. An occurrence of polyneuritis by n-hexane in the polyethylene laminating plants. *Jpn. J. Industr. Health* 6:192–194.

91. Sobue, I., Y. Yamamura, K. Ando, M. Iida, T. Takayanagi. 1968. N-Hexane polyneuropathy. *Clin. Neurol. (Jpn.)* 8:393–403.

92. Allen, N. 1979. Solvents and other industrial organic compounds. In *Handbook of Clinical Neurology: Intoxicants of the Nervous System*, Vol. 36, Part I, P. J. Vinken, G. M. Bruyn, eds., pp. 361–389. New York: Elsevier/North Holland.

93. Perbellini, L., F. Brugnone, I. Pavan. 1980. Identification of the metabolites of n-hexane, cyclohexane, and their isomers in men's urine. *Toxicol. Appl. Pharmacol.* 53:220–229.

94. American Conference of Governmental Industrial Hygienists. 1986. *Documentation of the Threshold Limit Values and Biological Exposure Indices*, 5th ed., p. 297. Cincinnati.

95. Lury, F., F. Zernik. 1931. *Schadliche Gase, Damfe, Nebel, Rauchund Staubarten*, pp. 257–284. Berlin: Springer.

96. Gerarde, H. W. 1963. *The Alicyclic Hydrocarbons Industrial Hygiene and Toxicology, Vol. 2.* New York: Interscience.

97. Waite, C. P., F. A. Patty, W. P. Yant. 1930. Acute response of guinea pigs to vapors of some new commercial organic compounds. IV. Ethylene oxide. *Pub. Health Rep.* 45:1832–1843.

98. Blackwood, J. D. Jr., E. B. Erskine. 1938. Carboxide poisoning. *U.S. Nav. Med. Bull.* 36:44–45.

99. Hopp, V., I. Henning, eds. 1983. *Handbook of Applied Chemistry*, pp. iv/8–24. Washington, DC: Hemisphere Publishing.

100. Hathaway, G. J., N. H. Proctor, J. P. Hughes, M. L. Fischman, eds. 1991. *Proctor and Hughes' Chemical Hazards of the Workplace*, 3rd ed., p. 14. New York: Van Nostrand Reinhold.

101. Elkins, H. B., eds. 1959. *The Chemistry of Industrial Toxicology*, 2nd ed., New York: John Wiley & Sons.

102. Fawcett, H. H. 1952. Carbon tetracholoride mixtures in the fire fighting. *Arch. Ind. Hyg. Occ. Med.* 6:435–440.

103. Von Oettingen, W. F. 1955. *Public Health Services Publication #414, pp.* 75–112, Washington, DC: U.S. Government Printing Office.

104. Fairhall, L. T. 1957. *Industrial Toxicology,* 2nd ed., pp. 183–185. Baltimore, MD: Williams & Wilkins.

105. Hardin, B. L. 1954. Carbon tetrachloride poisoning—A review. *Ind. Med. Surg.* 23:93–105.

106. Markham, T. N. 1967. Renal failure due to carbon tetrachloride. *J. Occup. Med.* 9:16–17.

107. Cornish, H. H., J. Adefuin. 1967. Potentiation of carbon tetrachloride toxicity by aliphatic alcohols. *Arch. Environ. Health* 14:447–449.

108. Hermann, H., C. B. Ford. 1941. Low concentrations of carbon tetrachloride capable of causing mild narcosis. *N.Y. Ind. Bull.* 20 (7):8.

109. Elkins, H. B. 1942. Maximal allowable concentrations. I Carbon tetrachloride. *J. Ind. Hyg. Toxicol.* 24 (8):233–235.

110. Industrial Hygiene Division, Illinois Department of Labor, 1947 Illinois Labor Bulletin, p. 10, May 31, 1947.

111. Kazanztis, G., R. R. Bomford. 1960. Dyspepsia due to inhalation of carbon tetrachloride vapour. *Lancet* 1:360–362.

112. Adams, E. N., H. C. Spencer, V. K. Rowe, D. D. McCollister, D. D. Irish. 1952. Vapor toxicity of carbon tetrachloride determined by experiments on laboratory animals. *AMA Arch. Ind. Hyg. Occup. Med.* 6:50–56.

113. Till, D. E., R. C. Reid, P. S. Schwartz, K. R. Sidman, J. R. Valentine, R. H. Whelan. 1982. Plasticizer migration from polyvinyl chloride film to solvents and foods. *Food Chem. Toxicol.* 20:95–104.

114. Goldman, S. M. et al. 2011. Solvent exposures and Parkinson disease risk in twins. *Ann. Neurol.* 71 (6): 776– 784.

115. Gash, D. M. et al. 2008. Trichloroethylene: Parkinsonism and complex 1 mitochondrial neurotoxicity. *Ann. Neurol.* 63 (2):184–192.

116. Guehl, D., E. Bezard, S. Dovero, T. Boraud, B. Bioulac, C. Gross. 1999. Trichloroethylene and parkinsonism: A human and experimental observation. *Eur. J. Neurol.* 6 (5):609–611.

117. Kochen, W., D. Kohlmuller, P. De Biasi, R. Ramsay. 2003. The endogeneous formation of highly chlorinated tetrahydro-beta-carbolines as a possible causative mechanism in idiopathic Parkinson's disease. *Adv. Exp. Med. Biol.* 527:253–263.

118. Liu, M., D. Y. Choi, R. L. Hunter, J. D. Pandya, W. A. Cass, P. G. Sullivan, H. C. Kim, D. M. Gash, G. Bing. 2010. Trichloroethylene induces dopaminergic neurodegeneration in Fisher 344 rats. *J. Neurochem.* 112 (3):773–783.

119. Braak, H., K. Del Tredici, U. Rub, R. A. de Vos, E.N. Jansen Steur, E. Braak. 2003. Staging of brain pathology related to sporadic Parkinson's disease. *Neurobiol. Aging* 24 (2):197–211.

120. Di Monte, D. A. 1991. Mitochondrial DNA and Parkinson's disease. *Neurology* 41 (5 Suppl 2):38–42. Discussion 42–43.

121. Sherer, T. B., J. R. Richardson, C. M. Testa, B. B. Seo, A. V. Panov, T. Yagi, A. Matsuno-Yagi, G. W. Miller, J. T. Greenamyre. 2007. Mechanism of toxicity of pesticides acting at complex I: Relevance to environmental etiologies of Parkinson's disease. *J. Neurochem.* 100 (6):1469–1479.

122. Miyazaki, Y., T. Takano. 1983. Impairment of mitochondrial electron transport by tetrachloroethylene. *Toxicol. Lett.* 18 (1–2):163–166.

123. Lash, L. H., W. Qian, D. A. Putt, S. E. Hueni, A. A. Elfarra, A. R. Sicuri, J. C. Parker. 2002. Renal toxicity of perchloroethylene and S-(1,2,2- trichlorovinyl)glutathione in rats and mice: Sex- and species-dependent differences. *Toxicol. Appl. Pharmacol.* 179 (3):163–171.

124. Boer, L. A., J. P. Panatto, D. A. Fagundes, C. Bassani, I. C. Jeremias, J. F. Daufenbach, G. T. Rezin, L. Constantino, F. Dal-Pizzol, E. L. Streck. 2009. Inhibition of mitochondrial respiratory chain in the brain of rats after hepatic failure induced by carbon tetrachloride is reversed by antioxidants. *Brain Res. Bull.* 80 (1–2):75–78.

125. Weber, L.W., M. Boll, A. Stampfl. 2003. Hepatotoxicity and mechanism of action of haloalkanes: Carbon tetrachloride as a toxicological model. *Crit. Rev. Toxicol.* 33 (2):105–136.

126. Manibusan, M. K., M. Odin, D. A. Eastmond. 2007. Postulated carbon tetrachloride mode of action: A review. *J. Environ. Sci. Health C. Environ. Carcinog. Ecotoxicol. Rev.* 25 (3):185–209.

127. Ou, J., Z. Ou, D. G. McCarver, R. N. Hines, K. T. Oldham, A. W. Ackerman, K. A. Pritchard Jr. 2003. Trichloroethylene decreases heat shock protein 90 interactions with endothelial nitric oxide synthase: Implications for endothelial cell proliferation. *Toxicol. Sci.* 73 (1):90–97.

128. Lam, H. R., G. Ostergaard, S. X. Guo, O. Ladefoged, S. C. Bondy. 1994. Three weeks' exposure of rats to dearomatized white spirit modifies indices of oxidative stress in brain, kidney, and liver. *Biochem. Pharmacol.* 47 (4):651–657.

129. Lopachin, R. M., T. Gavin, D. S. Barber. 2008. Type-2 alkenes mediate synaptotoxicity in neurodegenerative diseases. *Neurotoxicology* 29 (5):871–882.

130. Kim, M. S. et al. 2009. Neurotoxic effect of 2,5-hexanedione on neural progenitor cells and hippocampal neurogenesis. *Toxicology* 260 (1–3):97–103.

131. Al-Hajri, Z., M. R. Del Bigio. 2010. Brain damage in a large cohort of solvent abusers. *Acta Neuropathol.* 119 (4):435–445.

132. ATSDR. Agency for Toxic Substances and Disease Registry—Toxicological Profile for Trichlorethylene. United States Department of Health and Human Services; 1997.

133. Wu, C., J. Schaum. 2000. Exposure assessment of trichloroethylene. *Environ. Health Perspect.* 108 (Suppl 2):359–263.

134. EPA. United States Environmental Protection Agency (EPA). Toxic Release Inventory Program. http://www.epa.gov/tri/index.htm

135. ATSDR. *Agency for Toxic Substances and Disease Registry—Toxicological Profile for Carbon Tetrachloride.* United States Department of Health and Human Services; 2005.

136. Linn, B. 2009. Chemicals Used in Dry Cleaning Operations. Available from: http://www.drycleancoalition.org/chemicals/ChemicalsUsedInDrycleaningOperations.pdf

137. Lash, L. H., J. W. Fisher, J. C. Lipscomb, J. C. Parker. 2000. Metabolism of trichloroethylene. *Environ. Health Perspect.* 108 (Suppl 2):177–200.

138. Bringmann, G., R. God, D. Feineis, W. Wesemann, P. Riederer, W. D. Rausch, H. Reichmann, K. H. Sontag. 1995. The TaClo concept: 1-Trichloromethyl-1,2,3,4-tetrahydrobeta-carboline (TaClo), a new toxin for dopaminergic neurons. *J. Neural. Transm. Suppl.* 46:235–244.

139. Riederer, P., P. Foley, G. Bringmann, D. Feineis, R. Bruckner, M. Gerlach. 2002. Biochemical and pharmacological characterization of 1-trichloromethyl-1,2,3,4-tetrahydro-beta-carboline: A biologically relevant neurotoxin? *Eur. J. Pharmacol.* 442 (1–2):1–16.

140. Heim, C., K. H. Sontag. 1997. The halogenated tetrahydro-beta-carboline "TaClo": A progressively-acting neurotoxin. *J. Neural. Transm. Suppl.* 50:107–111.

141. Park, R. M., P. A. Schulte, J. D. Bowman, J. T. Walker, S. C. Bondy, M. G. Yost, J. A. Touchstone, M. Dosemeci. 2005. Potential occupational risks for neurodegenerative diseases. *Am. J. Ind. Med.* 48 (1):63–77.

142. McDonnell, L., C. Maginnis, S. Lewis, N. Pickering, M. Antoniak, R. Hubbard, I. Lawson, J. Britton. 2003. Occupational exposure to solvents and metals and Parkinson's disease. *Neurology* 61 (5):716–717.

143. Tanner, C. M. et al. 2009. Occupation and risk of parkinsonism: A multicenter case-control study. *Arch. Neurol.* 66 (9):1106–1113.

144. Dick, F. D. et al. Geoparkinson study group. 2007. Environmental risk factors for Parkinson's disease and parkinsonism: The Geoparkinson study. *Occup. Environ. Med.* 64 (10):666–672.

145. Firestone, J. A., J. I. Lundin, K.M. Powers, T. Smith-Weller, G. M. Franklin, P. D. Swanson, W. T. Longstreth Jr., H. Checkoway. 2010. Occupational factors and risk of Parkinson's disease: A population-based case-control study. *Am. J. Ind. Med.* 53 (3):217–223.

146. Lam, H. R., G. Ostergaard, O. Ladefoged. 1995. Three weeks' and six months' exposure to aromatic white spirit affect synaptosomal neurochemistry in rats. *Toxicol. Lett.* 80 (1–3):39–48.

147. Mattia, C. J., S. F. Ali, S. C. Bondy. 1993. Toluene-induced oxidative stress in several brain regions and other organs. *Mol. Chem. Neuropathol.* 18 (3):313–328.

148. Baydas, G., F. Ozveren, M. Tuzcu, A. Yasar. 2005. Effects of thinner exposure on the expression pattern of neural cell adhesion molecules, level of lipid peroxidation in the brain and cognitive function in rats. *Eur. J. Pharmacol.* 512 (2–3):181–187.

149. Mutti, A., I. Franchini. 1987. Toxicity of metabolites to dopaminergic systems and the behavioural effects of organic solvents. *Br. J. Ind. Med.* 44 (11):721–723.

150. Hubinette, A., S. Cnattingius, A. Ekbom, U. de Faire, M. Kramer, P. Lichtenstein. 2001. Birthweight, early environment, and genetics: A study of twins discordant for acute myocardial infarction. *Lancet* 357 (9273):1997–2001.

151. Hepworth, S. J., A. Bolton, R. C. Parslow, M. van Tongeren, K. R. Muir, P. A. McKinney. 2006. Assigning exposure to pesticides and solvents from self-reports collected by a computer assisted personal interview and expert assessment of job codes: The UK Adult Brain Tumour Study. *Occup. Environ. Med.* 63 (4):267–272.

152. Blair, A., S. H. Zahm. 1990. Methodologic issues in exposure assessment for case-control studies of cancer and herbicides. *Am. J. Ind. Med.* 18 (3):285–293.

153. McGuire, V., L. M. Nelson, T. D. Koepsell, H. Checkoway, W. T. Longstreth Jr. 1998. Assessment of occupational exposures in community-based case-control studies. *Annu. Rev. Public Health* 19:35–53.

154. Proctor, N. H., J. P. Hughes. 1978. *Chemical Hazards of the Workplace*, p. 505. Philadelphia: J. B. Lippincott.

155. Creech, J. L., M. N. Johnson. 1974. Angiosarcoma of the liver in the manufacture of polyvinyl chloride. *J. Occup. Med.* 16:150–151.

156. Hathaway, G. J. N. H. Proctor, J. P. Hughes, M. L. Fischman, eds. 1991. *Proctor and Hughes' Chemical Hazards of the Workplace*, 3rd ed., p. 581. New York: Van Nostrand Reinhold.

157. Benignus, V. A., A. M. Geller, W. K. Boyes, P. J. Bushnell. 2005. Human neurobehavioral effects of long-term exposure to styrene: A meta-analysis. *Environ. Health Perspect.* 113:532–538.

158. Baker, E. L. 1994. A review of recent research on health effects of human occupational exposure to organic solvents. A critical review. *J. Occup. Med.* 36 (10):1079–1092.

159. Ellingsen, D. G., M. Bekken, L. Kolsaker, S. Langard. 1993. Patients with suspected solvent-induced encephalopathy examined with cerebral computed tomography. *J. Occup. Med.* 35 (2):155–160.

160. Thuomas, K. A., C. Moller, L. M. Odkvist, U. Flodin, N. Dige. 1996. MR imaging in solvent-induced chronic toxic encephalopathy. *Acta Radiol.* 37 (2):177–179.

161. Filley, C. M., R. K. Heaton, N. L. Rosenberg. 1990. White matter dementia in chronic toluene abuse. *Neurology* 40 (3 Pt 1):532–534.

162. Yamanouchi, N., S. Okada, K. Kodama, S. Hirai, H. Sekine, A. Murakami, N. Komatsu, T. Sakamoto, T. Sato. 1995. White matter changes caused by chronic solvent abuse. *AJNR Am. J. Neuroradiol.* 16 (8):1643–1649.

163. Rosenberg, N. L., M. C. Spitz, C. M. Filley, K. A. Davis, H. H. Schaumburg. 1988. Central nervous system effects of chronic toluene abuse—Clinical, brainstem evoked response and magnetic resonance imaging studies. *Neurotoxicol. Teratol.* 10 (5):489–495.

164. Unger, E., A. Alexander, T. Fritz, N. Rosenberg, J. Dreisbach. 1994. Toluene abuse: Physical basis for hypointensity of the basal ganglia on T2-weighted MR images. *Radiology* 193 (2):473–476.

165. Ridgway, P., T. E. Nixon, J. P. Leach. 2003. Occupational exposure to organic solvents and long-term nervous system damage detectable by brain imaging, neurophysiology or histopathology. *Food. Chem. Toxicol.* 41 (2):153–187.

166. Seeber, A., T. Bruckner, G. Triebig. 2009. Occupational styrene exposure and neurobehavioural functions: A cohort study with repeated measurements. *Int. Arch. Occup. Environ. Health* 82 (8):969–984.

167. Gericke, C., B. Hanke, G. Beckmann, M. M. Baltes, K. P. Kuhl, D. Neubert, Toluene Field Study Group. 2001. Multicenter field trial on possible health effects of toluene. III. Evaluation of effects after long-term exposure. *Toxicology* 168 (2):185–209.

168. Haut, M. W., S. Leach, H. Kuwabara, S. Whyte, T. Callahan, A. Ducatman, L. J. Lombardo N. Gupta. 2000. Verbal working memory and solvent exposure: A positron emission tomography study. *Neuropsychology* 14 (4):551–558.

169. Tang, C. Y., D. M. Carpenter, E. L. Eaves, J. Ng, N. Ganeshalingam, C. Weisel, H. Qian, G. Lange, N. L. Fiedler. 2011. Occupational solvent exposure and brain function: An FMRI study. *Environ. Health Perspect.* 119 (7): 908–913.

170. American Psychiatric Association 1994. *Diagnostic and Statistical Manual of Mental Disorders (DSM-IV)*, 4th ed., Washington, DC: American Psychiatric Association.

171. Beck, A. T., R. A. Steer, G. K. Brown. 1996. *BDI-II, Beck Depression Inventory: Manual*. San Antonio, TX: Psychological Corporation.

172. Qian, H., N. Fiedler, D. F. Moore, C. P. Weisel. 2010. Occupational exposure to organic solvents during bridge painting. *Ann. Occup. Hyg.* 54 (4):417–426.

173. Kirchner, W. K. 1958. Age differences in short-term retention of rapidly changing information. *J. Exp. Psychol.* 55 (4):352–358.

174. Owen, A. M., K. M. McMillan, A. R. Laird, E. Bullmore. 2005. N-back working memory paradigm: A meta-analysis of normative functional neuroimaging. *Hum. Brain Mapp.* 25 (1):46–59.

175. Bockelmann, I., S. Darius, N. McGauran, B. P. Robra, B. Peter, E. A. Pfister. 2002. The psychological effects of exposure to mixed organic solvents on car painters. *Disabil. Rehabil.* 24 (9):455–461.

176. Colvin, M., J. Myers, V. Nell, D. Rees, R. Cronje. 1993. A cross-sectional survey of neurobehavioral effects of chronic solvent exposure on workers in a paint manufacturing plant. *Environ. Res.* 63 (1):122–132.

177. Kishi, R., I. Harabuchi, Y. Katakura, T. Ikeda, H. Miyake. 1993. Neurobehavioral effects of chronic occupational exposure to organic solvents among Japanese industrial painters. *Environ. Res.* 62 (2):303–313.

178. Morrow, L. A., N. Robin, M. J. Hodgson, H. Kamis. 1992. Assessment of attention and memory efficiency in persons with solvent neurotoxicity. *Neuropsychologia* 30 (10):911–922.

179. Ryan, C. M., L. A. Morrow, M. Hodgson. 1988. Cacosmia and neurobehavioral dysfunction associated with occupational exposure to mixtures of organic solvents. *Am. J. Psychiatry* 145 (11):1442–1445.

180. Callender, T. J., L. Morrow, K. Subramanian, D. Duhon, M. Ristovv. 1993. Three-dimensional brain metabolic imaging in patients with toxic encephalopathy. *Environ. Res.* 60 (2):295–319.

181. Fincher, C. E., T. S. Chang, E. H. Harrell, M. C. Kettelhut, W. J. Rea, A. Johnson, D. C. Hickey, T. R. Simon. 1997. Comparison of single photon emission computed tomography findings in cases of healthy adults and solvent-exposed adults. *Am. J. Ind. Med.* 31 (1):4–14.

182. Smith, E. E., J. Jonides, R. A. Koeppe. 1996. Dissociating verbal and spatial working memory using PET. *Cereb. Cortex* 6 (1):11–20.

183. Petrides, M., B. Alivisatos, E. Meyer, A.C. Evans. 1993. Functional activation of the human frontal-cortex during the performance of verbal working memory tasks. *Proc. Natl. Acad. Sci. U.S.A.* 90 (3):878–882.

184. Posner, M. I., S. E. Petersen. 1990. The attention system of the human brain. *Annu. Rev. Neurosci.* 13:25–42.

185. Chafee, M. V., P. S. Goldman-Rakic. 2000. Inactivation of parietal and prefrontal cortex reveals interdependence of neural activity during memory-guided saccades. *J. Neurophysiol.* 83 (3):1550–1566.

186. Jung, R. E., R. J. Haier. 2007. The Parieto-Frontal Integration Theory (P-FIT) of intelligence: Converging neuroimaging evidence. *Behav. Brain Sci.* 30 (2):135–154.

187. Haier, R. J., ed. 1993. *Cerebral Glucose Metabolism and Intelligence.* Norwood, NJ: Ablex.

188. Neubauer, A. C., A. Fink. 2009. Intelligence and neural efficiency. *Neurosci. Biobehav. Rev.* 33 (7):1004–1023.

189. Pfefferbaum, A., J. E. Desmond, C. Galloway, V. Menon, G. H. Glover, E. V. Sullivan. 2001. Reorganization of frontal systems used by alcoholics for spatial working memory: An fMRI study. *Neuroimage* 14 (1):7–20.

190. McAllister, T. W., L. A. Flashman, B. C. McDonald, A. J. Saykin. 2006. Mechanisms of working memory dysfunction after mild and moderate TBI: Evidence from functional MRI and neurogenetics. *J. Neurotrauma* 23 (10):1450–1467.

191. Chen, J. K., K. M. Johnston, S. Frey, M. Petrides, K. Worsley, A. Ptito. 2004. Functional abnormalities in symptomatic concussed athletes: An MRI study. *Neuroimage* 22 (1):68–82.

192. Johnson, S. C. et al. 2006. Activation of brain regions vulnerable to Alzheimer's disease: The effect of mild cognitive impairment. *Neurobiol. Aging* 27 (11):1604–1612.

193. Basser, P. J., S. Pajevic, C. Pierpaoli, J. Duda, A. Aldroubi. 2000. In vivo fiber tractography using DT-MRI data. *Magn. Reson. Med.* 44 (4):625–632.

194. Smith, E. E., J. Jonides. 1999. Storage and executive processes in the frontal lobes. *Science* 283 (5408):1657–1661.

195. Smith, E. E., J. Jonides, C. Marshuetz, R. A. Koeppe. 1998. Components of verbal working memory: Evidence from neuroimaging. *Proc. Natl. Acad. Sci. U.S.A.* 95 (3):876–882.

196. Raz, N., F. M. Gunning, D. Head, J. H. Dupuis, J. McQuain, S. D. Briggs, W. J. Loken, A. E. Thornton, J. D. Acker. 1997. Selective aging of the human cerebral cortex observed *in vivo*: Differential vulnerability of the prefrontal gray matter. *Cereb. Cortex* 7 (3):268–282.

197. Decarli, C., D. G. M. Murphy, J. A. Gillette, J. V. Haxby, D. Teichberg, M. B. Schapiro, B. Horwitz. 1994. Lack of age-related differences in temporal lobe volume of very healthy adults. *AJNR Am. J. Neuroradiol.* 15 (4):689–696.

198. Fuster, J. M. 2008. *The Prefrontal Cortex.* 4th ed., Boston: Academic Press.

199. Kondo, H., J. Huang, G. Ichihara, M. Kamijima, I. Saito, E. Shibata, Y. Ono, N. Hisanaga, Y. Takeuchi, D. Nakahara. 1995. Toluene induces behavioral activation without affecting striatal dopamine metabolism in the rat: Behavioral and microdialysis studies. *Pharmacol. Biochem. Behav.* 51 (1):97–101.

200. Williams, G. V., P. S. Goldman-Rakic. 1995. Modulation of memory fields by dopamine D1 receptors in prefrontal cortex. *Nature* 376 (6541):572–575.

201. Honma, T. 1983. Changes in acetylcholine metabolism in rat brain after a short-term exposure to toluene and n-hexane. *Toxicol. Lett.* 16 (1–2):17–22.

202. Tsuga, H., T. Honma. 2000. Effects of short-term toluene exposure on ligand binding to muscarinic acetylcholine receptors in the rat frontal cortex and hippocampus. *Neurotoxicol. Teratol.* 22 (4):603–606.

203. Stengard, K. 1995. Tail pinch increases acetylcholine release in rat striatum even after toluene exposure. *Pharmacol. Biochem. Behav.* 52 (2):261–264.

204. Bjornaes, S., L. U. Naalsund. 1988. Biochemical changes in different brain areas after toluene inhalation. *Toxicology* 49 (2–3):367–374.

205. Beckstead, M. J., J. L. Weiner, E. I. Eger, D. H. Gong, S. J. Mihic. 2000. Glycine and gamma-aminobutyric acid (A) receptor function is enhanced by inhaled drugs of abuse. *Mol. Pharmacol.* 57 (6):1199–1205.

206. Bowen, S. E., J. C. Batis, N. Paez-Martinez, S. L. Cruz. 2006. The last decade of solvent research in animal models of abuse: Mechanistic and behavioral studies. *Neurotoxicol. Teratol.* 28 (6):636–647.

207. Keski-Santti, P., R. Mantyla, A. Lamminen, H. K. Hyvarinen, M. Sainio. 2009. Magnetic resonance imaging in occupational chronic solvent encephalopathy. *Int. Arch. Occup. Environ. Health* 82 (5):595–602.

208. Rosenberg, N. L., J. Grigsby, J. Dreisbach, D. Busenbark, P. Grigsby. 2002. Neuropsychologic impairment and MRI abnormalities associated with chronic solvent abuse. *J. Toxicol. Clin. Toxicol.* 40 (1):21–34.

209. Rea, W. J. 1992. *Chemical Sensitivity*, Vol. 1, p. 221. Boca Raton, FL: Lewis Publishers.

210. Wallace, L. 1996. Environmental exposure to benzene: An update. *Environ. Health Perspect.* 104:1129–1136.

211. Rea, W. J. 1992. *Chemical Sensitivity,* Vol. 1, p. 86. Boca Raton, FL: Lewis Publishers.

212. Life Systems, Inc. 1989. *Toxicology Profile for Toluene,* p. 73. N. Manchester, IN: Heckman Bindery.

213. Verschueren, K., ed. 1983. *Handbook of Environmental Data on Organic Chemicals*, 2nd ed., p. 1103. New York: Van Nostrand Reinhold.

214. Life Systems, Inc. 1989. *Toxicology Profile for Toluene*, p. 1. N. Manchester, IN: Heckman Bindery.

215. Morata, T. C., D. E. Dunn, W. K. Sieber. 1994. Occupational exposure to noise and ototoxic organic solvents. *Arch. Environ. Health* 49 (5):359–365.

216. Rybak, L. P. 1992. Hearing: The effects of chemicals. *Otolaryngol. Head Neck Surg.* 106:677–686.

217. Abbate, C., C. Giorgianni, F. Munaò, R. Brecciaroli. 1993. Neurotoxicity induced by exposure to toluene. An electrophysiologic study. *Int. Arch. Occup. Environ. Health* 64 (6):389–392.

218. Vrca, A., V. Karacić, D. Bozicević, V. Bozikov, M. Malinar. 1996. Brainstem auditory evoked potentials in individuals exposed to long-term low concentrations of toluene. *Am. J. Ind. Med.* 30 (1):62–66.

219. Vrca, A., D. Bozicević, V. Bozikov, R. Fuchs, M. Malinar. 1997. Brain stem evoked potentials and visual evoked potentials in relation to the length of occupational exposure to low levels of toluene. *Acta Med. Croatica.* 51 (4–5):215–219.

220. Lataye, R., P. Campo, B. Pouyatos, B. Cossec, V. Blachère, G. Morel. 2003. Solvent ototoxicity in the rat and guinea pig. *Neurotoxicol. Teratol.* 25 (1):39–50.

221. Witter, H. L., R. C. Deka, D. M. Lipscomb, G. E. Shambaugh. 1980. Effects of prestimulatory carbogen inhalation on noise-induced temporary threshold shifts in humans and chinchilla. *Am. J. Otol.* 1 (4):227–232.

222. Pryor, G. T., R. A. Howd, E. T. Uyeno, A. B. Thurber. 1985. Interactions between toluene and alcohol. *Pharmacol. Biochem. Behav.* 23 (3):401–410.

223. Pryor, G. T., C. S. Rebert, J. Dickinson, E. M. Feeney. 1984. Factors affecting toluene-induced ototoxicity in rats. *Neurobehav. Toxicol. Teratol.* 6 (3):223–238.

224. Campo, P., D. Waniusiow, B. Cossec, R. Lataye, B. Rieger, F. Cosnier, M. Burgart. 2008. Toluene-induced hearing loss in phenobarbital treated rats. *Neurotoxicol. Teratol.* 30 (1):46–54.

225. Waniusiow, D., P. Campo, B. Cossec, F. Cosnier, S. Grossman, L. Ferrari. 2008. Toluene-induced hearing loss in acivicin-treated rats. *Neurotoxicol. Teratol.* 30 (3):154–160.

226. Sullivan, M. J., K. E. Rarey, R. B. Conolly. 1988. Ototoxicity of toluene in rats. *Neurotoxicol. Teratol.* 10:525–530.

227. Johnson, A. C., L. Juntunen, P. Nylén, E. Borg, G. Höglund. 1988. Effect of interaction between noise and toluene on auditory function in the rat. *Acta Otolaryngol* 105 (1–2):56–63.

228. Nylen, P., M. Hagman, A. C. Johnson. 1994. Function of the auditory and visual systems, and of peripheral nerve, in rats after long-term combined exposure to n-hexane and methylated benzene derivatives. *I. Toluene. Pharmacol. Toxicol.* 74 (2):116–123.

229. Rebert, C. S., S. S. Sorenson, R. A. Howd, G. T. Pryor. 1983. Toluene-induced hearing loss in rats evidenced by the brainstem auditory-evoked response. *Neurobehav. Toxicol. Teratol.* 5 (1):59–62.

230. Johnson, A. C., P. R. Nylen. 1995. Effects of industrial solvents on hearing. *Occup. Med.* 10 (3):623–640.

231. Johnson, A. C., B. Canlon. 1994. Progressive hair cell loss induced by toluene exposure. *Hear Res.* 75 (1–2):201–208.

232. Pryor, G. T., J. Dickinson, E. Feeney, C. S. Rebert. 1984. Hearing loss in rats first exposed to toluene as weanlings or as young adults. *Neurobehav. Toxicol. Teratol.* 6 (2):111–119.

233. Campo, P., R. Lataye, B. Cossec, V. Placidi. 1997. Toluene-induced hearing loss: A mid-frequency location of the cochlear lesions. *Neurotoxicol. Teratol.* 19 (2):129–140.

234. Lataye, R., K. Maguin, P. Campo. 2007. Increase in cochlear microphonic potential after toluene administration. *Hear Res.* 230 (1–2):34–42.

235. Campo, P., V. Blachère, J.P. Payan, B. Cossec, P. Ducos. 1993. No interaction between noise and toluene on cochlea in the guinea pig. *Acta Acustica* 1:35–42.

236. Schaper, M., P. Demes, M. Zupanic, M. Blaszkewicz, A. Seeber. 2003. Occupational toluene exposure and auditory function: Results from a follow-up study. *Ann. Occup. Hyg.* 47 (6):493–502.

237. Schaper, M., A. Seeber, C. van Thriel. 2008. The effects of toluene plus noise on hearing thresholds: An evaluation based on repeated measurements in the German printing industry. *Int. J. Occup. Med. Environ. Health* 21 (3):191–200.

238. Morata, T. C., D. E. Dunn, L. W. Kretschmer, G. K. Lemasters, R. W. Keith. 1993. Effects of occupational exposure to organic solvents and noise on hearing. *Scand. J. Work Environ. Health* 19 (4):245–254.

239. Chang, S. J., C. J. Chen, C.H. Lien, F. C. Sung. 2006. Hearing loss in workers exposed to toluene and noise. *Environ. Health Perspect.* 114 (8):1283–1286.

240. Lataye, R., P. Campo. 1997. Combined effects of a simultaneous exposure to noise and toluene on hearing function. *Neurotoxicol. Teratol.* 19 (5):373–382.

241. Brandt-Lassen, R., S. P. Lund, G. B. Jepsen. 2000. Rats exposed to toluene and noise may develop loss of auditory sensitivity due to synergistic interaction. *Noise Health* 3 (9):33–44.

242. Johnson, A. C., P. Nylén, E. Borg, G. Höglund. 1990. Sequence of exposure to noise and toluene can determine loss of auditory sensitivity in the rat. *Acta Otolaryngol.* 109 (1–2):34–40.

243. Lund, S. P., G. B. Kristiansen. 2008. Hazards to hearing from combined exposure to toluene and noise in rats. *Int. J. Occup. Med. Environ. Health* 21 (1):47–57.

244. U.S. Environmental Protection Agency. 1981. *Human Exposure to Atmospheric Concentrations of Selected Chemicals, Vols. I and II.* Research Triangle Park, NC: U.S. Environmental Protection Agency Office of Air Quality Planning and Standards.

245. Bonnichsen, R., A. C. Maehly, M. Moeller. 1966. Poisoning by volatile compounds. I. Aromatic hydrocarbons. *J. Forensic Sci.* 11 (2):186–204.

246. Verschueren, K., ed. 1983. *Handbook of Environmental Data on Organic Chemicals*, 2nd ed., p. 1191. New York: Van Nostrand Reinhold.

247. Rea, W. J., Y. Pan, A. R. Johnson. 1987/88. Clearing of toxic volatile hydrocarbons from human. *Clin. Ecol.* 5 (4):166–170.

248. Gaitan, E. 1986. Environmental goiterogens. In *The Thyroid Gland—A Practical Clinical Treatise*, L. Van Middlesworth, ed., p. 264. Chicago: Year Book Medical Publishing.

249. Hopp, V., I. Hennig, eds. 1983. *Handbook of Applied Chemistry*, pp. iv/4–iv31. Washington, DC: Hemisphere Publishing.

250. Emmett, E. A. 1986. Toxic responses of the skin. In *Casarett and Doull's Toxicology: The Basic Science of Poisons*, 3rd ed., C. D. Klaassen, M. O. Amdur, J. Doull, eds., New York: Macmillan.

251. Melzer, D. et al. 2012. Urinary bisphenol A concentration and risk of future coronary artery disease in apparently healthy men and women. *Circulation* 125 (12):1482–1490.

252. Ritter, S. 2011. Debating BPA's toxicity. *Chem. Eng. News* 89:5–13.

253. Dodds, E., W. Lawson. 1936. Synthetic estrogenic agents without the phenanthrene nucleus. *Nature* 137:996.

254. Diamanti-Kandarakis, E., E. Palioura, S. A. Kandarakis, M. Koutsilieris. 2010. The impact of endocrine disruptors on endocrine targets. *Horm. Metab. Res.* 42:543–552.

255. Lakind, J. S., D. Q. Naiman. 2008. Daily intake of bisphenol A and potential sources of exposure: 2005–2006 National Health and Nutrition Examination Survey. *J. Expo. Sci. Environ. Epidemiol.* 21:272–279.

256. Calafat, A. M., Z. Kuklenyik, J. A. Reidy, S. P. Caudill, J. Ekong, L. L. Needham. 2005. Urinary concentrations of bisphenol A and 4-nonylphenol in a human reference population. *Environ. Health Perspect.* 113:391–395.

257. Ye, X. et al. 2008. Urinary metabolite concentrations of organophosphorous pesticides, bisphenol A, and phthalates among pregnant women in Rotterdam, the Netherlands: The Generation R study. *Environ. Res.* 108:260–267.

258. Melzer, D., N. E. Rice, C. Lewis, W. E. Henley, T. S. Galloway. 2010. Association of urinary bisphenol a concentration with heart disease: Evidence from NHANES 2003/06. *PLoS One* 5:e8673.

259. European Food Standards Agency. 2010. European Food Standards Agency Scientific Opinion on Bisphenol A: Evaluation of a Study Investigating Its Neurodevelopmental Toxicity and Review of Recent Scientific Literature on Its Toxicity. *EFSA J.* 8:1829–1945.

260. Hengstler, J. G., H. Foth, T. Gebel, P. J. Kramer, W. Lilienblum, H. Schweinfurth, W. Volkel, K. M. Wollin, U. Gundert-Remy. 2011. Critical evaluation of key evidence on the human health hazards of exposure to bisphenol A. *Crit. Rev. Toxicol.* 41:263–291.

261. Lang, I. A., T. S. Galloway, A. Scarlett, W. E. Henley, M. Depledge, R. B. Wallace, D. Melzer. 2008. Association of urinary bisphenol A concentration with medical disorders and laboratory abnormalities in adults. *JAMA* 300:1303–1310.

262. Melzer, D., T. S. Galloway. 2011. Bisphenol A and adult disease: Making sense of fragmentary data and competing inferences. *Ann. Intern. Med.* 155:392–394.

263. Mahalingaiah, S., J. D. Meeker, K. R. Pearson, A. M. Calafat, X. Ye, J. Petrozza, R. Hauser. 2008. Temporal variability and predictors of urinary bisphenol A concentrations in men and women. *Environ. Health Perspect.* 116:173–178.

264. Nepomnaschy, P. A., D. D. Baird, C. R. Weinberg, J. A. Hoppin, M. P. Longnecker, A. J. Wilcox. 2009. Within-person variability in urinary bisphenol A concentrations: Measurements from specimens after long-term frozen storage. *Environ. Res.* 109:734–737.

265. Ye, X., L. Y. Wong, A. M. Bishop, A. M. Calafat. 2011. Variability of urinary concentrations of bisphenol A in spot samples, first-morning voids, and 24-hour collections. *Environ. Health Perspect.* 119:983–988.

266. Völkel, W., T. Colnot, G. A. Csanády, J. G. Filser, W. Dekant. 2002. Metabolism and kinetics of bisphenol A in humans at low doses following oral administration. *Chem. Res. Toxicol.* 15:1281–1287.

267. Sieli, P. et al. 2011. Comparison of serum bisphenol A concentrations in mice exposed to bisphenol A through the diet versus oral bolus exposure. *Environ. Health Perspect.* 119:1260–1265.

268. Stahlhut, R. W., W. V. Welshons, S. H. Swan. 2009. Bisphenol A data in NHANES suggest longer than expected half-life, substantial nonfood exposure, or both. *Environ. Health Perspect.* 117:784–789.

269. Dekant, W., W. Volkel. 2008. Human exposure to bisphenol A by biomonitoring: Methods, results and assessment of environmental exposures. *Toxicol. Appl. Pharmacol.* 228:114–134.

270. Biedermann, S., P. Tschudin, K. Grob. 2010. Transfer of bisphenol A from thermal printer paper to the skin. *Anal. Bioanal. Chem.* 398:571–576.

271. Teeguarden, J. G., J. M. Waechter Jr., H. J. Clewell 3rd, T.R. Covington, H.A. Barton. 2005. Evaluation of oral and intravenous route pharmacokinetics, plasma protein binding, and uterine tissue dose metrics of bisphenol A: A physiologically based pharmacokinetic approach. *Toxicol. Sci.* 85: 823–838.

272. Taylor, J. A., F. S. Vom Saal, W. V. Welshons, B. Drury, G. Rottinghaus, P. A. Hunt, P. L. Toutain, C. M. Laffont, C. A. VandeVoort. 2010. Similarity of bisphenol A pharmacokinetics in rhesus monkeys and mice: Relevance for human exposure. *Environ. Health Perspect.* 119:422–430.

273. Sharpe, R. M. 2010. Bisphenol A exposure and sexual dysfunction in men: Editorial commentary on the article "Occupational exposure to bisphenol-A (BPA) and the risk of self-reported male sexual dysfunction" Li et al., 2009. *Hum. Reprod.* 25:292–294.

274. Michels, K. B., A. A. Welch, R. Luben, S. A. Bingham, N. E. Day. 2005. Measurement of fruit and vegetable consumption with diet questionnaires and implications for analyses and interpretation. *Am. J. Epidemiol.* 161:987–994.

275. Bonefeld-Jorgensen, E. C., M. Long, M. V. Hofmeister, A. M. Vinggaard. 2007. Endocrine-disrupting potential of bisphenol A, bisphenol A dimethacrylate, 4-n-nonylphenol, and 4-n-octylphenol *in vitro*: New data and a brief review. *Environ. Health Perspect.* 115:69–76.

276. Mastin, J. P. 2005. Environmental cardiovascular disease. *Cardiovasc. Toxicol.* 5:91–94.

277. Okada, H., T. Tokunaga, X. H. Liu, S. Takayanagi, A. Matsushima, Y. Shimohigashi. 2008. Direct evidence revealing structural elements essential for the high binding ability of bisphenol A to human estrogen-related receptor-gamma. *Environ. Health Perspect.* 116:32–38.

278. Melzer, D. H., L. Harries, R. Cipelli, W. Henley, C. Money, P. McCormack, A. Young, J. Guralnik, L. Ferrucci, S. Bandinelli, A. M. Corsi, T. Galloway. 2011. Bisphenol A exposure is associated with in-vivo estrogenic gene expression in adults. *Environ. Health Perspect.* 119:1788–1793.

279. Lee, H. J., S. Chattopadhyay, E. Y. Gong, R. S. Ahn, K. Lee. 2003. Antiandrogenic effects of bisphenol A and nonylphenol on the function of the androgen receptor. *Toxicol. Sci.* 75:40–46.

280. Guillemette, C., E. Levesque, M. Beaulieu, D. Turgeon, D. W. Hum, A. Belanger. 1997. Differential regulation of two uridine diphospho-glucuronosyltransferases, UGT2B15 and UGT2B17, in human prostate LNCaP cells. *Endocrinology* 138:2998–3005.

281. Kandaraki, E., A. Chatzigeorgiou, S. Livadas, E. Palioura, F. Economou, M. Koutsilieris, S. Palimeri, D. Panidis, E. Diamanti-Kandarakis. 2011. Endocrine disruptors and polycystic ovary syndrome (PCOS): Elevated serum levels of bisphenol A in women with PCOS. *J. Clin. Endocrinol. Metab.* 96:E480–E484.

282. Basaria, S. et al. 2010. Adverse events associated with testosterone administration. *N. Engl. J. Med.* 363:109–122.

283. Okuda, K., M. Takiguchi, S. Yoshihara. 2010. In vivo estrogenic potential of 4-methyl-2,4-bis (4-hydroxyphenyl) pent-1-ene, an active metabolite of bisphenol A, in uterus of ovariectomized rat. *Toxicol. Letts.* 197:7–11.

284. Brenner, R., G. J. Perez, A. D. Bonev, D. M. Eckman, J. C. Kosek, S. W. Wiler, A. J. Patterson, M. T. Nelson, R. W. Aldrich. 2000. Vasoregulation by the beta1 subunit of the calcium-activated potassium channel. *Nature* 407: 870–876.

285. Asano, S., J. D. Tune, G. M. Dick. 2010. Bisphenol A activates Maxi-K (K(Ca)1.1) channels in coronary smooth muscle. *Br. J. Pharmacol.* 160:160–170.

286. Bindhumol, V., K. C. Chitra, P. P. Mathur. 2003. Bisphenol A induces reactive oxygen species generation in the liver of male rats. *Toxicology* 188:117–124.

287. Alonso-Magdalena, P., S. Morimoto, C. Ripoll, E. Fuentes, A. Nadal. 2006. The estrogenic effect of bisphenol A disrupts pancreatic beta-cell function *in vivo* and induces insulin resistance. *Environ. Health Perspect.* 114:106–112.

288. Ropero, A. B., P. Alonso-Magdalena, E. Garcia-Garcia, C. Ripoll, E. Fuentes, A. Nadal. 2008. Bisphenol-A disruption of the endocrine pancreas and blood glucose homeostasis. *Int. J. Androl.* 31:194–200.

289. Wright, H. M., C. B. Clish, T. Mikami, S. Hauser, K. Yanagi, R. Hiramatsu, C. N. Serhan, B. M. Spiegelman. 2000. A synthetic antagonist for the peroxisome proliferator-activated receptor gamma inhibits adipocyte differentiation. *J. Biol. Chem.* 275:1873–1877.

290. American Conference of Governmental Industrial Hygienists. 1976. *Cresol (All Isomers). Documentation of the TLVs for Substances in Workroom Air*, 3rd ed., p. 61. Cincinnati.

291. M.C.A., Inc. 1952. *Chemical Safety Data Sheet*. SD-48. Cresol, pp. 13–16. Washington, DC.

292. Curley, A., R. E. Hawk, R. D. Kimbrough, G. Nathenson, L. Finberg. 1971. Dermal absorption of hexa-chlorophene in infants. *Lancet* 2:296–297.

293. Ulsamer, A. G., F. N. Marzulli, R. W. Coen. 1973. Hexachlorophene concentrations in blood associated with the use of products containing hexachlorophene. *Food Cosmet. Toxicol.* 11:625–633.

294. Shuman, R. M., R. W. Lecch, E. C. Alvord Jr. 1974. Neurotoxicity of hexachlorophene in the human. I. A clinicopathologic study of 248 children. *Pediatrics.* 54:689–695.

295. Halling, H. 1979. Suspected link between exposure to hexachlorophene and malformed infants. *Ann. N. Y. Acad. Sci.* 320:426–435.

296. Larson, D. L. 1968. Studies show hexachlorophene causes burn syndrome. *Hospitals* 42:63–64.

297. Butcher, H. R., W. F. Ballinger, D. L. Gravens, N. E. Dewar, E. F. Ledlie, W. F. Barthel. 1983. Hexachlorophene concentrations in the blood of operating room personnel. *Arch. Surg.* 107:70–74.

298. Panel on Hazardous Trace Substances. 1972. Polychlorinated biphenyls—Environmental impact. *Environ. Res.* 5:249–362.

299. Kuwabara, K., T. Yakushiji, I. Watanabe, S. Yoshida, K. Yoyama, N. Kunita. 1979. Increase in the human blood PCB levels promptly following ingestion of fish containing PCBs. *Bull. Environ. Contam. Toxicol.* 21:273–278.

300. Finklea, J., L. E. Priester, J. P. Creason, T. Hauser, T. Hinners, D. I. Hammer. 1972. Polychlorinated biphenyl residues in human plasma expose a major urban pollution problem. *Ann. J. Public Health* 62:645–651.

301. National Institute for Occupation Safety and Health. 1977. *Occupational Exposure to Polychlorinated Biphenyls (PCBs)*. Cincinnati: National Institute for Occupation Safety and Health.

302. Matthews, H. B., M. W. Anderson. 1975. Effect of chlorination on the distribution and excretion of polychlorinated biphenyls. *Drugs Met. Disp.* 3:371–380.

303. Yobs, A. R. 1972. Levels of polychlorinated biphenyls in adipose tissue of the general population of the nation. *Environ. Health Perspect.* 1:79–81.

304. Fukano, S., M. Doguchi. 1977. PCT, PCB and pesticide residues in human fat and blood. *Bull. Environ. Contam. Toxicol.* 17:613–617.

305. Watanabe, I., T. Yakushiji, N. Kumita. 1980. Distribution differences between polychlorinated terphey-nyls and polychlorinated bipheynyls. *Bull. Environ. Contam. Toxicol.* 25:810–815.

306. Wickizer, T. M., L. B. Brilliant. 1981. Testing for polychlorinated biphenyls in human milk. *Am. J. Public Health* 68:132–137.

307. Hathaway, G. J., N. H. Prtoctor, J. P. Hughes, M. L. Fischman, eds. 1991. *Proctor and Hughes' Chemical Hazards of the Workplace*, 3rd ed., p. 166. New York: Van Nostrand Reinhold.

308. Fischpein, A., M. S. Wolff, R. Lilis, J. Thornton, I. J. Selikoff. 1979. Clinical findings among PCB-exposed capacitor manufacturing workers. *Am. N. Y. Acad. Sci.* 320:703–714.

309. Calabrese, E. J., ed. 1980. *Nutrition and Environmental Health, Vol. I. The Vitamins*, p. 51. New York: John Wiley & Sons.

310. Combs, G. F. Jr., M. L. Scott. 1975. Polychlorinated biphenyl-stimulated selenium deficiency in the chick. *Poult. Sci.* 54:1152–1158.

311. Siami, G., A. R. Schulber, R. A. Neal. 1972. A possible role for the mixed function oxidase enzyme system in the requirement for selenium in the rat. *J. Nutr.* 102:857–862.

312. Wassermann, M., D. Wassermann, S. Cucos, H. J. Miller. 1979. World PCBs map: Storage and effects in man and his biologic environment in the 1970s. *Am. N. Y. Acad. Sci.* 320:69–124.

313. Bastomsky, C. H. 1977. Goitres in rats fed polychlorinated biphenyls. *Can. J. Physiol. Pharmacol.* 55:288–292.

314. Letz, G. 1982. *The Toxicology of PCB's. An Overview with Emphasis on Human Health Effects and Occupational Exposure. Health Hazard and Information Service.* State of California, Department of Health Services.

315. Anderson, H. A., M. S. Wolff, R. Lilis, E. C. Holstein, J. A. Valciukas, K. E. Anderson, M. Petrocci, L. Sarkozi, I. J. Selikoff. 1979. Symptoms and clinical abnormalities following ingestion of polybrominated-biphenyl-contaminated food products. *Ann. N. Y. Acad. Sci.* 320:684–702.

316. Kimbrough, R., B. Burse, J. Liddle. 1977. Toxicity of polybrominated biphenyl. *Lancet* 2:602–603.

317. Meester, W. D., D. J. McCoy, Sr. 1977. Human toxicology of polybrominated biphenyls. In *Management of the Poisoned Patient*, B. H. Rumack, A. R. Temple, eds., pp. 32–61. Princeton: Science Press.

318. Meester, W. D. 1979. The effect of polybrominated biphenyls on man: The Michigan PBB disaster. *Vet. Hum. Toxicol.* 21:131–135.

319. Wolff, M. S., H. A. Anderson, I. J. Selikoff. 1982. Human tissue burdens of halogenated aromatic chemical in Michigan. *JAMA* 247 (5):2112–2116.

320. Kasza, L., M. A. Weinberger. 1978. Comparative toxicity of polychlorinated biphenyl and polybrominated biphenyl in the rat liver: Light and electron microscopic alterations after subacute dietary exposure. *J. Environ. Pathol. Toxicol.* 1:241–257.

321. Tilson, H. A., P. A. Cabe. 1979. Studies on the neurobehavioral effects of polybrominated biphenyls in rats. *Ann. N. Y. Acad. Sci.* 320:325–336.

322. Luster, M., R. E. Faith, J. A. Moore. 1978. Effects of polybrominated biphenyls (PBB) on immune response in rodent. *Environ. Health Perspect.* 23:227–232.

323. Kimbrough, R. D., D. F. Groce, M. P. Korver, V. W. Burse. 1981. Induction of liver tumors in female Sherman strain rats by polybrominated biphenyls. *J. Natl. Cancer Inst.* 66 (3):535–542.

324. Baselt, R. C., ed. 1982. *Disposition of Toxic Drugs and Chemicals in Man*, 2nd ed., pp. 649–650. Davis, CA: Biomedical Publications.

325. Wolff, M. S., H. A. Anderson, K. D. Roseman, I. J. Selikoff. 1979. Equilibrium of polybrominated biphenyl (PBB) residues in serum and fat of Michigan residents. *Bull. Environ. Contam. Toxicol.* 21:775–781.

326. Matthews, H. B., S. Kato, N. M. Morales, D. B. Tuey. 1977. Distribution and excretion of 2,4,5,2′, 4′, 5′ hexabromobiphenyl, the major component of firemaster BP-6. *J. Toxicol. Environ. Health* 3 (3):559–605.

327. Miceli, J. N., B. H. Marks. 1981. Tissue distribution and elimination kinetics of polybrominated biphenyls (PBB) from rat tissue. *Toxicol. Lett.* 9 (4):315–320.

328. Briliant, L. B., K. Wilcox, G. Van Amburg, J. Eyster, J. ISbister, A. W. Bloodmer, H. Humphrey, H. Price. 1978. Breast-milk monitoring to measure Michigan's contamination with polybrominated biphenyls. *Lancet* 2:643–646.

329. Meester, W. D., D. J. McCoy, Sr. 1977. Human toxicology of polybrominated biphenyls. In *Management of the Poisoned Patient*, B. H. Rumack, A. R. Temple, eds., pp. 32–61. Princeton, NJ: Science Press.

330. Goldstein, J. A., P. Hickman, D. L. Jue. 1974. Experimental hepatic porphyria induced by polychlorinated biphenyls. *Toxicol. Appl. Pharmacol.* 27:437–448.

331. Penning, C. H. 1930. Physical characteristics and commercial possibilities of chlorinated diphenyl. *Ind. Eng. Chem.* 22:1180–1182.

332. Warshaw, R., A. Fischbein, J. Thornton, A. Miller, I. J. Selikoff. 1979. Decrease in vital capacity in PCB-exposed workers in a capacitor manufacturing facility. *Ann. N. Y. Acad. Sci.* 320:277–283.

333. Wickizer, T. M., L. B. Brilliant. 1981. Testing for polychlorinated biphenyls in human milk. *Pediatrics* 68:411–415.

334. Matthews, H. B., M. Anderson. 1976. PCB chlorination versus PCB distribution and excretion. In *Conf. Proc. for National Conference on Polychlorinated Biphenyls*, pp. 50–56. EHP-560/6-75-004. Washington, DC: U.S. Environmental Protection Agency, Office of Toxic Substances.

335. Ecobichon, D. J., S. Hidvegi, A. M. Comcau, P. H. Cameron. 1983. Transplacental and milk transfer of polybrominated biphenyls to perinatal guinea pigs from treated dams. *Toxicology* 28 (1–2):51–63.

336. Root, D. E., D. B. Katzin, D. W. Schnare. May 14–16, 1985. Diagnosis and treatment of patients present-ing subclinical signs and symptoms of exposure to chemicals which bioaccumulate in human tissue. In *Proceedings of the National Conference of Hazardous Wastes and Environmental Emergencies*, Cincinnati.

337. Oschry, Y., B. Shapiro. 1981. Fat associated with adipose lipase the newly synthesized fraction that is the preferred substrate for lipolysis. *Biochim. Biophys. Acta* 664:201–206.

338. Hopp, V., I. Henning, eds. 1983. *Handbook of Applied Chemistry: Facts for Engineers, Scientist, Technicians, and Technical Managers*, pp. IV/3–IV18. Washington, DC: Hemisphere Publishing.

339. Kalin, E. W., C. R. Brooks. 1963. Systemic toxic reactions to soft plastic food containers. A double-blind study. *Med. Ann. Dist. Columbia* 32 (1):1–8.

340. Cohen, A. J., P. Grasso. 1981. Review of the hepatic response to hypolipidaemic drugs in rodents and assessment of its toxicological significance to man. *Food Cosmet. Toxicol.* 19:585–605.

341. Levine, S. A., P. M. Kidd. 1985. *Antioxidant Adaption: Its Role in Free Radical Pathology*, p. 254. Sam Leandro, CA: Biocurrents Division, Allergy Research Group.

342. Schlueter, D. P., E. F. Banaszak, J. N. Fink, J. Barboriak. 1978. Occupational asthma due to tetrachlo-rophthalic anhydride. *J. Occup. Med.* 20 (3):183–188.

343. Seth, P. K. 1982. Hepatic effects of phthalate esters. *Environ. Health Perspect.* 45:27–34.

344. Ecobichon, D. J. 1977. Hydrolytic transformation of environmental pollutants. In *Handbook of Physiology*, D. H. K. Lea, ed., Sect. 9, pp. 441–454. Baltimore, MD: Williams & Wilkins.

345. Gasgosian, R. B., E. T. Peltzer, O. C. Zafiriou. 1981. Atmospheric transport of continentally derived lipids to the tropical North Pacific. *Nature* 291:312–314.

346. Neff, J. M. 1979. *Polycyclic Aromatic Hydrocarbons in the Aquatic Environment*. London: Applied Science Publishers.

347. Buhler, D. R., D. E. Williams. 1989. Enzymes involved in metabolism of PAH by fishes and other aquatic animal: Oxidative enzymes (or phase I enzymes). In *Metabolism of Polycyclic Aromatic Hydrocarbons in Aquatic Environment*, U. Varanasi, ed., p. 155. Boca Raton, FL: CRC Press.

348. Williams, G. M., J. H. Weisburger. 1986. Chemical carcinogens. In *Casarett and Doull's Toxicology: The Basic Science of Poisons*, 3rd ed., C. D. Klaassen, M. O. Amdur, J. Doull, eds., p. 108. New York: Macmillan.

349. Conney, A. H. 1982. Induction of microsomal enzymes by foreign chemicals and carcinogenesis by polycyclic aromatic hydrocarbons. *Cancer Res.* 42:4875–4917.

350. Kraft, A. D., G. J. Harry. 2011. Features of microglia and neuroinflammation relevant to environmental exposure and neurotoxicity. *Int. J. Environ. Res. Public Health* 8 (7):2980–3018.

351. Hesterberg, T. W., W. B. Bunn 3rd, G. R. Chase, P. A. Valberg, T. J. Slavin, C. A. Lapin, G. A. Hart. 2006. A critical assessment of studies on the carcinogenic potential of diesel exhaust. *Crit. Rev. Toxicol.* 36:727–776.

352. Hartz, A. M., B. Bauer, M. L. Block, J. S. Hong, D. S. Miller. 2008. Diesel exhaust particles induce oxi-dative stress, proinflammatory signaling, and P-glycoprotein up-regulation at the blood-brain barrier. *FASEB J.* 22:2723–2733.

353. Block, M. L., X. Wu, Z. Pei, G. Li, T. Wang, L. Qin, B. Wilson, J. Yang, J. S. Hong, B. Veronesi. 2004. Nanometer size diesel exhaust particles are selectively toxic to dopaminergic neurons: The role of microglia, phagocytosis, and NADPH oxidase. *FASEB J.* 18:1618–1620.

354. Carson, M. J., C. R. Reilly, J. G. Sutcliffe, D. Lo. 1998. Mature microglia resemble immature antigen-presenting cells. *Glia* 22:72–85.

355. Aloisi, F. 2001. Immune function of microglia. *Glia* 36:165–179.

356. Becher, B., J. P. Antel. 1996. Comparison of phenotypic and functional properties of immediately ex vivo and cultured human adult microglia. *Glia* 18:1–10.

357. Long, T. C., J. Tajuba, P. Sama, N. Saleh, C. Swartz, J. Parker, S. Hester, G. V. Lowry, B. Veronesi. 2007. Nanosize titanium dioxide stimulates reactive oxygen species in brain microglia and damages neurons *in vitro*. *Environ. Health Perspect.* 115:1631–1637.

358. Campbell, A, M. Oldham, A. Becaria, S. C. Bondy, D. Meacher, C. Sioutas, C. Misra, L. B. Mendez, M. Kleinman. 2005. Particulate matter in polluted air may increase biomarkers of inflammation in mouse brain. *Neurotoxicology* 26:133–140.

359. Guastadisegni, C., F. J. Kelly, F. R. Cassee, M. E. Gerlofs-Nijland, N. A. Janssen, R. Pozzi, B. Brunekreef, T. Sandstrom, I. Mudway. 2010. Determinants of the proinflammatory action of ambient particulate matter in immortalized murine macrophages. *Environ. Health Perspect.* 118:1728–1734.

360. Gerlofs-Nijland, M. E., D. van Berlo, F. R. Cassee, R. P. Schins, K. Wang, A. Campbell. 2010. Effect of prolonged exposure to diesel engine exhaust on proinflammatory markers in different regions of the rat brain. *Part. Fibre Toxicol.* 7:12.

361. Kida, S., P. V. Steart, E. T. Zhang, R. O. Weller. 1993. Perivascular cells act as scavengers in the cerebral perivascular spaces and remain distinct from pericytes, microglia and macrophages. *Acta Neuropathol.* 85:646–652.

362. Brunssen, S. H., D. L. Morgan, F. M. Parham, G. J. Harry. 2003. Carbon monoxide neurotoxicity: Transient inhibition of avoidance response and delayed microglia reaction in the absence of neuronal death. *Toxicology* 194:51–63.

363. Calderon-Garciduenas, L. et al. 2011. Air pollution is associated with brainstem auditory nuclei pathology and delayed brainstem auditory evoked potentials. *Int. J. Dev. Neurosci.* 29:365–375.

364. Calderon-Garciduenas, L. et al. 2009. Immunotoxicity and environment: Immunodysregulation and systemic inflammation in children. *Toxicol. Pathol.* 37:161–169.

365. Finch, G. L. et al. 2002. Effects of subchronic inhalation exposure of rats to emissions from a diesel engine burning soybean oil-derived biodiesel fuel. *Inhal. Toxicol.* 14:1017–1048.

366. Jensen, L. K., H. Klausen, C. Elsnab. 1989. Organic brain damage in garage workers after long-term exposure to diesel exhaust fumes. *Ugeskr. Laeger.* 151:2255–2258.

367. Calderon-Garciduenas, L. et al. 2008. Long-term air pollution exposure is associated with neuroinflammation, an altered innate immune response, disruption of the blood-brain barrier, ultrafine particulate deposition, and accumulation of amyloid beta-42 and alpha-synuclein in children and young adults. *Toxicol. Pathol.* 36:289–310.

368. Takenaka, S., E. Karg, C. Roth, H. Schulz, A. Ziesenis, U. Heinzmann, P. Schramel, J. Heyder. 2001. Pulmonary and systemic distribution of inhaled ultrafine silver particles in rats. *Environ. Health Perspect.* 109(Suppl 4):547–551.

369. Calderon-Garciduenas, L. et al. 2009. Effects of a cyclooxygenase-2 preferential inhibitor in young healthy dogs exposed to air pollution: A pilot study. *Toxicol. Pathol.* 37:644–660.

370. Calderon-Garciduenas, L. et al. 2008. Air pollution, cognitive deficits and brain abnormalities: A pilot study with children and dogs. *Brain Cogn.* 68:117–127.

371. Hesterberg, T. W., C. M. Long, W. B. Bunn, S. N. Sax, C. A. Lapin, P. A. Valberg. 2009. Non-cancer health effects of diesel exhaust: A critical assessment of recent human and animal toxicological literature. *Crit. Rev. Toxicol.* 39:195–227.

372. Campen, M. J., N. S. Babu, G. A. Helms, S. Pett, J. Wernly, R. Mehran, J. D. McDonald. 2005. Nonparticulate components of diesel exhaust promote constriction in coronary arteries from ApoE-/- mice. *Toxicol. Sci.* 88:95–102.

373. Cherng, T. W., M. L. Paffett, O. Jackson-Weaver, M. J. Campen, B. R. Walker, N. L. Kanagy. 2011. Mechanisms of diesel-induced endothelial nitric oxide synthase dysfunction in coronary arterioles. *Environ. Health Perspect.* 119:98–103.

374. Mills, N. L. et al. 2005. Diesel exhaust inhalation causes vascular dysfunction and impaired endogenous fibrinolysis. *Circulation* 112:3930–3936.

375. Lehmann, A. D., F. Blank, O. Baum, P. Gehr, B. M. Rothen-Rutishauser. 2009. Diesel exhaust particles modulate the tight junction protein occluding in lung cells *in vitro*. *Part. Fibre Toxicol.* 6:26.

376. Amara, N., R. Bachoual, M. Desmard, S. Golda, C. Guichard, S. Lanone, M. Aubier, E. Ogier-Denis, J. Boczkowski. 2007. Diesel exhaust particles induce matrix metalloprotease-1 in human lung epithelial cells via a NADP(H) oxidase/NOX4 redox-dependent mechanism. *Am. J. Physiol. Lung Cell Mol. Physiol.* 293:L170–L181.

377. Bayram, H., J. L. Devalia, R. J. Sapsford, T. Ohtoshi, Y. Miyabara, M. Sagai, R. J. Davies. 1998. The effect of diesel exhaust particles on cell function and release of inflammatory mediators from human bronchial epithelial cells *in vitro*. *Am. J. Respir. Cell Mol. Biol.* 18:441–448.

378. Joris, I., T. Zand, J. J. Nunnari, F. J. Krolikowski, G. Majno. 1983. Studies on the pathogenesis of atherosclerosis. I. Adhesion and emigration of mononuclear cells in the aorta of hypercholesterolemic rats. *Am. J. Pathol.* 113:341–358.

379. Lippmann, M., T. Gordon, L. C. Chen. 2005. Effects of subchronic exposures to concentrated ambient particles in mice. IX. Integral assessment and human health implications of subchronic exposures of mice to CAPs. *Inhal. Toxicol.* 17:255–261.

380. Streit, W. J., D. L. Sparks. 1997. Activation of microglia in the brains of humans with heart disease and hypercholesterolemic rabbits. *J. Mol. Med. (Berl.)* 75:130–138.

381. Sama, P., T. C. Long, S. Hester, J. Tajuba, J. Parker, L. C. Chen, B. Veronesi. 2007. The cellular and genomic response of an immortalized microglia cell line (BV2) to concentrated ambient particulate matter. *Inhal. Toxicol.* 19:1079–1087.

382. Donaldson, K. 2003. The biological effects of coarse and fine particulate matter. *Occup. Environ. Med.* 60:313–314.

383. Proctor, N. H., J. P. Hughes. 1978. *Chemical Hazards of the Workplace,* p. 368. Philadelphia: J. B. Lippincott.
384. Williams, G. M., J. H. Weisburger. 1986. Chemical carcinogens. In *Casarett and Doull's Toxicology: The Basic Science of Poisons*, 3rd ed., C. D. Klaassen, M. O. Amdur, J. Doull, eds., p. 109. New York: Macmillan.
385. Nelson, S. D., W. L. Nelson, W. F. Trager. 1978. N-hydroxyamide metabolites of lidocaine, synthesis, characterization, quantitation and mutagenic potential. *J. Med. Chem.* 21:721–725.
386. Piper, J. M., J. Tonascia, G. M. Matanoski. 1985. Heavy phenacetin use and bladder cancer in women aged 20 to 49 years. *N. Engl. J. Med.* 313:292–295.
387. Hathaway, G. J., N. H. Proctor, J. P. Hughes, M. L. Fischman, eds. 1991. *Proctor and Hughes' Chemical Hazards of the Workplace*, 3rd ed., p. 79. New York: Van Nostrand Reinhold.
388. Hathaway, G. J., N. H. Proctor, J. P. Hughes, M. L. Fischman, eds. 1991. *Proctor and Hughes' Chemical Hazards of the Workplace*, 3rd ed., p. 81. New York: Van Nostrand Reinhold.
389. Williams, G. M., J. H. Weisburger. 1986. Chemical carcinogens. In *Cassarett and Doull's Toxicology: The Basic Science of Poisons*, 3rd ed., C. D. Klaassen, M. O. Amdur, J. Doull, eds., pp. 115–116. New York: Macmillan.
390. Casarett, L. J., J. Doull, eds. 1975. *Toxicology: The Basic Science of Poisons.* New York: Macmillan.
391. Hopp, V., I. Henning, eds. 1983. *Handbook of Applied Chemistry,* pp. iv/9-6–37. Washington, DC: Hemisphere Publishing.
392. Williams, G. M., J. H. Weisburger. 1986. Chemical carcinogens. In *Cassarett and Doull's Toxicology: The Basic Science of Poisons*, 3rd ed., C. D. Klaassen, M. O. Amdur, J. Doull, eds., p. 125. New York: Macmillan.
393. Rea, W. J. 1992. *Chemical Sensitivity*, Vol. 1, p. 342. Boca Raton, FL: Lewis Publishers.
394. Hopp, V., I. Henning, eds. 1983. *Handbook of Applied Chemistry: Facts for Engineers, Scientist, Technicians, and Technical Managers*, pp. 11/2–1113. Washington, DC: Hemisphere Publishing.
395. Geiger, L., L. L. Hogy, F. P. Guengerich. 1983. Metabolism of acrylonitrile by isolated rat hepatocytes. *Cancer Res.* 43:3080–3087.
396. Yamada, S. 1964. An occurrence of polyneuritis by n-hexane in the polyethylene laminating plants. *Jpn. J. Industr. Health* 6:19.
397. Williams, G. M., J. H. Weisburger. 1986. Chemical carcinogens. In *Cassarett and Doull's Toxicology: The Basic Science of Poisons*, 3rd ed., C. D. Klaassen, M. O. Amdur, J. Doull, eds., p. 124. New York: Macmillan.
398. Williams, G. M., J. H. Weisburger. 1986. Chemical carcinogens. In *Cassarett and Doull's Toxicology: The Basic Science of Poisons*, 3rd ed., C. D. Klaassen, M. O. Amdur, J. Doull, eds., p. 111. New York: Macmillan.
399. Hopp, V., I. Henning, eds. 1983. *Handbook of Applied Chemistry*, pp. iv/6–iv16. Washington, DC: Hemisphere Publishing.
400. Canaries in the Kitchen: Teflon Toxicosis. EWG. Retrieved February 24, 2016.
401. Daniels, M. 1987. Health debate; non-stick drip pans catch heat. *Chicago Tribune*. March 29, 1987.
402. Daniels, M. 1986. Stove fumes killing cages birds; overheating coated pans can bring quick death, *Chicago Tribune*. March 9, 1986.
403. Hopkins, S. 2001. Bird deaths linked to Teflon coating. *Waikato Times*. Hamilton, New Zealand. Independent Publishers Ltd. July 11, 2001. Copyright 2001 Independent Publishers Ltd.
404. Kreger, T. 2003. Teflon deaths. Email correspondence to EWG. April 2003.
405. Shively, C. 2003. PTFE fumes kill family's pet birds! Accessed online at www.quakerville.com/qic/ezine/96Issue5/qteflon.htm. April 2003.
406. Grahme. 2003. Teflon-related bird information. Email correspondence to Environmental Working Group. April 24, 2003.
407. Anonymous. 2003. Email correspondence to Environmental Working Group. April 2003.
408. Anonymous. 2003. Email correspondence to Environmental Working Group. April 2003.
409. DuPont. 2003. Consumer products help: Cookware safety. Will cooking fumes generated while cooking with non-stick cookware harm people or animals, especially pet birds? Accessed May 10, 2003. http://www.teflon.com.
410. Boucher, M., T. J. Ehmler, A. J. Bermudez. 2000. Polytetrafluoroethylene gas intoxication in broiler chickens. *Avian Dis.* 44:449–453.
411. Waritz, R. S. 1975. An industrial approach to evaluation of pyrolysis and combustion hazards. *Environ. Health Perspect.* 11:197–202.
412. Odegaard, J. I., A. Chawla. 2013. Pleiotropic actions of insulin resistance and inflammation in metabolic homeostasis. *Science* 339 (6116):172–177.

413. Finucane, M. M. et al., Global Burden of Metabolic Risk Factors of Chronic Diseases Collaborating Group (Body Mass Index). 2011. National, regional, and global trends in body-mass index since 1980: Systematic analysis of health examination surveys and epidemiological studies with 960 country-years and 9.1 million participants. *Lancet* 377 (9765):557–567.

414. Adams, K. F., A. Schatzkin, T. B. Harris, V. Kipnis, T. Mouw, R. Ballard-Barbash, A. Hollenbeck, M. F. Leitzmann. 2006. Overweight, obesity, and mortality in a large prospective cohort of persons 50 to 71 years old. *N. Engl. J. Med.* 355 (8):763–778.

415. Rosen, E. D., B. M. Spiegelman. 2006. Adipocytes as regulators of energy balance and glucose homeostasis. *Nature* 444:847–853.

416. Qatanani, M., M. A. Lazar. 2007. Mechanisms of obesity-associated insulin resistance: Many choices on the menu. *Genes Dev.* 21:1443–1455.

417. Samuel, V. T., G. I. Shulman. 2012. Mechanisms for insulin resistance: Common threads and missing links. *Cell* 148:852–871.

418. Cinti, S., G. Mitchell, G. Barbatelli, I. Murano, E. Ceresi, E. Faloia, S. Wang, M. Fortier, A. S. Greenberg, M. S. Obin. 2005. Adipocyte death defines macrophage localization and function in adipose tissue of obese mice and humans. *J. Lipid Res.* 46:2347–2355.

419. Hirosumi, J., G. Tuncman, L. Chang, C. Z. Görgün, K. T. Uysal, K. Maeda, M. Karin, G. S. Hotamisligil. 2002. A central role for JNK in obesity and insulin resistance. *Nature* 420:333–336.

420. Yuan, M., N. Konstantopoulos, J. Lee, L. Hansen, Z. W. Li, M. Karin, S. E. Shoelson. 2001. Reversal of obesity- and diet-induced insulin resistance with salicylates or targeted disruption of Ikkbeta. *Science* 293:1673–1676.

421. Hotamisligil, G. S. 2010. Review endoplasmic reticulum stress and the inflammatory basis of metabolic disease. *Cell* 140:900–917.

422. Nakamura, T., M. Furuhashi, P. Li, H. Cao, G. Tuncman, N. Sonenberg, C. Z. Gorgun, G. S. Hotamisligil. 2010. Double-stranded RNA-dependent protein kinase links pathogen sensing with stress and metabolic homeostasis. *Cell* 140:338–348.

423. Olefsky, J., C. Glass. 2010. Review macrophages, inflammation, and insulin resistance. *Annu. Rev. Physiol.* 72:219–246.

424. Pal, D., S. Dasgupta, R. Kundu, S. Maitra, G. Das, S. Mukhopadhyay, S. Ray, S. S. Majumdar, S. Bhattacharya. 2010. Fetuin-A acts as an endogenous ligand of TLR4 to promote lipid-induced insulin resistance. *Nat. Med.* July 29.

425. Tremaroli, V., F. Backhed. 2012. Review functional interactions between the gut microbiota and host metabolism. *Nature* 489:242–249.

426. Rosenbaum, M., H. R. Kissileff, L. E. Mayer, J. Hirsch, R. L. Leibel. 2010. Review energy intake in weight-reduced humans. *Brain Res.* 1350:95–102.

427. Chawla, A., K. D. Nguyen, Y. P. Goh. 2011. Review macrophage-mediated inflammation in metabolic disease. *Nat. Rev. Immunol.* 11 (11):738–749.

428. Lumeng, C. N., J. L. Bodzin, A. R. Saltiel. 2007. Obesity induces a phenotypic switch in adipose tissue macrophage polarization. *J. Clin. Invest.* 117:175–184.

429. Odegaard, J. I. et al. 2007. Macrophage-specific PPARgamma controls alternative activation and improves insulin resistance. *Nature* 447 (7148):1116–1120.

430. Weisberg, S. P., D. McCann, M. Desai, M. Rosenbaum, R. L. Leibel, A. W. Ferrante Jr. 2003. Obesity is associated with macrophage accumulation in adipose tissue. *J. Clin. Invest.* 112 (12):1796–1808.

431. Xu, H. et al. 2003. Chronic inflammation in fat plays a crucial role in the development of obesity-related insulin resistance. *J. Clin. Invest.* 112 (12):1821–1830.

432. Feuerer, M. et al. 2009. Lean, but not obese, fat is enriched for a unique population of regulatory T cells that affect metabolic parameters. *Nat. Med.* 15:930–939.

433. Nishimura, S. et al. 2009. CD8+ effector T cells contribute to macrophage recruitment and adipose tissue inflammation in obesity. *Nat. Med.* 15 (8):914–920.

434. Winer, S. et al. 2009. Normalization of obesity-associated insulin resistance through immunotherapy. *Nat. Med.* 15 (8):921–929.

435. Wu, D., A. B. Molofsky, H. E. Liang, R. R. Ricardo-Gonzalez, H. A. Jouihan, J. K. Bando, A. Chawla, R. M. Locksley. 2011. Eosinophils sustain adipose alternatively activated macrophages associated with glucose homeostasis. *Science* 332 (6026):243–247.

436. Liu, J. et al. 2009. Genetic deficiency and pharmacological stabilization of mast cells reduce diet-induced obesity and diabetes in mice. *Nat. Med.* 15 (8):940–945.

437. Talukdar, S. et al. 2012. Neutrophils mediate insulin resistance in mice fed a high-fat diet through secreted elastase. *Nat. Med.* 18 (9):1407–1412.

438. Odegaard, J. I., A. Chawla. 2012. Leukocyte set points in metabolic disease. *F1000 Biol. Rep.* 4:13.

439. Kang, K., S. M. Reilly, V. Karabacak, M. R. Gangl, K. Fitzgerald, B. Hatano, C. H. Lee. 2008. Adipocyte-derived Th2 cytokines and myeloid PPARdelta regulate macrophage polarization and insulin sensitivity. *Cell Metab.* 7 (6):485–495.

440. Odegaard, J. I., R. R. Ricardo-Gonzalez, A. Red Eagle, D. Vats, C. R. Morel, M. H. Goforth, V. Subramanian, L. Mukundan, A. W. Ferrante, A. Chawla. 2008. Alternative M2 activation of Kupffer cells by PPARdelta ameliorates obesity-induced insulin resistance. *Cell Metab.* 7 (6):496–507.

441. Liao, X. 2011. Krüppel-like factor 4 regulates macrophage polarization. *J. Clin. Invest.* 121 (7): 2736–2749.

442. Usher, M. G., S. Z. Duan, C. Y. Ivaschenko, R. A. Frieler, S. Berger, G. Schütz, C. N. Lumeng, R. M. Mortensen. 2010. Myeloid mineralocorticoid receptor controls macrophage polarization and cardiovascular hypertrophy and remodeling in mice. *J. Clin. Invest.* 120 (9):3350–3364.

443. Lynch, L., M. Nowak, B. Varghese, J. Clark, A. E. Hogan, V. Toxavidis, S. P. Balk, D. O'Shea, C. O'Farrelly, M. A. Exley. 2012. Adipose tissue invariant NKT cells protect against diet-induced obesity and metabolic disorder through regulatory cytokine production. *Immunity* 37 (3):574–587.

444. Patsouris, D., P. P. Li, D. Thapar, J. Chapman, J. M. Olefsky, J. G. Neels. 2008. Ablation of CD11c-positive cells normalizes insulin sensitivity in obese insulin resistant animals. *Cell Metab.* 8 (4):301–309.

445. Weisberg, S. P., D. Hunter, R. Huber, J. Lemieux, S. Slaymaker, K. Vaddi, I. Charo, R. L. Leibel, A. W. Ferrante Jr. 2006. CCR2 modulates inflammatory and metabolic effects of high-fat feeding. *J. Clin. Invest.* 116 (1):115–124.

446. Kamei, N. et al. 2006. Overexpression of monocyte chemoattractant protein-1 in adipose tissues causes macrophage recruitment and insulin resistance. *J. Biol. Chem.* 281 (36):26602–26614.

447. Huang, W., A. Metlakunta, N. Dedousis, P. Zhang, I. Sipula, J. J. Dube, D. K. Scott, R. M. O'Doherty. 2010. Depletion of liver Kupffer cells prevents the development of diet-induced hepatic steatosis and insulin resistance. *Diabetes* 59 (2):347–357.

448. Eguchi, K. et al. 2012. Saturated fatty acid and TLR signaling link β cell dysfunction and islet inflammation. *Cell Metab.* 15 (4):518–533.

449. Zhang, X., G. Zhang, H. Zhang, M. Karin, H. Bai, D. Cai. 2008. Hypothalamic IKKbeta/NF-kappaB and ER stress link overnutrition to energy imbalance and obesity. *Cell* 135 (1):61–73.

450. Li, P. et al. 2010. Functional heterogeneity of CD11c-positive adipose tissue macrophages in diet-induced obese mice. *J. Biol. Chem.* 285 (20):15333–15345.

451. Hevener, A. L. et al. 2007. Macrophage PPAR gamma is required for normal skeletal muscle and hepatic insulin sensitivity and full antidiabetic effects of thiazolidinediones. *J. Clin. Invest.* 117 (6):1658–1669.

452. Rocha, V. Z., P. Libby. 2009. Obesity, inflammation, and atherosclerosis. *Nat. Rev. Cardiol.* 6 (6):399–409.

453. Shoelson, S. E., J. Lee, A. B. Goldfine. 2006. Inflammation and insulin resistance. *J. Clin. Invest.* 116 (7):1793–1801.

454. Asterholm, I. W., D. I. Mundy, J. Weng, R. G. Anderson, P. E. Scherer. 2012. Altered mitochondrial function and metabolic inflexibility associated with loss of caveolin-1. *Cell Metab.* 15 (2):171–185.

455. Hotamisligil, G. S., R. S. Johnson, R. J. Distel, R. Ellis, V. E. Papaioannou, B. M. Spiegelman. 1996. Uncoupling of obesity from insulin resistance through a targeted mutation in aP2, the adipocyte fatty acid binding protein. *Science* 274 (5291):1377–1379.

456. Martin, S. L. 2008. Mammalian hibernation: A naturally reversible model for insulin resistance in man? *Diab. Vasc. Dis. Res.* 5 (2):76–81.

457. Bogardus, C., S. Lillioja, D. Mott, G. R. Reaven, A. Kashiwagi, J. E. Foley. 1984. Relationship between obesity and maximal insulin-stimulated glucose uptake *in vivo* and *in vitro* in Pima Indians. *J. Clin. Invest.* 73 (3):800–805.

458. Samocha-Bonet, D., D. J. Chisholm, K. Tonks, L. V. Campbell, J. R. Greenfield. 2012. Insulin-sensitive obesity in humans — A 'favorable fat' phenotype? *Trends Endocrinol. Metab.* 23 (3):116–124.

459. Lehrke, M., M. A. Lazar. 2005. The many faces of PPARgamma. *Cell* 123 (6):993–999.

460. Power, M. L., J. Schulkin. 2012. Maternal obesity, metabolic disease, and allostatic load. *Physiol. Behav.* 106 (1):22–28.

461. Cranford, J. A. 1983. Body temperature, heart rate and oxygen consumption of normothermic and heterothermic western jumping mice (*Zapus princeps*). *Comp. Biochem. Physiol. A Comp. Physiol.* 74 (3):595–599.

462. Arinell, K., B. Sahdo, A. L. Evans, J. M. Arnemo, U. Baandrup, O. Fröbert. 2012. Brown bears (*Ursus arctos*) seem resistant to atherosclerosis despite highly elevated plasma lipids during hibernation and active state. *Clin. Transl. Sci.* 5 (3):269–272.

463. Mominoki, K., M. Morimatsu, M. Karjalainen, E. Hohtola, R. Hissa, M. Saito. 2005. Elevated plasma concentrations of haptoglobin in European brown bears during hibernation. *Comp. Biochem. Physiol. A Mol. Integr. Physiol.* 142 (4):472–477.

464. Hall, J. E. *Guyton and Hall Textbook of Medical Physiology.* Saunders. 2010. p. 12

465. Saltiel, A. R. 2012. Insulin resistance in the defense against obesity. *Cell Metab.* 15 (6):798–804.

466. Tseng, Y. H., A. M. Cypess, C. R. Kahn. 2010. Cellular bioenergetics as a target for obesity therapy. *Nat. Rev. Drug Discov.* 9 (6):465–482.

467. Ricardo-Gonzalez, R. R., A. Red Eagle, J. I. Odegaard, H. Jouihan, C. R. Morel, J. E. Heredia, L. Mukundan, D. Wu, R. M. Locksley, A. Chawla. 2010. IL-4/STAT6 immune axis regulates peripheral nutrient metabolism and insulin sensitivity. *Proc. Natl. Acad. Sci. U. S. A.* 107 (52):22617–22622.

468. Nguyen, K., Y. Qiu, X. Cui, Y. P. Goh, J. Mwangi, T. David, L. Mukundan, F. Brombacher, R. M. Locksley, A. Chawla. 2011. Alternatively activated macrophages produce catecholamines to sustain adaptive thermogenesis. *Nature* 480 (7375):104–108.

469. Ravichandran, K. S. 2011. Beginnings of a good apoptotic meal: The find-me and eat-me signaling pathways. *Immunity* 35 (4):445–455.

470. Gordon, S., P. R. Taylor. 2005. Monocyte and macrophage heterogeneity. *Nat. Rev. Immunol.* 5 (12):953–964.

471. Cipolletta, D., M. Feuerer, A. Li, N. Kamei, J. Lee, S. E. Shoelson, C. Benoist, D. Mathis. 2012. PPAR-γ is a major driver of the accumulation and phenotype of adipose tissue Treg cells. *Nature* 486 (7404):549–553.

472. Gautier, E. L. et al., Immunological Genome Consortium. 2012. Gene-expression profiles and transcriptional regulatory pathways that underlie the identity and diversity of mouse tissue macrophages. *Nat. Immunol.* 13 (11):1118–1128.

473. Tremblay, M. E., R. L. Lowery, A. K. Majewska. 2010. Microglial interactions with synapses are modulated by visual experience. *PLoS Biol.* 8 (11):e1000527.

474. Ichimura, A. et al. 2012. Dysfunction of lipid sensor GPR120 leads to obesity in both mouse and human. *Nature* 483 (7389):350–354.

475. O'Brien, P. E. et al. 2006. Treatment of mild to moderate obesity with laparoscopic adjustable gastric banding or an intensive medical program: A randomized trial. *Ann. Intern. Med.* 144 (9):625–633.

476. Chiang, S. H. et al. 2009. The protein kinase IKKepsilon regulates energy balance in obese mice. *Cell* 138 (5):961–975.

477. Oh, D. Y., S. Talukdar, E. J. Bae, T. Imamura, H. Morinaga, W. Fan, P. Li, W. J. Lu, S. M. Watkins, J. M. Olefsky. 2010. GPR120 is an omega-3 fatty acid receptor mediating potent anti-inflammatory and insulin-sensitizing effects. *Cell* 142 (5):687–698.

478. Hartman, A. 1995. Diagrammatic assessment of family relationships. Families in society. *J. Contemp. Human Ser.* 1:111–122.

479. Wolff, M. S., H. A. Anderson, K. D. Roseman, I. J. Selikoff. 1979. Equilibrium of polybrominated biphenyl (PBB) residues in serum and fat of Michigan residents. *Bull. Environ. Contam. Toxicol.* 21:775–781.

480. Rea, W. J., Y. Pan, J. L. Laseter, A. R. Johnson, E. J. Fenyves. 1987. Toxic volatile organic hydrocarbons in chemically sensitive patients. *Clin. Ecol.* 5(2):70–74.

6 Formaldehyde

INTRODUCTION

Owing to its prevalence and toxicity, formaldehyde is discussed separately from other toxic chemicals. This is because it is ubiquitous in the chemically sensitive environment and has been found to propagate chronic degenerative disease as well as chemical sensitivity. The majority of chemically sensitive patients are triggered by formaldehyde challenge and do not do well in environments with much formaldehyde. Formaldehyde is the third most common environmental trigger of disease after natural gas and pesticides experienced in indoor air.

CHEMISTRY

Formaldehyde ($H-\underset{\underset{O}{\|}}{C}-H$) is an aliphatic hydrocarbon that is usually derived from petroleum, but it can be generated naturally at low levels in humans. It is widely distributed in products and industry, with uses in commerce and the home. Formaldehyde, being the number 3 pollutant in the home among other indoor air pollutants after natural gas and pesticides, can cause much discomfort and dysfunction of human physiology. Formaldehyde is obtained in pure crystals or in a liquid form called formalin, which is about 37% formaldehyde, 10% methyl alcohol, and 53% inert ingredients. Formaldehyde has the following physical properties: it is a colorless gas with a molecular weight of 30.0, a melting point of $-92°C$, and a boiling point of 19°C. Its characteristic odor is hay- or straw-like, and at high concentrations, it is pungent. For air pollution measurements, we consider 1 mg/m^3 = 0.815 ppm or 1 ppm = 1.248 mg/m^3. The threshold limit value (TLV) for the industrial environment is 2 ppm. There is no known safe level for 24-hour human exposure, and this is emphasized by reactions in the chemically sensitive who react at much lower levels in the lower parts per billion levels found in some indoor air samples. Table 6.1 shows an air analysis from a home concentrated with formaldehyde and other aldehydes. It also shows the total home load filled with other aldehydes and associated toxics. The metabolism of formaldehyde is discussed elsewhere. Its detoxification involves the aldehyde dehydrogenase noncytochrome enzyme systems, with a conversion to alcohol which requires alcohol dehydrogenase for its detoxification; both of these are zinc-dependent enzymes.

Furfural: Except for occasional use in perfume, furfural remained a relatively obscure chemical until 1922, when the Quaker Oats Company began mass-producing it from oat hulls. Today, furfural is still produced from agricultural by-products like sugarcane, bagasse, and corn cobs. The main countries producing furfural today are South Africa and China.

Furfural is an important renewable, nonpetroleum-based, chemical feedstock. Hydrogenation of furfural provides furfuryl alcohol (FA), which is a useful chemical intermediate and which may be further hydrogenated to tetrahydrofurfuryl alcohol (THFA). THFA is used as a nonhazardous solvent in agricultural formulations and as an adjuvant to help herbicides penetrate the leaf structure. Furfural is used to make other furan chemicals, such as furoic acid via oxidation[1] and furan itself via palladium-catalyzed vapor-phase decarbonylation[2]. Furfural is also an important chemical solvent.

Acetic acid is one of the simplest carboxylic acids. It is an important chemical reagent and industrial chemical, mainly used in the production of cellulose acetate, especially for photographic film and polyvinyl acetate for wood glue, as well as synthetic fibers and fabrics. In households, diluted acetic acid is often used in descaling agents. In the food industry, acetic acid is used under the food

TABLE 6.1

Volatile Organic Compounds (VOCs) and Aldehydes: A Home with High Levels of Aldehydes and Other Toxics

VOCs and Aldehydes	Test Results ($\mu g/m^3$)	Reference Levels ($\mu g/m^3$)	Comparison to Reference Levels (%)
Formaldehyde	80	20	400.0
Acetic acid	33.8	25	30
Furfuraldehyde	10.3	8	10
Crotenaldehyde	1	0.9	25
Acetaldehyde	42	45	93.3
Hexaldehyde[a]	30	80	37.5
Decanal	1.0	4	25.0
Butyraldehyde	9	74	12.2
d-Limonene	11.6	110	10.5
N-Butyl acetate	3.4	36	9.4
Nonyl aldehyde	12.9	150	8.6
α-Pinene	26.9	350	7.7
Valeraldehyde	12	180	6.7
Hexanoic acid	2.5	48	5.2
Glycol ether EB	1.3	36	3.6
Octylaldehyde	5.0	150	3.3
Methyl isobutyl ketone	1.8	82	2.2
Myrcene	1.6	100	1.6
N-Pentane	4.6	350	1.3
β-Pinene	3.5	350	1.0
N-Hexane	1.5	200	0.8
Dodecane	2.5	350	0.7
Isopentane	2.4	350	0.7
Isopropyl alcohol	3.0	492	0.6
Acetone	3.3	590	0.6
2,6,7-Trimethyl decane	1.2	245	0.5
Glycol ether DPM	1.2	310	0.4
2-Methylpentane	1.1	350	0.3
Toluene	2.9	1200	0.2
2-Heptanone	1.8	840	0.2
Decane	2.1	1000	0.2
Methyl ethyl ketone	0.7	590	0.1
2-Pentyl furan	5.9	n/l	n/l
Butyl butyrate	3.2	n/l	n/l
Total other VOCs as toluene	93		
Total VOCs and aldehydes	410.9	<200	

Source: Environmental Health Center-Dallas, January 2013.

Note: n/l, normal limits.

[a] Short-term ESL.

additive code E260 as an acidity regulator and as a condiment. As a food additive, it is approved for usage in the EU,[3] the United States,[4] Australia, and New Zealand.[5]

In the air, acetic acid can convert isoprene into camphor from α- and β-pinene.

The global demand of acetic acid is around 6.5 million tons per year (Mt/a), of which approximately 1.5 Mt/a is met by recycling; the remainder is manufactured from petrochemical feedstock.[6]

TABLE 6.2

Aldehydes Sampling Method: Collection on DNPH/Silica Gel Analytical Method HPLC-UV

Compound	Test Results (μg/m³)	Ppbv	Recommended Maximum Chronic Concentration (μg/m³)	Typical Sources
Formaldehyde	80	66	20	Paint, particleboard, plywood, adhesives, fiberglass insulation, and auto exhaust
Acetaldehyde	42	23	45	Food products, perfumes, tobacco smoke, paints, and auto exhaust
Acrolein	<1	<1	0.23	Plastics, perfumes, cooking animal fats, and laminate wood products
Propionaldehyde	<1	<1	46	Food products, paints, and laminate
Crotenaldehyde	1	<1	0.9	wood products
Butyraldehyde	9	3	74	Food products, degradation of fats and oils
Benzaldehyde	<1	<1	9	Oil alkyd paints, coatings, and adhesives
Tolualdehyde, *o*, *m*, and *p*	<1	<1	9	
Valeraldehyde	12	3	180	
Hexaldehyde[a]	30	7	80	
Heptaldehyde	<1	<1	40	

[a] Short-term ESL.

As a chemical reagent, biological sources of acetic acid are of interest but generally uncompetitive. Vinegar is dilute acetic acid often produced by fermentation and subsequent oxidation of ethanol (Table 6.2).

SOURCES OF FORMALDEHYDE POLLUTION

Formaldehyde is a common air contaminant in urban areas and usually accounts for about 50% of the total aldehydes in polluted air (Table 6.1). The highest level of formaldehyde is measured in urban air in Los Angeles[7] and total aldehydes in Washington DC is 0.1 ppm.[8] In urban air, levels typically range from 0.005 to 0.015 ppm. Normal humans can perceive the odor of formaldehyde at about 0.2 ppm. Often, the chemically sensitive can detect it at a lesser level; however, our experience is that the average chemically sensitive individual cannot detect any formaldehyde at a level less than 0.2 ppm due to the masking phenomenon. Although unmasked, they can perceive levels as low as 0.02 ppb. The response is usually unknown, causing pain, fibromyalgia, and severe fatigue. Nonetheless, many chemically sensitive patients do not do well in major cities, probably because of an additive effect from formaldehyde exposure along with other toxic exposures, such as nitrogen dioxide, carbon monoxide, ozone, particulates, and hydrocarbons such as car exhaust, gasoline, pesticides, etc. Formaldehyde can damage the olfactory nerve endings and thereby decrease an individual's ability to perceive its odor for several other toxic odors. Other aldehydes are found in air analysis of homes, including acetaldehyde, benzaldehyde, tolualdehyde, hexaldehyde, propional-dehyde, valeraldehyde, furfuraldehyde, butyraldehyde, crotenaldehyde, nonyl aldehyde, etc. (Table 6.2). Often, aldehydes, especially formaldehyde, are found in breath analysis. Formaldehyde is the third most common offender of toxics in the home. This is after the two most common offenders—natural gas and pesticides.

The primary source of formaldehyde in urban air is the incomplete combustion of hydrocarbons in gasoline and diesel engines, burning of fuels, and incineration of waste. The concentration formaldehyde—in diesel exhaust is 18.3 ppm, and in gasoline exhaust, it is 11.3–14.9 ppm.[9]

Combustion processes account directly or indirectly for most of the formaldehyde entering the environment. Direct combustion sources include power plants, incinerators, refineries, wood stoves, kerosene heaters, and cigarettes. Formaldehyde is produced indirectly by photochemical oxidation of hydrocarbons or other formaldehyde precursors that are released from combustion processes.[8] During smog episodes, indirect production of formaldehyde may be greater than direct emissions.[10] Oxidation of methane is the dominant source of formaldehyde in regions remote from hydrocarbon emissions.[11] Other anthropogenic sources of formaldehyde in the environment include vent gas from formaldehyde production; exhaust from diesel and gasoline-powered motor vehicles; emissions from the use of formaldehyde as a fumigant, soil disinfectant, embalming fluid, and leather tanning agent; emissions from resins in particleboard and plywood; emissions from resin-treated fabrics and paper; waste water from the production and use of formaldehyde in the manufacture of various resins and as a chemical intermediate; and waste water from the use of formaldehyde-containing resins.[8,9,12,13] Natural sources of formaldehyde include forest fires, animal wastes, microbial products of biological systems, and plant volatiles.

Formaldehyde has been identified in at least 26 of the 1428 current or former EPA National Priorities List (NPL) hazardous wastes sites.[14] However, the number of sites evaluated for formaldehyde is not known.

Although formaldehyde is found in remote areas, it is not probably transported there but is generated from longer-lived precursors that have been transported there.[8] Formaldehyde is soluble and will transfer into rain and surface water. Based upon the Henry's law constant for formaldehyde, volatilization from water is not expected to be significant. No experimental data were found concerning the adsorption of formaldehyde to soil, but because of the low octanol/water partition coefficient (log $K_{ow} = 0.35$),[15] little adsorption to soil or sediment is expected to occur. No evidence of bioaccumulation has been found.

The input of formaldehyde into the environment is counterbalanced by its removal by several pathways. Formaldehyde is removed from the air by direct photolysis and oxidation by photochemically produced hydroxyl and nitrate radicals. Measured or estimated half-lives for formaldehyde in the atmosphere range from 1.6 to 19 hours, depending upon estimates of radiant energy, the presence and concentrations of other pollutants, and other factors.[16–20] When released to water, formaldehyde will biodegrade to low levels in a few days.[21] In water, formaldehyde is hydrated; it does not have a chromophore that is capable of absorbing sunlight and photochemically decomposing.[22]

Levels of formaldehyde in the atmosphere and in indoor air are well documented. In a survey of ambient measurements of hazardous air pollutants, a median formaldehyde concentration of 2.5 ppb was found for a total of 1358 samples collected at 58 different locations.[23] In several separate studies involving rural and urban areas in the United States, atmospheric concentrations ranged from 1 to 68 ppb.[24–27] Generally, indoor residential formaldehyde concentrations are significantly higher than outdoor concentrations causing mild to severe chemical sensitivity in many cases. Formaldehyde concentrations in complaint homes (homes where people have complained of adverse symptoms), mobile homes, and homes containing large quantities of particleboard or urea-formaldehyde foam insulation (UFFI) have been measured at 0.02–0.8 ppm, with levels as high as 4 ppm, sufficient to cause irritating symptoms, observed in some instances.[28] Since the time, many of the above monitoring studies were performed; plywood and particleboard manufacturing methods have been changed to reduce the formaldehyde emission levels in the finished product.[29] However, changes are not significant enough to render building safe offices. Similarly, home construction methods have changed and the use of UFFI has been greatly reduced since the mid-1980s.[30] A recent pilot study on a newly constructed home reported localized formaldehyde concentrations of 0.076 ppm.[31] Approximately 30 days after the installation of pressed wood products, the average indoor concentration attained a level of 0.035–0.45 ppm. Older conventional homes tend to have the lowest indoor concentrations of formaldehyde, with values typically less than 0.05 ppm,[28] and mobile homes the highest due to their low rate of air exchange.[32] Few chemically sensitive patients can tolerate mobile homes.

Although pressed wood products may be a source of formaldehyde in indoor air, there are numerous others. These include permanent-press fabrics, fiberglass products, decorative laminates, paper goods, paints, wallpaper, foam mattresses, and cosmetics.[33] Its presence in indoor air also results from combustion sources, such as stoves, heaters, or burning cigarettes.[8,34]

Formaldehyde may also arise from the degradation of volatile organic chemicals commonly found in indoor air.[35,36]

Formaldehyde is unstable in water; however, it has been detected in municipal and industrial aqueous effluents, rainwater, lake water, and some waterways.[37,38] Formaldehyde levels in rainwater collected in California are low, ranging from not detectable to 0.06 µg/mL.[39] Measured concentrations of formaldehyde range from 0.12 to 6.8 mg/L in fogwater[40,41]; from 1.4 to 1.8 mg/L in cloudwater[40]; and from 0.25 to 0.56 mg/L in mist samples.[39] No data on formaldehyde levels in soil could be found in the literature.

Formaldehyde was found in three types of chewing tobacco[42] and in cigarette smoke.[43] Formaldehyde has also been found at levels ranging from 1 to 3517 ppm in fabric samples.[44]

A major route of formaldehyde exposure for the general population is inhalation of indoor air; releases of formaldehyde from new or recently installed building materials and furnishings may account for most of the exposure. Environmental tobacco smoke may contribute 10%–25% of the exposure. Since formaldehyde in food is not available in free form, it is not included in estimated exposures.[10] Consumers can be exposed to formaldehyde gas through its use in construction materials, wood products, textiles, home furnishings, paper, cosmetics, and pharmaceuticals. Dermal contact with formaldehyde-containing materials, including some paper products, fabrics, and cosmetics, may also lead to consumer exposure. Commuters may be exposed to formaldehyde while riding in automobiles or subways, walking, and biking.[45]

Occupational exposure to formaldehyde can occur during its production and its use in the production of end products, in the garment industry, in the building materials industry, and in laboratories. Healthcare professionals may be exposed to formaldehyde vapors during preparation, administration, and/or cleanup of various medicines. Pathologists, histology technicians, morticians, and teachers and students who handle preserved specimens may also be exposed. The National Occupational Exposure Survey (NOES), conducted from 1981 to 1983, indicated that 1,329,332 workers in various professions were exposed to formaldehyde in the United States.[46]

Members of the general population who come in contact with a large amount of unwashed permanent-press fabrics treated with formaldehyde-releasing resins may also be exposed to high levels.

RELEASES TO THE ENVIRONMENT

According to the Toxics Release Inventory (TRI), in 1996, 21 million pounds (9.6 million kg) of formaldehyde were released to the environment from 674 domestic manufacturing and processing facilities.[47] This number represents the sum of all releases of formaldehyde to air, water, soil, and underground injection wells. An additional 1.8 million pounds (0.8 million kg) were transferred to publicly owned treatment works (POTWs), and 1.3 million pounds (0.6 million kg) were transferred off-site.[47] Table 6.3 lists amounts released from these facilities. The TRI data should be used with caution because only certain types of facilities are required to report.[48] This is not an exhaustive list.

AIR

Formaldehyde is released to outdoor air from both natural and industrial sources. Combustion processes account directly or indirectly for most of the formaldehyde entering the atmosphere. One important source of formaldehyde is automotive exhaust from engines not equipped with catalytic converters.[49] Automobiles were found to emit about 610 million pounds (277 million kg) of formaldehyde each year.[12] Emissions were reduced with the introduction of the catalytic converter in

TABLE 6.3

Releases to the Environment from Facilities That Manufacture or Process Formaldehyde

Total of Reported Amounts Released in Pounds per Year[a]

State[b]	Number of Facilities	Air[c]	Water	Land	Underground Injection	Total Environment[d]	POTW[e] Transfer	Off-Site Waste Transfer
AK	1	375	0	0	0	375	0	0
AL	31	477,346	1312	361	0	479,019	2854	23,887
AR	15	204,464	735	5	0	205,204	1015	5229
AZ	3	12,873	0	0	0	12,873	13,000	13,140
CA	25	417,661	250	769	0	418,680	68,609	3658
CO	2	2062	0	0	0	2062	170	0
CT	6	27,833	4581	0	0	32,414	29,641	16,967
DE	1	1965	0	0	0	1965	0	0
FL	6	95,126	1522	37	0	96,685	0	1000
GA	36	702,021	714	500	0	703,235	4600	12,600
IA	4	30,736	400	0	0	31,136	580	1605
IL	24	37,944	2084	204	0	40,232	22,900	67,527
IN	15	76,532	0	0	0	76,532	47,761	5171
KS	8	278,316	0	0	27,000	305,316	10,320	1198
KY	8	65,275	21,902	0	0	87,177	1510	27,180
LA	31	330,423	15,674	382	8,601,956	8,948,435	0	76,529
MA	10	60,059	10	1500	0	61,569	809,791	17,273
MD	2	5517	0	0	0	5517	0	6175
ME	3	121.198	0	0	0	121,198	5229	58
MI	30	205,766	2396	12,553	250	220,965	493,193	227,079
MN	15	536.241	0	0	0	536,241	17,250	3945
MO	12	441,774	1127	5	0	442,906	19,343	67,062
MS	16	477,785	1102	2	0	478,889	0	4671
MT	4	100,214	0	0	0	100,214	0	250
NC	39	1,048,939	6689	1201	0	1,056,829	15,905	38,161
NH	4	5582	9419	4100	0	19,101	6372	512
NJ	18	52,595	3977	250	0	56,822	42,613	2509
NM	1	4570	0	0	0	4570	0	0
NV	1	4001	0	0	0	4001	0	802
NY	23	280,861	8409	40	0	289,310	8103	56,005
OH	49	1,031,374	87,225	87,335	13,000	1,218,934	126,617	173,090
OK	4	64,911	4	0	0	64,915	0	13,642
OR	25	1,070,119	3600	20	0	1,073,739	24,928	15,676
PA	21	274,854	1331	0	0	276,185	0	16,703
PR	4	2766	0	0	0	2766	20,827	530
RI	4	4753	0	0	0	4753	2042	0
SC	39	752,317	57,542	3800	0	813,659	16,718	217,365
SD	1	55,731	0	0	0	55,731	0	0
TN	8	295,461	1170	397	0	297,028	8329	5493
TX	55	996,970	31,770	500	761,069	1,790,309	4557	60,341
UT	4	18,313	0	0	0	18,313	23,568	285
VA	25	369,447	956	232	0	370,635	15,059	31,235
VT	1	333	0	0	0	333	0	0

(Continued)

TABLE 6.3 (*Continued*)

Releases to the Environment from Facilities That Manufacture or Process Formaldehyde

Total of Reported Amounts Released in Pounds per Year[a]

State[b]	Number of Facilities	Air[c]	Water	Land	Underground Injection	Total Environment[d]	POTW[e] Transfer	Off-Site Waste Transfer
WA	8	109,080	45,720	0	0	154,800	3028	760
WI	22	138,117	7422	213	0	145,752	17,204	53,649
WV	10	128,600	960	0	0	129,560	5136	14,154
	Totals	11,419,200	320,003	114,406	9,403,275	21,256,884		

Source: TRI96. 1998. Toxic Chemical Release Inventory. National Library of Medicine, National Toxicology Information Program, Bethesda, MD.

a Data in TRI are maximum amounts released by each facility.

b Post office state abbreviations used.

c The sum of fugitive and stack releases is included in releases to air by a given facility.

d The sum of all releases of the chemical to air, land, water, and underground injection wells; and transfers off-site by a given facility.

e POTW, publicly owned treatment works.

1975;[50] although they have been found to rise again with the introduction of oxygenated fuels.[51] Gaffney and coworkers found that in urban areas, the introduction of oxygenated fuels led to increased anthropogenic emissions of formaldehyde during the winter, the season these fuels are used.[52] Formaldehyde in vehicle emissions in 1994 were found to increase by 13% within 2 months after the average oxygen content of fuels sold in the San Francisco Bay area increased from 0.3% to 2.0% by weight.[51]

Formaldehyde concentrations in jet engine exhaust have been found to range from 0.761 to 1.14 ppm.[53] Formaldehyde is formed in large quantities in the troposphere by the oxidation of hydrocarbons,[49,54] leading to elevated formaldehyde levels shortly after periods of high vehicular traffic.[55]

Statistical analyses of formaldehyde data from four sites in New Jersey have been used to evaluate the effects of automobile traffic and photochemical formation on formaldehyde concentrations.[56] Integrated formaldehyde concentrations during the hours 5:00 a.m. to 8:00 p.m. decreased from workdays to Saturdays to Sundays, corresponding to a decrease in motor vehicle traffic. On workdays, formaldehyde concentrations were higher on days with more photochemical activity.

Altshuller[57] investigated the sources of aldehydes in the atmosphere during the night and early morning hours (between 9:00 p.m. and 9:00 a.m.). At night, the predominant sources of aldehydes should be the reaction of alkenes with O_3 and NO_3; during the early daylight hours, OH radical reactions with alkenes and alkanes will also contribute to aldehyde production. Altshuller[57] found that although the emissions of formaldehyde from vehicular exhaust are substantially relative to emissions of alkenes from vehicular exhaust, the secondary atmospheric production of aldehydes from the alkenes emitted from all vehicular sources during the period 9:00 p.m. to 9:00 a.m. can exceed the primary emissions of formaldehyde. However, if there is a large shift in the future to vehicles fueled with methanol and/or natural gas, formaldehyde emissions from the exhaust could predominate over the secondary emissions of formaldehyde during the 9:00 p.m. to 9:00 a.m. period. It should be noted that the rate of secondary production of aldehydes during the period 9:00 p.m. to 9:00 a.m. is much less than during the late morning and afternoon hours.[57]

Grosjean et al.[58] estimated the relative contributions of direct emissions and atmospheric photochemistry to levels of formaldehyde and other carbonyls in Los Angeles using measurements carried out simultaneously at a near-source site and at a site where the air quality was dominated by transport of polluted air masses from the downtown area (downwind smog receptor site). They found that the formaldehyde/carbon monoxide ratios were substantially higher at the downwind locations (average values, 3.2–11.7) than at the near-source site (average value, 1.8), indicating that photochemical production predominates over direct emissions in controlling formaldehyde levels in Los Angeles air. Using two models, their data were translated into formaldehyde photochemical production rates of 12–161 tons per day.

The amount of formaldehyde released to the atmosphere in 1996 by the U.S. industrial facilities sorted by state is given in Table 6.3.[47] According to TRI96,[47] an estimated total of 11.4 million pounds (5.2 million kg) of formaldehyde, amounting to approximately 54% of the total environmental release, was discharged to the air from 674 manufacturing and processing facilities in the United States in 1996. The TRI data should be used with caution since only certain types of facilities are required to report. This is not an exhaustive list.

Dempsey[59] estimated the masses of selected organic emissions from hazardous waste incinerators (HWIs) on a nationwide scale using "reasonable worst-case" assumptions. Formaldehyde emissions formed during combustion of hazardous wastes were estimated to be 892 ng/L, which would result in a release of 7.8 tons of formaldehyde to the air per year. When compared to the 1990 TRI air release data from the U.S. manufacturing operations, formaldehyde emissions from HWIs were found to be very small (0.12%).

There is a potential for release of formaldehyde to air from hazardous waste sites. Formaldehyde has been detected in air samples collected at 5 of the 26 hazardous waste sites where formaldehyde has been detected in some environmental medium.[14]

Pressed wood products contribute to indoor formaldehyde levels. Combustion sources and phenol-formaldehyde resin bonded products generally are weak emitters to indoor air. Common indoor combustion sources include gas burners and ovens, kerosene heaters, and cigarettes.[34]

Formaldehyde also arises in the atmosphere from natural sources. In monitoring studies performed in New Mexico, 1993–1994, Gaffney and coworkers looked at total (average) formaldehyde concentrations and formaldehyde:acetaldehyde ratios.[52] These researchers reported that if formaldehyde and acetaldehyde were being formed solely from the atmospheric oxidation of naturally occurring alkenes, the ratio of the two chemicals would be expected to be about 10. In this study, the formaldehyde:acetaldehyde ratio was lowest during the winter months and highest in the summer months. Gaffney et al.[52] concluded that atmospheric formaldehyde in urban areas resulted from both anthropogenic emissions and natural sources in the summer and primarily from anthropogenic sources during the winter.

Indirect production of formaldehyde may occur through the photochemical oxidation of airborne hydrocarbons from vehicle exhausts, the incomplete combustion of hydrocarbons in fuels, and from various other sources. In 1985, an estimated 253,201 metric tons/year of formaldehyde was released into the air from combustion (mobile, stationary, natural), petroleum, catalytic cracking, and phthalic anhydride production from mobile sources.[60] In 2010, these releases occurred primarily in urban and industrial areas. The EPA estimated formaldehyde production from this source at 127×10^6 lb/year.[61] Other sources of formaldehyde in the atmosphere include cigarette smoke, which has been measured at levels greater that 0.2 ppm,[62] and anaerobic decomposition of methane by microbes.[9]

Formaldehyde is widely used in industrialized societies. Its major uses are listed in Table 6.4. Because of its ubiquitousness, it often has a significant, negative impact on the chemically sensitive.

Formaldehyde is produced in the United States by 14 chemical companies in 48 locations encompassing 21 states.[60] Almost all (99%) of the 2710 million kg of formaldehyde directly produced in the United States in 1979 was consumed domestically.[63]

FORMALDEHYDE IS USED UBIQUITOUSLY IN THE INDOOR ENVIRONMENT

Lundqvist and Molhave[64] reported that formaldehyde levels in 25 recently constructed houses where particleboard had been used extensively in floors and walls ranged from 0.07 to 1.8 ppm, with a

---

TABLE 6.4

Major Uses of Formaldehyde in Industrialized Societies

1. To make permanent-press and wash-and-wear fabrics
2. As a tanning agent; therefore, will be in leather products
3. In the formulation of slow-release nitrogen fertilizers
4. In destroying microorganisms responsible for plant and human disease
5. As an additive to make concrete and plaster impermeable to liquids
6. As an antiperspirant and as an antiseptic in dentifrices, mouthwashes, and germicidal and detergent soaps
7. In hair-setting lotions and in shampoos
8. As air deodorant in public places and industrial environments
9. In synthesis of dyes, stripping agents, and various specialty chemicals in the dye industry (improves the color stability of dyed fabrics)
10. In embalming fluids
11. Preservative in waxes, polishes, adhesives, fats, oils, and anatomical specimens
12. To prepare fireproof compositions to apply to fabrics
13. In insecticidal solutions for killing flies, mosquitoes, and moths
14. To improve the wet strength and water resistance of paper products
15. As a preservative and accelerator for photographic developing solutions
16. To make natural and synthetic fibers crease resistant, wrinkle resistant, crush proof, water repellent, dye-fast, flame resistant, water resistant, shrink proof, moth proof (wool), and more elastic (wool)
17. One of the component parts of wallboard used in construction of houses and apartments
18. As a resin in nail polish and undercoating of nail polish
19. In building materials such as plywood, particleboard, fiberboard (especially in mobile homes), and urea-formaldehyde (UF) insulation

---

median value of 0.50. In 1977 and 1978, Breysse[65,66] reported his findings of excessive formaldehyde levels in the U.S. residences, and Sundin[67] observed formaldehyde levels in Swedish conventional homes, 75% of which contained unique fiberboard ceiling panels, to an average of 0.58 ppm.

In the period from 1978 to 1985, a significant number of residential formaldehyde measurements were carried out by state health departments in response to consumer complaints. States involved in these investigations included Connecticut,[68] Wisconsin,[69,70] New Hampshire,[71] Minnesota,[72] Texas,[73] New York,[74] California,[75] and Indiana.[76] Also, the Consumer Product Safety Commission[77] investigated residential formaldehyde levels. Both conventional and mobile homes were inspected.

In addition to state health investigations, epidemiological studies and studies designed to determine formaldehyde levels in specific structure types based on random selection have been conducted. Formaldehyde levels reported for epidemiological studies include those of Broder et al.,[78] Sterling et al.,[79] and a study of mobile homes in Texas,[80] which found that formaldehyde levels varied considerably on the basis of geographic location. Studies of mobile homes at various locations in the Southeast, Texas, California, and in the north central states,[81] and of conventional homes in eastern Tennessee[82] and Houston,[83] again recorded a variety of residential formaldehyde levels. A whole group of government studies reported recently developed mobile homes which were developed as a substitute large area after a hurricane were deemed unlivable due to the extraordinarily high levels of formaldehyde.[76]

For a basis of comparison and discussion, formaldehyde levels from these studies are summarized in Tables 6.5 through 6.8. With the exception of formaldehyde levels reported for conventional homes in Denmark and Sweden, it is obvious that the highest formaldehyde levels, and thus exposures, occur in mobile homes built in the United States. Further, mobile homes consistently appear to have a broader range of formaldehyde with some levels well in excess of 1.0 ppm. Relative to other states, levels in mobile homes in California appear to be unusually low. These differences may be due to climatic factors, lifestyle factors, or differences in sampling techniques and study protocol. In general, the highest concentrations occur in mobile homes sampled prior to 1982 and

TABLE 6.5

Family of Mother, Father, and Two Daughters with Formaldehyde Sensitivity Causing Other Chemical Sensitivity (Double-Blind Inhaled Challenges after 4 Days Deadaptation with Total Load Reduced in ECU, EHC-Dallas)

Incitant	PPM	Reaction—Patient Initials			
		CT	ST	BT	MT
Formaldehyde	<0.2	4+	4+	4+	4+
Phenol	<0.002	−	−	−	−
Pesticide (2,4-DNP)	<0.0034	4+	4+	4+	4+
Ethanol (petroleum derived)	<0.50	+	+	+	+
Chlorine	<0.33	−	−	−	−
Placebo #1			−	−	−
Placebo #2			−	−	−

Source: Modified from Rea, W.J. 1994. *Chemical Sensitivity, Volume II*, page 948, table 6.

in complaint-related investigations as compared with noncomplaint studies. An example of the devastating effects of formaldehyde-contaminated air on the occupants of a mobile home is shown in the following case report.

Case study: In 1980, when the mother, aged 36 years, was 6 months pregnant, she and her family moved into a new double-wide mobile home, which was subsequently shown to have contained a high level of formaldehyde contamination, for 2½ years. They began to have unexplained medical problems.

TABLE 6.6

Formaldehyde Emissions from a Variety of Construction Materials, Furnishings, and Consumer Products

Product	Range of Formaldehyde Emission Rates ($\mu g/m^2$/day)
Medium-density fiberboard[a]	17,600–55,000
Hardwood plywood paneling[b]	1500–34,000
Particleboard[b,c]	2000–25,000
Urea-formaldehyde foam insulation[c]	1200–19,200
Softwood plywood[c]	240–720
Paper products[b]	260–680
Fiberglass products[b]	400–470
Clothing[b]	35–570
Resilient flooring[b]	<240
Carpeting[b]	NP–65
Upholstery fabric[b]	NP–7

Source: Godish, T. 1988. Residential formaldehyde contamination: Sources and levels. *Comments Toxicol.* 2(3):1.15–134. with permission.

[a] Grot, R. A., S. Silberstein, K. Ishigars. 1985. Validity of models for predicting formaldehyde concentrations in residences due to pressed wood products, Phase I NBSIR 85-3255. National Bureau of Standards.

[b] Pickrell, J. A., C. Grifis, C. H. Hobbs. 1984. LMF-93, UC-48. U.S. Department of Energy.

[c] Matthews, T. G. et al. 1985. Consumer Product Safety Commission. CPSC-IAG-84-1103.

TABLE 6.7

Formaldehyde Levels in Urea-Formaldehyde Foam-Insulated Houses

Study	Concentration (ppm)			
	Number	Range	Mean	Median
Washington State	39	0.005–2.99		0.19
New Hampshire	71	0.01–0.17	0.06	0.05
Ontario	450		0.045	
Quebec	266			0.05
Consumer Product Safety Commission	636	0.01–3.40	0.12	
Indiana	33	0.02–0.17	0.07	0.06
New York State	1954	0.00–0.49	0.06	

Source: From Godish, T. 1988. Residential formaldehyde contamination: Sources and levels. *Comments Toxicol.* 2(3):115–134. With permission.

During her 7th month of pregnancy, this mother became ill with a series of infections thought to be scarlatina and later streptococcus. She was given an antibiotic during her 8th month of pregnancy. She still had, however, a sore throat and developed tunnel vision, eye irritation, an elevated blood pressure. She was put to bed. She subsequently complained of headache, numbness, and memory loss. She underwent double-blind inhaled challenge and was found to be sensitive to formaldehyde, ethanol, chlorine, and pesticides (Table 6.5). Her skin testing revealed that she had sensitivity to rhizopus, trichoderma, histamine, serotonin, estrone, luteinizing hormone, sterile progesterone, fluogen, and bacterial mixed respiratory vaccine (MRV), as well as to ethanol and formaldehyde. She was diagnosed with cephalgia, chemical sensitivity, dermatitis, irritable bowel syndrome, myalgia, rhinosinusitis, excessive urination, and vasculitis.

TABLE 6.8

Formaldehyde Levels in Mobile Homes

Study	Concentration (ppm)			
	Number	Range	Mean	Median
Washington	74	0.03–2.54		0.35
Minnesota	397	0.02–3.69	0.42	
Clayton	250		0.3 (0.54)[a]	
Indiana	54	0.02–0.75	0.18	0.15
New York	161		0.18	
Consumer Product Safety Commission	431	0.01–2.93	0.38	
Wisconsin				
Complaint	65	<0.10–3.68		0.47
Noncomplaint	137	<0.10–2.84	0.46	0.39
Texas	159	<0.02–0.78	0.15	
California	663		0.09	0.07[b]

Source: From Godish T. 1988. Residential formaldehyde contamination: Sources and levels. *Comments Toxicol.* 2(3):1154–134. With permission.

[a] Standardized to 78°F. 50% RH.

[b] Geometric mean.

The father, aged 36 years, had complaints of headaches and numbness of his feet. His eyes were sensitive to light. He complained of stiff joints and fatigue. The results of his double-blind inhaled challenge showed that he had sensitivity to formaldehyde, pesticides, and ethanol. He did not react to phenol, chlorine, or two placebos (Table 6.5). Intradermal tests confirmed these results. His skin tests revealed that he had sensitivity to dust, mite, rhizopus, trichoderma, histamine, serotonin, trees, and cigarette smoke. He was diagnosed with cephalgia, chest pain, chest wall syndrome, fatigue, irritable bowel syndrome, myalgia, rhinosinusitis, vasculitis, and chemical sensitivity.

The older daughter, aged 10 years, had the chief complaints of constant nasal drainage, congestion, sore throat, fatigue, dark circles under her eyes, sleeplessness, and headaches. She underwent double-blind inhaled challenge and was found to be sensitive to formaldehyde, ethanol, pesticide, phenol, and chlorine rhizopus, sporobolomyces, trichoderma, dust, mite, histamine, serotonin, fluogen, MRV, and cow's milk. She was diagnosed with chest wall syndrome, cephalgia, fatigue, irritable bowel syndrome, myalgia, rhinosinusitis and eczema.

The younger daughter, with whom the mother was pregnant while living in the mobile home, was the sickest when she arrived at 6 years of age with her family at the EHC-Dallas. She had the chief complaints of bladder dribbling and infection, constipation, and recurrent virus-like symptoms. She had been ill throughout her life. She experienced chronic, recurrent bladder infections and upper respiratory infections. She had been evaluated by numerous urologists who suggested a urinary diversion procedure to correct the urinary problems.

She underwent double-blind inhaled chemical challenges in the chemical-free booth and was found to be sensitive to formaldehyde, pesticides, chlorine, and phenol percent (Table 6.6). Intradermal tests confirmed these results. She had intradermal skin testing for chemicals and food, was also found to be sensitive to 10 foods, and was assigned a rotary diet.

She was diagnosed with severe urinary frequency and recurrent bladder infections with incontinence, rhinosinusitis, myalgia, irritable bowel syndrome, toxic brain syndrome, fatigue, and food, inhalant, and chemical sensitivity.

After a detoxification program, including a formaldehyde-free oasis, all four were doing well. All of their symptoms resolved, especially the bladder problems of the younger daughter, which completely subsided. No surgery was performed.

In a study conducted at the Inhalation Toxicology Research Institute, formaldehyde release rate coefficients were measured for six types of consumer products.[84] Release rates calculated per unit surface area ($\mu g/m^2/day$) were used to rank the products in the following order: pressed wood products $\gg$ clothes $\sim$ insulation products $\sim$ paper products $>$ fabric $>$ carpet. Release rates from pressed wood products ranged from below the limit of detection for an exterior plywood to 36,000 $\mu g/m^2/day$ for some paneling. Other release rates were: for articles of new clothing not previously washed, 15–550 $\mu g/m^2/day$; for insulation products, 52–620 $\mu g/m^2/day$; for paper plates and cups, 75–1000 $\mu g/m^2/day$; for fabrics, from below the limit of detection to 350 $\mu g/m^2/day$; and for carpets, from below the limit of detection to 65 $\mu g/m^2/day$. In a follow-up to Pickrell's study[85] performed as a result of changes to product manufacturing processes, many of these release rates were reinvestigated. Formaldehyde release rates from a variety of bare UF wood products (one-fourth to three-fourth) were reported to range from 8.6 to 1578 $\mu g/m^2/hour$, coated UF wood products from 1 to 461 $\mu g/m^2/hour$, permanent-press fabrics from 42 to 214 $\mu g/m^2/hour$, and bare phenol-formaldehyde wood products from 4 to 9 $\mu g/m^2/hour$.[33] Paper grocery bags and towels had emission rates of 0.4 and <0.3 $\mu g/m^2/hour$, respectively. For wet products, the emission rates were: latex paint, 591 $\mu g/m^2/hour$; more expensive latex paint, 326 $\mu g/m^2/hour$; fingernail hardener, 215,500 $\mu g/m^2/hour$; nail polish, 20,700 $\mu g/m^2/hour$; and commercially applied UF floor finish, 421 and 1,050,000 $\mu g/m^2/hour$ for base and topcoats, respectively.[33]

Formaldehyde may also arise in indoor air through the degradation of other compounds. Naturally occurring unsaturated hydrocarbons, such as limonene and pinene (which may also be released from consumer products), and anthropogenic compounds, such as 4-vinyl cyclohexene (an emission from carpet padding), and other alkenes commonly found in indoor air have been found to produce formaldehyde via their initial reaction with ozone.[35,36] Reiss and coworkers estimated that the amount of formaldehyde released by this process is 0.87 µg/second in winter months and 2.43 µg/second in summer (Reiss et al. 1995[86]).

In another study on indoor formaldehyde emissions, quasi-steady-state emission rates of formaldehyde from new carpets were measured in a large-scale environmental chamber.[87] The emission rates were 57.2 and 18.2 µg/m²/hour at 24 and 168 hours, respectively, after the start of each experiment. Similar results were observed in a Swedish study where indoor formaldehyde levels were found to be higher in homes having wall-to-wall carpeting.[88] Another recent Swedish study on indoor emissions reported that oil-based skin care products known to contain formaldehyde precursors (donors) released formaldehyde to the air even if the material had been in storage for 1 year.[89]

Formaldehyde release from pressed wood products is due to latent formaldehyde. During the pressing process, hot steam from moist wood particles transfers heat, formaldehyde, and other volatiles from the surface of the mat to the core of the board where unreacted UF resin components accumulate. The resulting formaldehyde concentration in the core is approximately twice that of the surface. Release of formaldehyde is diffusion controlled and gradually decreases over time.[90] Formaldehyde can also be produced by hydrolytic cleavage of unreacted hydroxy-methyl groups in the formaldehyde resins. Melamine formaldehyde resins generally are not stable, and the amounts of formaldehyde emitted from them are much lower.[49]

A formaldehyde emission rate of 0.48 µg/kJ has been determined for normal operation of unvented gas ranges; however, this emission rate leads to relatively low indoor formaldehyde concentrations.[91] Formaldehyde emission rates ranging from 0.43 to 4.2 µg/kJ were measured from eight well-tuned, unvented gas-fired space heaters operated at full fuel input in an environmental chamber with low ventilation.[92] In another study, formaldehyde emissions factors from unvented kerosene heaters ranged from 0.18 to 0.47 µg/kJ.[93]

Using an average cigarette consumption rate of approximately 10 cigarettes per indoor compartment per day with a measured formaldehyde emission rate of $0.97 \pm 0.97 \pm 0.06$ mg/hour, Matthews et al.[34] calculated an average formaldehyde emission rate of 0.4 ± 0.03 mg/hour over 24 hours. Triebig and Zober[94] report that the level of formaldehyde in sidestream cigarette smoke is 50 times higher than main stream smoke, while the National Research Council (NRC)[95] put the value at five to eight times more formaldehyde in sidestream smoke. Levels of formaldehyde in nonsmoking office buildings ranged from not detected to 0.22 ppm, while they ranged from not detected to 0.6 ppm where smoking was permitted.[96]

Formaldehyde can also be emitted into indoor air from fish during cooking. Amounts of formaldehyde that formed in a headspace when various kinds of fish flesh were heated at 200°C ranged from 0.48 µg/g of mackerel to 5.31 µg/g of sardine.[97]

Despite the enormous publicity that has been associated with UFFI houses, average formaldehyde levels are a fraction of those reported in mobile homes. With the exception of Washington State and the U.S. Consumer Product Safety Commission (CPSC) reports, average formaldehyde levels in UFFI houses typically appear to be in the range of 0.05–0.06 ppm. We have seen much higher levels (up to 25 ppm) in the mobile homes of some of our chemically sensitive patient, which made them ill and the home uninhabitable. Higher average levels reported in Washington State and CPSC reports may reflect the effect of product age at the time of sampling since there was a larger percentage of recently foam-insulated households in their ample population. Later studies tend to show a smaller range of concentration in UFFI houses, with a smaller maximum concentration reported.

The conventional home studies summarized in Table 6.9 represent a wide range of housing stock. As compared with results of studies conducted in the United States, formaldehyde levels reported for Denmark and Sweden are usually high. These, most likely, reflect unique products or unique usage patterns and the relatively early period (early to mid-1970s) in the history of the recognition of the formaldehyde contamination problem. At this time, chemical sensitivity increased partially due to these higher levels.

TABLE 6.9
Formaldehyde Levels in Conventional Houses

Study	Concentration (ppm)			
	Number	Range	Mean	Median
Denmark	25	0.07–1.8		0.50
Sweden	319	0.07–1.8	0.58	
Ontario	225		0.03	
Consumer Product Safety Commission	41	0.01–0.08	0.03	
Tennessee	40		0.6	
New York				
Single family	153	0.01–2.60	0.03	
Multifamily	50	0.01–0.11	0.03	
Texas				
Single family	45	0.0–0.14	0.05	
Multifamily	33	0.0–0.29	0.09	
Indiana				
Particleboard subflooring	30	0.01–0.46	0.11	0.09
Nonparticleboard subflooring	58	0.00–0.14	0.06	0.06
California	51	0.01–0.09	0.04	
Minnesota	489	0.01–5.52	0.14	

Source: From Godish T, 1988. Residential formaldehyde contamination: Sources and levels. *Comments Toxicol.* 2(3):115–134. With permission.

Conventional homes vary in kinds and quantities of formaldehyde-releasing products present. If conventional residences are classified as source type (note Indiana data), formaldehyde levels are seen to be significantly higher in residences that contain particleboard subflooring. These types of domiciles have been seen to severely exacerbate and at times cause chemical sensitivity. Average levels in the so-called typical house (as opposed to UFFI or mobile homes) depend on what sources are present. Conventional homes without particleboard subflooring appear to have average formaldehyde concentrations in the range of 0.03–0.06 ppm.

FACTORS AFFECTING INDOOR FORMALDEHYDE LEVELS

Knowing the source of environmental factors affecting indoor formaldehyde levels is very important in treating chemical sensitivity. Accurate evaluation of the home conditions under which the chemically sensitive live, including identification of any sources of formaldehyde with which they might come in contact, is essential to providing them with a safe environment in which they can improve. Outdoor levels of formaldehyde must be also accounted for in order to make a less polluted environment in which to recover. Indoor air is 60% outdoor air; city air results in a much higher indoor air level than country air.

SOURCE FACTORS

Common sources of formaldehyde emissions in indoor air include medium-density fiberboard (MDF), plywood, particleboard, sheetrock, new carpeting, foam insulation, and varnish-like surface coatings formulated from UF/melamine-formaldehyde resin mixtures. All of these have been observed to exacerbate chemical sensitivity.

MDF is the most potent source of formaldehyde. It is used on a low-volume basis in residential spaces for cupboards, counters, and subflooring. Its contribution to contamination of indoor air is not well known. However, the majority of chemically sensitive patient's studies at the EHC-Dallas complain that they become ill each time they open one of the cupboards. In source combinations, MDF is suspected of causing an increase in formaldehyde levels beyond those normally expected.

Harwood plywood is made of wood plies bonded with UF resin. It is most commonly used as a three-ply decorative wall paneling. It is also used in the construction of cabinets and furniture. Soft plywood is distinct from hardwood plywood in that it is bonded by chemically stable phenol-formaldehyde resins. It is used in flooring and roofing materials in new home construction. Both types of plywood are sufficiently strong emitters to keep the formaldehyde-sensitive patient ill.

Particleboard is a wood by-product manufactured from fine (ca. 1 mm) wood particles that are mixed with 6–8 wt% UF resin and pressed into panels at a temperature of 150–180°C.[98] It is used in residential construction for subflooring, shelving, and cabinetry. It is also used in the construction of furniture and is one of the more severe triggers of chemical sensitivity.

New carpeting is a significant source of air contamination with formaldehyde because of the use of glue which holds the fibers to the carpet backing and to the synthetic as an antiwrinkle fixative. Frequently, these have been shown to exacerbate and trigger chemical sensitivity.

From 1974 to 1982, UFFI was used to insulate buildings, and it caused many people to become chemically sensitive. Foam used for mattresses and furniture stuffing is another source of formaldehyde emissions.

Varnish-like surface coatings formulated from UF/melamine-formaldehyde resin mixtures are a relatively unknown source of indoor contamination. Imported from Europe, these products are intended for use on a variety of wood surfaces and concrete.

Levels of formaldehyde in indoor air are the result of three variables: source strength, loading factor (LF), and the presence of source combinations. The greater the potency of the formaldehyde emitting source, the higher is the indoor air level of formaldehyde (see Table 6.2 for the potency of formaldehyde released from specific products).

Another factor affecting the level of formaldehyde in indoor air is the LF. This is the ratio of formaldehyde-releasing surfaces to air volume. In restricted air space, a high LF will produce high formaldehyde levels.[99] For example, the LF in mobile homes is high as a direct result of the products used to construct these homes. As much as 916 ft of particleboard is used for the decking, shelving, counter tops, and cabinets in a single-wide mobile home,[100] it is important to note here that the relationship between the LF and formaldehyde levels is not linear. In fact, where there is increased airspace formaldehyde levels, formaldehyde emission rates decrease.[101] Also, formaldehyde emissions based on molecular diffusion cease for a particular product once a critical formaldehyde level in the air is reached. Thus, pressed wood products are capable of varying both in terms of type of product and within a product category as to the levels of formaldehyde required to cause formaldehyde emissions to cease.[102] However, as one source is removed in an effort to depollute a home for the chemically sensitive, the remaining source may emit enough to continue the same level, thus keeping the chemically sensitive ill.

The third variable affecting levels of formaldehyde in indoor air is source combinations. In conventional homes, the highest levels of formaldehyde in the air occur where particleboard underlayment has been used as subflooring.[65,76] However, these levels can be exacerbated by formaldehyde emissions from products used in cabinetry, shelving, wall paneling, and furniture. Often, hardwood plywood, particleboard, and/or MDF are used separately, or in combination, as base materials in the making of these items. Both Godish[103] and Berk et al.[104] found a significant increase in formaldehyde levels in indoor air after pressed wood furniture was introduced into a conventional residence. Waterbed frames constructed of particleboard can further contribute to elevated formaldehyde levels when their mattress, heated to greater than 90°F, is affixed to the frame.

At the EHC-Dallas and Buffalo, we have observed that most chemically sensitive patients are exacerbated by exposure to formaldehyde emitted from any source. Further, we have demonstrated that total formaldehyde exposures can have profound effects on the severity of illness experienced by these patients and on their prospects for recover. We, therefore, believe that successful treatment necessitates an examination of these patients' homes in order to identify and eradicate any source that might be formaldehyde contaminated. While some homes can be easily modified to reduce formaldehyde emissions and accommodate the needs of the chemically sensitive, other dwellings are moderately difficult or impossible to clean up depending on the various types of building materials that may have been used in the construction of the home and its furnishings. Regardless of the difficulty of the task, creating a formaldehyde-free residence may ultimately be essential to improving the health of some chemically sensitive patients.

Environmental Factors: Influence on Formaldehyde Levels

Although source factors are the most important aspect of formaldehyde pollution, levels of emission are further influenced by several environmental variables, including fluctuations in indoor and outdoor temperature, humidity, and ventilation. Gammage et al.,[105] Meyers et al.,[106] and Meyer and Hermanns[107] reported on the effects of diurnal variations on formaldehyde levels, noting these coincided with changes in indoor temperature. A rise in formaldehyde levels accompanied a rise in temperature; conversely, a drop in temperature coincided with a decrease in formaldehyde concentrations. Changes in temperature appear to affect both the hydrolysis and diffusion rate of UF products. An approximate 5–6°C rise in temperature produces a doubled formaldehyde concentration.[108]

As changes in temperature alter formaldehyde levels, the well-being of the chemically sensitive is also influenced. For those living in a house containing formaldehyde-treated products in a warm climate, summer can be a particularly difficult period, as both temperature and formaldehyde levels increase. In contrast, there are some chemically sensitive patients who marked improvement with dramatic drops in temperature.

Godish et al.[71] reported a significant positive correlation between formaldehyde levels in UFFI and outdoor temperature. Godish[109] has further observed that formaldehyde levels in UFFI houses and mobile homes are strongly correlated with outdoor average temperature, with the relationship between the two variables accounting for 85% of the variation in formaldehyde levels.

Changes in outdoor temperature cause a change in the pressure difference between the inside and outside of a structure. Pressure differences associated with temperature differences serve as one (the other is wind speed) of the main forces that cause air infiltration into a building. This "stack effect" draws air into houses and other buildings, diluting and removing formaldehyde and other contaminants, which helps the chemically sensitive. Infiltration by this means is directly related to ΔT, the difference between the inside and outside temperatures. The largest change in T conditions occurs during the winter time. However, the tighter the building is sealed, the lesser the help there is for the chemically sensitive.

Another exterior cause of increased interior formaldehyde levels that is independent of indoor air temperature is solar heating of the sidewalls of mobile homes internally clad with a potent formaldehyde source.[107] Godish[109] has demonstrated that air temperature and solar radiation are so closely linked that the independent effect of solar radiation cannot be demonstrated.

Formaldehyde levels are also sensitive to levels of both absolute and relative humidity. An increase of relative humidity from 30% to 70% is associated with an approximate 40% rise in indoor formaldehyde levels.[108]

Temperature and humidity changes in indoor environments can cause formaldehyde levels to vary by a factor of as much as five to six times.[108]

Because of the effect of temperature and humidity on formaldehyde levels, a single formaldehyde test result is not as meaningful (relative to that structure) unless it can be interpreted in the context of temperature and humidity conditions existing at the time the sample was collected. As a consequence, model equations have been developed to convert a measured formaldehyde concentration to one at a standard temperature and relative humidity. Though as many as a dozen have been developed, the most widely used standard equation has been that of Berge et al.[110] In its 1983 rule-making relative to new mobile homes, the U.S. Department of Housing and Urban Development required the use of the Berge equation in conjunction with "the large chamber method" to determine compliance with product standards.[111] As such, the Berge equation has regulatory status, even if it is not totally accurate in determining indoor formaldehyde levels. The Berge equation has the following form:

$$C_X = \frac{C}{[1 + A(H - H_0)e^{-R(1/T - 1/T_0)}}$$

C_X = corrected concentration (ppm)
C = test concentration (ppm)
e = natural log base
R = coefficient of temperature (9799)
T = test temperature (K)
T_0 = standardized temperature (K)
A = coefficient of humidity (0.0175)
H = test relative humidity (%)
H_0 = standardized relative humidity (%)

Based on mobile home climate control studies conducted by Godish and Rouch,[112] the application of the Berge equation in the temperature/humidity range of 20–30°C and 30%–70% RH gives an error rate of ±12% at two standard errors confidence interval. Those constructing less polluted rooms for the chemically sensitive should keep this equation in mind, but, in addition, no known formaldehyde emitters should be used. A chemically sensitive patient who is also formaldehyde sensitive generally does not improve unless formaldehyde is eliminated from his home.

It has been shown that the combination of toxics along with formaldehyde can be quite devastating for the chemically sensitive patient. Table 6.10 shows a house that has numerous other chemicals, both natural and synthetic. The pinenes and limonenes and other terpenes can cause bad indoor air as can the other petrochemical products. The total environmental pollutant load is shown in the table which made the patient ill (Table 6.10).

Formaldehyde levels are significantly affected by ventilation, both unintended and intended. Factors that cause the entry of more air will result in lower concentrations and lower exposures. Formaldehyde levels will be higher under closed conditions (assuming indoor temperature and humidity levels are the same) than when windows and doors are open. Some of the variability in the data summarized in Tables 6.2 through 6.4 is no doubt due to differences in sampling protocols that emphasize closure as compared with those that attempt to determine average exposures under "normal living conditions." Lower formaldehyde levels reported for California mobile homes may in part be explicable by the absence of closure conditions at the time of sampling. Information gathered at the EHC-Dallas and Buffalo emphasizes that no matter how good the ventilation is, formaldehyde emitters must be kept to a minimum, or be absent, to be satisfactory for the chemically sensitive. We have also found that the final test of a safe room for the formaldehyde chemically sensitive patient is for them to evaluate a room with no ventilation. If they deem it satisfactory, it will usually be safe under any conditions.

Morris[113] found 1.7 ppm in a biology wet lab, 0.60 ppm in fabric stores, 0.13 ppm in clothing stores, and 0.003 ppm in the outside air. It is interesting that they could tell when a clothing store had unpacked new clothing by a rise in formaldehyde levels from 0.14 to 0.15 ppm after unpacking. They found that patients who were very sensitive to formaldehyde had problems in clothing stores. Less sensitive patients would more likely have symptoms in fabric stores, and mildly sensitive patients would only have symptoms in biology wet lab or similar environment where the level was close to 2 ppm. These observations are similar to our findings at the EHC-Dallas.

TABLE 6.10

Votatile Organic Compounds (VOCs) and Aldehydes: In a Home That Made People Chemically Sensitive

VOCs and Aldehydes	Test Results (μg/m³)	Reference Levels (μg/m³)	Comparison to Reference Levels	
			Health (%)	Odor (%)
Formaldehyde	51.0	20	255.0	
Acetic acid	26.7	25	106.8	
Camphene*	1.0	2	50.0	
d-Limonene*	30.9	100	30.9	
Benzene*	1.1	4.5	24.4	
Ethyl alcohol	18.6	100	18.6	
Acetaldehyde	26.0	140	18.6	
d-Carene*	11.4	100	11.4	11.4
Glycol ether EB	1.7	36	4.7	
Mycrene*	3.0	100	3.0	
N-Butyl acetate	2.6	111	2.3	
Terpinol*	2.0	100	2.0	
Ethyl benzene*	3.9	200	2.0	
Isopentane*	5.7	350	1.6	
Isopropyltoluene/p-cymene	3.6	275	1.3	
Toluene	8.1	1200	0.7	
o-, m-, and p-Xylenes	1.4	208	0.7	
N-Butane*	10.9	1900	0.6	
Glycol ether DPM	0.7	300	0.2	
α-Pinene*	16.5	6		275.0
Propionaldehyde	2.0	2		100.0
Hexaldehyde	7.0	8		87.5
Butyraldehyde	1.0	1.4		71.4
β-Pinene	4.0	6		66.7
Benzaldehyde	1.0	2.2		45.5
Tolualdehyde, o, m, and p	1.0	2.2		45.5
Cyclohexanone	1.8	48		3.8
Ethyl acetate	0.5	1440		0.0
Linalool	2.6			
Eukaryotic	6.9			
Menthol	2.4			
Total other VOCs as toluene	92			
Total VOCs and aldehydes	349	<200		

Source: Environmental Health Center-Dallas, 2012.

DECAY OF FORMALDEHYDE LEVELS

Formaldehyde levels decrease significantly with time. As a consequence, formaldehyde measurements are only indicative of contamination that is occurring within the time frame of the measurement. They do not indicate either past contamination or those that will occur in the future. The chemically sensitive can usually tell if exposures are, or are not, constant.

Actual estimates of formaldehyde decay time vary considerable. This variability reflects differences in statistical approaches and decay models used to assess it. It also reflects variations in the data that are influenced by factors other than time. These factors include product emission strength,[114] ventilation, and factors such as local climate and occupant behavior. Where windows are often open or where average temperatures and humidity are high, the decay rate is usually rapid. Also, because emission rates are an exponential function of temperature and a linear function of relative humidity and formaldehyde concentrations, decay rates are seen to vary from one residential structure to the next.

In some cases, formaldehyde decay may occur indefinitely, while in others, it may be finite. As levels of this decay fluctuate, the exposed chemically sensitive individual may exhibit a spectrum of responses.

Several recent epidemiologic studies[115–119] have been conducted regarding the link between formaldehyde exposure and cancer. All of these studies have weaknesses in the exposure data, since often exposures were not measured, but only estimated. The power of detecting the rather rare nasopharyngeal cancer, which in humans is the type of cancer that had been found in rodents, was small. Controversy still exists regarding the carcinogenic role of formaldehyde in humans.[120] The rather extended discussion of the role of formaldehyde in animal cancers has been included here because we strongly suspect that a role in human cancer persists, despite the somewhat equivocal and contradictory evidence from various epidemiologic studies.

The molecular/cellular mechanism of formaldehyde toxicity is not yet entirely clear. Evidence exists that formaldehyde is electrophilic for macromolecules, including DNA, RNA, and protein, and it forms reversible adducts, as well as irreversible cross-linking.[121–123] Once cross-linking occurs, the chemically sensitive have a much more difficult time clearing.

EFFECTS OF FORMALDEHYDE EXPOSURE ON BIOLOGICAL RESPONSES AND DIAGNOSTIC TECHNIQUES

EPIDEMIOLOGICAL HISTORY: PHYSICAL

Clinical and epidemiologic data indicate considerable variation in human response to formaldehyde, which but when enough to disturb physiology vary from chronic, fatigue, fibromyalgia, arthritis, to GI upset, including hypersensitive reactions. Ranges and median responses to short-term exposure are listed in Table 6.11. This list does not include responses of immunosensitive populations. This list has not changed recently since people get the same or similar symptoms and signs to excess

TABLE 6.11

Effects of Formaldehyde in Humans after Short-Term Respiratory Exposure (Concentrations in mg/m³)

Reported Ranges	Estimated Median	Effect
0.06–1.20	0.1	Odor threshold 50% of people. Chemical sensitivity much lower
0.01–1.90	0.5	Eye irritation threshold. Chemical sensitivity much lower
0.10–3.10	0.6	Throat irritation threshold. Chemical sensitivity much lower
2.50–3.70	3.1	Burning sensation in nose and eye. Chemical sensitivity much lower
5.00–6.70	5.6	Tearing eyes, long-term lung effects. Chemical sensitivity much lower
12.00–25.00	17.8	Tolerable or 3 minutes with strong flow of tears lasting 1 hour. Chemical sensitivity much lower
37.00–60.00	37.5	Inflammation of lung (pneumonitis), edema
		Respiratory distress and danger to life. Chemical sensitivity much lower
60.00–125.00	125.0	Death

Source: Modified from National Center for Toxicology Research. 1984. Report on the consensus workshop on formaldehyde. *EHS Environ. Health Perspec.* 58:323–381. With permission.

formaldehyde exposures. However, with the continued and varied contamination of our environment, people may succumb to illness at levels much less than in 1989.

We have seen 5000 patients at the EHC-Dallas and Buffalo who have experienced significant formaldehyde exposure. After all formaldehyde sources were removed from their homes, they usually improved. However, prolonged re-exposure has always resulted in renewed sensitivity and severe chronic disease such as arthritis, vasculitis, and GI and GU diseases.

In a series of 200 chemically sensitive physicians seen at the EHC-Dallas, formaldehyde exposure was found in those who had sensitivity to this chemical. Some had developed their sensitivity in the anatomy, pathology, and postmortem laboratories or various other areas of the medical school or hospital containing high formaldehyde levels. These patients usually cleared their symptoms with avoidance and became able to function again.

Andersen and Proctor[124] showed decreased mucociliary clearance rates for human nasal epithelium exposed to formaldehyde. Some chemically sensitive patients exhibit slow clearing rates, while others develop total anosmia to formaldehyde due to damage of the olfactory nerve. These patients have trouble clearly for they have no mechanism to avoid it. Irritant effects of formaldehyde include increased cell membrane permeability, inflammation, and edema which at times can be irresistible. There have recently been reported that olfactory receptors do occur in the skin, but in today's human, they are usually covered. Therefore, they are not used efficiently as much.

In some individuals, sensitivity to "low concentrations" can cause a reaction, resulting in an exacerbation of the symptoms of the chemically sensitive. The health effects of acute exposure to gaseous formaldehyde at low or moderate concentrations include eye, nose, and throat irritation; olfactory fatigue; thirst; headaches; dizziness; lethargy; inability to concentrate; paranoia; irritability; disturbed sleep, moodiness; crying without cause; a crawling sensation of the skin; and hemicorporeal elevation of body temperature. Chronic exposure to formaldehyde can cause chronic rhinitis, chronic pharyngitis, hypertrophic or subatrophic nasal mucosa, and subatrophic or atrophic pharynx.[125] "Toxicity" was reported in the Wisconsin Epidemiology Bulletin in February 1979.[126] Eighty-seven cases were reported in 56 houses where the mean formaldehyde level was 0.88 ppm, with a range of 0.02–4.15 ppm. Symptoms were reported as eye irritation (69%), upper respiratory irritation (53%), lower respiratory difficulty (26%), headache (25%), and fatigue (20%). Harris[125] reported similar symptoms in 48 occupants of UF-insulated homes. They pointed out that allergic or sensitized individuals may have severe reactions to formaldehyde levels below odor threshold, which has been our experience at the EHC-Dallas in over 5000 inhaled challenges.

The "logical regression analysis" of enzyme levels monitored in blood fractions of organophosphate (OP)-sensitive, formaldehyde-sensitive, and chemical-sensitive individuals. These were developed and performed by Professors Jerry Alder and Dan Organiziac of the Wright State University Medical School.

The method looks for the most sensitive measurements that can used to differentiate between sensitive and normal individuals. rPon 1 and Wald were used as monitors. These were found in most formaldehyde-sensitive patients.

Their results suggest that in several of the enzyme levels they measured, aldehyde dehydrogenase (Wald) and peroxinase (rPon) in blood samples can distinguish between chemical-sensitive and normal individuals. Results showing formaldehyde-sensitive and normal individuals are shown in the attached graph. Individuals with no identified chemical sensitivity are plotted as filled squares. Results from individuals with demonstrated chemical sensitivities are plotted using triangular symbols. Filled triangles indicate enzyme levels from individual with one type of sensitivity (e.g., sensitivity to one class of compounds). Open symbols indicate enzyme levels from individuals with sensitivity to formaldehyde and at least one other class of compounds.

As you can see, the majority of points representing normal individuals are above and to the right of the line on the attached graph; while the points from blood enzyme levels of chemically sensitive individuals are below and to the left of the line. In fact, the line was drawn as a result of statistical analysis of the data from the various groups. Points on the line would have the same probability of being data collected from chemically sensitive and normal individuals.

The symptoms of imbalance in this group were always triggered upon exposure.

Formaldehyde has been described as an irritant in a study of morticians working in funeral homes. The investigators noted, however, a wide variance in the levels of formaldehyde in the air that caused irritation. Many experienced embalmers felt that they were not bothered at all, but this observation was colored by the fact that they may have had olfactory nerve damage. Also, three out of seven individuals bothered by formaldehyde suffered from asthma or sinus problems.[53]

INHALED CHALLENGE

The second modality for diagnosis after history and the physical exam as well as the epidemiology studies is the inhaled challenge.

Over the past 20 years at the EHC-Dallas, double-blind, inhaled studies performed on patients in the readapted state who had at least 4 days of reduction of total pollutant load (burden) and total formaldehyde avoidance in the environmental control units have reproduced neurologic, vascular, cardiac, respiratory, gastrointestinal, genitourinary, and skin symptoms at levels of less than 0.20 ppm (Table 6.12, Figure 6.1).

TABLE 6.12

Signs and Symptoms Reproduced after Double-Blind Inhaled Challenge of Formaldehyde (<0.20 ppm) after 4 Days Deadaptation with the Total Load Reduced in the ECU

Cardiovascular	Atrial and ventricular arrhythmia, peripheral vascular spasm, cyanosis, spontaneous bruising, petechiae, edema
Respiratory	Cough, wheezing, shortness of breath, rhinitis
Gastrointestinal	Bloating, belching, gas, diarrhea
Genitourinary	Frequency, urgency, recurrent infections
Skin	Rash (erythematous and maculopapular)

Source: Environmental Health Center-Dallas, 1994. No formaldehyde.

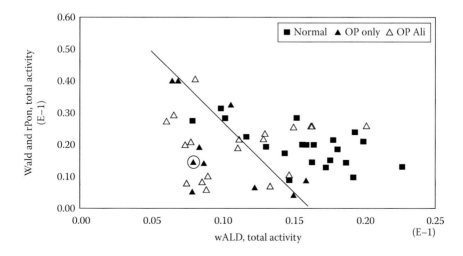

FIGURE 6.1 Predictors of formaldehyde sensitivity. (Adler, J. and Organiziac, D. Wright State Medical School, Department of Biochemistry, Dayton, Ohio.)

TABLE 6.13

Percentage of Skin Testing Reactions to Different Dilutions of Formaldehyde[a]

Formaldehyde Dilution	Volume Injection	Normal Control (*n* = 14)				Patients (*n* = 49)			
		Positive Reaction		No Reaction		Positive Reaction		No Reaction	
		No.	%	No.	%	No.	%	No.	%
#1	0.05 cc	1	7.1	13	92.9	1	2.0	1	2.0
(1:15 or 0.148%)	0.01 cc					1	2.0		
#2	0.5 cc					1	2.0		
(1:125 or 0.0296%)	0.01 cc					5	10.2		
#3	0.05 cc					2	4.1		
(1:625 or 0.00592%)	0.01 cc					18	36.7		
#4	0.05 cc					4	8.2		
(1:3125 or 0.001184%)	0.01 cc					16	32.7		
Total		1	7.1	13	92.9	48	98.0	1	2.0

Source: Rea, W.J. 1994. *Chemical Sensitivity, Volume II*, page 964, table 9. With permission.

[a] Tests performed in an environmentally controlled formaldehyde-free area.

Some investigators have reported negative bronchial challenge studies; however, these usually measured gross parameter changes or the wrong parameters. Further, these studies never took into account the masking phenomenon nor did they have sufficient, if any, environmental controls in their testing areas.[127] Most of their challenge areas were not noted to be formaldehyde free. Even with these flaws in experimental design, however, most had a subset of patients react to formaldehyde challenge.

Results of formaldehyde inhalation test (FIT): The signs and symptoms that were present before FIT are given in Table 6.13. Of the 49 patients, 46 had placebo inhalation testing (PIT). Thirty-one patients had one placebo inhaled test (PIT), nine patients had two PITs, eight patients had three PITs, and one patient had six PITs. All of these patients produced negative results with no symptom or sign induced.

Formaldehyde inhalation testing: Inhalation challenge testing was done in a steel and glass airtight booth (free of formaldehyde and other toxic volatile organic chemicals), in a double-blind fashion.

An open 4-oz glass jar with 30 mL of 0.74% formalin was put in the booth. After 10 minutes, the challenge concentration of formaldehyde in the air measured by gas chromatography/mass spectrometry (GC/MS) was less than 0.2 ppm. This was below the reported odor threshold.[128] No patients could tell what was being tested. There was no detectable level of methyl alcohol in the air of the booth, as measured by GC/MS. The placebo was spring water in a glass bottle with the lid open. Patients and controls were stabilized before testing, by means of 4 days of deadaptation in a formaldehyde-free environment. The interval between placebo testing and FIT was at least 24 hours.

The patients and controls sat in the booth with the bottle closed for 5 minutes before testing; if no symptoms occurred, formaldehyde exposure was done for 15 minutes. Patients and controls were attached to cardiac monitoring equipment for the entire inhaled booth testing procedure. Blood pressure and pulmonary function—peak flow rate (PFR)—were taken before and after the test. Pulse, symptoms, and signs were monitored at 5-minute intervals. Any symptoms and signs were noted prior to the start of the chemical booth test, and for 24 hours after the challenge, and scores were kept for these.

According to the severity of a patient's reaction, some therapies were used to try to prevent a prolonged course of symptoms. These methods included some form of neutralization of symptoms by means of a neutralizing dose of histamine: 0.05 mL of 0.004%, 0.05 mL of 0.0008%, 0.10 mL of 0.0004%, 0.10 mL of 0.0008%, etc., which was given subcutaneously, or serotonin given in the same manner as histamine. If further needed to clear symptoms, vitamin CV, 14 g in 200 mL of normal saline, was used intravenously. Also, oxygen inhaled for 15 minutes at 3–4 L/minute was used.

Formaldehyde exposure cannot be exactly related to the level of formic acid measured in the blood. Formic acid is also a metabolite of endogenously produced formaldehyde.

Formaldehyde oxidase normally rapidly converts aldehydes into acids, since aldehydes are harmful to the human body in promoting cross-linking.[129] But formaldehyde oxidase is limited in its manner and rate of production, and with ambient overload, production is unable to keep up with the increased demand. Once production is exceeded, the biochemistry switches from an oxidation reaction to a reduction reaction with alcohol dehydrogenase, resulting in the production of chloral hydrate. This switch with subsequent drug production may explain the preponderance of cerebral or toxic brain symptoms seen in some chemically sensitive patients as the aldehydes are reduced to alcohols.[129–132] Many of these reactions result in sluggishness and sleepy reaction which would be compatible with chloral hydrate. We have observed this reaction hundreds of times in the oppressed chemically sensitive patients. At times, it is difficult to keeping them awake upon a severe formaldehyde exposure.

Since oxidation skin reactions require folic acid,[133] often, folic acid deficiency is observed as well. Certainly, as deficiencies progressed with continual exposures, other biochemical systems would be adversely affected by a domino effect. This pattern may explain one type of spreading phenomenon whereby the chemically sensitive develop other sensitivities and other target organs become involved.

The diversity of symptoms of chemically sensitive patients is more easily appreciated with the understanding of the extent of the damage that is rendered by inhaled xenobiotics or toxic chemicals and especially formaldehyde. Toxic chemicals interfere with cellular energy metabolism by inhibiting glycolysis and mitochondrial respiration. They inhibit ATP synthesis and other enzymes, decrease the efficiency of the sodium pump, disrupt cell membranes, produce free radicals, overload the cytochrome P-450 detoxication system, and damage DNA.[134] Each person's biochemical uniqueness serves to amplify the possibilities.

We do not know the percentage of patients sensitive to formaldehyde nor do we understand all the mechanisms involved in the development of this sensitivity. We do know that beside the IgE and IgG mechanisms, a nonimmune reaction occurs. This involves cell membrane disturbance. The formaldehyde can make the membrane rest pores with K^+ leaking out and Ca^{2+} and N^+ entering the cells, Ca^{2+} combines with Kinase A and C which is then phosphorylated. This increases sensitivity up to 1000 times.[135] This likely is the mechanism of the hypersensitivity. In testing over 1000 patients with symptoms, however, we found that those who react positively to challenge have usually improved after being shown how to reduce their environmental chemical overload through both cleaning up their environment and changing their lifestyle in order to reduce their exposures and hence their total body load. ATP supplementation appears to help the chemically sensitive's energy.

SELECTED CASE EXAMPLES

The following are several selected case studies of patients who developed formaldehyde sensitivity, as reported by Rogers.[129]

Case study: A 39-year-old consulting engineer traveled extensively. Two years previous to treatment at the Northwest Environmental Center, he had moved into a new home in the Syracuse, New York area. New carpeting and particleboard subflooring had been used throughout the house. Six months after moving into his house, he experienced an insidious onset of joint pain. He consulted an internist and a rheumatologist, and in spite of their treatments, he reported 1½ years later that he had the same symptoms. He also indicated that he ached more after he had been at home for the weekend, but felt well whenever he was out of town for a few days.

His blood serum level of formic acid (a metabolite of formaldehyde was 10 μg/mL after a week-end at home, and 6 μg/mL after a day at work). A passive (badge) monitor showed an ambient 24-hour formaldehyde level of 0.06 ppm in his home. Current recommendations for maximum ambient air formaldehyde exposure levels range from 0.25 ppm (National Academy of Sciences) to 0.12 ppm (American Society of Heating, Refrigeration, and Air Conditioning Engineers), while concentrations below 0.06 ppm are considered of limited or no concern.[126]

Single-blind testing with normal saline produced no symptoms. An injection of 0.01 cc of dilution 3 (0.15% formaldehyde) produced wheal growth and "a warm feeling"; 0.05 cc of dilution 4 (0.03%) produced "ringing in the ears and achy joints." Ten minutes after an injection of a 0.05 cc of dilution 5 (0.006% formaldehyde), all of his symptoms were cleared, and there was no wheal growth. Another normal saline produced no wheal growth or symptoms. This patient was placed on an avoidance program and gradually cleared his symptoms.

Case study: M. B. was a 41-year-old teacher who had worked in the same school for 8 years. Over summer vacation, renovations were done in the school. When this teacher reentered the building in the fall, she started having symptoms that with each subsequent entry began more quickly and more severely. She would eventually lose her voice, as it gradually became more hoarse over the first few hours of work. She also experienced a sore throat and tender submandibular lymphadenopathy. She would have a feeling of achiness as though a flu were starting, and she became exhausted. These symptoms persisted for a day or two after leaving the building and were proportional in duration and severity to the amount of time she spent there. At home, she was without symptoms. Her serum level of formic acid was 10 μg/mL after a day at school and 6 μg/mL after a weekend at home. This measurement was repeated with the same results on subsequent days. The 24-hour level of form-aldehyde in the school air, measured with a passive (badge) monitor, was 0.06 ppm. Single-blind testing to formaldehyde duplicated her symptoms in the office, with the administration of 0.05 mL of dilution 5 (0.006% formaldehyde) producing visible facial flushing and weakening of the patient's voice. The next dose, 0.05 mL of dilution 6, cleared the symptoms. This patient was placed on a massive avoidance level and gradually lost her sensitivity.

At the EHC-Dallas and Buffalo, many patients have presented with systemic complaints, includ-ing vascular spasm, gastrointestinal upset, bladder spasm, premenstrual syndrome, asthma, cardiac arrhythmias, edema, and headaches.

After an adequate history has been obtained, the precise diagnosis of formaldehyde sensitivity can be confirmed through the use of sublingual drops, intradermal injection, inhaled challenges, and plotting sign and symptom curves as well as immune parameters. Examples of these plots are shown in Figures 6.1 and 6.2.

The following study performed by Pan[136] at the EHC-Dallas shows our technique of diagnosing formaldehyde sensitivity.

The line was calculated using formaldehyde-only sensitive individuals. The statistical analysis indicated the distinctions are significant (*p*-values less than 0.05). Another indication of reliability is that we correctly assigned individual as formaldehyde sensitive or normal 78% of the time.

Patients: Subjects were 49 selected patients, who were highly suspected of being sensitive to formaldehyde according to their symptoms, environmental exposures, and history. All had food, inhalant, or chemical sensitivity. Twenty-two were outpatients and 27 were inpatients. Thirteen were males and 36 females. Their ages ranged from 14 to 69 years, with an average age of 48.4 years.

Controls: Controls were 14 nonsmoking, healthy volunteers with no history of formaldehyde sensitivity, including 3 males and 11 females, aged 16–52 years, with an average age of 30.6 years.

This study was conducted between October 1983 and December 1988 in a formaldehyde-free, below analytical detection limit, less chemically polluted environment constructed of porcelain

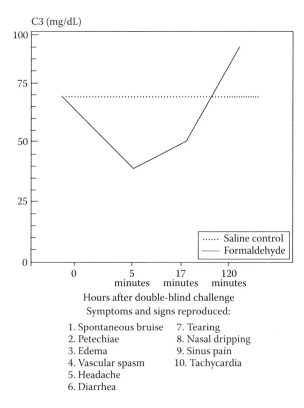

C3 (mg/dL)

Hours after double-blind challenge
Symptoms and signs reproduced:

1. Spontaneous bruise   7. Tearing
2. Petechiae   8. Nasal dripping
3. Edema   9. Sinus pain
4. Vascular spasm   10. Tachycardia
5. Headache
6. Diarrhea

FIGURE 6.2 Forty-five-year-old white female—inhaled double-blind formaldehyde challenge (<0.2 ppm, 15-minute exposure) after 4 days deadaptation in the ECU with total load decreased. (From Environmental Health Center-Dallas and Rea, W.J. 1994. *Chemical Sensitivity, Volume II*, page 958, Figure 1. With permission.)

steel. The patients were in the deadapted state with a reduced total body load when challenge was performed.

Formaldehyde skin test: An intracutaneous injection test was used. Four types of solutions were tested:

1. Saline stored in glass bottles (0.05 cc of preservative-free 0.9% intravenous saline solution) was used for placebo skin testing.
2. Histamine stored in glass bottles (0.01 cc of 0.022 mg/mL) was used for testing the positive control during FST.
3. Methyl alcohol (which is contained in the FST solution but bound to the formaldehyde) was tested to find if it might cause false-positive FSTs. Solutions of 0.2%, 0.04%, 0.008%, 0.0016%, 0.00032%, 0.000064%, 0.0000128%, 0.0000025%, 0.0000005%, and 0.0000001% methyl alcohol (which are in #1, #2, #3, #4, #5, #6, #7, #8, #9, #10 formaldehyde solution, respectively) were available. The concentration used for testing a patient was same as the methyl alcohol concentration in the formalin solution, which had previously induced a positive skin reaction in that patient.
4. Using 1:5 dilutions, formaldehyde solutions were prepared as follows: The formaldehyde concentrate consisted of 1 mL of USP, 37% formalin (containing 37% formaldehyde, 10% methyl alcohol, and 53% inert ingredients), and 49 mL of preservative-free isotonic sterile saline to make a 1:50 or 0.74% formaldehyde solution. One milliliter of concentrate was added to 4 mL of isotonic sterile saline to make dilution #1, a 1:250 or 0.148%

formaldehyde solution. One milliliter of #1 solution was added to 4 mL of isotonic sterile saline to make dilution #2, a 1:1250 or 0.0296% formaldehyde solution. One milliliter of #2 solution was added to 4 mL of isotonic sterile saline to make dilution #3, a 1:6250 or 0.00592% formaldehyde solution. Fivefold dilutions were thus prepared, out to #10 for very sensitive people.

Initially, the test dosage was 0.01 cc of the #4 dilution C1/3000, to make a wheal of approximately 5 mm × 5 mm. After 10 minutes, if no signs or symptoms and no growth of the wheal size were obtained, 0.05 cc of this dilution was injected, creating a 7 mm × 7mm wheal. If after 10 minutes, both parameters were again negative, 0.01 cc of #3 dilution (C1/625) was injected. If after 10 minutes, there were no signs or symptoms or wheal growth, 0.05 cc of #3 dilution was injected. If after 10 minutes both parameters were again negative, 0.01 cc of #2 dilution (C1/25) was injected. If after 10 minutes both parameters were negative, 0.01 cc of #1 dilution,(1/5) was injected. If after 10 minutes both parameters were negative, the test was considered negative. If wheal growth occurred and/or symptoms and signs were produced from testing, the test was considered positive. Delayed onset of wheal growth was also considered positive.

All injection tests were performed in a double-blind fashion. Neither patients nor controls knew what they were being tested with until all tests were finished. All of the patients were withdrawn from antihistamines 48 to 7 before testing.

The growth in wheal size was assessed by measuring the average diameter, being the sum of the width and height divided by 2.

Results of formaldehyde skin test: One hundred percent of patients (9/9) and all the normal controls had no skin or symptom reaction to the normal saline or dilute methyl alcohol. All of both groups had positive skin reactions to histamine.

Of the 48 patients with reactions to formaldehyde skin testing, 40 (83.3%) had positive reactions to the #3 (1/625) and #4 (1/300) dilutions. The rest were at either the #1 or #2 dilution. The mean increase of the average diameter of the wheal was 2.2 mm (range: 1–4 mm).

Of the 14 normal controls, 13 (92.9%) had no reaction to formaldehyde skin testing, and 1 patient (7.11) had a positive reaction to the #1 dilution (Table 6.13). Our study showed only immediate skin reactions, and no delayed reactions occurred. The symptoms and signs of patients are presented in Table 6.13. All of the patients and controls had a local burning or stinging sensation. Because all experienced this sensation, it was not considered a reaction.

Of the 49 patients who had formaldehyde inhalation challenge, 31 (63.3%) had positive reactions, 1 (2.0%) had a questionable responses, and 17 (34.7%) had negative symptom responses. The type reactions are shown in Table 6.14. None of the controls had any reaction to placebo inhalation or formaldehyde inhalation.

There was a relationship between past history of FST and FIT. Of 19 patients with formaldehyde sensitivity by history, 19 (100%) had positive reactions to formaldehyde skin testing, and 11 (57.9%) had positive inhalation testing.

Relationship between FST and FIT: Of the 48 patients with a positive skin test, 31 (64.6%) had a positive inhalation test. One hundred percent (31/31) of the patients with positive inhalation test had a positive skin test. The main results of FST and FIT are summarized in Tables 6.15 through 6.17.

We have performed over 2000 double-blind inhaled challenges with less than 0.20 ppm of formaldehyde in our center under rigid environmentally controlled conditions. Patients were studied in the deadapted state of 3–5 days of fasting in a formaldehyde-free environment. Seventy-five percent of the chemically sensitive patients had positive challenge reactions versus none when these patients were exposed to at least three placebos. Sign reproduction in these patients was similar to that in the previously described tests, but with more cardiovascular signs. These reactions involved all the smooth muscle systems, including respiratory, cardiovascular, gastrointestinal, and genitourinary systems. ALS, skin, and neurological reactions were seen (Table 6.18). Most patients had one system

TABLE 6.14
Reactions Present before Formaldehyde Inhalation Test (FIT)

Signs and Symptoms	Patients (66)	
	No.	%
None	44	
Light headache	8	14
Light head pressure	4	6.0
Light chest pain	6	9
Sore throat	4	6

Source: Pan et al. 2013. EHC-Dallas formaldehyde sensitivity.

Note: After FIT, signs and symptoms are shown in Table 6.18. The average duration of symptoms after FIT was 50 minutes (the range was 15 minutes to 3 hours and 45 minutes).

TABLE 6.15
Results of FST and FIT (Formaldehyde Inhalation Test)

		Patients (n = 49)				Control (n = 14)			
		Positive		Negative		Positive		Negative	
	Test	No.	%	No.	%	No.	%	No.	%
FST	Normal saline	0	0	9	100[a]	0	0	14	100
	Histamine	49	100	0	0	14	100	0	0
	Formaldehyde	48	98	1	2	1	7.1	13	92.9
	Methyl alcohol	0	0	9	100[a]	0	0	14	100
FIT	Formaldehyde	31	63.6	18	36.7[b]	0	0	14	100
	Spring water	0	0	46	100	0	0	14	100

Source: Pan, Y. et al. 1989. Formaldehyde sensitivity. *Clin. Ecol.* 6(3):79–84. With permission. Also from Rea, W.J. 1994. *Chemical Sensitivity, Volume II*, page 965, table 12. With permission.

[a] Nine patients were tested.
[b] The one patient with a questionable result was included in the negative category.

TABLE 6.16
Ratio of Patients with Positive FIT to Positive FST

Formaldehyde Dilution	Volume of Injection	No. of Patients with Positive FST	No. of Patients with Positive FIT	Patients with Positive FIT to Positive FST (%)
#1	0.05 cc	2	2	100
	0.01 cc	5	4	80
#2	0.05 cc	4	3	75
	0.01 cc	9	5	56
#3	0.05 cc	12	9	75
	0.01 cc	12	7	58
#4	0.05 cc	2	1	50
	0.01 cc	2	0	0
Total		48	31	65

Source: Pan, Y. et al. 1989. Formaldehyde sensitivity. *Clin. Ecol.* 6(3):79–84. With permission. Also from Rea, W.J. 1994. *Chemical Sensitivity, Volume II*, page 967, table 13. With permission.

TABLE 6.17
Reactions during FIT (Formaldehyde Inhalation Test)

Signs and Symptoms	No. of Patients
Neurological (headache, mental confusion dizziness, depression, head pressure, sleepiness, poor concentration)	16
Upper respiratory (ear pressure, ears ringing, running nose, itchy nose, sore throat, itchy throat)	14
Lower respiratory (tight chest, heavy feeling in chest, shortness of breath, coughing)	11
Cardiovascular (arrhythmia pulse increase, blood pressure increase)	12
Gastrointestinal (nausea)	2
Musculoskeletal (pain, tremor, arms feeling heavy)	4
Eyes (tearing, pain, burning, eyelids feeling heavy)	9
Skin (itching, dry lips, flushed)	5
Delayed reaction (night sweats)	1
Greater than 20% fall in PRF	2

Source: Pan, Y. et al. 1989. Formaldehyde sensitivity. *Clin. Ecol.* 6(3):79–84. With permission. Also from Rea, W.J. 1994. *Chemical Sensitivity, Volume II*, page 968, table 14. With permission.

Note: None of the controls had any reaction to placebo inhalation or formaldehyde inhalation.

TABLE 6.18
Signs and Symptoms during Formaldehyde Skin Test

Signs and Symptoms	No. of Patients (66)
Neurological (tired, headache, dizziness, sleepy, tight head, foggy)	13
Cardiovascular (pulse increase, swelling)	7
Musculoskeletal (muscle tightness, myalgia, arthralgia)	10
Respiratory (sore throat, coughing, burning in mouth nasal, membrane ache, bad taste)	12
Eyes (tearing, burning)	2
Skin (itching, flushed)	4
No reactions, only positive wheals	26

Source: Pan, Y. et al. 1989. Formaldehyde sensitivity. *Clin. Ecol.* 6(3):79–84. With permission. Also from Rea, W.J. 1994. *Chemical Sensitivity, Volume II*, page 965, table 10. With permission.

predominantly involved. It is clear that a combination of intradermal skin testing and inhaled formaldehyde challenge in the deadapted state will give significant findings that allow the diagnosis of formaldehyde sensitivities (Tables 6.15 and 6.16).

Sometimes, immune parameters can be altered by formaldehyde challenge and plotted in order to make a diagnosis (Figures 6.3 and 6.4).

The following case report further emphasizes the importance of diagnosing and treating environmental overload:

Case study: A patient was well until he decided to build a new house. He moved into a mobile home next to the building site. Shortly after moving into this mobile home, he developed a cough. In retrospect, he realized, this stopped when he was outside. He gradually developed severe asthma over a period of 2 months, which rapidly became refractory to medication. He entered the EHC-Dallas where he was placed in a formaldehyde-free environment, and all his symptoms cleared. His laboratory work was normal, but he had developed sensitivities to phenol and chlorine. He also developed confusion and increased bone pain. Double-blind inhaled challenges reproduced all his signs, including decreased pulmonary flow, as can be seen in Figure 6.5. He had to alter his plans

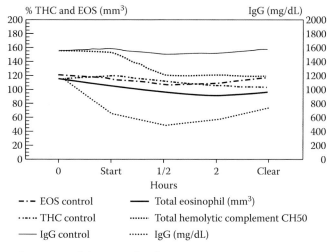

FIGURE 6.3 Thirty-five-year-old white female—inhaled, double-blind formaldehyde challenge, Ambient dose (<0.2 ppm, 15-minute exposure) after 4 days deadaptation in the ECU with total load decreased. (From Rea, W.J. 1994. *Chemical Sensitivity, Volume II*, page 961, figure 2. With permission.)

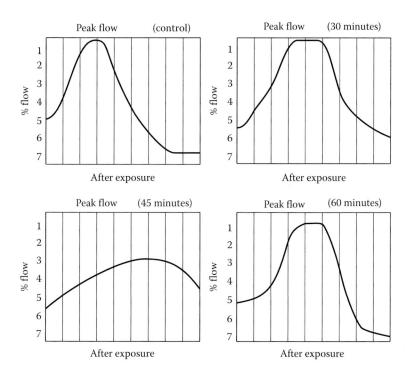

FIGURE 6.4 Peak flow after a formaldehyde challenge in ECU-Dallas after 4 days deadaptation. (From Rea, W.J. 1994. *Chemical Sensitivity, Volume II*, page 970, figure 5. With permission.)

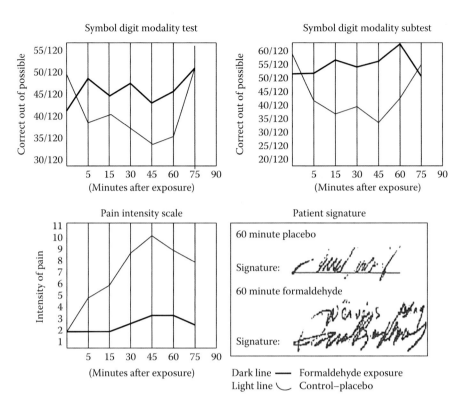

FIGURE 6.5 Thirty-eight-year-old white male—inhaled, double-blind formaldehyde challenge (<0.2 ppm, 15-minute exposure) after 4 days deadaptation in the ECU with total load decreased. (From Rea, W.J. 1994. *Chemical Sensitivity, Volume II*, page 971, figure 5. With permission.)

and build a formaldehyde-free house in order to remain symptom free. Like this patient, most formaldehyde-sensitive patients become sensitive to small doses of other toxic chemicals (Figures 6.6 through 6.8).

TREATMENT OF FORMALDEHYDE SENSITIVITY

The treatment for formaldehyde sensitivity is one of the most difficult problems in environmental medicine. Although extremely difficult, it is possible to construct a formaldehyde-free room, which is essential to the treatment of formaldehyde sensitivity. We have accomplished this by using porcelain, ceramic tile, aluminum, glass, hard wood, and stone. Care must be taken that there is no formaldehyde or synthetic grout used in this room (picture of porcelain and tile rooms). In addition, natural-fiber washable clothes must be used, and permanent-pressed fabrics must be avoided.

1. Avoidance as much as possible
   a. Outdoor air—Charcoal ceramic filters
   b. Indoor air—Charcoal ceramic filters
2. Prescription after an appropriate intradermal skin dose is found (be careful, some patients cannot tolerate).
3. Adequate nutritional supplement information
4. Oxygen supplementation—2 hours serially at the rate of 4–8 L/minute of PvO_2 is above 28 mmHg from antecubital fossa and is using a tourniquet.
5. Immune boosters if

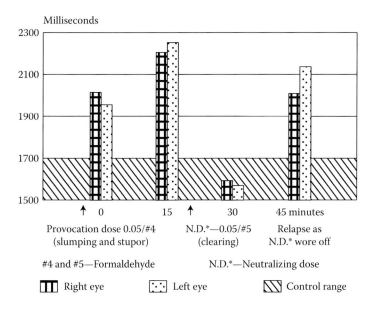

FIGURE 6.6 Formaldehyde provocation and neutralization by intradermal injection of 0.05 cc of formaldehyde (T5 pupillary response time as measured by the iris corder—patient deadapted and environmental control). (From Rea, W.J. 1994. *Chemical Sensitivity, Volume II*, page 972, figure 6. With permission.)

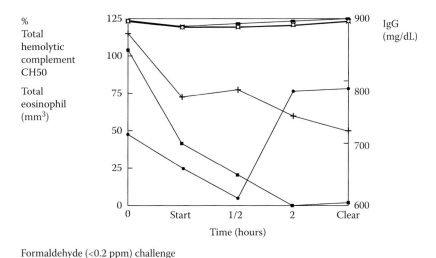

FIGURE 6.7 Thirty-seven-year-old white female—inhaled, double-blind formaldehyde challenge (<0.2 ppm, 15-minute exposure) after 4 days deadaptation in the ECU with total load decreased. (From Rea, W.J. 1994. *Chemical Sensitivity, Volume II*, page 968, figure 3. With permission.)

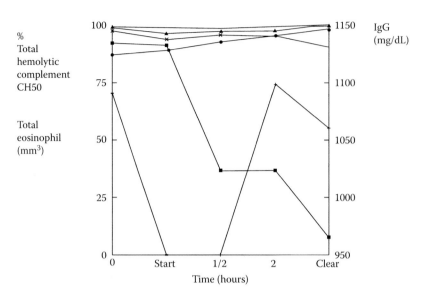

Formaldehyde (<0.2 ppm) challenge
Saline control

Symptoms produced:
1. Nausea
2. Lightheadedness
3. Pain of foot
4. White blotching of skin of legs

- THC   - Control THC
- EOS   - Control EOS
- IgG   - Control IgG

FIGURE 6.8   42-year-old white male—inhaled, double-blind formaldehyde challenge (<0.2 ppm, 15-minute exposure) after 4 days deadaptation in the ECU with total load decreased. (From Rea, W.J. 1994. *Chemical Sensitivity, Volume II*, page 969, figure 4. With permission.)

   a.   Low T and B lymphocytes or low T and B function use autogenous lymphocytic factor
   b.   Low gamma globulin subsets—prescription with gamma globulins
   c.   Autogenous whole-blood vaccine

AVOIDANCE OF WATER

Formaldehyde is released to water from the discharges of both treated and untreated industrial waste water from its production and use in the manufacture of formaldehyde-containing resins. Formaldehyde can also be formed in seawater by photochemical processes.[137] Calculations of sea–air exchange have indicated that this process is probably a minor source of formaldehyde in the sea.[137]

The amount of formaldehyde released to surface water and POTWs in 1996 by the U.S. industrial facilities sorted by state is shown in Table 6.17.[47] According to TRI96,[47] an estimated total of 320,003 pounds (145,153 kg) of formaldehyde, amounting to 2% of the total environmental release, was discharged to surface water in 1996. An additional 1.9 million pounds (0.8 million kg) of formaldehyde were discharged to POTWs.[47] The TRI data should be used with caution since only certain facilities are required to report.[138] This is not an exhaustive list. As a result of secondary treatment processes in POTWs, only a fraction of the formaldehyde that enters POTWs is expected to be released subsequently to surface water; however, this percentage is not known for formaldehyde. Experiments conducted at three full-scale drinking water treatment plants and a pilot plant provided evidence that ozone treatment resulted in the production of measurable levels of formaldehyde in all of the plants studied.[139]

There is a potential for release of formaldehyde to water from hazardous waste sites. Formaldehyde has been detected in surface water samples collected at 5 of the 26 hazardous waste sites and in groundwater samples collected at 4 of the 26 hazardous waste sites where formaldehyde has been detected in some environmental medium.[14]

When released to water, formaldehyde will biodegrade to low levels in a few days.[140] In nutrient-enriched seawater, there is a long lag period (40 hours) prior to measurable loss of formaldehyde by presumably biological processes.[137] Formaldehyde in aqueous effluent is degraded by activated sludge and sewage in 48–72 hours.[12,141–143] In a die-away test, using water from a stagnant lake, degradation was complete in 30 hours under aerobic conditions and 48 hours under anaerobic conditions.[12] Bhattacharya and Parkin[144] used anaerobic chemostats to study fate and kinetic effects of sludge and continuous additions of formaldehyde to acetate and propionate enrichment systems. The high reduction of formaldehyde with continuous addition is indicative of biodegradation, since the combination of volatilization, adsorption, and chemical transformation should account for less than 25% of the removal. Up to 80% of the formaldehyde was removed, with biodegradation accounting for 55%–60%.

Chameides and Davis[22] postulated that formaldehyde dissolved in cloudwater should not photolytically decompose because $CH_2(OH)_2$ is not a chromophore, and that the more probable fate of dissolved formaldehyde is oxidation by OH with the ultimate formation of formic acid. Experiments performed by Mopper and Stahovec[137] suggest that formaldehyde is formed and consumed in seawater as a result of a number of interacting photochemical, biological, and physical processes. Diurnal fluctuations of formaldehyde ranging from 15 to 50 nM were measured in humic-rich waters off the west coast of Florida over a 3-day sampling period.

Concentrated solutions containing formaldehyde are unstable, both oxidizing slowly to form formic acid and polymerizing.[145] In the presence of air and moisture, polymerization takes place readily in concentrated solutions at room temperature to form paraformaldehyde, a solid mixture of linear polyoxymethylene glycols containing 90%–99% formaldehyde.[146]

Avoidance of Outdoor Air Formaldehyde

Formaldehyde is removed from the atmosphere by direct photolysis and oxidation by photochemically produced hydroxyl radicals. Formaldehyde absorbs ultraviolet (UV) radiation at wavelengths of 360 nm and longer[17]; therefore, it is capable of photolyzing in sunlight. A half-life of 6 hours has been measured for photolysis in simulated sunlight.[20] There are two photolytic pathways, one producing H_2 and CO, and the other producing H and HCO radicals.[19,54] When the rates of these reactions are combined with estimates of actinic irradiance, the predicted half-life of formaldehyde due to photolysis in the lower atmosphere is 1.6 hours at a solar zenith angle of 40°.[54] Based on its rate of reaction with photochemically produced hydroxyl radicals, formaldehyde has a predicted half-life of approximately 19 hours in clean air and about half that time in polluted air.[16–18] Lowe et al.[19] report the lifetime of formaldehyde in the sunlit atmosphere, due to photolysis and reaction with hydroxyl radicals, is 4 hours. Singh et al.[27] report an estimated daily loss rate of formaldehyde of 88.2% on the basis of hydroxyl radical activity and photolysis. The hydroxyl-radical-initiated oxidation of formaldehyde also occurs in cloud droplets to form formic acid, a component of acid rain.[22,147] Calculations by Benner and Bizjak[148] suggest that removal of formaldehyde by H_2O_2 is probably negligible in atmospheric droplets. When formaldehyde is irradiated in a reactor, the half-life is 50 minutes in the absence of NO_2 and 35 minutes in the presence of NO_2.[12,149] The primary products formed are formic acid and CO.[20] The reaction of formaldehyde with nitrate radicals, insignificant in the daytime, may be an important removal mechanism at night.[150] Formaldehyde reacts with the NO_3 radical by H-atom extraction with a half-life of 12 days, assuming an average nighttime NO_3 radical concentration of 2×10^9 molecules per cm^3 (Table 6.19).[151]

Formaldehyde is released to the atmosphere in large amounts and is formed in the atmosphere by the oxidation of hydrocarbons. However, the input is counterbalanced by several removal paths.[140] Because of its high solubility, there will be efficient transfer into rain and surface water, which may be important sinks.[150] One model has predicted dry deposition and wet removal half-lives of 19 and

TABLE 6.19

Environmental Transformation Products of Formaldehyde by Medium

Reaction	Comments	References
Air		
$CH_2O + h\nu \bullet\bullet HCO + H$	Photolysis, pathway 1	Calvert et al.[54]
$CH_2O + h\nu \bullet\bullet H_2 + CO$	Photolysis, pathway 2	Calvert et al. [54]
$CH_2O + NO_3 \bullet\bullet HCO + HNO_3$	H-atom abstraction by NO_3 radical	Kao[152]
$CH_2O + HO \bullet\bullet CH_2(OH)_2$	H-atom abstraction by HO radical	NRC[150]
Dilute Aqueous Solution		
$CH_2O + H_2O \bullet\bullet CH_2(OH)_2$	Formation of gem-diol	Kumar[153]
	Methylene glycol; $k_{298\bullet\bullet} = 7.0 \times 10^3$ M atm^{-1}	
Concentrated Solution		
$CH_2O \bullet\bullet H(CH_2O)_nOH + C_3H_3O_3$	Formation of	EPA[154]
	Paraformaldehyde and trioxane	
Cloudwater		
$CH_2(OH)_2 + OH \bullet\bullet CH(OH)_2 + H_2O$ (1)	Formation of formic acid; $k_1 = 2 \times 10^9$ M^{-1} s^{-1}	Chameides and
$CH(OH)_2 + O_2 \bullet\bullet HO_2 + (HCOOH)_{aq}$ (2)	$k_2 = 4.5 \times 10^9$ M^{-1} s^{-1}	Davis[22]

50 hours, respectively.[19] Although formaldehyde is found in remote areas, it probably is not transported there, but is generated from longer-lived precursors that have been transported.[150]

Plants, such as kidney beans and barley, can absorb gaseous formaldehyde through their leaves.[12] Experiments performed on a variety of fish and shrimp showed no evidence of the bioaccumulation of formaldehyde.[155,156] Because formaldehyde is rapidly metabolized,[157] bioaccumulation is not expected to be important.

A recent survey of emission data from stationary and mobile sources was used as input for an atmospheric dispersion model to estimate outdoor toxic air contaminant concentrations for 1990 for each of the 60,803 census tracts in the contiguous United States.[158] The average long-term background concentration estimated for formaldehyde was 0.2 ppb (Table 6.19).[158]

In a survey of ambient measurements of hazardous air pollutants, a median formaldehyde concentration of 2.5 ppb was found for a total of 1358 samples collected at 58 different locations.[23] Air samples collected daily in Schenectady, New York, during the months of June through August 1983 had formaldehyde concentrations ranging from 1 to 31 ppb. There was a significant daily variation that appeared to correlate with traffic conditions.[26] In the same study, formaldehyde levels measured on the summit of Whiteface Mountain in Wilmington, New York, ranged from 0.8 to 2.6 ppb. Ambient formaldehyde concentrations at the California State University, Los Angeles campus ranged from 2 to 40 ppb during the period from May to June 1980; and concentrations in Claremont, California ranged from 3 to 48 ppb from September 19 to October 8, 1980.[24] Formaldehyde was measured in urban ambient air in 8 cities for 2–3-day periods from June 1980 to April 1984. The average concentrations were 11.3 ppb in St. Louis, Missouri (June 5–7, 1980); 12.3 ppb in Denver, Colorado (June 23–24, 1980); 2.3 ppb in Denver, Colorado (April 1–2, 1984); 19 ppb in Riverside, California (July 8–10, 1980); 14.3 ppb in Staten Island, New York (April 3–4, 1981); 18.5 ppb in Pittsburgh, Pennsylvania (April 15–16, 1981); 11.3 ppb in Chicago, Illinois (April 27–28, 1981); 15.5 ppb in Downey, California (February 28–March 1, 1984); and 3.8 ppb in Houston, Texas (March 18–19, 1984). The maximum concentration in each city ranged from 5.5 ppb in Denver in April to 67.7 ppb in Downey.[25,27]

Formaldehyde was detected in 99% of 48 ambient air samples obtained in Ohio urban centers, June–July 1989, at a mean and maximum concentration of 3.0 and 15.5 ppb, respectively.[159] The diurnal changes in concentration were found to be consistent with initial direct emissions from vehicles followed by secondary photochemical production and, ultimately, atmospheric removal. These data indicate that formaldehyde concentrations in urban atmospheres are expected to be the highest during, or shortly after rush hour, or other periods of high vehicular traffic. Similar results were obtained when temporal formaldehyde concentrations were measured during a smog event in California, September 1993.[156] In central Los Angeles, higher formaldehyde concentrations were found to correlate with vehicular traffic while at a downwind location, the concentration was found to spike later in the day. The average atmospheric formaldehyde concentration for all sites was 5.3 ppbv (parts per billion by volume) in this study, while the background concentration from San Nicolas Island (off the Southern California coast) was 0.8 ppmv (parts per million by volume). Average annual formaldehyde concentrations in California have been reported to vary from a minimum of 3.2 ppbv in the San Francisco Bay area to 4.9 ppbv in the South Coast Air Basin.[160]

INDOOR AIR AVOIDANCE

Several monitoring studies have been conducted in the United States to measure the concentration of formaldehyde in indoor environments.[161–164] The results for a variety of housing types and ages have been compiled by Gold et al.[28] and are presented in Table 6.20. Much of the data was collected in older homes, in homes that had UFFI, or in homes in which occupants had filed complaints of formaldehyde irritant symptoms. Since the time, many of these monitoring studies were performed; plywood and particleboard manufacturing methods have been changed to reduce the formaldehyde emission levels in the finished product.[29] Similarly, home construction methods have changed, and the use of UFFI has been greatly reduced since the mid-1980s.[30] A recent pilot study on a newly constructed and unoccupied house set up to measure formaldehyde emissions from construction materials had a maximum localized formaldehyde concentration of 0.076 ppm, which occurred shortly after a high loading of pressed wood materials, such as kitchen cabinets.[31] The average indoor concentrations measured in this study were 0.035–0.45 ppm, which was attained approximately 30 days after either high or low loadings of formaldehyde-releasing materials were installed. Porcelain, ceramic, plaster, and hardwood are the best for building formaldehyde-free home (Table 6.20).

The range of formaldehyde concentrations measured in complaint homes, mobile homes, and homes containing large quantities of particleboard or UFFI were 0.02–0.8 ppm, with levels as high as 4 ppm, sufficient to cause irritating symptoms, observed in some instances. Formaldehyde levels in more recently built (<1-year-old) conventional homes generally were within the range of 0.05–0.2 ppm, with few measurements exceeding 0.3 ppm. Older conventional homes had the lowest indoor concentrations of formaldehyde with values typically less than 0.05 ppm,[28] consistent with the expected decrease in latent formaldehyde release from wood-based building materials as they age.[165,166]

The Texas Department of Health measured formaldehyde in 443 mobile homes between April 1979 and May 1982 at the request of the occupants. Concentrations ranged from below detectable limits (<0.5 ppm) to 8 ppm.[72] Of the homes #1-year-old, 27% had mean concentrations .2 ppm, while 11.5% of older homes had concentrations .2 ppm. The concentration of formaldehyde in mobile homes would be expected to be higher than that found in conventional homes due to their lower rate of air exchange.[32]

Sexton et al.[167] selected an age-stratified random sample of 470 mobile homes, from the more than 500,000 in California, for measurement of 1-week average indoor formaldehyde concentrations during the periods July–August 1984 and February–March 1985. They observed relatively little variation in formaldehyde concentrations between summer and winter, with average 1-week formaldehyde values of 0.07–0.09 ppm. Of the homes, 31% exceeded the maximum concentration of 0.1 ppm formaldehyde recommended at the time of the study by AIHA, EPA, and the American Society of Heating, Refrigerating, and Air Conditioning Engineers. The investigators noted that formaldehyde levels appeared to have been decreasing in mobile homes manufactured since about 1980, probably as a result of increased use of low-formaldehyde-emitting building materials.

TABLE 6.20

Indoor Concentrations of Formaldehyde in U.S. Homes

Building Type	Concentration (ppm)			References
	Number	Range	Mean	
With UFFI	>1200	0.01–3.4	0.05–0.12	EPA[160]; Gammage and Hawthorne[162]
Without UFFI	131	0.01–0.17	0.025–0.07	
Complaint				
Mobile homes	>500	0.00–4.2	0.1–0.9	Gammage and Hawthorne[162]
Noncomplaint				
Conventional,				
randomly selected	560	<0.005–0.48	0.027–0.091	EPA[161]; Stock[164]
Mobile homes,	••1200	<0.01–2.9	0.091–0.62	EPA[161]
randomly selected				
By age				
Mobile homes				
New	260		0.86	Gammage and Hawthorne[162]
Older, occupied	–		0.25	Gammage and Hawthorne[162]
Conventional homes				
0–5 years	18		0.08	Gammage and Hawthorne[162]; Hawthorne et al.[163]
5–15 years	11		0.04	Gammage and Hawthorne[162]; Hawthorne et al.[163]
>15	11		0.03	Gammage and Hawthorne[162]; Hawthorne et al.[163]
Overall	40	<0.02–0.4	0.06	Gammage and Hawthorne[162]; Hawthorne et al.[163]

Note: UFFI, urea-formaldehyde foam insulation.

    The Indiana State Board of Health measured formaldehyde in four specific office and commercial establishments that had poor ventilation. The concentrations ranged from 0.01 to 1.01 ppm. In one case, the source of formaldehyde was UF foam. In the others, it was particleboard, plywood subflooring, and furniture.[168]

    Shah and Singh[169] collected indoor and outdoor data for volatile organic chemicals from both residential and commercial environments. The average daily outdoor concentration of formaldehyde for all outdoor site types (remote, rural, suburban, urban, and source-dominated) was 8.3 ppbv; the average daily indoor concentration of formaldehyde was 49.4 ppbv (Table 6.21).

    Zhang et al.[36] carried out simultaneous indoor and outdoor measurements of aldehydes at six residential houses in suburban New Jersey during the summer of 1992. Formaldehyde was the most abundant aldehyde, with a mean outdoor concentration of 12.53 ppb (60% of the total outdoor aldehyde concentration) and a mean indoor concentration of 54.56 ppb (87% of the total indoor aldehyde concentration).

    Krzyzanowski et al.[170] measured formaldehyde concentrations in 202 households in Pima County, Arizona, and found an average value of 26 ppb. Concentrations varied slightly with locations in the house, with the highest levels generally found in the kitchens. Only a few concentrations exceeded 90 ppb, with a maximum value of 140 ppb. The average indoor formaldehyde concentrations measured in homes in Pullman, Washington, ranged from approximately 5–72 ppb (Table 6.21).[171]

    A study was conducted in Boston to examine the commuter's exposure to six gasoline-related volatile emissions, including formaldehyde, in four different commuting modes.[45] The mean formaldehyde concentrations (in $\mu g/m^3$) measured while driving private cars, riding in subways, walking, and biking were 5.1 ($n = 40$), 4.5 ($n = 38$), 5.5 ($n = 31$), and 6.3 ($n = 11$), respectively. The maximum concentrations in all commuting modes were usually three to five times higher than the mean concentrations. A similar study in the New York/New Jersey area found that the mean in-vehicle concentration of formaldehyde during commutes was 0.3 $\mu g/m^3$.[172,173]

TABLE 6.21
Home and Work place Formaldehyde Levels

Source	mg/day
Air	
Outdoor air (10% of time)	0.02
Indoor Air	
Home (65% of time)	
Conventional	0.5–2.0
Prefabricated (chipboard)	1.0–10.0
Workplace (25% of Time)	
Without occupational exposure	0.2–0.8
With 1 mg/m^3 occupational exposure	5
Environmental tobacco smoke	0.1–1
Smoking (20 cigarettes/day)	1

Occupational exposure can occur during the production of end products in which formaldehyde is used, in the garment industry, during various preservation processes, and in laboratories. Healthcare professionals (pharmacists, physicians, veterinarians, dentists, nurses, etc.) may be exposed to vapors during the preparation, administration, and/or cleanup of various medicines. Pathologists and histology technicians, morticians, and teachers and students who handle preserved specimens may also be exposed.[174–178] The laser cutting of felt, woven fabrics, formica, plexiglass, and acrylic materials has been found to release formaldehyde.[179] Formaldehyde exposure for workers at a fiberglass insulation manufacturing plant were found to range from 49 to 516 µg/m^3.[180] Midrange photocopiers (30–135 copies per minute) have also been found to emit formaldehyde.[181]

The NOES, conducted from 1981 to 1983, indicated that 1,329,332 workers employed in various professions were potentially exposed to formaldehyde in the United States.[46] The NOES database does not contain information on the frequency, concentration, or duration of exposure; the survey provides only estimates of workers potentially exposed to the chemical in the workplace. OSHA has estimated that in the late 1980s, over 2 million workers in over 112,000 firms were exposed to formaldehyde; about 45% of these workers are estimated to be in the garment industry. About 1.9 million were exposed to levels of formaldehyde between 0.1 and 0.5 ppm (mainly in apparel, furniture, paper mills, and plastic molding); approximately 123,000 were exposed to levels of formaldehyde between 0.5 and 0.75 ppm (mainly in apparel, textile finishing, furniture, laboratories, and foundries); and about 84,000 were exposed to between 0.75 and 1 ppm (mainly in apparel, furniture, and foundries).[182]

OSHA has estimated that in the United States, approximately 107,000 employees are exposed to formaldehyde concentrations greater than 1 ppm, and approximately 430,000 employees are exposed to concentrations ranging from 0.5 to 1 ppm.[10] An initial evaluation of formaldehyde exposures in a sewing plant using fabrics with a postcure resin found time-weighted average exposure levels 1.2 ppm, with a mean of 0.9 ppm.[183] A modification that decreased the amount of residual formaldehyde in the fabric reduced worker exposure by 80%–85%. Area concentrations of formaldehyde in a plywood company ranged from 0.28 to 3.48 ppm; the average personal exposure was 1.13 ppm formaldehyde.[184] Airborne formaldehyde concentrations ranging from 0.187 to 0.783 ppm have been measured during particleboard-sanding operations.[185] Formaldehyde concentrations of 0.5–7 ppm have been measured in leather tanning facilities.[186] An average airborne formaldehyde level of 0.36 ± 0.19 ppm was measured during 22 embalming procedures.[175] Fire fighters are exposed to formaldehyde concentrations as high as 8 ppm during knockdown (bringing the main body of fire under control) and 0.4 ppm during overhaul (searching for and extinguishing hidden fire).[187] Formaldehyde levels of

0.3 ppm have been measured inside a fire fighter's self-contained breathing apparatus.[187] All of these exposures must be eliminated for the chemically sensitive to stay well.

Children are exposed to formaldehyde mainly from its presence in air. Formaldehyde levels are typically higher indoors[28] where younger children may spend a significant amount of time. Exposure for children outdoors will be similar to adults. It is likely to be greatest during rush hour commutes[159] or near known sources of formaldehyde release, such as factories using formaldehyde or during the use of products[169] that emit formaldehyde. Children may also be dermally exposed to formaldehyde as a result of its release from permanent-press fabrics or its presence in cosmetic products. Only a limited number of studies that address formaldehyde exposure to children or body burden measurements have been identified.[169,188]

In the home, formaldehyde sources include household chemicals, pressed wood products (especially when new),[29] combustion sources,[95] and some new fabrics[44] and garments. A number of common household products may release formaldehyde to indoor air, including antiseptics, medicines, dish-washing liquids, fabric softeners, shoe-care agents, carpet cleaners, glues, adhesives, and lacquers.[33] If children use or play with some of these products, or are present when they are used, additional exposure to formaldehyde may occur. Many cosmetic products contain formaldehyde and some, such as nail polish and nail hardeners, even contain high levels.[33] If children place these products in their mouth or on their skin, or sniff them, they will be exposed to elevated levels of formaldehyde.

New carpets have been found to release formaldehyde.[87] Older carpets, especially wall-to-wall carpets, have been found to be a sink for formaldehyde if there are other indoor sources.[88] In addition, some carpet cleaners may contain formaldehyde. Infants may be exposed to formaldehyde while crawling on carpets or on newly cleaned carpets.[49,189] Similarly, young children may be exposed while sitting or playing on indoor carpeting.

Formaldehyde is typically not found in water or soil, and children are not expected to be exposed by these routes. Because it is a gas, formaldehyde is not brought home on a parent's work clothes or tools. Occupants of newly constructed homes, including children, may be exposed to formaldehyde due to its release from pressed wood construction materials (Section "Populations with Potentially High Exposures"), a process that slowly decreases with time. As discussed above, formaldehyde is released to indoor air from many sources. Children that live in mobile homes may be exposed to higher levels of formaldehyde compared with those that live in conventional homes because mobile homes have lower air exchange rates. Children that live in households that have a cigarette, cigar, or pipe smoker will also be exposed to higher levels of formaldehyde due to its presence in sidestream smoke.[94]

Formaldehyde is released from many pressed wood products used in the construction of furniture.[165] When placed in a new crib manufactured from these materials, infants may be exposed because of their proximity to the furniture's structural components. Also, small rooms that have new furniture manufactured from pressed wood products installed may have localized, elevated concentrations of formaldehyde because of their low total volume.

Formaldehyde is highly water soluble, very reactive, and is rapidly metabolized by tissues at portals of entry. Thus, parental exposure at typical indoor, outdoor, or occupational levels is not expected to result in exposure to parental germ cells or the developing fetus (see Section "Children's Susceptibility" for additional information).

Since formaldehyde is typically found in the air, and since its concentration in indoor air is typically higher than that found outdoors, formaldehyde exposure to children can be reduced by bringing fresh air into the home. This can be accomplished by opening windows or using ventilation fans. It has been established that coated or laminated pressed wood products release less formaldehyde than those that are uncoated,[33,84] so sealing these surfaces would be expected to reduce formaldehyde levels in the home. Since formaldehyde is also formed in indoor air by the degradation of other volatile organic chemicals, such as solvents,[35] commonly found in the home, removing the source of these materials or using them with adequate ventilation will reduce indoor levels of formaldehyde.

Formaldehyde concentrations measured on two different days inside a tavern during normal smoking conditions were 85–72 ppb.[190] In the same study, the average airborne formaldehyde yield of a cigarette was found to be 2 mg. Levels of formaldehyde in nonsmoking office buildings ranged from not detected to 0.22 ppm, while it ranged from not detected to 0.6 ppm where smoking was permitted.[96]

Material that acts as a sink for formaldehyde, such as carpets,[88] can also be removed from the home to lower levels. Securing cosmetic products and other materials that have higher formaldehyde concentrations away from children's reach and not allowing individuals to smoke in the house will also lower levels of exposure.

Environmental fate: The environmental fate of formaldehyde in air has been well studied.[12,17,19,20,22,23,54,149,152] Formaldehyde is removed from the atmosphere by direct photolysis and oxidation by photochemically produced hydroxyl and nitrate radicals. Solutions of formaldehyde are unstable, both oxidizing slowly to form formic acid and polymerizing. When released to water, formaldehyde will biodegrade to low levels in a few days, with little adsorption to sediment.[140,191] No significant volatilization from water is expected to occur.[191] No experimental or estimated values for the half-life of formaldehyde in ambient water were found in the literature. Aqueous solutions of formaldehyde that are released to soil may leach through the soil.[15,191,192] Although formaldehyde is known to biodegrade under both aerobic and anaerobic conditions, the fate of formaldehyde in soil is still unknown.[140] There is a need for data on the fate and transport of formaldehyde in soil, including half-life values. The environmental fate of formaldehyde's predominant degradation product, formic acid, is well documented. In air, formic acid is expected to rapidly degrade (half-life approximately 1 month) through its reaction with hydroxyl radicals or it is expected to undergo wet deposition to the earth's surface.[193] In water or soil, formic acid is expected to rapidly biodegrade.

1. Prescription of appropriate intradermal neutralization dose is found—4 times/day to 1 injection every 4 days is used.
2. Adequate nutrients supplementation is used daily.
   a. Vitamin C—5 g/day
   b. Glutathione—800–1000 mg/day
   c. 1 multimineral capsule/day
   d. 1 multivitamin capsule/day
   e. Other nutrients as needed
3. Oxygen supplementation—4–8 L/minute for 2 consecutive hours to keep PvO_2 below 28 mmHg/minute in the antecubital fossa not using a tourniquet.
4. Immune modulators
   a. Autogenous lymphocytic factor for low T cell numbers or low T cell function
   b. Gamma globulin supplementation for low gamma globulin subsets or total g-globulin
   c. Autogenous whole-blood vaccine daily two times for 4 days

Pictures of different rooms:

1. Porcelain

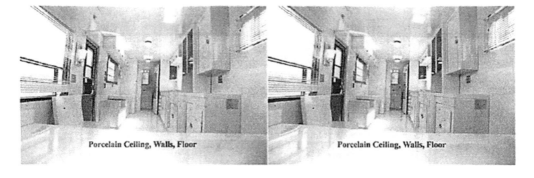

Porcelain Ceiling, Walls, Floor   Porcelain Ceiling, Walls, Floor

2. Glass

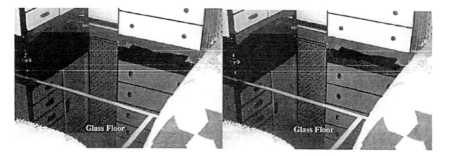

3. Aluminum

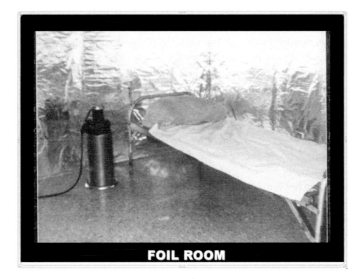

4. Hardwood

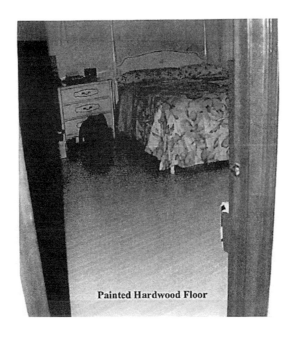

5. Stone

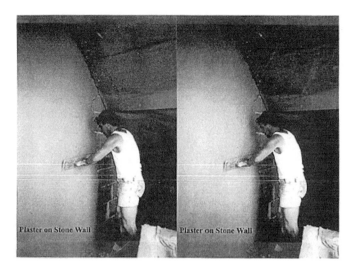

Plaster on Stone Wall   Plaster on Stone Wall

SOIL

Formaldehyde is released to soils through industrial discharges and through land disposal of form-aldehyde-containing wastes. The amount of formaldehyde released to land in 1996 by the U.S. industrial facilities sorted by state is shown in Table 6.22.[47] According to TRI96,[47] an estimated total of 114,406 pounds (51,894 kg) of formaldehyde, amounting to 0.54% of the total environmental release, was discharged to land from the U.S. manufacturing or processing facilities in 1996. An additional 9.4 million pounds (4.3 million kg), constituting about 44% of total environmental emissions, were released via underground injection.[47] Also, some of the estimated 1.3 million pounds of formaldehyde wastes transferred off-site (Table 6.1) may be ultimately disposed of in land. The TRI data should be used with caution since only certain facilities are required to report.[138] This is not an exhaustive list.

There is a potential for the release of formaldehyde to soil from hazardous waste sites. Formaldehyde has been detected in soil samples collected at 1 of the 26 hazardous waste sites and in sediment samples collected at 1 of the 26 hazardous waste sites where formaldehyde has been detected in some environmental medium.[14]

OTHER ENVIRONMENTAL MEDIA

Fresh shrimp from four local commercial markets in Atlanta, Georgia were found to have formalde-hyde levels ranging from 0.39 to 1.44 mg/kg.[194] In the same study, shrimp kept live in the laboratory were found to contain 0.99 mg/kg immediately after sacrifice, and the level rose to 2.15 mg/kg after refrigeration for 6 days.

Chou and Que Hee[42] measured the concentrations of carbonyl compounds in artificial saliva leachates of three chewing tobaccos. They found formaldehyde concentrations of 110, 670, and 530 ng/mL (0.11, 0.67, and 0.53 μg/mL, respectively) in three different commercial brands. Mansfield et al.[43] used liquid chromatography to measure formaldehyde as a combustion product in tobacco smoke from six different brands of American filter-tip cigarettes. The average amount of formaldehyde by brand ranged from 45.2 to 73.1 μg/cigarette and from 5.1 to 8.9 μg/puff. Triebig and Zober[94] report that the level of formaldehyde in sidestream cigarette smoke is 50 times higher than main stream smoke[94] while the NCR put the value at five to eight times more formaldehyde in sidestream smoke.[95]

Formaldehyde has also been found at levels ranging from 1 to 3517 ppm in 112 fabric samples, with 18 of the samples having a free formaldehyde concentration greater than 750 ppm (mg/kg).[92]

TABLE 6.22

Ongoing Studies on the Potential for Human Exposure to Formaldehyde

Investigator	Affiliation	Research Description	Sponsor
K. Knapp, D. Pahl, and F. Black	EPA-AREAL, Research Triangle Park, NC	Characterization of emissions, including formaldehyde, from motor vehicles using both traditional and alternative fuels	EPA
B. J. Collier	Louisiana State University, Baton Rouge, LA	Development of textile materials for environmental compatibility and human health and safety	USDA
D. V. Sandberg and R. D. Ottmar	Pacific Northwest Forest and Range Experiment Station, Portland, OR	Assessment of firefighter exposures to potential health hazards, including formaldehyde	USDA
T. Shibamoto	University of California, Davis, CA	Isolation and identification of mutagens and carcinogens in foods	USDA
J. S. Gaffney	Argonne National Laboratory, Argonne, IL	Atmospheric chemistry of organic oxidants and aldehydes	USDOE
P. Davidovits	Boston College, Chestnut Hill, MA	Laboratory studies of heterogeneous gas–liquid interaction of atmospheric trace gases, including formaldehyde	NSF
R. C. Bales and M. Conklin	University of Arizona, Tucson, AZ	Determination of the atmosphere-to-snow transfer function for peroxide and formaldehyde, whose deposition is reversible	NSF
R. C. Bales and M. Conklin	University of Arizona, Tucson, AZ	Distribution of reactive chemical species, including formaldehyde, in ice and snow.	NSF
V. A. Mohnen	State University of New York, Albany, NY	Examination of the involvement of natural hydrocarbons for the formation of peroxide and formaldehyde in air.	NSF
B. G. Heikes	University of Rhode, Island Kingston, RI	Background atmospheric measurements of hydrogen peroxide, organic hydroperoxides, and formaldehyde.	NSF
S. S. Que Hee	UCLA School of Public Health, Los Angeles, CA	Carbonyl compounds air sampling method	NIOSH
R. R. Fall	University of Colorado Boulder, Boulder, CO	Biogenic sources of oxygenated hydrocarbons in the troposphere	NSF

Note: EPA, Environmental Protection Agency; NSF, National Science Foundation; USDA, United States Department of Agriculture; USDOE, United States Department of Energy; NIOSH, National Institute for Occupational Safety and Health.

Injection therapy[195,196]

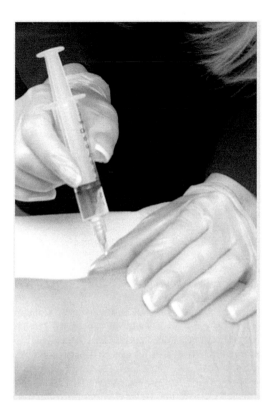

Nutrient therapy

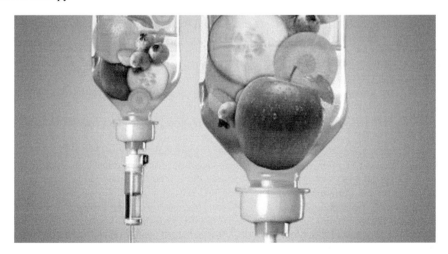

Immune modulators

1. Autogenous lymphocytic factor
2. Gamma globulin when IgGs 2, 3, 4 are low
3. Antigen therapy
4. Nutrition
5. Sauna

REFERENCES

1. Harrison, R. J., M. Moyle. *Org. Synth. Coll.* 4:493 (1963); 36:36 (1956).
2. Ozer, R. 2011. Vapor phase decarbonylation process. WIPO Patent Application WO/2011/026059.
3. UK Food Standards Agency. Current EU approved additives and their E numbers. https://www.food.gov.uk/science/additives/enumberlist. Last updated July 21, 2016.
4. U.S. Food and Drug Administration. Listing of Food Additives Status Part I. Archived from the original on January 17, 2012. Retrieved October 27, 2011.
5. Australia New Zealand Food Standards Code. Standard 1.2.4—Labeling of ingredients. Retrieved October 27, 2011.
6. Cheung, H., R. S. Tanke, G. P. Torrence. 2005. Acetic acid. In *Ullmann's Encyclopedia of Industrial Chemistry*. Weinheim: Wiley-VCH. doi: 10.1002/14356007.a01_045.pub2
7. Scott Research Laboratories. 1969. *Atmospheric Reaction Studies in the Los Angeles Basin*, Phase I. Vol. 2, pp. 143–149, 310–314. Washington, DC: U.S. Department of Health, Education and Welfare, Public Health Service, National Air Pollution Control Administration.
8. National Research Council. 1981. *Formaldehyde and Other Aldehydes*, p. 42. Washington, DC: National Academy Press.
9. Verschueren, K. 1983. *Handbook of Environmental Data on Organic Chemicals*, 2nd ed., pp. 678–679. New York: Van Nostrand Reinhold.
10. Fisbein, L. 1992. Exposure from occupational versus other sources. *Scand. J. Work Environ. Health* 18:5–16.
11. Staffelbach, T., T. Neftel, B. Stauffer, D. Jacob. A record of the atmospheric methane sink from formaldehyde in polar ice cores. *Nature* 349:603–605.
12. EPA. 1976. Investigation of Selected Potential Environmental Contaminants: Formaldehyde. U.S. Environmental Protection Agency, Office of Toxic Substances. PB 256 839, EPA 560/2-76-009.
13. Kleindienst, T. E., P. B. Shepson, E. O. Edney, L. D. Claxton, L. T. Cupitt. 1986. Wood smoke: Measurement of the mutagenic activities of its gas- and particulate-phase photooxidation products. *Environ. Sci. Technol.* 20:493–501.
14. HazDat. 1996. Database. *Agency for Toxic Substances and Disease Registry (ATSDR)*, Atlanta, GA.
15. SRC. 1995. Syracuse Research Corporation. *Octanol-Water Partition Coefficient Program (KOWWIN, Version 1.37, Serial L0148)*. Chemical Hazard Assessment Division, Environmental Chemistry Center, Syracuse, NY.
16. Atkinson, R., J. N. J. Pitts. 1978. Kinetics of the reactions of the OH radical with HCHO and CH_3CHO over the temperature range 299-426K. *J. Chem. Phys.* 68:3581–3584.
17. DOT. 1980. *Chemical Kinetic and Photochemical Data Sheets for Atmospheric Reactions*. Washington, DC: U.S. Department of Transportation. AD A 091 631, FAA-EE-80-17.
18. EPA. 1982. *Atmospheric Chemistry of Several Toxic Compounds*. Research Triangle Park, NC: U.S. Environmental Protection Agency, Environmental Sciences Research Laboratory, Office of Research and Development. PB83-146340, EPA-600/3-82-092.
19. Lowe, D. C., U. Schmidt, D. H. Ehhalt. 1980. A new technique for measuring tropospheric formaldehyde [CH_2O]. *Geophys. Res. Lett.* 7:825–828.
20. Su, F., G. Calvert, J. H. Shaw. 1979. Mechanism of the photooxidation of gaseous formaldehyde. *J. Phys. Chem.* 83:3185–3191.
21. Kamata, E. 1966. Aldehydes in lake and sea waters. *Bull. Chem. Soc. Jpn.* 39:1227–1229.
22. Chameides, W. L., D. D. Davis. 1983. Aqueous-phase source of formic acid in clouds. *Nature* 304:427–429.
23. Kelly, T. J., R. Mukund, C. W. Spicer, A. J. Pollack. 1994. Concentrations and transformations of hazardous air pollutants. *Environ. Sci. Technol.* 28:378A–387A.
24. Grosjean, D. 1982. Formaldehyde and other carbonyls in Los Angeles ambient air. *Environ. Sci. Technol.* 16:254–262.
25. Salas, L. J., H. B. Singh. 1986. Measurements of formaldehyde and acetaldehyde in the urban ambient air. *Atmos. Environ.* 20:1301–1304.
26. Schulam, P., R. Newbold, L. A. Hull. 1985. Urban and rural ambient air aldehyde levels in Schenectady, New York and on Whiteface Mountain, New York. *Atmos. Environ.* 19:623–626.
27. Singh, H. B., L. J. Salas, R. E. Stiles. 1982. Distribution of selected gaseous organic mutagens and suspect carcinogens in ambient air. *Environ. Sci. Technol.* 16:872–880.
28. Gold, K. W., D. F. Naugle, M. A. Berry. 1993. Indoor concentrations of environmental carcinogens. In *Environmental Carcinogens: Methods of Analysis and Exposure Measurement* (IARC Scientific Publications No. 109), B. Seifert, H. J. van de Wiel, I. K. O'Neill, eds., pp. 41–71. Lyon: International Agency for Research on Cancer.

29. EPA. 1996. *Sources and Factors Affecting Indoor Emission from Engineered Wood Products: Summary and Evaluation of Current Literature.* Research Triangle Park, NC: U.S. Environmental Protection Agency, National Risk Management Research Laboratory, Office of Research and Development. PB96183876, EPA-600/R-96-067.

30. CPSC. 1997. *An update on Formaldehyde.* Washington, DC: U.S. Consumer Product Safety Commission.

31. Hare, D. A., W. J. Groah, L. G. Schweer, M. D. Koontz. 1996. Evaluating the contribution of UF-bonded building materials to indoor formaldehyde levels in a newly constructed house. *Presented at Washington State University 30th Annual Particleboard/Composite Materials Symposium*, Pullman, WA.

32. Wolff, G. T. 1991. Air pollution. In *Kirk-Othmer Encyclopedia of Chemical Technology*, M. Howe-Grant, ed., pp. 711–749. New York: John Wiley & Sons, Inc.

33. Kelly, T. J., J. R. Satola, D. L. Smith. 1996. Emission rates of formaldehyde and other carbonyls from consumer and industrial products found in California homes. In *Measurement of Toxic and Related Air Pollutants, Proceedings of International Specialty Conference on Air and Waste Management Association*, pp. 521–526. Pittsburgh, PA.

34. Matthews, T. G., T. J. Reed, B. J. Tromberg, A. R. Hawthorne. 1985. Formaldehyde emission from combustion sources and solid formaldehyde-resin-containing products: Potential impact on indoor formaldehyde concentrations. In *Indoor Air and Human Health*, R. B. Gammage, S. V. Kaye, V. A. Jacobs, eds., 131–150. Chelsea, MI: Lewis Publishers, Inc.

35. Weschler, C. J., H. C. Shields. 1996. Production of the hydroxyl radical in indoor air. *Environ. Sci. Technol.* 30:3250–3258.

36. Zhang, J., W. E. Wilson, P. J. Lioy. 1994. Indoor air chemistry: Formation of or acids and aldehydes. *Environ. Sci. Technol.* 28:1975–1982.

37. EPA. 1976. *Frequency of Organic Compounds Identified in Water.* Athens, GA: U.S. Environmental Protection Agency, Environmental Research Laboratory, Office of Research and Development. EPA600/4-76-062.

38. Hushon, J., R. Clerman, R. Small, S. Sood, A. Taylor, D. Thoman. 1980. *An Assessment of Potentially Carcinogenic Energy-Related Contaminants in Water.* McLean, VA: Prepared for US Department of Energy and National Cancer Institute.

39. Grosjean, D., B. Wright. 1983. Carbonyls in urban fog, ice fog, cloudwater and rainwater. *Atmos. Environ.* 17:2093–2096.

40. Igawa, M., W. J. Munger, M. R. Hoffman. 1989. Analysis of aldehydes in cloud- and fogwater samples by HPLC with a postcolumn reaction detector. *Environ. Sci. Technol.* 23:556–561.

41. Muir, P. S. 1991. Fogwater chemistry in a wood-burning community, Western Oregon. *J. Air Waste Manage. Assoc.* 41:32–38.

42. Chou C.-C., S. S. Que Hee. 1994. Saliva-available carbonyl compounds in some chewing tobaccos. *J. Agric. Food Chem.* 42:2225–2230.

43. Mansfield, C. T., B. T. Hodge, R. B. Hege, W. C. Hamlin. 1977. Analysis of formaldehyde in tobacco smoke by high performance liquid chromatography. *J. Chromatogr. Sci.* 15:301–302.

44. Schorr, W. F., E. Keran, E. Plotka. 1974. Formaldehyde allergy: The quantitative analysis of American clothing for free formaldehyde and its relevance in clinical practice. *Arch. Dermatol.* 110:73–76.

45. Chan, C.-C., J. D. Spengler, H. Ozkaynak, M. Lefkopoulou. 1991. Commuter exposures to VOCs in Boston, Massachusetts. *J. Air Waste Manage. Assoc.* 41:1594–1600.

46. NIOSH. 1995. Formaldehyde numbers of potentially exposed employees. NOSE-based Job Exposure Matrix. *Am. J. Ind. Med.* 20:163–174.

47. TRI96. 1998. Toxic Chemical Release Inventory. National Library of Medicine, National Toxicology Information Program, Bethesda, MD.

48. EPA. 1975. U.S. Environmental Protection Agency, Code of Federal Regulations. 40 CFR 180.1032.

49. WHO. 1989. *World Health Organization. Formaldehyde: Environmental Health Criteria.* Geneva: World Health Organization.

50. Zweidinger, R. B., J. E. Sigsby, S. B. Tejada, F. D. Stump, D. L. Dropkin, W. D. Ray, J. W. Duncan. 1988. Detailed hydrocarbon and aldehyde mobile source emissions from roadway studies. *Environ. Sci. Technol.* 22:956–962.

51. Kirchstetter, T. W., B. C. Singer, R. A. Harley, G. R. Kendall, W. Chan. 1996. Impact of oxygenated gasoline use on California light-duty vehicle emissions. *Environ. Sci. Technol.*, 30:661–670.

52. Gaffney, J. S., N. A. Marley, R. S. Martin, R. W. Dixon, L. G. Reyes, C. J. Popp. 1997. Potential air quality effects of using ethanol-gasoline fuel blends: A field study in Albuquerque, New Mexico. *Environ. Sci. Technol.* 31:3053–3061.

53. Miyamoto, Y. 1986. Eye and respiratory irritants in jet engine exhaust. *Aviat. Space Environ. Med.* 57:1104–1108.

54. Calvert, J. G., J. A. Kerr, K. L. Demerjian, R. D. McQuigg. 1972. Photolysis of formaldehyde as a hydrogen atom source in the lower atmosphere. *Science* 175:751–752.

55. Grosjean, E., D. Grosjean M. P. Fraser, G. R. Cass, R. Bernd, T. Simonet. 1996. Air quality model evaluation data for organics. 2. C_1C_{14} carbonyls in Los Angeles air. *Environ. Sci. Technol.* 30:2687–2703.

56. Cleveland, W. S., T. E. Graedel, B. Kleiner. 1977. Urban formaldehyde: Observed correlation with source emissions and photochemistry. *Atmos. Environ.* 11:357.

57. Altshuller, A. P. 1993. Production of aldehydes as primary emissions and from secondary atmospheric reactions of alkenes and alkanes during the night and early morning hours. *Atmos. Environ.* 27:21–32.

58. Grosjean, D., R. D. Swanson, C. Ellis. 1983. Carbonyls in Los Angeles air: Contribution of direct emissions and photochemistry. *Sci. Total Environ.* 29:65–85.

59. Dempsey, C. R. 1993. A comparison of organic emissions from hazardous waste incinerators versus the 1990 Toxics Release Inventory air releases. *J. Air Waste Manage. Assoc.* 43:1374–1379.

60. Carey, P. M. 1987. *Air Toxic Emissions from Motor Vehicles*, p. 35. Washington, DC: U.S. Environmental Protection Agency. EPA-AA-TSS-PA-86-5.

61. Kitchens, J. F., R. E. Casner, G. S. Edwards, W. E. Harward, B. J. Macri. 1976. *Investigation of Selected Potential Environmental Contaminants: Formaldehyde*, p. 75. Washington, DC: U.S. Environmental Protection Agency. EPA-560/2-76-009.

62. Sawyer, C., P. McCarty. 1978. *Chemistry for Environmental Engineering*. New York: McGraw-Hill. 532 p.

63. Feinman, S. E. 1988. *Formaldehyde Sensitivity and Toxicity*, p. 18. Boca Raton, FL: CRC Press.

64. Anderson, I., G. R. Lundqvist, L. Molhave. 1975. Indoor air pollution due to chipboard used as a construction material. *Atmos. Environ.* 9:1121–1127.

65. Breysse, P. A. 1977. Formaldehyde in mobile and conventional homes. *Environ. Health Safety News* 26:19.

66. Breysse, P. A. 1978. Formaldehyde exposure following urea-formaldehyde insulation. *Environ. Health Safety News* 26:13.

67. Sundin, B. 1978. Formaldehyde emission from particleboard and other building materials: A study from the Scandinavian countries. *Proceedings of 12th International Washington State University Symposium on Particleboard/Composite Material*, T. Mahoney, ed., pp. 251–273. Pullman, WA.

68. Sardinas, A. V., R. S. Most, M. A. Guiletti, P. Honchar. 1979. Health effects associated with urea-formaldehyde foam insulation in Connecticut. *J. Environ. Health* 41:270–272.

69. Dally, K. A., L. P. Hanrahan, M. A. Woodburg, M. S. Kanarek. 1981. Formaldehyde exposure in nonoccupational environments. *Arch. Environ. Health* 367: 277–284.

70. Hanrahan, L. P., H. A. Anderson, K. A. Dally, A. D. Eckmann, M. S. Kanarek. 1985. Formaldehyde concentrations in Wisconsin mobile homes. *J. Air Pollut. Control Assoc.* 35(11):1164–1167.

71. Godish, T., J. Fell, P. Lincoln. 1984. Formaldehyde levels in New Hampshire urea-formaldehyde foam insulated houses, relationship to outdoor temperature. *J. Air Pollut. Control Assoc.* 34:1051–1052.

72. Ritchie, I. J., R. G. Lehnen. 1985. An analysis of formaldehyde concentrations in mobile and conventional homes. *J. Environ. Health* 47(6):300–305.

73. Norsted, S. W., C. A. Kozinetz, J. F. Annegars. 1985. Formaldehyde complaint investigations in mobile homes by the Texas Department of Health. *Environ. Res.* 37(1):93–100.

74. Syroitynski, S. 1985. Indoor air quality in cold climates: Hazards and abatement measures. *J. Air Pollut. Control Assoc.* 127–136.

75. Sexton, K. K., S. Lin, M. S. Petreas. 1986. Formaldehyde concentrations inside private residences: A mail-out approach to indoor air monitoring. *J. Air Pollut. Control. Assoc.* 36(6):698–704.

76. Godish, T. 1988. Residential formaldehyde contamination: Sources and levels. *Comments Toxicol.* 2(3):115–134.

77. Ulsamer, A. G., K. C. Gupta, M. S. Cohn, P. W. Preuss. 1982. Formaldehyde in indoor air: Toxicity and risk. *Proceedings of the 75th Annual Meeting on Air Pollution Control Association.* New Orleans.

78. Broder, I., P. Corey, S. Mintz, M. L. Pa, J. Nethercott. 1985. Indoor air quality in cold climates: Hazards and abatement measures. *J. Air Pollution Control Assoc.* 155–166.

79. Sterling, T. D., A. Arundel, C. W. Collett, A. J. Nantel. 1986. Dose-response effects of UFFI. *Proceedings of the 79th Annual Meeting on Air Pollution Control Association.* Minneapolis.

80. University of Texas School of Public Health. 1984. Texas indoor air quality study. *Environ. Monitor.* 3:38.

81. Walcott, R. J., C. C. St Pierre, T. W. Ferrel. 1983. *Formaldehyde Exposures in Mobile Homes: Recent Experience in Newly Constructed Homes Using Pararosaniline Analysis.* Southfield, MI: Clayton Environmental Consultants.

82. Hawthorne, A. R., R. B. Gammage, C. S. Dudney, D. R. Womack, S. A. Morriss, R. R. Westley, K. C. Gupta. 1983. Proceedings measurement and monitoring of noncriteria (toxic) contaminants in air. *J. Air Pollut. Control Assoc.* 12:514–526.

83. Stock, T. H., S. R. Mendez. 1985. Survey of typical exposures to formaldehyde in Houston area residences. *Am. Ind. Hyg. Assoc. J.* 46(6):313–317.

84. Pickrell, J. A., B. V. Mokler, L. C. Griffis, C. H. Hobbs, A. Bathija. 1983. Formaldehyde release rate coefficients from selected consumer products. *Environ. Sci. Technol.* 17:753–757.

85. Pickrell, J., L. Griffis, B. Mokler, G. M. Kanapilly, C. H. Hobbs. 1984. Formaldehyde release from selected consumer products: Influence of chamber loading, multiple products, relative humidity, and temperature. *Environ. Sci. Technol.* 18(9):682–686.

86. Reiss, R., P. B. Ryan, S. J. Tippets, P. Koutrakis. 1995. Measurement of organic acids, aldehydes, and ketones in residential environments and their relation to ozone. *J. Air Waste Manage. Assoc.* 45:811822.

87. Hodgson, A. T., J. D. Wooley, J. M. Daisey. 1993. Emissions of volatile organic compounds from new carpet measured in a large scale environmental chamber. *J. Air Waste Manage. Assoc.* 43:316–324.

88. Norback, D., E. Bjornsson, C. Janson, J. Widström, G. Boman. 1995. Asthmatic symptoms and volatile organic compounds, formaldehyde, and carbon dioxide in dwellings. *Occup. Environ. Med.* 52:388–395.

89. Karlberg, A.-T., L. Skare, I. Lindberg, E. Nyhammar. 1998. A method for quantification of formaldehyde in the presence of formaldehyde donors in skin-care products. *Contact Dermatitis.* 38:20–28.

90. Meyer, B., K. Hermanns. 1985. Reducing indoor air formaldehyde concentrations. *J. Air Pollut. Control Assoc.* 35:816–821.

91. Moschandreas, D., S. Relwani, D. Johnson, I. Billick. 1986. Emission rates from unvented gas appliances. *Environ. Int.* 12:247–253.

92. Traynor, G. W., J. R. Girman, M. G. Apte, J. F. Dillworth, P. D. White. 1985. Indoor air pollution due to emissions from unvented gas-fired space heaters. *J. Air Pollut. Control Assoc.* 35:231–237.

93. Woodring, J. L., T. L. Duffy, J. T. Davis, R. R. Bechtold. 1985. Measurement of combustion product emission factors of unvented kerosene heaters. *Am. Ind. Hyg. Assoc. J.* 46:350–356.

94. Triebig, G., M. A. Zober. 1984. Indoor air pollution by smoke constituents—A survey. *Prev. Med.* 13:570–581.

95. NRC. 1986. *National Research Council. Environmental Tobacco Smoke: Measuring Exposures and Assessing Health Effects.* Washington, DC: National Academy Press. 337 p.

96. Sterling, T. D., C. W. Collett, E. M. Sterling. 1987. Environmental tobacco smoke and indoor air quality in modern office work environments. *J. Occup. Med.* 29:57–61.

97. Yasuhara, A., T. Shibamoto. 1995. Quantitative analysis of volatile aldehydes formed from various kinds of fish flesh during heat treatment. *J. Agric. Food Chem.* 43:94–97.

98. Myer, C. B. 1979. *Urea-Formaldehyde Resins*, p. 423. Reading, MA: Addison Wesley.

99. Myers, G. E. 1985. The effects of temperature and humidity on formaldehyde emission from UF-bonded boards: A literature critique. *For. Prod. J.* 35:20–31.

100. Groah, W. J., G. D. Gramp, S. B. Garrison, R. J. Walcott. 1985. Factors that influence formaldehyde air levels in mobile homes. *For. Prod. J.* 35:11–181.

101. Matthews, T. G., A. R. Hawthorne, C. R. Daffron, T. J. Reed, M. D. Corey. 1983. Formaldehyde release from pressed wood products. *Proceedings of the 17th International Washington State University Symposium on Particleboard/Composite Material.* Pullman, WA.

102. Grot, R. A., S. Silberstein, K. Ishigars. 1985. Validity of models for predicting formaldehyde concentrations in residences due to pressed wood products, Phase I NBSIR 85-3255. National Bureau of Standards. 131 p.

103. Godish, T. 1983. Proceedings measurement and monitoring of noncriteria (toxic) contaminants in air. *J. Air Pollut. Control Assoc.* 463–467.

104. Berk, J. V., C. D. Hollowell, J. H. Pepper, R. A. Young. 1980. The Impact of Reduced ventilation on indoor air quality in Residential Buildings. 2013 EEB-Vent-80-5. *LBL-10507.* Berkeley, CA: Lawrence Berkeley Laboratory.

105. Gammage, R. B., B. E. Hingerty, D. R. Womack, R. R. Westley. 1983. Proceedings measurement and monitoring of noncriteria (toxic) contaminants in air. *J. Air Pollut. Control Assoc.* 453–462.

106. Meyers, G. E., J. W. Seymour, T. Khan. 1983. *Formaldehyde Air Contamination in Mobile Homes: Variation with Interior Location and Time of Day.* Madison. WI: Forest Products Laboratory.

107. Meyer, C. B., and K. Hermanns. 1985. Diurnal variations of formaldehyde exposure in mobile homes. *J. Environ. Health* 48:57–61.
108. Godish, T., J. Rouch. 1986. Mitigation of residential formaldehyde contamination by indoor climate control. *Am. Ind. Hyg. Assoc. J.* 47(12):792–797.
109. Godish, T. 1987. Unpublished manuscript.
110. Berge, A., B. Milligaard, P. Hanetho, E. B. Ormstad. 1980. Formaldehyde release from particleboard-evaluation of a mathematical model. *Holz Roh Werkst.* 38: 251–255.
111. Department of Housing and Urban Development. *Federal Register* 486, 37136–37141, 37150–37151, 37168–37169.
112. Godish, T., and J. Rouch. 1985. An assessment of Berge equation applied to formaldehyde measurements under controlled conditions of temperature and humidity in a mobile home. *J. Air Pollut. Control Assoc.* 35(11):1186–1187.
113. Morris, D. L. 1982. Recognition and treatment of formaldehyde sensitivity. *Clin. Ecol.* 1(1):27–30.
114. Matthews, T. G., T. J. Reed, B. R. Tromberg, K. W. Fung, C. V. Thompson, J. O. Simpson, A. R. Hawthorne. 1985. *Modeling and Testing Formaldehyde Emission Characteristics of Pressed Wood Products.* Consumer Product Safety Commission. CPSG-IAG-84-1103.
115. Olsen, J. H., S. P. Jensen, M. Hink, K. Faurbo, O. M. Jensen, N. O. Breum. 1984. Occupational formaldehyde exposure and increased nasal cancer risk in man. *Int. J. Cancer* 34:639.
116. Swenberg, J. A., W. D. Kerns, R. J. Mitchell, E. J. Gralla, K. L. Pavkov. 1980. Induction of squamous cell carcinomas of the rat nasal cavity by inhalation exposure of formaldehyde vapor. *Cancer Res.* 40:3398.
117. Hayes, R. B., J. W. Raatgever, A. de Bruyn, M. Gerin. 1986. Cancer of the nasal cavity and paranasal sinuses and formaldehyde exposure. *Int. J. Cancer* 37:487.
118. Marcus, S. C., S. E. Feinman. 1988. Formaldehyde and cancer epidemiology. In *Formaldehyde Sensitivity and Toxicity*, S. E. Feinman, ed., pp. 187–196. Boca Raton FL: CRC Press.
119. Blair, A., P. A. Stewart, R. N. Hoover, J. F. Fraumeni, J. Walrath Jr., M. O'Berg, W. Gaffery. 1987. Cancers of the nasopharynx and oropharynx and formaldehyde exposure. *J. Natl. Cancer Inst.* 78:191.
120. Sun, M. 1986. Formaldehyde poses little risk, study says. *Science* 231:1365.
121. Feldman, M. Y. 1973. Reaction of nucleic acids and nucleoproteins with formaldehyde. In *Progressive Nucleic Acid Research and Molecular Biology*, J. N. Davidson and W. E. Coihn, eds., p. 4. New York: Academic Press.
122. Casanova-Schmitz, M., T. B. Starr, H. D. Heck. 1984. Differentiation between metabolic incorporation and covalent binding in the labeling of macromolecules in the rat nasal mucosa and bone marrow by inhaled [14C] and [3H] formaldehyde. *Toxicol. Appl. Pharmacol.* 76(1):26–44.
123. Schwenberg, J. A., E. A. Gross, J. Martin, J. A. Popp. 1983. Mechanisms of formaldehyde toxicity. In *Formaldehyde Toxicity*, J. E. Gibson, ed., p. 310. New York: McGraw-Hill.
124. Andersen, I., D. F. Proctor. 1982. The fate and effects of inhaled materials. In *The Nose*, D. F. Proctor and I. Andersen, eds., pp. 423–455. New York: Elsevier.
125. Harris, J. C. 1981. Toxicology of urea-formaldehyde and polyurethane foam insulation. *JAMA* 245:243–246.
126. Wisconsin State Board of Health. 1979. *Wisconsin Epidemiol. Bull.* 1(2).
127. Day, J. H., R. E. J. Lees, R. H. Clark, P. O. Pattee. 1984. Respiratory response to formaldehyde and off-gas of urea formaldehyde foam insulation. *Can. Med. Assoc. J.* 131:1061–1065.
128. National Institute of Occupational Safety and Health. 1976. *Criteria for a Recommended Standard. Occupational Exposure to Formaldehyde (NIOSH) 77-126*, pp. 21–81. Washington, DC: U.S. Department of Health, Education and Welfare.
129. Rogers, S. A. 1987. Diagnosing the tight building syndrome. *Environ. Health Perspect.* 76:195–198.
130. Rea, W. J. 1994. *Chemical Sensitivity, Volume II.* pp. 534–1104. Boca Raton: CRC Press/Lewis Publisher.
131. Reeves, R. A. 1981. *Toxicology: Principles and Practice.* New York: Wiley and Sons. pp. 10–11.
132. Jacoby, W. B. 1980. *Enzymatic Basis of Detoxication*, Vol. 1. New York: Academic Press. p. 289.
133. Billings, R. E., T. R. Tephly. 1979. Studies on methanol toxicity and formate metabolism in isolated hepatocytes. *Biochem. Pharmacol.* 28:2985–2991.
134. Parke, D. V. 1982. Mechanisms of chemical toxicity—A unifying hypothesis. *Regul. Toxicol. Pharmacol.* 2:267–286.
135. Hennies, K., H. P. Neitzke, H. Voigt. 2000. Mobile Telecommunications and Health.
136. Pan, Y. 1987. Formaldehyde sensitivity in China. *Environ. Med.*, 9(1).
137. Mopper, K., W. L. Stahovec. 1986. Sources and sinks of low molecular weight organic carbonyl compounds in seawater. *Mar. Chem.* 19:305–321.

138. EPA. 1995. *Drinking Water Regulations and Health Advisories*. U.S. Environmental Protection Agency, Office of Water.

139. Glaze, W. H., M. Koga, D. Cancilla. 1989. Ozonation by-products. 2. Improvement of an aqueous phase derivatization method for detection of formaldehyde and other carbonyl products formed by the ozonation of drinking water. *Environ. Sci. Technol.* 23:838–847.

140. Howard, P. H. 1989. Formaldehyde. In *Handbook of Environmental Fate and Exposure Data for Organic Chemicals*, P. H. Howard, ed., pp. 342–350. Chelsea, MI: Lewis Publishers.

141. Hatfield, R. 1957. Biological oxidation of some organic compounds. *Ind. Eng. Chem.* 42:192–196.

142. Heukelekian, H., M. C. Rand. 1955. Biochemical oxygen demand of pure organic compounds. *Sewage Ind. Waste.* 27:1040–1053.

143. Verschueren, K. 1983. *Handbook on Environmental Data on Organic Chemicals*, 2nd ed., New York, NY: Van Nostrand Reinhold.

144. Bhattacharya, B. K., G. F. Parkin. 1988. Fate and effects of methylene chloride and formaldehyde in methane fermentation systems. *J. Water Pollut. Fed.* 70:531–536.

145. Gerberich, H. R., A. L. Stautzenberger, W. C. Hopkins. 1980. Formaldehyde. In *Kirk-Othmer Encyclopedia of Chemical Technology*, pp. 231–250. New York, NY: John Wiley and Sons.

146. EPA. 1984. U. S. Environmental Protection Agency, Code of Federal Regulations. 40 CFR 125.

147. Chameides, W. L. 1986. Photochemistry of the atmospheric aqueous phase. In *Chemistry of Multiphase Atmospheric Systems*, W. Jaeschke, ed., pp. 369–413. Berlin: Springer-Verlag.

148. Benner, W. H., M. Bizjak. 1988. Pseudo first-order reaction rate constant for the formation of hydroxymethyl hydroperoxide from formaldehyde and hydrogen peroxide. *Atmos. Environ.* 22: 2603–2605.

149. Bufalini, J. J., H. T. Lancaster, G. R. Namie, B. W. Gay Jr. 1979. Hydrogen peroxide formation from the photooxidation of formaldehyde and its presence in rainwater. *J. Environ. Sci. Health A* 14:135–141.

150. NRC. 1981. Hydrogen peroxide formation from the photooxidation of formaldehyde and its presence in rainwater. *J. Environ. Sci. Health A* 14:135–141.

151. Atkinson, R., C. N. Plum, W. P. L. Carter, A. M. Winer, J. N. Pitts Jr. 1984. Rate constants for the gas-phase reactions of nitrate radicals with a series of organics in air at 298 +/− 1K. *J. Phys. Chem.* 88:1210–1215.

152. Kao, A. S. 1994. Formation and removal reactions of hazardous air pollutants. *J. Air Waste Manage. Assoc.* 44:683–696.

153. Kumar, S. 1986. Reactive scavenging of pollutants by rain: A modeling approach. *Atmos. Environ.* 20:1015–1024.

154. EPA. 1991c. *Locating and Estimating Air Emissions from Sources of Formaldehyde (revised)*. Research Triangle Park, NC: U.S. Environmental Protection Agency. PB91-181842, EPA-450/4-91-012.

155. Hose, J. E., D. V. Lightner. 1980. Absence of formaldehyde residues in Penaeid shrimp exposed to formalin. *Aquaculture* 21:197–201.

156. Sills, J. B., J. L. Allen. 1979. Residues of formaldehyde undetected in fish exposed to formalin. *Prog. Fish Cult.* 41:67–68.

157. Casanova M., H. D. Heck, J. I. Everitt J. I. et al. 1988. Formaldehyde concentrations in the blood of rhesus monkeys after inhalation exposure. *Food Chem Toxicol.* 26:715–716.

158. Woodruff, T. J., D. A. Axelrad, J. Caldwell, J. Cogliano. 1998. Public health implications of 1990 air toxics concentrations across the United States. *Environ. Health Perspect.* 106:245–251.

159. Spicer, C. W., B. E. Buxton, M. W. Holdren, D. L. Smith, T. J. Kelly, S. W. Rust, A. D. Pate, G. M. Sverdrup, J. C. Chuang. 1996. Variability of hazardous air pollutants in an urban area. *Atmos. Environ.* 30:3443–3456.

160. Seiber, J. N. 1996. Toxic air contaminants in urban atmospheres: Experience in California. *Atmos. Environ.* 30:751–756.

161. EPA. 1987d. Assessment of Health Risks to Garment Workers and Certain Home Residents from Exposure to Formaldehyde. U.S. Environmental Protection Agency, Office of Pesticides and Toxic Substances.

162. Gammage, R. B., A. R. Hawthorne. 1985. Current status of measurement techniques and concentrations of formaldehyde in residences. In *Indoor Air and Human Health*, V. A. Jacobs, ed., pp. 117–130. New York, NY: Lewis Publishers, Inc.

163. Hawthorne, A. R., R. B. Gammage, C. S. Dudney. 1986. An indoor air quality study of 40 east Tennessee homes. *Environ. Int.* 12:221–239.

164. Stock, T. H. 1987. Formaldehyde concentrations inside conventional housing. *J. Air Pollut. Control Assoc.* 37:913–918.

165. EPA. 1996. Sources and factors affecting indoor emission from engineered wood products Summary and evaluation of current literature. U.S. Environmental Protection Agency. National Research Risk Management Research Laboratory, Office of Research and Development. PB96-183876, EPA-600/R-96-067.

166. Zinn, T. W., D. Cline, W. F. Lehmann. 1990. Long-term study of formaldehyde emission decay 545 from particleboard. *Forest prod. J.* 40:15–18.

167. Sexton, K., M. X. Petreas, K. S. Liu. 1989. Formaldehyde exposures inside mobile homes. *Environ. Sci. Technol.* 23:985–988.

168. Konopinski, V. J. 1983. Formaldehyde in office and commercial environments. *Am. Ind. Hyg. Assoc. J.* 44:205–208.

169. Shah, J., H. B. Singh. 1988. Distribution of volatile organic chemicals in outdoor and indoor air. *Environ. Sci. Technol.* 22:1381–1388.

170. Krzyzanowski, M., J. J. Quackenboss, M. D. Lebowitz. 1990. Chronic respiratory effects of indoor formaldehyde exposure. *Environ. Res.* 52:117–125.

171. Lamb, B., H. Westberg, P. Bryant, J. Dean, S. Mullins. 1985. Air infiltration rates in pre- and post-weatherized houses. *J. Air Pollut. Control Assoc.* 35:541–551.

172. Lawryk, N. J., P. J. Lioy, C. P. Weisel. 1995. Exposure to volatile organic compounds in the passenger compartment of automobiles during periods of normal and malfunctioning operation. *J. Expo. Anal. Environ. Epidemiol.* 5:511–531.

173. Lawryk, N. J., C. P. Weisel. 1996. Concentrations of volatile organic compounds in the passenger compartments of automobiles. *Environ. Sci. Technol.* 30:810–816.

174. Fleisher, J. M. 1987. Medical students' exposure to formaldehyde in gross anatomy laboratories. *NY State J. Med.* 87:385–388.

175. Holness, D. L., J. R. Nethercott. 1989. Health status of funeral service workers exposed to formaldehyde. *Arch. Environ. Health* 44:222–228.

176. Korky, J. K., S. R. Schwarz, B. K. Lustigman. 1987. Formaldehyde concentrations in biology department teaching facilities. *Bull. Environ. Contam. Toxicol.* 18:907–910.

177. Perkins, J. L., J. D. Kimbrough. 1985. Formaldehyde exposure in a gross anatomy laboratory. *J. Occup. Med.* 27:813–815.

178. Skisak, C. M. 1983. Formaldehyde vapor exposures in anatomy laboratories. *Am. Ind. Hyg. Assoc. J.* 44:948–950.

179. Kiefer, M., C. E. Moss. 1997. Laser generated air contaminants released during laser cutting of fabrics and polymers. *J. Laser Appl.* 9:7–13.

180. Milton, D. K., M. D. Walters, K. Hammond, J. S. Evans. 1996. Worker exposure to endotoxin, phenolic compounds, and formaldehyde in a fiberglass insulation manufacturing plant. *Am. Ind. Hyg. Assoc. J.* 57:889–896.

181. Leovic, K. W., L. S. Sheldon, D. A. Whitaker, R. G. Hetes, J. A. Calcagni, J. N. Baskir. 1996. Measurement of indoor air emissions from dry-process photocopy machines. *J. Air Waste Manage. Assoc.* 46:821–829.

182. OSHA. 1996. Occupational Exposure to Formaldehyde. OSHA fact sheet no. 92-27. U.S. Department of Labor, Occupational Safety and Health Administration.

183. Luker, M. A., R. W. Van Houten. 1990. Control of formaldehyde in a garment sewing plant. *Am. Ind. Hyg. Assoc. J.* 51:541–544.

184. Malaka, T., A. M. Kodama. 1990. Respiratory health of plywood workers occupationally exposed to formaldehyde. *Arch. Environ. Health* 45:288–294.

185. Stumpf, J. M., K. D. Blehm, R. M. Buchan, B. J. Gunter. 1986. Characterization of particleboard aerosol—Size distribution and formaldehyde content. *Am. Ind. Hyg. Assoc. J.* 47:725–730.

186. Stern, F. B., J. J. Beaumont, W. E. Halperin, L. I. Murthy, B. W. Hills, J. M. Fajen. 1987. Mortality of chrome leather tannery workers and chemical exposures in tanneries. *Scand. J. Work Environ. Health* 13(S1):108–117.

187. Jankovic, J., W. Jones, J. Burkhart, G. Noonan. 1991. Environmental study of firefighters. *Ann. Occup. Hyg.* 35:581–602.

188. Wantke, F., C. M. Demmer, P. Tappler, M. Götz, R. Jarisch. 1996. Exposure to gaseous formaldehyde induces IgE-mediated sensitization to formaldehyde in school-children. *Clin. Exp. Allergy* 26:276–280.

189. IARC. 1982. IARC monographs on the evaluation of carcinogenic risk of chemicals to humans. In *Some Industrial Chemicals and Dyestuffs*, Vol. 29. Lyon, France: World Health Organization.

190. Lofroth, G., R. M. Burton, L. Forehand, S. K. Hammond, R. L. Seila, R. B. Zweidinger, J. Lewtas. 1989. Characterization of environmental tobacco smoke. *Environ. Sci. Technol.* 23:610–614.

191. Lyman, W. J. 1982. Adsorption coefficient for soils and sediments. In *Handbook of Chemical Property Estimation Methods: Environmental Behavior of Organic Compounds*, W. J. Lyman, W. F. Reehl, D. H. Rosenblatt, eds., pp. 4–1 to 4–33. New York: McGraw-Hill Book Company.

192. Swann, R. L., D. A. Laskowski, P. J. McCall, K. Vander Kuy, H. J. Dishburger. 1983. A rapid method for the estimation of the environmental parameters octanol/water partition coefficient, soil sorption constant, water to air ratio, and water solubility. *Residue Rev.* 85:17–28.

193. HSDB. 1999. *Hazardous Substance Data Bank*. National Library of Medicine, National Toxicology Information Program, Bethesda, MD. March 3, 1999.

194. Radford, T., D. E. Dalsis. 1982. Analysis of formaldehyde in shrimp by high pressure-liquid chromatography. *J. Agric. Food Chem.* 30:600–602.

195. Weber, A., C. Jermini, E. Grandjean. 1976. Irritating effects on man of air pollution due to cigarette smoke. *Am. J. Public Health* 66: 672–676.

196. World Health Organization Report 78. 1983. WHO: p. 24.

197. National Center for Toxicology Research. 1984. Report on the consensus workshop on formaldehyde. *EHS Environ. Health Perspec.* 58:323–381.

198. Pan, Y. et al. 1989. Formaldehyde sensitivity. *Clin. Ecol.* 6(3):79–84.

7 Pesticides and Chronic Diseases

INTRODUCTION

Pesticides and herbicides are considered as one of the main factors involved in environmental contamination of today's world and are one of the prime generators of chemical sensitivity and chronic degenerative disease. These chemicals are on purpose designed to be toxic to pest and vectors of diseases; unfortunately, they also incidentally harm humans. These compounds are among more than 1000 active ingredients that are marketed as insecticide, herbicide, and fungicide. Nevertheless, formulation of new and potent pesticides is increasingly on the order of researchers and manufacturers because of pest resistance, hygienic controls, and major human need for more food as the world population grows. Contact with pesticides can result in acute and chronic harming of human life and can disturb the function of different organs in the body, including immune, reproductive, nervous, endocrine, renal, cardiovascular, dermal, and respiratory systems. In this regard, there is mounting evidence on the link of pesticide's exposure with the incidence of human chronic diseases, including cancer, Parkinson, Alzheimer, multiple sclerosis, diabetes, aging, cardiovascular, chemical sensitivity, and chronic kidney disease.[1–4] These findings are why we strongly advocate organic agriculture and other less toxic living.

This first section deals with the acute and chronic effects of pesticides and then classification-specific effects are presented.

EVIDENCES FOR THE LINK BETWEEN PESTICIDE EXPOSURE AND INCIDENCE OF CHRONIC DISEASES

Chronic diseases are characterized by their generally slow progression and long-term duration, which are considered as the leading cause of morbidity and mortality in the world, representing over 60% of all deaths and a large portion of chronic illness. According to the WHO report, 36 million people died from chronic disease in 2008, of which 9 million were under 60, and 90% of these premature deaths occurred in low- and middle-income countries. Chemical sensitivity is one of the leading problems triggered by pesticides and is a growing entity often signaling the onset of chronic degenerative disease. Pesticide overload involves the hypersensitivity response to toxics as well as chronic poisoning either of which can eventually develop chronic disease. Neglect in treatment leads to a downhill course in degenerative disease until death. This may take months to many years to occur and is often causes misery in its process,[5] resulting in long-term gradual disability, including weakness, fatigue, loss of vigor, and brain function, especially short- and long-term memory loss.

CHEMICAL SENSITIVITY

Hypersensitive response to chemicals and particularly pesticides were originally described by Randolph[6] and Dickey[7] some 50 plus years ago. They developed the first less polluted environmental units that were pesticide free and particulate reduced in hospitals.[8] Abou-Donia[9] describes the problem and relation history of organophosphates (OPs) and chemical sensitivity. We and other members of the American Academy of Environmental Medicine have treated at least 10,000 patients who developed chemical sensitivity after pesticide exposure and several with chronic degenerative diseases.

Recent data have shown that pesticide exposure can damage the cell membrane, allowing Na^+ and Ca^{2+} to enter the cell. When Ca^{2+} is combined with protein kinase A and C and when this complex is phosphorylated, hypersensitivity is increased 1000 times,[10] accounting for chemical sensitivity. Thus, membrane damage not only occurs in the olfactory nerves and its brain end organs but also can damage gastrointestinal (GI) mucosa, respiratory system, the cardiovascular system, the endocrine system, the musculoskeletal system, and the genitourinary system.

Second, the ability to handle molds, food, mycotoxins, volatile organic chemicals and particulates, bacteria, viruses, parasites, etc. is damaged and these elements can not only propagate the chemical sensitivity but also develop into chronic degenerative disease.

Certainly, there can be pesticide damage to the mitochondria, clinically causing weakness and fatigue. These are the main sources of ATP and reactive oxygen species (ROS) in the cell and have important roles in Ca^{2+} metabolism and homeostasis, synthesis of steroid hormones and heme, metabolic cell signaling, and apoptosis. The mitochondria are part of innate immunity, making O_2 increase to 30 torr outside the cell from 0.2 in the cell in the mitochondria matrix. It activates proteins that shield the cell membrane from further attacks. NAPH oxidase activates protein to shield the free radicals triggered by pollutants, especially pesticides, but also accompany oils, solvents, additives, etc.

Oxidative stress increase, which results in side the mitochondria, can be a big problem as is the decrease in the antioxidant capacity. This abnormality is seen clinically in the chemically sensitive patient. This is why there is such a need for intravenous and oral nutritional supplementation in the chemically sensitive.

Pesticides can damage the cell membrane with Ca^{2+} entering and then damaging the endoplasmic reticulum in the cell where the Ca^{2+} is stored. Ca^{2+} combines with protein kinase A and C. The protein kinase activates phosphorylation cascades, giving an increased expression of genes which act as molecular chaperones to establish ER folding which promotes ER degradation of unfolded proteins which when folded properly can adapt to the changing environment. Failure of adaptation gives ER stress that gives ER possession which yields expression of genes and thus gives downward progression to cell death (apoptosis).

Protein degradation, ubiquitin, and degradation: Cells degrade and misfold or are damaged where their normal expression is essential for maintaining and regulation of the cell. The two main cellular mechanisms for protein degradation are the ubiquitin proteasome system (UPS) by proteases and the lysosomal degradation pathway by autophagia. In this way, chemical sensitivity may occur and be propagated.

Organochlorines, organophosphates, carbamate, pyrethrins, pyrethroid, and many other pesticides, herbicides (atrazine, glyphosate), and fungicides can trigger and propagate chemical sensitivity and or chronic degenerative disease.

The disruptions of the immune and enzyme detoxification systems are the connector on how the body handles pesticides. The immune system will be discussed first as the pesticides enter the body. However, they should and will be classified.

CLASSIFICATION OF SPECIFIC PESTICIDES

Insecticides are generally classified into several categories. Organochlorines include such products as lindane, chlordane, dieldrin, aldrin, hexachlorobenzene (HCB), heptachlor, heptachlor epoxide, endrin, endosulfan, dichlorodiphenyltrichloroethane (DDT), dichlorodiphenyldichloroethylene (DDE), benzene hexachloride (BHC), and others. OPs include parathion, malathion, diazinon, and many others.[11–13] Carbamates are similar to OPs in that they interfere with cholinesterase, and they include aldicarb, carbofuran, and carbaryl. Other classes are pyrethrums, pyrethroids, pyrethrins and their chemical relatives, which include permethrin, allethrin, fenothrin, and others. Arsenicals, which include cacodylic acid, monosodium methyl arsonate, methane arsenic acid, and many others, constitute another distinct group of pesticides. Further, pesticide families include pentachlorophenol (PCP), nitrophenolic herbicides, chlorophenoxy compounds, paraquat, diquat, thiocarbamates and dithiocarbamates, and others. There are approximately 100 pesticides; each general category of some common pesticides is discussed separately. The majority have been found to trigger chemical sensitivity or propagate it.

ORGANOCHLORINES

Organochlorine insecticides (Figure 7.1) are a group of chlorinated benzenes that tend to persist in nature due to their stability. Some common commercial pesticide products (listed approximately in order of decreasing toxicity) are endrin (highly toxic), aldrin, toxaphene, BHC, DDE, heptachlor, heptachlor epoxide, chlordane, *trans*-nonachlor, kepone, terpene polychlorinates, dicofol, chloro-benzilate, mirex, HCB, methoxychlor, and ethylan. All are insecticides or ascaricides, except HCB, which is a fungicide. Many are absorbed from the gut and across the skin, but they can also be inhaled.[14]

Chlorinated hydrocarbon pesticides are initially stimulants to the nervous system (NS), unlike the solvents and fumigants, which are depressants. When these chlorinated hydrocarbon pesticides are present in the body for a long period of time, however, depressant effects may occur. Regardless of whether or not they act to stimulate or depress bodily functions, these pesticides cause the NS, as well as the immune and nonimmune detoxification systems, to malfunction. Often, they are still present in the chemically sensitive for years after the exposure.

The toxic action of these pesticides is to interfere with axonal transmission of nerve impulses, thus disrupting the proper activation of NS function, particularly in the central nervous system (CNS).[15] The sensitivity pathway appears to involve both the CNS and autonomic nervous systems. There are indications that some DDT and DDE, for example, serve to change the electrophysiology and alter enzymatic properties of nerve cell membranes. Chlorinated pesticides also induce mixed-function oxidases and protein and lipid synthesis, with changes in hepatic enzymes. They are cleared from the body by oxidative dehalogenation as well as peptide, glucuronic, and sulfur conjugation. Frequently, these systems become overloaded, resulting in chemical sensitivity. The degree of toxicity and sensitivity appears to be a function of the extent of chlorination on the molecule. However, other factors enter into their adverse effects. Toxicity clearly varies with different formulas. Some organochlorines can damage the liver and kidneys, and can also be hemotoxic agents. Many have now been designated as mutagens and carcinogens.[16] Photolysis can produce compounds of greater toxicity than the original pesticides as can exposure to nonionizing radiation (Smith, C. W. 1989, personal communication). Chemical breakdown in the body can produce more toxic intermediates, such as the case of chlordane breaking down to heptachlor epoxide. Organochlorine pesticides can have a severe impact on immune and nonimmune systems (Chemicaly Sensitivity, Vol. I).

DDT (Chlorophenothane)

DDT (Figure 7.2) is found in imported meats, fruits, and vegetables, in old homes and businesses, in old orchards and farmlands in the United States, and as "inert ingredients" in other U.S. products.

Often, some chemically sensitive patients live or work in buildings that were built or in use after World War II. We see these patients still have the breakdown product of DDT, DDE in their blood contributing to their chemical sensitivity.

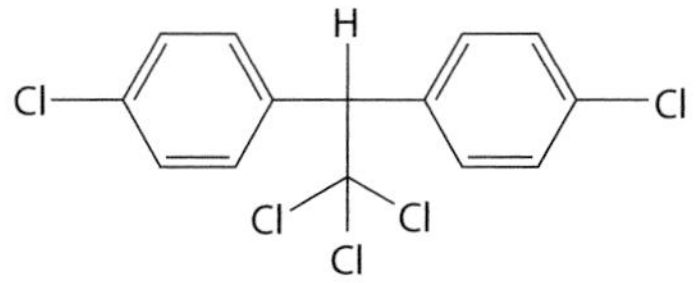

FIGURE 7.1 Organochlorines.

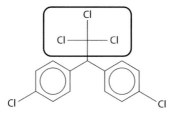

FIGURE 7.2   DDT (Chlorophenothane).

DDT and the other chlorinated hydrocarbons are stored in all tissues, but are particularly attracted to lipid-rich tissues such as the brain, liver, and all cell membranes, and can be deposited and sequestered there for extremely long periods of time.

While highest concentrations will be in the adipose tissues, substantial concentrations have been found in the blood and heart. As a general rule, ratios for DDT between blood and other organs have been worked out. Where there is 1 ppb DDT in the blood, there will be 5–10 ppb in the brain, 47 ppb in the liver, and 100 ppb in fat cells (Laseter, J. L. 1985, personal communication).

It should be remembered that every cell membrane in the body, including mitochondrial and rough and smooth endoplasmic reticulum, has a lipid component and, therefore, may be a target for organochlorine pesticides. However, as exposure and intake are reduced, the stored toxins will also reduce, although this reduction may take months to years in the chemically sensitive.

Pesticides may be ingested with food and water, inhaled through the air, or absorbed through the skin. The route of intake varies to some extent with the pesticide. For example, DDT is poorly absorbed through the skin, while some other organics are more readily absorbed transdermally.

Chlorinated hydrocarbons such as DDT are detoxified via activity of the hepatic microsomal hydroxylative enzymes.[17] Even though methylation is a conjugation pathway for toxic chemicals, it has been observed that methionine supplementation causes greater retention of DDT.[18] The reason for this effect is unclear, since supplementation of nutrient fuels for toxic chemical removal usually has a positive effect. B_3 in adequate quantities is needed for optimum chance of removal. DDT affects vitamin A utilization, while supplements of vitamin A diminish symptoms.[19] DDT affects $NADH_2$–NAD systems.[20] Ascorbic acid deficiency enhances pollutant effects of DDT, lindane, and other hydrocarbons.[21] The inadequate consumption of zinc enhances DDT toxicity.[22]

Immune dysfunction, including basophil degranulation, has been ascribed to DDT. Anaphylaxis is prevented with excessive exposure to DDT, but other effects are so severe that this phenomenon must be discounted. Organochlorine pesticides are readily and accurately measured in the blood in the ppb range by Laseter's method.[23]

To a slight extent, DDT is converted to much less toxic DDE by dehydrochlorination. DDE does not undergo further biotransformation. Instead, it is stored for an indefinite period of time in adipose tissue. Some opinion has held that most of the p-p'-DDE present in humans is preformed dietary from DDE, rather than endogenously produced from DDT breakdown. However, no really sound evidence exists to support this view. Having used chemically less contaminated DDT-free foods at the Environmental Health Center (EHC)-Dallas, we have come to believe that DDE is a breakdown product of DDT, since we frequently see DDE in the blood without the presence of DDT. We only see DDT when a patient has experienced an acute exposure.

The major detoxification pathway of DDT is via dechlorination to dichlorodiphenyl acetic acid (DDD), a water-soluble and a rapidly excreted detoxification product. We still see a lot of DDE residue in many chemically sensitive patients examined at the EHC-Dallas.

The following is a series of case studies showing one area in Oklahoma by one surgeon, showing the devastating effects of chlorinated pesticides on the local population which persists in the farming area of the United States.

The Oklahoma economy is based primarily on the oil and agriculture industries. Shortly after World War II, aerial crop-dusting using chlorinated pesticides was pioneered in Grady County. Today, the majority of acreage in the county is still devoted to agriculture and aerial crop-dusting continues.

Crowly noted a high incidence of cancer in the local population.[24] Although neither the state of Oklahoma nor Grady County maintained a tumor registry, the citizens in the area felt that they had a cancer problem in their community. Crowly's study was undertaken over a 1-year period to determine if chlorinated pesticides were playing a role in the development of head and neck cancer in the area.[24]

Even though the group is small and the two controls have toxics in them, it is clear that this group of people are prone to cancer due to long-term and rather massive exposure to toxic pesticides. The use of such large amount of pesticides is such a small area of the state is clearly in excess and no wonder that head and neck cancer rates and the rates of other cancers are so high.

Materials and Methods

Over a 12-month period from March 1997 to March 1998, Crowly diagnosed five patients with malignant tumors in the head and neck. All patients were female and had no history of alcohol consumption. Four of the five patients had no history of tobacco use. The fifth patient quit smoking 20 years prior to the diagnosis but had a 20-pack history of smoking previously. Three of the five had a positive family history for cancer.

Chlorinated pesticide levels in each patient's body were analyzed from adipose tissue. Sampling was formed at the time of diagnosis or immediately following completion of therapy. Using sterile technique, a left lower quandrant of abdominal incision 5 cm in length was made following injection of local anesthesia. A segment of adipose tissue measuring approximately $4 \times 3 \times 2$ cm was resected and the wound was closed in two layers. The adipose tissue was placed in an amber bottle supplied by the toxicology laboratory, refrigerated, and then sent by overnight courier to Accu-Chem Laboratories in Richardson, Texas. Accu-Chem Laboratories was a CLIA, Cap, and Medicare certified full-service toxicology lab. A panel of 21 chlorinated pesticides (Table 7.1) was analyzed for each specimen of adipose tissue. The method of analysis was high-resolution gas chromatography/ electron capture detector. In addition to the cancer patients, two normal controls (37-year-old white male, 40-year-old white female) with no past history of cancer, asthma, rhinitis, hypertension, vascular disease, or autoimmune disease were tested for pesticide residues. Both controls live in Grady County and both had a family history of cancer. Their levels are shown in Tables 7.2 and 7.3, with the averages shown in Table 7.4.

TABLE 7.1

Chlorinated Pesticides

Hexachlorobenzene	*Trans*-nonachlor
Endrin	Endosulfan II
α-Benzene hexachloride	Endosulfan sulfate
β-Benzene hexachloride	Aldrin
γ-Benzene hexachloride	Dieldrin
δ-Benzene hexachloride	DDE
Heptachlor	DDD
Heptachlor epoxide	DDT
α-Chlordane	Methoxychlor
γ-Chlordane	Mirex
Oxychlordane	

TABLE 7.2
Case 1—Chlorinated Pesticides—Type of Specimen: Tissue

Compound	Blood	Tissue Results ng/g (ppb)
HCB		33.1
Endrin		<10.0
α-BHC	<10.0	
β-BHC		<10.0
γ-BHC	<10.0	
δ-BHC		<10.0
Heptachlor	<10.0	
Heptachlor epoxide		32.2
α-Chlordane	<10.0	
γ-Chlordane	<10.0	
Oxychlordane		80.8
Trans-nonachlor		>100 (117)
Endosulfan II		<10.0
Endosulfan sulfate		<10.0
Aldrin		<10.0
Dieldrin		24.3
DDE		>100 (1296)
DDD		<10.0
DDT		37.0
Mehoxychlor		<10.0
Mirex	<10.0	

Source: John Laseter (PhD), Accu-Chem Labs.
Results: Parts per billion of the analyzed compound—seven pesticides positive.
Important: Although these compounds are detected in the general population, they are foreign and serve no recognized beneficial function to the human body. In certain medical or legal instances, serial testing may be advisable.

Case 1: A 51-year-old white female with no significant past medical history and no history of alcohol or tobacco use noted a mass in the right side of the neck 6 months prior to evaluation. Two days prior to consultation, she noted an abnormality in the right tonsillar region. She had no family history of cancer. Physical examination revealed a 3.5 cm mass involving all the right tonsillar fossa and pillars and abutting the uvula. A 3 × 2 cm right level II neck mass was palpated. Biopsy of the tonsil revealed a poorly differentiated invasive squamous cell carcinoma. This was staged T2N1MO.

TABLE 7.3
Case 2—Chlorinated Pesticides—Type of Specimen: Tissue Biopsy

Compound	Blood	Tissue Results ng/g (ppb)
HCB		29.6
Heptachlor epoxide		19.4
Oxychlordane		41.6
Trans-nonachlor		53.1
DDE		>100 (939)
DDT		15.5

TABLE 7.4

Case 3—Blood Chlorinated Pesticides: Adipose Tissue Biopsy

Compound		Results ng/g (ppb)
Heptachlor epoxide	41.4	
Trans-nonachlor	81.8	
DDE		>100 (540.2)
DDD		
DDT		20.9
Mirex	49.6	

Adipose tissue was obtained from the abdomen. Residues detected in the sample included HCB, heptachlor epoxide, oxychlordane, *trans*-nonachlor, dieldrin, DDE, and DDT.

Case 2: Six different chlorinated pesticides were studied. A 64-year-old white female with a past medical history of hypertension and no history of tobacco or alcohol use, noted a rash in the right preauricular skin 4 months prior to evaluation. Two months prior to evaluation, she felt a slight loss of hearing in the right ear. Family history was positive for cancer; the patient has a daughter who developed breast cancer at age 25 after a life-threatening episode of acute pesticide poisoning following a crop-dusting misadventure. Physical examination revealed an erythematous skin lesion 2 cm anterior and inferior to the right tragus extending circumferentially 2 cm below the lobule and into the postauricular crease. There was right facial and external auditory canal edema. A right 1 cm level IV neck mass was palpable. Biopsy of the skin revealed a moderate to poorly differentiated metastatic adenocarcinoma involving the reticular dermis. Extensive evaluation failed to reveal a primary source for the tumor. This was staged TXN2M1. Adipose tissue was obtained from the abdomen. Residues detected in the sample included HCB, heptachlor epoxide, oxychlordane, *trans*-nonachlor, DDE, and DDT.

Case 3: Five different pesticides were found in a 70-year-old white female with no significant past medical history and no history of alcohol or tobacco use noted a rapid growth of a left parotid mass without pain or facial paralysis 2 months prior to evaluation. Family history was positive for cancer. Physical examination revealed a left parotid mass measuring 3 cm, which was rubbery and nontender. Full facial function was present and no neck nodes were palable. A left lateral parotidectomy with facial nerve dissection was performed. Pathology consultation on the parotid specimen was obtained from Dr. John Batsakis of M.D. Anderson Cancer Hospital. Final consultation revealed a carcinosarcoma of the parotid gland with osteosarcoma as the sarcomatous element and squamous carcinoma as the carcinoma element. This was staged T20M0. Adipose tissue was obtained from the abdomen following completion of radiation therapy. Residues detected in the specimen included heptachlor epoxide, *trans*-nonachlor, DDE, DDT, and mirex.

Case 4: Five different chlorinated pesticides in a 77-year-old white female were seen in consultation for a 1–2 month history of a sore throat and globus symptoms (Table 7.5). She had been treated for a right breast carcinoma 3.5 years prior to evaluation and a left axillary malignant lymphoma 4.5 years prior to evaluation. Past medical history was also positive for CHF and osteoporosis. She had no history of alcohol or tobacco use. Family history was positive for cancer. She remembered being exposed to pesticides when she treated her house for termites in the past. Physical examination revealed a 2–3 cm smooth mass in the right tonsillar region with a negative neck evaluation. Biopsy of the tonsillar mass revealed a diffuse, lymphocytic, intermediate-grade malignant lymphoma consistent with a Mantle cell lymphoma. She was a stage II following complete evaluation. Adipose

TABLE 7.5
Case 4—Blood Chlorinated Pesticides: Adipose Tissue Biopsy

Compound		Results ng/g (ppb)
HCB		>100 (207)
Heptachlor epoxide	68.2	
Trans-nonachlor		>100 (173)
DDE		>100 (1530)
Mirex	90.8	

tissue was obtained from the abdomen. Residues detected in the sample included hexachloroben-zene, heptachlor epoxide, *trans*-nonachlor, DDE, and mirex.

Case 5: Extremely high DDE; a 70-year-old white female presented with a 4-month history of right aural pressure, autophony, and hearing loss with intermittent epistaxis (Table 7.6). She had no sig-nificant past medical history and had never used alcohol. She had been a 20-pack-year history of smoking but quit smoking 20 years prior to evaluation. Physical examination revealed a right serous otitis media. An ulcerated mass was seen in the nasopharynx occupying their posterior wall extend-ing onto the roof and laterally into the Eustachian tube orifice. The neck revealed no masses. Biopsy revealed a poorly differentiated squamous cell carcinoma. CT scanning revealed an erosion of the skull base, so the lesion was staged T4NOMO. Adipose tissue was obtained from the abdomen. Residues detected in the specimen included *trans*-nonachlor and DDE. Chlorinated hydrocarbon

TABLE 7.6
Case 5—Blood Chlorinated Pesticides: Adipose Tissue Biopsy

Compound	Results ng/g (ppb)
HCB	
Endrin	
α-BHC	
β-BHC	
γ-BHC	
Heptachlor	
Heptachlor epoxide	
α-Chlordane	
γ-Chlordane	
Oxychlordane	
Trans-nonachlor	
Endosulfan I	
Endosulfan II	
Endosulfan sulfate	
Aldrin	
Dieldrin	
DDE	>100 (2816)
DDD	
DDT	
Endrin aldehyde	
Methoxychlor	
Mirex	

pesticides are used worldwide for agriculture purposes, with the DDT family being the best known of a large number of related compounds. Their primary toxic effects are on nervous tissues and muscle membranes. These compounds affect the CNS, causing headaches, vertigo, anorexia, nausea, vomiting, sleep disturbances, irritability, thirst, dermatographia, paresthesias, myoclonus, seizures, and involuntary movements. Other toxic effects from human and animal studies include changes in CNS biogenic amine levels, induction of mixed function oxidase activity in the liver, and changes in enzymes associated with gluconeogenesis.[24] These compounds are lipophilic and have an affinity for adipose tissue and other lipid rich tissue. Humans are exposed through ingestion of contaminated food and water, inhalation of dust and vapors, and cutaneous absorption from direct skin contact. A number of factors have been known to influence metabolism and storage of these compounds, including vitamin levels, drug use, multiple pesticide interactions, and other hydrocarbon exposure.

Chlorinated pesticides are lipophilic compounds with body sequestration sites high in lipid content. Adipose tissue has the highest concentration of chlorinated pesticides, followed by liver, white matter, gray matter, and then blood. For every 1 ppb of DDE in the blood, there are 306 ppb in fat, 27 ppb in liver, 3.9 ppb in white matter, and 2.6 ppb in gray matter[24] of the NS.

In evaluating the data from this cohort of patients, the small sample size precludes drawing any valid statistical conclusions. However, the data are disturbing. In all five cancer patients, levels of HCB, heptachlor epoxide, oxychlordane, *trans*-nonachlor, dieldrin, DDE, DDT, and mirex in various combinations, and values were clearly elevated above the control values for at least one pesticide. In addition, only heptachlor epoxide, oxychlordane, *trans*-nonachlor, and DDE were present in the controls and in our opinion should not be. The presence of DDT in three cancer patients is particularly disturbing since DDT has been banned in the United States since 1973. The presence of DDT is usually only seen following an acute exposure. The source of this contamination could come from contaminated produce from countries still using DDT. But since there was such heavy use in this country, there may have been enough residual in the soil to cause the presence in these humans. It is theoretically possible for the normal xenobiotic detoxification mechanisms in the body to be overloaded, thus causing the compound to persist with any metabolism to partially dechlorinated derivatives.

The source of these pesticides could not be directly traced. Two of the five patients had known exposures, but they were ignorant to the types of pesticides used. The remaining three patients had no idea of where the compounds could have originated. The local environment in Grady County is contaminated with pesticides due to their widespread use in the agricultural industry. Therefore, the exact date and time of exposure could not be traced. Ingestion of contaminated produce has been mentioned previously as a source, but inhalation of dust and vapors as well as dermal absorption must be considered. It has been hypothesized that skin absorption is the primary site for systemic absorption for most chlorinated pesticides, exclusive of HCB, DDT, and mirex. Variables involved in dermal absorption of pesticides include increased temperature and hydration, skin injury, and location of the skin contamination. With the high heat and humidity in Oklahoma coupled with sun injury, small amounts of pesticide getting onto the skin could be readily absorbed. Physical and chemical properties (pH, lipophilicity, solubility, etc.) as well as the vehicles and accelerants present in the mixture play a role as well. Finally, individual variability (age, sex, ratio of body fat, nutritional status, previous exposure, and type and amount of skin exposure) can affect absorption.

Four of the five patients were over age 60 and all were female. Females have a higher ratio of body fat than males and when living in a highly contaminated environment, such as Grady County, these female patients could sequester a higher concentration of chlorinated pesticides in their bodies. Finally, genetic variables involving the metabolism and detoxification of xenobiotics in the body need to be considered in light of the fact that three of the five patients had a positive family history of cancer and the fact that all the cancer patients' pesticide levels were higher than the control patients who lived in the same environment.

The findings from this study elicit more questions than answers. Other than the source of contamination, the metabolism and excretion differences for chlorinated pesticides between the cancer patients and the controls could not be explained. Of course, if the controls were followed long enough due to their excess body burden they may develop cancer or some other degenerative disease. Differences between these rates could be related to the development of cancer. It is also unknown what level of which pesticide or combinations of pesticides can induce tumors in humans. The presence of other environmentally acquired carcinogens such as herbicides, polychlorinated biphenyls (PCBs), toxic volatile organic hydrocarbons, and OP pesticides were not evaluated in this study; any contributory role they may have been playing is unknown. Finally, the exact mechanism of tumor induction from chlorinated pesticides is unknown as well as how it can induce a variety of malignancies in a variety of locations. Since the concentrates are so high in this country many individuals developed cancer in other organs.

As a footnote, other patients not included in this study had other malignancies resulting in lymphoma of the groin, sarcoma of the back, breast carcinoma, and testicular seminoma were also noted to have elevated levels of chlorinated pesticides above the control values (Table 7.7).

Organochlorine pesticides have been generally phased out in the United States. However, due to their long half-life, they may still be around. For example, DDT has a half-life of over 50 years. We still find it as its breakdown products such as DDE still in the patient's blood. Of course, this substance and others will be part of the total body pollutant load and can contribute to the patients' illness.

Some of the exposures from around the world and the abnormal findings are shown in Table 7.8.

The CHAMACOS report on infants at age 6, 12, and 24 months[27] found significant reductions in the Bayley MDI at ages 12 and 24 months with increasing prenatal DDT exposure ($p < .01$). An important clinical point is that despite high DDT exposure levels in the cohort, breastfeeding was positively associated with Bayley developmental scores.

Two studies report on a cohort of 244 children with normal pregnancies and deliveries in Mexico. The study was conducted in an area with no known occupational exposure to DDT, but it was a malaria-prone area where DDT had been used. Torres-Sanchez[25] measured material DDE levels prepregnancy and in each trimester. The children were assessed using the Bayley Developmental Scales four times over the first year of life, that is, at 1, 3, 6, and 12 months of age. The first trimester DDE levels were negatively associated with performance on the Bayley Psychomotor Development Index (PDI) throughout the first year of life, each 10-fold increase in DDE levels being associated with a two-point reduction of the PDI ($p < 0.01$). Lead levels were measured and did not confound the association between DDE and neurodevelopmental deficits. Breastfeeding improved the Bayley MDI scores by 1.14 (confidence interval [CI] = 0.08–2.2), and an enriched home environment ($p < 0.05$) and higher birth weight ($p < 0.05$) were associated with significant increases in both PDI and MDI independent of DDE levels.

TABLE 7.7
Control Averages

Panel 1	Blood Chlorinated Pesticides	Adipose Tissue
Compound		Results ng/g (ppb)
Heptachlor epoxide		<10.0 (8.9)
Oxychlordane	23.1	
Trans-nonachlor	54.1	
DDE	231	

TABLE 7.8

Episodes of Chlorinated Exposure Disease by Year

Reference	Study Design	Population Description	Exposure Index	Pesticide	Exposure Window	Outcome	Result	Mean Score
Torres-Sanchez[25]	Birth cohort—Morelos, Mexico	244 mother–infant pairs residing in a malaria-endemic zone of Mexico; infants assessed at 1, 2, 6, and 12 months of age	Maternal serum levels of DDE before pregnancy and in each trimester, and interview	DDE		Neurodevelopment—Bayley Scales of Infant Development (BSID-II)	Increased levels of DDE in maternal blood during first trimester of pregnancy associated with decreased scores on the Psychomotor Scale of the BSID ($p < 0.02$). Breastfeeding was associated with higher BSID, although not significantly.	19
Torres-Sanchez[26]	Birth cohort—Morelos, Mexico	270 mother–infant pairs residing in a malaria-endemic zone of Mexico; infants assessed at 12, 18, 24, and 30 months of age	Maternal serum levels of DDE before pregnancy and in each trimester, and interview	DDE		Neurodevelopment—Bayley Scales of Infant Development (BSID-II)	Prenatal exposure to DDE is not associated with infant neurodevelopment beyond 12 months of age. Breastfeeding also had no influence on BSID scores at this age.	18.5
Eskenazi[27]	Birth cohort—CHAMACOS	330 infants at 6 months of age, 327 at 12 months, and 309 at 24 months from predominately Latino farm worker families in California	Serum levels of p,p-DDT, o,p-DDT, and p,p-DDE with interview	Organochlorines (DDE and DDT)		Neurodevelopment—Bayley Scales of Infant Development	A 10-fold increase in p,p-DDT levels at 6 and 12 months was associated with a decrease of 2 points on the PDI scale ($p < 0.05$). Breastfeeding was associated with higher scores.	18
Ribas-Fito[28]	Birth cohort—Menorc and Cataloni, Spain	475 children aged 4 years living in Catalonia and Menorca, Spain	Cord blood tested from HCB, delivery and postnatal maternal interview	Hexachlorobenzene (organochlorine)		Neurobehavioral—California Preschool Social Competence Scale, ADHD	Increased prenatal exposure to HCB was associated with decreased Social Competence scores (RR = 4.04; 95% CI = 1.76–9.58) and increased risk of ADHD (RR = 2.71; 95% CI = 1.05–6.96). No association was found with cognitive or motor performance.	18

(Continued)

TABLE 7.8 (Continued)
Episodes of Chlorinated Exposure Disease by Year

Reference	Study Design	Population Description	Exposure Index	Pesticide	Exposure Window	Outcome	Result	Mean Score
Ribas-Fitó[29]	Birth cohort—Menorca and Catalonia, Spain	475 children aged 4 years living in Catalonia and Menorca, Spain	Cord blood tested for DDT, delivery and postnatal maternal interview	Organochlorines (DDE and DDT)		Neurodevelopment—McCarthy Scales of Children's Abilities (MSCA)	Increased prenatal exposure to DDT was significantly associated with a decrease in verbal and memory scores on the MSCA ($p < 0.01$). DDE was not significantly associated.	18
Sagiv[30]	Birth cohort—Massachusetts	542 neonate–mother pairs residing near a PCB-contaminated harbor in Massachusetts	Cord blood tested for PCBs and DDE	Organochlorines (DDE and PCB)		Neurobehavioral—Neonatal Behavioral Assessment Scale (NBAS)	Neonates exposed to prenatal PCB and DDE showed decreased scores on the NBAS, particularly on alertness and attention-associated measures.	17
Sagiv[31]	Birth cohort—Massachusetts	607 children aged 7–11 years residing near a polychlorinated biphenyl (PCB)-contaminated harbor in Massachusetts	Cord blood tested for PCBs and DDE	Organochlorines (DDE and PCB)		ADHA—Conners' Rating Scale for Teachers (CRS-T)	Higher levels of p,p-DDE associated with higher risk of ADHD-like behaviors as assessed by the CRS-T, particularly in the highest quartile of exposure ($p < 0.05$).	17.5
Ribas-Fitó[32]	Birth cohort—Catalonia, Spain	92 infants aged 13 months living in Catalonia, Spain	Cord blood tested for OC, delivery and postnatal maternal interview	Organochlorines (hexachlorobenzene and DDE)		Neurodevelopment—Bayley Scales of Infant Development and Griffith Mental Development Scales	Prenatal exposure to DDE was associated with delayed mental and psychomotor development at 13 months ($p < 0.05$). Short-term breastfeeding (<16 weeks) was associated with lower scores while long-term breastfeeding was protective (associated with higher scores).	16.5
Saiyed[33]	Case–control	117 exposed and 90 unexposed male schoolchildren residing in 2 villages in India	Residing in the village below the cashew plantation	Endosulfan (insecticide)	Unknown	Male reproductive development ascertained by physician examination. Tanner stages of sexual maturity (SMR) and serum samples in a subset ($n = 70$ exposed and $n = 25$ controls)	Sexual maturity was negatively associated with serum levels of endosulfan ($p < 0.01$).	12

(Continued)

TABLE 7.8 (*Continued*)
Episodes of Chlorinated Exposure Disease by Year

Reference	Study Design	Population Description	Exposure Index	Pesticide	Exposure Window	Outcome	Result	Mean Score
Schenker[34]	Cross-sectional—Study of Agricultural Lung Disease (SALUD)	380 Costa Rican farm workers aged 40 years and older	Interviewer-administered questionnaire	Paraquat (Herbicide)		Respiratory function measures—TLC, DLCO, FVC, FEV$_1$, FEV$_1$/FVC, respiratory symptoms	Each 1-unit increase in paraquat index associated with a 1.8 × (1.0–3.1) increase in odds of chronic cough and a 2.3 × (1.2–5.1) increase in odds of shortness of breath with wheeze. However, no clinically significant increase in interstitial thickening or restrictive lung disease was noted for any pulmonary function tests.	17
Bhalia[35]	Nested case–control—Child Health and Development Studies (CHDS)	76 cases of cryptochidism, 66 cases of hypospadias, 4 cases of both, and 283 control infants enrolled in the CHDS in California	Blood samples in women	Organochlorines DDT/DDE	After delivery or during pregnancy	Cryptorchidism and hypospadias determined through medical records obtained for original cohort	No significant associations were found between maternal serum concentrations of DDT/DDE and congenital defects in male offspring.	19
Villanueva[36]	Cross-sectional	3510 births during the study period in Brittany, France	Maternal municipality of residence on date of birth	Altrazine in drinking water	Used measurements from 1990–1998 (not just pregnancy)	Preterm birth, low birth weight, and small for gestational age determined through birth records	No significant association was found between levels of atrazine in the drinking water and studied birth outcomes.	13
Rauh[37]	Birth cohort—Columbia Center for Children's Environmental Health	254 children, an aged 12, 24, and 36 months of nonsmoking black and Dominican mothers aged 18–35 years living in low-income neighborhoods in New York City	Cord blood tested for chlorpyrifos, pre- and postnatal maternal interview	Chlorpyrifos		Neurodevelopment—Bayley Scales of Infant Development (Child), Child Behavior Checklist (Mother)	Prenatal exposure to chlorpyrifos was associated with decreased scores in motor development, mental development, ADHD problems, and pervasive developmental disorder (OR = 6.5; 9% CI = 1.09–38.69; OR = 5.39; 95% CI = 1.21–24.11).	16.5
Fenster[38]	Birth cohort—CHAMACOS	303 neonates and their mothers from predominately Latino farm worker families in California	Prenatal (maternal) DDT/DDE serum samples and interview	Organochlorines (DDE and DDT)		Neurobehavioral–Brazelton Neonatal Behavioral Assessment Scale (BNBAS)	No association between *in utero* exposure and performance on Brazelton scale.	17.5

(Continued)

TABLE 7.8 (Continued)
Episodes of Chlorinated Exposure Disease by Year

Reference	Study Design	Population Description	Exposure Index	Pesticide	Exposure Window	Outcome	Result	Mean Score
Eggesbo[39]	Birth cohort—Norwegian Human Milk Study (HUMIS)	300 mother–infant pairs enrolled in the HUMIS cohort in Norway	Material milk and self-administered questionnaire	Hexachlorobenzene (HCB)	Infants <2 months age; 8 samples	Birth weight, birth length, small for gestational age, head circumference, ponderal index, and fetal growth restriction determined through the Medical Birth Registry of Norway	Increased levels of HCB in maternal milk were associated with decreased birth weight, head circumference and crown-heel length in addition to small-for-gestational-age among women who smoked ($p = 0.01$).	18
Sunyer[40]	Prospective cohort—Menorca, Spain	468 mother–infant pairs presenting for antenatal care in Menorca, Spain, with complete outcome data at 4 years	Maternal interview and DDE/DDT in cord serum	Organochlorines DDE/DDT		Maternal report of wheezing at age 4, maternal report of doctor-diagnosed asthma at age 4	Diagnosis of wheeze at age 3 years increased with serum DDE levels at birth (RR = 2.63; 95% CI = 1.19–4.69).	18
Sunyer[40]	Prospective—Menorca, Spain	462 mother–infant pairs presenting for antenatal care in Menorca, Spain	Maternal interview and DDE/DDT in cord serum and in blood at birth and at 4 years	Organochlorines DDE/DDT		Maternal report of wheezing at any age, maternal report of doctor-diagnosed asthma at age 6.5	Diagnosis of asthma at age 6.5 and wheeze at age 4 years associated with serum DDE levels at birth, but not with serum DDE levels at 4 years of age (OR = 1.18 and 1.14, respectively). Breastfeeding increased the mean DDE level, but protected against asthma diagnosis at age 6.	18
Sunyer[41]	Birth cohort	520 mother–infant pairs recruited prenatally in Catalonia, Spain	Interviewer-administered questionnaire during 6- and 14-month follow-up	Organochlorines DDE/DDT		Maternal report of doctor diagnosis of lower respiratory tract infections (LRTIs) including bronchitis, bronchiolitis, or pneumonia during an interviewer-led questionnaire	DDE levels above the first tertile of exposure were associated with LRTI at 6 months (OR = 1.68; 95% CI = 1.06–266) and 14 months (OR = 1.52; 95% CI 1.05–2.21) as well as recurrent LRTIs (OR = 2.40; 95% CI = 1.19–4.83).	17

(Continued)

TABLE 7.8 (Continued)
Episodes of Chlorinated Exposure Disease by Year

Reference	Study Design	Population Description	Exposure Index	Pesticide	Exposure Window	Outcome	Result	Mean Score
Dallaire[42]	Prospective cohort—Nunavik, Canada	199 Inuit infants up to 12 months of age living in Nunavik, Canada	4 maternal interviews (pre- and 3 postnatally), maternal blood, cord blood and infant blood at 7 months	Organochlorines DDT/DDE and PCBs		Chart review by nurses for any lower or upper respiratory tract infection (LTRI, UTRI)	Infants in the second quartile of prenatal DDE exposure were significantly more likely to develop an URTI at 6 and 12 months of follow-up (RR = 1.05 and 1.0, respectively) then were infants in the lowest quartile of exposure.	16
Glynn[43]	Prospective cohort—Uppsala, Sweden	190 primiparous women seeking prenatal care in Uppsala, Sweden who presented for follow-up with their infants at 3 months of age	Interviewer-administered questionnaires; two prenatal and one postnatal; maternal breast milk, and pre/postnatal blood sample, infant blood sample	Organochlorine DDE		Interview-administered questionnaire, maternal report of respiratory symptoms in infant, or doctor diagnosis of respiratory infection	No association was found between prenatal serum levels DDE and respiratory infections in the infants. Postnatally, all associations were null with the exception of the second quartile of exposure, which was reported to have a protective effect against respiratory infection (RR = 0.18; 95% CI = 0.06–0.60).	16
Venners[44]	Cohort	388 newly married textile workers aged 20–34 years working in Anhui, China	Maternal blood	Organochlorine DDT	Baseline—prior to stopping contraception	Pregnancy loss determined through daily urine sample for 1 year	Women in the highest fertile of serum DDT had increased odds of spontaneous abortions relative to the lower two fertile (OR = 2.12; 95% CI = 1.26–3.57).	19
Carmichael[45]	Case–control	20 cases and 28 controls in California	Maternal blood sampled midpregnancy	PCBs, HCB, DDT, and DDE	15–18th week of pregnancy	Hypospadias as determined through linkage with medical records reviewed by the California Birth Defects Monitoring Proram	No significant associations were found between levels of studied pesticides in maternal blood and infant hypospadia.	18

(Continued)

TABLE 7.8 (Continued)
Episodes of Chlorinated Exposure Disease by Year

Reference	Study Design	Population Description	Exposure Index	Pesticide	Exposure Window	Outcome	Result	Mean Score
Harley[46]	Cross-sectional analysis—CHAMACOS	402 pregnant women, enrolled in the CHAMACOS cohort in California	Maternal serum in subset ($n = 289$ women) and questionnaire	Organochlorines DDT/DDE	Serum sample in 2nd trimester and questionnaire asked for information 6 months prior to conception	Report of time to pregnancy during interview (face-to-face) at 13 weeks gestation	No association was seen with serum levels of DDT/DDE and fecundability. Maternal occupational exposure to pesticides, residence within 200 ft of an agricultural field, and home pesticide use were all associated with significantly increased time to pregnancy.	15
Toft[47]	Cohort	678 pregnant women, with at least one prior pregnancy, and their spouses residing in Poland, Ukraine, and Greenland	Maternal blood	DDE and CB-153	During pregnancy (approximately 33 weeks for Polish cohort and 24 weeks for others)	Self-report of fetal loss (miscarriage or stillbirth) in previous pregnancies during interview	Increased concentration of CB-153 in maternal blood was associated with increased odds of ever experiencing fetal loss when all countries were analyzed together (OR = 2.4; 95% CI = 1–5.5).	15
Axmon[48]	Cohort	778 women and 1505 women residing in Ukraine, Poland, Sweden, and Greenland	Blood samples in pregnant women and their partners	Persistent organochlorine pollutants (OPOs) including DDE	Variable	Self-report of time to pregnancy	In Greenland cohort, serum concentration of DDE and CB-153 in both men and women were associated with increased time to pregnancy.	14
Brucker-Davis[49]	Cohort	86 mothers of healthy male infants in southern France	Cord blood and maternal milk 2–5 days postpartum	DDE, linuron, lindane, vinclozolin, procymidone, and hexachlorobenzene (HCB)	Milk 2–5 days postpartum	Birth weight, head circumference, and birth length determined through unspecified source	Increased concentration of HCB in cord blood and maternal milk showed a negative correlation with infant head circumference ($p = 0.037$ and $p = 0.013$, respectively).	14
Salazar-Garcia[50]	Cross-sectional	2033 male antimalarial workers, providing information about 9187 pregnancies, working in Mexico	Interviewer-administered questionnaire	Organochlorines DDT/BBE	Not specified	Spontaneous abortions and stillbirths, sex ratio, and congenital anomalies determined through interviewer-administered questionnaire	Children born after paternal exposure to DDT had a higher risk of birth defects relative to those born before first exposure (OR = 3.77; 95% CI = 1.19–9.52).	10

(Continued)

TABLE 7.8 (Continued)
Episodes of Chlorinated Exposure Disease by Year

Reference	Study Design	Population Description	Exposure Index	Pesticide	Exposure Window	Outcome	Result	Mean Score
Sugiura-Ogassawara[51]	Case–control	45 cases of miscarriage and 30 controls presenting for care in Nagoya, Japan	Maternal blood	18 types of PCBs, HCB, and DDE	Unknown	Recurrent miscarriage defined as three or more consecutive 1st trimester miscarriages (method of ascertainment not specified)	No significant associations were found between concentration of studies pesticides and recurrent miscarriage.	10
Waliszewski[52]	Case–control	30 cases and 30 controls presenting for care at a hospital in Mexico	Maternal blood	Organochlorines DDE/DDT, HCH, and HCB	Post-partum (not specified)	Cyptorchidism identified through hospital diagnosis	Increased concentration of HCB, DDE, and DDT in maternal blood was associated with an increased risk of having a child with undescended testes.	10
Bianca[53]	Case–control	68 cases and 211 controls residing in an industrial and agricultural area in Southeastern Sicily, Italy	Neonatologist-administered questionnaire and parental occupation	Pesticides commonly used in hothouses.	Unknown	Physician confirmation of hypospadias reported through a surveillance system (EUROCAT)	Parental work in a hothouse was associated with an increased risk of hypospadia in offspring (OR = 2.9; 95% CI 1.01–8.55).	9
Fernandez[54]	Nested case–control	50 cases and 114 controls in a mother-infant cohort in Southern Spain	Placenta tissues and interviewer-administered questionnaire (face-to face)	Organochlorines (16 types) and TEXB (total effective xenoestrogen burden)	At delivery	Cyptorchidism or hypospadias identified through physician examination	Detectable levels of TEXB, DDT, lindane, and mirex in addition to maternal agricultural and paternal occupational exposure to xenoestrogens was association with increased risk of infant urogenital malformations.	19
Sagiv[55]	Prospective cohort—New Bedford, Massachusetts	722 mother–infant pairs residing near a PCB-contaminated harbor in New Bedford	Cord blood and interviewer-administered questionnaire	Organochlorine pesticides DDT/DDE/HCB, and PCBs	At delivery	Birth weight, length and head circumference determined through medical records	Small negative associations were seen between maternal serum levels of PCBs and infant birth weight.	19
Weiss[56]	Unknown	21 couples reporting to infertility clinic in Germany	Maternal blood, follicular fluid, and semen	Organochlorines DDT/DDE	Day of oocyte pickup	Pregnancy rates, semen mobility and morphology (method of ascertainment not specified)	No significant association was found between DDT/DDE and studies outcomes.	8
Tadevosyan[57]	Cross-sectional/prevalence	30 mothers who had recently given birth residing in rural Amenia	Maternal milk	Organochlorines (DDT, DDE, and HCH)	2–3 days post delivery	Self-repot of complications, preterm, stillbirth, miscarriage, and birth defects	Increased concentration of DDT in maternal milk was associated with an increased risk of infertility (OR = 2.14; 95% CI = 1.29–3.54).	7

(Continued)

TABLE 7.8 (Continued)
Episodes of Chlorinated Exposure Disease by Year

Reference	Study Design	Population Description	Exposure Index	Pesticide	Exposure Window	Outcome	Result	Mean Score
Cocco[58]	Retrospective cohort	98 spouses of men exposed to DDT in a 1956–1950 antimalarial campaign in Italy	Retrospective estimate based on the amount of DDT used in the antimalarial campaign	DDT—occupational exposure during antimalarial campaign	Unknown	Self-report of number of children, sex distribution, time to pregnancy, number of spontaneous abortions, and number of stillbirths; information from public registrars	Spouses of exposed DDT applicators had an increased rate of stillbirth pregnancies.	6
Cioroiu[59]	Cross-sectional	63 mothers living Iasi, Romania	Maternal milk (colostrums)	Organochlorines DDE, DDT, and HCH	1st week postpartum	Self-report of preterm birth	No significant association was seen between OC levels in colostrums and giving birth to a preterm infant.	11
Giordano[60]	Case–control	80 cases and 80 controls recruited from mothers receiving care at two hospitals in Rome, Italy	Maternal interview, job exposure matrix and maternal serum for small subset	Pesticides including hexachlorobenzene (HCB) DDE and PCBs	From 3 months before to 3 months after conception	Hypospadias identified through medical records	Maternal serum HCB above the median was associated with an increased risk of infant hypospadia (OR = 5.50; 95% CI = 1.24–24.31).	13
Pathak[61]	Case–control	23 cases and 23 control women who gave birth to full-term babies in India	Maternal and cord blood	Organochlorines	At delivery	Preterm birth determined through medical records	Maternal and cord blood levels of B-hexachlorocyclohexane (B-HCH) significantly correlated with preterm labor ($p < 0.05$).	12
Siggiqui[62]	Case–control	30 cases of intrauterine growth retardation and 24 controls presenting for antenatal care in Lucknow, India	Maternal blood, placenta and cord blood	Organochlorines DDT, HCH	At delivery	Intrauterine growth retardation (IUGR) identified through physical examination and ultrasound	Increased concentrations of HCH and DDE in maternal blood, and HCH in cord blood, were associated with an increased risk of IUGR ($p < 0.05$). Body weight of the newborn was negatively correlated with DDE in maternal blood, and with HCH and DDE in cord blood ($p < 0.05$).	16
Torres-Arreola[63]	Case–cohort	100 cases and 133 controls presenting for care in three hospitals in Mexico City	Maternal blood	Organochlorines DDT/DDE, HCH, and HCB	Shortly after delivery	Preterm birth defined as <37 weeks gestation identified through hospital cohort	No significant association was found between OC levels in maternal blood and preterm birth.	16

(Continued)

TABLE 7.8 (Continued)
Episodes of Chlorinated Exposure Disease by Year

Reference	Study Design	Population Description	Exposure Index	Pesticide	Exposure Window	Outcome	Result	Mean Score
Wojtyniak[64]	Cohort	1322 singleton births in Greenland ($n = 547$), Ukraine ($n = 577$), and Poland ($n + 198$)	Maternal blood	DDE and CB-153	During pregnancy (approximately 33 weeks for Polish cohort and 24 weeks for others)	Birth weight, gestational age, and preterm birth determined through questionnaire completed by medical staff	Increase in CB-153 in the serum of fruit mothers of one unit (log scale) was associated with a decrease in birth weight of 59 g and in birth age of 0.2 weeks ($p = 0.01$ and 0.02, respectively).	16
Gladen[65]	Cohort	197 singleton infants born in two cities in Ukraine	Maternal milk and self-administered questionnaire	Organochlorines (7 types)	At 4th or 5th day postbirth	Birth weight abstracted from medical records	No significant associations were found between concentrations of OC pesticides in maternal milk and infant birth weight.	18
Jusko[66]	Cohort—Child Health and Development Studies (CHDS)	399 women with pregnancies over 35 weeks gestation enrolled in the CHDS in California	Maternal serum	Organochlorine DDT	During pregnancy	Fetal growth (birth weight, gestational age, length, and head circumference) determined through medical records and 5-year growth assessed by a physician	No significant associations were found between maternal serum concentrations of DDT and any studied growth outcomes.	18
Neta[67]	Cross-sectional	300 singleton babies born at the Johns Hopkins Hospital in Baltimore	Cord blood	Permethrin and chlordane	After delivery	Birth weight, length, head circumference, ponderal index and gestational age abstracted from medical records	No significant associations were found between cord serum concentrations of chlordane or permethrin and studied birth outcomes.	18
Pierik[68]	Nested case–control	219 mothers of cases and 564 controls enrolled in a U.S. birth cohort study of pregnancies (1959–1966)	Maternal serum	Organochlorines (HCE, HCB, and b-HCCH)	Every 8 weeks during pregnancy at delivery and 6 weeks postpartum	Cryptorchidism as determined by records obtained for original cohort study	No significant association was found between maternal serum levels of OC and cryptorchidism in infants.	18
Farhang[69]	Cohort—Child Health and Development Studies (CHDFS)	420 mother-infant pairs enrolled in the CHDS in California	Maternal serum sample and interview at enrollment	Organochlorines DDT/DDE	Primarily postpartum	Preterm birth, small for gestational age, birth weight and gestational age determined from medical records	Weak association between preterm birth and DDE (OR $= 1.28$; 95% CI $= 0.73$, 2.23). No statistically significant results in study.	15

(Continued)

TABLE 7.8 (*Continued*)
Episodes of Chlorinated Exposure Disease by Year

Reference	Study Design	Population Description	Exposure Index	Pesticide	Exposure Window	Outcome	Result	Mean Score
Brucker-Davis[70]	Case–control	78 cases and 86 controls born in Nice area, France	Breast milk (colostrums) in 56 cases and 69 controls and cord blood in 67 cases and 84 controls	DDE, PCBs	Breast milk 3–5 days postpartum	Cryptorchidism determined by physician diagnosis at birth and confirmed at 3 and 12 months postnatal	Increased scores for exposure at birth (colostrums + cord blood) were associated with an increased risk of cryptorchidism ($p = 0.02$).	17
Cole[71]	Cohort	41 couples having their first pregnancy and residing in Ontario, Canada	Each couple completed a questionnaire(self-report) and provided a blood sample at delivery	Organochlorines	At time of delivery	Self-report of time to pregnancy (TTP)	Maternal benzene hexachloride exposure in the highest tertile was associated with increased time to pregnancy and lower fecundability (OR = 0.30; 95% CI = 0.10–0.89) relative to couples in lowest 2 tertiles.	17
Fenster[72]	Cohort—CHAMACOS	385 low-income Latina women living in the agricultural area of Salinas Valley, California	Maternal serum and maternal interview	Organochlorines (11 types)	Approximately 26 weeks and at delivery	Gestational age, birth weight and birth length as determined by through hospital records	Increased concentration of HCB in maternal blood associated with decreased gestational age ($p = 0.05$) but not with decreased birth weight or length.	17
Gesink Law[73]	Cohort- Collaborative Perinatal Project	390 pregnant women enrolled at 12 U.S. sites as part of the Collaborative Perinatal Project	Maternal serum	DDE and PCBs	3rd trimester	Self-report of time to pregnancy	No significant associations were found between maternal serum concentrations of DDE or PCBs, and time to pregnancy.	17
Longnecker[74]	Cross-sectional	781 mothers and new born males in Chiapas, Mexico	Maternal serum	Organochlorines DDT/DDE	Postpartum period	Anogenital distance and penile dimensions measured by study team within 1–2 days postpartum	No significant associations were found between concentration of DDT or DDE in maternal serum and reduced androgen action in male offspring.	17

(Continued)

TABLE 7.8 (*Continued*)
Episodes of Chlorinated Exposure Disease by Year

Reference	Study Design	Population Description	Exposure Index	Pesticide	Exposure Window	Outcome	Result	Mean Score
Damgaard[75]	Nested case–control	62 cases and 68 controls born in Finland and Denmark	Maternal milk	27 organochlorine pesticides	Between 1 and 3 months postpartum	Physician diagnosis of cryptorchidism at birth and confirmation at 3 months of age	No association was found between individual pesticides; however, combined exposure to the top eight pesticides was associated with an increased risk of cryptorchidism ($p = 0.032$).	16
Khanjani[76]	Cross-sectional	815 primiparous breastfeeding mothers of singleton babies in Victoria Australia	Maternal milk	Organochlorines (cyclodienes, HCB, β-BHC)	6–12 weeks postpartum	Birth weight, head circumference, prematurity, miscarriage, stillbirth, sex ratio determined through medical records	No significant associations were found between OC concentrations in maternal milk and any of the studied outcomes.	16
Khanjani[77]	Retrospective cohort	815 primiparous, breastfeeding mothers of singleton babies in Victoria, Australia	Maternal milk	Organochlorines DDT/DDE	6–12 weeks postpartum	Birth weight, head circumference, prematurity, miscarriage, stillbirth, sex ration and small for gestation age	A weak correlation was reported between DDT in material milk and low birth weight in female babies only ($p = 0.03$) No other associations.	16
Levairo-Carillo[78]	Case–control	79 cases and 292 controls from singleton pregnancies born to mothers in agricultural communities in Mexico	Interviewer-administered questionnaire, maternal blood sample after delivery and cord blood	Organophosphate insecticides	During gestation (not specified)	Intrauterine growth retardation (IUGR) identified through hospital records	Presence of acetylcholinesterase activity in mother or cord blood was associated with increased risk of IUGR ($p = 0.04$).	16
Ochoa-Acuna[79]	Retrospective cohort	24,154 infants in Indiana	Altrazine levels in drinking water collected through three data bases	Altrazine in drinking water	Entire pregnancy	Small for gestational age (SGA) and preterm birth determined through medical records	No significant associations were found between levels of atrazine in the drinking water and SGA or preterm birth.	16

The next report on this cohort[26] examined development in children between 12 and 30 months. There was no longer any association between DDE levels and Bayley scores in this age group, but early home stimulation (measured using the HOME Inventory) was a significant factor in improving the scores of 24- and 30-month-olds ($p < 0.001$).

A Spanish dual-cohort study enrolled children from a small town that had background contamination with organochlorines and PCBs from previous industrial production; a second cohort came from an area free of known industrial sources.[32] The children were assessed at age 13 months using Bayley Developmental Scales. Significant score reductions in the mental and physical scales were associated with increasing cord serum DDE levels, where each doubling of DDE caused a decline of 3.5 points on the MDI and 4.01 points on the PDI (both $p < 0.05$). When the effects of breastfeeding were analyzed, the worst Bayley outcomes were for highly exposed babies breastfed for short periods, and the best for low-exposure babies breastfed for long periods (>16 weeks) ($p < 0.05$). This suggests that breastfeeding is protective only when a longer duration can neutralize some of the impacts of toxin transfer in the breast milk.

Two studies report on the association between the organochlorine pesticide DDT/DDE and newborn behavior.[30,38] In the Mexican-American agricultural cohort (CHAMOCOS), there was no relationship between prenatal DDT/DDE exposure and the Brazelton Neonatal Behavioral Assessment Scale (BNBAS) scores for babies under 2 months old.[38]

A birth cohort from New Bedford, Massachusetts, an area known to have high PCB levels, was also studied. Cord serum PCB and DDE levels were measured and BNBAS assessments conducted at 2 weeks of age.[30] Measures of alertness and attention declined with higher cord levels of PCBs ($p < 0.01$). For DDE, irritability increased with exposure quartile after adjusting for cord blood lead level ($p < 0.03$). The DDE levels were presented in different units in each paper, but the New Bedford cohort was considered to have generally low DDE exposure.

A birth cohort in Granada, Spain, was randomly sampled when the children were aged 4 years to acquire 104 mother–child pairs with complete data on mirex levels in the placentas, and a full panel of other measured social and educational factors.[80] Mirex is an organochlorine pesticide long banned but very persistent in the environment, including in the Great Lakes, and highly bioaccumulative in the aquatic food chain. It is considered a human endocrine disruptor. The children were assessed by psychologists blinded to their exposure status using the McCarthy Scales of Children's Abilities (MSCA). Exposed children had lower scores on the MSCA working memory scale (−5.1; 95% CI = −0.83 to −9.4, $p < 0.02$) and quantitative scale (−7.33; 95% CI = −0.30 to −14.36, $p < 0.04$). Both these scales are considered important for mathematical ability and school success.[80] The motor development scores were not affected by mirex exposure.

More recently, a report on the same cohort at age 4 years found inverse relationships between cord DDE levels and the MSCA verbal and memory scales.[29] Cord DDE levels above 0.2 ng/mL were associated with declines of 7.86 points ($p < 0.05$) on the verbal scale and 10.86 points on the memory scale ($p < 0.01$) in an analysis, including both genders. The declines were much greater for girls and not statistically significant for boys. Another report on this cohort examined the relationship between cord serum HCB levels and social behavior in 4-year-olds.[28] When adjusted for PCB, DDE, and DDT, children in the highest 33% of HCB exposure (>1.459 ng/mL in cord serum) still had a higher probability of scoring <80 on the McCarthy Scales of cognitive function (MSCA) Social Competence Scale (relative risk = 5.63, 95% CI = 2.13–14.88). The Social Competence Scale was scored by the children's teachers only. The HCB levels were not associated with the MSCA.

DDT Breakdown Chemical Alters Thyroid Hormone Function in Pregnant Women

Researchers report that a woman's DDE exposure during early pregnancy is associated with altered thyroid hormone levels, a condition that could affect fetal brain development.

Pregnant women with higher blood levels of a long-lived pesticide residue were more likely to have skewed thyroid hormone levels, finds a study conducted in Spain.

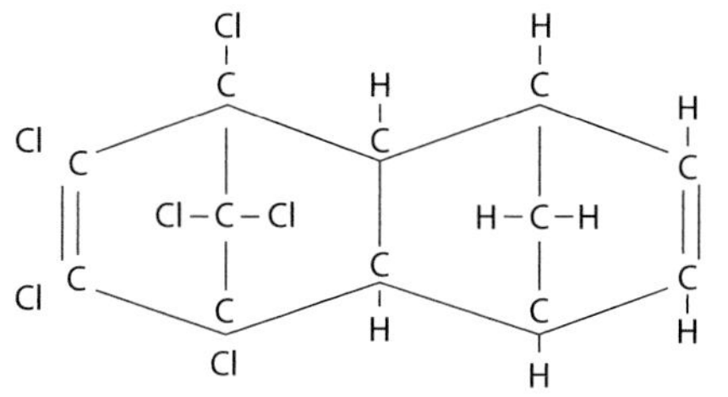

FIGURE 7.3 Chemical structure of aldrin.

Researchers found that women with higher DDE blood concentrations were 2.5 times more likely to have high thyroid-stimulating hormone (TSH). Increasing DDE exposure was also associated with reduced thyroxine (T4) levels.

Potential effects of chemicals on thyroid function during pregnancy are of concern because thyroid hormones play a crucial role in fetal brain development. A previous report found high TSH and low T4 in pregnant women to be associated with reduced cognitive abilities in children aged between 10 months and 8 years.

DDT was banned internationally following the 2001 Stockholm Convention on Persistent Organic Pollutants with an exception for malaria control.

DDE and thyroid hormone were measured in blood collected from 157 women during the 12th week of pregnancy. Researchers also measured the concentration of PCBs in maternal blood but contrary to some previously published reports, found no associations with thyroid hormone levels.

Aldrin (octalene): Aldrin (Figure 7.3) is a chlorinated naphthalene derivative that has been used as an insecticide since 1950. It is related to dieldrin and endrin and has been banned in some countries due to its persistence in the environment and potential for chronic toxicity. Aldrin is metabolized to dieldrin, which is its epoxide form. Aldrin is slowly eliminated from the body, as unknown hydrophilic metabolites in feces and a little in urine. Aldrin produces CNS stimulation with excitation characterized by nausea, dizziness, headaches, involuntary movements, convulsions, and loss of consciousness.

Dieldrin diminishes the storage of vitamin A in the liver. It accelerates an essential fatty acid deficiency in rats and induces foot-pad lesions. A deficiency of thiamine enhances pollutant toxicity, and pollutant toxicity enhances thiamine deficiency. An example of apparent dieldrin sensitivity, in combination with other insecticides, is shown in the following case.

Case study: A 58-year-old woman with a history of paroxysmal atrial tachycardia, bronchitis, sinusitis, and headache noted that in November 1983, her symptoms worsened significantly after she turned on her gas furnace. In March 1983, she underwent a chlorinated-pesticide screening test that revealed the presence of dieldrin (1.8 ppb), heptachlor epoxide 0.6 ppb), and DDE (0.5 ppb). By the following spring, she described her headaches as excruciating and pulsating. She was admitted to an environmental control unit (ECU) for evaluation. During her stay in a porcelain room, she fasted on spring water. She experienced detoxification symptoms of weakness and nausea, but within 3 days of admittance to the ECU, her headache, which had been almost constant for months, completely cleared.

Food testing in the ECU showed the usual development of food sensitivities that tend to occur from chemical overload. Tomatoes, bananas, cashews, tuna, cabbage, and eggs caused reactions, as did exposure to orris root, perfume, newsprint, cotton, auto exhaust, molds, dust, and dust mite. After hospitalization in the environmental unit, her blood dieldrin level reduced from 1.8 ppb to <0.1 ppb, and heptachlor epoxide went from 0.6 ppb to nondetectable.

Air analysis of her home showed concentrations in the parts per billion of a large variety of organic contaminants, including dieldrin, benzene compounds, naphthalene, other cyclic hydrocarbons, tetrachloroethylene, ethane, propane, pentane, octane, and other acyclic hydrocarbons. Her

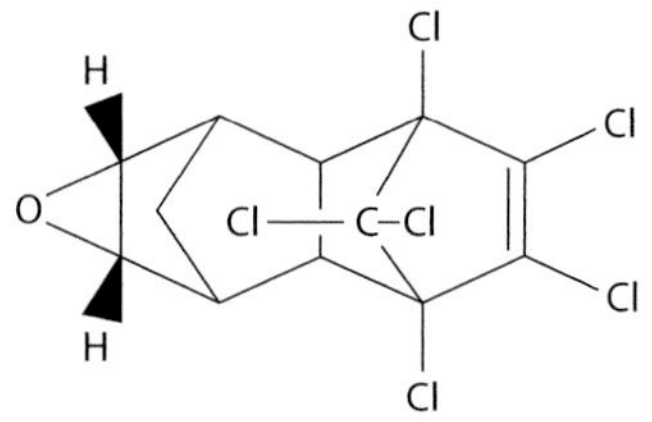

FIGURE 7.4 Chemical structure of dieldrin.

house was also found to have chlordane in the attic. Double-blind inhaled exposure to pesticide reproduced all of her symptoms.

The patient was found to have a low level of erythrocyte glutathione peroxidase (EGPx) of 2.13 (normal range: 4.23–07.23 μmol NADPH). This enzyme is specifically involved in the conjugation and detoxification of xenobiotics and free radicals, and her apparent deficiency might explain why she would be much more sensitive to chemicals than other patients were.

On a program of antigen injection therapy, chemically less contaminated food, and environmental clean-up (including removal of pesticides from her home), and with the conversion from gas to electric heat, this patient made substantial improvement, although she remains environmentally sensitive.

Dieldrin: Dieldrin (Figure 7.4) is the epoxide of aldrin, which has been developed over the last 30 plus years. Technical grades contain at least 85% dieldrin, with the rest being contaminants. Dieldrin, a stereoisomer of endrin, has been banned from most use in the United States due to its persistence and accumulation in the environment. It is still legal in many other countries, however, and the United States banned beef from Australia in 1988 due to its content of dieldrin. Many Australian patients have high levels of dieldrin in their blood.[81]

Blood concentrations in some U.S. residents averaged 0.0015 mg/L, with approximately 25% of the dieldrin being present in erythrocytes[82] and with similar results being reported in whole blood.[83] Plasma levels of dieldrin in exposed worker were found to average 0.0094–0.0270 mg/L.[84] Half-lives of 1 year[84] to 50–97 days have been reported.[85,86] In our experience, the half-life depends on the amount of dieldrin stored in the total body pool, a patient's total load of pollutants and state of nutrition, and the efficiency of an individual's enzyme detoxification system. Blood clearing will be much slower if there is a constant infusion from different tissue stores in the body or if metabolism is impaired.

Dieldrin has not been thought to undergo appreciable metabolic degradation, but this notion may be erroneous. Oxidative dechlorination is now thought to occur.[87] The average fat concentration in the general population in southern England was 0.21 mg/kg[88] while the mean value in the United States was 0.14 mg/kg.[89] Industry-exposed workers had an average fat concentration of 6.12 mg/kg.[90]

Clinical signs of dieldrin poisoning are similar to many of those signs seen in patients with chemical sensitivity who, in fact, have dieldrin in their blood. These include headache, dizziness, nausea, sweating, myoclonic limb movements, and convulsive seizures. Several dieldrin fatalities have occurred.[91–95]

Endrin: Endrin (Figure 7.5) is the stereoisomer of dieldrin and is one of the most toxic chlorinated hydrocarbon insecticides. Since 1950, it has had widespread use in agriculture against soil and foliage pests. It has been banned in some countries due to its environmental persistence. Endrin is not found in the plasma, fat, or urine of members of the general population.[96] Its metabolism is unsure, but it is thought to be through oxidation to 9-hydroxyendrin and then to ketoendrin and out the feces. A glueferonide conjugate has also been found in the urine.

The contamination of food stuffs by endrin has resulted in several mass poisonings with multiple fatalities. Usually vomiting, convulsions, and unconsciousness occurred.[97,98] Survivors were probably left with chemical sensitivity.

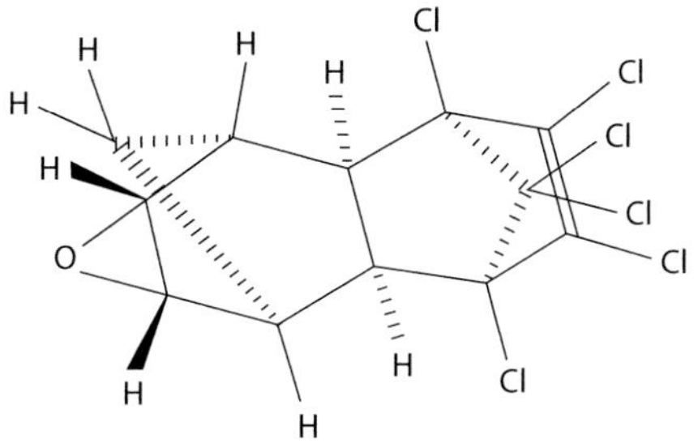

FIGURE 7.5 Chemical structure of endrin.

Chlordane, heptachlor, nonachlor, heptachlor epoxide, and trans-nonachlor: These substances (Figure 7.6) are extremely toxic. They have been widely used in agriculture. They have also been extensively used for termite-proofing of buildings, including much of the housing in the Southern United States. Chlordane (octachlor) is an organochlorine insecticide that was commercially available from 1979 to 1989. This commercial product is a mixture of 2 chlordane isomers (60%–75%) and related products, chlorodene, heptachlor, and nonachlor. Chlordane is readily absorbed via inhalation, ingestion, or dermal contact.

Metabolism is described in Chapter 4 of *Chemical Sensitivity Vol. I*[99] and, such as dieldrin, involves the oxidative dechlorination pathways.

Chlordane is a persistent fat-soluble CNS stimulant that causes confusion, delirium, nausea, convulsions, and if exposure is great enough, death. Continued exposure causes liver and kidney damage. People have been reported to have symptoms 36–48 hours after their water supply had been contaminated with chlordane.[100] Several cases have been reported in which the victims had monocytic leukemia[101] or megaloblastic anemia.[102] Chlordane has been shown to suppress the immune system.

Heptachlor, a chlorinated cyclodiene pesticide, was registered in 1952 as a commercial pesticide for foliage, soil, and structural applications. After 1960, it was used primarily in soil applications against agricultural pests and termites. As a result of positive findings in carcinogenicity assays, the U.S. Environmental Protection Agency (EPA) suspended all uses of products containing heptachlor in 1976, except for the treatment of seeds, control of ants on Hawaiian pineapple plants, and control of termites and the narcissus bulb fly. More recently, in August 1987, the EPA and the sole U.S. manufacturer of heptachlor entered into an agreement whereby all sales of chlordane and heptachlor would cease until safer methods of its application could be demonstrated.[103] Chlordane compounds have long half-lives and do persist. The EHC-Dallas knows of at least 50 homes that were made uninhabitable due to chlordane extermination. We have seen at least 200 patients damaged by termite proofing their homes with chlordane and heptachlor. The following is an example of the deleterious effects of chlordane.

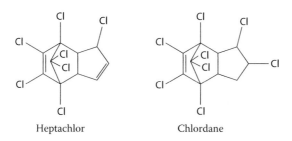

Heptachlor   Chlordane

FIGURE 7.6 Chemical structures of heptachlor and chlordane.

Case study: A 55-year-old female presented with chronic fatigue, myalgia, memory loss, insomnia, restlessness, recurrent respiratory infections, and pleurisy. Significant in her past history was a carcinoma of the left breast that had resulted in a radical mastectomy. Her main complaint of insomnia seemed to date from major pelvic surgery and appendectomy and, specifically, from an episode of high fever that she had had 2 days after surgery, which had been thought to be an anesthetic reaction.

She was evaluated in the hospital in an environmental unit, where she was fasted on spring water under controlled conditions. Here, she experienced hyperactivity, itching skin, insomnia, aching limbs, nausea, and fatigue. After the fast, these symptoms improved, but did not clear completely.

She was found to react with positive skin and clinical responses to 36 chemically less contaminated foods. In addition, regular commercial foods produced itchy nose, abdominal bloating, nausea, chills, itchy hands, ears, and feet, and GI bleeding.

In an inert glass and stainless-steel testing booth, the patient underwent double-blind exposure to ambient doses of gas, <0.005 ppm phenol, <0.20 formaldehyde, <0.0034 ppm 2,4-DNP insecticide, and <0.50 ppm petroleum-derived alcohol, all of which she reacted to. She did not react to <0.33 ppm of chlorine or three placebos of normal saline.

Two years after this hospitalization, because the patient was not improving as had been hoped and because she had reacted to insecticide on inhaled chemical challenge, she underwent a newly available blood chlorinated-pesticide screening test. Analysis revealed the presence of chlordane at 6 ppb, β-BHC at 0.5 ppb, DDE at 2.6 ppb, *trans*-nonachlor at 0.7 ppb, and HCB at 0.6 ppb and an absence of OPs. Her white cell parameter, including T and B lymphocytes, was normal. Serum zinc levels, however, were at times, low at 73.6 mcg/dL (C = 100–160 mcg/dL). Zinc deficiency seems to be associated with pesticide toxicity.[104] Subsequent analysis of the carpeting in the patient's home by the Texas Department of Health confirmed the presence of chlordane (53 ppm), heptachlor (3.1 ppm), DDT (4.9 ppm), and 210 ppm of diazinon (OP). Air samples from under her house confirmed the presence of lindane as well. These toxins had remained from the treatment for pest control that her home had received previously.

She had the carpet removed, made changes to ensure the house was more ecologically secure, and had the crawl space beneath the home ventilated and the impregnated ground sealed. Subsequent substantial reduction of the concentration of these pollutants was accompanied by improvement in her symptoms. Her recurrent infections stopped completely, and she became comfortable in her home. The pesticide levels disappeared from her blood chlordane contamination was first recognized in mid-1985 and continued to be noticed for a 1-year period. Chlordane compounds from contaminated mash have now been found in dairy products and in the blood and tissue of the farmers working with them. Heptachlor epoxide (a known carcinogen) was found to be as high as 12.6 ppm in milk sold at various grocery stores.[105] Farm family members who consumed dairy products from contaminated cows clearly showed an adversely different pattern of pesticide residue body burden that those people surveyed by the Second National Health and Education Survey (Brewster, M. 1988, personal communication).

Hexachlorobenzene

HCB (Figure 7.7) is used as a fungicide for control of smut in cereal grains, primarily wheat. This chemical is not to be confused with BHC (lindane, hexachlorocyclohexane BHC), which is actually a cyclohexane derivative. HCB is an aromatic benzene derivative. Environmental exposure occurs as the result of ingestion of contaminated food and water. At one time, the feeding of HCB-treated seed grain to livestock or its incorporation into bread via treated wheat was a common occurrence in certain areas of the world. HCB has no safe threshold value.

A disaster occurred in Turkey when 3000 people sustained damage following ingestion of wheat contaminated by HCB. The survivors of this exposure were left with chemical sensitivity. Several other episodes of mass contamination of food have occurred.[106,107] HCB has been found in German schoolchildren,[108] New Zealand adults,[109] and the U.S. adults.[110–112] The primary toxic

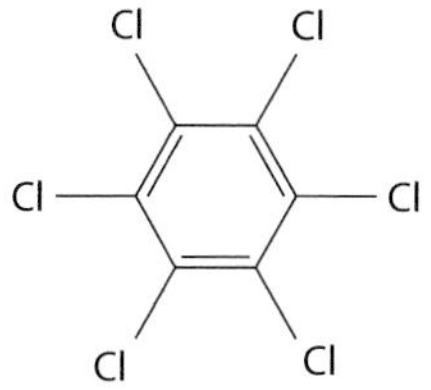

FIGURE 7.7 Chemical structure of hexachlorobenzene.

effect is cutaneous porpheria which involves blistering and epidermolysis of the skin of the face and hands.[113–117] HCB is stored in the fat. In rats, 7% comes out in urine, and 27% in feces. Known metabolites, including PCP, pentachlorobenzene, tetrachlorohydroquinone, tetrachlorophenol, and trichlorophenol (TCP), are toxic[115–118] and can exacerbate chemical sensitivity (Table 7.9).

A case report of a patient whose blood contained high levels of several organochlorine insecticides, including extremely high counts of BHC and HCB, is now presented.

Case study: A 41-year-old woman had a history of being unwell for several years, with symptoms of facial pain, headache, abdominal pain and bloody diarrhea, joint and muscle pain, skin flushing and burning, spontaneous bruising, and bladder spasms. She had consulted many physicians, with no resolution of her multiple symptoms.

In 1978, she had moved into a new home, which had been treated with chlordane and which was subsequently treated for pests and termites (inside and outside the home) for 53 consecutive months. The common agents used were chlorpyfos, diazinon, and chlordane. She had an episode of apparent herpes zoster, with general debilitation requiring hospitalization in April 1982.

Several times, her symptoms improved significantly while she was away from home on trips to Canada and Mexico, but consistently she worsened when she returned home. She also began to exhibit severe emotional liability with nervousness, agitation, and mental confusion. Eventually the state health authority tested her home and found significant levels of pesticides in the air, water, soil, foundation of the house, carpeting, and wallpaper (Tables 7.10 through 7.12).

The patient had a blood analysis performed that confirmed high levels of β-BHC, DDE, and HCB as well as three other organochlorine pesticides. She was also found to have nine organic solvents detectable in her blood, including xylene, tetrachloroethylene, and carbon tetrachloride. Viral cultures were negative for herpes.

She was found, further, to have evidence of immune suppression, with hypogammaglobulinemia (IgG-680 mg/dL [normal = 800–1800 mg/dL]), lymphopenia at $1306/mm^3$ (C < $1500/mm^3$), depressed T-cells of 45% (normal = 60%–80%), absolute T-cells at $891/mm^3$ (normal > $1000/mm^3$), depressed

TABLE 7.9
Water Samples (July 12, 1983)

Compounds	Home Water[a]	Office Water[a]
Dieldrin	0.014	0.008
Triluralin	0.014	ND[b]
p,p'-DDE	0.008	ND
Trans-Chlordane	0.004	ND
Cis-Chlordane	0.002	ND

[a] Concentrations are given in micrograms of compound per kilogram of water.
[b] ND = none detected.

TABLE 7.10
Air Samples (July 12, 1983)

Compounds	Breakfast Nook[a]	Living Room[a]	Carport Steps[a]	Bedroom[a]	Backyard[a]
Diazinon	0.527	0.709	0.056	0.603	ND[b]
Dursban	0.259	0.369	Trace	0.237	ND
Trifluralin	0.004	0.011	ND	0.017	0.030
β-BHC	0.007	0.004	0.004	0.004	ND
Heptachlor	0.033	0.024	0.029	0.024	ND

[a] Concentrations are given in micrograms of the compounds per cubic meter of air.
[b] ND = none detected. Chemical sensitivity Volume II, page 865, table 4. With permission.

TABLE 7.11
Wallpaper and Closet Samples (July 12, 1983)

Compounds	Wallpaper[a]	Carpet
Diazinon	99.4	374.4
Dursban	24.1	30.7
Heptaclor	0.7	0.3
Trifluralin	1.5	ND[b]
Trans-Chlordane	0.1	ND
Cis-Chlordane	0.1	ND
Endrin	0.1	ND
Mirex	1.6	ND

[a] Concentrations are given in micrograms of compound per gram of sample.
[b] ND = none detected. Chemical sensitivity Volume II, page 865, table 5.
     With permission.

TABLE 7.12
Soil Samples (July 12, 1983)

Compounds[a]	Pillar Beneath Bedroom[a]	Pear Orchard	Kitchen Steps[a]	Pond[a]
Trans-Chlordane	6459	14	5112	8
Cis-Chlordane	3681	8	2745	5
Trans-Novachlor	3899	8	2756	4
Cis-Novachlor	813	3	714	1
Oxychlordane	56	ND[b]	ND	ND
1-Hydroxychlordane	321	ND	107	ND
Heptachlor	1971	4	1465	3
Heptachlor epoxide	1415	4	303	2
Diazinon	Trace	ND	ND	ND
Durseban	ND	ND	Trace	ND
p,p'-DDE	ND	2	ND	2
p,p'-DDT	ND	3	ND	2
Mirex	ND	7	ND	7
Trifluralin	ND	1	ND	ND
Dieldrin	ND	1	ND	ND

[a] Concentrations are in micrograms of compound per kilogram of soil.
[b] ND = none detected. Chemical sensitivity Volume II, page 865, table 6. With permission.

absolute B-cells at 415 (normal > 500/mm³), and depressed total complement of 67% (normal = 70%–120%). Also, pyridoxine and vitamin D deficiencies with amino acid deregulation were present.

This patient was placed in an environmentally controlled room and fasted on pure spring water for 4 days. During this time, she experienced detoxification symptoms of flushing, burning, facial and head pain, numbness, rectal bleeding, muscle aches, bruising, and temporary paralysis. She ate chemically less contaminated foods and a rotary diversified diet. Intradermal and oral challenge testing revealed sensitivities to nine foods, along with molds, weeds, terpenes, candida, trees, ethanol, and cigarette smoke.

She improved significantly while in the hospital in an uncontaminated environment, but she had a relapse within 2 days of moving back into her home, which had been professionally cleaned in an attempt to remove the pesticides.

She was finally forced to live in a smaller building that was constructed on the grounds of her home, and to this day she remains extremely sensitive to any chemical exposure, especially pesticides. She worsened substantially in May 1984 when a neighbor sprayed diazinon about 20 yards from where she was living. This exposure caused generalized swelling, severe lethargy and weakness, mucous membrane burning, and mental confusion.

Lindane: Lindane (Figures 7.8 and 7.9) is an insecticide used as a fumigant and for the control of body lice. It is commonly used for sheep dipping in the wool industry. Lindane accumulates in plants and animals. It is the gamma isomer of hexachlorocyclohexane (BHC). Lindane is one of eight isomers of BHC, and it is the most toxic. Technically, BHC contains 12%–15% lindane, which at one time was found in the blood of most of the U.S. population. It is found in workers who manufacture lindane.[83,119–121] Lindane has been found in the blood of eight infants who were treated with a total body application of 1% lindane lotion.[122] The average half-life for one application is 21 hours, but it accumulates in fat and may last much longer in the chemically sensitive. The ratio of fat concentration to blood (serum) for BHC isomers is 220:1.[121] Lindane is metabolized by oxidation and dehalogenation, to a series of chlorinated phenols similar to HCB. Overload is associated

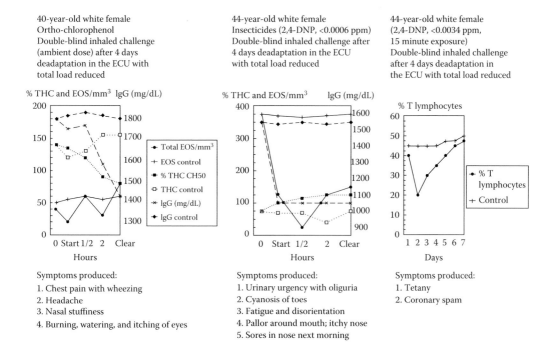

40-year-old white female
Ortho-chlorophenol
Double-blind inhaled challenge
(ambient dose) after 4 days
deadaptation in the ECU with
total load reduced

Symptoms produced:
1. Chest pain with wheezing
2. Headache
3. Nasal stuffiness
4. Burning, watering, and itching of eyes

44-year-old white female
Insecticides (2,4-DNP, <0.0006 ppm)
Double-blind inhaled challenge after
4 days deadaptation in the ECU
with total load reduced

Symptoms produced:
1. Urinary urgency with oliguria
2. Cyanosis of toes
3. Fatigue and disorientation
4. Pallor around mouth; itchy nose
5. Sores in nose next morning

44-year-old white female
(2,4-DNP, <0.0034 ppm,
15 minute exposure)
Double-blind inhaled challenge
after 4 days deadaptation in
the ECU with total load reduced

Symptoms produced:
1. Tetany
2. Coronary spam

FIGURE 7.8 Chlorinated pesticides screening. (From Chemical sensitivity Volume II, page 904, figure 33. With permission.)

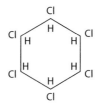

FIGURE 7.9   Chemical structure of lindane. (From Chemical sensitivity Volume II, page 858, figure 14. With permission.)

with neurological abnormalities, including EEG changes, muscular jerking, and emotional labil-ity.[123] Aplastic anemia occurred after chronic exposure from vaporizers.[124,125] Lindane was probably responsible for a mass-poisoning episode when it was absorbed dermally, producing mental confu-sion, weakness, anemia, convulsions, and death in six individuals (Table 7.13).[126]

Toxaphene: For several years, toxaphene insecticide ranked first in quantity used in the United States, with an estimated annual production of 75–95 million pounds.[127] The exact formula is

TABLE 7.13
Symptoms and Laboratory Analysis of 41-Year-Old White Female (1983)

1. Swelling and pain right side face
2. Edema—generalized
3. Spontaneous bruising—vasculitis
4. Recurrent cystitis
5. Recurrent GI upset

Positive Laboratory 5–83	Patient	Control Range
Phosphorus	4.8	($N = 4.0$–7.0 mg/dL)
Total eosinophil	0	($N = 150$–250/mm^3)
Cholesterol	356	($N = 150$–250 mg/dL)
Total complement (CH50)	67%	($N = 70\%$–130%)
C$_3$ activator	10.8	($N = 21 + 9$ mg/dL)
C$_4$	43	($N = 30 + 10$ mg/dL)
IgA	0	($N = 210 + 150$ mg/dL)
IgD	120	($N = 20 + 20$ mg/dL)
T lymphocyte	634	($N = 1900 + 500$/mm^3)
B lymphocyte	396	($N = 82$–500/mm^3)

Change after pesticide challenge
(<0.034 ppm 2,4 DNP, 15-minute exposure, after 4 days deadaptation in the ECU with total load decreased)

	Vasculitis	
Control	41%	T lymphocytes
Day 1	19%	T lymphocytes
Day 2	25%	T lymphocytes
Day 4	60%	T lymphocytes

Nutrition Laboratory

1. Pyridoxine—decreased
2. Vitamin D—decreased
3. Amino acid—deregulation
4. Oral herpes—H$_2$—1/400

TABLE 7.14

Correlation of Brain Function with Individual Organochlorine Pesticides in Chemically Sensitive Patients Admited to the ECU

Nervous System Complaint	% of Patients in Total Sample	% of Patients High in				
		Heptachlor Epoxide	HCB	β-BHC	Trans-Nonachlor	DDE
Sleepy	0	0	0	0	0	0
Physical fatigue[a]	54	51	46	40	49	50
Dizziness/light-headed	19	18	17	17	19	17
Brain fatigue[a]	30	25	22	29	26	26
Memory loss[a]	15	14	16	14	15	13
Speech defects	1	1	2	0	0	1
Seizures	4	4	5	5	2	3
Shaky	1	0	2	0	2	1
Fever	0	0	0	0	0	0
Headache[a]	69	56	54	48	60	55
Head pressure	9	8	10	7	9	8
Light sensitivity	2	1	2	2	0	1
Floaters	0	0	0	0	0	0
Blurred vision	4	3	3	2	2	3
Other	7	8	8	7	11	6

Source: Environmental Health Center Dallas Chemical Sensitivity Volume II, page 920, table 34. With permission.

Note: High chlorinated pesticide levels in the blood were found to be most common for heptachlor epoxide, HCB, β-BHC, *trans*-nonachlor, and DDE. The most common nervous system complaint for the total sample and for those high in chlorinated pesticides was headaches followed by physical fatigue, brain fatigue, dizziness/light-headedness, and memory loss. The nervous system complaints of those patients high in these five pesticides mirrored each other, as well as those of the total sample. Thus, pesticides do play a major role in environmental illness.

[a] Complaints were those presented upon first admission to the ECU. No postchemical booth inhaled complaints were gathered for this study.

unknown, but, empirically, it is listed as $C_{10}H_{10}Cl_{18}$. It appears to be a cytochrome P-450 stimulator and to be oxidized and gluconated. Its presence in the Fort Worth Rolling Hills water supply is discussed elsewhere. Toxaphens has been shown to cause liver tumors in mice and is mutagenic to salmonella (Tables 7.14 through 7.17, Figures 7.10 through 7.12).

In conclusion, pesticide overload is extremely common in the chemically sensitive, often acting as an initiator as well as an exacerbator. Pesticides are ubiquitous in our environment and must be minimized and hopefully eliminated from the chemically sensitive's surroundings in order to obtain optimal health. Numerous detoxification and metabolic systems can be damaged by these substances (Figure 7.13).

Pentachlorophenol

Commercially available substances containing PCP include Pentachlorophenol or Sodium Pentachlorophenate; PCP; Dow Pentachlorophenol; Dowicide EC-7; Penchlorol; Pentacon; Penwar; Veg-01-Ki11, penta; wood preserver; Wood Tox 140; Purina insect oil concentrate; GArdon Termi Tox; Usol Cabin Oil; Certified Kiltrol-74 Weed Killer; Ciba-Geigy Ontrack OS_3, OS_4, or OS_5; Ortho Triox Liquid Vegetation Killer; Black Leaf Grass Weed and Vegetation Killer Spray; DP-2 Antimicrobial; Priltox; and Sinituho.

PCP is used as a herbicide, defoliant, wood preservative, germicide, fungicide, and molluscicide. Over 50 billion pounds per year are produced. It is an ingredient of many formulated mixtures sold

TABLE 7.15

Changes in Cerebral Function after Unloading Chlorinated Pesticides in ECU

Test Analysis	Results
1. Sign and symptom score (lasting quantity and quality)	80% decrease ($p < 0.001$)
2. Composite brain function (Bender, WAIS, MMPI)	Change ($p < 0.001$)
3. Chlorinated blood pesticide (by Laester's method)	79% decrease ($p < 0.001$)

Objective Brain Evaluation

1. Bender–Gestalt: cerebral dysfunction
2. MMPI: personality measure neurotic versus psychotic
3. WAIS-R: intelligence test

Source: Chemical sensitivity Volume II, page 921, table 35. With permission.

TABLE 7.16

Change in Pesticides on Follow-Up Testing after Treatment[a]

Total No. of Patients	No. of Patients with Decreased or Absent Original Levels	No. of Patients with New Pesticides[b]
33	26	18 (16 with 1–3 kinds; 2 with 4–7 kinds)

Source: Chemical sensitivity Volume II, page 922, table 36. With permission.

[a] $p < 0.001$—Significant improvement clinically.

[b] May be due to reexposure or mobilization of pesticides from fat stores. The latter is more likely, since the patients continue to improve.

for one or more of these purposes. It has been used in leather for shoes. Its presence in the chemically sensitive appears to be very important in their pathologies. Since penta is often present in leather and home woods, the chemical sensitivity may be propagated.

PCP volatilizes from treated wood and fabric. Excessively treated interior surfaces may represent a source of intensive PCP exposure. PCP is often dissolved in hydrocarbon solvents for application by spraying, brushing, or pressure treatment, and it is known to be well absorbed after oral, inhalant, or dermal exposure.

TABLE 7.17

Improvement of Number of Blood Chlorinated Pesticides and the Number of Abnormal Immune Index in Six Patients after Treatment

No. of Patients	1		2		3		4		5		6	
	B[a]	A[b]	B	A	B	A	B	A	B	A	B	A
No. of abnormal immune index	7	0	4	0	4	0	1	0	1	0	7	0
No. of pesticides	6	2	4	1	5	1	5	1	5	1	5	1

Source: Rea, W. J., H.-C. Liang. 1991. Effects of pesticides on the immune system. *J. Nutr. Med.* 2:399–410. (From Chemical sensitivity Volume II, page 923, table 37. With permission.)

[a] Before treatment.

[b] After treatment.

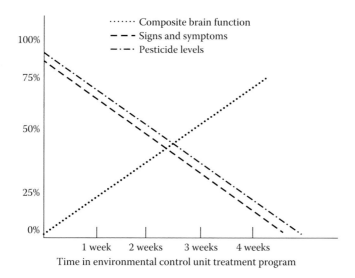

FIGURE 7.10   Percentage of change in composite brain functions, signs, and symptoms associated with pesticide levels—40 patients. (From Rea, W. J. et al. 1984. Pesticides and brain function changes. *Clinical Ecology* II(3):145–150; From Chemical sensitivity Volume II, page 921, figure 34. With permission.)

PCP is much used in Hawaii, where plasma concentrations of PCP have been found. Blood level ranges in individuals living in those areas of high spray were 0.05–1.0 mg/L, while levels in workers in a wood treatment plant were as high as 10 mg/L.

PCP is oxidized to tetrachloroquinone and is excreted in the urine both in the oxidized and conjugated forms. PCP is a highly toxic substance that produced delirium, weakness, flushing, hypo- or hyperpyrexia, tachypnea, coma, and death. Also, excessive sweating, facial flushing, fever, and weight loss occur after long exposure. Half-lives in poisoned humans range from 42 to 116 hours.[128] However, PCP appears to persist for years in some humans.[129]

PCP irritates the skin, eyes, and upper respiratory mucous membranes. It is efficiently absorbed across the skin, the lung, and the GI lining. Like nitrophenolic compounds, PCP stimulates cellular oxidative metabolism by uncoupling phosphorylation. This damage due to phosphorylation may well explain the energy loss seen in chemically sensitive patients with PCP in their blood. Like other

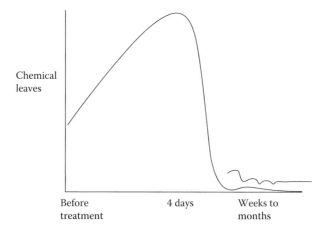

FIGURE 7.11   Pattern of clearing of chlorinated hydrocarbons from the body in patients in the ECU. (From Chemical sensitivity Volume II, page 922, figure 35. With permission.)

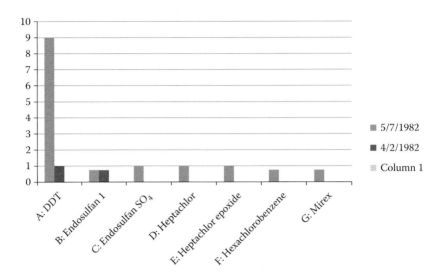

FIGURE 7.12 Toxicant (ppb) chemical. (From Chemical sensitivity Volume II, page 924, figure 36. With permission.)

phenols, PCP is toxic to the liver, kidney, and CNS. Impurities in the technical formulation of PCP may be responsible for chloracne in workers who are regularly exposed to it, which is certainly the case in the chemically sensitive.[130]

The most severe poisonings have occurred in workers exposed to penta while in hot environments, which volatize more toxic substances. However, a major epidemic of poisoning occurred in an American hospital among newborn infants who absorbed PCP from treated diapers. Dehydration and metabolic acidosis are important features of poisoning in children.[131,132]

Albuminuria, glycosuria, and elevated blood urea nitrogen (BUN) reflect renal injury. Liver enlargement has been observed in some cases. Anemia and leukopenia have occurred in some chronically exposed workers, but leukocytosis is more commonly found in acute poisoning.[133]

We have seen many patients severely damaged by exposure to PCP. Few patients have been able to live in houses treated with PCP. The following case is exemplary of this sensitivity.

Case study: A 30-year-old white female entered the EHC-Dallas with the chief complaint of diarrhea (up to 12 stools per day), swelling, and fatigue. She gave a history of her house having been treated with PCP. All four members of her family became ill with flu-like symptoms characterized by nausea, vomiting, muscle aches, and fatigue. These symptoms would improve after the family left the house and would exacerbate upon reentry. This exposure necessitated the family moving away from the home in order to survive. While living in another house, the father and children cleared all their symptoms, with the exception of recurrent respiratory infections. The mother developed a spreading phenomenon, becoming sensitive to more and more toxic chemicals on exposure to increasingly smaller amounts.

Upon entering the EHC-Dallas, she gradually cleared her symptoms, including the diarrhea. Double-blind inhaled reexposure to PCP in ambient doses reproduced all of her symptoms, including the diarrhea. This patient has remained well on an intense avoidance program (Table 7.18).

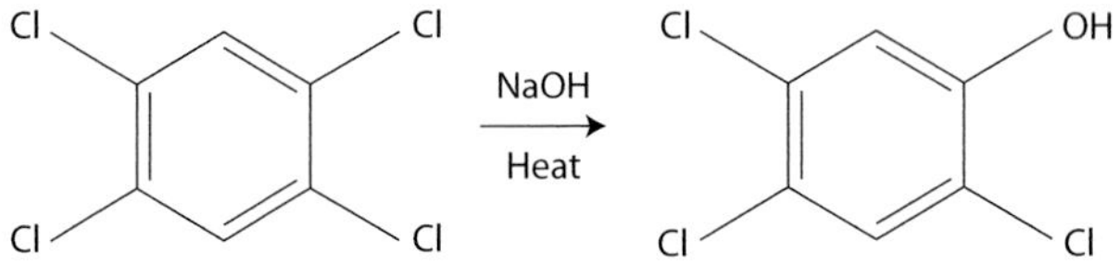

FIGURE 7.13 Chemical structure of chlorophenols.

TABLE 7.18

Inhaled Double-Blind Challenge after 4 Days Deadaptation in the ECU with the Total Load Reduced (15-Minute Exposure) 40-Year-Old White Female

Incitant	Dose (ppm)	Reactions
Pentachlorophenol	Ambient	4+[a]
Phenol	<0.002	2+[b]
Chlorine	<0.33	2+[b]
Pesticide (2,4-DNP)	<0.0034	1+[c]
Ethanol (petroleum derived)	<0.50	0
Formaldehyde	<0.20	1+[c]
Saline	Ambient	0
Saline	Ambient	0
Saline	Ambient	0

Source: Chemical sensitivity Volume II, page 861, table 8. With permission.

[a] Diarrhea for 1 day, generalized edema, muscle aches.

[b] Irritable bowel, generalized edema, muscle aches.

[c] Slight edema.

As discussed earlier, we studied 30 patients with proven chemical sensitivity who had PCP in their blood. The mean level was 12 ppm. All of these patients were extremely chemically sensitive. This pesticide was one of the most difficult to clear from the blood of our patients, but as it diminished, the patients did improve.

Mirex: Mirex (Figure 7.14) has been used in the southeast United States to control fire ants. The chronicity factor of mirex is greater than DDT.[134,135] Mice develop tumors, and rats develop megalocytosis, with an increase in hepatocellular carcinoma in males.[136,137] We are not certain about the effects in humans, but we have found this substance in the blood of some of the chemically sensitive we have treated. Mirex stimulates the hepatic microsomal system and causes proliferation of the smooth endoplasmic reticulum. There is evidence of a natural change in mirex to kepone.

Chlordecone (Kepone): Kepone (Figure 7.15) is a pesticide that is chemically closely related to mirex. Most of the kepone produced in the United States has been exported to control agricultural pests. Inadequate control during manufacturing led to many poisonings and large-scale environmental contamination.[138] The James River, which leads into the Chesapeake Bay, was the site of a disaster. A large amount of kepone was dumped into the James River, contaminating much of its sea life and leading to a ban on fishing. Positive levels of kepone were found in the blood of humans

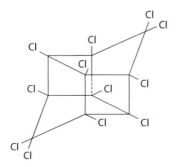

FIGURE 7.14 Structure of mirex. (From Chemical sensitivity Volume II, page 860, figure 16. With permission.)

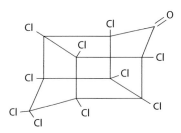

FIGURE 7.15   Chemical structure of chlorodecone (kepone). (From Chemical sensitivity Volume II, page 862, figure 17. With permission.)

living within a mile of the plant.[139] The half-life of kepone may be ~96 days (63–1148),[140] but this life span may depend on the amount stored in fat. Kepone may be metabolized through oxidation to alcohols and conjugation with glucuronic acids. Chronic problems associated with kepone poisoning include neurological, hepatic, and hormonal abnormalities. Kepone is carcinogenic in animals and potentially so in humans. Oral administration of cholestyramine (an ion exchange resin) for a month has been found to reduce the blood half-life by 50% in poisoned workers.[1216]

Table 7.19 shows a list of fat-soluble organochlorine insecticides all of which we have seen in selected chemically sensitive patients.

All PCB congeners are also lipophilic, as the corn oil was used to dissolve the mixture. The mixture, however, was not completely soluble in corn oil and 5% diethyl ether was used as a solvent to ensure complete solubility and homogeneity. Diethyl ether is a hydrophile with a K_{ow} of 0.89. It is not known what role the diethyl ether played in the mixture effects noted.

There is evidence that environmental pollution (car exhaust, gasoline, oil products, and pesticides) can trigger neurodegenerative disease such as Parkinson's disease (PD). Dutheil et al.[141] studied the association between PD and two polymorphisms in ABCB1 among subjects enrolled in the French health system for agricultural workers (Mutalite Sociale Agricole), as well as the interaction between ABCB1 and organochlorine insecticides.

The patients with PD were examined by a neurologist and were matched to a maximum of three controls. Participants were classified as never users, users for gardening, and professional users of pesticides. Detailed information on pesticides lifelong use was obtained for professional users by occupational health physicians.

DNA was obtained and 2 ABCB1 polymorphisms (exon 21: G2677[A,T]; exon 26: C3435T) associated with altered P-glycoprotein function were genotyped.

TABLE 7.19
Levels in ppb

Aldrin	6.50
DDT	6.91
DDE	6.51
Dieldrin	5.20
Heptachlor epoxide	4.98
Hexachlorobenzene	5.73
Mirex	7.18
Cis-Nonachlor	6.20
Trans-Nonachlor	6.20
Hexachlorocyclohexane	3.72
Oxychlordane	5.48

Among 207 cases and 482 matched controls, ABCB1 polymorphisms were not associated with PD (C3435T, $p = 0.43$; G2677[A,T], $p = 0.97$). Among 101 male cases and 234 matched controls, the odds ratio (OR) for organochlorines was 3.5 (95% CI = 0.9 –14.56) times higher among homozygous carriers of variant G2677(A,T) alleles than noncarriers. Among cases only, Dutheil et al.[141] found an association between carrying two variant G2677 (A,T) alleles and organochlorines (OR = 5.4, 95% CI = 1.1–27.5) as well as with the number of cumulative lifetime number of hours of exposure ($p = 0.005$; analyses restricted to subjects exposed to organochlorines, $p = 0.03$).

Their findings suggest that the ABCB1 gene and exposure to organochlorine insecticides interact to increase PD risk: in subjects professionally exposed to organochlorines, polymorphisms associated with a decreased ability of ABCB1 to clear xenobiotics from the brain increased the risk of PD. These findings support the hypothesis of gene × pesticides interactions in PD (Figure 7.16).

Endosulfan is a pesticide similar to DDT. The ban of endosulfan by the EPA is significant progress regarding health-damaging pesticides. Public and scientist's awareness of the problems caused by numerous pesticides and many other chemicals was started in 1962 by the great books of Rachel Carson[142] and Theron Randolph, MD[6] and continued by Dickey[7] and Rea.[31]

Most Americans still have significant levels of DDT and its by-products (DDE) in their blood and fat cells. Estrogen-increasing pesticides also help turn men into women.

Randolph[6] demonstrated that many people develop delayed allergic reactions to pesticides and petrochemicals that contribute to numerous common symptoms. These people need to carefully avoid even trace amounts of toxins and eat organically grown foods. Randolph's[6] discoveries were expounded in his scientific studies and articles and in his classic books.

The EPA, declaring that endosulfan is unsafe for farm workers, moved to ban one of the last organochlorine pesticides left in the United States, as endosulfan, like DDT, accumulates in the environment and in the bodies of people and wildlife, and is transported around the world to remote places.

Endosulfan—used largely on vegetables, apples, melons, and cotton—"poses unacceptable risks" to farm workers and wildlife.

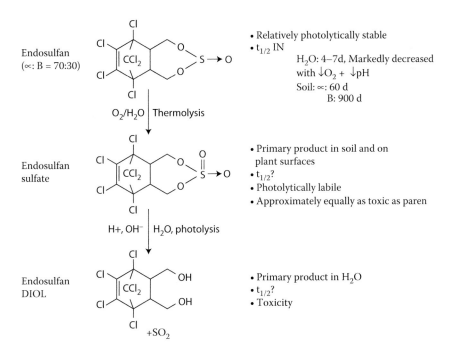

FIGURE 7.16   Chemical degradation of endosulfan in the environment.

The human effects are largely unknown but tests on laboratory animals have shown that endosulfan is toxic to the NS and can damage the kidney, liver, and male reproductive organs.

In late 2007, the EPA updated its assessment of endosulfan's risks based largely on new research showing effects on the developing brains of laboratory animals and studies of farm workers that showed their exposure was greater than previously believed despite use of protective equipment.

California officials determined that the amounts found in the air near some fields and orchards posed a public health risk to bystanders. The state declared endosulfan as a toxic air contaminant in 2008, which triggered efforts to reduce people's exposure.

In 2008, the EPA launched a review of the economic benefits of endosulfan, which is required before banning a substance under federal pesticide law. Its conclusion: While a few crop uses have relatively high benefits for growers, the nationwide benefits to society as a whole are low for all uses of endosulfan and do not exceed the risks.

The top crops that use endosulfan are tomatoes, cucurbits (which include melons, cucumbers, and squashes), potatoes, apples, and cotton. Usage has been decreasing since 2002, when new restrictions were added. In California, about 60,000 pounds were applied to crops in 2008,[143] compared with 151,000 pounds in 2002, according to the California Department of Pesticide Regulation.

First registered for use in the United States in the 1950s, endosulfan is one of the most abundant pesticides found in the global atmosphere. And unlike most other organochlorines, which were banned in the 1970s, its concentrations have been increasing since the 1980s in the Arctic and in other remote ecosystems, according to a 2009 study by British and Canadian researchers.[143]

Traces of endosulfan are found on food crops, but EPA officials say the risk from consuming the residue are low. Since organochlorines accumulate in fatty tissue, those who eat high on food chains—such as the Inuit who eat marine mammals—are the most highly exposed.

The ban on endosulfan will leave dicofol as the last major chlorinated pesticide allowed today in the United States, where it is used to kill mites, mostly on cotton and citrus crops. Pentachlorophenol is also used as a pesticide, although its use is restricted to treatment of railroad ties and utility poles, not food crops. Lindane is banned from crops but continues to be used in prescription shampoos for treating lice.

ORGANOPHOSPHATES

According to LD_{50} studies, which are accurate only for studies of acute exposures and, hence, invalid for approximating levels of chronic exposure, the order of descending toxicity for OPs (Figure 7.17) is tetraethyl pyrophosphate, phorate, disulfoton, fensulfothion, demeton, terbufor, meviphos, methidathion, chlormephos, sulfotep, chlorthiophos, monocrotophos, fonofos, prothoate, fenamiphos, phosfolan, methyl parathion, schradan, chlorfenvinphos, ethyl parathion, azinphos-methyl, phosphamidon, methamidophos, dicrotophos, isofenphos, bomy, carbophenothion, ethyl parathion (EPN), famphur, fenophosphon, dialifor, cyanofenphos, bromophos-ethyl, leopohos, dichlorvos, coumaphos, ethoprop, quinalphos, traizophos, demton-methyl, propetamphos, chlorpyrifos, sulprofos, dioxathion, isoxation, phosalone, thiometon, heptenophos, crotoxyphos, cythioate, phencapton, DEF, ethion, dimethoate, fenthion, dichlofenthion, and EPBP.[144] Survival from these exposures can cause chemical sensitivity.

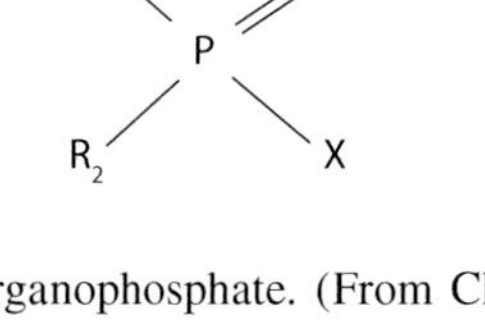

FIGURE 7.17 Chemical structure of organophosphate. (From Chemical sensitivity Volume II, page 862, figure 18. With permission.)

The order of toxicity and sensitivity for chronic exposure may be similar, parallel, or in some cases, in direct opposition to acute poisoning. However, we do know that in the long run, chronic exposure may in some cases create chemical sensitivity, and certainly, chemical sensitivity will be the result of an acute exposure in some patients, if they initially survive. Chronic exposure can also create not only chemical sensitivity but also chronic degenerative diseases such as atherosclerosis, PD, and Alzheimer's disease (AD). Generally, the more toxic the substance, the greater the likelihood that the exposed individual will develop chemical sensitivity after recovery from the acute symptoms. Since they have a much shorter half-life, OPs are used as replacements for organochlorine pesticides to insure safety. However, the presence of their breakdown products may be just as harmful or worse since they become incorporated into the phosphate pool, damaging the cytochrome P-450 system and producing antibodies against it. Our experience at the EHC-Dallas and the EHC-Buffalo is the OPs are just as toxic and highly sensitizing as organochlorines. According to recent EPA studies,[145] they, along with other pesticides and herbicides, are now found in virtually 85% of the food sold at commercial markets, excluding the organic market. It is well known that OP insecticides can now cause a hypersensitive response to molds, foods, and other chemicals which makes them extremely dangerous because they not only cause chronic toxicity but also trigger the hypersensitivity responses. It is estimated that now 50% of the population has some type of a hypersensitivity response to some element of the environment. These substances are one of the prime causes of chemical sensitivity. The Gulf War Veterans are examples of chronic effects of OP insecticides since their uniforms were impregnated from the beginning.

According to the study of various authors, Table 7.20 reviews many episodes of OP insecticide exposures.

The routine use of OP pesticides in homes and office buildings has been extremely dangerous to our patients and also to the public at large. We have seen numerous families made permanently ill by using OP insecticides in and/or around their homes, which have been made toxic by chronic spraying year in and year out. Owing to the process, much of the population has some brain or other neurological and vascular damage or dysfunction. Many have been incapacitated with chemical sensitivity.

The basis for toxicity in man from this class of pesticide (which is also used as a herbicide and fungicide) is most probably dependent on the inhibition of acetylcholinesterase (AChE) activity by phosphorylation which produces a more direct cholinergic action (seen in 40% of chemically sensitive patients), that is, neurologically mediated from an accumulation of acetylcholine. OP pesticides produce many effects through the inhibition (by phosphorylation OP cholinesterase). The resulting accumulation of acetylcholine at nerve synapses at parasympathetic and myoneural junctions in the autonomic nervous ganglia and in the brain initially over stimulates, and later paralyzes, neural transmission.[179,180] Heart rate variability and pupilliography in those chemically sensitive patients which can be measured then anatomically. These changes may account for many of the symptoms seen in some chemically sensitive patients. Both tolerance and toxic effects may be exhibited as a result of exposure to the same compound though at different dose levels. Certainly, the entering of Ca^{2+} inside the cell and assault on the mitochondria when combined with protein kinase A and C and then phosphorylated increases sensitivity up to 1000 times.[10] This can account for much of the hypersensitivity to foods, molds, and other chemicals seen in the chemically sensitive patient through the coherence principle. Poisoning may also be cumulative, inhibiting blood cholinesterase in a matter of days. The mechanisms of sensitization are presently unknown other than the Ca^{2+} protein-kinase phosphoralization phenomenon, but antibodies have not been shown to be generated to the cytochrome P-450 system. However, we believe that the anticholinesterase enzyme production is damaged, and then at times of repeated "low-level" exposure, nerve malfunction occurs. This phenomenon is demonstrated on the autonomic nervous system measurements by the heart rate variability or pupilliography in the thousands of chemically sensitive patients studied at the EHC-Dallas and EHC-Buffalo. The OPs may be trapped in the phosphorus pool of the body, causing continued disruption of intermediary metabolism.[87] Potentiative effects have now been shown

TABLE 7.20

Episodes of OP and Other Insecticide Exposures Creating Disease

Reference	Study Design	Population Description	Exposure Index	Pesticide	Exposure Window	Outcome	Result	Mean Score
Greenlee[146]	Case–control	322 case couples and 322 control couples residing in Wisconsin	Telephone questionnaire	Herbicides, insecticides, and fungicides	2 years before pregnancy attempt date	Female infertility determined through medical record review of patients seeking infertility treatment	Women mixing and applying herbicides 2 years before attempting conception or using fungicide had an increased risk of infertility (27; 95% CI = 1.9–380 and OR = 3.3; 95% CI 0.8–13).	15
Eskenazi[147]	Cohort—CHAMACOS	601 low-income Latina women living in the agricultural area of Salinas Valley, California	Maternal interview, maternal urine, maternal blood during pregnancy and delivery and umbilical cord blood	Organophosphates, malathion, chlorpyrifos, and parathion	Approximately 13 weeks, 26 weeks, and at delivery	Birth weight, length, head circumference, ponderal index and gestational age determined through hospital records	Increased maternal exposure to organophosphate pesticides was associated with a decrease in gestational duration ($p = 0.02$).	18
Mekonnen[148]	Cross-sectional	102 male agricultural pesticide sprayers and 69 nonsprayers working on four different farms in Ethiopia	Occupation (job title)	Agricultural pesticides, primarily organophosphate insecticides chlorpyrifos, diazinon, and malathion		Respiratory function measures: FVC, FEV, FEV/FVC, PEFR, and MMF	No significant association between farmers who sprayed and decreased or abnormal respiratory function was found relative to farmers who were not pesticide sprayers.	12
Ruckart[149]	Retrospective cohort	147 exposed and 218 unexposed children in Mississippi, 104 exposed, and 183 unexposed children in Ohio aged 6 or younger	Urinary metabolite of Methyl parathion (MP) (para-nitrophenol levels) and environmental wipe samples for MP	MP, an organophosphate		Neurobehavioral—Pediatric Environmental Neurobehavioral Test Battery (PENTB)	Exposed children showed decreased performance on tests of short-term memory and attention; however, results were not consistent between geographic sites.	12

(Continued)

TABLE 7.20 (Continued)
Episodes of OP and Other Insecticide Exposures Creating Disease

Reference	Study Design	Population Description	Exposure Index	Pesticide	Outcome	Exposure Window	Result	Mean Score
Whyatt[150]	Prospective cohort—Columbia Center of Children's Environmental Health (CCCEH)	314 African-American or Dominican mother–infant pairs aged 18–35 years in New York	Interviewer-administered questionnaire, cord blood, and personal air sample	Organophosphate and carbamate insecticides	Birth weight, birth length, and head circumference abstracted from medical records		For each log unit increase in cord plasma levels of chlorpyrifos by 42.6 g and birth length decreased by 0.24 cm ($p = 0.03$ and $p = 0.04$, respectively).	18
Salameh[151]	Cross-sectional	62 exposed and 19 unexposed pesticide factory workers in Lebanon	Interviewer-administered questionnaire	Pyrethroid and carbamate pesticides	Respiratory function measures: FEV, FEF25%–75%, FEV$_1$/FVC ratio, and FVC		Exposed workers had a $5.6 \times$ higher risk of abnormal FEV$_1$/FVC ratio and a $16.5 \times$ higher risk of abnormal FEF 25%–75% ($p < 0.001$). Acute exposure did not show any effect.	13
Peiris-John[152]	Repeat cross-sectional	25 occupationally exposed farmers, 22 environmentally exposed fishermen and 40 controls in Sri Lanka	Occupation self-report of pesticide exposure, residential proximity to agricultural areas. And AChE levels	Organophosphate pesticides (not specified)	Respiratory function measures—FEV, observed to predicted FVC ratios FEV$_1$, FEF25%–75%, FEV$_1$/FVC ratio—both between exposure periods and between study groups		FVC and FEV$_1$ was found to be significantly lower in farmers than in controls ($p < 0.001$ and $p < 0.05$, respectively) and FVC ratio was decreased during the exposure season. The FEV$_1$/FEV ratio did not differ between groups.	16
Young[153]	Birth cohort-CHAMACOS	381 infants ≤ 62 days old from predominately Latino farm worker families in California	Urinary DAP metabolite levels (both DMAP and DEAP concentrations) and interview	Organophosphates	Neurobehavioral—Brazelton Neonatal Behavioral Assessment Scale (BNBAS)		An increase in prenatal OP metabolite levels was associated with an increased number of abnormal reflexes in infants older than 3 days of age ($p < 0.05$). No association with postnatal OP metabolite levels was found.	17.5

(Continued)

TABLE 7.20 (Continued)
Episodes of OP and Other Insecticide Exposures Creating Disease

Reference	Study Design	Population Description	Exposure Index	Pesticide	Exposure Window	Outcome	Result	Mean Score
Grandjean[154]	Cross-sectional	35 exposed and 37 control subjects in 2nd and 3rd grades in northern Ecuador (up to 9 years of age)	AChE measured in blood samples, DAP metabolites measured in urine in children; questionnaire to mothers	30 pesticides, primarily organophosphates and diethyldithiocarbamates		Neurodevelopment—Wechsler Intelligence Scale for Children (IV) Santa Ana Form Board Reaction time. Stanford Binet copying test	Prenatal exposure associated with decreased visuospatial performance current exposure associated with increased reaction time.	12
Duramad[155]	Birth cohort-CHAMACOS	412 children born to mothers in Salinas Valley, California, with follow-up at both 12 and 24 months of age	Six maternal interviews including two during pregnancy, one at birth, and at 6, 12, and 24 months postpartum, and environmental home inspections	Organophosphate pesticides		Medical records used to determine diagnosis of asthma, eczema, bronchitis, bronchiolitis, or pneumonia	Maternal employment in agriculture as associated with a 25.9% ($p = 0.04$) increase in Th2 cytokines, biomarkers o allergic asthma.	14
Wolff[156]	Prospective cohort—Mount Sinai Hospital, NYC	404 singleton infants born to primiparous multiethnic mothers in New York City	Interviewer-administered questionnaire, cord blood, and maternal blood and urine in a random subset ($n = 194$)	Organophosphates PCBs and DDE	3rd Trimester	Birth weight, length, head circumference, ponderal index and gestational age determined from medical records	Increased concentration of DDE in maternal blood was associated with decreased infant head circumference ($p = 0.03$).	16
Engel[157]	Birth cohort-Mount Sinai Children's Environmental Health Study	311 neonates ages 1–3 days in New York	Urinary DAP and MDA metabolite levels, DDE in blood sample, and questionnaire in 3rd trimester of pregnancy	Organophosphates and DDE		Neurobehavioral—Brazelton Neonatal Behavioral Assessment Scale (BNBAS)	Total DAP levels and MDA levels were both associated with an increase in abnormal reflexes (RR = 1.32; 95% CI 0.99–1.77; RR = 2.24; 95% CI = 1.55–3.24, respectively). No association found for DDE	17

(Continued)

TABLE 7.20 (*Continued*)
Episodes of OP and Other Insecticide Exposures Creating Disease

Reference	Study Design	Population Description	Exposure Index	Pesticide	Exposure Window	Outcome	Result	Mean Score
Eskenazi[158]	Birth cohort-CHAMACOS	396 infants at 6 months of age, 395 at 12 months and 372 at 24 months from predominately Latino farm worker families in California	Urinary DAP, MDA, and chlorpyrifos metabolite levels and five interviews (two prenatal, three postnatal)	Organophosphates		Neurodevelopment—Bayley Scales of infant Development (child) Child Behavior Checklist (mother)	Pre- and postnatal DAPs associated with pervasive developmental disorder at 24 months (OR = 2.25; 95% CI = 0.99–5.16, 1.71;95% CI 1.02–2.87, respectively)	18.5
Hernandez[159]	Cross-sectional	89 exposed (pesticide sprayers) and 25 unexposed farm workers in southern Spain	Interviewer-administered questionnaire (face-to-face) and serum measurement of PChE and AChE levels	10 agricultural pesticides including endosulfan, neonicothoids, bipyridilium-class herbicides, fungicides, and carbamates		Respiratory function measures—FVC, FEV₁, FEV₁;FVC ratio, FEF25%–75%, TLC, and RV—in addition to physical examination and questionnaire	Restrictive lung disease was found to be associatd with exposure to neonicotinoid insecticides (TLC, RV, and FRC) and decreased diffusing capacity with exposure to bipyridilium-class herbicides (p < 0.05) Carrying the PON1R isoform found to be protective against abnormal respiratory symptoms (OR = 0.31; 95% CI = 0.10–0.92).	15
Sanchez Lizardi[160]	Cross-sectional	48 Hispanic children (mean age 7 years) from Children's Pesticide Survey in agricultural communities in Arizona	Urinary DAP metabolite levels (both DMAP and DEAP concentrations	Organophosphates		Neurodevelopment—Wechsler Intelligence Scale for Children (Children's Memory Scale, Wisconsin Card Sorting Test, Trail Making Test (children), Children's Behavior Checklist (parents) Teacher Report Form (teacher)	Exposed children performed more poorly on the trail making test (p < 0.01) but did not show significant differences on any other test.	14

(*Continued*)

TABLE 7.20 (Continued)
Episodes of OP and Other Insecticide Exposures Creating Disease

Reference	Study Design	Population Description	Exposure Index	Pesticide	Exposure Window	Outcome	Result	Mean Score
Handal[161]	Cross-sectional	121 infants aged 2–23 months living in rural Ecuador	Interview with mother to determine prenatal exposure	Organophosphate and carbamate pesticides (prenatal)		Neurodevelopment—Ages and Stages Questionnaire, Prehension and Visual Skills	Maternal employment in the flower industry associated with lower infant scores for communication, and fine motor skills and with poor visual acuity.	8.5
Boers[162]	Cross-sectional— EUROPIT study	248 exposed and 231 unexposed farmers and greenhouse workers in the Netherlands, Italy, Finland, and Bulgaria	Job title and ethylenethiourea in urine	Ethylene bisdithiocarbamates (EBDCs), fungicides and other pesticides (not specified)		Self-administered questionnaire using elements of the International Union Against Tuberculosis and Lung Disease (UATLD) Questionnaire	Exposure to EBDCs and other pesticides was not found to be associated with the development of asthma and asthmatic symptoms	12
Abdel Rasoul[163]	Cross-sectional	50 exposed and 50 unexposed male pesticide applicators aged 9–18 years in Egyptian cotton industry	AChE measured in blood samples, occupational history questionnaire	Organophosphate (primarily chlorpyrifos)		Neurodevelopment— Wechsler Adult Intelligence Scale (WAIS), age appropriate version	In both younger (aged 9–15 years) and older (16–18 years) subjects increased OP exposure was associated with lower WAIS scores ($p < 0.05$).	18.5
Lu[164]	Cross-sectional	35 children, 18 exposed, and 17 unexposed whose parents work on traditional and organic coffee plantations in Costa Rica	Two urine samples to test for organophosphate and pyrethroid metabolites	Organophosphates and pyrethroid insecticides		Neurobehavioral— Behavioral Assessment and Research System (BARS)	Exposed and unexposed children did not differ in levels of urinary pesticide metabolites; however, they did differ in BARS performance. This was attributed to differences in SES.	9.5
Barr[165]	Prospective Cohort	150 mother–infant pairs delivering at term by cesarean section in New Jersey	Self-administered questionnaire, maternal blood sample collected, at birth and cord blood	Pyrethroid, carbamate, OP insecticides, herbicides, repellents, fungicides	Samples collected at birth	Birth weight, birth length, abdominal and head circumference obtained through medical records	Increased concentrations of metolachlor in cord blood were associated with decreased birth weight ($p = 0.05$), while increased concentrations of dichloran were related to increased abdominal circumference ($p = 0.03$).	16

(Continued)

TABLE 7.20 (Continued)
Episodes of OP and Other Insecticide Exposures Creating Disease

Reference	Study Design	Population Description	Exposure Index	Pesticide	Exposure Window	Outcome	Result	Mean Score
Eskenazi[166]	Birth cohort CHAMACOS	371 children at 2 years of age from predominately Latino farm worker families in California	Urinary DAP (2 × during pregnancy), maternal blood, cord blood and six interviews	Organophosphates		Neurodevelopment—Bayley Scales of Infant Development	PON1 (108T) allele associated with poor Bayley MDI scores ($p < 0.05$), however, PON1 enzyme levels not significate associated with neurobehavioral outcomes.	19
Abu Shamn'a[167]	Cross-sectional	250 male Palestinian farmers aged 22–77 years	Interview-administered questionnaire	Agricultural pesticides including organophosphates		Interview-administered ATS-DLD and respiratory function measures; FVC, FEV1, and FEF25%–75%	No significant association was found between exposure to agricultural pesticides and lung function	12
Marks[168]	Birth cohort—CHAMACOS	348, 3.5 and 5-year-old children from predominately Latino farm worker families in California	Urinary DP metabolite levels (both DMAP and DEAP concentrations) 2 × prenatal	Organophosphates		ADHD-NEPSY-II visual attention (3.5 years), Conners' Kiddie Continuous Performance Test 5 years). Child Behavior Checklist mother), Hillside Behavior Rating Scale (psychometrist)	Prenatal DAPS not significantly associated with ADHD at 3.5 years. Prenatal DAPS associated with lower scores on the KCPT and increased risk of ADHD behaviors (OR = 3.5; 95% CI = 1.1–10.7). Postnatal DAPS were associated to a lesser extent.	17.5
Bouchard[169]	Cross-sectional data from NHANES	1139 participants and 119 cases of ADD (all subtypes) aged 8–15 years from general U.S. population	Urinary DAP metabolite levels (both DMAP and DEAP concentrations)	Organophosphates		ADHD-Diagnostic Interview Schedule for Children IV (DISC-IV)	A 10-fold increase in di-methyl containing OPs was associated with increased odds of any ADHD subtype (OR = 1.55; 95% CI = 1.14–2.10)	15.5

(Continued)

TABLE 7.20 (Continued)
Episodes of OP and Other Insecticide Exposures Creating Disease

Reference	Study Design	Population Description	Exposure Index	Pesticide	Exposure Window	Outcome	Result	Mean Score
Harari[170]	Cross-sectional	84 children aged 6–8 years living in Northern Ecuador and attending public school	Prenatal exposure interview (mother) and postnatal (child) OP metabolites in urine and AChE activity in blood	Organophosphates		Neurodevelopment—Wechsler Intelligence Scale for Children (IV), Santa Ana Form Board, Reaction time, Stanford Binet copying test	Prenatal exposure was associated with decrease in motor speed functions and visual memory ($p < 0.05$); current exposure was associated with increased reaction time ($p < 0.10$).	14.5
Xu[171]	Cross-sectional data from NHANES	200 cases of ADHD and 2339 controls aged 6–15 years from general U.S. population	Measurement of 2,4,5-TCP and 2,4,6-TCP in child's urine	Trichlorophenols (organochlorine compounds)		ADHD—Parental report	An increase in urinary levels of 2,4,6-TCP was associated with an increased odds of parent-reported ADHD (OR = 1.77; 95% CI = 1.18–2.66).	14.5
Horton[172]	Birth cohort—Columbia Center for Children's Environmental Health	Nonsmoking black and Dominican mothers aged 18–35 years and newborns aged 3–6 months living in low-income neighborhoods in New York City; 342 completed permethrin air samples, 272 completed blood tests and 230 completed piperonyl butoxide air samples	Air samples, cord blood, and plasma samples; maternal questionnaire	Pyrethroid insecticides (primarily permethrin) including piperonyl butoxide (PBO) a pyrethroid synergist		Neurodevelopment—Bayley Scales of Infant Development	Permethrin in air and blood not associated with Bayley Scale scores. Increased exposure to PBO in air associated with decreased Mental Development Index scores (OR = 2.49; 95% CI = 0.95–6.54).	16.5
Bouchard[173]	Birth cohort—CHAMACOS	329 children aged 6 months. 1, 2, 3.5, 5, and 7 years from predominately Latino farm worker families in California	Prenatal (mother) and postnatal (child) urinary DAP metabolites (DMAP, DEAP)	Organophosphates		Neurodevelopment-Wechsler Adult Intelligence Scale (WAIS) at 76 years of age	Prenatal DAP concentration associated with poorer intellectual development in 7-year-old children ($p < 0.01$).	17.5

(Continued)

TABLE 7.20 (Continued)
Episodes of OP and Other Insecticide Exposures Creating Disease

Reference	Study Design	Population Description	Exposure Index	Pesticide	Exposure Window	Outcome	Result	Mean Score
Rauh[174]	Birth cohort—Columbia Center for Children's Environmental Health	265 children at aged 7 years of nonsmoking black and Dominican mothers aged 18–35 years living in low-income neighborhoods in New York City	Cord blood tested for chlorpyrifos, pre- and postnatal maternal interview	Chlorpyrifos		Neurodevelopment—Wechsler Intelligence Scale for Children (IV) at 7 years of age	Prenatal exposure to chlorpyrifos was associated with decreased IQ and working memory score on the WISC ($p < 0.05$)	17.5
Engel[175]	Birth cohort-Mount Sinai Children's Environmental Health Study	200 infants at 1 year 276 at 2 years, 169 children aged 6–9 years in New York	Prenatal urinary DAP metabolite levels in 3rd trimester of pregnancy	Organophosphates		Neurodevelopment—Bayley (1 and 2 years) and Wechsler (6—9 years)	Increased levels of prenatal DAP are associated with lower neurodevelopment scores at 12 months (Bayley test) ($p < 0.01$).	17
Handal[176]	Cross-sectional	153 Ecuadorian mothers with two or more pregnancies	Interviewer-administered questionnaire (face-to-face)	Pesticides used in cut-flower industry including organophosphates, carbamates, and dithiocarbamates	Previous 6 years	Maternal report of spontaneous abortion	Women employed in the cut-flower industry had an increased risk of spontaneous abortion that increased with duration of employment (OR = 2.6; 95% CI = 1.03–6.7 increasing to OR = 3.4; 95% CI = 1.3–8.8 if worked 4–6 years) relative to women who did not.	8

(Continued)

TABLE 7.20 (Continued)
Episodes of OP and Other Insecticide Exposures Creating Disease

Reference	Study Design	Population Description	Exposure Index	Pesticide	Exposure Window	Outcome	Result	Mean Score
Waller[177]	Case–control	805 cases of gastroschisis and 3616 controls selected from singletons born in Washington State	Maternal residence and surface water concentrations of atrazine as determined through the United States Geological Survey Data	Atrazine in drinking water	Unknown	Gastroschisis identified through linkage with hospital records (ICD-9 codes)	Inverse relationship between maternal residence within 25 km of high-atrazine-concentrations areas and fetal gastroschisis ($p = 0.014$).	13
Chevrie[178]	Case–cohort—PELAGIE	579 pregnant women residing in Brittany, France	Maternal urine	Atrazine	Prior to 19 weeks gestation	Fetal growth restriction, head circumference, and congenital anomalies identified through hospital records by pediatricians	Presence of atrazine metabolites in maternal urine was associated with increased odds of fetal growth restriction and decreased head circumference ($OR = 1.5$; 95% $CI = 1.0–2.2$ and 1.7; 95% $CI = 1.0–2.7$, respectively).	19

between natural substances and OP pesticides. For example, Miyata et al.[181] have shown a strong potentiation of mountain cedar conjunctivitis in animals after exposure to very small doses of OP pesticides, suggesting one of the reasons that biological inhalant and food sensitivities occur in the chemically sensitive. Many of these chemically sensitive patients develop this entity in the course of their chemical sensitivity. The terpenes of natural products such as mountain cedar, pine, and other atophorus plants can trigger chronic illness, when combined with OP in this phosphorus pool. These terpenes make up one-third of the natural pollutant emanating from the earth, and therefore, are a very significant part of hypersensitivity illness, if they become sensitive.

OPs are absorbed through the respiratory and GI tracts and slowly through the skin. The process is often prolonged since the chemicals are difficult to remove. Dermatitis and high temperatures exacerbate the process and can lead to much more serious poisoning.[182] OP toxicity and sensitivity may be heightened by the presence of hydrocarbon solvents such as toluene and xylene, both of which are usually contained in commercial preparations.[4] These compounds are frequently found in the blood and breath of chemically sensitive patients who fell ill by OP exposures. Furthermore, many of these compounds are synergistic with each other resulting in more hypersensitization and chemical sensitivity. The combined neurotoxicity of the solvents and the OPs can cause axonal and myelin degeneration in distal fibers,[183] resulting in more damage and sensitivity. OP binds to the membrane-bound protein, resulting in degeneration.[184]

The characteristic signs and symptoms of OP pesticide exposure are the result of inhibition of cholinesterase and in the case of phosphorylcholines, direct cholinergic activity. Ninety-three percent of 2000 chemically sensitive patients studied at the EHC-Dallas had sympathetic cholinergic cholinolytic or sympatholytic responses when the autonomic nervous systems was measured by the iris corder and/or heart rate variability. In an ordinary case of chronic poisoning, blurred vision, giddiness, and headache will be followed by nausea, cramps, discomfort in the chest, and muscular twitching. Similar symptoms are seen in many chemically sensitive patients. Lapses in attention and impaired judgment may also be experienced, and these are often seen in a large subset of the chemically sensitive. In a few cases delirium, combativeness, depression, hallucinations, and other psychotic behavior may occur.[182] Similar symptoms occur with some patients' chemical sensitivity. These have been seen in brain damage due to OP in the war. Very rarely, damage to the myelin sheath of peripheral nerves has been reported. However, resultant numbness, pain, and weakness in extremities can last for weeks to years.[185] Chabra et al.[186] and Khandekar[187] have reported cardiac arrhythmias, heart block, and cardiac arrest associated with OP poisoning. We have seen arrhythmias in the OP chemically sensitive patient. Ludomirsky et al.[188] also report Q–T interval prolongation and ventricular arrhythmias. According to Hayes,[189] a massive oral dose of one of these compounds has resulted in death in 5 minutes. Diarrhea, cramps, and GI stress may also occur if the patient survives.

Signs and symptoms of OP toxicity and even sensitivity do not always correlate with biological measurements of poisoning (cholinesterase activity in the blood). In an episode reported by Xintaras et al.,[190] workers in a Texas manufacturing plant who were exposed to leptophos, an OP pesticide, showed normal cholinesterase activity. Before the correct diagnosis was made, physicians suspected encephalitis and other diseases, since the signs and symptoms included impaired memory, disorientation, drowsiness, headache, tremulousness, dizziness, anxiety, hallucinations, etc. We have had similar experiences of normal cholinesterase in some sensitive patients exposed to OP pesticides at the EHC-Dallas. Xintaras et al.[190] suggested that baseline data are imperative to accurately monitor the effects of these chemicals.[190]

OP levels are usually absent from the blood within 24–48 hours after exposure. However, they do appear in the urine many days to weeks after exposure. However, we at the EHC-Dallas, and Laseter[23] speculates that the breakdown products last much longer. It is evident from our series of over 1000 patients made ill by proven OP exposure that those tested often have no measurable evidence of cholinesterase deficiency. Nevertheless, these patients often have chemical sensitivity as severe as, or more severe than, those with organochlorine exposure. (Immunological data are presented.) Supposed maximally tolerated levels have been established for pirimiphos-methyl and chloropyrifos-methyl in some agricultural commodities. Of course, there appear to be no safe levels for these substances in some segments of the population, especially the chemically sensitive. This experience shows the widespread potential of contamination in the food chain.

Acute OP intoxication is important because of its high morbidity and long-term mortality and occurrence of muscular paralysis associated with the inhibition of AChE activity at the neuro-muscular junction. Cholinergic crisis, intermediate syndrome (IMS), and OP-induced delayed neu-ropathy (OPIDN) are the evidences that can be observed in OP intoxication. The main cause of morbidity due to OP poisoning is IMS that occurs 24–96 hours after poisoning. Mechanisms under-lying the IMS are not fully known. Although the electrophysiological aspects of delayed neuropathy are found.

In addition to malignancy and birth defects, neuropathy is known to occur due to pesticide expo-sure.[191–209] Also, Ishikawa et al.[210] have observed that the use of pesticides in Japan paralleled the occurrence of Behcet disease.

Pesticide contamination is now a global problem. Often, spraying in one area of the world will result in pesticides ending up someplace else. The spray used to kill grasshoppers in Africa, for instance, may end up in Key West, Florida, 5 days after spraying. It may then be carried up the East Coast via the Gulf Stream, across Bermuda, and into Europe (Seba, D. 1987, personal communica-tion). A few days after spraying was done in Lubbock, Texas, pesticides appeared in Cincinnati, ~1500 miles to the northeast.[211] Toxaphene pesticide sprayed in Greenville, Mississippi, has been shown to be deposited in St. Louis and 900 miles to the north in Northern Lake Michigan, and Isle Royale in Lake Superior.[211] This drift is truly a toxic wind.

Basic Mechanism of Chronic OP Exposure

Organophosphorus Ester-Induced Chronic Neurotoxicity

According to Abou-Donia et al.,[9] organophosphorus compounds are chemicals that contain both carbon and phosphorus atoms.[212] They are derivatives of phosphoric (H_3PO_4), phosphorus or phos-phonic (H_3PO_3), and phosphinic (H_3PO_2) acids (Figure 7.1). The biological action of organophospho-rus compounds is related to their phosphorylating abilities. This is dependent on the electrophilicity (positive character) of the phosphorus atom, which is determined by its substituent groups. Steric factors of substituents also play a major role in determining the biological activity of these chem-icals. Lipid solubility is important because it enhances the ability of these compounds to cross biological membranes and the blood–brain barrier, leading to increased biological activity to the detriment of the individual. This is where chemical sensitivity in some cases originates and at times propagates. Organophosphorus compounds are an economically important class of chemical com-pounds with numerous uses, such as in pesticides, industrial fluids, flame retardants, therapeutics, and nerve gas agents. They can cross membranes with holes punched or enlarged in the chemically sensitive. They combine with protein kinase A and C and when phosphorylated increase hypersen-sitivity up to 1000 times. This phenomenon can be the origin of many cases of chemical sensitivity.

Most modern synthetic organophosphorus compounds are tailor-made to inhibit AChE, an enzyme essential for life in humans and other animal species as previously stated. Tetraethylpyrophosphate was the first OP synthesized as an AChE inhibitor in 1854.[213] Later, dimethyl and diethyl phospho-rofluoridates were synthesized.[213] During World War II, organophosphorus compounds were devel-oped primarily as agricultural insecticides, and later as chemical warfare agents. The majority of organophosphorus insecticides are organophosphorothioates; nerve agents are organophosphonates or organophosphonothioates; industrial chemicals are typically OPs[214] (Table 7.21).

According to Abou-Donia et al.,[9] biologically, organophosphorus compounds are neurotoxic to humans and other animals via three distinct actions: (1) cholinergic neurotoxicity, (2) organo-phosphorus ester-induced delayed neurotoxicity (OPIDN), and (3) organophosphorus ester-induced chronic neurotoxicity (OPICN) (Figure 7.18).

TABLE 7.21

Compounds Cited in the Text and Their IUPAC Designations

Compound	IUPAC Designation
Chlorpyrifos	*O,O*-diethyl *O*-3,5,6-trichloro-2-pyridylphosphorothioate
Cyclosarin (GF)	*O*-cyclohexyl methylphosphonofluoridate
DFP	*O,O*-diisopropyl phosphorofluoridate
DEET	*N,N*-diethyl-*m*-toluamide
Diazinon	*O,O*-diethyl *O*-2-isopropyl-6-methylpyrimidin-4-yl phosphorothioate
Fenthion	*O,O*-dimethyl *O*-4 methylthio-*m*-tolyl phosphorothioate
Malathion	*S*-1,2-bis(ethoxycarbonyl)ethyl *O,O*-dimethylphosphorodithioate
Methamidophos	*O,S*-dimethyl phosphoramidothioate
Permethrin	3-phenoxybenzl (1*RS*)-*cis*-*trans*-3-(2,2-dichlorovinyl)-2,2-dimethylcyclopropanecarboxylate
Quinalphos	*O,O*-diethyl *O*-quinoxalin-2-yl phosphorothioate
Tabun (GA)	*O*-ethyl *N,N*-dimethylphosphoamidocyanidate
Sarin (GB)	*O*-isopropyl methylphosphonofluoridate
Soman (GD)	*O*-2,2-trimethypropyl methylphosphonofluoridate
TOCP	Tri-*ortho*-cresylphosphate
VX	*O*-ethyl *S*-2-diisopropylaminoethylmethylphosphonothioate
VR	*O*-isobutyl *S*-2-diethylaminoethylmethylphosphonothioate

Source: Abou-Donia, M. B. *Organophosphorus Ester-Induced Chronic Neurotoxicity.* [Accessed March 23, 2016] http://www.mindfully.org/Pesticide/2003/Organophosphorus-Neurotoxicity1aug03.html

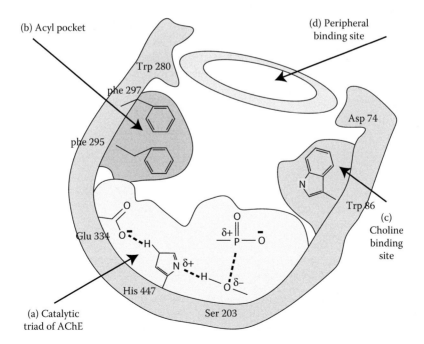

FIGURE 7.18 Sarin aged phosphonyl enzyme: methylphosphonyl acetylcholinesterase (AChE). (From Abou-Donia, M. B. *Organophosphorus Ester-Induced Chronic Neurotoxicity.* [Accessed March 23, 2016] http://www.mindfully.org/Pesticide/2003/Organophosphorus-Neurotoxicity1aug03.html.)

Cholinergic Neurotoxicity of Organophosphorus Compounds

According to Abou-Donia et al.,[9] organophosphorus compounds cause cholinergic neurotoxicity by disrupting the cholinergic system that includes AChE and its natural substrate, the neurotransmitter acetylcholine.[214] Acetylcholine is released in response to nerve stimulation and binds to postsynaptic acetylcholine receptors, resulting in muscle contraction or gland secretions. Its action is rapidly terminated by hydrolysis with AChE via the serine hydroxyl in the catalytic triad of AChE.[213] The three-dimensional structure of AChE reveals an active center located at the base of a narrow gorge about 20 μm in depth.[215] The active center includes the following sites (Figure 7.17): (1) the catalytic triad; Glu 334, His 447, and Ser 203; (2) an acyl pocket: Phe 295 and Phe 297; (3) a choline subunit: Trp 86, Glu 202, and Tyr 337; and (4) a peripheral site: Trp 286, Tyr 72, Tyr 124, and Asp 74 (Figure 7.19).

Organophosphorus ester inhibition of AChE: Organophosphorus esters inhibit AChE by phosphorylating the serine hydroxyl group at the catalytic triad site (Figure 7.17). The phosphoric or phosphonic acid ester formed with the enzyme is extremely stable and is hydrolyzed very slowly. If the phosphorylated enzyme contains methyl or ethyl groups, the enzyme is regenerated in several hours by hydrolysis. On the other hand, virtually no hydrolysis occurs with an isopropyl group (e.g., sarin) and the return of AChE is dependent upon synthesis of a new enzyme. Phosphorylated AChE undergoes aging—a process that involves the loss of an alkyl group, resulting in a negatively charged monoalkyl enzyme (Figure 7.18).[214] Organophosphorus compounds undergo detoxification by binding to other enzymes that contain the amino/acid serine. These enzymes include plasma butyrylcholinesterase (BChE)[216,217] and paraoxonase.[218,219]

Inhibition of AChE results in the accumulation of acetylcholine at both the muscarinic and nicotinic receptors in the CNS and the peripheral nervous system (PNS). Excess acetylcholine initially causes excitation, and then paralysis, of cholinergic transmission, resulting in some or all of the cholinergic symptoms, depending on the dose size, frequency of exposure, duration of exposure, and route of exposure, as well as other factors such as combined exposure to other chemicals and individual sensitivity and susceptibility.

Human exposure: According to Abou-Donia et al.,[9] human exposure mostly via inhalation to the organophosphorus nerve agent *sarin* was recently documented in two terrorist incidents in Japan. At midnight on June 27, 1994, sarin was released in Matsumoto City.[220] Of the 600

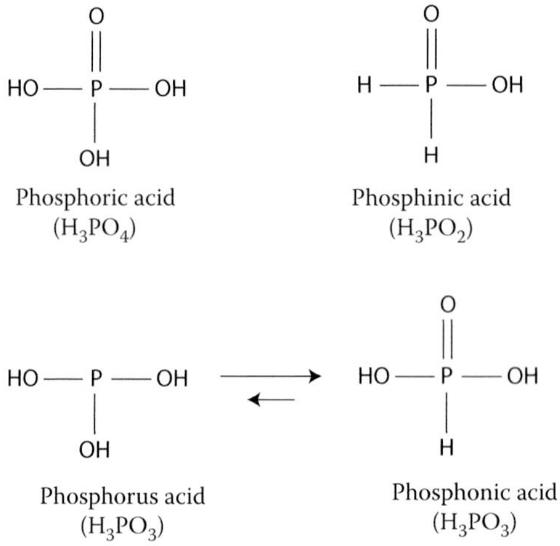

FIGURE 7.19 Chemical structures of phosphoric acid, phosphinic acid, phosphorus acid, and phosphonic acid. (From Abou-Donia, M. B. *Organophosphorus Ester-Induced Chronic Neurotoxicity*. [Accessed March 23, 2016] http://www.mindfully.org/Pesticide/2003/Organophosphorus-Neurotoxicity1aug03.html.)

persons who were exposed, 58 were admitted to hospitals, where 7 died. Although miosis was the most common symptom, severely poisoned patients developed CNS symptoms and cardio-myopathy. A few victims complained of arrhythmia and showed cardiac contraction. The second terrorist attack by *sarin* was in the Tokyo subway trains, at 3.20 a.m., 1995, when a total of 5000 persons were hospitalized and 11 died.[221] Patients with high exposure to sarin, in the Tokyo sub-way incident, exhibited marked muscle fasciculation, tachycardia, high blood pressure (nicotinic responses), sneezing, rhinorrhea, miosis, reduced consciousness, respiratory compromise, sei-zures, and flaccid paralysis.[222] Patients with mild exposure complained of headaches, dizziness, nausea, chest discomfort, abdominal cramps, and miosis. Interestingly, patients had pupillary constriction, even when their cholinesterase activity was normal. Furthermore, inhibition of red blood cell AChE activity was a more sensitive indicator of exposure than serum BChE activity.[223] The absence of bradycardia and excessive secretions which are common in dermal or ingestion exposures suggested that the major route of exposure to the sarin gas in these instances was via inhalation. The patients were treated with atropine eye drops for marked miosis, and with prali-doxime iodide (2-PAM).

Organophosphorus Ester-Induced Delayed Neurotoxicity (OPIDN) Type II

Characteristics of OPIDN: OPIDN is a neurodegenerative disorder characterized by a delayed onset of prolonged ataxia and upper motor neuron spasticity as a result of a single or repeated exposure to organophosphorus esters.[224–227] The neuropathological lesion is a central-peripheral distal axonopa-thy caused by a chemical transaction of the axon (known as Wallerian-type degeneration), followed by myelin degeneration of distal portions of the long- and large-diameter tracts of the CNS and PNS.[228] Incidents of OPIDN have been documented for over a century. The earliest recorded cases were attributed to the use of tri-*o*-cresyl phosphate (TOCP) containing creosote oil for treatment of pulmonary tuberculosis in France in 1899.[224,226,227] Later, it was used for jet engine oil which is then pumped into the cabin, causing neuropathy in jet pilots and flight attendants. In 1930, TOCP was identified as the chemical responsible for an estimated 50,000 cases of OPIDN in the Southern and Midwestern regions of the United States.[224,226,227] More recently, Himuro et al.[229] reported that a 51-year-old man who was exposed to sarin during the Tokyo subway incident and survived its acute toxicity, then died 15 months later. Neuropathological alterations and neurological deficits observed in this individual were consistent with the dying back degeneration of the NS characteris-tic of OPIDN. This incident indicated that humans are more sensitive than experimental animals to sarin-induced OPIDN, inasmuch as it required 2–28 daily doses of LD50 (25 μg/kg, intramuscular) sarin to produce OPIDN in the hen.[230] OPIDN has been divided into three classes: Type I is caused by the pentavalent phosphates and phosphonates, as well as their sulfur analogs; Type II is induced by phosphines.[231,232] All three OPIDN types are produced by organophosphorus compounds and characterized by central peripheral distal axonopathy. Type II differs from Type I in terms of the susceptibility of rodents and the presence of neuropathological lesions in neuronal cell bodies.[233] Type III OPIDN is not accompanied by inhibition of the neurotoxicity target esterase (NTE), thus casting further doubt on this enzyme as the target for OPIDN.[231,232]

Mechanisms of OPIDN: Early studies on the mechanisms of OPIDN centered on the inhibition of the esterases AChE[234] and BChE[235] by organophosphorus esters. Subsequent studies eliminated both enzymes as targets for OPIDN.[236] Johnson[237] reported an NTE an enzymatic activity preferen-tially inhibited by organophosphorus compounds capable of producing OPIDN as its target. Despite numerous studies since the introduction of this concept 35 years ago, the NTE hypothesis has not advanced our understanding of the mechanism of OPIDN because: (1) evidence for the involvement of NTE in the development of OPIDN is only correlative; (2) it has not been shown how inhibition and aging of NTE leads to axonal degeneration; (3) NTE, which is present in neuronal and non-neuronal tissues and in sensitive and insensitive species, has no known biochemical or physiological function; (4) some organophosphorus pesticides that produce OPIDN in humans do not inhibit or age NTE[238–241]; and (5) phosphines that produce Type III OPIDN do not inhibit NTE.[231,232] However, the most convincing evidence against this hypothesis is the recent finding that NTE-knockout mice are sensitive to the development of OPIDN,[242,243,1217] indicating that this enzyme is not involved in the mechanisms of OPIDN.

Protein kinases as targets for OPIDN: Because research on esterases did not increase our understanding of the mechanisms of OPIDN. Abou-Donia et al.[9] have been studying the involvement of protein kinase-mediated phosphorylation of cytoskeletal proteins in the development of OPIDN. These studies were prompted by the following observations: (1) Since organophosphorus compounds are effective phosphorylating agents, it is reasonable to expect that they would interfere with normal kinase-mediated phosphorylation of a serine or threonine group at the target protein. (2) The earliest ultrastructural alterations in OPIDN are seen mostly as aggregation and accumulation of cytoskeletal proteins, microtubules, and neurofilaments, followed by their dissolution and disappearance. (3) The structural and functional status of cytoskeletal proteins are affected significantly by protein kinase-mediated phosphorylation.

This process when Ca^{2+} goes into the cell causes hypersensitivity up to 1000 times as well as structural and functional influences.[10]

Anomalous hyperphosphorylation of cytoskeletal elements is associated with OPIDN, a neurodegenerative disorder characterized by distally located swellings in large axons of the CNS and PNS, with subsequent axonal degeneration. Central to Abou-Donia's hypothesis is the observation that increased aberrant protein kinase-mediated phosphorylation of cytoskeletal proteins could result in the destabilization of microtubules and neurofilaments, leading to their aggregation and deregulation in the axon.[244] This unstability phenomena has been observed in some chemically sensitive patients who when neutralized interdermally do not hold precise end points and due to this instability deter proper treatment. Protein kinases are able to amplify and distribute signals because a single protein kinase can phosphorylate many different target proteins. Several protein kinases are turned on by secondary messengers. For example, calcium/calmodulin-dependent protein kinase II (CaM Kinase II) is inactive until it is bound by the calcium-calmodulin complex that induces conformational changes and causes the enzyme to unfold an inhibitory domain from its active site.[245] Abou-Donia et al.[9] have demonstrated substantial increases in the autophosphorylation,[246,247] enzymatic activity,[248] protein levels, and mRNAs of CaM kinase II in hens treated with diisopropylphosphorofluoridate (DFP).[249] These aberrant alterations have resulted in increased phosphorylation of the following cytoskeletal proteins: tublin, neurofilaments, microtubule associated proteins (MAP-2),[213] and tau proteins.[249–252] Increased activity of CaM kinase II can affect the stability of cytoskeletal proteins through posttranslational modification. Phosphorylation of these proteins interrupts their interaction, polymerization, and stabilization, leading to their degeneration.[249,253,254] This is probably the reason that intradermal end points are constantly changing in some chemically sensitive patients making their hypersensitivity treatment difficult for their intradermal mold, food, and chemical end points to stabilize. The coherences of the molds, foods, and chemicals makes it possible for the treatment end points to work.

On the other hand, early studies identified transcription factors as critical phosphoproteins in signaling cascades. Immediate early genes control gene expression and therefore affect long-term cellular responses. Abou-Donia et al.[9] have demonstrated that the transcription of c-fos is elevated in OPIDN, perhaps through the activation of cAMP (adenosine monophosphate) response element binding (CREB) which is phosphorylated by CaM kinase II. Subsequent to c-fos activation,[255] they observed altered gene expression of CaM kinase II,[253] neurofilaments,[256] glial fibrillary acidic protein (GFAP), and vimentin.[257] Their results also showed an increase in medium (NF-M) and a decrease in low (NF-L) and high (NF-H) molecular weight neurofilaments in the spinal cords of hens treated with DFP.[256] This imbalance in the stoichiometry of neurofilament proteins interferes with their interaction with microtubules and promotes neurofilament dissociation from microtubules, leading to the aggregation of both cytoskeletal proteins.[258] Immunohistochemical studies in NS tissues from TOCP- and DFP-treated hens demonstrated aberrant aggregation of phosphorylated neurofilament, tubulin, and CaM kinase II.[259] This process may occur in the OP-stimulated chemically sensitive patient where we see changes in the spinal cords of some long-standing chemically sensitive patients who are exposed to OP.

Organophosphorus Ester-Induced Chronic Neurotoxicity (OPICN) Type III

Various epidemiological studies have demonstrated that individuals exposed to a single large toxic dose or too small subclinical doses of organophosphorus compounds have developed a chronic neurotoxicity that persists for years after exposure and is a distance from both cholinergic and OPIDN effects[260] which can occur by the coherence principle seen to be common for foods, molds, chemicals, and EMF mechanisms as seen in the chemically sensitive. This disorder has been variously referred to in the literature as "chronic neurobehavioral effects."[222] There are also "chronic organophosphate-induced neuropsychiatric disorder (COPIND),"[260] "psychiatric sequelae of chronic exposure,"[261] "CNS effects of chronic exposure,"[262] "psychological and neurological alterations,"[263] "long-term effects,"[264] "neuropsychological abnormalities,"[265] "central cholinergic involvement in behavioral hyperreactivity,"[266] "chorea and psychiatric changes,"[267] "chronic central nervous effects of acute OP pesticide intoxication,"[268] "chronic neurological sequelae,"[269,270] "neuropsychological effects of long-term exposure,"[271] "neurobehavioral effects,"[272] and "delayed neurologic behavioral effects of subtoxic doses."[273] The review of the literature by Abou-Dunia et al.[9] indicated that these studies describe an NS disorder induced by organophosphorus compounds which involves neuronal degeneration and subsequent neurological, neurobehavioral, and neuropsychological consequences. They will next define and describe this disorder, and refer to it as OPICN which we often observed in the OP sensitive patient with cerebral symptoms of chemical sensitivity.

Characteristics of OPICN: OPICN is produced by exposure to large, acutely toxic or small subclinical doses of organophosphorus compounds. Clinical signs, which continue for a prolonged time ranging from weeks to years after exposure, consist of neurological and neurobehavioral abnormalities. Damage is present in both the PNS and CNS, with greater involvement of the latter although involvement of the autonomic nervous systems also occurs frequently. Within the brain, neuropathological lesions are seen in various regions, including the cortex, hippocampal formation, and cerebellum. The lesions are characterized by neuronal cell death resulting from early necrosis or delayed apoptosis. Neurological and neurobehavioral alterations are exacerbated by concurrent exposure to stress or to other chemicals that cause neuronal cell death or oxidative stress. Since CNS injury predominates, improvement is slow and complete recovery at times is unlikely. However, with our rigid avoidance program, intradermal neutralization, treatment, nutritional supplementation, immune augmentation with autogenous lymphocytic factor supplementation, we see many chemically sensitive patients with these cerebral manifestations to clear their symptoms.

OPICN following large toxic exposure to organophosphorus compounds: Several studies have reported that some individuals who were exposed to large toxic doses of organophosphorus compounds, and who experienced severe acute poisoning and subsequently recover, eventually developed the long-term and persistent symptoms of OPICN. Many of the adverse effects produced by organophosphorus compounds are not related to AChE inhibition.[274] Individuals with a history of acute OP exposure reported an increased incidence of depression, irritability, confusion, and social isolation.[275] This condition is seen in some chemically sensitive patients. Such exposures resulted in decreased verbal attention, visual memory, motoricity, and affectivity.[276] Rosenstock et al.[268] reported that even a single exposure to OPs requiring medical treatment was associated with a persistent deficit in neuropsychological functions. A study of long-term effects in individuals who experienced acute toxicity with organophosphorus insecticides indicated dose-dependent decreases in sustained visual attention and vibrotactile sensitivity.[269] In another study, one-fourth of the patients who were hospitalized following exposure to methamidophos exhibited an abnormal vibrotactile threshold between 10 and 34 months after hospitalization.[277] When they develop their chemical sensitivity, these patients show imbalance and cannot stand on their toes with their eyes open or closed and cannot walk a straight line.

Case report: Callender et al.[270] have described a woman with chronic neurological sequelae following acute exposure to a combination of an organophosphorothioate insecticide, pyrethrin, piperonyl butoxide, and petroleum distillates. Initially, she developed symptoms of acute cholinergic toxicity. One month after exposure, she experienced severe frequent headaches, muscle cramps, and diarrhea. After 3.5 months, she developed numbness in her legs, tremors, memory problems, anxiety, depression, and insomnia. One year following exposure, she developed weakness, imbalance, and dizziness, and was confined to a wheelchair. Her symptoms were all characteristic of OPIDN. Twenty-eight months after exposure, she developed "delayed sequelae of gross neurologic symptoms," consisting of coarse tremors, intermittent hemiballistic movements of the right arm and leg, flaccid fasiciculations of muscle groups, muscle cramps, and sensory disturbances.

According to Abou-Donia et al.,[9] some victims of the Tokyo subway sarin incident, who developed acute cholinergic neurotoxicity, also developed long-term, chronic neurotoxicity characterized by CNS neurological deficits and neurobehavioral impairments.[222] Six to eight months after the Tokyo poisoning, some victims showed delayed effects on psychomotor performance, the visual NS, and the vestibular-cerebellar system.[278] It is noteworthy that females were more likely than males to exhibit delayed effects on the vestibular-cerebellar system, many showing imbalance and dizziness. Three years after the Matsumoto attack in Japan, some patients complained of fatigue, shoulder stiffness, weakness, and blurred vision.[220] Others complained of insomnia, bad dreams, husky voice, slight fever, and palpations. Colosio et al.[272] reviewed the literature on the neurobehavioral toxicity of pesticides, and reported that some individuals who were acutely poisoned with organophosphorus compounds developed long-term impairment of neurobehavioral performance. They also concluded that these effects were only "a specific expression of damage and not of direct neurotoxicity."

OPICN following subclinical exposures to organophosphorus compounds: Reports on OPICN in individuals following long-term, subclinical exposures, without previous acute poisoning, have been inconsistent, mostly because of difficulty in the quantitative determination of exposure levels, but also because of problems with selection of controls. Several studies of workers exposed to low subclinical doses of organophosphorus insecticides failed to show neurobehavioral alterations between pre- and postexposure measurements.[279–285] It has been suggested that the levels of exposure of subjects in these reports might have been below the threshold level needed to cause neurobehavioral deficits, and that studies of prolonged low-level exposures may eventually reveal neurobehavioral deficits.[272] Consistent with this opinion are the reports of impairment, in neurobehavioral performance in individuals exposed to low-levels of organophosphorus insecticides. Professional pesticide applicators and farmers who had been exposed to organophosphorus pesticides showed elevated levels of anxiety, impaired vigilance, and reduced concentration.[286] Kaplan et al.[287] reported persistent long-term cognitive dysfunction and defects in concentration, word finding, and short-term memory in individuals exposed to low subclinical levels of the organophosphorus insecticide chlorpyrifos. A significant increase in hand vibration threshold was reported in a group of pesticide applicators,[288] and significant cognitive and neuropsychological deficits have been found in sheep dippers who had been exposed to organophosphorus insecticides.[282,283] Male fruit farmers who were chronically exposed to organophosphrous insecticides showed significant slowing of their reaction time.[289] Female pesticide applicators exhibited longer reaction times, reduced motor steadiness, and increased tension, depression, and fatigue compared with controls.[284] Workers exposed to the organophosphorus insecticide quinalphos during its manufacture exhibited alterations in CNS function that were manifested as memory, learning, vigilance, and motor deficits, despite having normal AChE activity.[290] Rescue workers and some victims who did not develop any acute neurotoxicity symptoms nevertheless complained of a chronic decline in memory 3 years and 9 months after the Tokyo attack.[291] Pilkington et al.[265] reported a strong association between chronic low-level exposure to OP concentrates in sheep dips and neurological symptoms in sheep dippers, suggesting that long-term health effects may occur in at least some sheep dippers exposed to these insecticides over their working lives.

Neurological and neurobehavioral alterations: Although the symptoms of OPICN are a consequence of damage to both the PNS and CNS, they are related primarily to CNS injury and resultant neurological and neurobehavioral abnormalities. Studies on the effects of exposure to organophosphorus compounds over the past half century have shown that chronic neurological and neurobehavioral symptoms include headache, drowsiness, dizziness, anxiety, apathy, mental confusion, restlessness, labile emotions, anorexia, insomnia, lethargy, fatigue, inability to concentrate, memory deficits, depression, irritability, confusion, generalized weakness, and tremors.[261,262,292,293] Respiratory, circulatory, and skin problems may be present as well in cases of chronic toxicity.[212] It should be noted that not every patient exhibits all of these symptoms. Gershon and Shaw[261] reported that most of the symptoms that develop after OP exposure resolve within 1 year. We have not found this to be true for the chemically sensitive patient who lives next to or in a farm where OP are sprayed or a home that is frequently sprayed. Jamal[260] conducted an extensive review of the health effects of organophosphorus compounds and concluded that either acute or long-term, low-level exposure to these chemicals produces a number of chronic neurological and psychiatric abnormalities that he called "chronic organophosphate-induced neuropsychiatric disorder," or COPIND. Jamal recommended a multifaceted approach to the evaluation of the toxic effects of chronic, subclinical, repeated, low-level exposures to organophosphorus compounds; included were structural and quantitative analyses of symptoms and clinical neurological signs. In the present article, the concept of OPICN encompasses structural, functional, physiological, neurological, and neurobehavioral abnormalities, including neuropsychiatric alterations or COPIND. OPICN may be caused by an acute exposure that results in cholinergic toxicity, or by exposure to subclinical doses that do not produce acute poisoning.

Neuropathological alterations: Petras[294] investigated the neuropathological alterations in rat brains 15–28 days following intramuscular injections of large, acutely toxic doses (79.4–114.8 μg/kg) of the nerve agent soman. He reported that the brain damage in all four animals that developed seizures was comparable to damage present in three of the four animals that exhibited only limb tremor. Neuropathological lesions were characterized by axonal degeneration seen in the cerebral cortex, basal ganglia, thalamus, subthalamic region, hypothalamus, hippocampus, fornix, septum, preoptic area, superior colliculus, pretectal area, basilar pontine nuclei, medullary tegmentum, and corticospinal tracts. Although the mechanism of soman-induced brain injury was not known, Petras noted that the lesions did not resemble those present in experimental fetal hypoxia[295] or OPIDN.[228] These results are consistent with later findings obtained after acute soman exposure,[296,297] exposure to the nerve agent sarin,[298] and neuronal necrosis induced by the organophosphorus insecticide fenthion.[299] Petras also indicated that soman-treated rats did not need to experience a seizure to develop lesions. Abdel-Rahman et al.[300] demonstrated neuropathological alterations in rat brain 24 hours after administration of an intramuscular LD_{50} dose (100 μg/kg) of sarin. Neuronal degeneration was present in the cerebral cortex, dentate gyrus, CA1 and CA3 subfields of the hippocampal formation, and the in Purkinje cells of the cerebellum. Neuronal degeneration of hippocampal cells is consistent with organophosphorus compound-induced alterations in behavior and cognitive deficits such as impaired learning and memory.[301–304] Furthermore, chronic exposure to organophosphorus compounds resulted in long-term cognitive deficits, even in the absence of clinical signs of acute cholinergic toxicity.[305,306] Shih et al.[307] demonstrated that lethal doses (2 × LD50) of all tested nerve agents (i.e., tabun, sarin, soman, cyclosarin, VR, and VX) induced seizures accompanied by neuropathological lesions in the brains of guinea pigs, similar to those lesions reported for other organophosphorus compounds in other species.[308–313] Recent reports have indicated that anticonvulsants protected guinea pigs against soman- and sarin-induced seizures and the development of neuropathological lesions.[314,315] Time-course studies have also reported that sarin-induced brain lesions exacerbated over time and extended into brain areas that are not initially affected.[298,316] Kim et al.[317] found that an intraperitoneal injection of 9 mg/kg (1.8 × LD50) DFP in rats protected with pyridostigmine bromide (PB) and atropine nitrate caused tonic–clonic seizures, followed by prolonged and mild clonic epilepsy accompanied by early necrotic and delayed apoptotic neuronal degeneration. Early necrotic brain injury in the hippocampus and piriform/entorhinal cortices was seen between 1 and 12 hours after dosing. On the other hand, typical apoptotic terminal deoxy-nucleotidyl transferase-mediated dUTP-X nick end labeling (TUNEL)-positive cell death began to appear at 12 hours in the thalamus. Daily dermal administration of 0.01 × LD50 of malathion for 28 days caused neuronal degeneration in the rat brain that was exacerbated by combined exposure to the insect repellent DEET and/or the insecticide permethrin.[318]

Correlation between neuropathological lesions and neurological and neurobehavioral altera-tions: According to Abou-Donia et al.,[9] neuropathological changes, the hallmark of OPICN, could explain the neurological, neurobehavioral, and neuropsychological abnormalities reported in humans and animals exposed to organophosphorus compounds. A subcutaneous dose of 104 μg/kg soman-induced status epilepticus in rats, followed by degeneration of neuronal cells in the piriform cortex and CA3 of the hippocampus.[313] Similar results have been reported in a variety of species.[308,319,320] In another study, only those mice treated with a subcutaneous dose of 90 μg/kg of soman which developed long-lasting convulsive seizures exhibited the neuropathological altera-tions.[321] Twenty-four hours after dosing, numerous eosinophilic cells and deoxyribonucleic acid (DNA) fragmentation (TUNEL-positive) cells were observed in the lateral septum, the endiopiri-form and entorhinal cortices, the dorsal thalamus, the hippocampus, and the amygdala. Animals that had only slight tremors and no convulsions did not show any lesions.[321] Guinea pigs given a subcutaneous dose of 200 μg/kg soman (2 × LD50) developed seizures and exhibited neuropatho-logical lesions in the amygdala; the substantia nigra; the thalamus; the piriform, entorhinal, and perirhinal cortices; and the hippocampus between 24 and 48 hours following injection.[314] Male guinea pigs developed epileptiform seizures after receiving 2 × LD50 subcutaneous doses of the following nerve agents: tabun (240 μg/kg) sarin 84 μg/kg), soman (56 μg/kg), cyclosarin (11 μg/kg), VX (16 μg/kg), or VR (22 μg/kg). The seizures were accompanied by necrotic death of neuro-nal cells, with the amygdala having the most severe injury followed by the cortex and the caudate nucleus.[307]

An intraperitoneal injection of 9 mg/kg (1.8 × LD50) DFP caused severe early (15–90 minutes) tonic–clonic limbic seizures, followed by prolonged mild clonic epilepsy.[317] Necrotic cell death was seen 1 hour after DFP administration, primarily in the CA1 and CA3 subfields of the hippocampus and piriform/entorhinal cortices, and manifest as degeneration of neuronal cells and spongiform of neurophils. Whereas the severity of hippocampal injury remained the same for up to 12 hours, damage to the piriform/entorhinal cortices, thalamus, and amygdala continue to increase up to 12 hours. Furthermore, apoptotic death of neuronal cells (TUNEL-positive) was seen in the thala-mus at 12 hours, and peaked at 24 hours. Rats that survived 1 × LD50 sarin (95 μg/kg) exhibited persistent lesions, mainly in the hippocampus, pyriform cortex, and thalamus.[298] Furthermore, brain injury was exacerbated over time; at 3 months after exposure, other areas that were not initially affected became damaged. A recent study has described the early neuropathological changes in the adult male rat brain 24 hours after exposure to a single intramuscular dose of 1.0, 0.5, 0.1, or 0.01 × LD50 (100 μg/kg) sarin.[300] Sarin at 1.0 × LD50 caused extensive severe tremors, seizures, and con-vulsions accompanied by damage involving mainly the cerebral cortex, the hippocampal formation (dentate gyrus, and CA1, and CA3 subfields) and the cerebellum. Damage was evidenced by (1) a significant inhibition of plasma BChE, brain region AChE, and M2 M-acetylcholine receptor-ligand binding; (2) an increase in permeability of the blood–brain barrier; and (3) diffuse neuronal cell death coupled with decreased MAP-2 expression within the dendrites of surviving neurons. The 0.5 × LD50 sarin dose did not cause motor convulsions, and only moderate Purkinje neuron loss. The 0.1 and 0.01 × LD50 doses of sarin caused no alterations at 24 hours after dosing. These results indicate that sarin-induced acute brain injury is dose dependent. However, in the chemically sensi-tive humans who are sensitized to a whole host of chemicals, seizures and hippocampus charges may occur at lower levels.

In animals treated with 1 × LD50 sarin, both superficial layers (I–III) and deeper layers (IV–V) of the motor cortex and somatosensory cortex showed degeneration of neurons. In the deeper layers of the cortex, neuron degeneration was seen in layer V. Pyramidal neurons in layers III and V of the cortex are the source of the axons of the corticospinal tract, which is the largest descending fiber tract (or motor pathway) from the brain controlling movements of various contralateral muscle groups. Thus, sarin-induced death of layers III and V neurons of the motor cortex could lead to considerable motor and sensory abnormalities, ataxia, weakness, and loss of strength. Furthermore, disruption of the hippocampal circuitry because of the degeneration of neurons in different subfields can lead to learning and memory deficits. Lesions in the cerebellum could result in gait and coordination abnormalities which we often see in the severe chemically sensitive patient as seen in the autistic and other individuals with chemical sensitivity. Since the severely affected areas (e.g., the limbic system, corticofugal system, and central motor system) are associated with mood, judgment, motion, posture, locomotion, and skilled movements, humans exhibiting acute toxicity symptoms following exposure to large doses of OPs may also develop psychiatric and motor deficits. Inasmuch as the severely damaged areas of the brain do not usually regenerate, these symptoms are expected to persist long-term.[322–324] However, recent studies with pain in patients suggests that the brain can shrink one-third with pain and then expand where the pain is relieved. These findings are in agreement with a recent study by Kilburn[325] who evaluated the neurobehavioral effects of chronic low-level exposure to the organophosphorus insecticide chlorpyrifos in 22 patients. Kilburn demonstrated an association between chlorpyrifos sprayed inside homes and offices and neurophysiological impairments in balance, visual fields, color discrimination, hearing reaction time, and grip strength. These patients also had psychological impairment of verbal recall and cognitive function, and two-thirds of them had been prescribed antidepressant drugs. In addition, the patients exhibited severe respiratory symptoms, accompanied by airway obstruction. Other chlorpyrifos-induced neurotoxicity incidents in humans have been reported.[326] These results are consistent with the report that daily dermal application of 0.1 mg/kg chlorpyrifos to adult rats resulted in sensorimotor deficits.[327] Also, material exposure to a daily dermal dose of 0.1 mg/kg chlorpyrifos during gestational days 4–20 caused an increased expression of GFAP in the cerebellum and hippocampus of offspring on postnatal day 30.[328] A major component of astrocytic intermediate neurofilaments, GFAP is upregulated in response to reactive gliosis resulting from insults such as trauma, neurodegenerative disease, and exposure to neurotoxicants.[329]

Mechanisms of OPICN: Recent studies have shown that large toxic doses of organophosphorus compounds cause early convulsive seizures and subsequent encephalopathy, leading to the necrotic death of brain neuronal cells, whereas small doses produce delayed apoptotic death. Pazdernik et al.[313] have proposed the following five phases that result in organophosphorus compound-induced cholinergic seizures: (1) initiation, (2) limbic status epilepticus, (3) motor convulsions, (4) early excitotoxic damage, and (5) delayed oxidative stress. The mechanisms of neuronal cell death in OPICN that appear to be mediated through necrosis or apoptosis, which may involve increased AChE gene expression, are discussed below.

Necrosis: The large toxic doses of organophosphorus compounds which induce early seizures activating the glutamatergic system and involve the Ca^{2+}-related exicitotoxic process,[330,331] possibly mediated by the *N*-methyl-D-aspartate (NMDA) subtype of glutamate receptors.[332,333] This is where the initiation of chemical sensitivity occurs in many chemically sensitive patients. When this hypersensitivity occurs, food, molds, and other chemicals are introduced into the hypersensitivity, exacerbating and triggering more illness. deGroot[314] hypothesized that accumulated acetylcholine, resulting from acute inhibition of AChE by organophosphorus compounds, leads to activation of glutamatergic neurons and the release of the excitatory L-glutamate amino acid neurotransmitter. This in turn produces increased depolarization and subsequent activation of the NMDA subtype of glutamate receptors—and the opening of NMDA ion channels—resulting in massive Ca^{2+} fluxes into the postsynaptic cell and causing neuronal degeneration but also hypersensitivity. Thus, glutamate-induced neuronal degeneration during seizures may occur as a result of lowering of the threshold for glutamate excitation at NMDA receptor sites.

Activation of nitric oxide synthase, following stimulation of NMDA receptor sites, increases the level of nitric oxide (NO), which functions as a signaling or cytotoxic molecule responsible for neuronal cell death.[334] As a retrograde messenger, NO induces the release of several neurotransmitters, including excitatory amino acid L-glutamate[335] which alters neurotransmitter balance and affects neuronal excitability. The production of NO is enhanced in AChE-inhibitor-induced seizures.[336,337] Kim et al.[317] demonstrated the involvement of NO in OP-induced seizures and the effectiveness of NO synthesis inhibitors in preventing such seizures. Pall has elicited and elaborated on the presence of NO in chemical sensitivity. (In Chapter 5 Nitric Oxide section for more information.)

Apoptosis and oxidative stress: Neuronal degeneration caused by apoptosis or programmed cell death may have physiologic or pathologic consequences. Elimination of precancerous, old, or excess cells is carried out by apoptosis without injury to surrounding cells as seen in necrosis.[338] Small doses of organophosphorus compounds cause delayed neuronal cell death that involves free radical generation (i.e., ROS) as shown earlier in this book. OPs that cause mitochondrial damage/dysfunction also cause depletion of ATP and increased generation of ROS, which results in oxidative stress.[339,340] ROS can cause fatal depletion of mitochondrial energy (ATP), induction of proteolytic enzymes, and DNA fragmentation, leading to apoptotic death.[339,341,342] These results are consistent with the DNA damage detected in the lymphocytes in peripheral blood in eight individuals, following residential exposure to the organophosphorus insecticides, chlorpyrifos and diazinon.[343] This sequence appears to occur in many chemically sensitive patients that we have treated at the EHC-Dallas.

The brain is highly susceptible to oxidative stress-induced injury for several reasons: (1) its oxygen requirements are high; (2) it has a high rate of glucose consumption; (3) it contains large amounts of peroxidizable fatty acids; and (4) it has relatively low antioxidant capacity.[341,342] A single sublethal dose of $0.5 \times LD_{50}$ sarin, which did not induce seizures, nevertheless caused delayed apoptotic death of rat brain neurons in the cerebral cortex, hippocampus, and Purkinje cells of the cerebellum 24 hours after dosing.[300,343] Furthermore, rats treated with a single $0.1 \times LD_{50}$ dose of sarin, and which did not exhibit brain histopathological alterations 1,7, or 30 days after dosing, nevertheless showed apoptotic death of brain neurons in the same areas mentioned above, 1 year after dosing.[300,344] These results are consistent with the sensorimotor deficits exhibited by sarin-treated animals 3 months after exposure; the animals showed continued deterioration when tested 6 months after dosing.

Increased AChE gene expression: Recent studies have suggested that AChE may play a role in the pathogenesis of OPICN similar to that reported for AD.[345,346] Abou-Donia et al.[9] have demonstrated that sarin induced the AChE gene in the same regions of the brain that underwent neuronal degeneration.[347] AChE has been shown to be neurotoxic *in vivo* and *in vitro*; it accelerates the assembly of amyloid peptide in Alzheimer's fibrils, leading to cell death via apoptosis.[348] Some studies have demonstrated increased AChE expression in apoptotic neuroblastoma SK-N-SH cells after long-term culturing.[348] Brain AChE has been shown to be toxic to neuronal (neuro 2a) and glial-like (B12) cells.[346] There are also reports that transgenic mice overexpressing human AChE in brain neurons undergo progressive cognitive deterioration.[349] These results suggest that sarin may provoke an endogenous cell suicide pathway cascade in susceptible neurons (e.g., in the caspase-3 pathway), resulting in the release of AChE into adjacent brain tissues. The aggregation of AChE intiates more apoptotic neuronal death. Amplification of this cascade thus may result in the progressive neuronal loss that is the hallmark of sarin-induced chronic neurotoxicity. It is noteworthy that a common symptom of both PIICN and AD is memory deficit, suggesting that the aging process may be accelerated following exposure to organophosphorus compounds in OPICN. We have observed this process in the long-term chemically sensitive patient.

Other factors: According to Abou-Donia et al.,[9] the occurrence and severity of OPICN is influenced by factors such as environmental exposure to other chemicals, foods, molds, virus, bacteria, stress, or individual genetic differences. For example, cholinotoxicants such as OPs or carbamates—which do not have a positive charge and are capable of crossing the blood–brain barrier—act at the same receptors and thus exacerbate OPICN. Individuals with low levels of the plasma enzymes BChE[216,217,350] or paraoxonase[218,219] that act as the first line of defense against neurotoxicity (by removing OPs from circulation through scavenging hydrolysis) are vulnerable to the development of persistent OPICN. All of these factors may be involved in the development of the "chemical sensitivity." Thus, prior chemical exposure stress, or genetic factors, might make individuals predisposed or susceptible to CNS injury upon subsequent exposure to other chemicals. This phenomenon is often seen in the chemically sensitive when their total pollutant load is increased.

According to Abou-Donia et al.,[9] combined exposure to other chemicals that cause oxidative stress can intensify OPICN which results from exposure to organophosphorus compounds.[318] The total body pollutant load thus increases the susceptibility to the OP, creating the chemical sensitivity and making those that have it more vulnerable. Furthermore, stress that also causes oxidative stress decreases the threshold level required to produce neuronal damage and results in increased OPICN following combined exposure to total body pollutant load, and to stress and OPs. Thus, OPICN may explain the reports that Persian Gulf War Veterans showed a higher than normal propensity toward persistent neurological complaints such as memory and attention deficits, irritability, chronic fatigue, muscle and joint pain, and poor performance on cognition tests.[351–355] A large number of these personnel were exposed to low levels of sarin during the demolition of Iraqi munitions at Khamisya,[356,357] as well as to other chemicals and total body pollutant load stress.[358,359] Also, OPICN may explain the recent report that Persian Gulf War Veterans are at an almost two-fold greater risk of developing amyotrophic lateral sclerosis (ALS) than other veterans,[360] which is consistent with Haley's[361] suggestion that the increase in ALS is "a war-related environmental trigger." Furthermore, OPICN induced by low-level inhalation of OPs, that is, tricresyl phosphate present in jet engine lubricating oils and the hydraulic fluids of aircraft[362] could explain the long-term neurologic deficits consistently reported by crewmembers and passengers, although OP levels may have been too low to produce OPIDN.[363]

Prognosis: Previous reports have indicated that, subsequent to exposure to organophosphorus compounds, an individual could develop acute cholinergic neurotoxicity, followed by OPICN. In a few cases, OPIDN may occur with or without the development of cholinergic neurotoxicity, with OPICN developing later. Furthermore, OPICN may occur following long-term, low-level exposure to organophosphorus compounds, and without the development of acute neurotoxicity. Since the long-term, persistent effects of OPICN result from neuronal degeneration of the PNS and CNS, induced by OPs, it is unlikely that improvement is the consequence of the regeneration of brain neurons, inasmuch as such repair is not typical of the CNS. However, repair may occur in the chemically sensitive with loss of mild edema, local oxidative stress, and repair of membrane integrity and internal cell elements. Clinical improvement may also occur, however, through the repair of the PNS. Also, reversible changes in the CNS that might be present initially (e.g., edema) could later subside, giving the appearance of repair. Furthermore, if damage is not too extensive, other neurons having the same function could meet the added demands and maintain normal activity. Apoptosis could be stopped by cessation of exposure not leading to necrosis. Also, healing may leave minsours which can lend to mini seizures. When the CNS is severely damaged, however, neither of these repair mechanisms is possible and some loss of function will likely occur.

Conclusions: Herein it has been described how the long-term persistent neurodegenerative disorder induced by exposure to organophosphorus compounds occurs. Numerous cases documenting this disorder have been reported since the extensive use of these chemicals in industry and agriculture began >50 years ago. Although largely characterized by chronic neurobehavioral alterations, OPICN involves other molecular neurochemical, neurophysiological, neuropathological, neuropsychological, and neurological changes, and chemical sensitivity being induced. The term "neurotoxicity" encompasses all of these, and adequately describes this neurodegenerative disorder.

Synergistic Effects of Pesticides

Some OP pesticides, foods, and other pesticides produce cancer, birth defects, neurotoxicity, and kidney and liver damage,[364] and chemical sensitivity due to their coherence effect. Synergistic effects of several pesticides may increase toxicity and definitely increase sensitivity. EPN and malathion, two OP pesticides, for example, have been found to have 50 times greater synergistic toxicity in rats.[365] A similar type of synergism may occur with solvent cohorts, which usually accompany pesticides as penetrating agents. Since studies for synergistic effects of pesticides are not required by the EPA for registration of these substances, they rarely undergo such testing except in the environmental medicine specialist's office. Owing to lack of study, public information on toxicity and sensitivity is limited. Our observations show that the higher the total pollutant load, the more toxic it is and the more sensitive the exposed individual becomes to the pesticide. Also, age has to do with the susceptibility. Children are more vulnerable.

Because of play behaviors, hand-to-mouth behaviors, type of clothing worn, and other habits, children are more likely than adults to spend time on treated turf and to have greater direct contact with the turf. In addition, children's breathing rates are higher, while they have smaller bodies with greater relative surface area, all of which make them likely to have higher relative exposure to lawn chemicals than adults.[364]

We have seen the graphic effects of the use of lawn chemicals on a 4-year-old child who presented at the EHC-Dallas with gangrene of her left foot (Figure 7.20). This patient had given a history of rolling and playing in a recently treated lawn for 1 day. She developed nausea, vomiting, and swelling of her left leg. She was admitted to a children's hospital in Florida and thought to have either a clot in the femoral artery and vein or extremely severe vasospasm. The attending physicians could not differentiate by their tests. She was tried with intravenous antibiotic and anticoagulants and transferred to the EHC-Dallas. This patient was placed on good environmental control and gradually cleared. She only lost the tips of three toes. Subsequent challenge showed this patient was sensitive to pesticides, petrochemicals, and chlorine. She also had multiple food sensitivities. She has done well for 2 years on injection therapy for food and inhalants and avoidance of toxic exposures (Figures 7.20 and 7.21). Now at 18 years past environmental treatment, she has remained free of vascular and other diseases.

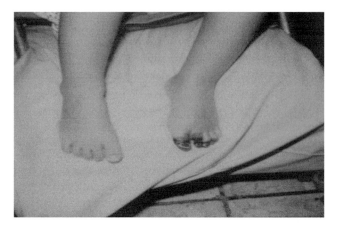

FIGURE 7.20   (See color insert.) Four-year-old white female. After exposure to lawn pesticides, gangrene of foot developed.

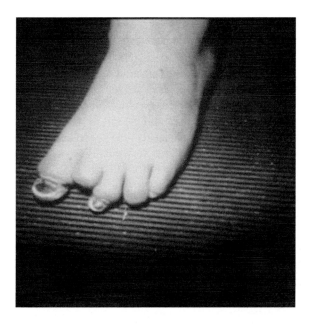

FIGURE 7.21 (**See color insert.**) Four-year-old white female. After ECU treatment: minimal loss of toes; foot and leg intact.

It appears that sensitivity may be triggered at any age. More serious acute effects appear to be produced by direct inhalation of pesticide sprays rather than by skin absorption or ingestion of contaminated foods and water, although pesticide residues in foods are almost certainly the most widespread source of exposure and are highly significant in many people. Glyphosate is one of the more common ones which occurs on genetically affected wheat. All pesticides can produce toxicity and sensitivity in humans. The chemically sensitive are particularly prone to pesticides in food and usually need to eat organic food.

Although acute, high-level exposure to some OP pesticides is known to result in delayed peripheral neuropathy as just shown[366]; the PNS effects of long-term exposure at levels insufficient to cause clinical toxicity are more controversial but quite evident. Most research has focused on the CNS effects of long-term OP pesticide exposure with a majority of studies of nonpoisoned individuals reporting increase in neurologic symptoms or impaired neurobehavioral function following OP exposure.[367] Few studies have examined associations among participants without prior pesticide poisoning.[368] The results of these studies vary, possibly due to differences in exposure characterization, comparison populations, measures of PNS function, and small sample sizes.[367,369]

Starks et al.[370] observed significant associations between the use of several OP pesticides and neurological physical examination (NPx) abnormalities among pesticide applicators. No single pesticide was uniformly associated with all neurological measures and no one measure was uniformly associated with all pesticides. Toe proprioception was the most responsive NPx outcome and was associated with 6 of 16 OP pesticides. Significant exposure–response relationships were observed for several pesticides, including those shown in Table 7.21 suggesting that associations between these pesticides and toe proprioception abnormality were not spurious. For most other outcomes, they observed mostly null associations and a few significant inverse associations between OP pesticide use and other PNS outcomes. Despite the inconsistency in finding across the outcome measures together results provide some evidence that long-term exposure to specific OP pesticides may adversely affect the PNS.

Published studies show considerable variability in association between OP pesticide exposure and PNS outcomes. Studies of PNS function among pesticide workers vary with respect to the populations studied (manufacturing workers to pesticide applicators), outcomes assessed (e.g., neurological signs and symptoms, electrophysiological tests, etc.), exposure characterization, inclusion of pesticide poisoned individuals, and age of participants. In a study of 123 OP pesticide applicators (mean age = 37 years) and 123 nonapplicators (mean age = 37 years), significantly elevated OPs were observed for motor coordination signs, deep tendon reflexes, and reduced muscle strength among the most heavily exposed applicators.[371] Contrary to Starks et al.[370] results, a borderline association was observed for vibrotactile threshold but not for toe vibration abnormality on NPx. In a study of 164 OP pesticide applicators (mean age = 34 years) and 83 unexposed controls (mean age = 33 years), neither vibrotactile threshold nor tremor was associated with pesticide exposure. In a study comparing 191 OP termiticide applicators (mean age = 39 years) to 106 unexposed friends (mean age = 38 years) and 83 unexposed workers (mean age = 3 years), no difference was observed between applicators and either comparison group on NPx outcomes or measures of great toe vibrotactile threshold.[368] However, mean sway path length was significantly longer among the applicators.

PNS symptoms were assessed with a questionnaire and quantitative measures of vibrotactile and thermal thresholds were administered to 612 "sheep dipping" farmers in the United Kingdom and exposed to OP pesticides (mostly younger than 55 years) and 160 unexposed referents.[372] Neurological symptoms were not associated with total number of dipping days or cumulative OP exposure. Cumulative OP exposure was not associated with cutaneous temperature perception or vibrotactile threshold. Handling of OP concentrate was associated with symptoms and marginally associated with cutaneous cold temperature perception.

Vibrotactile thresholds were measured among 68 male pesticide applicators in New York State (most 50 years of age) and 68 referents matched for age, sex, and county of residence.[373] Azinphosmethyl was the most commonly used insecticide. Poorer vibrotactile acuity of the fingers and toes was observed among the applicators.

Stark et al.[370] observed significant adverse associations between abnormal toe vibration on NPx and two OP pesticides (dichlorvos and tetrachlorvinphos) whereas they did not observe associations between quantitative toe vibrotactile thresholds and these chemicals.

In this study of 678 licensed pesticide applicators with well-characterized lifetime exposure to OP pesticides, their findings provide evidence that long-term exposure to some OP pesticides may be associated with selected indices of poorer NS function among pesticide applicators with no previous history of diagnosed pesticide poisoning. The most consistent associations were with the clinical NPx outcomes, particularly toe proprioception, which was significantly associated with ever use of chlorpyrifos, coumaphos, dichlorvos, fonofos, phosmet, and tetrachlorvinphos. Furthermore, monotonic increases in OPs were observed for abnormal toe proprioception and chlopyrifos, fonofos, and phosmet. Especially for this outcome, the number of pesticides with significant adverse associations and the observation of dose–response relationships suggest that they are the result of long-term pesticide exposure rather than chance alone.

AGENT ORANGE: DIOXIN HERBICIDE

Over the past 2 years, federal officials say an estimated 10,000 more veterans have sought medical compensation for diseases related to Agent Orange, a herbicide that contains a toxic chemical dioxin. In a recent report, the Institute of Medicine said there is sufficient evidence of an association between exposure to Agent Orange and illnesses, including soft-tissue sarcoma, non-Hodgkin lymphoma, chronic lymphocytic leukemia, Hodgkin lymphoma, and chloracne. The report recommended further research to determine whether there could be a link between Agent Orange exposure and other illnesses such as chronic obstructive pulmonary disorder, tonsil cancer, melanoma, and AD.

Even if data are limited to long-term human exposure to OP pesticides, without poisoning, results show that illness is associated with adverse PNS.

Starks et al.[370] investigated associations between OP pesticide use and PNS function. Starks et al.[370] administered Peripheral nerve studies (PNS) tests to 701 male pesticide applicators in the Agricultural Health Study (AHS). The participants completed an NPx, electrophysiological tests, and tests of hand strength, sway speed, and vibrotactile threshold. Self-reported information on lifetime use of 16 OP (Table 7.22) #8 pesticides were received from AHS interviews and a study questionnaire. Associations between pesticide use and measures of PNS function were estimated with linear and logistic regression controlling for age and outcome-specific covariates. Significantly increased ORs were observed for associations between ever use of 10 of the 16 OP pesticides and one or more of the six NPx outcomes. Most notably, abnormal proprioception was significantly associated with every use of six OP pesticides with ORs ranging from 2.03 to 3.06; monotonic increases in strength of association with increasing use was observed for three of the six pesticides Mostly null associations were observed between OP pesticide use and electrophysiological tests, hand strength, sway speed, and vibrotactile threshold. This study provides some evidence that long-term exposure to OP pesticides is associated with signs of impaired peripheral nerve function among pesticide applicators.

TABLE 7.22

Demographic Characteristics, Personal Health Information, and Occupational Exposure among 678 Male Licensed Pesticide Applicators in the Agricultural Health Study

Characteristic	Mean	SD	N	%
Age (years)	61.2	11.6	–	–
Height (cm)	179.1	6.4	–	–
BMI (kg/m^2)	28.7	4.0	–	–
Foot temperature (°C)	31.9	0.8	–	–
Testing location				
Iowa	–	–	342	50.4
North Carolina	–	–	336	49.6
Education				
≤High school	–	–	344	50.7
>High school	–	–	334	49.3
Smoking status				
Never smoked	–	–	390	57.5
Current smoker	–	–	43	6.3
Past smoker	–	–	245	36.1
Alcohol consumption[a]				
0 drinks	–	–	389	57.4
1–7 drinks	–	–	225	33.2
>7 drinks	–	–	64	9.4
Pesticide poisoning	–	–	8	1.2
Solvent exposure	–	–	279	41.2
Soldering exposure	–	–	34	5.0
Welding exposure	–	–	136	20.1
Inner ear surgery	–	–	14	2.1
Ear infection in the past 12 months	–	–	17	2.5

Source: Starks S. E. et al. 2012. Peripheral nervous system function and organophosphate pesticide use among licensed pesticide applicators in the agricultural health study. *Environ. Health Perspect.* 120(4):515–520.

[a] The average number of drinks/week during the past 12 months.

Genetically Engineered

A new problem has occurred with OP pesticide. This is genetically engineered (GE) soy, corn, cotton, and alfalfa to tolerate more OP pesticides. Regulators have known since 1980 that Roundup, an OP herbicide manufactured by the U.S. company Monsanto (glyphosate), causes birth defects, and have done nothing to make the information public.[374]

This is not the first instance of accusations against the world's best-selling herbicide. Earlier this year, researchers found that genetically modified (GM) crops used in conjunction with Roundup contain a pathogen that may cause animal miscarriages (Huber, D., professor emeritus at Purdue).[374]

GMO and Peripheral Neuropathy: OPs

GMO OPs are now being used on American farm land. They have many dangers not only for the future food production but for the health and disability of humans.

Dow Agro Sciences (a subsidiary of Dow Chemicals) have developed a new generation of GM crops—soybeans, corn, and cotton—that are engineered to resist weeds. The herbicide is called 2,4-dichlorophenoxyacetic acid (2,4-D), which was a major ingredient in Agent Orange. Once the 2,4-D-resistant seeds are released, it means farmers will be spraying massive amounts of the herbicide onto the U.S. farmland; health effects linked to 2,4-D include birth defects, blood, liver, and kidney toxicity. The 2,4-D-resistant crops are being touted as a solution to Monsanto's Roundup Ready (RR) crops, which have triggered the creation of super weeds; however, the new crops will likely only add to the problem of herbicide farmland, exposing millions to their harmful effects.

Many protests have occurred against GMO products. France and England have led the protest. However, India and many of the other European countries are lining up against GMO foods. Peru went so far as a 10-year ban on them. Europe also banned them.[374] One study has shown that 99.8% dilution of "RR" (glyphosate) can still cause DNA damage. Tens of thousands of toxics have been applied worldwide. Polyoxyethylene amine, a surfactant in the Roundup coupled with glyphosate the active ingredient causes a synergetic effect.

Increased risk of malignant lymphoma has been found in farmers in California,[375] Iowa,[376,377] Minnesota, Utah,[378] Wisconsin,[379] and New Zealand,[380] and in grain mill workers.[18] Increased risk of leukemia,[379,381–388] multiple myeloma,[376,377,379,380,386,389–393] testicular cancer,[379,394–398] liver and pancreatic cancer,[375,376,379,387,399–406] lung cancer,[375,392,404,406–409] and brain cancer[375,379,385,397,407,409–411] has also been reported.

A major new scientific study has confirmed growing conviction that the world's most widely used chemical herbicide, Monsanto Corporation's Roundup is toxic and a danger to human as well as animal organisms. The latest scientific research carried out by a multinational scientific team headed by Professor Andres Carrasco, head of the Laboratory of Molecular Embryology at the University of Buenos Aires Medical School and member of Argentina's National Council of Scientific and Technical Research, presents alarming demonstration that Monsanto and the GMO agribusiness industry have systematically not divulged the toxicity and the safety of Roundup. Roundup in far lower concentrations than used in agriculture is linked to birth defects. The health implications are huge. All major GMO crops on the market today are genetically manipulated to "tolerate" the herbicide Roundup.

Glyphosate was patented by Monsanto in the 1970s well before GMO was commercialized, as a so-called broad-spectrum weed killer. It is typically sprayed and absorbed through the leaves, or used as a forestry herbicide. It was initially patented and sold by Monsanto under the trade name *Roundup*, which also contains nondisclosed added chemicals the company refuses to divulge for "trade secret" reasons. As of 2005, 87% of all U.S. soybean fields were planted with glyphosate-resistant varieties of GMO soybeans and sprayed with Roundup.

Because the seeds of Monsanto RR GMO soybeans or other crops have been manipulated solely to be "resistant" to Roundup herbicide, while all other plant life in the field is killed by Roundup, farmers using RR seeds must also purchase Roundup herbicide, making a captive market for both seed and chemicals.

The problem with this cozy arrangement, aside from the fact that Roundup-resistant "super-weeds" are emerging as a new biological catastrophe, is that glyphosate has now been demonstrated to be linked to birth defects as one of the most highly toxic substances in agriculture. The U.S. Government's EPA, nonetheless continues to regard Roundup as "relatively low in toxicity, and without carcinogenic or teratogenic effects." Of course nothing is said about the hypersensitive response which results in chemical sensitivity.

Now, a new international scientific team headed by Professor Andres Carrasco and including researchers from the United Kingdom, Brazil, the United States, and Argentina have demonstrated that glyphosate, the main active ingredient in Roundup, causes malformations in frog and chicken embryos at doses far lower than those used in agricultural spraying and well below maximum residue levels (MRLs) in products presently approved in the European Union.[412] The Carrasco group was led to research the embryonic effects of glyphosate by reports of high rates of birth defects in rural areas of Argentina where Monsanto's GM "RR" soybeans are grown in large monocultures sprayed from airplanes regularly. RR soy is engineered to tolerate Roundup, allowing farmers to spray the herbicide liberally to kill weeds while the crop is growing. The result of and use of glyphosate has skyrocketed since 1996.[413–416]

Widespread reports of human malformations began to be reported in Argentina beginning 2002, 2 years after widespread aerial spraying of Roundup and planting of RR soybeans was begun. The test animals used by Carrasco's group share similar developmental mechanisms with humans. The authors concluded that the results "raise concerns about the clinical findings from human offspring in populations exposed to Roundup in agricultural fields." Carrasco added, "The toxicity classification of glyphosate is too low. In some cases this can be a powerful poison."

The MRL allowed for glyphosate in soy in the EU was raised 200-fold from 0.1 mg/kg to 20 mg/kg in 1997 after genetically manipulated RR soy was commercialized in Europe. Carrasco found malformations in embryos injected with 2.03 mg/kg glyphosate. Soybeans can typically contain glyphosate residues of up to 17 mg/kg (Figure 7.22).

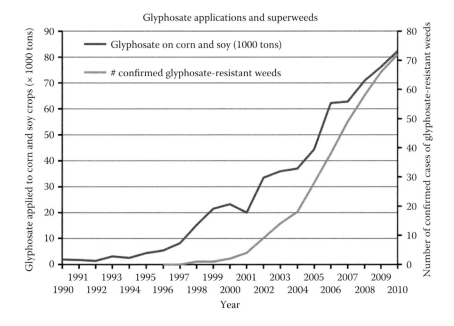

FIGURE 7.22 Glyphosate applications to corn, soy, and cotton along with the advent of glyphosate-resistant weeds. (From Earth to Seattle Times: Glyphosate Is an Endocrine Disruptor. http://www.examiner.com/article/earth-to-seattle-times-glyphosate-is-an-endocrine-disruptor.)

GM Food

After being slammed with a lawsuit by concerned farmers, GMO crops have been banned in China and most of the Europe.

The active ingredient in the pesticides is usually inactive to make them more water soluble. Various salt formations include isopropylamine, diamonine, and monammonium for potassium calcium. One adjusts to overcome glyphosate-resistant weeds is garlic, acid, or salt which increases cell membrane permeability, suppresses oxidative base, or increases expression of hydroxyproline-richglycoproteins. Hoy has been documenting malformation for 19 years in wildlife in Western Montana.[416]

In their paper they present documentation of wildlife deformation and evidence of organ damage. In addition, they obtained corresponding data for human congenital malformation and diseases in newborn infants, along with diseases in children 0–15 years and all age groups (except newborn) from hospital discharge data. Finally, they obtained pesticide application data on selected crops from the USDA. They show that congenital malformation and wildlife diseases follow trends for dicamba, 2,4-D, chlorothalonil to glyphosate use. They also show that congenital malfunction and other human diseases follow trends in glyphosate use. They hypothesized that the exposure to air, water, as well as food contributes to these diseases.

Glyphosate-Based Herbicides: Teratogenic Effects Produced on Vertebrates by Impairing Retinoic Acid Signaling Reports of neural defects and craniofacial malformations from regions where glyphosate-based herbicides (GBH) are used lead people to undertake an embryological approach to explore the effects of low doses of glyphosate in development. *Xenopus laevis* embryos were incubated with 1/5000 dilutions of a commercial GBH. The treated embryos were highly abnormal with marked alterations in cephalic and neural crest development and shortening of the anterior posterior (A–P) axis. Alterations on neural crest markers were later correlated with deformities in the cranial cartilages at tadpole stages. Embryos injected with pure glyphosate showed very similar phenotypes. Moreover, GBH produced similar effects in chicken embryos, showing a gradual loss of rhombomere domains, reduction of the optic vesicles, and microcephaly. This suggests that glyphosate itself was responsible for the phenotypes observed, rather than a surfactant or other component of the commercial formulation. A reporter gene assay revealed that GBH treatment increased endogenous retinoic acid (RA) activity in *Xenopus* embryos and cotreatment with a RA antagonist rescued the teratogenic effects of the GBH. Therefore, they conclude that the phenotypes produced by GBH are mainly a consequence of the increase of endogenous retinoid activity. This is consistent with the decrease of Sonic hedgehod (Shh) signaling from the embryonic dorsal midline, with the inhibition of OTX2 expression and with the disruption of cephalic neural crest development. The direct effect of glyphosate on early mechanisms of morphogenesis in vertebrate embryos opens concerns about the clinical findings from human offspring in populations exposed to GBH in agricultural fields.

According to Huber,[417] "it is well-documented that glyphosate promotes soil pathogens and is already implicated with the increase of more than 40 plant diseases," Huber also adds that the pathogen is implicated in spontaneous abortions in cattle at rates as high as 45%.[417]

Based on a review of the data, it is in much higher concentrations in RR soybeans and corn–suggesting a link with the RR gene or more likely the presence of Roundup.[417]

Earth Open Source's study is only the latest report to question the safety of glyphosate. Exact figures are hard to come by because the U.S. Department of Agriculture stopped updating its pesticide use database in 2008. According to its Pesticide Industry Sales and Usage Report for 2006–2007 published in February, 2011, the EPA estimates that the agricultural market used 180–185 million pounds of glyphosate between 2006 and 2007, while the nonagricultural market used 8–11 million pounds between 2005 and 2007.[418]

The Earth Open Source study also reports that by 1993, the herbicide industry, including Monsanto, knew that visceral anomalies such as dilation of the heart could occur in rabbits at low- and medium-sized doses. The report further suggests that since 2002, regulators with the European

Commission have known that glyphosate causes developmental malformations in laboratory animals. Glyphosate has now been banned in Europe.[418]

While Roundup has been associated with deformities in a host of laboratory animals, its impact on humans remains unclear. One laboratory study done in France in 2005 found that Roundup and glyphosate caused the death of human placental cells.[418] Another study, conducted in 2009 found that Roundup caused total cell death in human umbilical, embryonic, and placental cells within 24 hours.[418] Yet, researchers have conducted few follow-up studies.

Obviously, there is a limit to what is appropriate in terms of testing poison on humans.[418]

Glyphosate has been shown in several recent studies to be an endocrine disruptor. According to the National Institutes of Health, endocrine disruptors could have long-term effects on public health, especially reproductive health. The "dose makes the poison" rule does not apply to endocrine disruptors, which wreak havoc on our bodies at low doses.

A June 2013 study concluded that glyphosate "exerted proliferative effects in human hormone-dependent breast cancer." An April 2013 study by an MIT scientist concluded that "glyphosate enhances the damaging effects of other food-borne chemical residues and environmental toxins," and pointed out that glyphosate's "negative impact on the body is insidious and manifests slowly over time as inflammation damages cellular systems throughout the body."[419]

According to Samsel and Seneff,[419] glyphosate is possibly "the most important factor in the development of multiple chronic diseases and conditions that have become prevalent in Westernized societies, "including but not limited to: autism, GI diseases such as inflammatory bowel disease, chronic diarrhea, colitis, and Crohn's disease, obesity, allergies, cardiovascular disease, depression, cancer, infertility, AD, PD, multiple sclerosis, ALS, and more.[419]

Seneff and Samsel's research on glyphosate residues, found in most commonly consumed foods in the Western diet, courtesy of GE sugar, corn, soy, and wheat "enhance the damaging effects of other food-borne chemical residues and toxins in the environment to disrupt normal body functions and induce disease."[419]

Interestingly, *gut bacteria* are a key component of glyphosate's mechanism of harm. Monsanto has steadfastly claimed that Roundup is harmless to animals and humans because the mechanism of action it uses (which allows it to kill weeds), called the shikimate pathway, is absent in all animals. However, the shikimate pathway is present in bacteria, and that is the key to understanding how it causes such widespread systemic harm in both humans and animals.[419]

The bacteria in the body outnumber cells by 10 to 1. For every cell in the body, the individuals have 10 microbes of various kinds, and all of them have the shikimate pathway, so they will all respond to the presence of glyphosate.

Glyphosate causes extreme disruption of the microbe's function and lifecycle.[420] What is worse, glyphosate preferentially affects beneficial bacteria, allowing pathogens to overgrow and take over. At that point, the body also has to contend with the toxins produced by the pathogens. Once the chronic inflammation sets in, the patient is well on the way toward chronic and potentially debilitating disease.

Overlooked Component of Toxicity

The research reveals that glyphosate inhibits cytochrome P450 (CYP) enzymes, of enzymes that catalyze the oxidation of organic substances. This, the authors state, is "an overlooked component of its toxicity to mammals." One of the functions of CYP enzymes is to detoxify xenobiotic chemical compounds found in a living organism that are not normally produced or consumed by the organism in question. By limiting the ability of these enzymes to detoxify foreign chemical compounds, glyphosate enhances the damaging effects of chemicals and environmental toxins that the individual may be exposed to.

Interference with CYP enzymes acts synergistically with disruption of the biosynthesis of aromatic amino acids by gut bacteria, as well as impairment in serum sulfate transport. These facts may be significant in the chemically sensitive who not only usually has GI upset but also often food sensitivity which triggers the symptoms.

Consequences are most of the diseases and conditions associated with a Western diet, which include GI upset and food sensitivity, obesity, diabetes, heart disease, depression, autism, infertility, cancer, and AD.[420] The recent alarming increase in all of these health issues can be traced back to a combination of gut dysbiosis, impaired sulfate transport, and suppression of the activity of the various members of the CYP family of enzymes. Chemical sensitivity and food sensitivity prevails.

U.S. Trends in Pesticide Usage

With the exception of glyphosate, pesticide use on crops decreased for the first 5 or 6 years after the introduction of GE crops in 1996. Survey data from the U.S. Department of Agriculture[421] show that the use of 2,4-D and dicamba on corn steadily decreased starting about 1996 as shown in Figure 7.23. Applications of EPTC and alachlor also decreased, but the use of atrazine has remained constant. The use of 2,4-D on soy also started decreasing in 1996 as shown in Figure 7.24. In the meantime, glyphosate was being promoted as a preharvest treatment to grain, dried pea and bean, and potato crops for more even ripening, dry-down, and preharvest weed control.[422] The use of 2,4-D and dicamba on wheat decreased, being replaced by glyphosate starting in early to mid-1990s (Figures 7.25 through 7.27). With the exception of fungicides used for potato blight, pesticide applications to potatoes were also decreasing (Figure 7.28).

After about 2002, there was a steep increase in glyphosate and 2,4-D applications on all of these crops, along with an increase in dicamba on wheat. This coincides with a steep increase in the number of confirmed cases of glyphosate-resistant weeds as shown in Figure 7.29.

As seen in the figures, not all crop data were reported for all years. Data for glyphosate applications to corn, soy, and wheat were interpolated[423] and the results are shown in Figure 7.30.

Pesticide Use in the Region of Interest

Prior to 1994, there was extensive use of multiple herbicides and other pesticides, especially 2,4-D and dicamba, on wheat, potato, and other crops in Idaho, Washington, Oregon, and other states

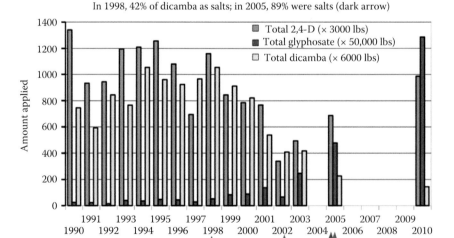

FIGURE 7.23 Herbicide applications to corn. Scale varies for each as indicated in the legend. Glyphosate salts were first applied in 2002, almost exclusively applied by 2005. Dicamba salts were first applied in 1998, almost exclusively by 2005. EPTC and alachlor applications have steadily decreased, becoming negligible by 2002 (not shown). Atrazine applications to corn crops have remained approximately constant at about 52.5 million pounds (also not shown).

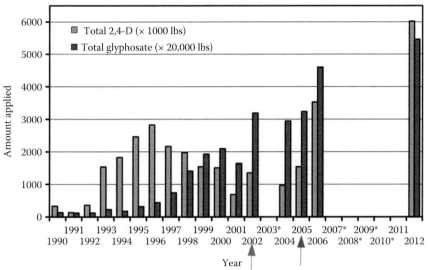

FIGURE 7.24 Glyphosate and 2,4-D applications to soy. Scale varies for each as indicated in the legend. Glyphosate salt formulations began to be applied to soy in 2002, almost exclusively by 2005.

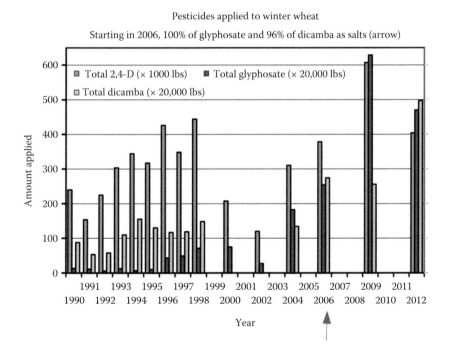

FIGURE 7.25 Glyphosate, dicamba, and 2,4-D applications to winter wheat. By 2006, nearly all of the glyphosate and dicamba were salt formulations. Scale varies for each as indicated in the legend.

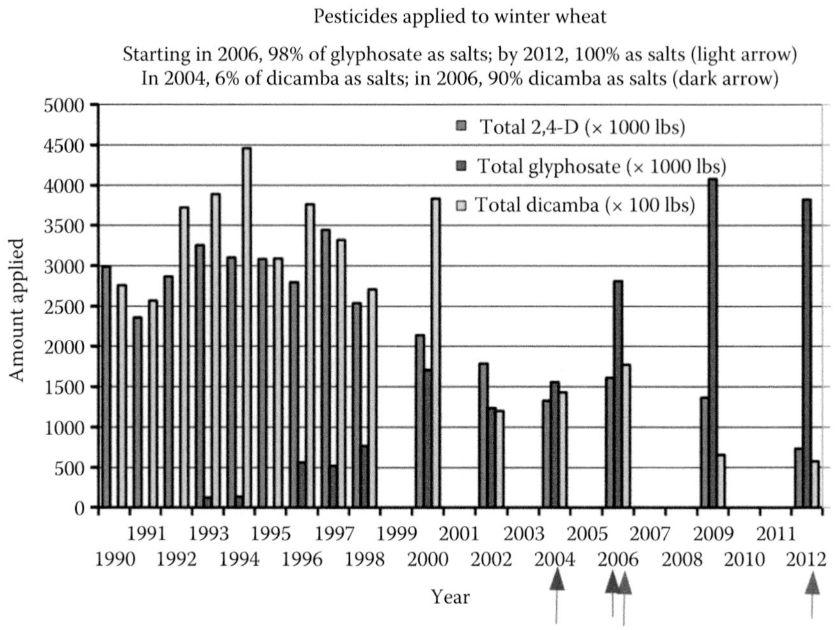

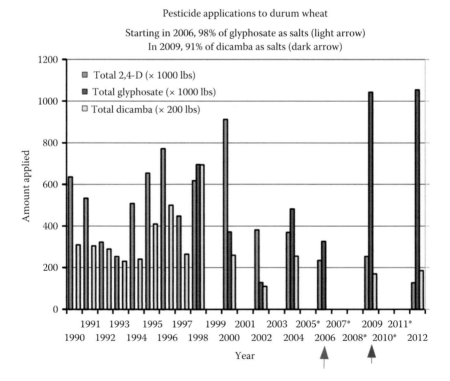

FIGURE 7.26 Glyphosate, dicamba, and 2,4-D applications to spring wheat (except durum). By 2006, nearly all of the glyphosate and dicamba were salt formulations. Scale varies for each as indicated in the legend.

FIGURE 7.27 Glyphosate, dicamba, and 2,4-D applications to durum wheat. By 2005, nearly all of the glyphosate and dicamba were salt formulations. Scale varies for each as indicated in the legend.

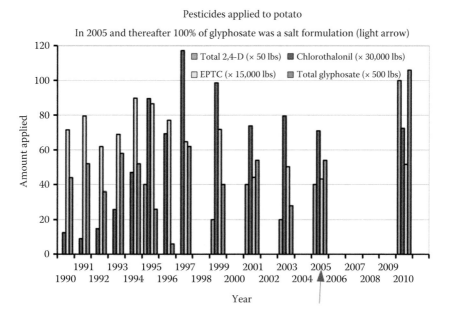

FIGURE 7.28 Pesticides applied to potato crops. By 2005, all of the glyphosate was a salt formulation. Scale varies for each as indicated in the legend.

upwind of Western Montana as shown in Figures 7.28 and 7.29. Glyphosate was also being used prior to 1994, and its use has increased significantly since 1996. The formulation for glyphosate and other commonly used herbicides applied during the growing seasons in 2006 and 2007 was changed to salt formulations[424] (we hypothesize that oxalic acid was introduced with these salts as an adjuvant, but this cannot be confirmed).

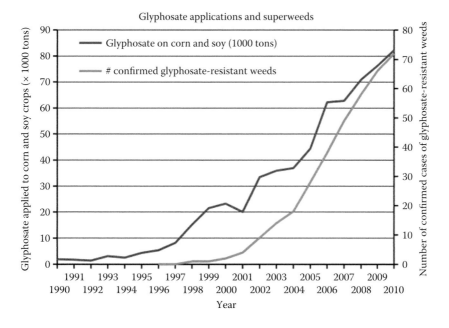

FIGURE 7.29 Glyphosate applications to corn, soy, and cotton along with the advent of glyphosate-resistant weeds.

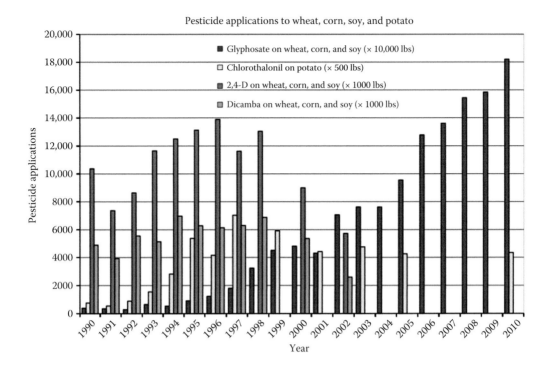

FIGURE 7.30　Total glyphosate, 2,4-D, and dicamba applied to wheat, corn, and soy crops; chlorothalonil applied to potato crops. Glyphosate data have been interpolated. Data for dicamba and 2,4-D were not added in the years when data were not reported.

In addition to glyphosate, 2,4-D, and dicamba as shown in Figure 7.30, other pesticides were widely used in Western United States prior to 1994, including picloram, atrazine, and several organochlorine herbicides. Multiple fungicides were used on over 500,000 acres of potato fields in Idaho, Washington, and Oregon. Many types of insecticides were also used in Western Montana and states upwind long before 1994. Even with this extensive exposure to multiple wind drift and locally applied pesticides, almost no birth defects were observed or reported on developing young in Western Montana until 1995. An epidemic of multiple birth defects began being observed on many individuals of domestic and wild animals born that spring,[422,425] with a significant increase in many of the birth defects over the study period, despite substantial annual variability.

Development and Health Issues in Wild Animals and Humans

In the case of the ungulates, they tabulated frequencies of multiple developmental defects, and noted a general pattern consisting of a high rate of disease early in the study period, a gradual decline until around 2006 and then a generally rising trend subsequently. This is consistent with the trends in pesticide use shown in Figures 7.20 through 7.27. They hypothesize that chlorothalonil on potatoes, along with dicamba and 2,4-D on the other crops, may contribute significantly to the early disease patterns in wildlife, whereas glyphosate is a major factor in the later rise in observed frequency.

Hoy et al.[426] sought human data on disease trends in the hospital discharge data that would correspond as much as possible with the observed defects in the wild animals. This was not always easy, as jaw malocclusion is not reported explicitly in the database, nor are genital malformations. However, there are several malformations of the lower face that are tracked, such as dent-facial anomalies (ICD 526), diseases of the jaws (ICD 527), diseases of the salivary glands (ICD 527), and diseases of the oral soft tissues (ICD 528), whose trends can be compared with those observed in the animals with jaw malformations. The plot they obtained for human urogenital disorders encompasses hydrocele (watery fluid around one or both testicles, ICD 778.6); hypospadias (ICD 752.6); and hydronephrosis—obstruction of urine flow (ICD 591), and other disorders of the kidney and ureter (ICD 593). Thyme involution and dysfunction, notable in postmortem examination of the wild animals, is not normally indicated in ICD-9. Although a code exists for diseases of the thymus (254.8), it is almost never used (only two cases among the infant and newborn data in our data set). However, T lymphocytes mature within the thymus gland, so its impairment can be reasonably linked to immune system disorders. In most other cases, such as the organ tumors, eye deformities, skin disorders, liver cancer, and metabolic issues documented on wild and domestic animals, a more direct comparison was possible.

Their results are discussed. In addition to plots where they superimpose time trends for human data or wild animal data with pesticide usage, they also provide photos taken of a variety of wild and domestic animals exhibiting pathologies (Figures 7.31 through 7.39).

Congenital Head and Facial Malformations

Brachygnathia superior (BS), the underdevelopment of the upper facial bones of ungulate species, has been photographed in countries around the world and posted on the Internet, usually labeled as underbite. In Montana and throughout the United States, wild and domestic ungulate species appear to have an extremely high prevalence of BS, including our main study species, white-tailed deer[425] as shown in the photos in Figure 7.28. The percentage of white-tailed deer with BS has increased significantly in this region since 1995, as shown in Figure 7.37. Figure 7.40 also shows the prevalence of head, face, and musculoskeletal anomalies in newborn infants superimposed with glyphosate applications to wheat, corn, and soy crops. The newborn data correlate with glyphosate usage with a Pearson correlation coefficient of $R = 0.947$.

They also noticed that trends in hypothyroidism in children aged 0–15 were rising, and that these patterns aligned very well with the data on brachygnathia in wild animals, both exhibiting a sharp

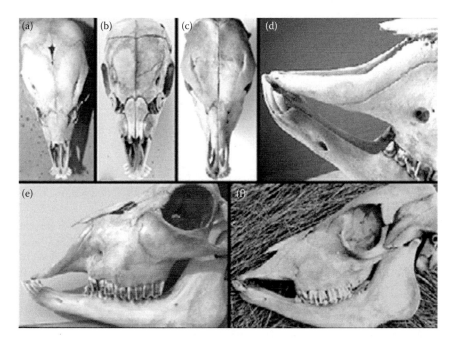

FIGURE 7.31 (**See color insert.**) Brachygnathia superior and wide lower incisors on ruminant species. (a) White-tailed deer fawn skull. (b) Mule deer fawn skull. (c) Elk calf skull. (d) Adult male bighorn sheep skull, showing short narrow premaxillary bone. (e) Domestic beef calf skull. (f) Skull of an adult male domestic goat.

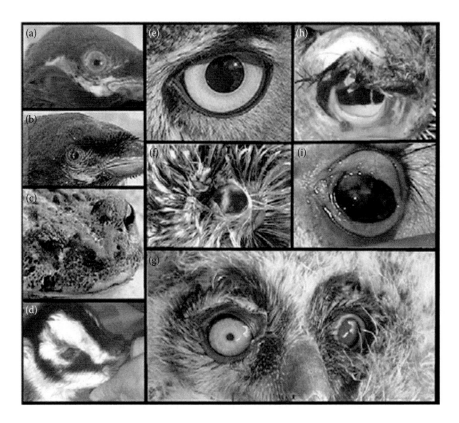

FIGURE 7.32 **(See color insert.)** Recent eye malformations in vertebrates. (a) Black-billed magpie fledgling showing a normal-sized eye. (b) Blind black-billed magpie fledgling right eye, both eyes were underdeveloped. (c) Adult 2014 western toad with right eye not formed and left eye normal. (d) Pygmy goat born in 2015 with small eye, malformed external ear and BS. (e) The normal left eye and eyelids of a Great Horned Owl (GHOW). (f) Underdeveloped left eye with malformed eyelids and pupil on 2014 hatch year GHOW. (g) Face of a 2013 fledgling GHOW showing the malformed left pupil and malformed eyelids on both eyes. (h) The malformed left pupil and eyelids of another 2014 hatch year GHOW. (i) The inflamed conjunctiva of a female WTD fawn after exposure to environmental toxins.

peak in 2007 (Figure 7.38) approximately coincident with the changeover to salt formulations in the herbicides. Congenital hypothyroidism is common, and it is linked to other congenital disorders, for example, hearing loss[427] and renal and urinary tract disorders (Figure 7.41).[428] According to Kumar et al.,[428] "Congenital hypothyroidism is the most common congenital endocrine disorder, affecting 1 in 3000–4000 newborns. Its incidence has increased 138% from 1978 to 2005 in New York State and 73% in the United States from 1987 to 2002."

Congenital Thymus Malformations and Impaired Immune System

On examined fawns of white-tailed deer, newborn domestic goats, and other newborn ruminants, BS and congenital defects of the thymus increased in spring of 2007 and have remained high since then.

Newborn Skin Disorders

In recent years, observation of skin disorders, rash, blistering, and skin tumors have been increasing on birds and wild and domestic mammals (Figure 7.34). Figure 7.42 shows newborn skin disorders and skin disorders for the general population superimposed with glyphosate applications to wheat, corn, and soy crops. The newborn skin disorders include atopic dermatitis (ICD 691); pilonidal

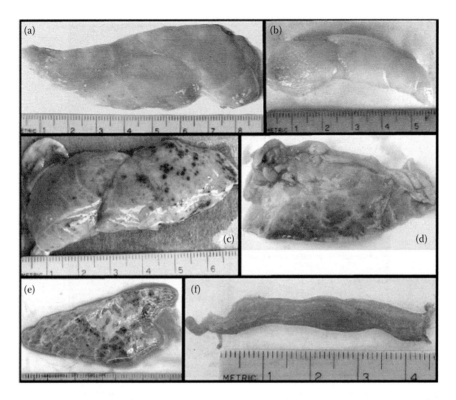

FIGURE 7.33 **(See color insert.)** Newborn white-tailed deer thymus conditions. (a and b) Normal thymus color and shape. (c and d) Thymus with red spots throughout. (e) Odd shaped, mostly red thymus. (f) Undersized thymus, red throughout.

cyst (ICD 685); erythema and urticarial (ICD 778.8); vascular hamartomas (benign tumors) (ICD 757.32); pigment anomalies (ICD 757.33); unspecified deformities of hair, skin, and nails (ICD 757.9); and meconium staining (ICD 779.84). The Pearson correlation coefficient with glyphosate usage is $R = 0.963$. Skin disorders for the general population include rash, swelling, and changes in skin tone and texture (ICD 782); eczema (ICD 692); and psoriasis (ICD 696). The Pearson correlation coefficient with glyphosate usage is $R = 0.899$.

Lymphatic Disorders in the Nonnewborn Populations

The thymus regulates the immune system; therefore, any problems with the thymus will result in a compromised immune system. The human lymphatic disorders, in particular, dramatically increased in 2007 at the same time that almost all of the glyphosate was being used as a salt formulation.

In conjunction with the increase in birth defects after the spring of 1995, necropsied wildlife and domestic ruminants of all ages had various degrees of dilation of the lymphatic vessels on the surface of their hearts. The lymphatic vessels on hearts, especially of newborns, were more severely affected beginning in 2007. Data for humans were examined for similar effects on the lymphatic system. The increase in lymphatic disorders among humans is not restricted to the infant population. Figure 7.41 shows the hospital discharge rate for children aged 0–15 with lymphatic disorders, superimposed with glyphosate applications to wheat, corn, and soy crops. The disorders include lymphedema (ICD 457), lymphocytosis (ICD 288.6), and Castleman's disease (angiofollicular lymph node hyperplasia) (ICD 202). The correlation coefficient is $R = 0.861$ (Figure 7.43). Figure 7.44 also shows the hospital discharge rate of these same lymphatic disorders over the full age range (except newborn). The correlation coefficient between this and glyphosate applications to wheat, corn, and soy crops is $R = 0.885$.

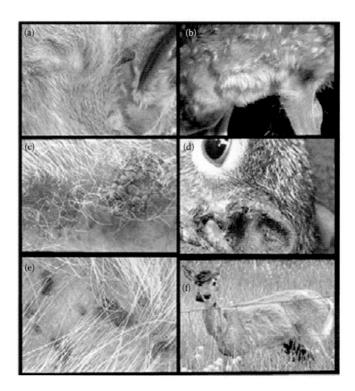

FIGURE 7.34 (**See color insert.**) Skin disorders on wild and domestic mammals. (a) Large blisters at the base of the right ear on a male WTD fawn, born 2013. (b) Hair loss on shoulders, sides, and hind legs of a female WTD fawn after exposure to environmental toxins, born 2003. (c) Male WTD fawn inner ear skin with chemical blistering, born 2010. (d) Young male eastern fox squirrel's left ear showing severe chemical skin blisters in 2005. (e) Adult female dog with chemical blisters, summer 2013. (f) Adult female WTD with multiple skin growths in May 2010.

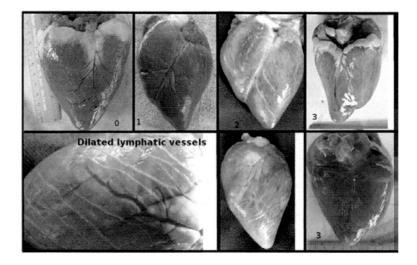

FIGURE 7.35 (**See color insert.**) White-tailed deer heart conditions ranked from 0 to 3. 0. Normal heart. (1) Slightly enlarged right ventricle. (2) Moderately enlarged right ventricle. (3) Severely enlarged right ventricle. Dilated lymphatic vessels on heart surface of newborn fawn and close-up of dilated lymphatic vessels on newborn fawn. Corresponding numbers were used in the field to record the presence or severity of any abnormal heart condition observed.

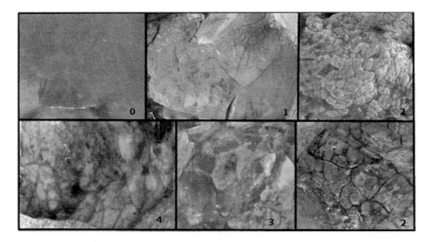

FIGURE 7.36 (**See color insert.**) White-tailed deer lung conditions ranked 0–4. 0. Normal lungs. (1) Slightly bumpy on outer lobes. (2) Raised alveoli on much of lung area. (3) Raised alveoli and white areas in lungs. (4) Raised alveoli and bleeding lungs. Corresponding numbers were used in the field to record the presence or severity of any adverse lung conditions observed.

Diseases and Malformations of the Heart and Lung

On necropsied deer of all ages, the prevalence and severity of enlarged right heart ventricle (Figure 7.35) and emphysema-like symptoms on lungs (Figure 7.36) were high in 1998 and 1999, and then decreased until 2005, when these unusual conditions of the heart and lung increased dramatically, as shown graphically in Figure 7.44. Again, the increase after 2005 is approximately coincident with the switchover to salt formulations in the herbicides.

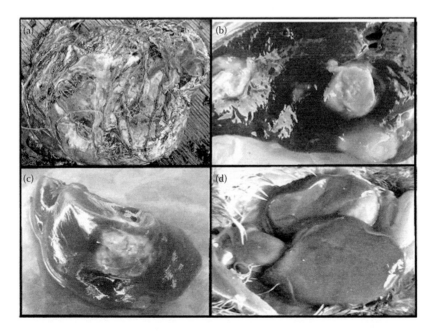

FIGURE 7.37 (**See color insert.**) Liver conditions in wildlife. (a) Large tumor verified as cancer, 18 cm. (7 in.) in diameter, removed from the outside of the liver on a female gray wolf. (b) Tumorlike growths in the liver of an adult female domestic goat. (c) Tumorlike growths in the liver of a fledgling Rock Pigeon. (d) A black-billed magpie fledgling's enlarged, discolored liver.

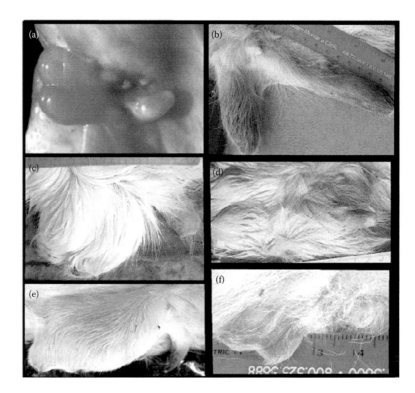

FIGURE 7.38 (See color insert.) Normal and abnormal white-tailed deer male genitalia. (a) White-tailed deer fetus, normal genitalia. (b) One-year-old white-tailed deer, normal genitalia. (c) One and half-year-old white-tailed deer with misaligned hemiscrota and short penis sheath. (d) One and half-year-old white-tailed deer, no scrotum formed on external skin, testes ectopic under the skin (see bumps), short penis sheath. (e) Two-year-old white-tailed deer, horizontal misaligned hemiscrota, penis sheath normal. (f) Newborn white-tailed deer with misaligned hemiscrota and short penis sheath.

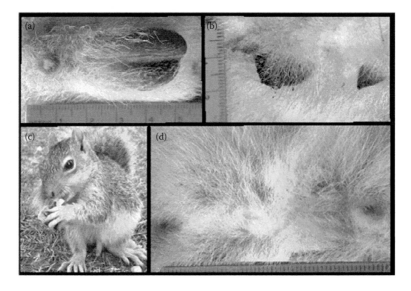

FIGURE 7.39 (See color insert.) Normal and abnormal eastern fox squirrel male genitalia. (a) Normal scrotum, very short penis sheath. (b) Scrotum is misaligned with short empty skin flaps, penis sheath very short. (c) White spot where scrotum should be formed, penis sheath very short. (d) Live juvenile male with normal penis sheath for comparison.

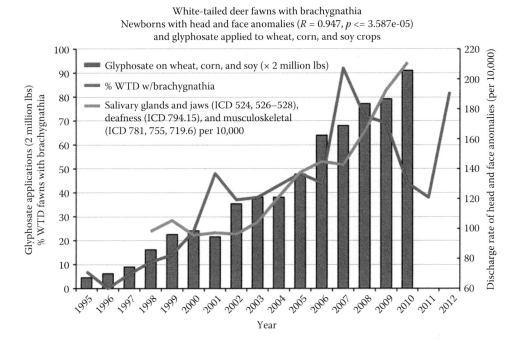

FIGURE 7.40 Comparison of hospital discharge rates for congenital facial anomalies with glyphosate applications. The graph shows the percentage of white-tailed deer fawns with brachygnathia superior from 1995 to 2012; congential facial and musculoskeletal anomalies; and glyphosate applications to wheat, corn, and soy crops. The Pearson correlation coefficient between the newborn anomalies and glyphosate applications is $R = 0.947$.

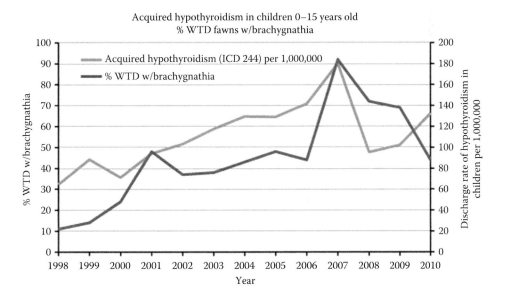

FIGURE 7.41 Hospital discharge rates for hypothyroidism in children superimposed with the percentage of WTD with brachygnathia superior.

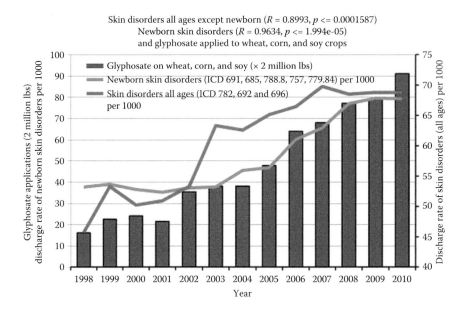

FIGURE 7.42 (**See color insert.**) Hospital discharge rates for newborn skin disorders and skin disorders in the general population superimposed with glyphosate applications to wheat, corn, and soy crops. The newborn skin disorders are: atopic dermatitis (ICD 691); pilonidal cyst (ICD 685); erythema and urticaria (ICD 778.8); vascular hamartomas (ICD 757.32); pigment anomalies (ICD 757.33); unspecified deformities of hair, skin, and nails (ICD 757.9); and meconium staining (ICD779.84). The Pearson correlation coefficient is $R = 0.9634$. Skin disorders for the general population include rash, swelling, and changes in skin tone and texture (ICD 782); eczema (ICD 692); and psoriasis (ICD 696). The Pearson correlation coefficient is $R = 0.8993$.

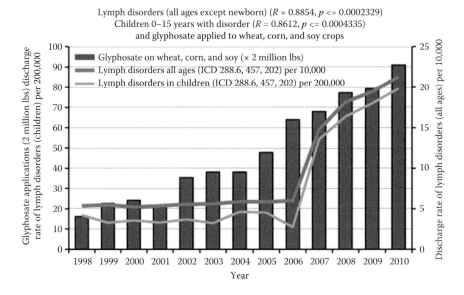

FIGURE 7.43 (**See color insert.**) Hospital discharge rates for children with lymphatic disorder and lymphatic disorder in the general population superimposed with glyphosate applications to wheat, corn, and soy crops. The lymphatic disorders for children are: lymphedema (ICD 457); lymphocytosis (ICD 288.6); Castleman's disease (angiofollicular lymph node hyperplasia, ICD 202). The Pearson correlation coefficient is $R = 0.8612$. The lymphatic disorders for the general population are: lymphedema (ICD 457); lymphocytosis (ICD 288.6); Castleman's disease (angiofollicular lymph node hyperplasia, ICD 202). The Pearson correlation coefficient is $R = 0.8854$.

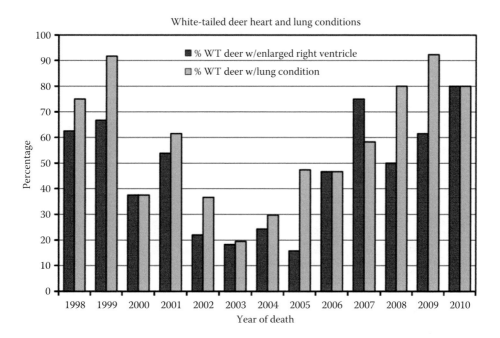

FIGURE 7.44 **(See color insert.)** Percentage of white-tailed deer with heart and lung conditions, 1998–2010.

They compared this trend with human data in Figure 7.45. Both newborn data for congenital heart disorders and data for all ages (except newborn) on enlarged right ventricle show remarkable correspondence with glyphosate usage on core crops. The tabulated newborn heart conditions include heart murmur (ICD 785.2); ostium secundum-type atrial septal defect (ICD 745.5); patent ductus arteriosus (ICD 747.0); pulmonary artery anomalies (ICD 747.3); other congenital anomalies of circulatory system (ICD 747.8); other heart/circulatory conditions originating in the perinatal period (ICD 779.89); and bradycardia (ICD 779.81,427.89). The Pearson correlation coefficient between congenital heart defects and glyphosate applications is $R = 0.983$, and for enlarged right ventricle, it is $R = 0.955$.

Figure 7.46 shows newborn lung conditions superimposed with pulmonary bleeding and edema for all ages (except newborn), and with glyphosate usage on wheat, corn, and soy crops. The newborn lung conditions include asphyxia and hypoxemia (ICD 799); pulmonary artery anomalies (ICD 747.3); meconium passage during delivery (ICD 763.84); and other respiratory conditions of fetus and newborn (ICD 770). The ICD codes for the full population data are pulmonary congestion and accumulation of fluid (ICD 514); extrinsic allergic alveolitis (e.g., "farmer's lung," ICD 495); and other diseases of the lung (ICD 518, excluding 518.5, surgery following trauma). The Pearson correlation between the newborn data and glyphosate applications is $R = 0.949$, and for all ages (except newborn), $R = 0.971$.

Liver disease An increasing number of mammals and birds have been observed with liver tumors, enlarged liver, or liver involution. Liver cancer in humans has also been increasing in frequency in the United States over the past two decades, with a shift toward relatively younger ages.[429] Similar trends are seen in China.[430] Figure 7.47 shows the hospital discharge rates of liver cancer in all ages (except newborn), alongside glyphosate usage on core crops. The Pearson correlation coefficient is $R = 0.932$.

Congenital urogenital malformations Birth defects of the male reproductive organs (Figures 7.38 and 7.39) have become common on mammals in Montana and appear to be occurring in some

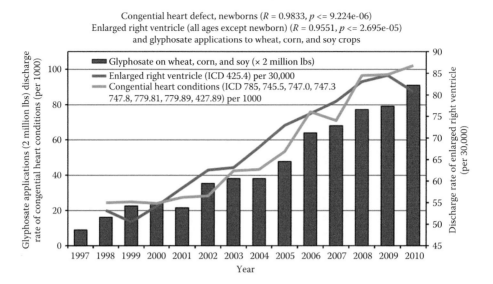

FIGURE 7.45 Hospital discharge rates for congenital heart conditions; enlarged right ventricle (ERV) for all ages (except newborn); superimposed with glyphosate applications to wheat, corn, and soy crops. The congential heart conditions include heart murmur (ICD 785.2); ostiumsecundum-type atrial septal defect (ICD 745.5); patent ductus arteriosus (ICD 747.0); pulmonary artery anomalies (ICD 747.3); other congenital anomalies of circulatory system (ICD 747.8); other heart/circulatory conditions originating in the perinatal period (ICD 779.89); and bradycardia (ICD 779.81,427.89). The Pearson correlation coefficient between congenital heart defects and glyphosate applications is $R = 0.9833$. The Pearson correlation coefficient between the ERV for all ages and glyphosate applications is $R = 0.9551$.

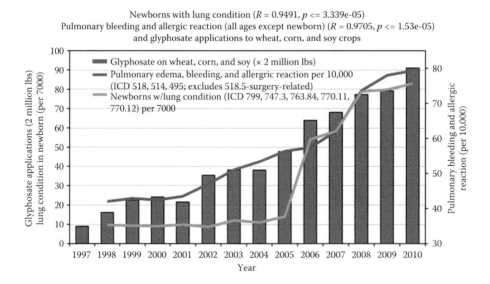

FIGURE 7.46 Hospital discharge rates for newborn lung conditions; pulmonary bleeding and edema for all ages (except newborn); superimposed with glyphosate applications to wheat, corn, and soy crops. The Pearson correlation coefficient between the pulmonary disorders and glyphosate is $R = 0.9705$. The newborn lung conditions include asphyxia and hypoxemia (ICD 799); pulmonary artery anomalies (ICD 747.3); other respiratory conditions of fetus and newborn (ICD 770); meconium passage during delivery (ICD 763.84); meconium aspiration with and without respiratory symptoms (770.11 and 12). The Pearson correlation coefficient between the newborn lung conditions and glyphosate applications is $R = 0.9491$.

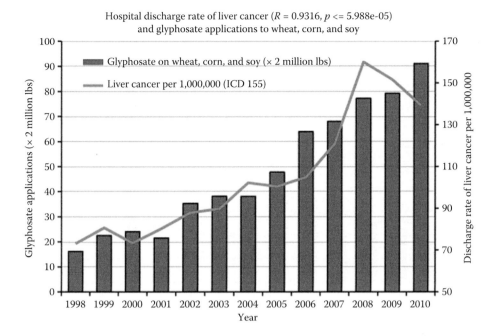

FIGURE 7.47 Hospital discharge rates of liver cancer for all ages (except newborn) along with glyphosate applications to wheat, corn, and soy crops. The Pearson correlation coefficient between the prevalence of liver cancer and glyphosate applications is $R = 0.9316$.

wildlife populations over much of the United States.[431,432] The decrease in penis sheath length, scrotum size, and the change in testes position in Montana are depicted. Several of the reproductive malformations have not been well studied, especially misplacement forward of the inguinal lymph node and the left spermatic cord, resulting in misalignment of the testes and corresponding hemis-crota during fetal formation of the scrotal sac.

Failure to Thrive

Failure to thrive, observed on multiple species of wild newborns, is a recognized problem in live-stock, and may well be related to human failure to thrive. For example, porcine periweaning failure-to-thrive syndrome (PFTS) is an increasingly recognized syndrome in the swine industry in North America.[432] It is characterized by anorexia developing within 1 week of weaning followed by leth-argy and, in some cases, death (Figure 7.48).

They examined the data in human newborns for comparison and found that a number of meta-bolic disorders have been increasing in frequency in human newborns, as illustrated in Figure 7.49, in step with glyphosate applications to wheat, corn, and soy crops. Included are disorders of fluid electrolyte and acid/base balance (ICD 276); underweight, feeding problems and fetal malnutrition (ICD 783); disorders of mineral metabolism (ICD 275); slow fetal growth and fetal malnutrition (ICD 764); and other congenital anomalies of the upper alimentary tract (ICD 750). The Pearson correlation coefficient between these two plots is $R = 0.949$.

Discussion

Hoy[426] has been documenting health status of wild animals in the mountains of Western Montana for over 40 years (Figure 7.50). She has noticed a significant degradation in health over the past two decades, mainly consistent with mineral deficiencies and thyroid hormone disruption, and she surmises that the health issues are related to exposure to various pesticides being applied to crops in close proximity to the animals' habitat. Besides exposure from nearby applications, many pesticides

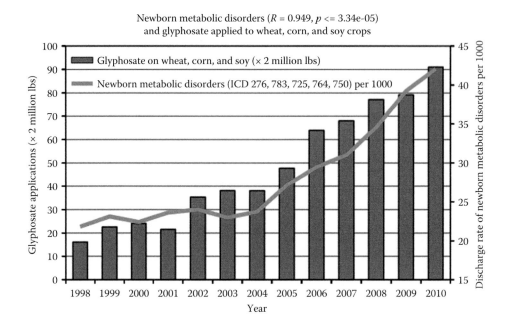

FIGURE 7.48 Hospital discharge rates for newborn metabolic disorders compared to glyphosate applications to wheat, corn, and soy crops. The metabolic disorders include disorders of fluid electrolyte and acid–base balance (ICD 276); underweight, feeding problem, and fetal malnutrition (ICD 783); disorders of mineral metabolism (ICD 275); slow fetal growth and fetal malnutrition (ICD 764); other congenital anomalies of upper alimentary tract (ICD 750). The Pearson correlation coefficient is $R = 0.949$.

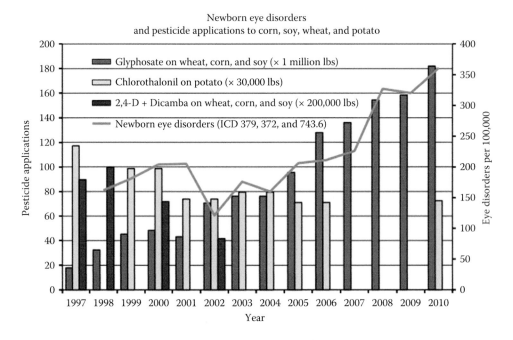

FIGURE 7.49 Hospital discharge rate for congenital eye disorders superimposed with pesticide applications to wheat, corn, and soy crops. Eye disorders include congenital anomalies of eyelids lacrimal system and orbit (ICD 743.6); disorders of conjunctiva (ICD 372); other disorders of the eye (ICD 379).

Immune-related newborn blood disorders ($R = 0.9216$, $p <= 8.204e-05$)
and glyphosate applied to wheat, corn, and soy crops

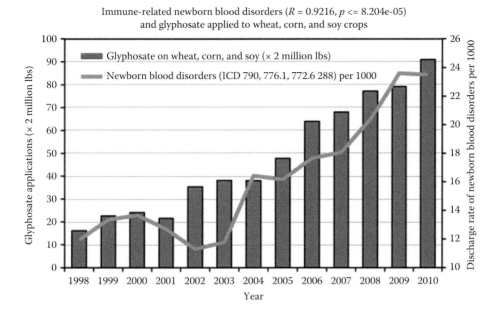

FIGURE 7.50 Hospital discharge rates for newborn blood disorders superimposed with glyphosate applications to wheat, corn, and soy crops. The blood disorders are transient neonatal thrombocytopenia (ICD 776.1); cutaneous hemorrhage of fetus or newborn (ICD 772.6); diseases of white blood cells (ICD 288); and nonspecific findings on examination of blood (ICD 790). The Pearson correlation coefficient is $R = 0.9216$.

have been shown to travel on fast-moving weather fronts to come down in rain or snow many hundreds of miles from the application site.[433,434] Low-level exposure to 60% of all herbicides applied in the United States are known to interfere with thyroid function, in particular 2,4-D.[435] Glyphosate, another thyroid hormone-disrupting herbicide,[436] has also been shown to chelate multiple minerals essential to normal fetal development and health of adult animals, and to disrupt RA.[437,438] A large number of field studies have "found an association between exposure to environmental contaminants and alterations in thyroid gland structure, circulating thyroid hormones and vitamin A (retinoid) status" in multiple populations of wild vertebrates.[438] The proper quantity of minerals, RA and thyroid hormones are essential to normal development and growth as well as sustaining health during the life of the animal. Thus, exposure to environmental contaminants often results in "reproductive and developmental dysfunction" in all vertebrate classes.[439]

While the animals' exposure is likely mostly through water and air, it is believed that human exposure is predominantly through food, as the majority of the population does not reside near agricultural fields. Government data have been obtained on pesticide usage from the USDA and on human disease patterns over time from the CDC's hospital discharge data, available from 1998 to 2010. Since glyphosate is by far the most widely used herbicide, we believe it to be a major source of contamination for the humans, and any correlations between glyphosate usage over time and specific health issues is likely to reflect a causal relationship. The research literature can help to clarify whether conditions whose incidence is rising in step with rising glyphosate usage could plausibly be caused by glyphosate, given its known toxicology profile.

Most of our graphs illustrating human disease patterns involve infants, but we also present evidence from children aged 0–15 and from the full population excepting newborns. They found many diseases and conditions whose hospital discharge rate over the 12-year period match remarkably well with the rate of glyphosate usage on corn, soy, and wheat crops. These include head and face anomalies ($R = 0.95$; Figure 7.40), newborn eye disorders (Figure 7.49), newborn blood disorders (Figure 7.47; $R = 0.92$), newborn skin disorders ($R = 0.96$), and skin disorders in the general population ($R = 0.90$), lymph disorders in children aged 0–15 ($R = 0.86$) and in the general population ($R = 0.89$), congenital heart conditions in newborns ($R = 0.98$) and enlarged right ventricle in all age groups except newborn ($R = 0.96$; Figure 7.45), newborn lung problems ($R = 0.95$) and pulmonary bleeding and edema for all age groups except newborn ($R = 0.97$; Figure 7.46), liver cancer ($R = 0.93$; Figure 7.47), newborn genitourinary disorders ($R = 0.96$; Figure 7.51), and newborn metabolic disorders ($R = 0.949$; Figure 7.48).

Glyphosate's established mode of action in killing weeds is through disruption of the *shikimate pathway*[437,440] whose products, the essential aromatic amino acids, are important precursors to multiple biologically important molecules, including the neurotransmitters dopamine, serotonin, melatonin, and epinephrine, vitamin B, foliate, molecule nicotinamide dinucleotide (NAD) involved in many redox reactions, and tanning pigment, melanin.[439,441] Gut microbes produce the aromatic amino acids using the shikimate pathway, so this ability is impaired in the presence of glyphosate. A general mode of action of glyphosate is that it chelates the soluble ions of many mineral nutrients, including calcium, copper, iron, magnesium, nickel, and zinc, which are essential cofactors in many specific biochemical reactions.[440,442] Glyphosate has been shown to disrupt the gut microbiome in animals, probably in part through disrupting mineral bioavailability, including manganese, iron, zinc, and cobalt.[437,439] Impaired manganese homeostasis can explain many features of disorders whose incidence is rising in the human population, including autism, AD, PD, osteoporosis, and rheumatoid arthritis.[443] Multiple pathogenic infections due to gut dysbiosis are a major factor in the decline in orcas (*Orcinus orca*) along the North Pacific coast of the United States,[444] and glyphosate exposure is a likely contributor.

The newborn is highly susceptible to oxidative stress produced by free radicals.[445–447] An excess of free radicals is implicated in neonatal chronic lung disease,[448] which rose sharply in the newborn population in 2006 and was highly correlated with glyphosate usage. Inflammation, hypoxia,

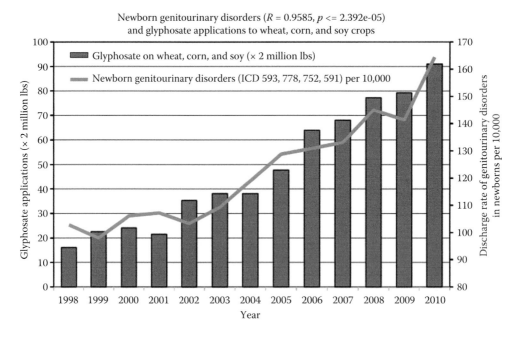

FIGURE 7.51 Hospital discharge rates for newborn genitourinary disorders compared to glyphosate applications to wheat, corn, and soy crops. The genitourinary disorders include other disorders of the kidney and ureter (ICD 593); hydrocele (watery fluid around one or both testicles, ICD 778.6); hypospadias (ICD 752.6); and hydronephrosis—obstruction of urine flow (ICD 591). The Pearson correlation coefficient between the genitourinary disorders and glyphosate use is $R = 0.9585$.

ischemia, glutamate, and free iron magnify the effect of free radicals.[445] Glyphosate suppresses the first step in the synthesis of the pyrrole ring, a core structural component of heme,[449–451] leading to excess bioavailability of free iron. Glyphosate also, through its chelation of manganese, disrupts the synthesis of glutamine from glutamate, because the enzyme glutamine synthase depends on manganese as a catalyst.[443] Glyphosate can be expected to induce hypoxia by interfering with hemoglobin synthesis. Furthermore, melatonin is a highly effective antioxidant,[447] but its synthesis depends on the shikimate pathway. Melatonin appears to be both safe and effective as a supplement to treat oxidative stress in newborns,[447] and it is possible that melatonin deficiency due to poor bioavailability of its precursor molecule, the shikimate pathway product tryptophan, is contributing to increased oxidative stress in newborns.

Many pesticides, including chlorothalonil and glyphosate, have been shown to work synergistically to more quickly damage vital biological processes in the cells of plants and animals.[452,453] Combinations of pesticides that chelate minerals and disrupt endocrine functions can easily have synergistic effects at extremely low doses that are not predicted by the effects found at higher doses in common toxicity studies. The National Toxicology Program defines the low-dose effects of pesticides we have commonly observed on wildlife as those effects that occur in the range of human exposures or effects observed at doses below those used for traditional toxicological studies.[454] Epidemiological studies present strong evidence that exposures to far lower levels than the concentrations of environmental toxins now found in most air and water samples are associated with diseases and birth defects in all vertebrate classes.[430,455] Glyphosate has been shown to be an endocrine-disrupting hormone, able to induce growth of breast cancer tumor cells in concentrations of parts per trillion. This is well below the level usually studied in toxicology investigations.[454,456] Estrogenic compounds such as glyphosate can cause sexual reversal during development in alligators, as demonstrated in studies in Florida, particularly if exposure occurs during a critical period of gestation.[457]

The patterns over time for the wild animals and the humans are distinctly different. It is believed that the explanation for the high levels of defects in the early years in the wild animals, as contrasted with the humans, are due to exposure to other pesticides besides glyphosate. Between 1997 and 2006, the use of chlorothalonil and other fungicides on potato crops for blight steadily decreased in states directly upwind of our wildlife study area. There was a corresponding observable decrease in the birth defects in mammals and birds in Western Montana. When the more severe birth defects that cause mortality went down, more wild young began to survive, especially those of wild ruminant species in serious decline. By spring of 2006, the facial malformations on grazing animals had decreased to approximately half the 2001 prevalence, and the populations of white-tailed deer and other wild ungulates were steadily going up from 2002 through 2006. However, the wild ungulate populations declined sharply in subsequent years, closely corresponding with the increase in the use of glyphosate after 2006 (Figures 7.23 through 7.30).

In addition to the well-documented effect of disrupting normal hormone functions,[454] many toxic chemicals, including commonly used herbicides such as 2,4-D, picloram, and glyphosate as well as some fungicides, including chlorothalonil, adversely affect the mitochondria of the cells and disrupt energy metabolism.[456,458] Manganese is a cofactor in the important antioxidant enzyme in mitochondria, manganese superoxide dismutase (Mn-SOD). Mn-SOD plays an important role in defense against inflammation,[459] known to be a major factor in cancer. Undoubtedly, such deficits in metabolism would seriously affect the ability of a pregnant female to maintain normal weight and health and would inhibit normal fetal growth, as well as a newborn's ability to maintain heat, energy, and normal growth.

Evidence of Increased Toxicity of Glyphosate Formulations   The toxicology experiments used by regulatory agents to decide whether to approve a new chemical explicitly require that the active ingredient be evaluated only in isolation.[460] Glyphosate formulations are trade secrets, but they often contain other ingredients that either make glyphosate itself more toxic to cells or are themselves innately toxic.[461,462] Polyethyoxylated tallow amine (POEA) is used in many formulations as a common surfactant to improve glyphosate's effectiveness. By 2006, nearly all of the glyphosate usage was in the form of the salt formulations. Other herbicides were also converted to salt formulations, including 2,4-D and dicamba. With continuously increasing use of the herbicide salt formulations, the symptoms of fetal hypothyroidism and multiple mineral deficiencies have increased alarmingly in wildlife.

Studies on rat liver mitochondria revealed that Roundup at 15 mM concentration collapsed the transmembrane potential, caused mitochondrial swelling, and depressed respiration by 40%.[463] Glyphosate alone did not exhibit this effect. *In vitro* studies showed that only 1–3 ppm of POEA is enough to produce toxic effects on cellular respiration and membrane integrity.[464] The lipophilic character of POEA gives it the ability to penetrate cell membranes, and probably also enables glyphosate to gain access to cells. In addition, the salt-based formulations are suspected to be much more deadly to humans who attempt suicide through glyphosate ingestion.[464]

Both glyphosate and chlorothalonil suppress CYP enzyme activity, resulting in a gradual depletion of the vital functions in the liver performed by the CYP enzymes.[441,465] CYP enzymes are responsible for the activation of vitamin D, and they play a role in the production of bile acids and the synthesis and/or metabolism of cholesterol, testosterone, estrogen, progesterone, and other corticosteroids. The suppression of CYP enzymes in the liver can be expected to greatly increase the toxicity of all xenobiotics to the liver, but it also has serious adverse effects on the immune system and other organ functions, including the reproductive organs.[443] While the fatality rate for glyphosate attempted suicide or accidental exposure had been relatively low in earlier reports, a paper published in 2008 claimed a fatality rate of nearly 30%.[466] Symptoms associated with human acute poisoning with glyphosate included respiratory distress, altered consciousness, pulmonary edema, shock, dysrhythmia, and renal dysfunction. Pulmonary and renal toxicity lead to mortality in humans, following metabolic acidosis and tachycardia.[464] Exposure of glyphosate to piglets in controlled experiments showed that the POEA-based formulation was much more toxic to the piglets.[467] Multiple adverse cardiovascular effects were observed, including pulmonary hypertension, circulatory collapse, and acute metabolic acidosis.

Additionally, in spring of 2006, a relatively new class of neonicotinoid insecticides, which bear a chemical resemblance to nicotine, began being used throughout the United States and in other countries. These may well have synergistic effects with glyphosate, due to glyphosate's suppression of CYP enzymes, which are needed for detoxification of neonicotinoids.[468] Our own observations on multiple disease trends in the U.S. population reveal a sharp increase in hospital discharge rates for the health problems addressed herein around the 2006 time frame, which we hypothesize, may be connected to the widespread switch to glyphosate salt-based formulations, as well as the introduction of neonicotinoids.

There was a corresponding increase after 2005 of birth defects and serious health problems on white-tailed deer fawns and other animals. This included a significant increase in enlarged right heart ventricle, lung damage, dilated lymphatic vessels on the heart surface, and underdeveloped or damaged thymus on newborn white-tailed deer necropsied by Hoy.[426] The original formulation of glyphosate had been shown to cause dilated heart on rabbit fetuses, and the percentage of rabbit fetuses with dilated heart was significantly elevated at all dose levels along with skeletal variations, anomalies, and malformations.[469] We also observed congenital heart conditions in newborns as well as impaired lung function and enlarged right ventricle in human data (Figures 7.42 and 7.43), trending upward in step with glyphosate usage.

An extremely serious health issue with the hooves of wild ruminants began around 2007 in many areas of the United States and Canada. Moose, elk, deer, bighorn sheep, and possibly other wild ungulates were observed to have disrupted growth of the keratin of the hooves, causing malformed hooves, severe lameness, and resultant mortality. Laminitis has been increasing in horses throughout the United States. The keratin of the hooves of ungulates has a significant amount cholesterol sulfate in its composition, as shown in tests of horse hooves.[470] Impaired cholesterol sulfate synthesis appears to be a primary toxicity path of glyphosate.[441]

Below, we will discuss some of our specific findings in more detail and link them to the research literature on animal exposures and on the effects of glyphosate and other pesticides on biological systems.

Conclusion

Something is causing alarming increases in diseases and birth defects in wildlife as well as in humans. Our graphs illustrating human disease patterns over the 12-year period correlate remarkably well with the rate of glyphosate usage on corn, soy, and wheat crops.

Glyphosate is known to chelate vital minerals (U.S. Patent #3160632 A). Glyphosate is an antimicrobial and biocide (U.S. Patent #20040077608 A1). Glyphosate has been classified as an endocrine disruptor by the Endocrine Society. Glyphosate has been classified as "probably carcinogenic" by the World Health Organization and by the American Cancer Society. Glyphosate interferes with the shikimate pathway, essential to healthy gut microbes. Glyphosate inhibits the CYP enzyme activity, which is vital to a healthy functioning liver.

The strong correlations between glyphosate usage and disease patterns, the highly significant p-values and the known toxicological profile of glyphosate indicate that glyphosate is likely a major factor in the increases in the serious issues with human health documented here.

Our overreliance on chemicals in agriculture is causing irreparable harm to all beings on this planet, including the planet herself. Most of these chemicals are known to cause illness, and they have likely been causing illnesses for many years. But until recently, the herbicides have never been sprayed directly on food crops, and never in this massive quantity. We must find another way.

The Roundup-Autism Connection

Environmental Toxicants and Autism Spectrum Disorders: A Systematic Review   Although the involvement of genetic abnormalities in autism spectrum disorders (ASD) is well accepted, recent studies point to an equal contribution by environmental factors, particularly environmental toxicants. However, these toxicant-related studies in ASD have not been systematically reviewed to date. Rossignol[471] compiled publications investigating potential associations between environmental toxicants and ASD, and arranged these publications into the following three categories: (1) studies examining estimated toxicant exposures in the environment during the preconceptional, gestational, and early childhood periods; (2) studies investigating biomarkers of toxicants; and (3) studies examining potential genetic susceptibilities to toxicants. A literature search of nine electronic scientific databases through November 2013 was performed, in the first category examining ASD risk and estimated toxicant exposures in the environment, the majority of studies (34/37; 92%) reported an association. Most of these studies were retrospective case–control, ecological or prospective cohort studies, although a few had weaker study designs (e.g., case reports or series). Toxicants implicated in ASD included pesticides, phthalates, PCBs, solvents, toxic waste sites, air pollutants, and heavy metals, with the strongest evidence found for air pollutants and pesticides. Studies at the EHC-Dallas have defined all of these. Gestational exposure to methylmercury (through fish exposure, one study) and childhood exposure to pollutants in water supplies (two studies) were not found to be associated with SD risk. In the second category of studies investigating biomarkers of toxicants and ASD, a large number was dedicated to examining heavy metals. Such studies demonstrated mixed findings, with only 19 of 40 (47%) case–control studies reporting higher concentrations of heavy metals in blood, urine, hair, brain, or teeth of children with ASD compared with controls. Other biomarker studies reported that solvent, phthalate, and pesticide levels were associated with ASD, whereas PCB studies were mixed. Seven studies reported a relationship between autism severity and heavy metal biomarkers, suggesting evidence of a dose–effect relationship. Overall, the evidence linking biomarkers of toxicants with ASD (the second category) was weaker compared with the evidence associating estimated exposures to toxicants in the environment and ASD risk (the first category) because many of the biomarker studies contained small sample sizes and the relationships between biomarkers and ASD were inconsistent across studies. Regarding the third category of studies investigating potential genetic susceptibilities to toxicants, 10 unique studies examined polymorphisms in genes associated with increased susceptibilities to toxicants, with eight studies reporting that such polymorphisms were more common in ASD individuals (or their mothers, one study) compared with controls (one study examined multiple polymorphisms). Genes implicated in these studies included paraoxonase (PON1, three of five studies), glutathione *S*-transferase (GSTM1 and GSTP1, three of four studies), δ-aminolevulinic acid dehydratase (one study), SLC11A3 (one study), and the metal regulatory transcription factor 1 (one of two studies). Notably, many of the reviewed studies had significant limitations, including lack of replication, limited sample sizes, retrospective design, recall and publication biases, inadequate matching of cases and controls, and the use of nonstandard tools to diagnose ASD. The findings of this review suggest that the etiology of ASD may involve at least in a subset of children, complex interactions between genetic factors and certain environmental toxicants that may act synergistically or in parallel during critical periods of neurodevelopment, in a manner that increases the likelihood of developing ASD. Owing to the limitations of many of the reviewed studies, additional high-quality epidemiological studies concerning environmental toxicants and ASD are warranted to confirm and clarify many of these findings.

For the past 30 years, Seneff[441] has been passionate about testing out potential causes of autism, after seeing what it was like for a close friend whose son was diagnosed. She points out the clear correlations between increased glyphosate use over recent years (the result of GE crops causing weed resistance, necessitating ever-larger amounts to be used) and skyrocketing autism rates.

The rate of autism has risen so quickly; there can be no doubt that it has an environmental cause. Genes simply cannot mutate fast enough to account for the rapid rise we are now seeing. The latest statistics released by the CDC show that 1 in 50 children in the United States now fall within the autism spectrum[472,473] with a 5:1 boy to girl ratio. Just last year, the CDC reported a rate of 1 in 88, which represented a 23% increase since 2010, and 78% since 2007. Meanwhile, remember when previously the incidence of autism in the United States was only 1 in 100,000 just 30 years ago.

Seneff[441] identified two key problems in autism that are unrelated to the brain, yet clearly associated with the condition both of which are linked with glyphosate exposure:

1. Gut dysbiosis (imbalances in gut bacteria, inflammation, leaky gut, food allergies such as gluten intolerance)
2. Disrupted sulfur metabolism/sulfur and sulfate deficiency

Interestingly, certain microbes in the body actually break down glyphosate. However, a by-product of this action is ammonia, and children with autism tend to have significantly higher levels of ammonia in their blood than the general population. Ditto for those with AD. In the brain, ammonia causes encephalitis.

Another devastating agent is formaldehyde, which a recent nutritional analysis discovered is present in GE corn at a level that is 200 times the amount that animal studies have determined to be toxic to animals. Formaldehyde destroys DNA and can cause cancer. Formaldehyde and other aldehydes are seen in air analyses of many indoor environments (indoor air in Chapter 2). The combination with formaldehyde in pesticides and food will increase chemical sensitivity, making the individual very ill. This has been observed in the autistic child.

Other research backing up the Roundup-autism link is that from Swanson.[474] Ten years ago, she became seriously ill, and in her journey to regain her health, she turned to organic foods. Not surprisingly (for those in the know), her symptoms dramatically improved. This prompted her to start investigating GE foods.

She has meticulously collected statistics on glyphosate usage and various diseases and conditions, including autism. To access her published articles and reports, visit Sustainable Pulse,[474] a European website dedicated to exposing the hazards of GE foods.

What the biotech industry, spearheaded by Monsanto, has managed to do is turn food into poison. Here, we are just talking about the effects of Roundup. There are plenty of indications that the genetic alteration of a crop itself can pose significant health concerns. So, with the vast majority of GE crops, you have no less than two potentially hazardous factors ammonia and formaldehyde to contend with, glyphosate toxicity being just one part of the equation.

As discussed above, glyphosate has a number of devastating biological effects. So much so that it may very well be one of the most important factors in the development of a wide variety of modern diseases and conditions, including autism. In summary, these detrimental effects include:

Nutritional deficiencies: Glyphosate immobilizes certain nutrients and alters the nutritional composition of the treated crop.

Disruption of the biosynthesis of aromatic amino acids: There are essential amino acids not produced in the body that must be supplied via your diet.

Increased toxin exposure: This includes high levels of glyphosate and formaldehyde in the food itself.

Impairment of sulfate transport and sulfur metabolism; sulfate deficiency.

Systemic toxicity a side effect of extreme disruption of microbial function throughout the body; beneficial microbes in particular, allowing for overgrowth of pathogens.

Gut dysbiosis: Imbalances in gut bacteria, inflammation, leaky gut, food allergies such as gluten intolerance.

Enhancement of damaging effects of other food-borne chemical residues and environmental toxins as a result of glyphosate shutting down the function of detoxifying enzymes.

Creation of ammonia: A by-product created when certain microbes break down glyphosate, which can lead to brain inflammation associated with autism, chemical sensitivity, and AD.

It is important to understand that the glyphosate sprayed on conventional and GE crops actually becomes systemic throughout the plant, so it cannot be washed off. It is inside the plant. For example, GE corn has been found to contain 13 ppm of glyphosate, compared with zero in non-GMO corn. At 13 ppm, GMO corn contains more than 18 times the "safe" level of glyphosate set by the EPA. Organ damage in animals has occurred at levels as low as 0.1 ppm. That is reason enough to become a label reader to avoid anything with corn in it, such as corn oil or high fructose corn syrup.

Until the United States requires GE foods to be labeled, the only way to avoid GE ingredients is to make whole, fresh organic foods the bulk of the diet, and to only buy 100% USDA-certified organic processed foods. Meats need to be grass fed or pasteurized to make sure the animals were not fed GE corn or soy feed.

Last but not least, do not confuse the "natural" label with organic standards.

The natural label is not based on any standards and is frequently misused by sellers of GE products. Growers and manufacturers of organic products bearing the USDA seal, on the other hand, have to meet the strictest standards of any of the currently available organic labels. In order to qualify as organic, a produce must be grown and processed using organic farming methods that recycle resources and promote biodiversity. Crops must be grown without synthetic pesticides, bioengineered genes, petroleum-based fertilizers, or sewage sludge-based fertilizers.

GMOs in Infant Formula

Nobody should be eating GMO foods, especially babies. GMOs have not been adequately tested for safety, and results from a number of animal studies point to potential harm. What is especially troubling is that long-term safety tests are nonexistent.

Given that 92% of soybeans used in processed food are now GMO, soy-based infant formula is extremely likely to contain GMOs. Dairy-based formula contains soy oil, also likely derived from GMO soy. A sure way to avoid GMOs in infant formula is to buy organic brands—GMOs are prohibited in organics.

Until infant formula makers such as Abbott Laboratories stop using GMO ingredients, hundreds of thousands of newborns and infants will be unwilling participants in a huge uncontrolled experiment with the health of the next generation.

(1) Autism can be characterized as a chronic low-grade encephalopathy, associated with excess exposure to NO, ammonia, and glutamate in the CNS, which leads to hippocampal pathologies and resulting cognitive impairment, and (2) encephalitis is provoked by a systemic deficiency in sulfate, but associated seizures and fever support sulfate restoration. The impaired synthesis of cholesterol sulfate in the skin and red blood cells (RBCs), catalyzed by sunlight and NO synthase enzymes, creates a state of colloidal instability in the blood manifested as a low zeta potential and increased interfacial stress. Encephalitis, while life-threatening, can result in partial renewal of sulfate supply, promoting neuronal survival. Research is cited showing how taurine may not only help protect neurons from hypochlorite exposure, but also provide a source for sulfate renewal. Several environmental factors can synergistically promote the encephalopathy of autism, including the herbicide, glyphosate, aluminum, mercury, lead, nutritional deficiencies in thiamine and zinc, and yeast overgrowth due to excess dietary sugar. Given these facts, dietary and lifestyle changes, including increased sulfur ingestion, organic whole foods, increased sun exposure, and a avoidance of toxins such as aluminum, mercury, and lead, may help alleviate symptoms or, in some instances, to prevent autism altogether.

Theoretical inferences, based on biophysical, biochemical, and biosemiotic consideration, are related here to the pathogenesis of cardiovascular disease, diabetes, and other degenerative conditions. Endothelial nitric oxide synthase (eNOS), when sunlight is available, is to catalyze sulfate production. There is a striking alignment between cell types that produce either cholesterol sulfate or sulfated polysaccharides and those that contain eNOS. The signaling gas, NO, a well-known product of eNOS, produces pathological effects not shared by hydrogen sulfide, a sulfur-based signaling gas. Sulfate plays an essential role in HDL-A1 cholesterol trafficking and in sulfation of heparin sulfate proteoglycans (HSPGs), both critical to lysosomal recycling (or disposal) of cellular debris. HSPGs are also crucial in glucose metabolism, protecting against diabetes, and in maintaining blood colloidal suspension and capillary flow, through systems dependent on water-structuring properties of sulfate, an anionic kosmotrope. When sunlight exposure is insufficient, lipids accumulate in the atheroma in order to supply cholesterol and sulfate to the heart, using a process that depends upon inflammation. The inevitable conclusion is that dietary sulfur and adequate sunlight can help prevent heart disease, diabetes, and other disease conditions.

The contributing factor in autism is a deficiency in cholesterol sulfate supply. There is a link between preeclampsia and subsequent autism in the child, and it is hypothesized that both conditions can be attributed to a severe depletion of cholesterol sulfate. Through studies on the Vaccine Adverse Event Reporting System (VAERS) database, it is demonstrated that a strong statistical relationship exists among the signs and symptoms associated with autism and those associated with preeclampsia, pernicious anemia, and serious adverse reactions to vaccines.[475] They show that VAERS reports associated with symptoms typical of pernicious anemia produce both a set of symptoms that are highly correlated with preeclampsia and another set highly correlated with autism. In a severe reaction, the cascade of events subsequent to vaccination reflects a profuse production of NO and consequential destruction of both RBCs and cobalamin.[475] This may explain the diverse signs and symptoms associated with both preeclampsia and severe vaccine adverse reactions. Excess NO synthesis induced by the aluminum and antigen in vaccines results in hemolysis of RBCs, which allows hemoglobin to scavenge the excess NO, converting it to nitrate. The NO is also scavenged by cobalamin, leading to its inactivation and contribution to subsequent pernicious anemia. Finally, it is demonstrated that severe adverse reactions to vaccines can be associated with life-threatening conditions related to the heart and brain, as well as stillbirth, when the vaccine is administered to a woman in the third trimester of pregnancy, as demonstrated by statistical analysis of the Gardasil records.

Autism is a condition characterized by impaired cognitive and social skills, associated with compromised immune function. The incidence is alarmingly on the rise, and environmental factors are increasingly suspected to play a role. There is strong evidence supporting a link between autism and the aluminum in vaccines. A literature review showing toxicity of aluminum in human physiology offers further support.[476] Mentions of autism in VAERS increased steadily at the end of the last century, during a period when mercury was being phased out, while aluminum adjuvant burden was being increased. Using standard log-likelihood ratio techniques, they identify several signs and symptoms that are significantly more prevalent in vaccine reports after 2000, including cellulitis, seizure, depression, fatigue, pain, and death, which are also significantly associated with aluminum-containing vaccines. Children with the autism diagnosis are especially vulnerable to toxic metals such as aluminum and mercury due to insufficient serum, sulfate, and glutathione.[476] A strong correlation between autism and the measles, mumps, rubella (MMR) vaccine is also observed, which may be partially explained via an increased sensitivity to acetaminophen administered to control fever.

In reviewing the literature pertaining to interfacial water, colloidal stability, and cell membrane function, it appears that a cascade of events that begins with acute exogenous surfactant-induced interfacial water stress can explain the etiology of sudden death syndrome (SDS), as well as many other diseases associated with modern times. A systemic lowering of serum zeta potential mediated by exogenous cationic surfactant administration is the common underlying pathophysiology. The cascade leads to subsequent inflammation, serum sickness, thrombohemorrhagic phenomena, colloidal instability, and ultimately even death. A sufficient precondition for sudden death is lowered bioavailability of certain endogenous sterol sulfates, sulfated glycolipids, and sulfated glycosaminoglycans, which are essential in maintaining biological equipoise, energy metabolism, membrane function, and thermodynamic stability in living organisms. A literature review provides the basis for the presentation of a novel hypothesis as to the origin of endogenous biosulfates which involves energy transduction from sunlight. The hypothesis is amply supported by a growing body of data showing that parenteral administration of substances that lowers serum zeta potential results in kosmotropic cationic and/or chotropic anionic interfacial water stress, and the resulting cascade.

The documented effects of glyphosate and its ability to induce disease, is that glyphosate is the "textbook example" explaining what exogenous semiotic entropy is the disruption of homeostasis by environmental toxins.

Other GMO Products

In 2012, The Cornucopia Institute unearthed a vast body of scientific literature, spanning four decades, pointing to serious harmful health effects from consuming an additive common in food marketed as organic and natural. Carrageenan, the science revealed, contributes to intestinal inflammation, ulcerations in the colon, and even colon cancer in laboratory animals. Derived from seaweed, carrageenan is used as a thickener and stabilizer in many types of foods.[477]

Eden Foods was one of the first companies to immediately commit to removing carrageenan; now it has only two products containing this additive. Oregon Ice Cream, which has one flavor of Julie's ice cream remaining with carrageenan vowed to have it reformulated. Turtle Mountain is currently in the taste-testing phase of its newly formulated, carrageenan-free So Delicious coconut milk line.[477]

GE Salmon Mounts

Nearly 1.5 million citizens have registered their opposition to the FDA's proposal to approve the commercialization of GE salmon.[477] AquaBounty Technologies, the developer of the fish, has engineered a variant of Atlantic salmon that is reputed to grow twice as fast as its natural counterpart. The company inserted a growth hormone gene from Pacific Chinook salmon and another promoter gene from ocean trout into the Atlantic salmon.

Washington and Maine are the two states that currently allow ocean fish farming. Washington State, in 2002, enacted a ban on the rearing of GE fish in state waters.

The Argentine Model

Years after Argentine scientists and residents targeted glyphosate, they argued that it caused health problems and environmental damage.[419]

Farmers and others in Argentina use the weed killer primarily on GM RR soy, which covers nearly 50 million acres, or half of the country's cultivated land area. In 2009, farmers sprayed that acreage with an estimated 200 million liters of glyphosate.[419]

The Argentine government helped pull the country out of a recession in the 1990s in part by promoting GM soy. Though it was something of a miracle for poor farmers, several years after the first big harvests, residents near where the soy crop grew began reporting health problems, including high rates of birth defects and cancers as well as the losses of crops and livestock as the herbicide spray drifted across the countryside.

Such reports gained further traction after an Argentine government scientist Andres Carrasco conducted a study, "Glyphosate-Based Herbicides Produce Teratogenic Effects on Vertebrates by Impairing Retinoic Acid Signaling" in 2009.[419]

The study, published in the journal *Chemical Research in Toxicology* in 2010, found that glyphosate causes malformations in frog and chicken embryos at doses far lower than those used in agricultural spraying. It also found that malformations caused in frog and chicken embryos by Roundup and its active ingredient glyphosate were similar to human birth defects found in GM soy-producing regions.

"The findings in the laboratory are compatible with malformations observed in humans exposed to glyphosate during pregnancy" (Carrasco, director of the Laboratory of Molecular Embryology at the University of Buenos Aires).

In March 2010, a regional court in Argentina's Santa Fe province banned the spraying of glyphosate and other herbicides near populated areas. A month later, the provincial government of Chaco province issued a report on health statistics from La Leonesa. The report showed that from 2000 to 2009, following the expansion of GM soy and rice crops in the region, the childhood cancer rate tripled in La Leonesa and the rate of birth defects increased nearly four fold over the entire province.

The growth in adoption of GM crops has exploded since their introduction in 1996. According to Monsanto, an estimated 89% of domestic soybean crops were RR in 2010, and as of 2010, there were 77.4 million acres of RR soybeans planted, according to the Department of Agriculture.

Other data recently showed brain damage in children exposed to pesticides. Three studies found that children exposed *in utero* to substantial levels of neurotoxic pesticides have somewhat lower IQs by the time they enter school than do kids with virtually no exposure.[478]

The researchers screened women for exposure to OP compounds such as chlorpyrifos, diazinon, and malathion. These bug killers, which can cross the human placenta, work by inhibiting brain-signaling compounds. Although the pesticides' residential use was phased out in 2000, spraying on farm fields remains legal.[478]

All three studies began in the late 1990s and followed children through age 7. In more than 300 low-income Mexican-American families, exposures came mostly from farmwork, and the report of researchers from the University of California at Berkeley and their colleagues.[478] In two comparably sized New York City populations, exposures were probably traced to bug spraying of homes or eating treated produce.[478]

Among the California families, the average IQ for the 20% of children with the highest prenatal OP exposure was seven points lower compared with the least-exposed group.[478]

A Columbia University study followed low-income black and Hispanic mothers. Each additional 4.6 pg of chlorpyrifos per gram of blood in a woman during pregnancy correlated with a drop of 1.4% in her youngster's IQ and 2.8% in a measure of the child's working memory.

A more diverse group of New York City families recruited by the Mount Sinai School of Medicine points to genetics as a major determinant of risk. Children who showed the biggest cognitive impacts tended to have mothers carrying a gene variant for a slow-acting version of the enzyme that breaks down OPs.[478] This variant is present in roughly one-third of all Americans.

Of course, genetics is not a problem, the environmental exposures, for example, pesticides, solvents, natural gas, and mycotoxins are the real problems.

There was an amazing degree of consistency in the findings across all three studies that is concerning, because a drop of seven IQ points. In fact, half of seven IQ points would be a big deal, especially when it is seen across a population.

Each IQ-point drop will add up to extra costs in lost earnings over an individual's lifetime, mainly to higher education and other costs, to deal with behavioral and learning problems that may occur during childhood.

Other OPs can cause neurological damage. The study by Koc et al.[479] shows the importance of agriculture and widespread use of pesticides, and intoxication due to OP insecticides is common in Turkey. Organophosphorus compounds may cause late-onset distal polyneuropathy occurring 2 or more weeks after the acute exposure. An 18-year-old woman and a 22-year-old man were admitted to the hospital with weakness, paresthesia, and gait disturbances at 35 and 22 days, respectively, after ingesting dimethyl-2,2-dichloro vinyl phosphate (DDVP). Neurological examination revealed weakness, vibration sense loss, bilateral dropped foot, brisk deep tendon reflexes, and bilaterally positive Babinski sign. Electroneurography demonstrated distal motor polyneuropathy with segmental demyelination associated with axonal degeneration prominent in the distal parts of both lower extremities.

According to Johnson, exposure of an environmental toxicant as a risk factor in the development of ALS was first hinted at (demonstrated) in the Chamorro indigenous people of Guam.[480] During the 1950s and 1960s, these indigenous people presented an extremely high incidence of ALS which was presumed to be associated with the consumption of flying fox and cycad seeds. No other strong association between ALS and environmental toxicants has since been reported, although circumstantial epidemiological evidence has implicated exposure to heavy metals such as lead and mercury, industrial solvents, and pesticides, especially OPs and certain occupations such as playing professional soccer.[480] Given that only ~10% of all ALS diagnosis have a genetic basis, a gene–environment interaction provides a plausible explanation for the other 90% of cases.

Israelis living close to areas in which pesticides are heavily used are suffering long-term nerve damage.[480]

The figures came out of a study conducted by a public committee on reducing damage caused by pesticide, headed by former Supreme Court Justice Yaakov Turkel.[480]

Finkelstein said that recent years have seen an upswing in the use of organic pesticides containing phosphorus, which can harm the human NS (Table 7.23).[481]

The studies that have been done illustrate the risk that long-term exposure, even to a low level of pest control substances, leads to damage, not only to those using the substances but also to individuals living in agricultural communities. Such communities show a higher than normal rate of children afflicted with attention disorders.

There are many neurotoxic pesticides. A list of these is shown in Table 7.24. Table 7.25 shows a list of other neurotoxic chemicals.

Table 7.26 shows the structure and area changes in the neurotoxic chemicals.

Table 7.27 shows solvent-based paint that can cause neurotoxicity.

Table 7.28 shows a partial list of neurotoxic chemicals all of which we have seen in chemically sensitive patients.

Neurodevelopmental/Behavioral Health Outcomes and Pesticide Exposure in Children

As pesticides are known to cross the placenta and blood–brain barrier and are found in cord blood and amniotic fluid, there is concern about their potential effects on the developing brain as a result of prenatal and early childhood exposure.

The systematic review included 32 studies of pesticide exposure and neurodevelopmental or behavioral outcomes in children. The range of outcomes, from primitive neonatal reflexes through age-specific developmental testing, to complex cognitive and behavioral outcomes such

TABLE 7.23
List of Pesticides

Reference	Study Design	Population Description	Exposure Index	Pesticide	Exposure Window	Outcome	Result	Mean Score
Petrelli[482]	Cross-sectional	184 male greenhouse workers aged 20–55 years in Italy	Interviewer-administered questionnaire	10 Pesticides	During and preceding pregnancy in spouse (not specified)	Self-report of spontaneous abortion in spouse	Spouses of exposed greenhouse workers had a significantly increased risk of spontaneous abortion (OR = 11.8; 95% CI 2.3–59.6).	10
Hanke[483]	Retrospective cohort	104 women delivering singleton infants and residing in an agricultural district in Poland	Interviewer-administered questionnaire (face-to-face)	24 Pesticide categories	From 3 months prior to conception and throughout pregnancy (but this was generated from history of over 7 years of questions)	Birth weight abstracted from medical records	Maternal exposure to pyrethroid pesticides was associated with a decrease in infant birth weight ($p = 0.02$).	14
Dabrowski[484]	Case-control	117 cases and 377 controls delivering infants in rural Poland	Physician-administered questionnaire 1–2 days post	Pesticide (not specified)	During 1st and 2nd trimesters	Birth weight as determined by physician interview	Women exposed to pesticides in 1st and 2nd trimester delivered infants with lower birth weight by 189 g ($p < 0.01$).	13
Sallmen[485]	Cross-sectional	578 couples (families of male greenhouse workers) in Finland	Self-administered questionnaire, exposure assessment by occupational hygienist pesticide data collected from employers and the exposure results of previous studies in the population	11 Categories of pesticides	Unknown	Self-report of time to pregnancy and calculation of fecundability density ratio (FDR)	Paternal occupational exposure to pyrethroids was associated with decreased fecundability as measured by the FDR (OR = 0.40; 95% CI = 0.19–0.85). In addition, men who used PPE correctly were as fertile as unexposed men.	13
Pierik[486]	Nested case-control	78 cases of cyptochidism, 56 cases of hypospadia, and 313 control infants visiting child health care centers in Netherlands	Interviewer-administered questionnaire (face-to-face) and job exposure matrix	Pesticides (not specified)	Year before delivery	Cyptorchidism or hypospadias as determined by records obtained from original cohort study (physician diagnosis)	Paternal occupational exposure to pesticides was associated with an increased odds of cryotorchidism in infants (OR = 3.8; 95% CI = 1.1–13.4).	12

(Continued)

TABLE 7.23 (Continued)
List of Pesticides

Reference	Study Design	Population Description	Exposure Index	Pesticide	Exposure Window	Outcome	Result	Mean Score
Berkowitz[487]	Prospective cohort—Mount Sinai Hospital, NYC	404 singleton infants born to primiparous, multiethnic mothers in New York City	Interview-administered questionnaire, maternal blood sample collected in the 3rd trimester and cord blood	Indoor use pesticides	Questionnaire administered "during pregnancy," biomarkers in 3rd trimester	Birth weight, birth length, head circumference, and gestational age determined through linkage with a perinatal database at Mount Sinai Hospital	With the exception of an association between decreased maternal PON1 activity and decreased infant head circumference ($p = 0.014$), no significant associations were found between indoor pesticide use and birth outcomes.	16
Salam[488]	Nested case-control—Children's Health Study (CHS)	691 children, including 279 cases and 4112 controls, enrolled in the CHS in Southern California	Telephone interview with mother	Pesticides (not specified)		Maternal report of physician-diagnosed asthma by age 5	Every exposure to pesticides was significantly associated with development of asthma before age 5, particularly if exposure occurred in the first year of life (OR = 4.58; 95% CI = 1.36–15.43).	14
Newman[489]	Case-control	706 cases of sarcoidosis over 18 years of age and 706 matched controls residing in the United States	Interviewer-administered questionnaire	Insecticides (not specified) and employment in agriculture		Tissue confirmation of noncaseating granulomas within 6 months of enrollment and clinical symptoms consistent with sarcoidosis upon presentation to the medical clinic	Exposure to insecticides at work was associated with an increased risk of sarcoidosis in a multivariate model controlling for other exposures (OR = 1.61; 95% CI = 1.13–2.28). Employment in agriculture was positively associated with sarcoidosis in the univariate analysis (OR = 1.46; 95% CI = 1.13–1.89).	13
Idrovo[490]	Cross-sectional	2085 primiparous women workers from flower production companies in Colombia	Maternal interview	Pesticides (not specified)	1 year before pregnancy, 2 years before, >2 years before	Self-report of time to pregnancy	Maternal employment in the flower industry was associated with an increased time to pregnancy with a trend toward increased TTP with increased duration of employment (OR = 0.86; 95% CI = 0.75–0.98 working <24 months and OR = 0.73; 95% 0.673–0.84 >2 years	12

(Continued)

TABLE 7.23 (Continued)
List of Pesticides

Reference	Study Design	Population Description	Exposure Index	Pesticide	Exposure Window	Outcome	Result	Mean Score
Ronda[491]	Cross-sectional	587,360 records from the Stillbirth and Birth National Register of Spain (SBNRS)	Paternal occupation	Pesticides (not specified)—agricultural exposure	At conception	Fetal death from congenital anomalies as determined by the SBRS	Housewives of male agricultural workers had an increased risk of fetal death (OR = 1.68; 95% CI = 1.03–2.73).	11
Lacasana[492]	Case-control	151 cases of anencephaly and 151 controls of >20 weeks gestation in three Mexican states	Interviewer-administered questionnaire (both parents)	Pesticides (not specified) agricultural exposures	Last 6 months before and 1 month after last period, and 2 prior to this	Anencephaly (type of neural tube defect) identified through death certificates and the Epidemiological Surveillance System of Neural Tube Defects in Mexico	Maternal employment in agriculture was associated with increased odds of having an anencephalic child (OR = 4.57; 95% CI 1.05–19.96).	14
Meyer[493]	Case-control	354 cases and 727 controls in Arkansas	Estimate of pounds of pesticides applied through the National Agricultural Statistics Service (NASS) and geographic information systems (GIS)	38 Types of pesticides	Gestational weeks 6–16	Hypospadias identified through the Arkansas Reproductive Health Monitoring System (ARHMS)	For every 0.05-pound increase in estimated exposure to diclofop-methyl use, the odds of hypospadia increased by 8% (OR = 1.08; 95% CI = 1.01–1.15). Negative associations were found with alachlor and permethrin, while all other studied pesticides had null results.	14
Zhu[494]	Prospective cohort—Danish National Birth Cohort (DNBC)	225 pregnancies in gardeners, 214 pregnancies in farmers, and 214 reference pregnancies in the DNBC	Interviewer-administered questionnaire	Pesticides (not specified)—agricultural and horticultural exposure	3 Months prior to conception and during pregnancy	Late fetal loss, congenital abnormalities, preterm birth, small for gestational age, sex ratio, and multiple births ascertained through medical records	Maternal occupational exposure as a gardener was associated with an increased risk of very preterm birth (OR = 2.6; 95% CI = 1.1–5.9).	12
Brouwers[495]	Case-control	232 case-control pairs in Netherlands	Self-administered questionnaire	Pesticides (not specified)	3 Months preconception or 1st trimester	Confirmed cases of hypospadia treated at a pediatric urology center identified through hospital records	No significant associations were found between parental pesticide exposure and infant hypospadia.	11

(Continued)

TABLE 7.23 (Continued)
List of Pesticides

Reference	Study Design	Population Description	Exposure Index	Pesticide	Exposure Window	Outcome	Result	Mean Score
Handal[496]	Cross-sectional	142 children aged 2–5 years living in rural Ecuador	Interview with mother to determine prenatal exposure	Pesticide not specified; agricultural pesticides used in flower industry		Neurodevelopment— Ages and Stages Questionnaire, Visual Motor Integration Test	Maternal employment in the flower industry associated with increased developmental scores.	8.5
Eckerman[497]	Cross-sectional	38 rural (exposed) and 28 urban (unexposed) schoolchildren aged 10–18 years	Self-report of exposure collected by interview	Unspecific agricultural pesticide		Neurobehavioral— Behavioral Assessment and Research System (BARS)	Motor and attention deficits shown in adolescents engaged in farming ($p < 0.01$).	4.5
Roberts[498]	Case–control	465 cases of autism spectrum disorder (ASD) and 6975 controls born between 1996 and 1998 residing in California	Residential proximity (radius and temporal window to pesticide applications during small area geocodes)	Wide range of agricultural pesticides and fungicides (Appendix 1, p. 1487 of study)		Autism-Spectrum Disorder (ASD)— diagnostic codes and service usage records.	Maternal proximity within 500 m of organochlorine pesticide application was associated with increased odds of ASD (OR = 6.1; 95% CI 2.4–15.3) particularly during gestation weeks 1–8.	12.5
Weselak[499]	Retrospective cohort—Ontario Farm Family Health Study (OFFHS)	3412 pregnancies of farm women in the OFFHS in Ontario, Canada	Self-administered questionnaires (3)	Specific chemical names	3 months prior to conception and 1st trimester	Self-report of birth defects	Farm women exposed to cyanazine and diamba before conception had an increased risk of birth defects in male offspring (OR = 4.99; 95% CI = 1.64–15.27 and OR = 2.442; 95% CI = 1.06–5.53, respectively).	14
Zuskin[500]	Cross-sectional	82 exposed (pesticide plant) and 60 unexposed (bottling plant) workers in Croatia	Duration of employment and job title from employment records	Pesticides (not specified)		Respiratory function measures—MEFV, FFVC, FEV$_1$, FEF$_{50}$, and FEF$_{25}$—and chronic respiratory symptoms as recorded by physicians using the British Medical Research Council questionnaire on respiratory symptoms	Female pesticide workers had increased odds of chronic cough, and both sexes had increased odds of dyspnea and nasal catarrh ($p < 0.05$). Pesticide workers had significantly decreased FVC, FEV$_1$, and FEF$_{25}$ compared with predicted ($p < 0.01$). No difference in FEV$_1$ was noted.	13

(Continued)

TABLE 7.23 (Continued)
List of Pesticides

Reference	Study Design	Population Description	Exposure Index	Pesticide	Exposure Window	Outcome	Result	Mean Score
Settimi[501]	Cross-sectional	717 women greenhouse workers in Italy with a total of 973 pregnancies	Interviewer-administered questionnaire (face-to-face)	Work in a greenhouse (five different categories of exposure)	At least 1 month in 1st trimester	Self-report of spontaneous abortion	Occupationally exposed women who reported reentering the greenhouse within 24 hours of pesticide application (OR = 3.2; 95% CI 1.37–7.7) or having applied pesticides (OR = 2.6; 95% CI = 1.0–6.6) had an increased risk of spontaneous abortion.	11
Hoppin[502]	Cross-sectional analysis—Agricultural Health Study (AHS)	20,175 farmers and pesticide applicators enrolled in the AHS in Iowa and North Carolina	Self-administered questionnaire	40 pesticides		Self-report of wheeze in the previous year based on the question "How many episodes of wheezing in your chest have you had in the past 12 months?"	Exposure to herbicide chlorimuron ethyl was associated increased risk of wheeze in a dose-dependent manner (OR = 1.62; 95% CI 1.25–2.10) in commercial pesticide applicators. Use of the OP insecticide chlorpyrifos for at least 20 days a year was associated with wheeze in both farmers and applicators ($p < 0.01$).	15
Hoppin[502]	Cross-sectional analysis—Agricultural Health Study (AHS)	20,908 farmers (20,400 male and 508 female), including 654 cases of chronic bronchitis, enrolled in the AHS (Iowa and North Carolina)	Self-administered questionnaire	50 pesticides		Self-report of doctor diagnosis of chronic bronchitis after age 20	Every use of 11 pesticides was associated with prevalent chronic bronchitis, with heptachlor having the highest odds ratio (OR = 1.50; 95% CI = 1.19–1.89 in adjusted model). Every use of 5 organochlorine and 5 organophosphate pesticides was also significantly related to prevalent chronic bronchitis.	15

(Continued)

TABLE 7.23 (Continued)
List of Pesticides

Reference	Study Design	Population Description	Exposure Index	Pesticide	Exposure Window	Outcome	Result	Mean Score
Hoppin[503]	Cross-sectional analysis—Agricultural Health Study (AHS)	21,393 farmers and 30,242 spouses enrolled in the AHS in Iowa and North Carolina	Self-administered questionnaire	50 pesticides		Self-report of doctor-diagnosed farmer's lung (hypersensitivity pneumonitis)	High pesticide exposure events (HPEE), carbamate and organochlorine insecticides were positively associated with a diagnosis of farmer's lung, with HPEE having the highest odds ratio (OR = 1.75; 95% CI = 1.39–2.231). A significant dose–response relationship was seen between increased pesticide exposure and report of farmer's lung ($p < 0.0005$).	14
Carbone[504]	Case–control	90 cases and 203 controls in agricultural area in the province of Ragusa, Italy	Interview-administered questionnaire	Pesticides (not specified)	From 3 months before to 3 months after conception	Hypospadias and cryptorchidism as determined by pediatric records and physician consultation	No significant associations were found between parental pesticide exposure and infant hypospadia or cryptorchidism.	12
Fear[505]	Case–control	594 cases and 526 controls living in England	Parental occupation abstracted by nurse from hospital records	Agricultural chemicals (not specified)	Unknown	Neural tube defects (NTD) identified through an NTD register	Paternal exposure to agricultural chemicals ("grochemicals") was associated with increased odds of NTD in offspring (OR = 2.69; 95% CI = 1.09–6.65).	11
Bretveld[506]	Case–control	4872 exposed greenhouse workers and 8133 controls in Netherlands	Self-administered questionnaire and job title	Pesticides (not specified)	6 months prepregnancy	Self-report of time to pregnancy (TTP), spontaneous abortion, preterm, LBW, sex ratio, and birth defects	Maternal employment as a greenhouse worker was associated with an increased TTP (OR = 1.9; 95% CI = 0.8–4.4) and increased risk of spontaneous abortion (OR = 4.0; 95% CI = 1.1–14.0).	10

(Continued)

TABLE 7.23 (*Continued*)
List of Pesticides

Reference	Study Design	Population Description	Exposure Index	Pesticide	Exposure Window	Outcome	Result	Mean Score
Felix[507]	Case–control	47 cases of esophageal atresia (EA) and 63 cases of congenital diaphragmatic hernia and 202 controls in Netherlands	Self-administered questionnaire (both parents)	Herbicides, insecticides	From 1 month before conception to end of 1st trimester	Congenital diaphragmatic hernia and esophageal atresia identified through medical records	Parental contact with herbicides or insecticides was associated with a diagnosis of EA (OR = 2.0; 95% CI = 1.0–4.1).	14
Hoppin[508]	Cross-sectional analysis—Agricultural Health Study (AHS)	25,112 farm women, including 702 cases of asthma, enrolled in the AHS (Iowa and North Carolina)	Self-administered questionnaire (81%) or telephone interview (19%)	48 pesticides		Self-report of doctor-diagnosed asthma after 19 years of age	Atopic asthma was significantly associated with use of 10 pesticides; 7 insecticides, 2 herbicides, and 1 fungicide. Exposure to the organophosphate insecticide parathion resulted in the highest odds ratio (OR = 2.88; 95% CI = 1.34–6.20).	16
Hoppin[509]	Cross-sectional analysis—Agricultural Health Study (AHS)	19,704 male farmers, including 441 cases of asthma, enrolled in the AHS (Iowa and North Carolina)	Self-administered questionnaire	48 pesticides		Self-report of doctor-diagnosed asthma after 19 years of age	High pesticide exposure events doubled risk of reporting both atopic and nonatopic asthma. Atopic asthma was associated with exposure to 12 pesticides including 3 herbicides and 6 insecticides. The organophosphate insecticide coumaphos showed the strongest association (OR = 2.34; 95% CI = 1.49–3.70).	16
Hougaard[510]	Observed versus expected rates	Comparison of women employed in agricultural versus general population in Denmark	Employment register	Pesticides (not specified)—horticultural exposure	Year preceding treatment for infertility	Infertility determined through national hospital register	No significant associations between employment in horticulture and female infertility seen at the ecological level.	9
Dugas[511]	Case–control	471 case and 490 control infants residing in Southeast England	Telephone questionnaire	Several domestic-use pesticides (e.g., insect repellent)	During pregnancy	Hypospadias cases as confirmed by surgeon's records and case notes	Maternal use of insect repellant during the first trimester was associatied with an increased risk of hypospadias (OR = 1.81; 95% CI = 1.06–3.11)	14

(Continued)

TABLE 7.23 (Continued)
List of Pesticides

Reference	Study Design	Population Description	Exposure Index	Pesticide	Exposure Window	Outcome	Result	Mean Score
Burdorf[512]	Prospective cohort—Generation R, Netherlands	6830 pregnant women (mean age 30 years) in Netherlands	Self-administered questionnaire and job-exposure matrix	Pesticide (not specified)	Unknown	TTP, preterm birth, and decreased birth weight determined through self-administered questionnaire and hospital registries	Maternal occupational exposure to pesticides as determined by the job-exposure matrix was associated with decreased birth weight (OR = 2.42; 95% CI = 1.10–5.34).	12
Sathyanarayana[513]	Cross-sectional analysis—Agricultural Health Study (AHS)	2246 farm women who gave birth to a singleton baby within 5 years of enrollment in the AHS (Iowa and North Carolina)	Self-administered questionnaire	27 pesticides	First 3 months of pregnancy	Self-report of infant birth weight	Every use of the insecticide carbaryl was significantly associated with a decreased birth weight.	12
Brender[514]	Case–control	184 Mexican-American case women and 255 comparison women residing in Texas	Interview-administered questionnaire	Home use, occupational use, and residential proximity to pesticides (not specified)	3 months preconception and 3 months postconception	Identification of neural tube defects (delivered or aborted) through a regional surveillance project including hospitals, clinics, birthing centers, and abortion clinics	Maternal exposure to pesticides in the home and living within 0.25 miles of crops was associated with an increased incidence of neural tube defects in offspring (OR = 2.0; 95% CI 1.2–3.1 and OR = 3.6; 95% CI 1.7–7.6, respectively).	15
Petit[515]	Prospective cohort—PELAGIE	3159 pregnant women residing in Brittany, France	Census records of agricultural activities at the municipal level	Pesticides (not specified)	Early pregnancy (not specified)	Birth weight, birth length, and head circumference abstracted from hospital records	No association was found between residential proximity to agriculture and birth weight or intrauterine growth. However, maternal resident in areas where peas were grown was associated with an increased risk of small head circumference (OR = 2.2; 95% CI = 1.2–3.6).	11

Source: Sanborn, M. 2012. *Systematic Review of Pesticide Health Effects*. Ontario College of Family Physicians.

TABLE 7.24
Neurotoxic Pesticides

Organophosphates	**Organochlorines**
Azinphos-methyl	DDT
Dichlorvos	Aldrin
Tetraethyl pyrophosphate	Dieldrin
Ethyl parathion	Toxaphene
Diazinon	Mirex
Ethion	Endrin
Chlorpyrifos	Lindane
Malahion	Heptachlor
Endothion	Chlordane
Chlorthipophos	
	Pyrethroids
Thiometon	Bathrin
	Tetramethrin
Carbamates	Cyfluthrin
Aldicarb	Fluvalinate
Propoxur	Resmethrin
Dimetan	
Bendiocarb	**Chlorophenoxy compounds**
Carbaryl	2,4-Dichlorophenoxyacetic acid (2,4-D)
	2,4,5-Trichlorophenoxyacetic acid (2,4,5-T)
	2-Methyl-4-chlorophenoxyacetic acid (MCPA)
	2,4,5-Trichlorophenoxyproprionic acid (Silvex)

Granted Permission by Elsevier. Human Toxicology of Chemical Mixtues. Harold Ziegler Pages 537–558

TABLE 7.25
Partial List of Neurotoxic Volatile Organic Chemicals

Aliphatic hydrocarbons	**Ketones**
n-Hexane	Acetone
Isomethylhexane	Methylethylketone
Propane	Methyl-*n*-butylketone
Butane	Methylisobutylketone
n-Hepatane	Methyl-*n*-amylketone
Aromatic hydrocarbons	**Halogenated compounds**
Toluene	Methylene chloride
Xylene	Chloroform
Styrene	1,1,1-Trichloroethane
	Trichloroethylene
Ethers	Perchloroethylene
2-Butoxyethanol	Chlorodifluoromethane
Diethyl ether	Dichlorodifluoromethane
	Trichlorofluoromethane
	Esters
	Ethyl acetate
	n-Butyl acetate

Granted Permission by Elsevier. Human Toxicology of Chemical Mixtues. Harold Ziegler Pages 537–558

TABLE 7.26

Indicators of Neurotoxic Poisoning and Their Symptoms

1. Structural or neuropathological
   Gross changes in morphology, including brain weight
   Histologic changes in neurons or glia (neuropathy, axonopathy, myelinopathy)
2. Neurochemical
   Changes in synthesis, release, uptake of vital molecular species, and/or neurotransmitter degradation
   Changes in membrane-bound enzymes regulating neuronal activity
   Inhibition and aging of neuropathy enzymes
   Increases in glial fibrillary acidic protein in adults
3. Neurophysiological
   Change in velocity, amplitude, or refractory period of nerve conduction
   Change in latency or amplitude or sensory-evoked potential
   Change in electroencephalographic pattern
4. Behavioral and neurological
   Changes in touch, vision (including color perception loss), auditory, taste, or smell sensations
   Speech impairment
   Changes in equilibrium
   Pain disorders
   Increased or decreased motor activity
   Abnormal movement
   Changes in motor coordination, weakness, twitching, paralysis, tremor, or posture
   Decreased occurrence or absence, magnitude or latency of sensorimotor reflex
   Changed magnitude of neurological measurement, including grip strength and hind limb splay
   Loss of coordination and unsteadiness
   Seizures and convulsions
   Changes in rate or pattern of activities
   Changes in learning, memory or attention span
   Confusion
   Sleep disturbances
   Headache
   Loss of appetite
   Excitability
   Depression
   Irritability
   Restlessness
   Nervousness
   Tension
   Depression
   Stupor
   Fatigue
   Delirium and hallucinations
5. Developmental
   Changes in the time of appearance or lack of expected behavior elements
   During development, or failure to develop as expected
   Onset of unexpected behavior patterns during development
   Changes in growth or organization of nervous system elements

Granted Permission by Elsevier. Human Toxicology of Chemical Mixtues. Harold Ziegler Pages 537–558

as intelligence testing and attention deficit disorder (ADD), reflects the various ways of assessing neurologic development depending on a child's age.

All studies were assessed for quality using the modified Downs and Black Quality Assessment Tool.

As a group, these are high-quality studies, reflecting biomarker exposure assessment and sophisticated measurement of neurodevelopmental outcomes and confounders. The mean assessment

TABLE 7.27

Organic Solvents Typically Found in Solvent-Based Paints and Their K_{ow} Values

Toluene	2.73
Xylene	3.15
C-6–C-9 aliphatic hydrocarbons	4.10–6.15
Ispropanol	0.05
n-Butanol	0.88
Acetone	−0.24
Methyl isobutyl ketone	1.19
Ethyl acetate	0.73
n-Butyl acetate	1.78

Granted Permission by Elsevier. Human Toxicology of Chemical Mixtues. Harold Ziegler Pages 537–558

score of all included studies was 15.5 out of 20 (range 4.5–19) and median score was 117. Twenty-two of the studies had assessment scores above 15.

Organophosphate Pesticides Linked to ADHD

In a representative sample of the U.S. children, those with higher levels of organophosphate pesticide metabolites in their urine were more likely to have attention-deficit hyperactivity disorder (ADHD) than children with lower levels, indicating less exposure to these compounds, researchers report in the *Pediatrics*, published on May 17, 2010.

Bourchard et al. found that "each 10-fold increase in urinary concentration of organophosphate metabolites was associated with a 55%–723% increase in the odds of ADHD". In previous similar investigations, Bouchard focused on "special groups with high levels of exposure, such as children from agricultural communities, and reported pesticides-related cognitive deficits (involving memory and attention), and behavioral problems". The present study is the first investigation on children's neurodevelopment to be conducted in a group with no particular pesticide exposure.

The findings are based on cross-sectional data on 1139 children, aged 8–15 years, from the National Health and Nutrition Examination Survey (NHANES) (2000–2004). One hundred nineteen of the children met current diagnostic criteria for ADHD. When children taking ADHD medication were included as case subjects, there were 148 cases.

Six urinary dialkyl phosphate (DAP) metabolites, resulting from the degradation of different organophosphates, were measured in urine to provide an indicator of the body burden of common organophosphates. The proportions of children with urinary DAP concentrations below the detection limit were between 35.7% and 80.0%. Most children (93.8%) had one or more detectable metabolites of the six DAPs measured. Sex, race/ethnicity, and fasting duration were not significantly associated with DAP metabolite concentrations (all $p > 0.3$).

For the most commonly detected pesticide metabolite, dimethyl thiophosphate (64.3%), those with levels higher than the median of detectable concentrations had nearly twice the odds of ADHD (adjusted OR = 1.93; 95% CI = 1.23–3.02) compared with children with undetectable levels. The adjusted OR was higher when children taking ADHD medication were included as case subjects (adjusted OR = 2.12; 95% CI: 1.32–0.43).

Several biological mechanisms might underlie an association between organophosphate pesticides and ADHD.

Approximately 40 organophosphate pesticides are registered with the U.S. EPA, the investigators note in their report. In 2001, 73 million pounds of organophosphates were used in both agricultural and residential settings. Diet is a major source of pesticide exposure for children. According to a

TABLE 7.28

Partial List of Known Developmental Neurotoxic Chemicals

Metals

Cadium	Learning disabilities
	Decreased IQ
Lead	Learning disabilities
	Hyperactivity and aggression
	Brain damage
	Memory impairment
Mercury	Motor dysfunction
	Learning and memory disabilities

Solvents

Ethanol	Attention deficits and behavioral disorders
	Memory impairment
Styrene	Decreased activity
	Behavioral disorders
Toluene	Speech and motor dysfunctions
	Learning disabilities
Trichloroethylene	Hyperactivity
	Behavioral disorders
Xylene	Learning and memory impairments
	Motor dysfunction

Pesticides

Bioallethrin	Hyperactivity
Chlorpyrifos	Decreased coordination
	Memory impairment
DDT	Hyperactivity
	Memory and coordination impairment
DDE	Motor dysfunction
Deltamethrin	Hyperactivity
Diazinon	Decreased coordination
	Memory impairment

Miscellaneous

Dioxins	Learning disabilities
Fluoride	Hyperactivity
	Decreased IQ
Nicotine	Hyperactivity
	Learning and cognitive disabilities
PCBs	Memory and learning impairments
	Psychomotor dysfunction
Carbon monoxide	Brain damage

Granted Permission by Elsevier. Human Toxicology of Chemical Mixtues. Harold Ziegler Pages 537–558

2008 U.S. report, detectable concentrations of the organophosphate malathion were found in 28% of frozen blueberry samples, 25% of strawberry samples, and 19% of celery samples.

The study by Bouchard et al.[169] showed "children with higher concentrations of urinary DAP, especially dimethyl alkyl phosphates (DMAP), were more likely to be diagnosed with ADHD. A 10-fold increase in DMAP concentration was associated with an OR of 1.55 (95% CI = 1.14–2.10), after adjusting for sex, age, race/ethnicity, poverty–income ratio, fasting duration, and urinary creatinine concentration. For the most commonly detected DMAP metabolite, dimethyl thiophosphate, children with levels higher than the median of detectable concentrations had double the odds of ADHD (adjusted OR = 1.93 [95% CI = 1.23–3.02]) compared with those with nondetectable levels."

Attention deficit hyperactivity disorder: It is one of the most common childhood disorders and can continue through adolescence and adulthood. Symptoms include difficulty staying focused and paying attention, difficulty controlling behavior, and hyperactivity (overactivity). About 3%–7% of school-aged children in the United States had ADHD in 2003, with 2.5 million children medicated for the condition. A study on organophosphate pesticides published in 2007 found a tentative link between the exposure to pesticides and brain development. The authors of the report noted: "more than 1 billion pounds of pesticides are used annually in the United States, three-quarters of which are used in agriculture". Recent biological monitoring studies indicate that pesticide exposures are widespread in the U.S. population, including pregnant women and children.

Organophosphate pesticides account for about half of the insecticides used in the United States. A large number of organophosphate pesticides metabolize to DAP metabolites and other specific metabolites. There are six DAP metabolites; each of these can be produced from the metabolism of more than one organophosphate pesticide.

Organophosphate pesticides act by interfering with the transmission of signals in the nervous systems of both insects and humans, if humans are exposed in high enough amounts. Organophosphate pesticides injure and even kill large numbers of people around the world every year, and have been associated with chronic NS damage in people who survive poisoning."

Exposure, says the Center for Disease Control, does not have to be direct. Eating foods that have organophosphates sprayed on them can contribute to the effect on an individual's health.

There are dozens of organophosphate pesticides on the market, including the better-known brands, Diazinon, Malathion, and Trichlorphon.

ADHD, a controversy in its own right, has just had some fuel added to the flames by Australia's Therapeutic Goods Administration. At least 30 kids had "psychotic episodes." About 827 children have had severe reactions to the drugs in the last 3 years.

The University of British Columbia (UVC) researchers report that well-known culinary herbs can be used as natural pesticides.

Traces of pesticides and herbicides have been found in the urine of pregnant women in France, even a long time after exposition to them. That is the conclusion of a report published by the French Institute of Health Surveillance, a government agency.[516]

A study of individuals who apply pesticides recently found that exposure to certain pesticides doubles one's risk of developing an abnormal blood condition.[516]

We have seen hundreds of chemically sensitive patients at the EHC-Dallas who had ADHD. Many could be corrected if the food, mold, and other chemical sensitivity could be intradermally neutralized, massive avoidance done, and nutrients replaced.

Five studies assess the association between pesticide exposure and ADHD. These studies are cohort reports[517–519] and two are cross-sectional studies using NHANES data from the United States.[169,520]

Organophosphates: The Columbia–New York City cohort study reported on the association between prenatal chlorpyrifos exposure and attention deficit in 3-year-olds.[518] Child behavior was assessed by maternal completion of the Child Behavior Checklist, which assesses behaviors in the previous 2 months. Compared with low-exposure children, high-exposure children were significantly more likely to have attention problems (10.6% vs. 1.1%; $p < 0.01$) and ADHD problems (10.6% vs. 2.2%, $p < 0.02$).

The follow-up on the CHAMACOS cohort at ages 3.5 and 5 years[517] focused on specific assessments for attention problems and clinical ADHD. Outcome measures included the Child Behavior Checklist, and also researcher-administered tests for ADHD at 3.5 and 5 years and psychometric assessments at age 5 using the Hillside Behavior Rating Scale. In 3.5-year-olds, prenatal organophosphate metabolite levels were positively associated with attention problems and ADHD, but the results reached statistical significance only for boys ($p < 0.05$). For the 5-year-old boys, there were significant positive associations between prenatal metabolite levels and two mother-reported ADD measures, that is, attention scale ($p < 0.05$) and ADHD scale ($p < 0.01$).

A highly generalizable study using NHANES data from the general population compared rates of ADD in children aged 8–15 years with organophosphate metabolite levels (indicating current exposure) above or below the study median.[169] ADHD was diagnosed using a standardized diagnostic interview (DISC-IV) or based on a report of having taken ADHD medication in the last year; 13% of 1139 children had an ADD diagnosis. For each 10-fold increase in urinary dimethyl, alkyl phosphate DMAP organophosphate metabolites, children had a 2.13 times higher risk of the hyperactive-impulsive subtype of ADHD (OR = 2.13, 95% CI = 1.08–3.27). The associations between exposure and the inattentive and combined subtypes of attention deficit were in the same direction but not statistically significant after adjusting for gender, race, and ethnicity. The metabolite that best predicted ADHD (all subtypes) for boys and girls was dimethyl thiophosphate, a DMAP group metabolite produced by organophosphate pesticides, such as malathion. Children whose levels were above the median for the national data had a significantly elevated risk of ADHD (OR = 1.93, 95% CI = 1.23–3.02).

Organochlorines: A second study using NHANES data[520] examined the association between urinary TCP, an organochlorine compound, and ADHD in 2539 children aged 6–15 years. TCP exposure occurs through multiple pathways, including chlorinated drinking water by-products, ingestion of food contaminated by the parent pesticides, exposure to pesticides in wood preservatives, and exposure to other fungicides. TCP was frequently found, 2,4,5-TCP in 29% and 2,4,6-TCT in 65% of children. ADHD was measured by parental report of physician diagnosis or taking medication for the condition. Only 2,4,6-TCP was associated with ADHD, and a dose–response relationship was found ($p < 0.006$). There was a nonsignificant trend for children with detectable levels below the national median for 2,4,6-TCP (<3.58 μg/g) to have more ADHD diagnoses than did children with nondetectable levels (RR = 1.54). Children with 2,4,6-TCP levels above the median were significantly more likely to have and ADHD diagnosis (OR = 1.77, 95% CI = 1.18–2.66, p for trend <0.006). The results were adjusted for lead exposure and environmental tobacco smoke, measured by whole blood lead and serum continued concentrations. This study is important for documenting the high rates of exposure to these chemicals and potential-associated health effects; however, because of the multiple routes of exposure to this chemical group, the exposure route that is clinically significant for these effects is not known, and could be drinking water and not pesticides.

The second study of organochlorine exposure and ADHD was from a Spanish cohort of 4-year-olds prenatally exposed to the organochlorine HCB.[521] The high-exposure tertile (cord blood levels >1.4 ng/mL) had a higher probability of having ADHD as assessed by the ADHD DSM-IV checklist administered by teachers (RR = 3.43, 95% CI = 1.24–9.51). The results were adjusted for the effects of other organochlorines.

The Columbia–New York City cohort tested IQ in 265 7-year-old children and assessed its relationship to prenatal chlorpyrifos exposure.[522] For each standard deviation increase in exposure, full-scale IQ declined 1.4% ($p < 0.02$) and working memory, an important predictor of school failure,[523] declined 2.8% ($p < 0.0001$). In a subset of children that had lead levels drawn, these levels were not correlated with chlorpyrifos levels or with IQ.

The studies included in this systematic review have a number of limitations. Although metabolite biomarkers have refined the exposure assessments in many studies, the organophosphate and pyrethrin metabolites have very short half-lives in the order of 24–48 hours, and the use of one sample could result in underrepresentation of true exposure. The consistent associations with neurodevelopmental outcomes found in the studies argue that this is not an absolute limitation. The metabolites currently measured for organophosphates do not differentiate exposure to the parent compounds from direct ingestion of the metabolites, which are frequently present on fruits and vegetables. This may be an important distinction, since the metabolites do not have cholinergic activity.[524]

The concept of a critical prenatal period for pesticide exposure is a potential limitation. Some researchers believe that first trimester exposures, as in traditional teratology, are most important. Others point to the period of rapid brain growth in the third trimester and early childhood as the most critical. This group of studies includes findings of positive associations with first and third trimester measures of prenatal exposure, with a trend toward the first trimester being more critical for organochlorines and third trimester for organophosphates. However, the cross-sectional studies also find that current exposures of older children are associated with neurodevelopmental outcomes, such as ADHD.

The longitudinal cohort design has much strength, but a weakness of the current cohorts is that they were recruited from areas where higher than normal exposure is expected. This limits their generalizability to cohorts with lower exposures, and at the same time may obscure important health effects that could occur at very low levels of exposure, as may be the case with the endocrine disruptors.[525–527]

Finally, in some cohorts, a decision was made to exclude children with autism or pervasive developmental delay from the cohorts upon diagnosis. This probably reflects the author's uncertainty about the etiology of these conditions, but may have reduced opportunities to find out whether pesticide exposures were associated with these conditions.

The studies in this systematic review show that prenatal pesticide exposure is associated with consistent measurable deficits in child neurodevelopment across a wide age range.

In neonates, this is manifest as abnormal reflexes and deficits in attentiveness to stimuli with organophosphate exposure and as irritability with organochlorine exposure. In pesticide-exposed children aged 12–24 months, there are consistent deficits in the Mental Development Index with organophosphates. For exposure to organochlorines such as DDT, there are deficits in both scales but with stronger effects for the PDI. For these early childhood deficits, the relative risks are usually in the 1.5–2.0 range. However, even a small increase in the incidence of such complex conditions may impact both the health care system and the learning and earning potential of affected individuals.

In older children, attention problems such as ADHD, reduced overall IQ, and other conditions including autism spectrum disorder and pervasive developmental disorder are more common in children who had higher levels of organophosphate or DDT/DDE exposure during pregnancy. Typically, statistically significant health effects are seen primarily in children with the highest 20%–25% of exposure. On the other hand, there are rarely unexposed control groups, which may result in underestimation of the risk of ADHD. Some studies of ADHD and autism associated with prenatal exposure have higher relative risks in the 6.0–7.0 range. Knapp[528] studied 30-year-olds from a birth cohort in the United Kingdom and found that both males and females diagnosed with attention deficit at age 10 had "lower employment rates, worse jobs, lower earnings if employed, and lower expected earnings overall." Children diagnosed with ADHD also have a much higher likelihood of engaging in criminal behavior as adults, with high attendant social costs.[529] They also suffer earlier death than those without ADHD, perhaps (as found in a longitudinal cohort, now in midlife) because they start smoking at a younger age and are more likely to continue binge drinking as they age.[530]

In multiscale IQ tests, working memory and verbal comprehension appear to be most consistently affected. The effects are modest, with relative risks usually <2.0. However, the reductions in total IQ found (2–7 points) will have substantial impacts on school performance and later earning potential when viewed from an economic population perspective. In 2001, Environment Canada scientists estimated the cost of a loss of 5 IQ points at CAD 30 billion dollars per year for Canada, and the cost of neurodevelopmental deficits and hypothyroidism at CAN 2 billion per year for Ontario alone. The proportion of those conditions (and costs) considered attributable to environmental exposures was at least 10% and as high as 50%.[531]

Our understanding of the association between pesticide exposure and child neurodevelopment has benefited from several large longitudinal studies of birth cohorts from the United States, Spain, and Mexico. These cohorts were all recruited from groups thought to have higher-than-average exposure to pesticides. In the future, it will be important to study the associations with health effects in cohorts with typical exposures. The NHANES data from the United States give us a cross-sectional snapshot of current childhood exposure, which is important, with the limitation that prenatal exposures may be more predictive of neurodevelopmental deficits.

For example, ADHD was associated with pesticide exposure in both types of study, and autism was associated with pesticide spraying within 500 miles of rural homes in the first trimester in a case–control study. Other studies made autism or pervasive developmental delay exclusion criteria, removing children (and potentially important information) from some of the longitudinal cohorts.

Taken as a whole, the results of the systematic review of pesticide exposure and child neurodevelopment suggest that children are experiencing neurodevelopmental problems of various types, starting in the newborn period and throughout childhood, that are associated with prenatal and childhood pesticide exposures. This suggests that vigilance is required to minimize the pesticide exposures of pregnant women and children from all potential sources, including dietary, indoor and outdoor air, water, and farm exposures. The current-use organophosphates are consistently implicated in neurodevelopmental deficits, as is use of the organochlorines, still heavily used as crop pesticides in agricultural settings (Tables 7.29 through 7.31).

CARBAMATE CHOLINESTERASE-INHIBITING PESTICIDES

The following common commercial pesticide products are listed approximately in order of decreasing toxicity:

- *Highly toxic (acute oral LD_{50} in the rat <50 mg/kg)*: aldicarb (this carbamate is a systemic, for example, it is taken up by the plant and translocated into foliage and sometimes into the fruit) (Temik), oxamyl (Vydate), carbofuran (Furadan), methomyl (Lannate, Nudrin), formetanate HCI (Carzol, Dicazol), aminocarb (Matacil), dimetilan (Ship Fly Bands)
- *Moderately toxic (acute oral LD_{50} in the rat above 50 mg/kg)*: promecarb (Carbamult), methiocarb (Mesurol, Draza), propoxur (Baygon), pirimicarb (Pirimor Aphox, Rapid), bufencarb (Bux), carbaryl (Sevin)

TABLE 7.29
Characteristics of Cohort Studies of Pesticide Exposure and Child Neurodevelopment

Name of Cohort	Location and Characteristics	Original Cohort Size	Retention Rate in Most Recent Publication
CHAMACOS	Agricultural Salinas Valley, California; Mexican-American farm workers' children	$n = 26$ newborns	62%, age 7
Mt. Sinai–New York City	Inner city	$n = 404$ newborns	42%, age 7
Columbia–New York City	Low-income black and Dominican	$n = 725$	74%, age 7
Mexican	Area with endemic malaria but no occupational DDT exposure	$n = 333$	81% at age 30 months
Spanish	Birth cohorts from a highly contaminated industrial area and a less contaminated area	$n = 102$ (organochlorine-contaminated area) $n = 482$ (no known industrial contaminants, 86% organochlorine pesticides in cord serum)	69%, age 4 98%, age 4
New Bedford, Massachusetts	Area highly contaminated with PCBs	$n = 788$	77%, age 8

TABLE 7.30

Maximum Safe Levels of Organophosphates[a] Found in Food Not Safe for the Chemically Sensitive

Commodity[b]	Parts per Million	Commodity[c]	Parts per Million
Corn	8.0	Barley, grain	6.0
Cattle, fat	0.2	Cattle, fat	0.50
Cattle, kidney and liver	2.0	Cattle, meat	0.5
Cattle	0.2	Cattle	0.5
Cattle, meat	0.2	Eggs	0.1
Eggs	0.5	Goats, fat	0.5
Goats, fat	0.2	Goats, meat	0.5
Goats, kidney and liver	2.0	Goats	0.5
Goats	0.2	Hogs, fat	0.5
Goats, meat	0.2	Hogs, meat	0.5
Hogs, fat	0.2	Hogs	0.5
Hogs, kidney and liver	2.0	Horses, fat	0.5
Hogs	0.2	Horses, meat	0.5
Hogs, meat	0.2	Horses	0.5
Horses, fat	0.2	Milk, fat (0.05 ppm [N] in whole milk)	1.25
Horses, kidney and liver	2.0	Oats, grain	6.0
Horses	0.2	Poultry, fat	0.5
Horses, meat	0.2	Poultry, meat	0.5
Kiwifruit	5.0	Poultry	0.5
Milk, fat (0.1 ppm [N] in whole milk)	3.0	Rice, grain	6.0
Poultry, fat	0.2	Sheep fat	0.5
Poultry	2.0	Sheep, meat	0.5
Poultry, meat	2.0	Sheep	0.5
Sheep, fat	0.2	Sorghum, grain	6.0
Sheep, kidney and liver	2.0	Wheat, grain	6.0
Sheep	0.2		
Sheep, meat	0.2		

Source: Federal Register 51. August 6, 1986. P. 28228.

[a] These levels will trigger chemical sensitivity.

[b] Pirimiphos-methyl; tolerances for residues. Tolerances are established for the combined residues of the insecticides pirimiphos-methyl, *O*-(2-diethylamino 6-methyl-pyrimidinyl), *O,O*-dimethyl phosphorothioate, the metabolite *O*-(2-ethylamino-6-methyl-pyrimidin-4-yl), *O,O*-dimethyl phosphorothioate and, in free and conjugated form, the metabolites 2-diethylamino-6-methylpyrimidin-4-ol), 2-ethylamino-6-methyl-pyrimdin-4-ol, and 2-amino-6-methyl-pyrimidin-4-ol in or on the above raw agricultural commodities.

[c] Chlorpyrifos-methyl. Tolerances are established for the combined residues of the insecticide chlorpyrifos-methyl *O,O*-dimethyl *O*-(3,5,6-trichloro-2-pyridyl) phosphorothioate and its metabolite (3,5,6-trichloro-2-pyridinol) in or on the above raw agricultural commodities.

Insecticides of this class cause reversible carbamylation of AChE enzyme, allowing accumulation of acetylcholine at cholinergic neuroeffector junctions (muscarinic effects) and at skeletal muscle myoneural junctions and in autonomic ganglia (nicotinic effects). This poison also impairs CNS function. The carbamyl–enzyme combination dissociates more readily than does the phosphorylated enzyme produced by organophosphate insecticides. This lability tends to mitigate the toxicity of carbamates, but also limits the usefulness of blood enzyme measurements in the diagnosis of

TABLE 7.31

Four Cross-Sectional Studies of Ecuadorian Children with Parents Employed in Floriculture

Grandjean[154] 12/20	Handal[532] 8.5/20	Handal[161] 8.5/20	Harari[170] 14.5/20
$n = 79$, grade 1–2 children	$n = 142$, children aged 24–61 months	$n = 121$, infants aged 3–23 months	$n = 87$, children's median age 6.5 years
• Prenatally exposed scored lower on design-copying test ($p < 0.05$) • Currently exposed had slower reaction times ($p < 0.01$)	• Children with mothers prenatally or currently in flower industry had better developmental scores (trend NS) • Children playing in irrigation water had decreased fine motor and problem-solving skills ($p < 0.05$) • Wide confidence intervals on many outcome measures	• Prenatally exposed children had a 13% decrease in fine motor scores ($p < 0.05$) and 9–18-month-olds had increased risk of visual problems (OR = 4.7, 95% CI = 1.1–20)	• Prenatally exposed children (maternal) showed deficits in simple motor speed, design coping, and visual memory recall (all $p < 0.05$) • For paternal only, prenatal exposure children showed visual memory deficits ($p < 0.05$) • Current exposure: no significant deficits

Note: Numbers behind the first author's names indicate quality assessment score out of 20.

poisoning. Carbamates are absorbed by inhalation, ingestion, and dermal penetration. They are actively metabolized by the liver, and the degradation products are excreted by the liver and kidneys.

A few carbamate insecticides are formulated in methyl (wood) alcohol. In cases of ingestion of these formulations, the toxicology of the methanol must be taken fully into consideration, including severe gastroenteric irritation, acidosis, CNS injury, and neuropathy.

Another group of carbamates are fungicides and herbicides. They do not deplete cholinesterase, but certainly can trigger chemical sensitivity. The mechanism of sensitivity probably lies in cell membrane damage, as shown in the OP section, but is unknown at the present.

Dithiocarbamates and Thiocarbamates

These functional classes include many fungicides and herbicides. There are several subclasses, including bisdithiocarbamates, metallodithiocarbamates, ethylene bisdithiocarbamates, and (mono) thiocarbamates.

The commercial products containing bisdithiocarbamates (Figure 7.52) include thiram (Arasan, Thiramad, Thirasan, Thylate, Pomarsol forte, TMTDS, Thiotex, Fernasan, Nomersan, TGersan, Thiuramin, Tuads, AAtack, Aules, Chipco Thiram 75, Fermide 850, Trametan, Hexathir, Mercuram, Polyram-Ultra, Spotrete, Tripomol, Tersan 75, Tetrapom, Thioknock). Thiram is a fungicide.

Commercial products containing metallobisdithiocarbamates (Figure 7.52) include ziram (Z-C Spray, Carbazinc, Corozate, Cuman, Drupina 90, Fuclasin Ultra, Fuklasin, Fungostop, Hexazir, Mezene, Pomarsol Z Forte, Prodaram, Tricarbamix Z, Triscabol, Zerlate, Vancide MZ-96, Zincmate, Ziram Technical, Ziramvis, Zirasan 90, Zirberk, Zirex 90, and Ziride), abam (Dithane D14, Chem

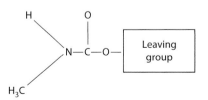

FIGURE 7.52 General chemical structure of carbamate cholinesterase-inhibiting pesticides. (From *Chemical sensitivity* Volume II, page 868, figure 19. With permission.)

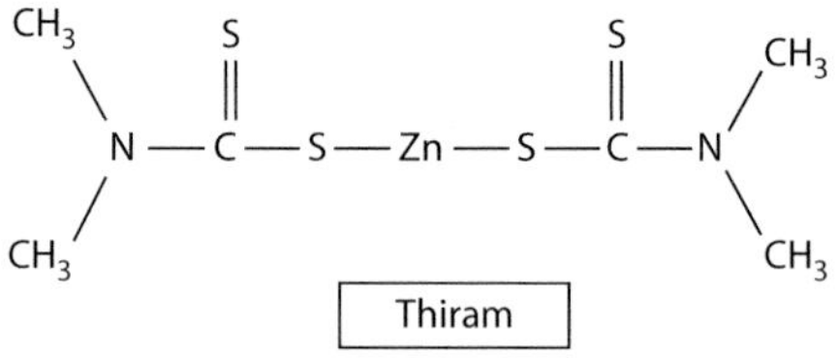

FIGURE 7.53 Chemical structure of bisdithiocarbamates. (From Chemical sensitivity Volume II, page 868, figure 20. With permission.)

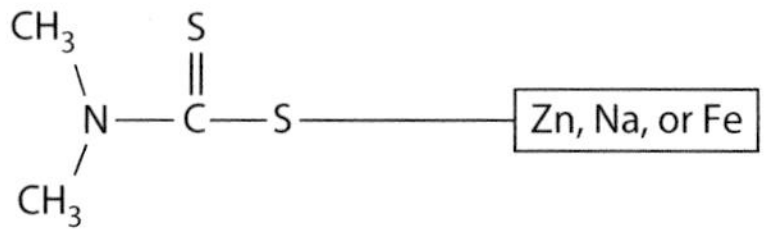

FIGURE 7.54 Chemical structure of metal bisdithiocarbamates. (From Chemical sensitivity Volume II, page 868, figure 21. With permission.)

Bam, DSE, Nabasan, Parzate, and Spring-Bak), and ferbam (Ferberk, Hexaferb, Knockmate, Trifungol and Vancide FE95). These chemicals are fungicides.

Commercial products containing ethylene bisdithiocarbamates (Figures 7.53 and 7.54) include maneb (Dithane M22, Griffin Manex, Kypman 80, Manebgan, Manesan, Manzate, Nespor, Manzeb, Polyram M, Manzin, Tersan LSR, Trimangol, Tubothane, and Vancide Maneb 80) and zineb (Aspor, Dipher, Dithane Z-78, Hexathane, Kypzin, Lonacol, Parzate, Polyram Z, Tiezene, Tritoftorol, Zebtox, and Zinosan).

These fungicides are often combined with thiram and with various inorganic salts of copper, manganese, and zinc in commercial preparations. Mancozeb (Dithane M45) is essentially a combination of maneb and zineb.

Commercial products containing (mono) thiocarbamates include butylate (Sutan), cycloate (Ro-Neet), pebulate (Tillam), vernolate (Vernam, Surpass), EPTC (Etpam), diallate (Avadex), and triallate (Far-Go, Avadex-BW). These chemicals are selective herbicides.

Although these agents have chemical similarities, the separate classes are metabolized differently by mammals, and effects on human health are also different. In general, mammalian toxicity, as measured by oral dosing studies in laboratory rodents, is low. Occupational exposures in humans, however, have caused acute adverse effects and laboratory investigations have suggested potential chronic effects from some agents. Chemical sensitivity has been observed after exposure. None of these agents is a cholinesterase inhibitor (Figure 7.55).

Thiram is irritating to skin and mucous membranes. It has sensitized some individuals, generally after contact with rubber products containing residues of thiram used as a curing agent.

The metallodithiocarbamates and ethylene dithiocarbamates are moderately irritating to skin and the respiratory mucous membranes following contact with sprays or dust.

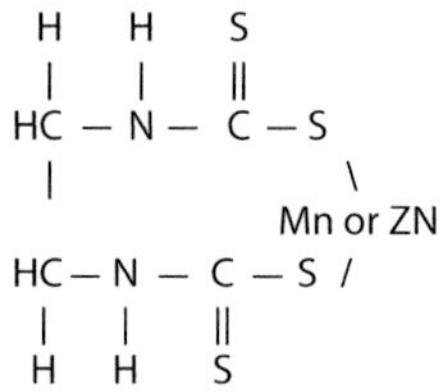

FIGURE 7.55 Structure of ethylene bisdithiocarbamates. (From Chemical sensitivity Volume II, page 869, figure 22. With permission.)

The ethylene bisdithiocarbamate class includes maneb, zineb, mancozeb, metiram, and nabam. According to the EPA, a common contaminant ethylene thiourea (ET) is a carcinogen in rats and has specific effects on the thyroid in three animal types. ET accumulates in processed and cooled foods. These thiocarbamates are all complexed with minerals, zinc, manganese, iron, and sodium. We have seen one farmer who worked with maneb who had extremely high levels of manganese and was extremely ill with chemical sensitivity.[171]

Thiram is the methyl analog of disulfiram (Antabuse), an agent used to condition alcoholics against ingested alcohol. Much more is known of the toxic effects of disulfiram than of thiram, although the acute toxicity of thiram in laboratory animals is substantially greater. Given to animals in extreme doses, disulfiram has caused GI irritation, demyelinization of CNS tissues, and necrosis of liver, splenic, and kidney tissues. Peripheral neuropathy and psychotic reactions have occurred in humans taking large doses of disulfiram regularly.

Functional and anatomic CNS damage has been demonstrated in rats on high chronic dosage regimens of iron and zinc dimethyldithiocarbamates. Because all of these agents are degraded partly to carbon disulfide in the body, a role of this metabolite in neurotoxic effects is suspected.

Both thiram and disulfiram inhibit aldehyde dehydrogenase and are therefore capable of inducing "Antabuse" reactions in persons who consume the beverage with alcohol following substantial absorption of dithiocarbamates. Reactions may have occurred rarely in workers who imbibed alcohol after extraordinary occupational exposure to thiram. Theoretically, the metallodithiocarbamates may also predispose to an "Antabuse" reaction. Peripheral vasodilation is the main pathophysiologic feature of the disulfiram–alcohol reaction, probably due to high tissue levels of acetaldehyde. This type of exposure may occasionally lead to shock and even more rarely to myocardial ischemia, cardiac arrhythmias, circulatory failure, and death. Animal experimentation has suggested certain other biochemical mechanisms of toxicity involving reaction products of ethanol and disulfiram. Frequently, a subset of chemically sensitive individuals has this peripheral dilation phenomenon. Possibly, inhalation, ingestion, or absorption of other nonliquor alcohols will trigger this response in them.

The ethylene bisdithiocarbamates do not inhibit aldehyde dehydrogenase, and evidence of neurotoxicity is unknown. In the environment and in mammalian tissues, however, dithiocarbamates do degrade to ET, a compound known as a goitrogen and carcinogen in laboratory animals. This feature mandates extra care in the protection of harvesters and in removal of residues from harvested crops.

Except for some moderate irritant effects on skin, respiratory tract, and eyes, the (mono) thiocarbamate herbicides do not appear to be highly toxic, but they do exacerbate chemical sensitivity. Extreme doses in laboratory animals do produce paralysis. There is a very remote possibility of "Antabuse" reactions from ethanol following extraordinary exposure to these (mono) thiocarbamates. They do not form ET on degradation.

Pyrethrum, which has been used as an insecticide for >60 years, is the partly refined extract of the chrysanthemum flower. It is an oleoresin. The extract contains about 50% active ingredients. Pyrethrins are the insecticidally active ingredients of pyrethrum, now known to consist of ketoalcohol esters of pyrethric and chrysanthemic acids. The alcohols are pyrethrolone, cinerolone, and jasmolone, whose respective esters are known as pyrethrins, cinerins, and jasmolins. Being light, heat, and moisture sensitive, they have a half-life in hours. Pyrethroids are synthetic compounds based structurally on the pyrethrin molecule but modified to improve stability in the natural environment for light, heat, etc. In general, they have been observed to cause more health problems than natural pyrethrums.[533]

Pyrethrins and pyrethroids are contained in several hundred commercial products. Commonly, these products combine pyrethrins or pyrethroids with a synergist, such as piperonal butoxide, and an additional pesticide for increased killing power. Many of these combinations are packaged with a propellant in a spray can or bomb.

Some commercial pyrethroids are found in the following: allethrin (Pynamin), bifenthrin, bioresmethrin, cypermethrin (Ripcord), decamethrin, fenothrin, fenpropanate, fenvalerate (Belmark, Pydrin), permethrin (Ambush, Ectiban, Pounce), phthalthrin or tetramethrin (Neo-Pynamin), and resmethrin (Synthrin, Chrysron).

These esters rapidly paralyze the insect nervous system, making them famous for their quick "knockdown" effect. Both pyrethrins and pyrethroids interfere with some conductors of nerve membranes by prolonging the sodium current. Mammalian toxicity, however, is extraordinarily low for pyrethrins, but not necessarily for pyrethroids. Oral LD_{50} values for these compounds in rats are several hundred or thousand mg/kg body weight. There is apparently less efficient absorption of pyrethrins across the GI lining and skin than across insect chitin, and much more rapid biodegradation (hydrolysis and oxidation) by the mammalian liver than by insect tissues.

Some of the less purified pyrethrum extracts contain allergenic substances that induce attacks of allergic rhinitis and asthma in humans. Rarely, hypersensitivity pneumonitis has followed pyrethrum inhalation. Chemical hypersensitivity does occur.

Administered orally to rodents in extraordinary dosage, pyrethrins and pyrethroids cause nervous irritability, tremors, and motor ataxia. Bloody tears and urinary incontinence have also been observed. Manifestations of toxicity occur at a much lower dosage after intravenous administration than after oral dosing. Chronic feeding of these chemicals induces an increase in liver size and bile duct hyperplasia. To date, neither pyrethrins nor pyrethroids have been identified as mutagenic, carcinogenic, or teratogenic. Again, one has to be extremely cautious about using animal data in humans, since there may be no relationship.

Pyrethrums are dermal and respiratory allergens resulting in dermatitis and asthma. There is a strong cross-reactivity with ragweed pollen. Large oral doses give NS excitation, convulsions, muscle fibrillation, and diarrhea.[534,535]

Piperonal butoxide inhibits the mixed-function oxidase enzymes of the liver, which catabolize pyrethrins and pyrethroids. The amount absorbed by humans during ordinary acute exposure is not likely to affect liver function measurably. However, chronic exposure combined with other toxic chemicals probably damages this system.

The behavior and fate of pesticides in the environment will determine their impact on both humans and nontarget organisms. Biochemical biomarkers are increasingly used in ecological risk assessment to identify the incidence of exposure to and effects caused by xenobiotics. This study was undertaken to investigate the potential toxic effect of a locally produced insect powder called "Rambo" (which contains 0.6% permethrin) on nontarget organisms exemplified with albino rats. The results obtained showed that glutathione S-transferase (GST) activity in the newly weaned rats (NWR) and middle-aged rats (MAR) groups were found to increase significantly ($p < 0.05$) in the liver homogenates at the concentrations used (1%, 5%, and 10%) compared with their parallel controls. In the plasma and brain homogenates, a decrease in GST activity was observed; this decrease was significant ($p < 0.05$) in the brain homogenates, but in the blood plasma, the decrease in GST activity was not significant ($p > 0.05$).

However, the highest GST activity (398.44 + 23.44) U/L was recorded in the liver homogenates while the least activity (9.07 + 3.44) U/L was obtained in the plasma sample. The significance of such a decrease in intracellular GST is that protection against reactive intermediates may be lost and thus affect vital metabolic processes that may result in death.

This shows that GST can be used as a biomarker in ecological risk assessment of pesticide-contaminated environment.

Pyrethroids are a widely used class of insecticides used for mosquito control and various insects in residential and agricultural settings. However, pyrethroids are highly neurotoxic and have been linked to cancer, endocrine disruption, suppression of the immune system, and various reproductive effects chemical sensitivity. This class of chemicals includes permethrin, bifenthrin, resmethrin, cyfluthrin, and scores of others. (Reference Read Beyond Pesticides factsheet Synthetic Pyrethroids.) Once the agency completes and approves the pyrethroid chemical assessment, it is likely that new uses of these pesticides will be added. The agency claims that more pyrethroid registrations may help combat recent pervasive pest problems, such as stink bugs and bed bugs, even though this class of chemicals is already known to be ineffective against these pests due to growing resistance issues compounded with continued pesticide use. However, serious issues such as the carcinogenic and endocrine-disrupting potential of several pyrethroids were not mentioned in the risk assessment even though a recent study published in *Environmental Health Perspectives* finds that low-dose, short-term exposure to esfenvalerate, a synthetic pyrethroid pesticide, delays the onset of puberty in at doses two times lower than EPAs stated no observable effect level.

Studies have found that certain pyrethroids, such as permethrin, are almost five times more toxic to the young compared with adults. Additionally, studies have shown that permethrin may inhibit neonatal brain development. In this new cumulative risk assessment, the agency even states, based on pharmacokinetic data, there is evidence that indicates an increase in sensitivity to pyrethroids of the young compared with adults, which is attributed to the difference in the ability of the adults and juveniles to metabolize pyrethroids.[4] EPA's modeling data also predict a threefold increase of pyrethroid concentrations in juvenile brains compared with adults. Similarly, researchers at Emory University and the Centers for Disease Control and Prevention (CDC) in a published study conclude that residential pesticide use represents the most important risk factor for children's exposure to pyrethroid insecticides.

With the phaseout of most residential uses of the common organophosphate insecticides, chlorpyrifos and diazinon, home use of pyrethroids has increased. Pesticide products containing synthetic pyrethroids are often described by pest control operators and community mosquito management bureaus as safe as chrysanthemum flowers. While pyrethroids are a synthetic version of an extract from the chrysanthemum plant, they are chemically engineered to be more toxic, take longer to break down, and are often formulated with synergists, increasing potency, and compromising the human body's ability to detoxify the pesticide.

As a consequence of their widespread use, many pests such as bed bugs are now becoming resistant to pyrethroids.

A recent study shows that modern bed bugs have developed the ability to defend themselves against pyrethroid pesticides, with a required dosage of as much as 1000 times the amount that should normally be lethal, due in part to the widespread use of such treatment methods. Due to the ability of these organisms to develop resistance to chemical agents, exposing these bugs to more pesticides would lead to higher rates of resistance among insect populations, a point that EPA does not acknowledge. Perhaps, washing and steaming them would be more efficacious.

Exposure to synthetic pyrethroids has been reported to lead to headaches, dizziness, nausea, irritation, and skin sensations. There are also serious chronic health concerns related to synthetic pyrethroids. EPA classifies permethrin and cypermethrin as possible human carcinogens, based on evidence of lung tumors in lab animals exposed to these chemicals. EPA also lists permethrin as a suspected endocrine disruptor. Synthetic pyrethroids have also been linked to respiratory problems such as hypersensitization, and may be triggers for asthma attacks. Material Safety Data Sheets, issued by the Occupational Safety and Health Administration (OSHA), for pyrethroid products often warn, "Persons with history of asthma, emphysema, and other respiratory tract disorders may experience symptoms with low exposures."

In addition to human health effects which this cumulative risk assessment addresses, pyrethroids are also persistent in the environment and adversely impact nontarget organisms. A 2008 survey found pyrethroid contamination in 100% of urban streams sampled in California. Researchers also find pyrethroid residues in California streams, although at relatively low concentrations (10–20 parts per trillion) in river and creek sediments that are toxic to bottom dwelling fish. Other studies find pyrethroids present in effluent from sewage treatment plants at concentrations just high enough to be toxic to sensitive aquatic organisms.

At the same time, there are clear established methods for managing homes and schools that prevent infestation of unwanted insects without the use of synthetic chemicals, including exclusion techniques, sanitation, and maintenance practices, as well as mechanical and least toxic controls (which include boric acid and diatomaceous earth). Based on the host of health effects linked to this chemical class, an increase in synthetic pyrethroid use is hazardous and unnecessary.

Corbel,[536] from the Institut de Recherche pour le Developpement in Montpellier, and Bruno Lapied, from the University of Angers, France, led a team of researchers who investigated the mode of action and toxicity of DEET (*N,N*-diethyl-3-methylbenzamide). Corbel found that DEET is not simply a behavior-modifying chemical but also inhibits the activity of a key CNS enzyme, acetyl-cholinesterase, in both insects and mammals.

DEET is the most common ingredient in insect repellent preparations. It is effective against a broad spectrum of medically important pests, including mosquitoes. Despite its widespread use, controversies remain concerning both the identification of its target sites at the molecular level and its mechanism of action in insects. In a series of experiments, Corbel et al.[536] found that DEET inhibits the AChE enzyme—the same mode of action used by organophosphate and carbamate insecticides.

These insecticides are often used in combination with DEET, and it was found that DEET interacts with carbamate insecticides to increase their toxicity. These findings question the safety of DEET, particularly in combination with other chemicals.

ARSENICALS

Arsenicals (Table 7.28) are pesticides containing many types of arsenic compounds (Figures 7.56 through 7.60). They can be both organic and inorganic compounds.

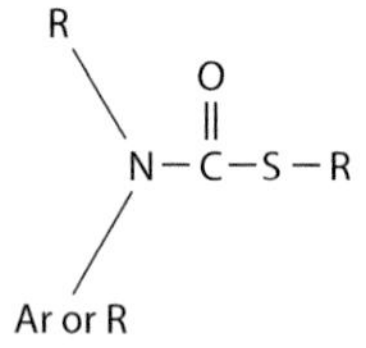

$$
\begin{array}{c}
R \\
\diagdown \\
 \overset{\displaystyle O}{\underset{\displaystyle \|}{N-C}}-S-R \\
\diagup \\
Ar\ or\ R
\end{array}
$$

FIGURE 7.56 Structure of (mono) thiocarbamates. (From Chemical sensitivity Volume II, page 868, figure 23. With permission.)

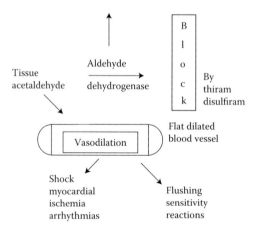

FIGURE 7.57 Inhibition of aldehyde dehydrogenases by thiram and disulfiram (Antabuse effect). (From Chemical sensitivity Volume II, page 870, figure 24. With permission.)

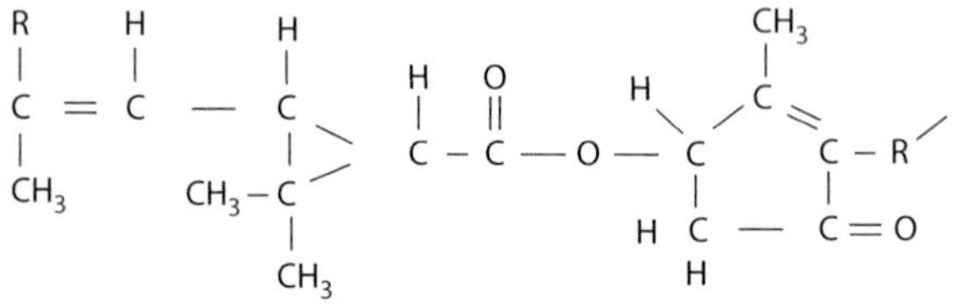

FIGURE 7.58 Pyrethrum, pyrethrins, pyrethroids, and piperonyl butoxide. (From Chemical sensitivity Volume II, page 871, figure 25. With permission.)

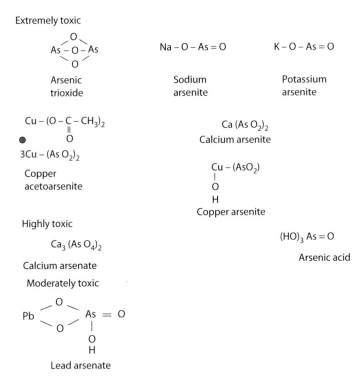

FIGURE 7.59 Chemical structure of inorganic arsenicals. (From Chemical sensitivity Volume II, page 873, figure 26. With permission.)

Although there may be some degrees of dermal and pulmonary absorption of arsenical liquids and sprays, ingestion is the route of intake involved in virtually all acute poisonings by the solid arsenicals. Many areas in the United States and around the world contain arsenics. Arsenic is used in chickens as a growth promoter. We are not sure about sensitivity, but probably either route will suffice, since we have seen many cases of patients who contained arsenic and were sensitive.

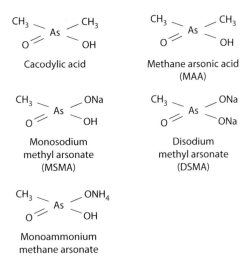

FIGURE 7.60 Chemical structure of arsenical pesticides. (From Chemical sensitivity Volume II, page 874, figure 27. With permission.)

Inhalation of arsine gas (sometimes generated inadvertently in pesticide manufacturing plants) has caused serious illness and death by hemolytic action.[537]

Generally, the organic (methylated) pentavalent arsenicals are considerably less toxic than the trivalent inorganic arsenicals. In fact, methylation is the principal mechanism of detoxification of inorganic arsenicals in mammals. To date, methylation is also the prime detoxification system that is malfunctioning in the chemically sensitive, though all others appear to be involved, and impairment of this process may make an individual more prone to arsenical sensitivity. The less soluble inorganic forms (notably lead arsenate and even arsenic trioxide) present less hazard than the more soluble salts such as sodium arsenite and copper acetoarsenite. But because gastric pH, GI motility, and gut bacterial action can enhance the absorption and toxicity of ingested compounds, it is safest to manage cases of arsenic ingestion though all forms of arsenic are highly toxic (Table 7.32).[4]

Trivalent arsenicals (or, more likely an arsenious acid metabolite) bind efficiently to the functional thiol groups of many tissue components, including enzymes. Its affinity for thiol groups in keratin accounts for the accumulation of arsenic in skin, nails, and hair in cases of chronic poisoning. When absorbed across the gut wall, these arsenicals injure the splanchnic vasculature, causing abdominal pain, colic, and diarrhea. Once absorbed into the blood, they cause toxic damage to the liver, kidneys, brain, bone marrow (BM), and peripheral nerves. Liver injury is manifest as hepatomegaly, jaundice, and an increase in circulating hepatocellular enzymes LDH and GOT. Renal damage is reflected in albuminuria, hematuria, pyuria, cylinduria, and then azotemia. Acute tubular necrosis may occur in severe poisoning. Injury to blood-forming tissues can take the form of agranulocytosis, aplastic anemia, thrombocytopenia, or pancytopenia. Toxic encephalopathy may manifest as speech and behavioral disturbances. Peripheral neuropathy occurs in both acute and chronic forms.

Sequelae of arsenic poisoning include cirrhosis, hypoplastic BM, renal insufficiency, and peripheral neuropathy. Excessive exposures to arsenicals have caused hyperkeratosis and skin cancers.

TABLE 7.32
Common Commercial Arsenic Products

1. Arsenic trioxide	"White arsenic," arsenious oxide, 90 registered only for ant pastes, veterinary medicinal, and marine antifouling preparations).
2. Sodium arsenite	Chem Pels C, Chem-Sen 56, Kill-All, Penite, Prodalumnol Double
3. Calcium arsenite	Monocalcium arsenite
4. Copper arsenite	Chemonite
5. Copper acetoarsenite	Paris green, Schweinfurt green, Emerald green, French green, Mitis green
6. Arsenic acid	Desiccant L-10, Hi-Yield Desiccant H-10
7. Sodium arsenate	Jones Ant Killer, Terro Ant Killer
8. Calcium arsenate	Pencal, Spra-cal, Security
9. Lead arsenate	Gypsine, Security, Soprabel, Talbot
10. Methane arsonic acid	MAA
11. Monosodium methyl arsenate	MSMA, Ansar 170HC, methane arsonate, Ansar 529HC, Arsonate liquid, Bueno 6, Daconate 6, Dal-E-Rad, Herb-All, Merge 823, Mesamate, Target MSMA, Trans-Vert, Weed-E-Rad, Weed-Hoe
12. Disodium methyl arsenate	DSMA, Ansar 8100, methane arsonate, Ansar DSMA liquid, Arrhenal, Arsinyl, Chipco Crab-Kleen, Crab-E-Rad, Dal-E-Rad 100, Di Tac, DMA, DMA 100, Methar, Namate, Sodar, Weed-E-Rad, Weed-E-Rad 360, Wee-E-Rad DMA Powder, Weed-Hoe
13. Monoammonium methyl arsenate	MAMA, monoammonium methanearsenate
14. Calcium acid methanearsenate	CAMA, Super Crab-E-Rad Calar, Super Dal-E-Rad Calar
15. Cacodylic acid	Dilic, Phytar 560, Rad-E-Cate 25, Salvo (Crystal Chemical Co.)

Source: U.S. Environmental Protection Agency. 1982. *Recognition and Management of Pesticide Poisonings*, 3rd ed., p. 48. Washington, DC: U.S. Environmental Protection Agency. EPA-540/9-80-005. (From Chemical sensitivity Volume II, page 875, table 10. With permission.)

Excessive inhalation of dusts may cause bronchitis and pneumonia; protracted inhalation has been associated epidemiologically with increased occurrence of lung cancer.

NATURE CHANGES DUE TO PESTICIDES

HONEYBEES AND CROPS

Researchers have found that exposure to two common pesticides can interfere with the growth and viability of both honeybee and bumblebee hives. The exposure, they say, may therefore contribute to the devastating loss of bee populations known as colony collapse disorder (CCD). Because of bees' role as crop pollinators, losses could cause a crisis for agriculture.

Since the CCD phenomenon was recognized in the mid-2000s, scientists have investigated possible causes, including fungal infection, viruses, and pesticides. But no study has been definitive. However, two new reports, one from entomologist Henry[538] at the French National Institute for Agricultural Research in Avignon and coworkers, and the other from biological sciences professor Goulson[539] at the University of Sterling, in Scotland, and colleagues, reinforce the pesticide theory.

The reports show that when exposed to pesticides known as neonicotinoids, honeybees have problems returning home after foraging, whereas bumblebee colonies grow poorly and produce fewer queens.[538,539]

The Henry group used radio frequency ID tags on individual bees to confirm known effects of pesticides on their foraging abilities. They tagged more than 600 free-range bees and then exposed some of them to sublethal doses of the neonicotinoid pesticide thiamethoxam. The exposed bees were twice as likely to die while foraging, implying that the bees' homing abilities were impaired.

Even more damning for pesticides, says University of Maryland entomologist vanEngelsdorp, is the Goulson research, in which colonies of bumblebees were exposed to sublethal doses of the neonicotinoid imidacloprid. Six weeks after exposure, colonies were 8%–12% smaller, and the number of queens produced dropped 85% compared with control hives. Pesticides are a big component of outside air and can cause many problems related to chemical overload and sensitivity. For example, a Colorado beekeeper recently obtained a leaked document revealing that the U.S. EPA knows a popular crop pesticide is killing off honeybees, but has allowed its continued approval anyway. Despite opposition from its own scientists, EPA official's first gave an approval to Bayer Crop Science's toxic pesticide clothianidin in 1993 based on the company's own flawed safety studies. But now, it has been revealed that the EPA knew all along about the dangers of clothianidin and decided to just ignore them.

By now, most people know that honeybees are dying off at an incredibly disturbing rate. CCD, a condition where bees stray from the hive and never find their way back, is nixing millions of nature's pollinators every year. Previous studies have pinpointed various environmental toxins as the primary culprits, including toxic pesticides such as clothianidin.[540]

The leaked document, which was written by the EPA's Office of Chemical Safety and Pollution Prevention, explains clearly that "clothianidin's major risk concern is nontarget insects (honeybees)" and that acute toxicity studies to honeybees show that clothianidin is highly toxic on both a contact and an oral basis."

To simulate pesticide exposures that bumblebees might encounter when a field of canola blooms, entomologist Goulson[539] of the University of Stirling in Scotland and his colleagues fed 50 *Bombus terrestris* laboratory colonies nonfatal doses of the pesticide imidacloprid. After 2 weeks of eating spiked pollen and sugar water, bees were set outside and allowed to forage around the Stirling campus at will. By season's end, the pesticide-dosed colonies were an average of 8%–12% smaller than 25 unexposed neighbor colonies.

More noticeably, the contaminated colonies managed to produce only about two young queens each. The other colonies averaged about 14. Pitiful production of new young queens bodes ill for bumblebees because all other colony members die at the end of the growing season. Young queens represent each group's sole hope for making new colonies the next year.

A drop in pollinator reproduction is the kind of finding that can get the attention of agencies regulating pesticide use, says Pettis,[541] a U.S. Department of Agriculture bee researcher in Beltsville,

Maryland. With these and previous studies, concerns are growing that usage rules for neonicotinoids may need to be tightened.

For honeybees, earlier tests have raised the possibility that chronic, nonfatal exposure to neonicotinoids impairs learning, memory, and other capacities that bees need for good flower hunting. To set up a test with bees flying freely outdoors, a research team in France used dental cement to fasten electronic identifiers onto more than 600 bees. Feeding bees low doses of the pesticide thiamethoxam in sugar water provided a realistic exposure, says coauthor Henry[538] of the French National Institute for Agricultural Research in Avignon.

After sipping the pesticide-tainted solution, the honeybees were moved up to a kilometer from their hives and released to find their way home. Researchers challenged bees with both familiar territory and landscapes the bees had never seen. Automated counters at hives logged the returnees.

By comparing the homing success of dosed versus untreated hives, researchers concluded that pesticides roughly doubled the risk on any given day that a forager would not make it home. Such a population drop substantially weakens a colony.

Mussen[542] emphasizes that poor pollination will not only reduce crop yields but, equally important, will also reduce the quality of some crops, such as melon and fruits. In experiments with melons, Atkins (Atkins, E. L. 1990, University of California, personal communication) reported that with adequate pollination, melon yields increased 10% and melon quality was raised 25% as measured by the dollar value of the melon crop.

Based on the analysis of honeybee and related pollination losses from wild bees caused by pesticides, pollination losses attributed to pesticides are estimated to represent about 10% of pollinated crops and have a yearly cost of about $210 million per year (Table 7.33). Clearly, the available evidence confirms that the yearly cost of direct honeybee losses, together with reduced yields resulting from poor pollination, is significant.

CROP AND CROP PRODUCT LOSSES

According to Pimental,[543] basically, pesticides are applied to protect crops from pests in order to increase yields, but sometimes the crops are damaged by the pesticide treatments. This occurs when (1) the recommended dosages suppress crop growth, development, and yield; (2) pesticides drift from the targeted crop to damage adjacent crops; (3) residual herbicides either prevent chemical sensitive crops from being planted; and/or (4) excessive pesticide residue accumulates on crops, necessitating the destruction of the harvest. Crop losses translate into financial loss for grower, distributors, wholesalers, transporters, retailers, food processors, and others. Potential profits as well as investments are lost. The costs of crop losses increase when the related costs of investigations, regulation, insurance, and litigation are added to the equation. Ultimately, the consumer pays for these losses in higher marketplace prices.

Data on crop losses due to pesticides are difficult to obtain. Many losses are never reported to the state and federal agencies because the parties settle privately.[544]

TABLE 7.33

Estimated Honeybee Losses and Pollination Losses from Honeybees and Wild Bees

List LOSS	Cost ($ million/per year)
Colony losses from pesticides	$13.3
Honey and wax losses	$25.3
Loss of potential honey production	$27.0
Bee rental for pollination	$ 8.0
Pollination losses	$210.0
Total	$283.6

Damage to crops may occur even when recommended dosages of herbicides and insecticides are applied to crops under normal environmental conditions. Recommended dosages of insecticides used on crops have been reported to suppress growth and yield in both cotton and strawberry crops.[545,546] The increase in susceptibility of some crops to insects and diseases following normal use of 2,4-D and other herbicides has been demonstrated.[547,548] Furthermore, when weather and/ or soil conditions are inappropriate for pesticide application, herbicide treatments may cause yield reductions ranging from 2% to 50%.[544]

Crops are lost when pesticides drift from the target crops to nontarget crops located as much as several miles downwind.[549] Drift occurs with most methods of pesticide application, including both ground and aerial equipment; the potential problem is greatest when pesticides are applied by aircraft. With aircraft, 50% to 75% of the pesticide applied never reaches the target acre.[544,550,551] In contrast, 10%–35% of the pesticide applied with ground application equipment misses the target area.[552] The most serious drift problems are caused by "speed sprayers" and ultralow-volume (ULV) equipment, because relatively concentrated pesticide is applied. The concentrated pesticide has to be broken into small droplets to achieve adequate coverage. Crop injury and subsequent loss due to drift are particularly common in areas planted with diverse crops. For example, in Southwest Texas in 1983 and 1984, nearly $20 million in cotton was destroyed from drifting 2,4-D herbicide when adjacent wheat fields were aerially sprayed with the herbicide.[553] Owing to the drift problem, most commercial applicators carry insurance that costs about $245 million year.[544]

When residues of some herbicides persist in the soil, crops planted in rotation are sometimes injured. This has happened with a corn and soybean rotation. When atrazine or Scepter herbicides were used in corn, the soybean crop planted after was seriously damaged by the herbicides that persist in the soil. This problem also has environmental problems associated. For example, if the herbicide treatment prevents another crop from being grown, soil erosion may be intensified.[544]

An average 0.1% loss in annual U.S. production of corn, soybeans, cotton, and wheat, which together account for about 90% of the herbicides and insecticides used in the U.S. agriculture, was valued at $35.3 million in 1987.[554] Assuming that only one-third of the incidents involving crop losses due to pesticides are reported to authorities, the total value of all crop lost because of pesticides could be as high as three times this amount, of $106 million annually.

However, this $106 million does not take into account other crop losses nor does it include major events such as large-scale losses that have occurred in one season in Iowa ($25–30 million), in Texas ($20 million), and in California's aldicarb/water melon crisis ($8 million) (Table 7.34).[544]

Additional losses are incurred when food crops are disposed of because they exceed the FDA and EPA regulatory tolerances for pesticide residue levels. Assuming that all the crops and crop products that exceed the FDA and EPA regulatory tolerances (reported to be 1%–5%) were disposed of as required by law, then about $11 billion in crops would be destroyed because of excessive pesticide contamination.

TABLE 7.34

Estimated Loss of Crops and Trees due to the Use of Pesticides

Impacts	Total Cost (in Millions of Dollars)
Crop losses	136
Crop applicator insurance	245
Crops destroyed because of excess pesticide contamination	1000
Governmental investigations and testing	10
Total	1391

Source: With permission from Springer Science+Business Media: *Environment, Development and Sustainability*, Environmental and economic costs of the application of pesticides primarily in the United States, 7(2), 2005, Pimentel, D., Table V.

Special investigations and testing for pesticide contamination are estimated to cost the nation more than $10 million each year.[544]

GROUND AND SURFACE WATER CONTAMINATION

Certain pesticides applied at recommended dosages to crops eventually end up in ground and surface waters. The three most common pesticides found in groundwater are aldicarb, alachlor, and atrazine.[555] Estimates are that nearly one-half of the groundwater and well water in the United States is or has the potential to be contaminated.[556,557] In 1990, EPA[558] reported that 10% of community wells and 4% of rural domestic wells have detectable levels of at least 1 pesticide of the 127 pesticides tested in a national survey. Estimated costs to sample and monitor well and groundwater for pesticide residues costs $1100 per well per year.[559] With 16 million wells in the United States, the cost of monitoring all the wells for pesticides would cost $17.7 billion per year.[560]

Two major concerns about groundwater contamination with pesticides are that about one-half of the human population obtains its water from wells and once groundwater is contaminated, the pesticide residues remain for long periods of time. Not only are there extremely few microbes present in groundwater to degrade the pesticides but the groundwater recharge rate is also <1% per year.[561]

Monitoring pesticides in groundwater is only a portion of the total cost of groundwater contamination. There is also the high cost of cleanup. For instance, at the Rocky Mountain Arsenal near Denver, Colorado, the removal of pesticides from the groundwater and soil was estimated to cost approximately $2 billion. If all pesticide-contaminated groundwater was to be cleared of pesticides before human consumption, the cost would be about $500 million per year. Note the cleanup process requires a water survey to target the contaminated water for cleanup. Thus, in addition to the monitoring and cleaning costs, the total cost regarding pesticide-polluted groundwater is estimated to be about $2 billion annually. The $17.7 billion figure shows how impossible it would be to expect the public to pay for pesticide-free well water.

FISHERY LOSSES

Pesticides are washed into aquatic ecosystems by water runoff and soil erosion. About 13 ha^{-1} year^{-1} is washed and/or blown from pesticide-treated cropland into adjacent locations, including rivers and lakes.[562] Pesticides also can drift during application and contaminate aquatic systems. Some soluble pesticides are easily leached into streams and lakes.

Once in aquatic ecosystems, pesticides cause fishery losses in several ways. These include high pesticide concentrations in water that directly kill fish; low doses that may kill highly susceptible fish fry; or the elimination of essential fish foods, such as insect and other invertebrates. In addition, because government safety restrictions ban the catching or sale of fish contaminated with pesticide residues, such fish are unmarketable and are an economic loss.

Only 6–14 million fish are reported killed by pesticides each year.[544] However, this is an underestimate because fish kills cannot be investigated quickly enough to determine accurately the cause of the kill. Also, if the fish are in fast-moving water in rivers, the pesticides are diluted and/or the pesticides cannot be identified. Many fish sink to the bottom and cannot be counted.

The best estimate for the value of a fish is $10. This is based on EPA fining Coors Beer $10 per fish when they polluted a river.[563] Thus, the estimate of the value of fish killed each year is only $10–24 million per year. This is an underestimate and estimates $100 million per year minimum.

WILD BIRDS AND MAMMALS

Wild birds and mammals are damaged and destroyed by pesticides and these animals make excellent "indicator species." Deleterious effects on wildlife include death from the direct exposure to pesticides or secondary poisonings from consuming contaminated food; reduced survival, growth, and reproductive rates from exposure to sublethal dosages; and habitat reduction through the elimination of food resources and refuges. In the United States, approximately 3 kg of pesticide is applied per hectare on about 160 million ha of cropland each.[544]

With such heavy dosages of pesticides applied, it is expected that wildlife would be significantly impacted.

The full extent of bird and mammal kills is difficult to determine because birds and mammals are often secretive, camouflaged, highly mobile, and live in dense grass, shrubs, and trees. Typical field studies of the effects of pesticides often obtain extremely low estimates of bird and mammal mortality.[564] This is because bird and small mammal carcasses disappear quickly, well before the dead birds and small mammals can be found and counted. Even when known numbers of bird carcasses were placed in identified locations in the field, from 62% to 92% of the animals disappeared overnight due to vertebrate and invertebrate scavengers.[565] In addition, field studies seldom account for birds that die a distance from the treated areas. Finally, birds often hide and die in inconspicuous locations.

Nevertheless, many bird kills caused by pesticides have been reported. For instance, 1200 Canada geese were killed in one wheat field that was sprayed with a 2:1 mixture of parathion and methyl parathion at a rate of 0.8 kg/ha.[566] Carbofuran applied to alfalfa killed more than 5000 ducks and geese in five incidents, while the same chemical applied to vegetable crops killed 1400 ducks in a single application.[567,568] Carbofuran is estimated to kill 1–2 million birds each year.[569] Another pesticide, diazinon, applied to three golf courses, killed 700 Atlantic brant geese of the wintering population of just 2500 birds.[570]

EPA reports that there are 1100 documented cases of bird kills each year in the United States.[571] Birds are not only killed in the United States but are also killed as they migrate from North America to South America. For example, more than 4000 carcasses of Swainson's hawks were reported poisoned by pesticides in late 1995 and early 1996 in farm fields of Argentina.[572] Although it was not possible to know the total kill, conservatively, it was estimated to be more than 20,000 hawks.

Several studies report that the use of some herbicides has a negative impact on some young birds. Since the weeds would have harbored some insects in the crops, their nearly total elimination shows herbicides to be devastating to particular bird populations.[573] This has led to significant reductions in the gray partridge in the United Kingdom and in the common pheasant in the United States. In the case of the partridge, population levels have decreased >77% because the partridge chicks (also pheasant chicks) depend on insects to supply them with needed protein for their development and survival.

Frequently, the form of a pesticide influences its toxicity to wildlife. For example, treated seed and insecticide granules, including carbofuran, fensulfothion, fonofos, and phorae, are particularly toxic to birds. Estimates are that from 0.23 to 1.5 birds were killed ha^{-1} year^{-1} by the pesticides.[574]

Pesticides also adversely affect the reproductive potential of many birds and mammals. Exposure of birds, especially predatory birds, to chlorinated insecticides has caused reproductive failure, sometimes attributed to eggshell thinning.[575] Most of the affected predatory birds, such as the bald eagle and peregrine falcon, have recovered since the banning of DDT and most other chlorinated insecticides in the United States.[562] Although the United States and most other developed countries have banned DDT and other chlorinated insecticides, other countries, such as India and China, are still producing, exporting, and using DDT.[576]

Habitat alteration and destruction can be expected to reduce mammal and bird populations. For example, when glyphosate (Roundup) was applied to forest clear-cuts to eliminate low-growing vegetation, such as shrubs and small trees, the southern red-backed vole population was greatly reduced because its food source and cover were practically eliminated.[577] Similar effects from herbicides have been reported on other mammals. Overall, the impacts of pesticides on mammal populations have been inadequately investigated.

Although the gross values for wildlife are not available, expenditures involving wildlife made by humans are one measure of the monetary value. Nonconsumptive users of wildlife spent an estimated $14.3 billion on their sport.[578] Yearly, the U.S. bird watchers spend an estimated $600 million on their sport and an additional $500 million on birdseed or a total of $1.1 billion.[578] For bird watching, the estimated cost is about 40 cents per bird. The money spent by hunters to harvest 5 million game birds was $1.1 billion or approximately $216 per bird.[578] In addition, the estimated cost of replacing a bird of an affected species of the wild, as in the case of the Exxon Valdez oil spill, was $800 per bird.[579]

If it is assumed that the damages that the pesticides inflict on birds occur primarily on the 160 million ha of cropland that receives the most pesticide, and the bird population is estimated to be 4.4 birds per ha of cropland,[580] then 720 million birds are directly exposed to pesticides. Also, if it is conservatively estimated that only 10% of the bird population is killed by the pesticide treatments, it follows that the total number of birds killed is 72 million birds. Note this estimate is at the lower range of 0.25–8.9 birds killed per ha per year mentioned earlier.

The American bald eagle and other predatory birds suffered high mortalities because of DDT and other chlorinated insecticides. The bald eagle population declined primarily because of pesticides and was placed on the endangered species list. After DDT and the other chlorinated insecticides were banned in 1972, it took nearly 30 years for the bird populations to recover. The American bald eagle was recently removed from the endangered species list.[581]

The assumed value of a bird is about $30 based on the information presented, plus the fact that the cost of a fish is about $10, even a 1 in. fish. Thus, the total economic impact of pesticides on birds is estimated to be $2.1 billion per year. This estimate does not include the birds killed due to the death of one of the parent and in turn the deaths of the nestlings. It also does not include nestlings killed because they were fed contaminated arthropods and other foods.

MICROBES AND INVERTEBRATES

Pesticides easily find their way into soils, where they may be toxic to arthropods, earthworms, fungi, bacteria, and protozoa. Small organisms are vital to ecosystems because they dominate both the structure and function of ecosystems.[582]

For example, an estimated 4.5 t/ha of fungi and bacteria exist in the upper 15 cm of soil. They, with the arthropods, make up 95% of all species and 98% of the biomass (excluding vascular plants). The microbes are essential to proper functioning in the ecosystem, because they break down organic matter, enabling the vital chemical elements to be recycled.[583,584] Equally important is their ability to "fix" nitrogen, making it available to plants and ecosystems.[584]

Earthworms and insects aid in bringing new soil to the surface at a rate of up to 200 t/ha.[544] This action improves soil formation and structure for plant growth and makes various nutrients more available for absorption by plants. The holes (up to 10,000 holes per m) in the soil made by earthworms and insects also facilitate the percolation of water into the soil.[585]

Insecticides, fungicides, and herbicides reduce species diversity in the soil as well as the total biomass of these biota. Stringer and Lyons[586] reported that where earthworms had been killed by pesticides, the leaves of apple trees accumulated on the surface of the soil and increased the incidence of scab in the orchards. Apple scab, a disease carried over from season to season on fallen leaves, is commonly treated with fungicides. Some fungicides, insecticides, and herbicides are toxic to earthworms, which would otherwise remove and recycle the fallen leaves.

On golf courses and other lawns, the destruction of earthworms by pesticides results in the accumulation of dead grass or thatch in the turf.[587] To remove this thatch, special equipment must be used and it is expensive.

Although these microbes and invertebrates are essential to the vital structure and function of both natural and agricultural ecosystems, it is impossible to place a money value on the damage caused by pesticides to this large group of organisms. To date, no relevant quantitative data on the value of microbe and invertebrate destruction by pesticides are available.

CONCLUSION

An investment of about $10 billion in pesticide control each year saves approximately $40 billion in the U.S. crops based on direct costs and benefits. However, the indirect costs of pesticide use to the

---

TABLE 7.35

Total Estimated Environmental and Social Costs from Pesticide in the United States

Costs	Millions of $ per Year
Public health impacts	1140
Domestic animals deaths and contaminations	30
Loss of natural enemies	520
Cost of pesticide resistance	1500
Honeybee and pollination losses	334
Crop losses	1391
Fishery losses	100
Bird losses	2160
Groundwater contamination	2000
Government regulations to prevent damage	470
Total	9645

Source: With permission from Springer Science+Business Media: *Environment, Development and Sustainability*, Environmental and economic costs of the application of pesticides primarily in the United States, 7(2), 2005, Pimentel, D., Table V.

---

environment and public health need to be balanced against these benefits. Based on the available data, the environmental and public health costs of recommended pesticide use totaled more than $9 billion each year. Users of pesticides pay directly only about $3 billion, which includes problems arising from pesticide resistance and destruction of natural enemies. Society eventually pays this $3 billion plus the remaining $98 billion in environmental and public health costs.

Our assessment of the environmental and health problems associated with pesticides was made more difficult by the complexity of the issues and the scarcity of data. For example, what is an acceptable monetary value for a human life lost or a cancer illness due to pesticides? Equally difficult is placing a monetary value on killed wild birds and other wildlife; on the dearth of invertebrates, or microbes lost; or on the price of contaminated food and groundwater.

In addition to the costs that cannot be accurately measured, there are many costs that were not included in the $12 billion figure. If the full environmental, public health, and social costs could be measured as a whole, the total cost might be nearly double the $12 billion figure. Such a complete and long-term cost/benefit analysis of pesticide use would reduce the perceived profitability of pesticides.

The efforts of many scientists to devise ways to reduce pesticide use in crop production while still maintaining crop yield have helped, but a great deal more needs to be done. Sweden, for example, has reduced pesticide use by 68% without reducing crop yields and/or the cosmetic standards.[588] At the same time, public pesticide poisonings have been reduced by 77%. It would be helpful, if the United States adopted a similar goal to that of Sweden. Unfortunately, with some groups in the United States, integrated pest management (IPM) is being used as a means of justifying pesticide use (Table 7.35).

MISCELLANEOUS PESTICIDES OF HIGH TOXICITY

The following pesticides are not similar in chemical structure or toxicologic action to the major classes of pesticidal toxicants (organophosphate, arsenicals, etc.). In general, they are not widely used, and opportunities for serious human exposure are rare. However, those included here are characterized by either high toxicity or an important unique mechanism of toxic action. Occasional poisonings by these chemicals have occurred in humans and domestic animals. Sensitivity can occur more frequently.

4-Aminopyridine (Avitrol, 4-AP): This chemical, now used as a bird repellant, has caused severe poisoning in adult humans at dosages no greater than about 60 mg. This dosage is only two to three times that employed clinically in managing certain rare neuromuscular disorders. The principal pharmacologic action of 4-AP is to facilitate the release of transmitter substances at neuroeffector junctions and at synapses throughout the nervous system.[589]

Human poisonings have been characterized by thirst, nausea, dizziness, weakness, and intense diaphoresis, followed by toxic psychosis, ataxia, tremors, dyspnea, and tonic–clonic convulsions. Metabolic acidosis, leukocytosis, and elevations of serum GOT, LDH, and alkaline phosphatase were notable laboratory findings. EKG may show nonspecific ST–T wave changes.

Chlordimeform (Acaron, Fundal, Fundex, Galecron, Spanone): Although the acute toxicity of this ovicidal agent is low (oral LD_{50} in the rat about 200 mg/kg, it is now known from an incident of excessive respiratory and dermal exposure to chlordimeform powder that it can cause acute illness and urinary bladder irritation. In all likelihood, the offending metabolite is 2-methyl-4-chloroaniline. Principal symptoms are dysuria, gross hematuria, urethral discharge, abdominal and back pain, and a hot sensation all over. Sleepiness, skin rash, anorexia, and a sweet taste in the mouth have also been reported. Cystoscopic examination of victims of excessive exposure demonstrated acute hemorrhagic cystitis. Methods are available for detecting 2-methyl-4-chloroaniline metabolite in the urine.

Copper salts and organic complexes (oxide, hydroxide, arsenite, carbonate, chloride, oxalate, phosphate, silicate, sulfate, zinc chromate, acetate, naphthenate, oleate, quinolinolate, and resinate): These are commonly used as *fungicides*, either alone or in combination with other agents. There are several dozen proprietary products. LD_{50} values vary from 6 to 1000 mg/kg, depending mainly on the solubility and degree of ionization of the copper compound. Toxicity of copper arsenite salts is due mainly to the arsenic content.[589]

All of these salts irritate the skin and eyes and damage mucous membranes. When ingested, they are powerfully emetic. The stomach usually empties promptly and automatically in fully conscious individuals. When retained and absorbed, these salts cause toxic injury that affects the GI lining, capillaries, brain, liver, kidney, and formed elements of the blood. Copper salts are hemolytic.[589]

Manifestations of poisoning include burning pain in the chest and abdomen, intense nausea, vomiting, diarrhea, headache, sweating, and shock. Later, the liver is enlarged. Jaundice may reflect hemolysis or liver damage or both. Anuria indicates kidney injury by copper and/or free hemoglobin. *Death* may occur from *convulsions*, coma, or hepatorenal failure. Elevated serum copper levels (maximum normal level is 125 µg per 100 mL) indicate severity of poisoning.

Cycloheximide (Naramycin, Acti-dione, Actispray, Hizarocin): This is an antibiotic fungicide of high toxicity. The oral LD_{50} in rats is 2 mg/kg. Dermal absorption is probably not efficient. When ingested, the agent causes excitement, tremors, salivation, diarrhea, and melena. Mechanisms of toxicity are not well defined, but probably include irritation of the gut, stimulation of sympathetic and parasympathetic nervous systems, renal injury, and damage to the adrenal cortex. There are no chemical tests to confirm cycloheximide poisoning.[589]

Endothall (Accelerate, Aquathol, Des-I-cate, Hydout, Hydrothol): Acute oral L_{50} of this herbicide is 51 mg/kg. Dermal absorption of the commonly used salts is probably slight. It is irritating to eyes, mucous membranes, and skin, but it is not sensitizing. Mechanisms of systemic toxicity are not clear, but the CNS, heart, blood vessels, and GI lining appear to be primary targets. Poisoned animals exhibit ataxia, convulsions, shock, and respiratory depression. Erosions and ulcers of the GI tract follow ingestion. There are no standard analytical methods for confirming poisoning.[589]

Nicotine sulfate (Black Leaf 40): This time-honored natural insecticide is still used in horticulture. The lethal dose in humans is about 60 mg. Nicotine preparations, especially those using the free alkaloid, are well absorbed across the gut wall, lung, and skin. Poisoning symptoms from excessive doses appear promptly. They are due to transient stimulation, then prolonged depression, of the CNS, autonomic ganglia, and motor end plates of skeletal muscle. Similar symptoms are seen in the chemically sensitive. CNS injury manifests as headache, dizziness, incoordination, and tremors, followed by clonic convulsions leading to tonic-extensor convulsions that are often fatal.

In some instances, convulsive activity is minimal, and death by respiratory arrest occurs within a few minutes. Effects on autonomic ganglia give rise to sweating, salivation, nausea, abdominal pain, diarrhea, and hypertension. The heart is usually slow and often arrhythmic. Block of skeletal muscle motor endplates causes profound weakness, then paralysis. Death may occur from respiratory depression or shock. Nicotine can be measured in blood and urine to confirm poisoning.[589]

Sorghum chlorate (*De-Fol-Ate, Drexel Defol, Drop-Leaf, Fall, Grain Sorghum Harvest-Aid, Klores, Kusatol, Tumbleaf*): Although the oral LD_{50} in the rat is high (1200 mg/kg), there have been several deaths from this herbicide defoliant in the past decade. The principal mechanisms of toxicity are irritation of the GI lining, CNS depression, hemolysis, oxidation of free hemoglobin to methemoglobin, and renal tubular injury. Dermal absorption is minimal. If ingested, chlorate causes swelling of the oral and pharyngeal membranes and pain in the chest and abdomen. The victim is first restless, then apathetic. On the third or fourth day after ingestion, lumbar pain, albuminuria, hematuria, then anuria with azotemia, reflect renal injury. Death may be due to hyperkalemia (hemolysis), tissue anoxia (methemoglobinemia), or renal failure.

Although chlorate itself is not readily measured in the blood, free hemoglobin and methemoglobin in the plasma point to poisoning by an oxidizing agent. In the experience of the EHC-Dallas, these patients, if they survive, may develop chemical sensitivity with the spreading phenomenon. Chlorine sensitivity occurs, and the patients may develop recurrent respiratory infections as well as learning disability.[589]

Sodium cyanide (*Cymag*): Occasionally, sodium cyanide is used as a rodenticide. Toxicity is extreme, similar to that of hydrogen cyanide gas used as a fumigant. Cyanide salts are not absorbed on activated charcoal.

HERBICIDES

Numerous herbicides are available on the market. Only a few of the most commonly used will be discussed here.

BHOPAL DISASTER: METHYL ISOCYANATE

The Bhopal disaster, also referred to as the Bhopal gas tragedy, was a gas leak incident in India, considered the world's worst industrial disaster.[590] It occurred on the night of 2–3 December 1984 at the Union Carbide India Limited (UCIL) pesticide plant in Bhopal, Madhya Pradesh. Over 500,000 people were exposed to methyl isocyanate gas and other chemicals. The toxic substance made its way in and around the shantytowns located near the plant.[591] Estimates vary on the death toll. The official immediate death toll was 2259. The government of Madhya Pradesh confirmed a total of 3787 deaths related to the gas release.[592] Others estimate that 8000 died within two weeks and another 8000 or more have since died from gas-related diseases.[593–595] A government affidavit in 2006 stated that the leak caused 558,125 injuries including 38,478 temporary partial injuries and approximately 3900 severely and permanently disabling injuries.[596]

Civil and criminal cases are pending in the District Court of Bhopal, India, involving Union Carbide Corporation (UCC) and Warren Anderson, UCC CEO, at the time of the disaster.[597,598] In June 2010, seven ex-employees, including the former UCIL chairman, were convicted in Bhopal of causing death by negligence and sentenced to 2 years imprisonment and a fine of about $2000 each, the maximum punishment allowed by Indian law. An eighth former employee was also convicted, but died before the judgment was passed.[590]

Several hundred commercial products contain chlorophenoxy herbicides (Figure 7.58) in various concentrations and combinations. The following are names of widely advertised formulations (in some cases, the same name is used for products with different ingredients; exact composition must, therefore, be determined from product labels): 2,4-D; Agrotec; Amoxone; Aqua-Kleen; BH 2,4-D; Chipco Turf Herbicide "D"; Chloroxone Crop Rider; D50; Dacamine 4D; Ded-Weed; Desoromone;

Dinoxol; DMA4, Dormone; Emulsamine BK; Emulsamine E-3; Envert DT or 171; Esteron 99 Concentrate; Esteron 4; Esteron Brush Killer; Estone; Fernoxone; Fernimine; Ferxone; Fernesta; Formula 40; Hedonal; Herbidal; Lawn-Keep; Macondray; Miracle; Netagrone 600; Pennamine D; Planotox; Plantgard; Rhodia; Salvo (a product of identical name marketed by the Crystal Chemical Company contains cacodylic acid as the active ingredient); Spritz-Hormin/2,4-D; Spritz-Hormit/2,4-D; Superoromone Concentre; Super D Weedone; Transamine; U46; Verton 2D; Visko-Rhap; Weed-B-Gon; Weedar; Weed-Rhap, Weed Tox; Weedtrol; De Broussaillant 600; Lithate; Dicotox; Field Clean Weed Killer. 2,4-DB is the butyric acid homolog of 2,4-D. Dichlorprop is the propionic acid homolog. 2,4,5-trichlorophenoxyacetic acid (2,4,5-T) (Brush-Rhap, Dacamine 4T, De Broussaillant Concentre, Ded-Weed Brush Killer, Esteron 245, Fence Rider, Forron, Inverton 245, Line Rider, Spontox, Super D Weedone, Transamine, Trinoxol, Trioxone, U46, Veon 245, Verton 2T, Weedar, Weedone Envert T).[4]

Common mixtures of 2,4-D and 2,4,5-T are Dacamine 2D/2T, Esteron Brush Killer, Rhodia Low Volatile Brush Killer No. 2 U46 Special, Tributon, Visko0Rhyap LV2D-2T, and Transamine.[4]

2,4,5-TP (Silvex) is the propionic acid homolog of 2,4,5-T. Kuron is a low-volatility ester of 2,4,5-TP. 2,4,5-TB is the butyric acid homolog of 2,4,5-T. Fenac or clorfenac is 2,3,6-trichlorophenylacetic acid. Dicamba (Banvel) is dichloroanisic acid. MCPA, MCPB, MCPB-ethyl, MCPCA, and MCPP (Mecoprop) are 2-methyl,4-chlorophenoxy aliphatic acids and esters.[4]

Some of the chlorophenoxy acids, salts, and esters are irritating to the skin, eyes, and respiratory and GI linings. In a few individuals, local depigmentation has apparently resulted from prolonged and repeated dermal contact with chlorophenoxy materials.[599]

The chlorophenoxy compounds are absorbed across the gut wall, lung, and skin. They are not significantly fat storable. Excretion occurs within hours or, at most, days, primarily through the urine. These hormonal agents produce their effects by overstimulating plant growth.

Given in large doses to experimental animals, 2,4-D causes vomiting, diarrhea, anorexia, weight loss, ulcers of the mouth and pharynx, and toxic injury to the liver, kidneys, and CNS. Myotonia (stiffness and incoordination of hind extremities) develops in some species and is apparently due to CNS damage. Demyelination has been observed in the dorsal columns of the cord, and EEG changes have indicated functional disturbances in the rains of heavily dosed experimental animals.[599] 2,4-D also has been shown to cause malignant lymphoma in dogs.[600]

Ingestion of large amounts of chlorophenoxy acids has resulted in severe metabolic acidosis in humans. Such cases have been associated with electrocardiographic changes, myotonia, muscle weakness, myoglobinuria, and elevated serum creatine phosphokinase (CPK), all reflecting injury to striated muscle. Because chlorophenoxy acids are weak uncouplers of oxidative phosphorylation, extraordinary doses may produce hyperthermia from increased production of body heat.[4] They also have been seen to initiate and exacerbate chemical sensitivity in some case studies at the EHC-Dallas.

Polychlorinated dibenzo-dioxin (CDD) compounds are generated in the synthesis of 2,4,5-T. The 2,3,7,8-tetra CDD form (TCDD) is extraordinarily toxic to multiple mammalian tissues and is the most toxic synthetic discovered. Hexa-, hepta-, and octa-compounds exhibit less systemic toxicity, but are the likely cause of chloracne (a chronic, disfiguring skin condition) seen in workers engaged in the manufacture of 2,4,5-T. Although toxic effects, notably chloracne, have been observed in manufacturing plant workers, they have not been observed in formulators or applicators regularly exposed to 2,4,5-T. They have been seen in veterans of the Vietnam War and many chemically susceptible people. TCDD causes degenerative changes in the liver and thymus, chloracne, porphyria, altered serum enzyme concentrations, loss of body weight, induction of microsomal enzymes, and cancer. Soldiers in Vietnam and local residents suffered long-term effects of dioxin. Epstine[601] has shown a high fetal abnormality of birth defects in Vietnamese residents of these sprayed areas. When delivered to pregnant rats, a very low dose of dioxin can not only demasculinize but it also can also feminize the sexual development of male offspring. Newborn males had 30%–50% the normal amount testosterone in their bloodstreams.[602]

The ingredients of Agent Orange were equal quantities of 2,4-D and 2,4,5-T, but in addition, TCDD was found in many of the samples. It was estimated that 44 million pounds were sprayed in South Vietnam from 1967 to 1970.[603,604] Many veterans had diffuse symptoms, including porphyria, liver damage, polyneuropathies, and psychiatric disturbances. Jennnings et al.[605] showed immunological abnormalities, such as high killer cells, in 15 workers exposed to 2,3,7,8-tetra-chlorodibenzo-p-dioxin 17 years after exposure. Autoimmune disease is a sequel of dioxin exposure along with chemical sensitivity.[4]

It has now been shown that 40% of 2,3,7,8-TCDD passes through a rat's skin when given at a dose of 0.3 μg/kg of body weight.[606] Absorption falls to less than half that of TCDD doses between 32 and 320 μg/kg.[607]

The medical literature contains several reports of peripheral neuropathy following what seemed to be minor dermal exposures to 2,4-D. It is not certain that exposures to other neurotoxicants were entirely excluded in these cases.[608,609]

Eighteen workers were reviewed 17 years after accidental exposure to 2,3,7,8-tetrachlorodibenzo-p-dioxin (TCDD; dioxin). Clinical assessment showed that they were in good health. A study of several biochemical and immunological parameters in these subjects and in 15 carefully matched controls showed no difference in serum concentrations of hepatic enzymes between exposed workers and controls. Although mean serum concentrations of cholesterol and triglyceride were higher in exposed subjects than in controls, the results did not reach statistical significance. Antinuclear antibodies and immune complexes were detected significantly more frequently in the peripheral blood of workers exposed to dioxin. This occurrence of autoantibodies is similar to those seen at the EHC-Dallas in chemically sensitive patients exposed to 2,4-D and other chlorinated components. There was no significant difference between exposed workers and controls in the number of T lymphocytes, B lymphocytes, and helper and suppressor T-cell counts in peripheral blood, but the number of natural killer cells identified by the monoclonal antibody Leu-7 was significantly higher in workers exposed to dioxin.[605]

Farmers and the food industry are asking the Obama administration to ease coming federal guidance that will advise consumers to minimize their intake of dioxins, chemicals that may be harmful at certain levels.

Beef cattle feeding on hay is one way dioxin enters the food chain.

Dioxins are a by-product of paper, metal, and cement production, but the primary source of exposure for people is food. Meat and dairy products in particular absorb the chemicals, which are ubiquitous in the environment and get into what livestock eat, especially if the animals graze. When ingested at high levels, dioxins are linked to human reproductive problems, acute skin conditions, and cancer.

Scientists generally agree that dioxins are poisonous, but some disagree with the EPA's conclusions that the small amounts people are exposed to through food today are dangerous.

Observers expect the dioxin limit to be similar to a preliminary one the agency set last year, which said people should not consume >0.7 pg of dioxin per kilogram of body weight a day. For example, a person who weighs 100 pounds would be limited to ingesting 32 pg of dioxin per day, and a person who weighs 200 lbs would be limited to about 64 pg per day. A picogram is one trillionth of a gram.

According to Schecter, a science advisory board member of a 2011 EPA dioxin review panel, children are more susceptible to dioxin than adults because they weigh less.[610]

The best way people can cut down on their dioxin intake is to eat more fruits and vegetables and less meat, especially meat with a high fat content. According to Schecter, cows, pigs, chickens, and fish consume dioxins when they feed, and the chemicals build up in the animals' fatty tissue.[610]

DIOXINS, ASSESSED AT LAST

After 21 years of contentious scientific analysis, the EPA has established a safe level of exposure to the most toxic form of dioxin.

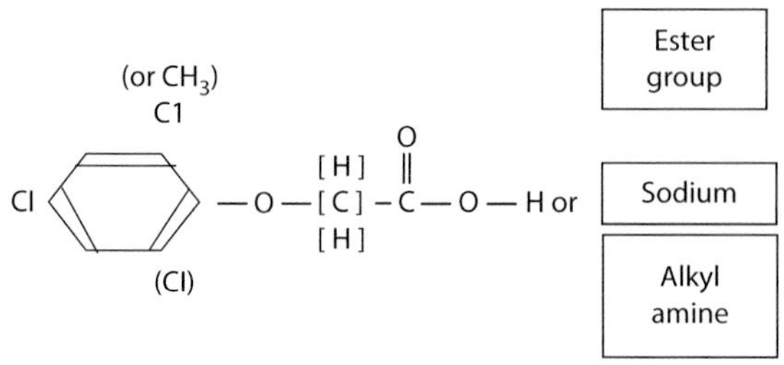

FIGURE 7.61 Chlorophenoxy compounds. (From Chemical sensitivity Volume II, page 879, figure 28. With permission.)

EPA set a safe daily dose of 0.7 pg of 2,3,7,8-TCDD per kilogram of body weight. TCDD is the most potent congener of the dioxins, which generally are unintentional by-products of manufacturing processes involving chlorine and burning of biomass or waste.

Eventually, this defined level of safe exposure will affect the degree and cost of cleanups of soil and of industrial air and water releases polluted with dioxins. This category of chemicals consists of chlorinated dioxins and durans and certain PCBs. These substances can trigger similar adverse health effects, but their potencies vary.

Data in EPA's annual Toxics Release Inventory indicate that the U.S. industry has slashed its releases of dioxins in the past two decades (C&EN, February 6, 2012, p. 26). Backyard waste burning is the major source of dioxins in the United States today.

The EPA limit is based on two studies. One found adverse reproductive effects in men exposed to TCDD as boys. The other found hormonal effects in infants born to mothers who had high levels of exposure.

People are exposed to dioxins mainly by eating meat, poultry, dairy products, fish, or eggs. However, EPA claims that "most Americans have only low-level exposure to dioxins," adding that this "does not pose a significant health risk."

The agency's document examines health effects other than cancer from TCDD exposure. They include chloracne, a severe skin disease producing acne-like lesions, developmental and reproductive effects, damage to the immune system, hormonal disruption, and possibly mild liver damage. The agency is still working on a second document focusing on cancer hazards of TCDD.

The assessment, which EPA launched in 1991 to update a 1985 document describing the cancer hazards of TCDD, has faced many delays. Throughout the years, polluting industries including chemical companies have faulted EPA's work. Community and public health groups, meanwhile, have pressured the agency to finish the review (Figures 7.61 and 7.62).

These herbicides include dinitrophenol (Chemox PE), dinitrocresol (DNOC, DNC, Sinox, Chemsect DNOC, Elgetol 30, Nitrador, Selinon, Trifocide), dinoseb (DNBP, Dinitro, Basanite, Caldon, Chemox General, Chemox PE, Chemsect DNBP, Dinitro-3, Dinitro General, Dow General Weed Killer, Dow Selective Weed Killer, Dynamyte, Elgetol 318, Gebutox, Kiloseb, Nitropone C, Premerge 3, Sinox General, Subitex, Unicrop DNBP, Vertac Dinitro Weed Killer), dinosam (DNAP), dinoprop, dinoterbon, dinosulfon, binapacryl (Morocide, Endosan, Ambox, Dapacryl), dinobuton (Acrex, Dessin, Dinofen, Drawinol, Talan), and dinopenton, dinocap (Crotone, Karathane). Several

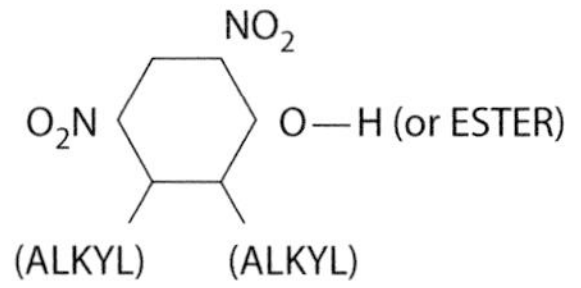

FIGURE 7.62 Nitrophenolic and nitrocresolic herbicides. (From Chemical sensitivity Volume II, page 881, figure 29. With permission.)

combinations are widely used: Dyanap and Klen Krop = dinoseb + naptalam; Ancrack = sodium salts of dinoseb + naptalam; Naptro = dinitrophenol + naptalam.

These materials should be regarded as highly toxic to humans and animals. Most nitrophenols and nitrocresols are well absorbed from GI tract, across the skin, and by the lung when fine droplets are inhaled. Except in a few sensitive individuals, aromatic nitro-compounds are only moderately irritating to the skin. Like other phenols, they are toxic to the liver, kidney, and nervous system. The basic mechanism of toxicity and probably sensitivity is a stimulation of oxidative metabolism in cell mitochondria, by interference with the normal coupling of carbohydrate oxidation to phosphorylation (ADP to ATP). Increased oxidative metabolism leads to pyrexia, tachycardia, and dehydration, and ultimately depletes carbohydrate and fat stores. Chemically sensitive patients exposed to these substances exhibit severe weakness that probably is due to a lack of ADP–ATP coupling. Most severe poisonings from absorption of these compounds have occurred in workers who were concurrently exposed to hot environments. Pyrexia and direct action on the brain cause cerebral edema and manifest clinically as a toxic psychosis and, sometimes, convulsions. Liver parenchyma and renal tubules show degenerative changes. Abuminuria, pyuria, hematuria, and increased BUN are often prominent signs of renal injury.[611]

Agranulocytosis has occurred in humans following large doses of dinitrophenol.[611] Cataracts have occurred in some chronically poisoned laboratory species, but this effect had not been observed in humans[611] until a case was seen at the EHC-Dallas. This man was poisoned by DNB and rapidly developed cataracts following his exposure. One can appreciate the exacerbation and onset of chemical sensitivity in patients such as this, as the patient became legally blind after repeated exposure. He worked in a state laboratory analyzing nitrophenols for the agriculture department.

Nitrophenols and nitrocresols are efficiently excreted by the kidneys, and there is some hepatic excretion into the bile. Unless the absorbed dose is extremely high, or kidney function is impaired, nearly complete elimination from the body might be expected within 3–4 days, except in some chemically sensitive or in individuals with impaired detoxification systems.

Death in nitrophenol poisoning is followed promptly by intense rigor mortis.

Yellow staining of skin and hair often signifies contact with a nitrophenolic chemical. Whether or not this is what is called the "chemical yellows" in the chemically sensitive patient is under study. However, our studies strongly suggest that phenolated and nitrophenolic compounds result in the chemical yellows. A patient with yellow skin who has neither jaundice nor carotinemia is likely chemically sensitive (Chapter 1). A complete work-up for this illness is indicated. Staining of the sclera and urine indicates absorption of potentially toxic amounts of chemicals, although often the sclera is clean in the chemically sensitive. Profuse sweating, headache, thirst, malaise, and lassitude are the common early symptoms of poisoning as well as sensitivity. Warm, flushed skin, tachycardia, and fever characterize a serious degree of poisoning as well as sensitivity. Apprehension, restlessness, anxiety, manic behavior, or unconsciousness reflects severe cerebral injury. Convulsions occur in the most severe poisonings. Cyanosis, tachypnea, and dyspnea result from stimulation of metabolism, pyrexia, and tissue anoxia. Weight loss occurs in persons chronically poisoned at low dosages. These symptoms are seen in the chemically sensitive.[612]

Unmetabolized nitrophenols and nitrocresols can be identified spectrophotometrically or by gas–liquid chromatography in the serum and urine at concentrations well below those necessary to cause poisoning, but certainly exacerbating sensitivity (Figure 7.63).

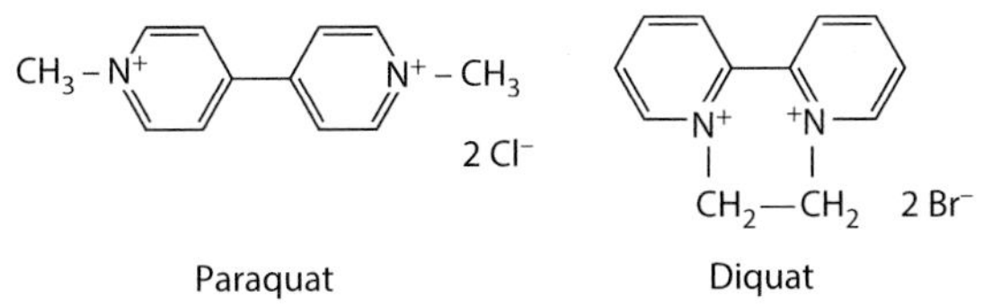

FIGURE 7.63   Paraquat and diquat. (From Chemical sensitivity Volume II, page 883, figure 30. With permission.)

Paraquat products are paraquat dichloride (usually as a 21% concentrate). Other names by which these products are identified are Ortho paraquat CL, Crisquat, Dextrone X, and Esgram; mixtures are Priglone, Preeglone, and Weedol with diquat; TerraClean with simazine; Gramonol and Mofisal with monolinuron; Pathclear with diquat and simazine; and TotaCol and Dexuron with diuron.[613]

Diquat products include diquat (Reglone, Reglox, Aquacide, Dextrone, Weedtrine-D). Mixtures are Priglone, Preeglone, and Weedol with paraquat; and Pathclear with paraquat and simazine.[613]

These dipyridyls injure the epithelial tissues: skin, nails, cornea, liver, kidney, and linings of the GI and respiratory tracts. In addition to direct irritant effects, injury may involve peroxidation of intracellular and extracellular phospholipids and inhibition of surfactant synthesis by lung tissue. These toxic properties may derive from the capacity of dipyridyls to generate free radicals in tissues. The injury is usually reversible; however, the pulmonary reaction that follows ingestion of paraquat is often fatal.

Certain injuries have followed occupational contact with paraquat. Contact with the concentrate may cause irritation and fissuring of the skin of the hands, and cracking, discoloration, and sometimes loss of fingernails. Splashed in the eye, paraquat concentrate causes conjunctivitis and, if not promptly removed, may result in protracted opacification of the cornea.

Although nearly all systemic intoxications by paraquat have followed ingestion of the chemical, occasional poisonings have resulted from excessive dermal contact. Absorption of toxic amounts is much more likely to occur if the skin is abraded. Persons who have experienced extraordinary dermal contact with paraquat (especially the concentrate) should be examined and tested for hazardous concentrations of the agent in the blood and urine.[613]

Inhalation of diluted spray mist may irritate the upper respiratory passages, causing a scratchy throat and nosebleed. Effects induced by dilute paraquat sprays ordinarily resolve promptly following withdrawal from exposure.[613]

If ingested, paraquat produces inflammation of the mouth and GI tract, sometimes progressing to ulceration within 1–4 days. Once absorbed, it damages the parenchymal cells of the liver and tubule cells of the kidney. In most instances, the victim survives these injuries. Paraquat is actively concentrated in the pneumocytes of lung tissue. Several days after ingestion, these cells die. After this event, there is rapid proliferation of connective tissue cells which fill the alveolar spaces. Although some victims have survived, death from asphyxia usually occurs once this degree of lung damage has been sustained. In survivors, recovery of normal lung function requires weeks or months. One patient had such damaged lungs that he received a lung transplant, which was successful. As he mobilized more paraquat from his peripheral tissues, he damaged his new lung until death occurred.[614] In a few instances, ingestion of large quantities of paraquat has induced protracted pulmonary edema. Myocardial injury has also been noted in some poisonings.

According to Spangenberg et al.,[615] Paraquat poisoning is rare. Since plasma levels do not necessarily match the ingested amount of paraquat, repeated measurement of plasma levels is imperative. There is a large potential in the prehospital phase to improve prognosis; further reabsorbing must be terminated by rigorous charcoal administration and early tracheal intubation if necessary. Since paraquat can be reabsorbed by dermal contact, steps to ensure sufficient protection of emergency medical personnel must be taken. As soon as further resorption has been prevented sufficiently, forced diaresis, renal replacement therapy, and hemoperfusion can be helpful, but still remain controversial. To reduce pulmonary fibrosis, inspiratory oxygen concentrations must be adjusted to their minimal amount needed to ensure satisfactory tissue oxygenation.[615]

FUMIGANTS

Chloroform, carbon tetrachloride, methyl bromide (MeBr; Fumigant-1, Kayafume, Meth-O-Gas, Pestmaster, ProFume), chloropicrin (Acquinte, Chlor-O-Pic, Pic-Clor, Picfume, Tri-Clor), ethylene dichloride (EDC), ethylene dibromide (EDB, Bromofume, Celmide, Dowfume W-85, Kop-Fume, Nephis, Pestmaster EDB-85, Soilbrom), dichloropropene and dichloropropane (Telone, D-D), sulfuryl fluoride (Vikane), and dibromochloropropane (DBCP) are known common fumigants (Figures 7.64 and 7.65).

The Dowfume fumigants manufactured by the Dow Chemical Company are mixtures of halocarbons, mainly EDC, EDB, carbon tetrachloride, MeBr, and chloropicrin (EIC, oxirane); propylene oxide (epoxypropane), formaldehyde (formalin is a 40% aqueous solution); propenal (Acrolein, Aqualin, Acrylaldehyde); carbon di- (or bi) sulfide; hydrogen cyanide (prussic acid, Cyclon); acrylonitrile (ingredient of fumigant mixtures Acrylofume, Acritet, Carbacryl); and aluminum phosphide (photoxin).

Fumigants have extraordinary power to penetrate the lining membranes of the respiratory and gastrointestinal tracts and the skin. They also penetrate the rubber and plastics used in protective garb, and they are not efficiently taken up by conventional absorbents used in ordinary respirators. These properties make the protection of applicator personnel very difficult, essentially mandating methods of use that do not require on-site operator handling.[616]

Since these chemicals are either gases or volatile liquids at room temperature, inhalation is the most common route of absorption. Dermal injury does follow contact with some fumigants, ranging in severity from a mild chemical burn to vesiculation and ulceration. Fumigant gases irritate the eyes; liquid fumigant may cause blindness from corneal ulceration. Penetration of the skin appears much more important, and we have seen fumigant gases in the blood of chemically sensitive patients.

Respiratory tract irritation is the most common and serious injury caused by fumigants, and chemical sensitivity easily develops. Some agents, such as sulfur dioxide, chloropicrin, formaldehyde, and acrolein, cause so much irritation of the upper respiratory tract that the exposed individual

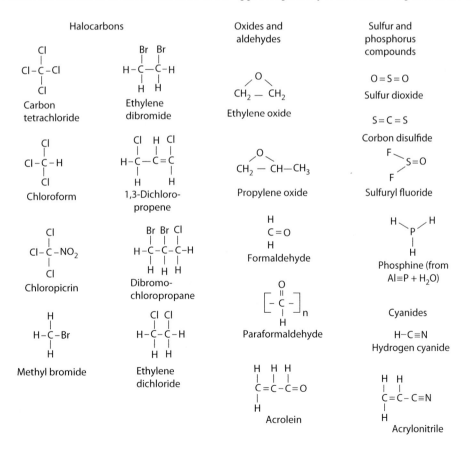

FIGURE 7.64 Chemical structures of fumigants. (From Chemical sensitivity Volume II, page 885, figure 331. With permission.)

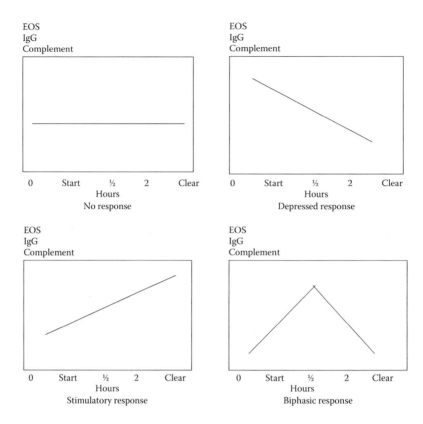

FIGURE 7.65 Type of immune response after pesticide-inhaled challenge. (From Chemical sensitivity Volume II, page 902 and 903, figure 32. With permission.)

is unlikely to inhale a quantity of fumigant capable of damaging the lung other than causing sensitivity. Laryngeal edema or bronchospasm results from inhalation of high concentrations.

Other gases, such as MeBr, phosphine, and ethylene oxide, are not so irritating to the nose, eyes, throat, and bronchi, but cause serious injury to the cells lining the alveoli of the lung. Thus, they are more likely than other fumigants to induce pulmonary edema, a major cause of death from fumigant exposure.

In varying degrees, these fumigants depress the CNS. As in the case of the anesthetic chloroform, adequate dosage may lead to unconsciousness. Depression or cessation of respiration is a major hazard of acute inhalation exposure to fumigants. Acute exposures to MeBr have induced convulsions. Absorbed in lower concentrations over several consecutive days, MeBr has impaired basal ganglion function in humans, causing ataxia for weeks or months after exposure. Protracted exposure to carbon disulfide has caused peripheral neuropathy and changes in CNS function (chronic encephalopathy of chronically exposed workers).[616]

The halocarbon fumigants increase the irritability of the heart muscle. Intensive exposures may lead to sudden death as a result of ventricular fibrillation. Some cases of sensitization have been seen with cardiac irritability in a chemically sensitive patient.

Liver and kidney damage occurs commonly following excessive exposure to fumigants. Liver injury may take the form of fatty infiltration, diffuse necrosis, or massive necrosis. Elevated serum levels of GOT, LDH, alkaline phosphatase, and bilirubin reflect hepatocellular injury. The fumigants may inflict direct injury on glomerular and tubular elements of the kidney, leading to functional proteinuria and glycosuria or to acute renal failure, depending on the severity of toxicant exposure. In addition, hyperbilirubinemia resulting from liver damage may compound the tubular injury (hepatorenal syndrome).

Inhaled phosphine gas (PH$_3$, a grain fumigant) and ingested metal phosphides cause pulmonary edema, CNS depression, toxic myocarditis, and circulatory collapse. Victims who survive these immediate reactions suffer liver injury (fatty degeneration and necrosis) and acute renal tubular necrosis. Unlike its analog arsine, phosphine is not hemolytic. Enzymatic mechanisms of toxicity are not known. Ingested metal phosphide (from which phosphine is generated) causes intense GI irritation followed by degenerative and necrotizing lesions of the liver, kidney, and heart. Death is often due either to cariogenic shock or pulmonary edema.

DIAGNOSIS OF PESTICIDE OVERLOAD

Acute toxicity is discussed in many toxicology textbooks and will not, therefore, be discussed here.

SIGNS AND SYMPTOMS OF PESTICIDE SENSITIVITY AND CHRONIC PESTICIDE OVERLOAD

Chronic significant pesticide effects on humans are frequently overlooked. While there is much overlap in symptomatology from pesticide poisoning and sensitivity, the kind and progression of symptoms will often differ. Generally, the effects of organochlorine pesticides, and probably others, initially have a stimulant effect on the nervous system, while solvents have a depressant effect. Some fumigants act as depressants. Any pesticide, however, may have a stimulating or depressive effect on the nervous system, the immune system, and/or the enzyme detoxification systems, depending on doses and virulence of the substance and the total load and state of nutrition of the individual at the time of exposure. Studies at the EHC-Dallas show that abnormalities of the autonomic NS also occur and are often the first signs seen of pesticide sensitivity overload. Cholinergic and/or sympatholytic effects are seen in 70% of the patients with pesticide sensitivity seen at the EHC-Dallas giving a sympathetic NS stimulant. In one study at the EHC-Dallas, the blood of 90% of the patients with organochlorine pesticides also contained solvents. These patients experienced depressant effects on their autonomic nervous system. However, another group containing solvent only showed cholinergic stimulating effects. Apparently, different amounts and combinations with different levels of exposure may show either part of the spectrum, from stimulation to depression. For example, DDT-poisoning symptoms will usually begin with tremors around the mouth and can progress through a wide variety of other manifestations, including vomiting, weakness, malaise, depression, convulsions, and even death. The chronic effects may be weakness, malaise, and depression. However, BHC symptoms can initially begin with convulsions, but long-term effects may be depression. It should be remembered that since many pesticides are designed to adversely affect all major parts of the CNS and PNS, any part of these systems or their related tissues, may be damaged. However, effects on the motor cortex and cerebellum have probably been the most frequently observed after autonomic NS involvement. A number of symptom consequences to various chlorinated hydrocarbons and to various pesticides are summarized in Tables 7.36 through 7.41.

As can be seen, there is a broad range of symptom complexes related to pesticide exposure. Each of these symptoms has been seen in some patients with chemical sensitivity at the EHC-Dallas. Our patients not only had these aforementioned symptom complexes but they also had organochlorine pesticides in their blood and reacted to inhaled double-blind challenges of so-called ambient doses of pesticides. The clinical responses to these challenges reproduced most of these symptoms in one individual or the other over the course of performing inhaled tests in 2000 patients. In addition, a systematic study by Rea et al.[190] of treatment effects in the ECU clearly showed that as pesticide blood levels decreased, there was a corresponding decrease in symptoms, with an increase in cognitive/cerebral functioning ability, thus showing the reversal of the neurotoxic effects of these pesticides.

The history of an acute exposure can be important and lead to the diagnosis of chemical and pesticide sensitivity. It has been observed that one large exposure or repeated exposures of not only pesticides but also other toxic chemicals may bring on pesticide sensitivity. The following case illustrates the development of long-term problems after an acute exposure.

TABLE 7.36

Index to Pesticide Poisonings and Sensitivity by Symptoms and Signs: 33-Year-Old Woman

Manifestations	Characteristic Chemical	Chemicals Known to Produce Symptoms on Inhaled Challenge
	General	
Breath odor of: Garlic	Arsenic, phosphorus, phosphides, phosphine	
Bitter almonds	Cyanide	
Rotten cabbage	Carbon disulfide	
Fever	Nitro-, chloro-, phenols	Chlorophenoxy compounds
Hypothermia	Vacor	
Myalgia		Chlorophenoxy compounds
Chills	Arsine, vacor	
Thirst	Nitro-, chloro-, phenols, aminopyridine, phosphine	
Anorexia	Organophosphates, carbamate insecticides, nicotine	Fumigants, nitro-, chloro-, phenols, arsenicals
Hot sensations	Chlordimeform, arsine	

Source:　From Chemical sensitivity Volume II, page 889, table 11A. With permission.

TABLE 7.37

Index to Pesticide Poisoning by Symptoms and Signs

Manifestations	Characteristic Chemical	Chemicals Known to Produce Symptoms on Inhaled Challenge
	Skin and Mucous Membranes	
Dry, cracked skin of hands	Paraquat, petroleum distillates, weed oil	
Loss of nails	Paraquat	
Brittle nails	Inorganic arsenicals	
Loss of hair	Thallium, inorganic arsenicals	
Sweating	Organophosphates, carbamate insecticides, nitro-, chloro-, phenols, nicotine, aminopyridine	
Pallor	Organochlorines	Anticoagulant rodenticides
Cyanosis	Paraquat, strychnine, crimidine nicotine, sodium fluoroacetate	Organophosphates, carbamate insecticides, organochlorines
Scratchy throat and irritated eyes	Sulfur dioxide, acrolein, chloropicrin, nitro-, chloro-, phenols, formaldehyde, pyrethins, copper compounds, endothall, sodium chlorate, methyl bromide	Paraquat, bisdithiocarbamates, ethylene bisdithiocarbamates, chloraliphatic acids
Blisters or burns	Phosphorus	Liquid methyl bromide or ethylene oxide
Rash	Sulfur, thiram, propachlor, barban	Picloram, difolatan, captan, chlorothalonil, nitro-, chloro-, phenols; many other herbicides and fungicides
Yellow stain		
	Nitrophenols	
Ecchymoses	Anticoagulant rodenticides, phosphorus, phosphides	
Keratoses	Inorganic arsenicals	
Jaundice	Phosphorus, phosphides, phosphine, halocarbon fumigants	Paraquat, inorganic arsenicals

Source:　From Chemical sensitivity Volume II, page 890, table 11B. With permission.

TABLE 7.38

Index to Pesticide Poisonings and Sensitivity by Symptoms and Signs

Manifestations	Characteristic Chemical	Chemicals Known to Produce Symptoms on Inhaled Challenge
Central Nervous System		
Headache	Organophosphates, carbamate insecticides, organochlorines, fumigants, nicotine, inorganic arsenicals	Nitrophenols, chlorophenols
Ataxia	Organophosphates, carbamate insecticides, endothall, nicotine, organochlorines, phenyl mercuric acetate	Fumigants, inorganic arsenicals,
Convulsions	Organochlorines, strychnine, crimidine, phosphorus, cyanide, sodium fluoroacetate, nicotine, aminopyridine, endothall	Nitro-, chloro-, phenols, organophosphates, carbamate insecticides, sulfuryl fluoride
Muscle twitching	Organophosphates, carbamate insecticides, sulfuryl fluoride	Chlorophenoxy compounds
Tremors	Organophosphates, carbamate insecticides, phosphine, aminopyridine, cycloheximide, nicotine	Strychnine, crimidine, nicotine, inorganic arsenicals
Mental confusion	Organophosphates, carbamate insecticides, chlorophenols, cyanide, organochlorines, vacor, sodium fluoroacetate, carbon disulfide, aminopyridine, cycloheximide	Strychnine, crimidine, nicotine, inorganic arsenicals
Sudden unconsciousness	Cyanide	Organophosphates, diquat, carbamate insecticides, halocarbon fumigants
Tingling and numbness in the extremities	Carbon disulfide, vacor, sodium fluoroacetate	Inorganic arsenicals
Tetany	Phosphorus, phosphides	
Myotonia		Chlorophenoxy compounds
Miosis	Organophosphates carbamate insecticides	

Source: From Chemical sensitivity Volume II, page 891, table 11C. With permission.

Case study: A 33-year-old white male was admitted to the ECU with the chief complaint of joint pain, muscle pain, and nerve pain with tremor of the right arm and hand.

The patient stated that 4 months prior to admission, he was involved in a plane crash investigation as an emergency medical technician. The plane had been crop-dusting with organochlorine and organic phosphate pesticides, and during the course of this evacuation and investigation, he was in the immediate area for approximately 2 hours. Following this, he developed fatigue, nausea, impairment of vision, and severe aching. The patient was hosed down with water in the middle of the street and taken to the hospital. His serum cholesterase was low. The patient was discharged from the hospital the following day, but he continued to experience severe symptoms after that time. The actual chemical found to be on the plane was Azodrin, a dimethylphosphate of 3-hydroxy-*N*-methylescrotonamide. However, the tank was apparently contaminated with organochlorine pesticides also.

This patient's history was significant. His problem began in 1976 when he met a motor vehicle accident and suffered a pharyngeal injury. Thereafter, between 1976 and 1978, he had many upper respiratory and pharyngeal infections and was told that his immune system was destroyed. He also had voice problems in the form of dysphonia. This patient had a history of asthma as an infant; he also had a tonsillectomy in 1957 and a myelogram in 1975. For a long period of time, he had been sensitive to sulfa drugs. His family history was negative for neurological disease, but positive for organic heart disease and cancer.

TABLE 7.39

Index to Pesticide Poisonings and Sensitivity by Symptoms and Signs

Manifestations	Characteristic Chemical	Chemicals Known to Produce Symptoms on Inhaled Challenge
Renal System		
Renal failure	Arsine, fumigants, cycloheximide chlorates	Paraquat, diquat, inorganic arsenicals, copper compounds
Urinary frequency, dysuria	Chlordimeform, vacor	
Renal colic	Anticoagulant rodenticides, chlorates	
Blood		
Anemia	Naphthalene, anticoagulant rodenticides	Inorganic arsenicals
Leukopenia		Nitrophenols; inorganic arsenicals
Hypoprothrombinemia	Anticoagulant rodenticides	
Depressed cholinesterase enzyme activities	Organophosphates	Carbamate insecticides (large dosage)
Methemoglobinemia	Chlorates	
Free hemoglobin in plasma	Naphthalene, arsine, copper compounds, sodium chlorate	
Elevated alkaline phosphatase, GOT, LDH	Halocarbon fumigants, inorganic arsenicals, diquat paraquat, aminopyridine	Endrin
Elevated blood bromide	Methyl bromide	
Hyperbilirubinemia	Paraquat, diquat, phosphine, phosphorus, Phosphides, copper compounds, inorganic arsenicals	Halocarbon fumigants
Elevated BUN, creatine	Paraquat, diquat, fumigants, chlorates, inorganic arsenicals	Sulfuryl fluoride, nitro-, chloro-, phenols
Hyperkalemia	Naphthalene, chlorates, copper compounds	

Source: From Chemical sensitivity Volume II, page 892, table 11D. With permission.

His physical examination was normal, except the extremities showed nonintentional tremor of the right hand and arm. Also, he dragged his left foot and had severe spasms in his erector spinae muscle.

He was admitted to the ECU after 4 months of the crop-dusting accident. During the hospital course, the patient was placed in two environmentally controlled rooms. The first room was constructed of plaster and the second room of porcelain. The patient fasted for 5 days. He did not completely clear his symptoms during the fast.

During the hospital course, he underwent chemical exposure in a steel and glass airtight booth. The chemicals that produced symptoms by double-blind inhaled challenge were <0.50 ppm alcohol, <0.20 ppm formaldehyde, <0.33 ppm chlorine, <0.002 ppm phenol, and <0.0034 ppm insecticide. Saline placebos were negative.

This patient was challenged with less chemically contaminated foods. He had sensitivity to 33 foods. He was further tested by intradermal injection and found to be sensitive to molds, dust, mite, weeds, trees, grasses, TOE Candida, terpenes, cigarette smoke, orris root, ethanol, newsprint, perfume, histamine, serotonin, and cotton.

His chest x-ray was normal ECG showed a sinus rhythm within normal limits. Brain resonance imaging and CAT scan of the head were normal. An x-ray of his lumbar spine revealed a mild form of bone dysplasia and probably lumbar spinal stenosis. The deformity of L-3 was possibly due to previous trauma.

Abnormal laboratory tests showed depressed white blood cell (WBC) at 4500/mm^3 (normal: 4800–10,800/mm^3), depressed lymphocytes at 28% (normal: 30–40/mm^3), and absolute number

TABLE 7.40

Index to Pesticide Poisonings and Sensitivity by Symptoms and Signs

Manifestations	Characteristic Chemical	Chemicals Known to Produce Symptoms on Inhaled Challenge
Urine		
Proteinuria	Diquat, paraquat, nitro-, chloro-, phenols, fumigants, cycloheximide, copper compounds, phenyl mercuric acetate, sodium chlorate	Endothall, sulfuryl fluoride
Hematuria	Anticoagulant rodenticides, sodium chlorate, cycloheximide, chordimeform	Chlordimeform, fumigants, paraquat, diquat
Ketonuria	Vacor, aminopyridine	Phosphorus, phosphides
Hemoglobinuria	Naphthalene, arsine, sodium chlorate	
Myoglobinuria		Chlorophenoxy compounds
Porphyrinuria	Hexachlorobenzene	
Bilirubinuria	Halocarbon fumigants, phosphorus, phosphides, phosphine	
Glycosuria	Vacor	
Feces		
Blood present (melena)	Diquat, sodium chlorate, anticoagulant rodenticides, phosphorus, phosphides, endothall, cycloheximide	Paraquat
Luminescence	Phosphorus	
Semen		
Low sperm count		Dibromochloropropane, kepone

Source: From Chemical sensitivity Volume II, page 893, table 11E. With permission.

of 1260/mm^3 (normal: 1440–4320/mm^3), depressed absolute T-cells at 781/mm^3 (normal: 1066–3197/mm^3), depressed absolute B-cells at 270/mm^3 (normal: >500/mm^3), and elevated 5HIAA at 12.0 mg/24 hours (normal: 0–10 mg/24 hours). The blood toxic chemicals analysis showed very high DDE at 5.09 ppb, heptachlor at 0.8 ppb, HCB at 0.7 ppb, β-BHC at 0.21 ppb, dieldrin at 0.15 ppb, DDT at 0.2 ppb, and *trans*-nonachlor at 0.24 ppb.

He was discharged with a diagnosis of chemical overexposure with resultant immune vascular syndrome, joint and muscle pain, and spasm not amenable to other forms of treatment. He then received immunotherapy injections for pollens, dust mite, and foods. He was discharged to an oasis where he had a less chemically contaminated room. He maintained a rotation diet of chemically less contaminated food and drank spring water over the next 5 years.

Recently, the patient developed hypertension refractory to antihypertensive agents. His blood pressure was 210/110 mmHg; however, after MgC1 IV treatment at our office, his blood pressure decreased to 122/80 mmHg, and his tremor also dramatically stopped completely for the first time in 4 years. Now, his WBC has increased at 5300/mm^3. His blood toxic chemicals have improved. DDE has decreased to 2.6 ppb. He has become much better than before his recent treatment.

The symptoms of chemical sensitivity due to pesticides are often similar to the toxic effects (Tables 7.39 through 7.44). At times, however, they may be quite different and blend with almost any type of chemical sensitivity symptoms. They involve any of the smooth muscle systems in addition to the brain and NS (Table 7.38).

Blood Levels

The diagnosis of pesticide overload is not always simple. If a patient has just survived a recent spraying, however, a clinical history is adequate. If an organophosphate exposure is seen within 48 hours,

TABLE 7.41

Index to Pesticide Poisonings and Sensitivity by Symptoms and Signs

Manifestations	Characteristic Chemical	Chemicals Known to Produce Symptoms on Inhaled Challenge
Gastrointestinal Tract		
Nausea, vomiting, abdominal cramps, diarrhea	Organophosphates, carbamate insecticides, diquat, phosphorus, phosphine, inorganic arsenicals, arsine, fumigants, red squill cycloheximide, endothall, nicotine, chlorates, copper compounds, organic arsenicals, paraquat	Organochlorines, chloro-, nitro-, phenols, bisdithiocarbamates, ethylenebisdithiocarbamates, chlorophenoxy compounds, bentazon, chloroaliphatic acids
Salivation	Organophosphates, carbamate insecticides, cycloheximide, nicotine	
Respiratory System		
Stuffy nose, wheezing	Pyrethrum, bisdithiocarbamates plus alcohol	
Nosebleed		Paraquat
Coughing froth sputum (pulmonary edema)	Methyl bromide, phosphine, phosphorus, phosphides, ethylene oxide	Organophosphates, carbamate insecticides, ANTU
Rhinorrhea	Organophosphates, carbamate insecticides, fumigants	
Tachypnea	Nitro-, chloro-, phenols	
Respiratory depression	Organophosphates, carbamate insecticides, fumigants, cyanide, acrylonitrile, nicotine, endothall, sodium chlorate	Organochlorines
Labored breathing	Methyl bromide, organophosphates, carbamate insecticides, phosphine, phosphides, phosphorus	Sulfuryl fluoride
Chest pain	Fumigants, sodium chlorate	Organophosphates, carbamate insecticides, chlorophenoxy herbicides, nitro-, chloro-, phenols, chloroaliphatic acids.
Cardiovascular System		
Bradycardia	Organophosphates, carbamate insecticides, cyanide	
Tachycardia	Nitrophenols, chlorophenols	Organochlorines
Hypotension, chock	Phosphorus, phosphides, phosphine, vacor, endothall, cyanide	Bisdithiocarbamates plus alcohol, inorganic arsenicals, anticoagulant rodenticides
Irregular heart beat	Sodium fluoroacetate, halocarbon fumigants, endothall	Organochlorines, red squill
Hypertension	Nicotine	

Source: From Chemical sensitivity Volume II, page 896 and 897, table 12. With permission.

blood levels for the active substance or its metabolites may be done. Usually, these substances will be present. Organochlorine levels can be drawn at almost any time, since they are present for days to years in a patient. Levels of other pesticides, such as PCPs, PCBs, and various phenoxy herbicides are available. Blood levels are not practically available for the rest of the pesticides.

At the EHC-Dallas, we have performed studies on the incidence of organochlorine pesticides in the chemically sensitive patient. Eighty-one consecutive chemically sensitive patients measured in 1981 contained organochlorine pesticides. Today, 2015, only a few have VOC in them (Table 7.45).

The highest percentages were of DDT and its breakdown products, HCBs and chlordane compounds. In 1986, a similar group of 200 chemically sensitive patients was studied and found to have measurable levels of organochlorine pesticides (Table 7.40).

TABLE 7.42

Organochlorine Pesticides in the Blood of 81 Hospitalized Chemically Sensitive Patients

Pesticide	% High
DDT, DDE, DDD	101
	(DDT 19%)
	(DDE 79%)
	(DDD 3%)
Heptachlor epoxide[a]	74
HCB[a]	64
Trans-nonachlor[a]	47
β-BHC[a]	42
Dieldrin	33
α-BHC	2
Endosulfan I	2
γ-BHC	1
Endosulfan II	1
Endrin	1
Heptachlor	1
Aldrin	0
δ-BHC	0
α-Chlordane	0
γ-Chlordane	0
Mirex	0

Source: Chemical sensitivity Volume II, page 898, table 13. With permission.

[a] Incidence of complaints involving the nervous system was reviewed in the total sample and in those patients with high heptachlor epoxide, HCB, β-BHC, *trans*-nonachlor, or DDE levels. The most common complaint was headache, followed by physical fatigue, brain fatigue, dizziness/ light-headedness, and memory loss. The order of incidence of these complaints is the same within each of the five pesticide groups as well as the total sample; that is, the nervous system complaints of those high in pesticides mirrored each other as well as the total sample.

The presence and levels of these organochlorine pesticides have evolved over the past several years, with much lower levels and decreased frequency than previously seen. This finding may well reflect the more cautious use of organochlorines and the banning of many. Laseter's studies of a much larger number of patients (2000) reveal similar elevation and similar percentages. However, fat biopsies of patients with "low blood levels" of organochlorine pesticides have revealed much higher levels of these pesticides in the fat. These higher levels in the fat suggest that there is a greater lipophilicity among organochlorine pesticides, and their damage to cell membranes may be higher, explaining some of the long-term problems experienced by the chemically sensitive who are exposed to these substances.

Inhaled Challenges

In addition to blood levels, inhaled exposure studies in so-called safe ambient dose ranges in the parts per billion can be done on the patient suspected of being sensitive to pesticides. At present, this type of inhaled challenge is the best diagnostic tool for pesticide sensitivity. It should only be done on the very stable chemically sensitive patient who is at a plateau in his stage of recovery. Only ambient doses generally accepted as safe in society can be used for exposure. Extremely fragile patients cannot be tested because testing makes them much worse. The patient must be removed from these ambient doses to a pesticide-free, controlled environment for at least 4 days to reduce their total pollutant

TABLE 7.43

Distribution of Chlorinated Pesticides in the Blood of 200 Environmentally Sensitive Patients

Pesticide	Number of Patients	% Distribution in 200 Patients
DDT and DDE (114)	124	62.0
Hexachlorobenzene	115	57.5
Heptachlor epoxide	108	54.0
β-BHC	68	34.0
Endosulfan I	68	34.0
Dieldrin	48	24.0
γ-Chlordane	40	20.0
Heptachlor	25	12.5
γ-BHC (Lindane)	18	9.0
Aldrin	13	6.5
Endrin	11	5.5
δ-BHC	8	4.0
α-BHC	7	3.5
Mirex	4	2.0
Endosulfan II	3	1.5

Source: Chemical sensitivity Volume II, page 889, table 14. With permission.

TABLE 7.44

Two Hundred Consecutive Patients with Chemical Sensitivity: 52 Sensitive by Double-Blind Inhaled Challenge

	Ambient Dose
Raid	2,22-DDVP and -2-(1-M)-PMC
Decon	
DDT	
Heptachlor	
Chlordane	
Pyrethrum	

Source: Chemical sensitivity Volume II, page 899, table 15. With permission.

TABLE 7.45

Pesticide-Related Immune Changes in Chemically Sensitive Patients

	%	Patients
Total low T- and B-cells	81	107
T-cell below 65%	56	61
T-cell below 1000	32	35
B-cell below 5%	24	26
B-cell below 60/cm³	48	52

Source: Chemical sensitivity Volume II, page 905, table 16. With permission.

load and allow deadaptation to occur. We have studied 1500 patients under controlled environmental conditions in the deadaptated state using double-blind techniques without any long-term effects. Levels challenged by inhalation were supposedly ambient doses that had been generally accepted as safe. Usually, the level challenged was in <0.0034 ppm range for a substance, such as 2,4-DNP, in one consecutive series of 200 (proven by inhaled challenge of pesticide (Table 7.47). This result suggests that at least one-fourth of chemically sensitive patients are sensitive to this type of pesticide. Since not all types of pesticide were challenged, we conclude that the incidence of pesticide sensitivity in the chemically sensitive must be much higher. This conclusion may be particularly likely, since another 80% of these people were sensitive to phenol and chlorine, on separate challenges.

For more accurate assessment, patients should be deadaptated in a pesticide-free environment for a minimum of 4 days and a maximum of 7 days before undergoing testing. There are four different possibilities of responses that can result from an inhaled ambient dose of <0.0034 ppm of 2,4-DNP challenge (Figure 7.66). First, of course, no change could occur. Second, third, and fourth,

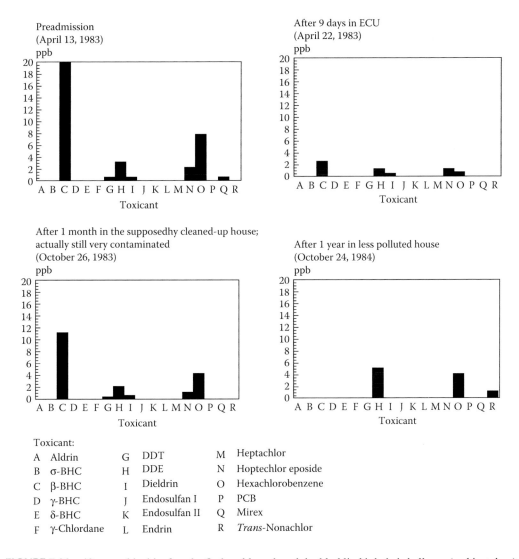

FIGURE 7.66   40-year-old white female. Ortho-chlorophenol double-blind inhaled challenge (ambient dose) after 4 days deadaptation in the ECU with total load decreased. (From Chemical sensitivity Volume II, page 858, figure 13. With permission.)

respectively, are stimulation, depression, or a biphasic response of the immune and nervous systems. At the EHC-Dallas, we have now seen hundreds of these various responses. Individual responses are seen to inhaled challenges of different pesticides, resulting in changes in eosinophils, total hemolytic complement, and IgG. Challenge can also show changes in T-cells (Figure 7.67).

Organophosphates

OP levels can be measured for malathion, parathion, sarin, and chlorpyrifos herbicides for atrazine; glyphosate can be measured in the blood.

Immune Correlation

In addition to direct blood analysis and challenge, immune parameter and antipollutant enzyme changes can also be measured.[99] Though these different immune changes appear to be nonspecific, there is some evidence that changes in immune parameters can be correlated with the presence or absence of chlorinated and OP pesticides and herbicides in an individual's blood. In a series of 107 consecutive chemically sensitive patients at the EHC-Dallas who were found to have organochlorine pesticides in their blood, 81% showed abnormally low T and B lymphocytes, when compared with our controls (Tables 7.49 and 7.50). In addition, different pesticides were shown to have more influence on the T-cells than others.

According to the literature, there are many different substances in pesticides, mitocides, herbicides, and fumigants, which alter the immune system. These include organochlorines, organophosphate, carbamate, pyrethroid, and arsenical pesticides as well as mitocides such as milibes (Table 7.52).

Pesticides can stimulate, suppress, or cause the immune system to malfunction, as was discussed in the previous section on challenge tests. Most can do all three, depending on the concentration and duration of the dose; the virulence of the pesticides, mitocides, herbicides, and fumigants on the immune system; and the total body pollutant load and state of nutrition of an individual at the time of exposure.

The simplest change that can be seen in the immune system is the altering of proteins that become haptens. The fumigant formaldehyde is known to trigger the IgE mechanism with hapten formation.[617] It is suspected by some that other pesticides may also alter proteins and cause a similar type of hapten complex.

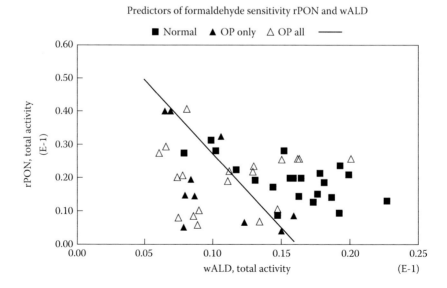

FIGURE 7.67   Predictors of formaldehyde sensitivity. (From Alter, S, Organiziak, D, Rea, W. Department of Biochemistry, University of Dayton School of Medicine and the Environmental Health Center: Dallas.)

Direct cytotoxic effects may be seen on cells. Mercurial-containing insecticides and fumigants may trigger this effect.[618]

Immune complexes between IgG and complement are known to occur with toxic chemicals. Many of the organochlorine and OP pesticides and herbicides are known to deregulate complements.

Direct T-cell triggering is found with many organochlorine pesticides. Often, they cause suppression of the suppressor T-cells.[619] Numerous substances such as DDT,[620–625] HCB,[626–628] and PCP may alter the bactericidal, virucidal, and phagocytic ability of the neutrophils.[629] They may also decrease the responder plasma cells in the lymph nodes.[630,631] Many pesticides such as DDT will deregulate the basophils, thus preventing histamine release and anaphylaxis, but they also suppress skin whealing capacity for immediate antigen reactions.[625,632–635] Ishikawa et al.[210] have shown a correlation of high levels of organochlorine and organophosphate pesticides with the changes of Behcet's disease. Other pesticides may alter the antigen recognition sites on cells, resulting in the spreading phenomenon seen in many chemically sensitive patients. Also, receptor sites for substances such as hormones may be altered, particularly by organochlorines.[636,637]

Organochlorine pesticides that are known to alter the immune system are DDT,[620,629] chlordane,[620] aldrin,[638] lindane,[638,639] HCB,[626–628] mirex,[640] and arochlor (a PCB).[619] Organophosphates that cause changes in the immune system are anthio,[641] malathion,[639] leptohos,[642] chlorophos,[629,643–646] chlorpyrifos,[647] and parathion.[620,624,648,649] Carbamates are known to cause immune changes,[620] as well as arsenicals[650] and mitocides such as chlorobenzylate[651] and milbex.[652] Other substances like herbicides and fumigants are known to cause immune dysfunction. These are the phenoxy herbicides barban,[652] TCD dioxin,[653–657] monum,[652] TEC fran,[658] nitrophenols, diquat, and paraquat.[652] Fumigants such as chloroform, carbon tetrachloride, and formaldehyde are known to be animal carcinogens, and we suspect that they are carcinogenic in humans as well.[659]

Several correlative studies have been performed at the EHC-Dallas. Rea and Liang[98] studied 66 patients with chemical sensitivity that had organochlorine pesticides in their blood.

In this group of 66 proven chemically sensitive patients, there were 9 males and 57 females who had environmentally triggered (essential) hypertension (17), porphyria (1), vasculitis (33), or multiple sclerosis (15). Eighty-seven percent of 23 patients who had 0 to <2 organochlorine pesticides in their blood had normal T- and B-cells; whereas 13% did not. Of the group that had >2 organochlorine pesticides in their blood, 40 (93%) had abnormal T and B lymphocytes (Table 7.55).

Significant differences in the frequencies of individual pesticides found in the blood were found in T and B changes in patients with BHC, DDE, dieldrin, heptachlor E, HCB, and *trans*-nonachlor versus those with two or less pesticides (Table 7.48).

Significant differences of the means of the individual levels were also seen in β-BHC, DDE, dieldrin, heptachlor E, HCB, and *trans*-nonachlor, as compared with those patients who had less than two pesticides in their blood (Table 7.48).

There was also a positive correlation between the frequency of abnormal immune parameters between the group with more than two organochlorine pesticides, in contrast to those with two or less. Abnormal WBC (C = 4800–10,000/mm^3), T_{11} (C = 1260–2650/mm^3), and T_4 (C = 670–1800/mm^3) were seen to the 0.001 significance level (Table 7.49).

Analysis of the means of the blood cell parameters reveals significant differences to the 0.001–0.005 levels in the WBC, lymphocyte count, T_{11}, T_4:T_8 ratio, and B lymphocytes count.

Comparison of the means of T and B lymphocytes in chemically sensitive patients with more than two pesticides identified in their blood versus 60 patients of a normal control group measured at the EHC-Dallas revealed a significant difference between 0.001 and 0.05 range, with the T and B being less than the control. WBCs, though in the normal range for both groups, were significantly lower (5520 vs. 7560/mm^3) in the group with more than two pesticides present in their blood, with resultant significance to the 0.001 level (Tables 7.51 and 7.52).

The blood levels of chlorinated pesticides and T and B lymphocyte parameters in 60 proven chemically sensitive patients were also studied. There was a significant decrease in T-cell parameters when correlated with individual organochlorine pesticides (Table 7.52). The simple regression results showed that α-BHC had a negative correlation with B lymphocyte ($R = 0.3136$, $p < 0.02$); β-BHC had a significant negative correlation with the absolute lymphocyte, T_{11} cell, T_8 cell, and B lymphocyte count ($R = -0.3875$ to -0.2558, $p < 0.003$–0.05) and a significant positive correlation with the percentage of T_{11} cell, T_4 cell, and T_4/T_8 ($p < 0.002$–0.008). DDT had a positive correlation with percentage of T_{11} cells ($R = 0.2547$, $p < 0.05$). *Trans*-nonachlor had a negative correlation with absolute lymphocytes ($R = 0.2578$, $p < 0.05$) and a positive correlation with the percentage of T_8 cells ($R = 0.3006$, $p < 0.02$). The multiple regression results showed that there was significant correlation between chlorinated pesticides and T and B lymphocyte parameters, including the absolute lymphocyte count, the percentage of T_{11} cells, the percentage of T_4 cells, the absolute T_8 cell count, T_4/T_8, and the absolute B lymphocyte count (multiple $R = 0.45$–0.60, adjusted $R = 0.36$–0.49, $p < 0.004$–0.03). These results indicate that chlorinated pesticides do have an immune deregulation effect on the T and B lymphocyte parameters in the chemically sensitive. According to these regression equations, a concept of critical reference value was defined and discussed by Liang et al. (Tables 7.52 through 7.56). If the pesticide level was elevated at 1 ppb, a consequential drop in T- or B-cells was seen. For example, this drop in B-cells for α-BHC would be 114/mm³ B-cells for each 0.1 ppb increase of the pesticide (Tables 7.46 through 7.48).

In addition to evaluating these parameters, we studied 66 proven chemically sensitive patients with blood level of chlorinated pesticides and correlated them with the cell-mediated immunity (CMI) parameters. The simple regression analysis showed DDE and DDT had a significant positive correlation with the CMI parameters, including the number of the reacted antigens and the sum of the average per millimeter ($p < 0.0001$–0.02). Heptachlor epoxide had a significant positive correlation with the sum of average of CMI ($p < 0.004$). Dieldrin and *trans*-nonachlor had a negative correlation with the CMI parameters ($p < 0.002$–0005), and β-BHC also showed a trend for negative correlation with the number of reacting antigens ($p < 0.05$). According to these simple regression equations, when dieldrin is 0.85–1.1 ppb, there is no CMI reaction. When *trans*-nonachlor is 2.8–2.9 ppb, there is also no CMI reaction. The multiple regression analysis showed a significant correlation between chlorinated pesticides and CMI parameters (multiple $R = 0.66$–0.68, adjusted $R = 0.60$–0.62, $p < 0.0001$). According to these equations, when the mean of each eight kinds of correlated pesticides is 0.26–0.36 ppb, there is no CMI reaction. These results indicate that chlorinated pesticides do have significant effects on the CMI. Some of them have an immunostimulation effect (DDE, DDT, and heptachlor epoxide), while some of them have an immunosuppression effect (β-BHC, dieldrin, and *trans*-nonachlor) (Tables 7.49 and 7.50).

In another series at the EHC-Dallas, 48 of 51 consecutive chemically and pesticide-sensitive patients with organochlorines in their blood had T lymphocytes below 1000 ($C = 1400$–2200/mm³).

TABLE 7.46

Chlorinated Pesticides versus Lymphocytes versus Brain Function in 107 Chemically Sensitive Patients

Pesticides	Change in Lymphocytes				Change in Brain Function % Patient
	% T	T_{abs}	%B	B_{abs}	
BHC	50	30	30	30	52.0
Dieldrin	60	30	20	45	61.0
Chlordane	60	32	32	40	77.0
DDT	49	35	27	45	44.0
Heptachlor epoxide	60	33	24	47	40.0
Hexachlorobenzene	58	35	20	41	44.4

Source: From Chemical sensitivity Volume II, page 906, table 17. With permission.

TABLE 7.47

Pesticides and Herbicides Known to Cause Immune Change

Organochlorines	Organophosphates	Carbamates	Herbicides
DDT[620–625,6]	Antio[16]	Sevin (Laseter, J. L. 1985, personal communication)[1,17,23]	Monum[7]
Clordane[7]	Malathion[9]	Carbaryl[5,14,21]	TEC furan[80]
Aldrin[8]	Leptophos (Smith, C. W. 1989, personal communication)	Carbofurun[5,14,21]	Nitrophenol, agranulocytosis—humans[29] Cataracts—animals[28]
Lindane[8,9]	Chlorophos (Laseter, J. L. 1985, personal communication)[17–20]	Agranulocytosis[27]	Diquat and paraquat[7]
Hexa chlorobenzene[10–12]	Parathion	Chlorobenzilate[7]	Dicresyl[24]
Mirex[13]		Milbex[7]	
			Pyrethroids[22]
Arochlor (a POCB)[10,11,14,15]			
			Arsenicals[27]
			Mitocides[7]
			Phenoxy
			Barban[7]
			TCD doxin[25,26,30,32,38]

Source: Modified from Rea, W. J., H.-C. Liang. 1991. Effects of pesticides on the immune system. *J. Nutr. Med.* 2:399–410. (From Chemical sensitivity Volume II, page 907, table 18. With permission.)

In addition, other studies done by Bertschler and Butler[659] at the EHC Dallas have shown specific brain function changes with exposure to specific pesticides. In addition to pesticides, inert ingredients, including over 270 organ substances are involved in covering up the odor of pesticides and herbicides. No one knows how the combination of these fragrances when added to the pesticides can respond to the chemically sensitive and chronic degenerative patient.

PESTICIDES AND IMMUNE FUNCTION

Pesticides are generally classified (discussed later) into insecticides, herbicides, fumigants, and miscellaneous categories. Each group is toxic in its own right, but some are more toxic than others, with resultant chemical sensitivity and/or chronic degenerative disease in many people who are exposed to them. The following discussion attempts to classify these substances as to their immune

TABLE 7.48

Relationship between the Number of Pesticides and T and B Count in 66 Patients

No. of Pesticides	No. of Patients	T and B Count	No. of Patients	%
0–2	23	Normal	20	87
		Abnormal	3	13
>2	43	Normal	3	7
		Abnormal	40	93

Source: Rea, W. J., H.-C. Liang. 1991. Effects of pesticides on the immune system. *J. Nutr. Med.* 2:399–410.

TABLE 7.49

Comparison of the Frequency of Chlorinated Pesticides between CP < 2 and CP > 2

Pesticides	CP < 2 Group			CP > 2 Group			
	No. of Patients	No. of Positive	No. of %	No. of Patients	Positive	%	p
α-BHC[a]	20	0	0	40	5	12.5	<0.02
β-BHC[a]	20	4	20	40	27	67.5	<0.001
DDT	20	2	10	40	9	22.5	>0.05
DDE[a]	20	13	65	40	40	100.0	<0.01
Dieldrin[a]	20	0	0	40	17	42.5	<0.001
Endosulfan I	20	0	0	40	2	5.0	>0.05
Heptachlor epoxide[a]	20	3	15	40	34	85.0	<0.001
HCB[a]	20	2	10	40	35	87.5	<0.001
γ-Chlordane	20	0	0	40	1	2.5	>0.05
Trans-nonachlor[a]	20	1	5	40	28	70.0	<0.001

Source: Rea, W. J., H.-C. Liang. 1991. Effects of pesticides on the immune system. *J. Nutr. Med.* 2:399–410. (From Chemical sensitivity Volume II, page 911, table 20. With permission.)

[a] Significant difference.

dysfunction. We give their general mode of action and potential routes of excretion or neutralization in the body. Some understanding of their chemistry will help the physician understand the reasons for the induction and exacerbation that are seen in the chemically sensitive upon exposure to these extremely toxic substances. Synthetic and natural pesticides have been developed. Both may be toxic to man. Immune deregulation starts with the immune deregulation followed by changes in the T lymphocytes (CD_3, CD_4, and CD_8) and also total B lymphocytes. There is a tendency for the low T lymphocytes, C_3–$D_{4,8}$, or their function to be low to be more common. Serum complements are either low or high in most sensitive patients exposed to pesticides. The clinician rarely finds a normal complement. Often, enzymes are changed as are auto-antibodies which are elevated. Gamma globulins and their subsets are also disrupted.

TABLE 7.50

Comparison of the Means of Chlorinated Pesticides between CP < 2 and CP > 2 Group

Pesticides	CP < 2 Group	CP > 2 Group	p
α-BHC	0	0.04	>0.05
β-BHC[a]	0.15	0.42	<0.01
DDT	0.03	0.04	>0.05
DDE[a]	1.27	5.31	<0.0005
Dieldrin[a]	0	0.13	<0.01
Endosulfan I	0	0.075	>0.5
Heptachlor epoxide[a]	0.055	0.561	<0.0001
HCB[a]	0.04	0.338	<0.0001
γ-Chlordane	0	0.015	>0.5
Trans-nonachlor[a]	0.03	0.28	<0.0001

Source: Chemical sensitivity Volume II, page 912, table 21. With permission.

[a] Significant difference.

INNATE IMMUNITY: METABOLIC RESPONSE TO CELLULAR ATTACK

This is one of the ancient functions of mitochondria. There are many mitochondrial changes and the net result of oxidative shielding is innate immunity which is to limit the replication and prevent the exit of the invading pathogen or toxic substance. Reactive oxidative substances (ROS) are produced.

The immune system can be interpreted as a true mobile nervous system (Tables 7.51 and 7.52).

In another series of patients at the EHC-Dallas, there was a direct correlation with the removal of organochlorine pesticides and the recovery of T-cells improved.

In a series of patients with pesticide sensitivity who were followed at the ECU, we saw a dramatic improvement in brain function as the pesticides cleared their blood. These results held even if autotransfusion reoccurred. However, each time more pesticides appeared in the blood, the patient had temporary brain dysfunction usually no matter the type and usually at the ambient dose. In a breakdown of pesticides cleared from the blood, we have found chlordane compounds and DDT compounds to clear more slowly, although they all clear with difficulty. In subsequent studies, we have shown clearing of all types of chlorinated pesticides. This clearing has paralleled the lessening of the chemical sensitivity. However, often the organochlorines, especially DDT and DDE, may take up to many years.

It has been observed that rapid treatment with avoidance and intravenous vitamin C (15–30 g daily for 1–2 weeks) will entirely reverse an acute chemically sensitive onset resulting from acute pesticide exposure. Long-term treatment is the same as discussed in the treatment chapters contained in Volume 5, Chapter 6, Tables 6.38–6.43 (Tables 7.53 through 7.61).

Enzyme changes: Many enzyme changes occur in selected chemically sensitive and chronic degenerative disease patients.

According to Mauck et al.,[660] exposure to the reversible cholinesterase inhibitor, PB, in conjunction with stress has been suggested as a possible cause of Gulf War Syndrome. This work explores the hypothesis that PB exposure coupled with stress will alter cholinergic receptor density based on the rationale that prolonged exposure to PB and stress will lead to increased stimulation of cholinergic

TABLE 7.51
Comparison of the Frequency of Abnormal Immune Parameters between CP < 2 and CP > 2 Group

Immune Parameters	CP < 2 Group			CP > 2 Group			
	No. of Patients	No. of Abonormal	%	No. of Patents	No. of Abnormal	%	*p*
WBC[a]	20	1	5	40	14	35.0	<0.001
Lym %[a]	20	0	0	40	8	20.0	<0.01
Lym C[a]	20	2	10	40	15	37.5	<0.01
T_{11} %[a]	20	2	10	40	12	30.0	<0.05
T_{11} C[a]	20	2	10	40	21	52.5	<0.001
T_4 %	20	1	5	40	18	45.0	<0.001
T_4 C[a]	20	1	5	40	14	35.0	<0.001
T_8 %	20	1	5	40	8	20.0	>0.05
T_8 C[a]	20	0	0	40	12	30.0	<0.001
T_4/T_8[a]	20	1	5	40	11	27.5	<0.01
B lym %	20	3	15	40	7	17.5	>0.05
B lym C[a]	20	1	5	40	12	30.0	<0.01

Source: Rea, W. J., H.-C. Liang. 1991. Effects of pesticides on the immune system. *J. Nutr. Med.* 2:399–410. (From Chemical sensitivity Volume II, page 913, table 22. With permission.)

[a] Significant difference for both OC and OP insecticides.

TABLE 7.52

Comparison of the Means of Immune Parameters between CP < 2 and CP > 2 Group

Immune Parameters	CP > 2 Group	CP < 2 Group	p
WBC[a]	5500	6685	<0.01
Lym %	36.3	33.6	>0.5
Lym C[a]	1949	2217	<0.05
T_{11}%[a]	78.1	74.4	<0.05
T_{11}C	1597	1666	>0.1
T_4%[a]	49.8	44.2	<0.05
T_4C	963	965	>0.1
T_8%	25.5	23.6	>0.1
T_8C	508	515	>0.1
T_4/T_8[a]	2.2	1.9	<0.05
B lym %	10.9	12.1	>0.1
B lym C[a]	211	272	<0.05

Source: Rea, W. J., H.-C. Liang. 1991. Effects of pesticides on the immune system. *J. Nutr. Med.* 2:399–410. (From Chemical sensitivity Volume II, page 914, table 23. With permission.)

[a] Significant difference.

receptors due to the reduced capacity to degrade acetylcholine, leading to changes in receptor levels. Male C57B16 mice were exposed to PB (3 or 10 mg/kg/day) or physostigmine (2.88 mg/kg/day) for 7 days via ALZET mini-osmotic pumps implanted subcutaneously. The mice were stressed by shaking at random intervals (average of 2 minutes/30 minutes) for 1 week, which was sufficient to increase blood cortisol levels. Brain tissue for autoradiographic analysis was collected on day 7 of

TABLE 7.53

Simple Regression Equation, Correlation Coefficients, and the Test of Correlation Significance between Chlorinated Pesticides and T and B Lymphocyte Parameters

Pesticides (X)	T and B (Y)	Regression Equation	Spearman R	p
α-BHC	B lym C	Y = 1/0.00644 + 0.0235a X	−0.3136	0.0147
β-BHC	Lym C	Y = 2222.6 − 474.8 X	−0.3875	0.0022
β-BHC	T_{11} %	Y = 74.8 + 6.6 X	0.3429	0.0073
β-BHC	T_{11} C	Y = 1683.3 − 263.7 X	−0.2558	0.0458
β-BHC	T_4 %	Y = 45.3 + 8 X	0.4059	0.0013
β-BHC	T_8 C	Y = 570.3 − 148.2 X	−0.2917	0.0237
β-BHC	T_4/T_8	Y = 1.93 + 0.7 X	0.366	0.004
β-BHC	B lym C	Y = 245.2 − 75.8 X	−0.3316	0.0097
DDT	T_{11} %	Y = 75.8 + 20.6 X	0.2547	0.0495
Trans-nonachlor	Lym C	Y = 2013 EXP (−0.12115 X)	−0.2578	0.0467
Trans-nonachlor	T_8 %	Y = 23.8 + 5.8 X	0.3006	0.0196

Source: Liang, H.-C. et al. 1992. Study on the critical reference value from the regression equations between chlorinated pesticides and immune parameters. *Environ. Med.* 9(1):10–16. (From Chemical sensitivity Volume II, page 915, table 24. With permission.)

TABLE 7.54

Significant Test for B Coefficients in Multiple Regression between Chlorinated Pesticides and T and B Lymphocyte Parameters

Parameters	α-BHC	β-BHC	DDE	DDT	Die	En I	HCB	HeE	γCh	TrN
Lym C	–	<0.005	>0.4	–	–	–	–	<0.02	>0.4	<0.04
T_{11} %	–	<0.01	–	>0.05	–	<0.04	–	–	–	–
T_4 %	>0.1	<0.02	>0.05	>0.3	>0.05	>0.3	>0.05	–	–	<0.04
T_8 C	<0.01	<0.007	>0.1	–	>0.5	>0.4	>0.1	<0.001	>0.6	>0.3
T_4/T_8	>0.1	<0.009	>0.5	–	–	–	<0.03	>0.5	>0.5	>0.2
B lym C	<0.04	<0.004	>0.2	>0.1	–	>0.2	–	<0.03	–	<0.03

Source: Liang, H.-C., W. J. Rea. *Chemical Sensitivity.* Vol. 2, p. 916. CRC Press, Inc. (From Chemical sensitivity Volume II, page 916, table 25. With permission.)

treatment. While Mauck et al.[660] examined many brain regions, analysis revealed that most of the significant changes ($p < 0.05$) were seen in cholinergic nuclei. Stress typically increased muscarinic receptor density, while PB and PHY generally decreased muscarinic receptor density.

Residents of the agricultural community of Cache County, Utah, who were aged 65 years and older as of January 1995, were invited to participate in the study. At baseline, participants completed detailed occupational history questionnaires that included information about exposures to various types of pesticides. Cognitive status was assessed at baseline and after 3, 7, and 10 years. Standardized methods were used for detection and diagnosis of dementia and AD. Cox proportional hazards survival analyses were used to evaluate the risk of incident dementia and AD associated with pesticide exposure. Among 3,084 enrollees without dementia, more men than women reported pesticide exposure ($p < 0.0001$). Exposed individuals ($n = 572$) had more years of education ($p < 0.01$) but did not differ from others in age. Some 500 individuals developed incident dementia, 344 with AD. After adjustment for baseline age, sex, education, APOE epsilon 4 status,

TABLE 7.55

Effects of Chlorinated Pesticides on the T and B Lymphocyte Parameters in 60 Chemically Sensitive Patients

Pesticides	Blood Level (ppb)	T and B	Change	Normal
α-BHC	0.1	B lym C		114/mm^3
	0.25			<82/mm^3
β-BHC	1.0	Lym C	Decrease	475/mm^3
	1.0	T_{11} %	Increase	6.6%
	1.0	T_{11} C	Decrease	264/mm^3
	1.0	T_4 %	Increase	8.0%
	1.0	T_8 C	Decrease	148/mm^3
	1.0	T_4/T_8	Increase	2.6
	1.0	B lym C	Decrease	76/mm^3
DDT	1.0	T_{11} %	Increase	20.6%
Trans-nonachlor	1.0	Lym C	Decrease	168/mm^3
	1.0	T_8 %	Increase	5.8%

Source: Liang, H.-C., and W. J. Rea. *Chemical Sensitivity.* Vol. 2, p. 916. CRC Press, Inc. (From Chemical sensitivity Volume II, page 916, table 26. With permission.)

TABLE 7.56
Critical Reference Value for Simple Regression between the Chlorinated Pesticides and T and B

	Lymphocyte Parameters in 60 Chemically Sensitive Patients			
Pesticides	**Blood Level (ppb)**	**T and B**	**Change**	**Normal Range**
α-BHC	0.25	B lym C	<82/mm^3	82–477/mm^3
β-BHC	1.1	T$_4$ %	>54%	32%–54%
	1.15	T$_4$/T$_8$	>2.7	1–2.7
	1.32	Lym C	<1600 mm^3	1600–4200/mm^3
	1.6	T$_{11}$ C	<1260/mm^3	1260–2650/mm^3
	1.6	T$_8$ C	<333/mm^3	333–1070/mm^3
	1.7	T$_{11}$ %	>86%	62%–86%
	2.16	B lym C	<82/mm^3	82–477/mm^3
DDT	0.5	T$_{11}$ %	>86%	62%–86%
Trans-nonachlor	1.4	Lym C	<1600/mm^3	1600–4200/mm^3
	2.0	T$_8$%	>35%	17%–35%

Source: Liang, H.-C. et al. 1992. Study on the critical reference value from the regression equations between chlorinated pesticides and immune parameters. *Environ. Med.* 9(1):10–16. (From Chemical sensitivity Volume II, page 917, table 27. With permission.)

TABLE 7.57
Critical Reference Value for Multiple Regression between the Chlorinated Pesticides and T and B Lymphocyte Parameters in 60 Chemically Sensitive Patients

T and B	**No. of Correlated Pesticides**	**Mean of Each Pesticides (ppb)**	**Change**	**Normal Range**
Lym C	5	0.28	<1600/mm^3	1600–4200/mm^3
T$_{11}$ %	3	0.22	<62%	62%–86%
T$_4$ %	8	0.9	<32%	32%–54%
T$_8$ C	9	0.251	<333/mm^3	333–1070/mm^3
T$_4$/T$_8$	7	0.65	<1	1–2.7
B lym C	7	0.126	<82/mm^3	82–477/mm^3

Source: Liang, H.-C. et al. 1992. Study on the critical reference value from the regression equations between chlorinated pesticides and immune parameters. *Environ. Med.* 9(1):10–16. (From Chemical sensitivity Volume II, page 918, table 28. With permission.)

and baseline risks among pesticide-exposed individuals for all-cause dementia, with hazard ratio (HR) 1.38 and 95% CI 1.09–1.76 and for AD (HR 1.42, 95% CI = 1.06–1.91). The risk of AD associated with organophosphate exposure (HR 1.53, 95% CI = 1.0–2.23) was slightly higher than the risk associated with organochlorines (HR 1.49, 95% CI = 0.99–2.24), which was nearly significant. Pesticide exposure may increase the risk of dementia and AD in late life.

Another example of enzyme deficiency from pesticide spraying occurred in France.

These chronic effects of pesticides have been shown in French winegrowers when a French winegrower, who died after contracting leukemia, became the first farmer to have his illness officially linked to the pesticides he used for years on his crops.

Y. C., 43, had cultivated vineyards and other crops for decades at his farm in Ruffec, in the Poitou-Charentes region of Southwestern France. His death has served to highlight the dangers of working in the vineyards.

TABLE 7.58
Effects of Chlorinated Pesticides on the Number of Reacted Antigens of CMI (Chemically Sensitive Patients)

Pesticides	Blood Level (ppb)	CMI-N (Y)	Change
β-BHC	3	Decrease	1
DDE	11	Increase	1
DDT	0.17	Increase	1
Dieldrin	0.85	Decrease Y = O	No reaction
Trans-nonachlor	2.8	Decrease Y = O	No reaction

Source: Liang, H.-C., W. J. Rea. *Chemical Sensitivity.* Vol. 2, p. 916. CRC Press, Inc. (From Chemical sensitivity Volume II, page 919, table 30. With permission.)

TABLE 7.59
Effects of Chlorinated Pesticides on the Sum of Average Reacted Diameters of CMI (Chemically Sensitive Patients)

Pesticides	Blood Level (ppb)	CMI-S (Y)	Change (mm)
DDE	1.0	Increase	0.37
Heptachlor epoxide	1.0	Increase	1.47
DDT	0.1	Increase	2.30
Dieldrin	1.1	Decrease Y = O	No reaction
Trans-nonachlor	2.9	Decrease Y = O	No reaction

Source: Liang, H.-C., W. J. Rea. *Chemical Sensitivity.* Vol. 2, p. 916. CRC Press, Inc. (From Chemical sensitivity Volume II, page 919, table 31. With permission.)

TABLE 7.60
Significance of Correlation between Chlorinated Pesticide Levels and the Number of Reacting Antigens CMI (Chemically Sensitive Patients)

Pesticide	F-Value	p
Dieldrin	13.85	<0.0001
β-BHC	4.71	<0.05
DDT	9.85	<0.0005
DDE	28.29	<0.0001
Trans-nonachlor	9.77	<0.005

Source: Liang, H.-C., W. J. Rea. *Chemical Sensitivity.* Vol. 2, p. 916. CRC Press, Inc. (From Chemical sensitivity Volume II, page 919, table 32. With permission.)

TABLE 7.61

Significance of Correlation between Chlorinated Pesticide Levels and the Sum of the Average Wheal Diameters of CMI Tests (Chemically Sensitive Patients)

Pesticide	F-Value	p
Dieldrin	13.94	<0.0005
DDT	5.95	<0.02
DDE	23.27	<0.0001
Heptachlor epoxide	9.09	<0.004
Trans-nonachlor	10.56	<0.002

Source: Liang, H.-C., W. J. Rea. *Chemical Sensitivity.* Vol. 2, p. 916. CRC Press, Inc. (From Chemical sensitivity Volume II, page 919, table 33. With permission.)

He is among 40 or so farmers in France whose illnesses have now been officially linked to their profession and the pesticides they have sprayed on the land, by the French agricultural public health body.

Another farmer and Mr. Chenet's close friend also suffers from severe health problems recognized as being linked to the products he used.

In April 2004, he inadvertently breathed in noxious fumes from his agricultural spraying machine without a mask on. Immediately admitted to hospital, he fell into a coma. Since then, his illness continues to affect his kidneys and NS and he has again fallen into comas on several occasions.

While no specific product has been singled out by the French agricultural public health body, they suspect benzene as well as the pesticide, a chemical frequently used as a solvent or thinner by farmers, also played a part in contracting blood cancer.

Other farmers have had PD and other cancers recognized as being linked to the chemical products.[660]

More than a quarter of the roughly 220,000 tons of pesticide used in Europe per year is sprayed onto French soil; some 65,000 tons and a fifth of that amount goes onto French vineyards, despite the fact, these only account for 5% of the country's total crop surface.

Aerial spraying can be most devastating to the worker and as well as to the bystander.

According to Hayden et al.,[661] commonly used organophosphate and organochlorine pesticides inhibit *AChE at synapses* in the somatic, autonomic, and CNS and may therefore have lasting effect on the NS as it did in those French farmers. This situation may account for chronic degenerative disease. Few studies have examined the relationship of pesticide exposure and risk of dementia or AD. Hayden et al.[661] sought to examine the association of occupational pesticide exposure and the risk of incident dementia and AD in later life.

According to tests by the consumer organization Environmental Working Group (EWG), seven most contaminated fruits with organophosphate pesticides among the foods are: peaches, strawberries, apples, domestic blueberries, nectarines, cherries, and imported grapes.

The EWG also found high pesticide levels in six vegetables: celery, sweet bell pepper, spinach, kale, collard greens, and potatoes. The good news is the EWG found 15 fruits and vegetables to be relatively low in pesticide residues: onions, avocado, sweet corn (frozen), pineapples, mango, sweet peas (frozen) asparagus, kiwi fruit, cabbage, eggplant, domestic cantaloupe, watermelon, grapefruit, sweet potatoes, and honeydew melon.

Weisskopf and colleagues report their findings in the May 17 online issue of *Pediatrics*.[662] Another enzyme that can be damaged is reported by Wang et al.[663] who examined the protective efficacy of paraoxonase-1 (PON1) against tissue damage caused by dichlorvos; purified rabbit PON1 was injected intravenously into rats 30 minutes before they were given dichlorvos, while dichlorvos administration group and corn oil administration group were conducted to compare. Blood was collected at different time points after dichlorvos administration to examine the acetyl cholinesterase (AChE) inhibition level and clinical signs were observed after poisoning. After 72 hours, animals were anesthetized and the hippocampus, liver, lung, and kidney were removed for observation of ultrastructure. AChE activities in PON1 pretreatment group were statistically significant from dichlorvos administration group ($p < 0.01$). The clinical signs were alleviated by PON1 significantly ($p < 0.05$). The most common change of organophosphorus poisoning damage to liver was small lipid-like structures could be seen throughout the liver structure. In kidney, dense bodies were seen. As the most significant changes of hippocampus, demyelination takes place after acute organophosphorus poisoning, but neural edema was not improved significantly in their study. In conclusion, PON1 can decrease the AChE inhibition, and alleviated clinical signs and tissue damage caused by dichlorvos.[663]

The graph (Figure 7.67) entitled "Predictors of Organophosphate Sensitivity" uses levels of the enzymes, arylesterase (rAE) and aldehyde dehydrogenase (wALD) to distinguish between OP-sensitive and normal individuals. The line in each graph divides it into regions where enzyme levels of normal individuals tend to cluster and regions where enzyme levels of chemically sensitive individuals tend to cluster. Enzyme levels measured in the blood sample were used to place a symbol corresponding on each graph. The position of the symbol is below the line in either figure; we would classify the patient as being chemically sensitive to the chemical agent referenced in that figure. If the results are above the line, we would classify the individual as normal.[663]

Alter, Organiziak, and Rea[664] used "logical regression analysis" of the enzyme levels monitored in blood fractions of OP-sensitive, formaldehyde-sensitive, and chemically sensitive individuals. The method looks for the most sensitive measurements that can be used to differentiate between sensitive and normal individuals.

Our results suggest that several of the enzyme levels measured in blood samples can distinguish between chemically sensitive and normal individuals. Results showing formaldehyde-sensitive, (Figure 7.67) OP-sensitive (Figure 7.68), and normal individuals (both figures) are shown in the attached graphs. Individuals with no identified chemical sensitivity are plotted as filled squares. Results from individuals with demonstrated chemical sensitivities are plotted using triangular symbols. Filled triangles indicate enzyme levels from individuals with one type of sensitivity (e.g., sensitivity to one class of compounds). Open symbols indicate enzyme levels from individuals with sensitivity to formaldehyde or OP and at least one other class of compounds. (Open symbols could represent sensitivity to both formaldehyde and OP, and may be other chemical classes.)

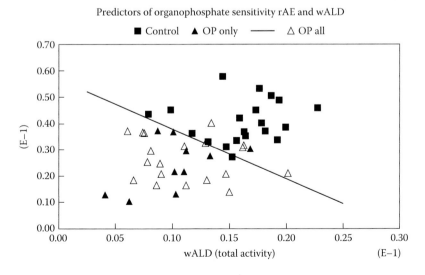

FIGURE 7.68 Predictors of organophosphate sensitivity. (From Alter, S, Organiziak, D, Rea, W. Department of Biochemistry, University of Dayton School of Medicine and the Environmental Health Center: Dallas.)

As you can see in Figures 7.67 and 7.68, the majority of points representing normal individuals are above and to the right of the line on both graphs; while the points from blood enzyme levels of chemically sensitive individuals are below and to the left of the line. In fact, the line was drawn as a result of statistical analysis of the data from the various points. Points on the line would have the same probability of being data collected from chemically sensitive and normal individuals. For distinguishing OP sensitive from normal individuals, the line was calculated based on individuals sensitive to OP only and OP in addition to other chemicals. In the case of formaldehyde sensitivity, the line was calculated using formaldehyde-only sensitive individuals. The statistical analysis indicates the distinctions are significant (p-values <0.05). Another indication of reliability is that we correctly assigned individual as OP sensitive or not chemically sensitive (normal) 82% of the time (Figure 7.68). Similarly, 78% of the time individuals are correctly assigned as chemically sensitive or normal when formaldehyde sensitivity is considered (Figure 7.67).

Acute and chronic exposures of OP pesticides can cause chemical sensitivity and chronic degenerative disease. An example of acute exposures to OP was shown by Yilmazlar and Özyurt in Buria, Turkey. They found that organophosphate poisonings cause substantial morbidity and mortality worldwide. Yilmazlar and Öyurt have studied cerebral perfusion to investigate neurotoxic effects.[665] Clinical effects, plasma cholinesterase activity, and brain single-photon emission computerization tomography (SPECT) data were investigated in 16 patients with organophosphate poisonings. The subjects were from an adult intensive care unit in a university hospital. Cholinesterase activity in plasma was determined upon admission and then every day in the morning. Brain SPECT studies were performed during the first week, at the end of therapy, and 3 months after discharge. Patients were classified into three groups using a modified Namba classification: latent poisoning (Group A), mild and moderate poisoning (Group B), or severe poisoning (Group C). None of the six patients in Group A showed any symptoms; three patients in Group B had muscarinic and nicotinic effects; five patients in Group C had muscarinic, nicotinic, and CNS symptoms. The average plasma cholinesterase for Groups A, B, and C were 54.16+/−9.10, 42.2+/−12.02, and 13+/−4.84 U/mL, respectively (normal range of plasma cholinesterase is 40–90 U/mL). Only one patient from Group A required treatment with oxime; two patients from Group B, and all patients in Group C were given oxime, atropine sulfate, and mechanical ventilation. In the brain SPECT studies, the patients in Group A showed fewer perfusion defect areas than did Group B and C patients. All cases showed perfusion defects especially in the parietal lobe. In addition, perfusion improvement took more time for Group C than for the other groups. The intensive care unit stays of Group C were statistically longer than for Groups A and B. They concluded that brain SPECT is a highly sensitive diagnostic method, together with clinical symptoms and plasma cholinesterase activity, for monitoring the clinical prognosis of organophosphate poisonings. These results are similar to what we have seen at the EHC-Dallas and EHC-Buffalo. As shown throughout this series of books, acute and chronic exposure of OP pesticides can cause neurologic dysfunction which can often be shown by not only chemical sensitivity but also those of the triple camera SPECT series (Figures 7.69 and 7.70).

OP poisoning continues to represent an important medical issue through its high prevalence among toxic pathologies and through its severity. In diagnosing this toxicological disorder, the most frequently utilized and available laboratory test remains the assessment of plasma cholinesterase— BChE—activity. Despite the reluctance of many researchers on the usefulness of serum BChE for kinetic analysis in OP intoxications they are used, Sorodoc et al.[666] have tested a recently proposed protocol, which is safe, non-expensive, easy to perform, appropriate to distinguish between an aged cholinesterase and a still reactivable one. Their aim was to validate the usefulness of this protocol, studying a series of 23 consecutive patients acutely intoxicated with OP, admitted in a regional emergency hospital, over a 1-year period. Introducing the proposed test in the routine of monitoring OP-intoxicated patients has resulted in the identification of a pattern with a funnel aspect, consequence of the initial possibility to increment the degree of BChE activity. This funnel shape defines the presence of reactivability, while its absence demonstrates the lack of obidoximes effect, due to

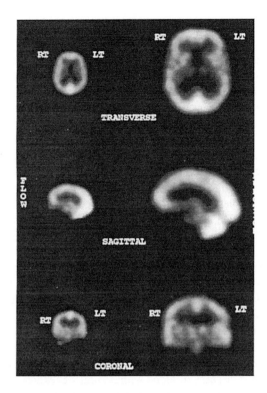

FIGURE 7.69   Normal SPECT scan.

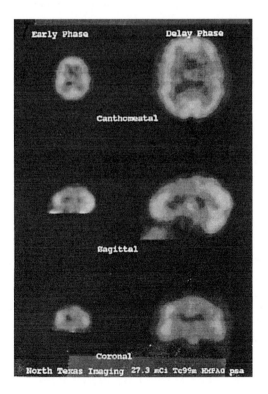

FIGURE 7.70   Abnormal SPECT scan.

cholinesterase's aging process. This method consisted in an advantage for the diagnosis, having the potential of improving prognostic evaluation and therapeutic orientation in OP intoxications.

Once these pesticides are allowed into the cells by either immune tolerance or enzyme loss or suppression, the chemically sensitive and chronic degenerative disease patients will have much intracellular dysfunction, including the mitochondria which allows oxidative stress to occur endoplasmic reticulum which stores calcium and unfolding of proteins and degradation to occur.

Taken together, chronic diseases discussed above are considered as the major disorders affecting public health in the twenty-first century. The relationship between these diseases and environmental exposures, particularly pesticides, increasingly continues to strengthen. Near to all studies carried out in the area of pesticides and chronic diseases are categorized in the field of epidemiologic evidence or experimental investigation with mechanistic insight into the disease process. Clearly, chemical sensitivity is one of these major problems. Some epidemiologic studies have been debated on their uncertainty in elicitation of a definite conclusion because of some restrictions. However, existence of more than a few dozen reports on the association of one case such as brain cancer with exposure to pesticide is enough to create concern even without finding a direct link. Thousands of cases of chemical sensitivity have now been reported and attempts have been taken to treat them. Abundance of evidence in this regard has promoted scientists to evaluate the mechanisms by which pesticides cause the development of chronic diseases. Although there remains a lot to do in this way, several mechanisms and pathways have been clarified for pesticide-induced chronic diseases. It should not be forgotten that these mechanisms work alongside or sequentially rather than singly in most cases, or they even can potentiate genetically susceptible individuals. However, the body of studies in this respect has become massive enough to consider pesticide exposure as a potential risk factor for developing chronic diseases. It along with natural gas exposure are tied for number 1 in induction of ill health. Considering chronic diseases as the most important global health problems, it is time to find a preventive approach in association with agrochemicals by logical reducing pesticide use or pesticide dependency and efficient alternatives for hazardous ones.

Interaction between OP Pesticide Exposure and PON1 Activity on Thyroid Function

Organophosphate pesticides are widely used in agricultural purposes. Recently, studies have demonstrated the ability of these chemicals to alter the function of the thyroid gland in humans. Moreover, the PON1 enzyme plays an important role in the toxicity of some OP pesticides, with low PON1 activity being associated with higher pesticide sensitivity. This study evaluates the interaction between exposure to OP compounds and PON1 enzyme activity on serum levels of TSH and thyroid hormones in a population of workers occupationally exposed to pesticides. A longitudinal study was conducted on a population of floriculture workers from Mexico during two periods of high- and low-intensity levels of pesticide application. A structured questionnaire was completed by workers containing questions on sociodemographic characteristics and other variables of interest. Urine and blood samples were taken, and biomarkers of exposure (dialkyl phosphates), susceptibility (PON1 polymorphisms and activity), and effect (thyroid hormone levels) were determined. Interaction between dialkyl phosphates and PON1 polymorphisms or PON1 activity on hormone levels was evaluated by generalized estimating equation (GEE) models. A significant interaction was found between serum diazoxonase activity and total dialkyl phosphates (Sigma DAP) on TSH levels. Thus, when PON1 activity was increased, they observed a decrease in the percentage of variation of TSH level for each increment in one logarithmic unit of the Sigma DAP levels. This interaction was also observed with the PON1 (192) RR genotype. These results suggest a stronger association between OP pesticides and thyroid function in individuals with lower PON1 enzyme.

BASIC MECHANISMS OF CELL CHANGE BY PESTICIDES

Pesticide injury to the cell wall causes irritation, enlargement of pores, new pores, and inflammation.

INFLAMMATION

One of the most ancient functions of the mitochondria is cellular defense (innate immunity) with apoptosis and stiffened membranes. Metabolic mismatch occurs with an increase in O_2 outside the cell and mitochondria membrane of 30 torr to 0.02 torr inside the membrane. Inflammation develops with the excess pollutants. This mismatch directs electron flow away from the mitochondria in the cell folds and intramitochondria electron flow and mitochondrial oxygen consumptions falls. Capillaries dilate bringing more O_2 to the cell. Cellular oxygen rises and the chemistry of polymer assembly (DNA, RNA), lipid, and protein synthesis is stopped because NADPH/NADP ratio falls. Under those oxidizing conditions, electrons are no longer available for carbon–carbon bond formation to build biomass for the viral or intracellular bacterial replication. Electrons are instead instructed by the rising tide of O_2 to make superoxide, other ROS, and reactive nitrogen species and form bonds between free thirds in amino acids such as cysteine and peptides such as glutathione (G-SSG). An increase in each intracellular O_2 also oxidizes Fe-S clusters and redox-responsive sites activating proteins, and inactivating protein for macromolecular synthesis and activity proteins that inhibit the cell membrane from further attack. These include lipoxgenases and NF-κB oxidase (NADPH), redox-sensitive, radical-sensitive signal systems in innate immunity such as purinergic, receptors, and transconformal regulators such as Keap/Nrf2 and sirtuin-FOXO. The net result of the oxidative shielding in innate immunity is to limit the replication and prevent the exit of the invading pathogen or toxic. Thus, inflammation occurs.

MITOCHONDRIAL DYSFUNCTION

According to Mostafalou and Abdollahi,[667] as dynamic multifunctional organelles, mitochondria are the main source of ATP and ROS in the cell and have important roles in calcium homeostasis, synthesis of steroids and heme, metabolic cell signaling, energy, and apoptosis. Abnormal function of the mitochondrial respiratory chain is the primary cause of imbalanced cellular energy homeostasis and has been widely studied in different types of human diseases, most of all diabetes[668–671] and neurodegenerative disorders.[672]

Perturbation of this organelle has been accepted as one of the crucial mechanisms of neurodegeneration since there is broad literature supporting mitochondrial involvement of proteins such as α-synuclein, Parkin, Dj-1, PINK1, APP, PS1 and 2, and SOD1 that have some known roles in major neurodegenerative disorders, including Parkinson, Alzheimer, and ALS.[673]

Some evidence even proposed the involvement of mitochondrial DNA and its alterations in development of these diseases[674]; Parkinson was almost the first disease in which the role of mitochondrial dysfunction was uncovered when the classical inhibitor of complex I electron transport chain, metabolite of MPTP, was reported to cause Parkinsonism in drug abusers.[675] In 2000, developing the symptoms of Parkinson was also reported for a broad-spectrum pesticide, rotenone, whose mechanism of action is selective inhibition of complex I mitochondrial respiratory chain so that it has been widely used to create a Parkinson model in laboratory animals.[676] In this regard, interfering with mitochondrial respiratory chain functions has made a pattern in development of different types of pesticides, and many agrochemicals are known to inhibit electron transport chain activity as their primary or secondary mechanism of action. Most of the pesticides interfering with mitochondrial respiratory chain activities are mainly inhibitors of complex I electron transport chain and some others partially inhibit complexes II, III, and V.[677]

Moreover, a wide variety of pesticides has been known as uncouplers of mitochondrial oxidative phosphorylation.[678] Nevertheless, impairment of normal oxidative phosphorylation has been reported in exposure to a large number of pesticides particularly neurotoxic agents through inhibition of a biosynthetic pathway essential for mitochondrial function or extramitochondrial generation of ROS.[679] The weakness and fatigue of the chemically sensitive can often be attributed to mitochondrial dysfunction. Often, ATP supplementation will help these patients to gain back energy (see Treatment in Volume 5, Chapter 6).

Likewise, there is enough evidence on the role of mitochondrial dysfunction in pathophysiological features of diabetes, including insulin deficiency and insulin resistance. Pancreatic beta cell failure has been reported to be associated with mitochondrial dysfunction and can be caused by exposure to pesticides.[680,681] On the other hand, exposure to pesticides inhibiting complex I and III mitochondrial respiratory chain can lead to a diminished oxygen consumption and cellular energy supply which in turn can result in reduced insulin signaling cascade. In this way, organochlorines, atrazine, and some dioxin-like pesticides have been shown to decrease mitochondrial capacity in beta oxidation of fatty acids resulting in accumulation of intracellular fat, a situation considered to develop obesity and insulin resistance.[682,683] The result can be seen in our society of those who are obese.

This weakness and fatigue phenomena is seen in the chemically sensitive patient who continuously fights to maintain energy. Other chemically sensitive patients do develop diabetes and insulin resistance while others eventually develop neuropathy, GI upset, and secondary food and mold sensitivity.

Oxidative stress: Oxidative stress is discussed earlier in this volume in Chapter 1. It is the precursor of inflammation and eventual end organ failure. It predisposes chemical sensitivity.

Increased production of ROS and/or decreased capacity of antioxidant defense can disrupt oxidative balance and result in damaging all components of the cell, including lipids, proteins, and DNA. Further, oxidative stress can disrupt various parts of cellular signaling because ROS are considered as one of the main messengers in redox signaling which is imbalanced in the chemically sensitive. However, the role of oxidative stress has been uncovered in induction and development of different kinds of human diseases, including cancer, diabetes, neurodegeneration, atherosclerosis, schizophrenia, chronic fatigue syndrome, chemical sensitivity, and renal and respiratory disorders.[684–688] On the other hand, there is a huge body of literature on induction of oxidative stress by pesticides, and it has been implicated in development of health problems mediated by exposure to pesticides.[689–692] It has been revealed that pesticides can disturb oxidative homeostasis through direct or indirect pathways, including mitochondrial or extramitochondrial production of free radicals, thiol oxidation, and depletion of cellular antioxidant receptors.[693–696] Considering the oxidative stress as a powerful promoter of other cellular pathways involved in disease process and as a unique attendant in inflammatory responses, it has been put in the spotlight of the most mechanistic studies regarding the association of pesticide's exposure with chronic disorders. Oxidative stress has been implicated in the onset and progression of pesticide-induced PD.[697] In this regard, organochlorine pesticides have been reported to cause degeneration of dopaminergic neurons by an oxidative-dependent pathway in the Parkinson model.[698,699] Additionally, disrupting effects of OPs on glucose homeostasis have been reportedly linked to oxidative damages and inflammatory cytokines and thought to be compensatory responses accompanied with reduced insulin signaling in insulin-sensitive organs such as liver, muscle, and adipose tissue.[700,701] As such, further disruption of glucose homeostasis in diabetic models of laboratory animals exposed to OP insecticides has been associated with enhanced lipid peroxidation and decreased activity of antioxidant enzymes.[702] Oxidative stress has also been reported to be involved in nephrotoxicity of some pesticides, including diazinon, acephate, and paraquat.[703–705] Clearly, oxidative stress plays a part in chemical sensitivity because when the chemically sensitive patient is exposed to pesticides, oxidative damage and inflammatory cytokines are liberated.

Oxidative defenses: See Chapter 1 of this volume for more details.

Endoplasmic Reticulum Stress and Unfolded Protein Response

According to Mostafalou and Abdollahi,[667] as the first compartment of secretory pathway, ER is specialized for synthesis, folding, and delivery of proteins in addition to its fundamental role in the storage of calcium. Any disturbance in calcium homeostasis, redox regulation, and energy supply can cause perturbation of ER normal function resulting in the accumulation of unfolded or misfolded proteins in this organelle, a situation which is called ER stress. Unfolded proteins occupy ER-resident chaperones, leading to release of transmembrane ER protein kinases which activate a series of phosphorylation cascades resulting in increased expression of genes, which act as molecular chaperones to reestablish ER folding capacity or promote ER-associated degradation (ERAD) to remove misfolded proteins. This process is called unfolded protein response (UPR) aiming to adjust with the changing environment. Also with the entry and release of Ca^{2+} protein kinase A and C, phosphorylation results in an increase in sensitivity to 1000 times and increased chemical sensitivity occurs.[10] In case if adaptation fails, ER stress results in expression of genes involved in programmed cell death pathways.[706] Certainly in this situation, inflammation occurs. Recent discoveries indicate that prolonged ER stress and UPR play an important role in the development of several human diseases, particularly chronic ones, including chemical sensitivity, insulin resistance, diabetes,[707–709] Parkinson, Alzheimer, ALS,[709–711] tumor formation and progression,[712,713] atherosclerosis, cardiomyopathy, chronic kidney diseases, and renal failure.[714,715] Usually, before these diseases develop, chemical sensitivity appears in a subset of patients warning of the eventual development of the aforementioned. However, many have no warning and just develop degenerative disease.

On the other hand, ER stress and related pathways have been reported to be involved in cytotoxicity by some pesticides. Paraquat, a bipyridyl herbicide, which is suspected to increase the risk of PD following chronic exposures, has been reported to induce ER stress and trigger dopaminergic cell death by enhanced cleavage of a small ER cochaperone protein, p23, and inhibition of ERAD.[716] Elevated level of ER stress biomarkers such as glucose-regulated protein 78 (GRP78), ER degradation-enhancing-α-mannosidase-like protein (EDEM), and C/EBP homologous protein (CHOP) has also been implicated in paraquat-induced toxicity in human neuroblastoma cells. Further, paraquat activated calpain and caspase 3 along with ER-induced cascade inositol-requiring protein 1 (IRE1)/apoptosis signal-regulating kinase 1 (ASK1)/c-jun N-terminal kinase (JNK).[717] In another study carried out on neuroblastoma cells, rotenone-induced ER stress has become evident by increased phosphorylation of protein kinase RNA-like endoplasmic reticulum kinase (PERK), protein kinase RNA-activated (PKR), and eukaryotic initiation factor 2-a (elF2a) as well as the expression of GRP78. Moreover, rotenone activates glycogen synthase kinase 3β (GSK3β), an ER-related multifunctional serine/threonine kinase implicated in the pathogenesis of neurodegeneration.[718] Deltamethrin, a pyrethroid pesticide, has been reported to induce apoptosis through ER stress pathway involving elF2α, calpain and caspase 12.[719] Induction of apoptosis by pyrrolidine dithiocarbamate (PDTC)/Cu complex, a widely used pesticide, has also been linked to the ER stress-associated signaling molecules, including GRP78, GRP94, caspase-12, activating transcription factor 4 (ATF4), and CHOP in lung epithelial cells.[720] Chloropicrin, an aliphatic nitrate pesticide, has been indicated to increase ER stress-related proteins including GRP78, IRE1α, and CHOP/GADD 153 in human retinal pigment epithelial cells.[721] Some other pesticides belonging to the organochlorines (endosulfan), carbamates (formetanate, methomyl, pirimicarb), and pyrethroids (bifenthrin) have been evaluated for their effects on stress proteins among which upregulation of the ER chaperone GRP78 and downregulation of the cytosolic chaperone HSP72/73 were significant. These effects can occur when ER is under stress and the UPR result in increased expression of ER chaperones and decreased protein synthesis in the cytosol.[722,723] The chemically sensitive patient can have problems with the endoplasmic reticulum but we do not know about the protein folding part. Certainly, the chemicals give ER stress and most likely problems with the folding problems. It is clear that the chemically sensitive and electrically sensitive patients have less and less adaptation as they progress in their disease which appears to be due to the proper folding phenomena.

Protein Aggregation

Degradation of misfolded, damaged, or unneeded proteins is a fundamental biological process which has a crucial role in the maintenance and regulation of cellular function including adaptation. There are two major cellular mechanisms for protein degradation; UPS that mainly targets short-lived proteins by proteases and autophagy that mostly clears long-lived and poorly soluble proteins through the lysosomal machinery.[724] These are used in the chemically sensitive and chronic degenerative disease patient by fasting for hours to days.

UPS is composed of ubiquitin for tagging and proteasomes for proteolysis of proteins which are to be degraded. Deregulation of this system has been implicated in the pathogenesis of several chronic diseases; most neurodegeneration and cancers evidenced by decreased and increased proteasome activity, respectively.[725] Environmental exposure to certain pesticides has been linked to proteasomal dysfunction in the development of neurodegenerative diseases. The organochlorine pesticide dieldrin has been reported to decrease proteasome activity along with enhanced sensitivity to occurrence of apoptosis in dopaminergic neuronal cells.[726] Dieldrin in the blood has been seen in chemically sensitive and when gone, the chemical sensitivity improves. Proteasome inhibition has also been shown in neuroblastoma cells exposed to rotenone, ziram, diethyldithiocarbamate, endosulfan, benomyl, and dieldrin.[727,728] Paraquat has also been noted to impair UPS given by decreased proteasome activity and increased ubiquitinated proteins in DJ-1 deficient mice and dopaminergic neurons.[729,730] Increased degradation of proteasome components has been presented as the mechanism of proteasome inhibition by rotenone, an inducer of Parkinson.[731] The lysomal degradation pathway of autophagy is known as a self-digestion process by which cells not only get rid of misfolded proteins, damaged organelles, and infectious microorganisms but also provide nutrients during fasting. Defect of this process has found an emerging role in many human diseases such as cancer, neurodegeneration, diabetes, aging, chemical sensitivity, and disorders of the liver, muscle, and heart.[732,733,1218] There are a few reports on the involvement of defective autophagy in toxic effects of pesticides. A relationship between autophagy and paraquat-induced apoptosis in neuroblastoma cells was shown by Gonzalez-Polo and colleagues in 2007.[734] This effect was confirmed in another study in which paraquat-induced autophagy was attributed to the occurrence of ER stress.[735] Lindane, a broad-spectrum organochlorine pesticide, has been reported to promote its toxicity through disruption of an autophagic process in primary rat hepatocytes[736] (Figure 7.9).

We have treated chemically sensitive patients who were exposed and made toxic by lindane. They had classic chemical sensitivity and were cleared with the removal of lindane and other chemicals and repaired by good extra nutrition. Fasting helped them markedly.

The lysosomal pathway manipulation has been extremely important in the treatment of many cases of chemical sensitivity. Often, fasting in a pollutant-free environment can clear the chemically sensitive patient out of debris and damaged tissue. This is performed by skipping a meal to 7 days of total food avoidance. The patient then rights the physiology and can return to equilibrium (see Volume 5, Chapter 6 on Treatment for more details). The UPS of degradation with the lysomonal degradation pathway of autophagy is probably at work with pesticide exposure in the chemically sensitive patient.

MECHANISMS OF ENVIRONMENT PESTICIDE EXPOSURE

Since protein aggregation is a major component of the adaptation phenomenon, it is often a determent to tissue repair when damaged by pesticides and other toxics (Figures 7.71 and 7.72). Here, the chemically sensitive patient and particularly the unaware patient with chronic degenerative disease gets used to the pesticide and the other toxic substances exposure. They continue to take in the toxics because of the adaptation (masking) phenomena; therefore, their toxic load gets so high that they develop chemical sensitivity and/or chronic degenerative disease at times until they are totally incapacitative and/or die.

CLINICAL EFFECTS OF PESTICIDES: NEUROLOGICAL

The neurological effects of OP pesticides, commonly used on foods and in households, are an important public health concern. Furthermore, subclinical exposure to combinations of OPs is implicated in Gulf War illness. Here, they characterized the effects of the broad used insecticide chlorpyrifos on dopamine and glutamatergic neurotransmission effectors in corticostriatal motor/reward circuitry as previously shown in this chapter. Chlorpyrifos potentiated PKA-dependent phosphorylation of the striatal protein DARPP-32 and the GLuR1 subunit of AMPA receptors in mouse brain

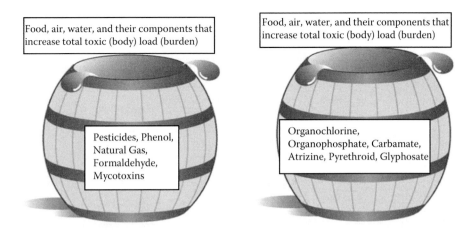

FIGURE 7.71   Mechanisms of environment pesticide exposure.

slices. It also increased GLuR 1 phosphorylation by PKA when administered systemically. This correlated with enhanced glutamate release from cortical projections in rat striatum. Similar effects were induced by the sarin congener, diisopropyl fluorophosphates, alone or in combination with the putative neuroprotectant, PB, and the pesticide DDT. This combination, meant to mimic the neurotoxicant exposure encountered by veterans of the 1991 Persian Gulf War, also induced hyper-phosphorylation of the neurofibrillary tangle-associated protein tau. Diisopropyl fluorophosphates and pyridostigmine bromide, alone or in combination, also increased the aberrant activity of the protein kinase, Cdk5, as indicated by conversion of its activating cofactor p35–p25. Thus, consistent with recent finding in humans and animals, OP exposure causes deregulation in the motor/reward circuitry and invokes chemical sensitivity and even cancer.

CANCER

The first reports on the association of pesticides with cancer were presented around 50 years ago regarding the higher prevalence of lung and skin cancer in the farmers using insecticides in grape fields.[737–739] During the past half century, a wide spectrum of population-based studies has been carried out in this respect leading to significant progress in understanding the relationship of pesticides to the incidence of different types of malignancies.[740,741]

Different types of neoplasm have been reported such as breast cancer, testicular cancer, pancreatic cancer, esophageal cancer, stomach cancer, skin cancer, and non-Hodgkin lymphoma.[742–744] Van Maele-Fabry et al.[745–747] pointed out exposure to pesticides as a possible risk factor for prostate cancer and leukemia by a meta-analysis of risk estimates in pesticide manufacturing workers. In a series of agricultural health studies, Lee et al.[748–750] found an association between exposure to pesticides and cancer incidence, particularly lymphohematopoietic cancers for alachlor, lung cancer for chlorpyrifos, and colorectal cancer for aldicarb. Nowadays, chronic low-dose exposure to pesticides is considered as one of the important risk factors for cancer expansion. According to a new list of Chemicals Evaluated for Carcinogenic Potential by EPA's Pesticide Program published in 2010, more than 70 pesticides have been classified as a probable or possible carcinogen.

However, carcinogenic mechanisms of pesticides can be explored in their potential to affect genetic material directly via induction of structural or functional damage to chromosomes, DNA, and histone proteins, or indirectly disrupting the profile of gene expression through impairment of cellular organelles such as mitochondria and endoplasmic reticulum, nuclear receptors, endocrine network, and the other factors involved in maintenance of cell homeostasis.[751,752] Table 7.62 is indicating data extracted from epidemiological studies implicating on the relation between exposure to specific pesticides and increased risk of some kind of cancers.

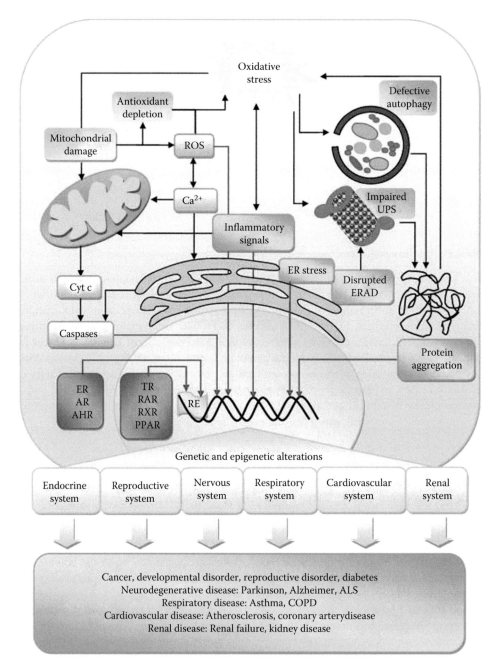

FIGURE 7.72 Simplified model for mechanisms by which pesticides induce and develop chronic disease, ROS: reactive oxygen species, Cyt c: cytochrome c, UPS: ubiquitin proteasome system, ER stress: endoplasmic reticulum stress, ERAD: endoplasmic reticulum associated degradation, ER: estrogen receptor, AR: androgen receptor, AHR: aryl hydrocarbon receptor, TR: thyroid receptor, RAR: retinoic acid receptor, RXR: retinoid X receptor, PPAR: peroxisome proliferator-activated receptor, RE: response element, ALS: amyotrophic lateral sclerosis, COPD: chronic obstructive pulmonary disease. (Modified from Mostafalou, S., Abdollahi, M. 2013. Pesticides and human chronic diseases: Evidences, mechanisms, and perspectives, *Toxicol. Appl. Pharmacol.* 268(2):157–77.)

TABLE 7.62

Pesticides Associated with Elevated Incidence of Cancer in Epidemiological Studies

Type of Cancer	Pesticide	Reference
Leukemia	Chlordane/heptachlor	Purdue et al.[753]
	Chlorpyrifos	Lee et al.[749]
	Diazinon	Beane Freeman et al.[754]
	EPTC	van Bemmel et al.[755]
	Fonofos	Mahajan et al.[756]
Non-Hodgkin's	Lindane	Purdue et al.[753]
Lymphoma	Oxychlordane/chlordane	Spinelli et al.[757]
Multiple myeloma	Permethrin	Rusiecki et al.[724]
Brain cancer	Chlorpyrifos	Lee et al.[749]
Prostate cancer	Fonofos	Mahajan et al.[756]
	Methyl bromide	Alavanja et al.[758]
	Butylate	Lynch et al.[759]
	Chlordecone	Multigner et al.[760]
	DDT, indane, simazine	Band et al.[761]
Colon cancer	Aldicarb	Lee et al.[750]
	Dicamba	Samanic et al.[762]
	EPTC	van Bemmel et al.[721]
	Imazethapyr	Koutros et al.[763]
	Trifluralin	Kang et al.[764]
Rectum cancer	Chlordane	Purdue et al.[753]
	Chlorpyrifos	Lee et al.[749]
		Lee et al.[750]
	Pendimethalin	Hou et al.[765]
Pancreatic cancer	EPTC pendimethalin	Andreotti et al.[766]
	DDT	Garabrant et al.[767]
Lung cancer	Chlorpyrifos	Lee et al.[714]
	Diazinon	Beane Freeman et al.[754]
	Dicamba	Alvanja et al.[768]
	Dieldrin	Purdue et al.[753]
	Metolachlor	Alvanja et al.[768]
	Pendimethalin	Hou et al.[765]
Bladder cancer	Imazethapyr	Koutros et al.[763]
Melanoma	Carbaryl	Mahajan et al.[756]
	Toxaphene	Purdue et al.[753]
	Carbaryl, parathion, maneb/mancozeb	Dennis et al.[769]

Source: Reprinted from *Toxicology and Applied Pharmacology*, 268(2), S. Mostafalou, M. Abdollah, Pesticides and human chronic diseases: Evidences, mechanisms, and perspectives, 157–177, Copyright 2013, with permission from Elsevier.

According to Mostafalou and Abdohi,[667] pesticides are associated with elevated incidence of cancer in epidemiological studies.

Cancer and Other Chronic Effects

According to Pimentel et al.,[770] ample evidence exists concerning the carcinogenic threat related to the use of pesticides. For example, some pesticides have been found to cause testicular dysfunction or sterility.[771]

The U.S. data indicate that 18% of all insecticides and 90% of all fungicides are carcinogenic.[772] Several studies have shown that the risks of certain types of cancers are higher in some people, such as farm workers and pesticide applicators, who are often exposed to pesticides.[771] Certain pesticides have been shown to induce tumors in laboratory animals and there is some evidence that suggest similar effects occur in humans.[771]

Cases of acquired aplastic anemia (AAA) in patients with a long history of pesticide exposure from agricultural fields have been investigated by Law et al. using an immunological approach.[773] These patients showed moderate to severe degrees of BM aplasia as a result of 9–12 years protracted exposure to pesticides which were mainly composed of organophosphorous and organochloride compounds.

Surprisingly, administration of cytokines in the first set and CBPF in the second set triggered CD34 + cell generation as revealed through flow cytometric analysis (FACS). The effect was more pronounced in the second set. Investigations carried out with non-pesticide aplastic anemia (NPAA) showed relatively insignificant effects with both cytokine and CBPF setup. The investigations indicated that AAA as induced by pesticides could be therapeutically manipulated by exogenous cytokines and growth factors and, more efficiently, by CBPF by way of immunopotentiation through microenvironmental supplementation.

Aplastic anemia, a disease characterized by moderate to severe degrees of BM aplasia, may account for the probable cellular component damage leading to immunological deficiency in the BM.[774–776] The acquired toxicity through pesticides causes damage to the BM-derived cellular organ system wherein the cell renewal system achieves aplastic condition.[777] The SAA patient is at immediate risk for catastrophe if left untreated.[778–780] This possibly maintains a difference with the inherited aplastic anemia, which has been described to be a BM deficient condition caused by stem cell defects that may have a genetic component.[781] Thus, the possible measures of recovery from stem cell defects still await meticulous efforts to formulate a therapeutic protocol.[782] Although it is true that the current therapy constituting immunosuppressive agents together with BM transplantation provides moderate survival benefits, this also involves several contraindications.[778,783–785] AAA, in many cases, is thought to occur accidentally by radiation insults, prolonged antibiotic use, chloramphenicol, and exposure to other toxic chemicals, which may well account for both direct/indirect BM damage followed by immunodeficiency.

This may involve the stem/stromal cell interrelationship and the microenvironment, including various cytokines and growth factors.[786–788]

Investigations on a number of patient suffering from hypoplastic/aplastic anemia in the outpatient department revealed that the disease accumulation was statistically high in the field workers engaged in agricultural work that have continuous exposure to different pesticides of organophosphorus/organochloride origin. Previous reports on this score were also found to bear supportive evidences.[789–791] Law et al.[773] attempted to investigate into the damages caused by the toxic pesticides within the BM organization causing aplastic anemia and also to look at the plausible therapeutic approaches for the disease distribution of the pesticide victims. These also involved two control groups, a healthy control (N) and a NPAA group for the purpose of comparison. The objectives of the present investigation were to (1) characterize the growth patterns of the BM-derived cells of the pesticide victims and the non-pesticide aplastic groups together with elucidation of their immune profiles, (2) evaluate the role of exogenous biomodulators, including stem cell factor (SCF), interleukin-3 (IL-3), and granulocyte-colony stimulation factor (G-CSF) on *ex vivo* culture systems of deficient marrow (set 1), (3) elucidate the role of CBPF (set 2) on the BM culture of the subjects from an immunological perspective, and (4) reveal the quantum of CD34 + cell generation in the *ex vivo* BM culture of the subjects modulated with cytokines (set 1) and CBPF (set 2).

Patients identified with aplastic anemia are classified as (1) those caused by stem cell disorders and (2) those due to accidental exposure to external agents, called AAA.[790,792] Both conditions present with severe to moderate degrees of immunological deficiency, principally due to qualitative and quantitative deterioration of BM cells. The present investigation found a significant amount of AAA among field workers who were chronically exposed to pesticides of different categories. The clinical features, hematological parameters, and the cellular pathophysiology were all in agreement with pesticide-mediated toxicity, mainly the OP and organochlorides, causing BM suppression with consequent alteration in hematological picture as well as immunological suppression. The profound degree of cytopenia and a severe suppression of hemoglobin levels were the typical findings in all cases including that of the present investigations.[777,789]

They suppose that the toxicity might have effects at the stem cell level resulting in inhibition of the stem cell renewal system, leaving a deserted BM.[773]

Thus, the reason behind induction of aplastic anemia with subsequent cytopenia has been suggested to be due to stem cell defects caused by the environmental contact.[790] Simultaneously, immunological parameters showed cellular deficiency under the event. The results therefore simulate the typical pathophysiological conditions in AAA involving the stem cell status, degree of immune suppression, depressed cellularity, and indication of impaired hematopoiesis.[792–795] The above parameters were compared with the NPAA group and the normal control (healthy) subjects. These revealed that the NPAA group also has a similar degree of suppression with respect to hemogram and functional parameters. The immunological functions are also suppressed simultaneously compared with the normal ($p < 0.001$).

As understood, severe BM default can be held responsible for the above which is indicated toward deficient or deceased stem cell renewal/regeneration system.[792,796,797]

This observation gained further support from the data of cytokine and CBPF-supplemented BM cells of AAA patients that showed an improved cellular generation system in *in vitro* model. It is presumed that the cells gathered necessary growth factors or the stimulatory cytokines, which were absent in the AAA patients that were pesticide-exposed victims. In case of NPAA, the cytokines and CBPF did not show significant improvement in cellular regeneration that might be due to an irreversible stem cell defect.

Flow cytometric analysis also demonstrated a poor CD34 positive cell generation in AAA patients (0.55%) as well as in non-pesticide (N) patients with an indication of microenvironmental inhibition or defective/deficient stem/stromal interaction leading to a "cold BM."[796,798] Previous studies carried out in their laboratory also revealed that stromal inhibitions has a direct bearing with the stem cell regeneration renewal process.[799] Indeed, it can be correlated with the marrow inhibition of AAA patients caused by pesticide exposure. Histopathological investigation of the BM of such patients also presented a typically suppressed BM feature with an insignificant number of stem/progenitor cells.[797] They also observed decreased growth kinetics under the event when the BM cells refused to grow and die off within a period of 24–96 hours. They presume that such observation may account for a qualitative damage of the pluripotent BM cells after exposure. Upon administration of CBPR, the CD34 + cell population was further increased up to 5.07% ($p < 0.001$). NPAA group, when compared, showed a similar degree of stem cell inhibition/suppression under the event. CBPF could, however, have elevated the stem cell percent but not to the same level as the AAA group. This suggests that stem cell regeneration is induced possibly more in pesticide-mediated AAA group than in the non-pesticide anemia (PAA) group.

Both observations concomitantly proved the stimulatory role of microenvironmental factors on the stem/progenitor cells by removing the blockade.[798] The higher CD34 positivity in supplemented BM culture pointed toward initiation of progenitor differentiation in the usual route. The CBPF constituting the microenvironmental requirement[800] renders a much better effectiveness under the event. It can further be resolved that CBPF contains some additive components responsible for negotiating the appropriate signal toward the differentiation mode with a greater efficacy.

The pluripotent BM cells express appropriate immunological functions under physiological emergency.[801–804] The observations also provided data that biological response modifiers (BRMs) could effectively induce functional efficacy in pluripotent cells. The question of receptivity of such cells with different stimulatory components reasonably correlate with the interaction of the stimulatory components with existing receptors culminating in effective signals from appropriate differentiation.[805]

The NPAA group, on the other hand, possibly lacks the receptors for the stimulatory components. It may further be that the recovery of NPAA group is irreversible, as they may have some existing stem cell defect at the genetic level.

A UFW (2002) study of the cancer registry in California analyzed the incidence of cancer among Latino farm workers and reported that per year. If everyone in the United States had a similar rate of incidence, there would be 83,000 cases of cancer associated with pesticides. The incidence of cancer in the U.S. population due to pesticides ranges from about 10,000 to 15,000 cases per year.[584] Now we think, there are more cases.

Drift depends on many factors, including wind velocity and direction, humidity, and size of the rain droplets. Studies have shown that drifts can range from 12 ft to 14.5 miles,[806] although dust from North Africa blows south to Florida, Alabama, Mississippi, Louisiana, and Texas from mid-May to mid-September carrying many pesticides. From 1% to 80% of a pesticide is estimated to be lost in the dispersal process.[807]

Widespread pesticide contamination of air, food, and water once led to speculation as to whether or not pesticide residues could be detected in humans.[808] Today, pesticide contamination of mother's milk and chemically sensitive people has been confirmed. Organochlorine pesticides have been found in the blood of chemically sensitive populations around the world, including patient populations in the United States, where some of the identified pesticides, such as DDT, have been banned for 25 years.[4]

Levels of pesticides in humans were worse in China, which had been isolated from world commerce for almost 40 years between 1949 and 1984. In England, Arabia, and Australia, high levels of pesticides were also found in humans.

Only one group of people was relatively free of organochlorine and OP pesticides and, incidentally, disease free. These were the killer Indians who lived at the headwaters of the Amazon. They had a dense jungle cover, fresh spring water from the Andes, and a constant supply of highly nutritious, fresh, chemically less contaminated food.[4]

The Japanese experience with these alternative pesticides is not much different from the American or British experience. As quickly as a new one is introduced, disease triggers are also identified. For example, Ishikawa et al.[210] have seen eye problems and neuropathy resulting from overexposure to OP pesticides in Japan. The American experience is similar with DDT and dieldrin, which have been banned and replaced by others such as the OPs and then when problems occurred with OP, carbamates and pyrethroids. At the EHC-Dallas, we have seen over 10,000 patients who were fallen ill from exposure to OP pesticides. Our data strongly support the idea that as a society, we must change our attitude toward known human toxins. We must stop their production and develop alternative methods of pest control.

Infants and children[809] have greater susceptibility to pesticide toxicity and sensitivity than do adults with certain chronic illnesses such as asthma, lupus erythematosus, vasculitis, and dermatitis. Children are particularly susceptible to lawn pesticides.[810-814] Those whose homes and gardens are treated with pesticides have a 6.5 times greater risk of childhood leukemia than do children living in untreated environments.[815]

OTHER CHRONIC DISEASES

However, there are sporadic reports on the association of exposure to pesticides with different types of human chronic diseases, including chronic fatigue syndrome,[816] autoimmune diseases such as systemic lupus erythematosus and rheumatoid arthritis[817-819] which need further investigations for more proof. Our group[585] has shown small vessel vasculitis can be triggered by pesticides.

According to Walsh,[820] women have a risk of developing rheumatoid arthritis and/or lupus which increases incrementally according to the frequency and duration of their exposure to insecticides. This is often preceded by chemical sensitivity. However, with the adaptation (making) phenomenon in alloy, the patients often do not appreciate the trigger agents. Further, they can be covered up by medication.

Women who had not lived on or worked on a farm, pesticide exposure through application by someone else (such as a lawn service) was not associated with a significant risk of autoimmune rheumatic disease but they do get ill with chronic fatigue, weakness, anxiety, and depression; fibromyalgia often occurs. Solvents, natural gas, and other toxics have been shown to trigger these diseases.[821] Women's risk of developing autoimmune rheumatic disease increase incrementally according to the frequency and duration of their exposure to insecticides, a large observational study suggested.

According to Parks, of the National Institute for Environmental Health Science in Durham, North Carolina, and colleagues, the study of almost 77,000 women found that those who personally mixed or applied insecticides has an adjusted hazard ratio for rheumatoid arthritis or systemic lupus erythematosus of 1.57 (95% CI = 1.18–2.11) when compared with women who reported no exposure to the chemicals.

Moreover, the adjusted hazard ratio rose to 1.97 (95% CI = 0.20–3.23, $p = 0.003$) with 20 or more years of exposure and to 2.04 (95% CI = 1.17–3.56, $p = 0.003$) with six or more exposures per year.

So, the researchers analyzed data from 76,648 enrollees in the Women's Health Initiative (WHI) observational study. All of the women were postmenopausal (age 50–79) and free of autoimmune rheumatic disease at baseline.

After 3 years, there were 186 incident cases of rheumatoid arthritis and 35 cases of lupus—for a total of 0.28% in the cohort.[820] The majority of women in the cohort were white, as were those with autoimmune disease.

More women with autoimmune disease than those without the diseases reported personal use of insecticides (45% vs. 38%, $p = 0.010$), and having lived on a farm (34% vs. 26%, $p = 0.025$).

Most of the cases (63%) reported their exposure to insecticides occurred in the home.

The 3-year risk of developing rheumatoid arthritis or lupus was 0.22% among women reporting no personal use of insecticides.

The risk among women whose exposure occurred at home was 0.30% and 0.31% among those reporting workplace exposures.

The 3-year risk of autoimmune disease was 0.50% in women reporting personal use of insecticides six times or more per year.

Living or working on a farm for 20 years or more was associated with a 3-year increased risk of 0.48% and an age-adjusted hazard ratio of 1.97 (95% CI = 1.14–3.42).

Among women who had not lived or worked on a farm, pesticide exposure through application by someone else (such as a lawn service) was not associated with a significant risk of autoimmune disease—with the age-adjusted hazard ratio for six or more applications per year being 0.34, but other chemicals have been shown to trigger them.[821]

But among women who also had a farm history, the age-adjusted hazard ratio for six or more pesticide applications by others was 2.95.

It is possible that pesticides, solvents, and persistent organic pollutants could have similar fundamental effects on susceptible genotypes, possibly through the aryl hydrocarbon receptor or toll-like receptors, predisposing to the development of autoimmunity in similar ways.

Limitations of the study included its observational design and reliance on self-reported data (Table 7.63).

MOLECULAR MECHANISMS LINKING PESTICIDE EXPOSURE TO CHRONIC DISEASES

Genetic Damages

Genetic damages are caused by direct interaction with genetic material resulting in DNA damage or chromosomal aberrations and considered as a primary mechanism for chronic diseases within the context of carcinogenesis and teratogenesis. They are studies in the field of genetic toxicology and can be detected by distinctive kinds of genotoxicity tests. Growing body of data concerning genetic toxicity of pesticides have been collected from epidemiological and experimental studies using

TABLE 7.63

List of Studies Whose Results Implicate on the Association of Exposure to Pesticides with Incidence of Chronic Diseases

Disease	Types	Case–Control	Cohort	Reports Ecological	Others
Cancer	Childhood leukemia	Alderton et al.[822]	Carozza et al.[823]	Turner et al.[824]	
		Alexander et al.[825]			
		Buckley et al.[826]			
		Buckley et al.[827]			
		Infante-Rivard et al.[828]			
		Lafiura et al.[829]			
		Laval and Tuyns[830]			
		Leiss and Savitz[831]			
		Lowengart et al.[815]			
		Ma et al.[832]			
		Magnani et al.[833]			
		Meinert et al.[834]			
		Menegaux et al.[835]			
		Monge et al.[836]			
		Mulder et al.[837]			
		Rau et al.[838]			
		Reynolds et al.[839]			
		Rudant et al.[840]			
		Rull et al.[841]			
		Shu et al.[842]			
		Soldin et al.[843]			
	Adult leukemia	Alavanja et al.[844]	Beane Freeman et al.[754]	Chrisman Jde et al.[845]	Cuneo et al.[846]
		Brown et al.[847]	Beard et al.[848]	Delzell and Grufferman[849]	Merhi et al.[850]
		Ciccone et al.[851]	Blair et al.[408]		Van Maele-Fabry et al.[852]
		Clavel et al.[853]	Bonner et al.[854]	Mills[855]	
		Miligi et al.[856]	Cantor and Silberman[857]		

(Continued)

TABLE 7.63 (Continued)
List of Studies Whose Results Implicate on the Association of Exposure to Pesticides with Incidence of Chronic Diseases

Disease	Types	Case-Control	Cohort	Ecological	Others
			Reports		
Hodgkin's lymphoma		Orsi et al.[858]	Flower et al.[859]	Carozza et al.[823]	
		Persson et al.[860]		Cerhan et al.[861]	
		Rudant et al.[840]			
		van Balen et al.[862]			
	Non-Hodgkin's lymphoma	Alavanja et al.[844]	Bonner et al.[854]	Khuder et al.[863]	
		Buckley et al.[864]	Kristensen et al.[865]	Mehri et al.[850]	
		Cantor[866]	Kross et al.[867]		
		Cantor et al.[868]	Morrison et al.[869]		
		Chiu et al.[870]	Purdue et al.[871]		
		De Roos et al.[872]	Ritter et al.[873]		
		Eriksson et al.[874]	Zhong and Rafnsson[875]		
		Hardell and Eriksson[876]			
		Hardell et al.[877]			
		Hoar et al.[878]			
		McDuffie et al.[879]			
		Meinert et al.[880]			
		Miligi et al.[881]			
		Nordstrom et al.[882]			
		Pearce et al.[883]			
		Rudant et al.[840]			
		Schroeder et al.[884]			
		t Mannetje et al.[885]			
		Vajdic et al.[886]			
		Woods et al.[887]			
		Zahm et al.[888]			
		Zahm et al.[889]			

(Continued)

TABLE 7.63 (*Continued*)
List of Studies Whose Results Implicate on the Association of Exposure to Pesticides with Incidence of Chronic Diseases

Disease	Types	Case–Control	Cohort	Ecological	Others
			Reports		
	Multiple myeloma	Burmeister et al.[890]	Kristensen et al.[865]	Cerhan et al.[891]	Mehri et al.[850]
		Pearce et al.[883]	Landgren et al.[892]		
			Lope et al.[893]		
	Neuroblastoma	Daniels et al.[894]	Feychting et al.[895]	Carozza et al.[823]	
		Walker et al.[896]	Giordano et al.[897]		
			Kristensen et al.[865]		
			Littorin et al.[898]		
Cancer	Soft tissue sarcoma	Kogevinas et al.[899]		Carozza et al.[823]	
		Leiss and Savitz[831]		Chrisman Jde et al.[845]	
		Magnani et al.[900]			
	Childhood brain cancer	Bunin et al.[901]	Kristensen et al.[865]		
		Cordier et al.[902]			
		Davis et al.[903]			
		Efird et al.[904]			
		Gold et al.[905]			
		Holly et al.[906]			
		Pogoda and Preston-Martin[907]			
		Rosso et al.[908]			
		Ruder et al.[909]			
		Searles Nielsen et al.[910]			
		van Wijngaarden et al.[1219]			
		Wilkins and Koutras[1220]			
		Wilkins and Sinks[912]			

(*Continued*)

TABLE 7.63 (Continued)
List of Studies Whose Results Implicate on the Association of Exposure to Pesticides with Incidence of Chronic Diseases

			Reports		
Disease	Types	Case–Control	Cohort	Ecological	Others
	Adult brain cancer	Lee et al.[713]	Blair et al.[911]	Delzell and Grufferman[849]	Smith-Rooker et al.[913]
		Musicco et al.[914]	Figa-Talamanca et al.[915]		
		Provost et al.[916]	Kross et al.[867]	Mills[855]	
		Rodvall et al.[917]	Viel et al.[918]	Wesseling et al.[919]	
		Samanic et al.[920]			
		Zheng et al.[921]			
	Bone cancer	Merletti et al.[922]	Holly et al.[923]	Carozza et al.[823]	
		Moore et al.[924]		Wesseling et al.[919]	
	Prostate cancer	Cerhan et al.[891]	Alavanja et al.[758]	Chrisman Jde et al.[845]	Keller-Byrne et al.[925]
		Dosemeci et al.[926]	Chamie et al.[927]	Delzell and Grufferman[849]	Sharma-Wagner et al.[928]
		Forastiere et al.[929]	Dich and Wiklund[930]		
		Meyer et al.[931]	Fleming et al.[932]	Mills[855]	
		Mills and Yang[933]	Kross et al.[867]		
		Settimi et al.[934]	MacLennan et al.[935]		
			Morrison et al.[936]		
	Breast cancer	Band et al.[937]	Dolapsakis et al.[938]		Ortega Jacome et al.[1221]
		Brophy et al.[939]			
		Duell et al.[940]			
		Mills and Yang[941]			
		Teitelbaum et al.[942]			
	Colorectal cancer	Cerhan et al.[861]	Kang et al.[764]	Wesseling et al.[919]	
		Forastiere et al.[943]	Koutros et al.[763]		
		Lo et al.[944]	Kross et al.[867]		
			Lee et al.[750]		
			Samanic et al.[762]		
			van Bemmel et al.[755]		
			Zhong and Rafnsson[875]		

(Continued)

TABLE 7.63 (*Continued*)

List of Studies Whose Results Implicate on the Association of Exposure to Pesticides with Incidence of Chronic Diseases

Disease	Types	Case–Control	Cohort	Ecological	Others
			Reports		
	Pancreatic cancer	Alguacil et al.[945] Forastierre et al.[943] Ji et al.[946] Kauppinen et al.[947] Lo et al.[948] Partanen et al.[949]	Andreotti et al.[766] Cantor and Silberman[857]		Chrisman Jde et al.[845]
	Kidney cancer	Buzio et al.[950] Fear et al.[951] Forastiere et al. Hu et al.[952] Karami et al.[953] Mellemgaard et al.[954] Olshan et al.[955] Sharpe et al. Tsai et al.[956]	Kristensen et al.[865]	Carozza et al.[823]	
	Lung cancer	Brownson et al.[957] Bumroongkit et al.[958] Pesatori et al.[959]	Alavanja et al.[768] Barthel[407] Beane Freeman et al.[754] Blair et al.[408] Lee et al.[749] Rusiecki et al.[960] Samanic et al.[762]	Wesseling et al.[919]	
	Stomach cancer	Forastiere et al.[943] Mills and Yang[962]			Van Leeuwen et al.[961]
	Esophageal cancer	Jansson et al.[963]			Chrisman Jde et al.[845] Wesseling et al.[919]

(Continued)

TABLE 7.63 (Continued)
List of Studies Whose Results Implicate on the Association of Exposure to Pesticides with Incidence of Chronic Diseases

Disease	Types	Reports			
		Case–Control	Cohort	Ecological	Others
	Liver cancer		Giordano et al.[897]		Carozza et al.[823] Wesseling et al. Mills[855]
	Testicular cancer	Mills et al.[964]	Fleming et al.[932]		Wesseling et al.[919]
	Bladder cancer	Forastiere et al.[943]	Koutros et al.[763]		Wesseling et al.[919]
	Gall bladder cancer		Giordano et al.[897]		Carozza et al.[823]
	Thyroid cancer		Ward et al.[965]		Carozza et al.[823]
	Melanoma	Fortes et al.[966]	Dennis et al.[769] Mahajan et al.[967]		Wesseling et al.[919]
	Eye cancer	Carozza et al.[823]	Kristensen et al.[865]		
	Lip cancer		Wiklund[968]	Cerhan et al.[861] Chrisman Jde et al.[845]	
	Mouth cancer		Tarvainen et al.[969]		
	Larynx cancer			Wesseling et al.[919]	
	Sinonasal cancer				Tisch et al.[970]
	Ovarian cancer	Donna et al.[971]		Wesseling et al.[919]	
	Uterine cancer			Wesseling et al.[919]	
	Cervical cancer		Fleming et al.[932]		
Birth defects		Brender et al.[972] Brucker-Davis et al.[975] Dugas et al.[978] Nassar et al.[982] Ren et al.[1222]	Chevrier et al.[178] Perera et al.[976] Petit et al.[979]	de Siqueira et al.[973] Garry et al.[977] Schreinemachers[980] Windchester et al.[983]	Banachour and Seralini[974] Enoch et al.[981] Greenlee et al.[984] Qiao et al.[985] Rauch et al.[986] Richard et al.[987] Rocheleau et al.[988] Sherman[1224]

(Continued)

TABLE 7.63 (Continued)

List of Studies Whose Results Implicate on the Association of Exposure to Pesticides with Incidence of Chronic Diseases

Disease	Types	Case–Control	Cohort	Reports Ecological	Others
Reproductive disorders		Greenlee et al.[146]	Saiyed et al.[33]	Swan et al.[989]	Anway et al.[990]
		Swan et al.[991]	Snijder et al.[992]		Cavieres et al.[993]
		Tiido et al.[994]			Fei et al.[995]
		Tiido et al.[996]			Gray et al.[997]
					Joshi et al.[998]
					Meeker et al.[999]
					Oliva et al.[1000]
					Orton et al.[1001]
					Stanko et al.[1002]
					Wang et al.[1003]
Neuro degenerative diseases	Parkinson	Baldi et al.[1004]	Ascherio et al.[1005]	Barbeau et al.[1006]	Barlow et al.[1007]
		Butterfield et al.[1008]	Baldi et al.[1009]	Ritz and Yu[1010]	Barlow et al.[1011]
		Chan et al.[1012]	Kamel et al.[367]	Schulte et al.[1013]	Caudle et al.[1014]
		Costello et al.[1015]	Petrovitch et al.		Chou et al.[727]
		Dick et al.[1016]	Tuchsen and Jensen		Jia and Misra[1017]
		Dutheil et al.[141]			Priyadarshi et al.[1018]
		Elbaz et al.[1019]			Priyadarshi et al.[1020]
		Fall et al.[1021]			Purisai et al.[1022]
		Firestone et al.[1023]			Richardson et al.[1024]
		Fong et al.[1025]			
		Figerio et al.[1026]			
		Gatto et al.[1027]			
		Gorell et al.[1028]			
		Hancock et al.[1029]			
		Hertzman et al.[1030]			
		Hubble et al.[1031]			
		Hubble et al.[1031]			

(Continued)

TABLE 7.63 (Continued)
List of Studies Whose Results Implicate on the Association of Exposure to Pesticides with Incidence of Chronic Diseases

Disease	Types	Reports			
		Case–Control	Cohort	Ecological	Others
	Alzheimer	Koller et al.[1032]	Baldi et al.[1009]	Parron et al.[1042]	
		Mantghripragada et al.[1033]	Hayden et al.[661]		
		Menegon et al.[1034]	Tyas et al.[1043]		
		Ritz et al.[1035]			
		Seidler et al.[1036]			
		Semchuk et al.[1037]			
		Stephenson[1223]			
		Tanner et al.[1038]			
		Tanner et al.[1039]			
		Wang et al.[1040]			
		Zorzon et al.[1041]			
	ALS	Bonvicini et al.[1044]	Burns et al.[1045]		Choy and Kim[1046]
		Das et al.[1047]			Doi et al.[1048]
		McGuire et al.[1049]			Kanavouras et al.[1050]
		Morahan and Pamphlett[1051]			
		Pamphlett[1052]			
		Qureshi et al.[1053]			
Cardiovascular diseases	Hypertension		Morton et al.[1054]		Antov and Aianova[1055]
	Atherosclerosis				Zamzila et al.[1056]
	Coronary artery disease				

(Continued)

TABLE 7.63 (Continued)

List of Studies Whose Results Implicate on the Association of Exposure to Pesticides with Incidence of Chronic Diseases

Disease	Types	Reports			
		Case-Control	Cohort	Ecological	Others
Respiratory diseases	Asthma	Salam et al.[1057]	Beard et al.[848] Hoppin et al.[1059] Hoppin et al.[1061] Slager et al.[1063]		Draper et al.[1058] Kolmodin-Hedman et al.[1060] Lessenger[1062] Moretto[1064] Salameh et al.[1065] Vandenplas et al.[1066] Wagner[1067] Weiner and Worth[1068]
	COPD	Arifkhanova et al.[1069] Ubaidullaeva[1072]	Chakraborty et al.[1070] Hoppin et al.[1073] LeVan et al.[1075] Valcin et al.[1076]		Barczyk et al.[1071] Faria et al.[1074]
Diabetes	Type 1, 2 and gestational	Lee et al.[1077]	Montgomery et al.[1078] Saldana et al.[1081]	Kouznetsova et al.[1079]	Everett and Matheson[1080] Patel et al.[1082]
Chronic renal diseases	Chronic renal failure				Peiris-John et al.[1083] Wanigasuriya et al.[1084]
	Chronic kidney disease				Siddarth et al.[1085]
Autoimmune diseases	Rheumatoid arthritis		Parks et al.[819]		Gold et al.[818]
	Systemic lupus erythematosus	Cooper et al.[1086]	Parks et al.[819]		Gold et al.[818]

Source: Reprinted from *Toxicology and Applied Pharmacology*, 268(2), S. Mostafalou, M. Abdollah, Pesticides and human chronic diseases: Evidences, mechanisms, and perspectives, 157–177, Copyright 2013, with permission from Elsevier.

different types of examinations, including chromosomal aberrations, micronucleus, sister chromatid exchanges (SCEs), and comet assay.[1087,1088]

Indeed, genetic damages are classified into three groups as follows: (1) premutagenic damages like DNA strand breaks, DNA adducts, or unscheduled DNA synthesis; (2) gene's mutation which means insertion or deletion of a couple of base pairs; (3) chromosomal aberrations, including loss or gain of whole chromosome (aneuploidy), deletion or breaks (clastogenicity), and chromosomal segments or rearrangements. Premutagenic damages may be repaired prior to cell division while the damages in the second and third groups are permanent and have the ability of transmission to daughter cells after cell division[1089] (Figure 7.73).

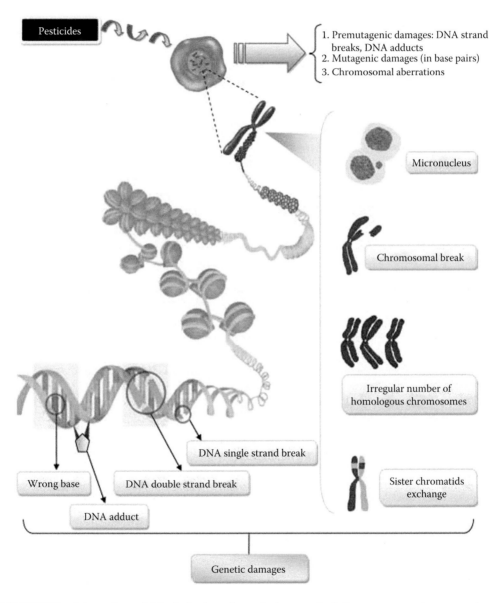

FIGURE 7.73 Schematic model for induction of genetic damages including premutagenic, mutagenic, and chromosomal effects by exposure to pesticides. (From Mostafalou, S., Abdollahi, M. 2013. Pesticides and human chronic diseases: Evidences, mechanisms, and perspectives, *Toxicol. Appl. Pharmacol.* 268(2):157–77.)

Between chromosomal assessments, micronucleus has been recognized as the most reliable and successful test as verified by the Organization for Economic Co-operation and Development (OECD). A micronucleus is referred to the third nucleus formed during the metaphase/anaphase transition of mitosis. The group of these cytoplasmic bodies is called micronuclei having a portion of acentric chromosome or whole chromosome, which does not integrate in the opposite poles during the anaphase. This results in the formation of daughter cells without a part or all of a chromosome. Regarding sensitivity, reliability, and cost-effectiveness of this test, it has been proposed as a biomarker for genotoxicity calculations, and has been used in different studies on pesticide-exposed populations. Most of these surveys implied on the increased level of micronucleus formation in people dealing with pesticides for a long time.[1090–1092]

SCE or exchange of genetic material between sister chromatids is another testing for chemicals suspected to be mutagenic. Elevated level of SCE has been observed in some diseases, including Bloom syndrome and Behcet's syndrome and may be tumor formation. There are some reports on increased frequency of SCE in pesticide applicators who worked in agricultural fields.[1092–1094]

Single-cell gel electrophoresis (SCGE) or comet assay is a simple and sensitive testing for the evaluation of DNA strand breaks in eukaryotic cells.[1095] This technique has been frequently used for biomonitoring genotoxic effect of pesticides in a large number of studies most of which implicate on induction of DNA damage by these chemicals.[1096–1099]

Although genotoxicity assays are among necessary tests applying for pesticides prior to introducing to the market, collected data from postmarket monitoring studies have been evident for potential of allowed pesticides in induction of genetic damages. Considering genetic damages as one of the main events for cancer induction or development, further studies focusing on genotoxicity of pesticides, of course in appropriate models such as exposure to their mixtures along with some other promoting factors, are required to understand the carcinogenic and tumorigenic mechanisms of pesticides (Table 7.64).

METABOLIC CHANGES: EPIGENETIC

Epigenetic is referred to the heritable changes in gene expression or cellular phenotype without any alterations in the DNA sequence, and its mechanisms include DNA methylation, histone modifications, and expression of noncoding RNAs. A growing body of evidence has been implicated on the role of environmental exposures, particularly in early development, in the induction of epigenetic changes that may be transmitted in subsequent generations or may serve as a basis of diseases developed later in life. Furthermore, it has become so likely that epigenetics contribute to the causes or transmission of chronic disorders from one generation to another[1115] (Figure 7.74).

Several evidences collected from animal studies during the past decade suggested that exposure to pesticides can induce epigenetic changes. Heritable alterations of DNA methylation in male germline along with testis and ovarian dysfunction have been reported after exposure to some pesticides such as vinclozolin and methoxychlor.[990,1116–1118] Exposure to dichloroacetic acid and trichloroacetic acid has been associated with decreased methylation in promoter regions of c-jun and c-myc in liver of mice.[1119,1120] Global DNA hypomethylation has also been reported in people who had an elevated blood level of pesticides and persistent organic pollutants in two surveys.[1121,1122] Furthermore, increased acetylation of core histones H3 and H4 has been reported by dieldrin, an organochlorine pesticide, in mouse models.[1123]

On the other hand, growing progress has been made in the recognition of epigenetic modifications in human chronic diseases, particularly cancer. Cancer is now considered as an epigenetic disease, the same as a genetic disease. There is tremendous evidence on the contribution of epigenetic events in the initiation, promotion, and progression of different types of cancers, mainly through silencing of tumor suppressor genes and/or activation of proto-oncogenes. These modifications have allocated such a fundamental role in cancer development that epigenetic therapy of cancer is rapidly growing in medical sciences.[1124] In addition, epigenetic changes currently have been a powerful tool

TABLE 7.64

Genotoxicity Biomarkers Determined in Populations Occupationally Exposed to Different Types of Pesticides

Genetic Damage	Pesticides	Reference
DNA strand breaks	Acephate, chlorpyrifos, dimethoate, monocrotophos, phorate, cypermethrin, fenvalerate, carbendazim	Grover et al.[1096]
	Dimethoate, ethephon, omethoate, oxydemeton-methyl, thiometon, bifenthrin, beta-cyfluthrin, deltamethrin, mancozeb, carbendazim, endosulfan, chlorothalonil, iprodione, diflufenicanil, L-cyhalothrin, pyrimethanil, fluroxypyr, cyproconazole, epoxyconazole, flutriafol, tebuconazole, atrazine	Lebailly et al.[1100]
DNA adducts	Glyphosate, methamidophos, monocrotophos, parathion methyl, methomyl, metam sodium, dazomet, zineb, benomyl, carbendazim, paraquat, captan, folpet, endosulfan	Peluso et al.[1101]
Chromosomal aberration	Acephate, chlorpyrifos, dimethoate, fenitrothion, fenthion, fosetyl, isofenphos, methamidophos, naled, pyrazophos, cypermethrin, deltamethrin, fenpropathrin, fenvalerate, methiocarb, methomyl, oxamyl, mancozeb, propineb, zineb, benomyl, diquat, paraquat, captan, folpet, procymidone, endosulfan, abamectin, kasugamycin, iprodione, oxadixyl, buripimate, metribuzin, linuron, methabenzthiazuron, triforine, vinclozolin, bitertanol, fenbutatin oxide, amitraz, propargite, dithiocarbamate	Carbonell et al.[1102]
	Diazinon, dichlorvos, dimethoate, malathion, ethylazinophos, monocrotophos, parathion, parathion methyl, phorate, prothoate, terbufos, trichlorofon, cypermethrin, fenpropathrin, permethrin, maneb, thiram, dazomet, mancozeb, zineb, ziram, thiabendazole, paraquat, captan, folpet, endosulfan, dodemorph, chlorothalonil, iprodione, acetic metaldehyde, barium polysulfide, copper oxychloride, copper sulfate, sulfur, white oil, dinocap, DNOC, alachlor, simazine, MCPA, linuron, vinclozolin, phenmedifam, methalaxyl, ethofumesate, 2,4-D, dicofol	De Ferrari et al.[1103]
	Dimethoate, mevinphos, monocrotofos, parathion, parathion methyl, aldicarb, maneb, dazomet, propineb, zineb, captan, endosulfan, aldrin, aramite, chlordimeform, heptachlor, tetradifon	Dulout et al.[1104]
	2,4-D	Garry et al.[1105]
	Chlorpyrifos, cypermethrin, deltamethrin, fenpropathrin, methomyl, thiram, pirimicarb, benomyl, carbendazim, endosulfan, chlorothalonil, iprodione, buprofezin, atrazine, triforine, vinclozolin, cyhexatin, fetin acetate, carboxin, 2,4-D, chloridazon, defenamide, oxadiazon, propargyl	Lander et al.[1106]
Micronucleus formation	Metham sodium, dodemorph, zineb, antracol, captan, dazomet, dichloropropane, dichloropropene	Bolognesi et al.[1107]
	Diazinon, dichlorvos, fosetyl-aluminum, malathion, ethamidophos, parathion methyl, cypermethrin, carbaryl, methomyl, mancozeb, pirimicarb, benomyl, captan, endosulfan, lindane, diuron, 2,4-D, aldrin, ametrina, BHC, DDT, dacomil, dieldrin, di-syxtox, endrin, furadan, gusathion, javelin, metalaxyl, nuvacron, oxidemeton methyl, talstar, tordon	Gomez-Arroyo et al.[1108]
	Deltamethrin, carbaryl, mancozeb, propineb, benomyl	Pasquini et al.[1109]
Sister chromatid exchange	Azinphos-methyl, dimethoate, malathion, methyl parathion, 2,4,5-T, 2,4-D	Laurent et al.[1110]
	Mancozeb-contained fungicide	Jablonicka et al.[1111]
	A complex mixture of pesticides (atrazine, alachlor, cyanazine, 2,4-dichlorophenoxyacetic acid, and malathion)	Zeljezic and Garaj-Vrhovac[1112]
	DDT, BHC, endosulfan, malathion, methyl parathion, phosphamidon, dimethoate, monocrotophos, quinalphos, fenvalerate, and cypermethrin	Rupa et al.[1113]
	DDT, BHC, malathion, parathion, dimethoate, fenitrothion, urea, and gromor	Rupa et al.[1114]

Source: Reprinted from *Toxicology and Applied Pharmacology*, 268(2), S. Mostafalou, M. Abdollah, Pesticides and human chronic diseases: Evidences, mechanisms, and perspectives, 157–177, Copyright 2013, with permission from Elsevier.

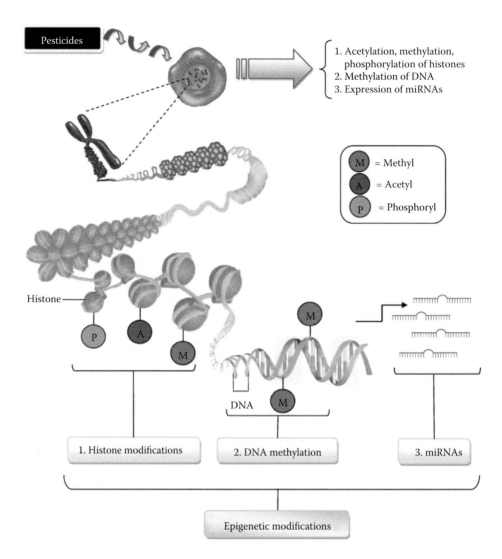

FIGURE 7.74 Schematic model for induction of epigenetic modifications including DNA methylation, histone modification, and expression of miRNAs by pesticides. (Reprinted from *Toxicology and Applied Pharmacology*, 268(2), S. Mostafalou, M. Abdollah, Pesticides and human chronic diseases: Evidences, mechanisms, and perspectives, 157–177, Copyright 2013, with permission from Elsevier.)

for studying the carcinogenesis mechanisms of occupational and environmental exposures.[1125] The first note on pesticide-induced carcinogenesis through epigenetic mechanisms was from a study carried out by Maslansky and colleagues in 1981. They reported hepatocarcinogenesis of organochlorine pesticides with no genotoxic effects in hepatocytes and suspected to epigenetic modifications disrupting intracellular communications.[1126] Later, reports presented about epigenetic actions of vinclozolin, a fungicide known to be an environmental endocrine disruptor, in association with adult-onset diseases, particularly tumor development.[1127] Pesticides were introduced as carcinogens acting through epigenetic or nongenotoxic mechanisms.[752]

Other than cancer, epigenetic alterations have increasingly been detected and investigated in neurodegenerative diseases, including Parkinson,[1128] Alzheimer,[1129] ALS,[1130] and multiple sclerosis.[1131] On the role of epigenetic changes in pesticide-induced neurodegenerative disorder, recently, neurotoxic insecticides were found to promote apoptosis in dopaminergic neurons through hyperacetylation of core histones H3 and H4.[1123]

Epigenetic alterations have also been reported to be involved in some other late-onset diseases such as diabetes,[1132] aging,[1133] chronic kidney disease,[1134] and atherosclerosis.[1135] Nevertheless, presenting epigenetic modifications as a mechanism by which pesticides develop these chronic diseases depends on the future studies.

However, epigenetics has opened a new field for studying the influence of environmental exposures on transcriptional regulation of genes in association with human diseases. There are a lot of findings about changing the pattern of gene expressions in exposure to pesticides which can be used as a tool in studying the process of human diseases,[1136] but further studies are still required to determine the role of epigenetic mechanisms in these variations.

OTHER MECHANISMS INVOLVED IN PESTICIDE-INDUCED CHRONIC DISEASES

Endocrine Disruption

Diabetes

Diabetes can be said that has become epidemic since 347 million people worldwide are appraised to be diabetic and based on WHO belief, diabetes deaths are expected to double between 2005 and 2030. Unlike diseases mentioned above, diabetes, particularly type 2, has some identified risk factors, including rich diet, obesity, and sedentary manner of living but the extent of reports implicating on the relation of exposure to environmental pollutants, particularly pesticides, and development of diabetes is rapidly growing.[665,1137] The possibility of studying diabetes in experimental models allowed researchers to investigate effects of exposure to pesticides on glucose homeostasis in laboratory animals. In this regard, there were lots of reports on disrupting effects of pesticides particularly OPs and organochlorines on glucose metabolism in association with imbalanced insulin secretion and response in animals.[646,1138,1139] A couple of epidemiological studies whose results published during the past few years indicated that exposure to pesticides can be a potential risk factor for developing diabetes.[1140–1142] It has also been suggested that exposure to some pesticides can be a promotor for other risk factors of diabetes such as obesity by distressing neural circuits that regulate feeding behavior or altering differentiation of adipocytes.[1143] Note all the populations who are obese are eating pesticide-contaminated food.

At a cellular level, endocrine disruption refers to a mechanism of toxicity that interferes the ability of the cells to communicate hormonally and results in a wide variety of adverse health effects including birth defects, reproductive, developmental, metabolic, immune, and neurobehavioral disorders as well as hormone-dependent cancers. The term "endocrine disruptor" was first introduced in 1991 referring to the substances that interfere with synthesis, secretion, transport binding, action, metabolism, or elimination of hormones in the body.[1144] Up to now, a huge body of evidence has brought up on endocrine-disrupting properties of pesticides so that currently a total of 101 pesticides have been listed as proven or possible EDs by the Pesticide Action Network UK.[1145] Most endocrine-disrupting pesticides mimic estrogen function by acting as a ligand for a receptor, converting other steroids to active estrogen, or increasing the expression of estrogen-responsive genes as shown by some organochlorines, OPs, carbamates, and pyrethroids. Antiandrogenic affects have also been reported for organochlorine and carbamate insecticides, as well as triazines, a group of herbicides through inhibition of binding natural ligand to receptors and androgen-binding receptors.

These pesticide and herbicide exposures may account for the rising amount of feminization in men in this world. Competitive inhibition of thyroid hormone receptors by OPs and inhibition of progesterone action by pyrethroids are other findings regarding endocrine disruption by pesticides.[1146] However, the results of various transactivation assays using mammalian and yeast cells indicated agonistic or antagonistic activity of pesticides toward aryl hydrocarbon receptors and some members of the nuclear receptor superfamily including RA receptors, pregnane X receptors, and peroxisome proliferator-activated receptors[1147,1148] (for more information, see the section

"Endocrine Disruption"). We find many males made impotent with the estrogen effect and the antitestosterum-type response, while the females get disruption of their menstrual cycle.

Rochman[1149] showed that in addition to big bellies, pregnant women are toting around dozens of chemicals, including some that have been banned for decades and others used in flame retardants, sunscreens, and nonstick cookware.

Woodruff looked at data on 163 chemicals, counted the number of chemicals that pregnant women are exposed to, and discovered that 43 of the 163 chemicals tracked were found in >99% of pregnant women.[1149]

Those chemicals included PCBs, organochlorine pesticides, perfluorinated compounds (PFCs), phenols, polybrominated diphenyl ethers (PBDEs), phthalates, polycyclic aromatic hydrocarbons (PAHs), and perchlorate. Benzophenone-3, an ingredient in sunscreen, was also found.[1149]

Woodruff crunched data on 268 pregnant women from the U.S. CDC, which collected blood and urine samples from participants in its NHANES 2003–2004.[1149]

Bisphenol A (BPA)—the controversial plastic-hardening chemical that baby bottle manufacturers have phased out in the wake of consumer protests—was found in 96% of the pregnant women. BPA, which is still used as a liner inside metal food and beverage cans, has been associated with hormonal disruption and adverse brain development (more on Time.com: Study: BPA Exposure May Reduce Chances of IVF).[1149]

Examination of Table 7.65 shows that contaminant levels of Canadians are comparable with those found in the review, except for HCB, where the Canadian 95 percentile levels are ~20% of the mean levels found in a dual Spanish cohort. The patterns of OP metabolite levels also differ from those in the United States. For the dimethyl metabolites (e.g., resulting from exposure to malathion), levels are very similar between Canada and the United States. For diethyl metabolites (e.g., resulting from exposure to diazinon), the detection frequency in Canada is lower, but the highest 5% of children have levels five times higher than the U.S. mean.

An alternate approach to determining Canadian contaminant burdens is the detection rates for chemicals of interest in the national health survey and in environmental monitoring data. Table 7.66 shows national detection frequencies in children for selected current-use pesticide metabolites from the Canadian Health Measures Survey. Concerning findings include the detection rate of nearly 100% for pyrethroid metabolites in Canadian children. Pyrethroids, or synthetic pyrethrins, are widely used for household insect control and on pets and livestock. Their main effect is axonal excitation, and they are considered likely carcinogens by the oral exposure route.[1152] They have suppressing effects on natural killer cells of the immune system in rats, which could have implications for carcinogenesis if similar effects occurred in humans. For OP insecticides, the 72% rate of detection of the dimethyl metabolites of current-use insecticides such as malathion raises concerns about child exposure. Malathion was associated with hypotonic or absent reflexes in newborns[157] and the dimethyl metabolites were the most highly correlated with ADHD in a U.S. cohort study,[485] as well as being linked to the development of atopic asthma and abnormal respiratory function in children and adults.

The Canadian biomonitoring data were collected year-round for 2 years. While DDT/DDE levels would be expected to have minimal seasonal fluctuation, the metabolite levels for current-use pesticides including OPs have very short half-lives and could vary seasonally if the dominant source was agricultural or lawn/garden use, and not diet or drinking water. Despite this limitation, there is a high rate of detection for OP and pyrethrin metabolites in Canadian children (Table 7.65). In addition, environmental sampling shows that several pesticides associated with adverse health effects are frequently found in surface waters across the country.[1153] For example, atrazine, a corn herbicide and endocrine disruptor with antiandrogenic and antiestrogenic effects, is consistently found in more than 90% of surface water samples in Ontario, while the current-use OPs malathion and diazinon are found in about 15%. In contrast, chlorpyrifos, which has been banned for most uses in Canada, is present in only 3% of Ontario water samples and azinphos-methyl (restricted use) in <2%.[1153]

TABLE 7.65

Comparison of Canadian Maternal/Child Contaminant Levels with those Reported in Reviewed Studies

Contaminant	Median (Review)	Median, CDN Women Age 20–39	Median, CDN Children or Cord Blood	95%/ile CDN F = Women C = Children
Organochlorines				
p,p-DDE (µg/L)	• 0.64 (United States) • 6.3 (Mexico) • 0.86, 1.03 (Spain, two cohorts) • All prenatal	• 0.55 • 0.76 (Calgary) • Women prenatal[1150] • Baffin Is.: Inuit • 2.2, Cauc.96[1151]	• Not measured[1152] • Cord blood, mean 0.03 (Calgary)[1150]	4.21-F
Hexachlorobenzene (µg/L)	• 0.73 (Spain)	• Not detected[1152] • 0.10 (Calgary)[1150]	• Not measured[1152] • Cord blood 0.14 (Calgary)[2]	0.19-F
p,p-DDE (ng/G lipid) lipid-adjusted DDE	• 1436 (United States, pregnant women) • 110 (United States, pregnant women) • 299 (Greenland, pregnant women) • 654 (Warsaw, pregnant women)	• Not detected[1152] • 109.9 (Calgary pregnant women)	• Not measured[1152] • Cord blood 76.5 (Calgary)[1150]	832-F
Organophosphate Metabolites				
Dimethyl thiophosphate (µmol/L)	• 0.0137 (United States, prenatal)	• 0.0127[1152]	• 0.0177[1152]	0.389-C
Diethyl thiophosphate (µmol/L)	• 0.0047 (United States)	• Not detected	• Not detected	0.0284-C

Sources of Canadian data: Common Menu Bar Links. 2012. Canada Health Act Annual Report 2010–2011 (Health Canada, 2011). [Accessed March 22, 2016] http://www.hc-sc.gc.ca/hcs-sss/pubs/cha-lcs/2011-cha-lcs-ar-ra/index-eng.php; Jarrell, J. et al. 2005. Longitudinal assessment of PCBs and chlorinated pesticides in pregnant women from Western Canada. *Environ. Health* 4:10; Butler Walker, J. et al. Organochlorine levels in maternal and umbilical cord blood plasma in Arctic Canada 2003. *Sci. Total Environ.* 302(1–3):27–52.

Reproductive Health Outcomes and Pesticide Exposure

The reproductive review examined 75 studies published since 2003. The strongest area of association is between current-use pesticides, including diazinon and atrazine, and fetal growth, with 7 of 10 studies positive. This is a concern in Canada, as detection rates for the two metabolites of diazinon are 36% and 77% for women aged 20–39. Atrazine is a high-volume agricultural herbicide used on corn crops and considered to be an endocrine disruptor. It has been banned in Europe for over a decade. There was no biomonitoring of atrazine in the 2007–2009 Canadian Health Measures Survey; based on health effects and its persistence in the environment, it would be a candidate for inclusion in the next survey.

Cardiovascular Diseases

About the relationship between pesticide's exposure and cardiovascular diseases, there is a growing number of reports carried out in varied forms. In addition to a report concerning hypertension in Oregon pesticide-formulating workers,[1054] there have been a few evidences on the link between

TABLE 7.66

Detection Rates of Pesticide Metabolites Found in the Canadian Health Measures Survey

Pesticide Metabolite	Parent Compound	Detection Rate, Age 6–11	Detection Rate, Age 12–19	Pesticide Class and Use
3-PBA	• Many, including permethrin deltamethrin, cypermethrin	99%	100%	• Pyrethroids—scabies Rx, pets household, livestock, mosquito nets and coils
cis-DCCA	• cis-Permethrin • cis-Cypermethrin	97%	99%	• Pyrethroids—agricultural and livestock
4-F-3-PBB	• Cyfluthrin • Flumethrin	42%	51%	• Pyrethroids—agricultural, indoor surfaces (for flying and crawling insects), insect-control strips in beehives
2,4-DCP (all from environment, not a human metabolite)	• 2,4-D herbicide • Pharmaceuticals • Wastewater chlorination	78%	83%	• Phenoxy herbicides—lawns and crops; also a metabolite of other processes
Dimethyl thiophosphate (DMTP)	• Malathion, azinphos-methyl (restricted), dimethoate, other insecticides	72%	72%	• Organophosphate insecticides—gardens, food crops, forestry
Diethyl thiophosphate (DETP)	• Diazinon (currently used in phaseout), terbufos, chlorpyrifos (banned)	55%	55%	• Organophosphate insecticides—garden, food crops

Source: Common Menu Bar Links. 2012. Canada Health Act Annual Report 2010–2011 (Health Canada, 2011). [Accessed March 22, 2016] http://www.hc-sc.gc.ca/hcs-sss/pubs/cha-lcs/2011-cha-lcs-ar-ra/index-eng.php.

Note: All results rounded to nearest whole percent.

exposure to pesticides and atherosclerosis.[1055,1154] Recently, it was reported that chronic exposure to OP pesticides can potentiate the risk of coronary artery disease presumably through diminished paraoxonase activity.[1056]

Pesticide Use and Myocardial Infarction Incidence among Farm Women in the Agricultural Health Study

Objective: To evaluate the relationship between pesticide use and myocardial infarction (MI) among farm women.

Methods: Dayton used logistic regression to evaluate pesticide use and self-reported incident non-fatal MI among women in the AHS.

Results: Of those MI free at enrollment ($n = 22,425$), 168 reported an MI after enrollment. They saw no association with pesticide use overall. Six of 27 individual pesticides evaluated were significantly associated with nonfatal MI, including chlorpyrifos, coumaphos, carbofuran, metalaxyl, pendimethalin, and trifluralin, which all had ORs >1.7. These chemicals were used by <10% of the cases, and their use was correlated, making it difficult to attribute the risk elevation to a specific pesticide.

Conclusion: Pesticides may contribute to MI risk among farm women.

Pesticide poisonings sometimes involve cardiac complications. For example, OP poisoning has been associated with arrhythmias and cardiac abnormalities[1155,1156]; however, little is known about the cardiac risks associated with low-level chronic exposure to pesticides. Studies of mortality among the U.S. crop and livestock farmers[1157] and licensed pesticide applicators[1158] have suggested increased risk of MI mortality, whereas other studies of other farming populations have shown deficits in MI mortality[1159,1160] or no evidence of an association.[1161] These studies, although focusing on agricultural populations, have generally not evaluated potential MI risk from specific pesticides. In an ecological analyses using crop patterns as a surrogate for pesticide exposure, Schreinemachers[1162] reported greater risk for acute fatal MIs in the U.S. counties with high wheat production. An analysis of both fatal and nonfatal MIs among male pesticide applicators in the AHS provided no evidence of an association of MI with pesticides.[1163] Little information is available regarding MI risk among farm women. In general, farm women have been historically underrepresented in health research.[1164] To better assess MI risk associated with pesticides among women, they used data from the AHS to investigate potential agricultural risk factors for MI among farm women.

The AHS is a prospective study of 52,395 licensed private pesticide applicators, mainly farmers, and 32,346 spouses of farmers from Iowa and North Carolina enrolled from 1993 to 1997.[1165] Spouses enrolled by using a self-administered questionnaire brought home by the enrolled applicator (81% returned the questionnaire by mail; 19% completed the interview by phone). In 1999–2003, 69% of applicators and 6% of spouses completed a follow-up phone interview.

Their study population consisted of all female participants in the AHS, including both female spouses of applicators ($N = 23{,}703$) and female applicators ($N = 912$), who completed both the enrollment questionnaire and the follow-up phone interview. Information on occurrence of MI was obtained at the follow-up phone interview. Women who had an MI before enrollment were excluded ($n = 193$). Also excluded were women missing information on smoking status ($n = 1234$), body mass index ($n = 719$), and age ($n = 1$). The final analytical sample included 22,425 farm women.

For their primary analysis, MI was defined as having a positive response to the question, "Has a doctor ever told you that you had (been diagnosed with) a MI (heart attack)?" Women who reported having had a diagnosis of MI were also asked "at what age?" Responses to the latter question were used to classify reported MIs as incident or prevalent based on woman's age at diagnosis and age at enrollment. Incident MI were defined as those occurring at an age greater than or equal to age at enrollment.

Information on demographic characteristics, medical history, and agriculture exposure history, including personal pesticide use and current farm activities, was obtained from the enrollment questionnaire. They focused on lifetime pesticide use history and current farm activities at enrollment. Women provided information on every use of 50 individual pesticides and overall lifetime use of pesticides. Because they included both spouses and applicators, the exposure assessment for pesticides was limited to the detail provided on the spouse questionnaire. Farm activities evaluated included contact with animals, operation of farm equipment, farm maintenance activities, and solvent use on the farm. Questionnaires are available at www.aghealth.org/questionnaires.html.

To assess the association between farming exposures and MI, they used logistic regression controlling for age, body mass index, smoking status, and state of residence. Logistic regression was suitable for this analysis because of the short duration from enrollment to MI (generally <5 years). Goodness-of-fit tests were used to identify covariates to be included in the model. Their model showed little change in fit when smoking status was modeled as a three-level variable (current, past, and never) when compared with combined past and current smokers; therefore, the two-level variable (ever and never) was used in the analysis. Other parameterizations of smoking (e.g., pack years) were evaluated, but none fit the model better than the two-level variable, probably because of the low frequency of smoking in the sample. They also considered alcohol consumption, education, and physical activity but did not include them in the final model because they did not affect the point estimates.

Using the individual pesticide variables, they created summary variables for pesticide functional categories (fumigants, fungicides, herbicides, and insecticides) and subclassifications of insecticide classes (carbamates, organochlorines, and OPs). They evaluated each group and pesticide individually. They limited their analysis to individual pesticides that had at least five reported cases of MI among those exposed.

Pesticide use can be correlated. To address potential confounding by correlated variables, they looked at the correlations between pesticides that were significant in the single pesticide models. For pairs of pesticides with a Spearman correlation of ≥ 0.3, they included both pesticides in the model to evaluate the impact on the ORs.

To assess possible misclassification of self-reported MI, they repeated our analyses, excluding women with self-reported angina or arrhythmia. In addition, to assess the overall risk of incident MI, they conducted an analysis including both fatal and nonfatal MIs. Fatal MIs were identified using ICD-10 codes (I21–I22) from death certificates for all women in the AHS who had died since time of enrollment until December 31, 2005. The number of MI deaths was too small ($N = 48$) to evaluate MI mortality alone.

SAS version 9.0 was used for all statistical analyses. The AHS data sets used were PIRELO506 and PIREL0612.01 releases.

A total of 168 incident nonfatal doctor-diagnosed MIs were reported among the 22,425 farm women who completed the follow-up interview (Table 7.63). Cases were older and had lived on farms longer. Women with incident MI were more likely to have reported a history of hypertension, diabetes, angina, and arrhythmia at enrollment. Alcohol consumption was more common among controls than cases (676% vs. 38%). Women who were licensed pesticide applicators were more likely to report MI (99% vs. 4%).

MI risk was not associated with ever use of any pesticide (OR = 0.9, 95% CI = 0.7, 1.2) nor was it associated with either number of days or number of years applied pesticides. Incident MI was associated with ever use of a few specific pesticides but not with use of specific chemical classes. Six of 27 specific pesticides were statistically significantly associated with increase MI: the insecticides chlorpyrifos (OR = 2.1, 95% CI = 1.2, 3.7), coumaphos (OR = 3.2, 95% CI = 1.5, 7.0), and carbofuran (OR = 2.5, 95% CI = 1.3, 5.0); the herbicides pendimethalin (OR = 2.5, 95% CI = 1.2, 4.9) and trifluralin (OR = 1.8, 95% CI = 1.0, 3.1); and the fungicide metalaxyl (OR = 2.4, 95% CI = 1.1, 5.3). There was no association between nonfatal MI and farming activities reported at enrollment (Tables 7.67 and 7.68), and these activities did not confound the pesticide associations.

The six chemicals significantly associated with MI were correlated with each other, particularly among cases ($r = 0.3–0.7$). To evaluate whether this correlation influenced the results, they built models that included two pesticides at a time. In doing this, the ORs for MI remained elevated but no longer statistically significant. Chlorpyrifos was correlated with all of the five other pesticides. When chlorpyrifos was included in a model with coumaphos, the estimates were both attenuated ($OR_{chlorpyrifos} = 1.4$, 95% CI = 0.7, 2.8 and $OR_{coumaphos} = 3.1$, 95% CI = 1.3, 7.1), but the number of exposed cases decreased as well due to missing exposure information for one of the pesticides in the model. The other pairwise models of pesticides suggested some evidence of potential confounding or interaction of the pesticides, but given the small number of exposed cases ($n = 5–14$), they lacked statistical power to explore this further. Women who used at least one of the six pesticides had an elevated risk of MI (OR = 1.6, 95% CI = 1.1, 2.4).

Female pesticide applicators may have greater pesticide exposure and may have used more toxic chemicals. To assess whether the results were driven by 3.7% of the women who were private pesticide applicators, they reran their main analyses excluding female applicators. With these women excluded ($n = 15$ cases), eight pesticides were significantly associated with MI, the six previously observed in addition to petroleum oil (OR = 1.9, 95% CI = 1.0, 3.8) and terbufos (OR = 2.1, 95% CI = 1.0, 4.4). The point estimates of all eight pesticides were very similar to those observed in the full sample with the exception of chlorpyrifos; the OR for chlorpyrifos reduced from 3.2 to 2.2 (95% CI = 1.2, 4.2).

Exclusion of women with self-reported angina ($n = 29$) or arrhythmia ($n = 26$) did not substantially change their results. With these women excluded, Dayton et al.[1165] observed significant risk for incident MI for coumaphos (OR = 3.7, 95% CI = 1.6, 8.6) and chlorpyrifos (OR = 2.3, 95% CI = 1.2, 4.3) and not significant, but elevated risks, for carbofuran (OR = 2.2, 95% CI = 1.0, 5.1), pendimethalin (OR = 2.1, 95% CI = 0.9, 4.8), and trifluralin (OR = 1.3, 95% CI = 0.6, 2.6). There were too few metalaxyl-exposed cases ($n = 3$) to estimate MI risk. When they included the 48 women with fatal MIs since enrollment, there were only 2 more cases who had ever applied pesticides and none

TABLE 7.67

Demographics of 22,425 Farm Women Enrolled in the Agricultural Health Study Completing Both Enrollment (1993–1997) and Follow-Up Questionnaires (1999–2003)

	Cases (*N* = 168)	Controls (*N* = 22,257)
Age at enrollment (year)		
17–39	8 (5)	6642 (30)
40–49	21 (13)	6529 (29)
50–59	51 (30)	5529 (25)
60–88	88 (52)	3557 (16)
State		
Iowa	95 (57)	16,003 (72)
North Carolina	73 (43)	6254 (28)
Licensed pesticide applicator		
Yes	15 (9)	815 (4)
No	153 (91)	21,442 (96)
Body mass index (kg/m²)		
15.0–25.0	60 (36)	10,705 (48)
25.1–30.0	58 (35)	7306 (33)
>30	50 (30)	4246 (19)
Smoking status		
Never	112 (67)	16,356 (73)
Ever	56 (33)	5901 (27)
Alcohol consumption at enrollment (drinks/month)		
Never	105 (64)	9662 (44)
1–10	53 (32)	10,621 (48)
>11	6 (4)	1715 (8)
Years lived on a farm (year)		
0–15	31 (18)	5240 (24)
15–30	30 (18)	5849 (26)
30–45	33 (20)	5897 (26)
>45	74 (44)	5271 (24)
Days per year mixing pesticides		
None	109 (65)	12,802 (58)
1–5	22 (13)	4712 (21)
5–9	15 (9)	2179 (10)
10–19	11 (7)	1612 (7)
>20	11 (7)	952 (4)
Year(s) spent mixing pesticides		
None	109 (65)	12,815 (58)
1–5	9 (5)	3406 (15)
6–10	13 (8)	1824 (8)
11–20	15 (9)	2214 (10)
>21	22 (13)	1998 (9)
Education		
High school or less	101 (656)	8762 (44)
More than high school	55 (35)	11,162 (56)
Strenuous exercise during leisure time (hour/week)[a]		
None	45 (35)	3452 (21)
<1	18 (14)	2969 (17)

(Continued)

TABLE 7.67 (*Continued*)

Demographics of 22,425 Farm Women Enrolled in the Agricultural Health Study Completing Both Enrollment (1993–1997) and Follow-Up Questionnaires (1999–2003)

	Cases (*N* = 168)	Controls (*N* = 22,257)
1–2	25 (20)	3289 (19)
3–5	26 (20)	4452 (26)
>6	13 (10)	2858 (17)
Medical history at enrollment		
Family history of a heart attack	25 (16)	2359 (11)
Angina[b]	29 (19)	423 (2)
Arrhythmia[b]	26 (17)	1278 (6)
Diabetes[b]	35 (23)	630 (3)
Hypertension [b]	73 (47)	3106 (14)

Source: From Shile, B. D. et al. 2010. *Pesticide Use and Myocardial Infarction Incidence Among Farm Women in the Agricultural Health Study*, Wolters Kluwer Health, Inc. Table 1. With permission.

Note: Values are represented as *N* (%).

[a] The highest level reported during summer or winter.

[b] Self-reported doctor diagnosis.

who reported using the pesticides associated with nonfatal MIs; hence, the results were essentially unchanged from the analysis including the nonfatal MIs only (data not shown).

Dayton et al.[1165] investigated the relationship between agricultural pesticide use and the incidence of MI among women in the AHS. Little is known about the effect of chronic low-dose pesticide exposure on cardiovascular outcomes because the majority of human data are from poisoning episodes. Six pesticides were positively associated with nonfatal MI among the farm women. The insecticide coumaphos had the highest OR. There were no associations between MI and total lifetime days of pesticide use or for various farm activities, such as operating farm equipment or solvent use. Although, they observed associations with use of specific chemicals for women in the AHS, no associations were seen for MI among the men in the cohort.[1163]

Their findings of an increased risk of MI associated with ever use of specific pesticides are intriguing, but the sample size is small and the exposure detail limited. The pesticides associated with MI were all registered with the EPA for at least 15 years before the collection of the exposure data. Coumaphos, registered in 1958, was the longest in use.[1166] The six pesticides associated with MI have no common use patterns, although among case women, the use of these pesticides was correlated. Of the six, three were insecticides, two herbicides, and one was a fungicide.

Chlorpyrifos and coumaphos are both OP insecticides; chlorpyrifos is used on both crops and livestock, but coumaphos is used exclusively on animals. Carbofuran, a carbamate insecticide, is used on crops. Pendimethalin and trifluralin are herbicides used on annual grasses and broadleaf weeds among crops, and metalazyl is a fungicide used on crops and in soil treatment for disease control. The acute toxicities of these pesticides vary from slightly toxic (pendimethalin) to highly toxic (coumaphos and carbofuran).[1167] Chlorpyrifos, coumaphos, and carbofuran all inhibit AChE to varying degrees.[1167] Thus, it is unlikely that the observations for these six chemicals could result from some common use pattern or toxicity. Although the findings for these unrelated pesticides make it difficult to speculate on a potential mechanism, the results do suggest that pesticide exposures that do not result in poisonings may be a risk factor for MI in women.

The most commonly used chemicals were the herbicide glyphosate (37%) and the insecticide carbaryl (33%). Given this low exposure prevalence and the lack of information on duration and frequency of use, they were limited in their ability to assess potential confounding by related exposures

TABLE 7.68

Odds Ratios for Incident Nonfatal Myocardial Infarction and Pesticide Use among 22,425 Farm Women in the Agricultural Health Study

	Cases (N = 168)	Controls (N = 22,254)	Odds Ratio[a]	95% Confidence Interval
Ever applied pesticides	92 (55)	13,357 (60)	0.9	0.7–1.2
Fumigants	7 (4)	522 (2)	1.5	0.7–3.2
Methyl bromide	5 (3)	347 (2)	1.7	0.7–4.3
Fungicides	16 (10)	1365 (6)	1.3	0.8–2.3
Captan	5 (3)	601 (3)	1.1	0.4–2.6
Maneb	6 (4)	376 (2)	1.7	0.7–3.9
Metalaxyl	7 (5)	385 (2)	2.4	1.1–5.3
Herbicides	54 (33)	8980 (41)	0.8	0.6–1.2
2,4-D	27 (17)	3652 (17)	1.1	0.7–1.7
Alachlor	9 (6)	1085 (5)	1.2	0.6–2.4
Atrazine	13 (8)	1192 (6)	1.5	0.8–2.7
Butylate	5 (3)	343 (2)	2.1	0.8–5.2
Chlorimuron-ethyl	5 (3)	424 (2)	1.8	0.7–4.5
Cyanazine	6 (4)	739 (3)	1.2	0.5–2.9
Dicamba	5 (3)	1019 (5)	0.8	0.3–1.9
Glyphosate	46 (29)	8096 (37)	0.8	0.6–1.2
Metolachlor	5 (3)	863 (4)	0.9	0.4–2.2
Metribuzin	5 (3)	452 (2)	1.5	0.6–3.7
Petroleum oil	10 (7)	852 (4)	1.8	0.9–3.4
Pendimethalin	9 (6)	592 (3)	2.5	1.2–4.9
Trifluralin	15 (10)	1360 (6)	1.8	1.0–3.1
Insecticides	77 (47)	9497 (43)	1.1	0.8–1.6
Carbamates	63 (38)	7576 (34)	1.1	0.8–1.5
Carbaryl	55 (36)	7087 (33)	1.0	0.7–1.4
Carbofuran	9 (6)	478 (2)	2.5	1.3–5.0
Organochlorines	21 (14)	1951 (9)	1.1	0.7–1.7
Chlordane	14 (10)	998 (5)	1.7	0.9–2.9
Dichlorodiphenyl trichloroethane	11 (8)	856 (4)	1.0	0.6–1.9
Organophosphates	49 (30)	6411 (29)	1.1	0.8–1.5
Chlorpyrifos	14 (9)	1056 (5)	2.1	1.2–3.7
Coumaphos	7 (4)	314 (1)	3.2	1.5–7.0
Diazinon	13 (9)	2388 (11)	0.8	0.4–1.4
Fonofos	5 (3)	448 (2)	1.7	0.7–4.3
Malathion	31 (21)	4639 (22)	0.9	0.6–1.3
Terbufos	9 (6)	735 (3)	1.9	1.0–3.8

Source: From Shile, B. D. et al. 2010. *Pesticide Use and Myocardial Infarction Incidence Among Farm Women in the Agricultural Health Study,* Wolters Kluwer Health, Inc. Table 2. With permission.

Note: Values are represented as *N* (%).

[a] Odds ratios adjusted for age, body mass index, smoking status, and state.

and were unable to assess dose–response. Nevertheless, when they controlled for correlated pesticides and when they excluded people with angina and arrhythmia, the associations remained elevated although no longer statistically significant.

They relied on self-reported MI as their primary outcome. Accuracy of self-reported MIs among middle-aged and elderly Americans generally ranges from 53% to 72%, validity decreases with

TABLE 7.69

Farm Exposures and Risk of Myocardial Infarction among 22,425 Farm Women Enrolled in the Agricultural Health Study

Exposure	Cases (N = 168)	Controls (N = 22,257)	Odds Ratio[a]	95% Confidence Interval
Animal activities				
Grind feed	11 (8)	1513 (7)	1.2	0.7–2.3
Contact with farm animals	19 (13)	2974 (14)	1.4	0.9–2.3
Milk cows	7 (5)	1051 (5)	1.1	0.5–2.3
Farm equipment operation				
Drive trucks	54 (37)	8205 (39)	1.2	0.8–1.6
Diesel tractors	46 (32)	7301 (35)	1.3	0.9–1.8
Gasoline tractors	44 (31)	5804 (28)	1.4	1.0–2.0
Maintenance activities				
Welding	6 (4)	567 (3)	1.3	0.6–2.9
Repair engines	5 (4)	640 (3)	1.0	0.4–2.5
Grind metal	7 (5)	615 (3)	1.4	0.7–3.1
Solvent exposures				
Clean with solvents	33 (23)	4595 (22)	1.2	0.8–1.8
Paint	40 (28)	7124 (34)	0.9	0.6–1.3

Source: From Shile, B. D. et al. 2010. *Pesticide Use and Myocardial Infarction Incidence Among Farm Women in the Agricultural Health Study*, Wolters Kluwer Health, Inc. Table 3. With permission.

Note: Values are represented as N (%).

[a] Odds ratios adjusted for age, body mass index, smoking status, and state.

age.[1168,1169] The inaccuracy of reporting of an MI is most commonly associated with diagnoses of other cardiac outcomes, such as unstable angina, especially among women older than 64 years when self-report was compared with hospital records.[1168,1169] Other investigators have used self-reported MI as an outcome.[1170,1171] When they repeated the analysis after removing women who reported arrhythmia and angina, their results were similar. Because they relied on self-reported data, they may have underestimated MI risk because women who had medical interventions that may have prevented MIs or undetected MIs were included in their comparison group. Inclusion of MI deaths, on the other hand, may include some overreporting of outcome resulting from inaccurate reporting of MIs as cause of death for women of advanced age.[1225] Nevertheless, their estimates were similar when we included fatal cases.

Farm women seem to be at low risk for MI death compared with other women.[1159,1172] Their estimate of 1.5 nonfatal MIs/1000 woman-years is lower than other U.S. populations.[1173,1174] In previous AHS analyses, cardiovascular disease mortality for farm women was 60% that of the general population in Iowa and North Carolina.[1159] Even in this low-risk population, Dayton et al.[1165] saw increased risk of incident MI among women who used specific pesticides. Among male applicators in the AHS cohort, they saw no association with pesticides and MI risk.[1163] In that analysis, they had a more highly exposed population with detailed pesticide use information with a larger number of cases. Thus, it is somewhat surprising that they would see associations between pesticide use and MI among farm women in their cohort but not among men, particularly given the large magnitude of the effect estimates. With their small numbers, chance may explain the findings; however, the results could suggest a different role for pesticides in MI risk for women than men. Although they lacked use information to evaluate exposure–response relationships, the prospective nature of the analysis adds strength to these findings. Although we cannot rule out chance, these results suggest the need for future investigation of pesticides and MI risk among farm women (Tables 7.69).

VIP Gene Deletion in Mice Causes Cardiomyopathy Associated
with Upregulation of Heart Failure Genes

Rationale: Vasoactive intestinal peptide (VIP), a pulmonary vasodilator and inhibitor of vascular smooth muscle proliferation, is absent in pulmonary arteries of patients with idiopathic pulmonary arterial hypertension (PAH). They previously determined that targeted deletion of the VIP gene in mice leads to PAH with pulmonary vascular remodeling and right ventricular (RV) dilation. Whether the left ventricle is also affected by VIP gene deletion is unknown. In the current study, they examined if VIP knockout mice (VIP$^{-/-}$) develop both RV and left ventricular (LV) cardiomyopathy, manifested by LV dilation and systolic dysfunction, as well as overexpression of genes conducive to heart failure.[1175]

Methods: They examined VIP$^{-/-}$ and wild type (WT) mice using magnetic resonance imaging (MRI) for evidence of cardiomyopathy associated with biventricular dilation and wall thickness changes. Lung tissue from VIP$^{-/-}$ and WT mice was subjected to whole-genome gene microarray analysis.

Results: Lungs from VIP$^{-/-}$ mice showed overexpression of cardiomyopathy genes; Myh1 was upregulated 224 times over WT and Mylpf was increased 72-fold. Tnnt3 was increased 105 times and tnnc2 by 181-fold. Hearts were dilated in VIP$^{-/-}$ mice, with thinning of LV wall and increase in RV and LV chamber size, though RV enlargement varied. Weights of VIP$^{-/-}$ mice were consistently lower.

Conclusions: Critically important heart failure-related genes are upregulated in VIP$^{-/-}$ mice associated with the spontaneous cardiomyopathy phenotype, involving both left and right ventricles, suggesting that loss of the VIP gene orchestrates a panoply of pathogenic genes which are detrimental to both left and right cardiac homeostasis.

CHRONIC NEPHROPATHIES

Higher incidence of the late-onset nephropathies such as chronic kidney disease and chronic renal failure has been reported in middle-aged people (40–60 years) living in the agricultural areas with more prevalence in men. The results of a survey in North Central Province of Sri Lanka have presented a significant relationship between chronic renal failure and environmental factors in farming areas.[1176] Exposure to AChE-inhibiting pesticides was associated with chronic renal failure.[1177] Furthermore, higher level of organochlorine pesticides was detected in chronic kidney disease patients along with a reduced glomerular filtration and increased oxidative stress.[1178]

CHRONIC RESPIRATORY DISEASE

Chronic respiratory asthma is considered as the most common disorder among chronic respiratory dysfunctions affecting both children and adults. Its close relationship with work-related exposures has been known from 18 countries so that occupational asthma is characterized as a disease in medicine. There have been several reports on increased rate of asthma in people occupationally exposed to pesticides.[1179] Moreover, the result of an AHS indicated that exposure to some pesticides may increase the risk of chronic obstructive pulmonary disease (COPD; in farmers).[1166]

Chemical sensitivity has been prominent in recent years. It is clear that the pesticides and herbicides also exposure to natural gas are the prime triggers for developing chemical sensitivity.

Respiratory Health Outcomes and Pesticide Exposure in Children and Adults

The respiratory tract is routinely exposed to many environmental chemicals, such as tobacco smoke, ozone, dust, and allergens, the inhalation of which is the leading cause of respiratory diseases. Exposure to pesticides, whether domestic or occupational, has been increasingly investigated for its effect on respiratory health after first being identified as a potential risk factor in agricultural populations over three decades ago. Exposure to pesticides, including herbicides, insecticides, and fungicides, has been hypothesized as leading to asthma, chronic obstructive respiratory conditions, decreased lung function, and increased respiratory tract infections in both children and adults.

This systematic review selected studies of pesticide exposure and several respiratory health outcomes, including asthma, COPDs, lung function changes and respiratory symptoms (e.g., cough and wheeze), respiratory tract infections, and interstitial lung diseases. Reactive airways dysfunction syndrome, a subtype of work-related irritant-induced asthma, was not assessed as only case series were found relating to pesticide exposures.[1180] A total of 40 articles investigating both children and adults were reviewed.

Asthma

The increasing incidence of asthma over the past three decades is coincident with increased pesticide exposure from occupational, environmental, and residential use.[1179,1181] In particular, OP pesticides were introduced in the 1970s and have been extensively used since then as a replacement for organochlorines.[1182] A significant association between asthma and pesticide use in farmers was first found in Saskatchewan in the 1980s, and has since been studied widely.[1183]

The review included 12 studies investigating pesticide exposure and asthma, both atopic and nonatopic. Of these studies, six investigated asthma in children and six addressed adult-onset asthma. Populations in Canada, the United States, Europe, Australia, and Lebanon were studied. All but two reviewed studies found positive associations between exposure to OP, carbamate, and organochlorine insecticides in particular, and diagnosis of asthma and wheeze in both children and adults.

Adult asthma: A diagnosis of adult-onset asthma was shown to be associated with exposure to insecticides in three of the six studies described in this section. Moreover, a retrospective cohort study of Australian outdoor workers exposed to insecticides found increased mortality from asthma relative to the general population (SMR 3.45; 95% CI = 1.39–7.10). Of the studies that showed a positive association, pesticide exposure was related primarily to the development of atopic asthma, with the strongest correlation with exposure to OP insecticides.

Two studies by Hoppin,[1061,1184] one of farm women and the other of male farmers, used cross-sectional data from the AHS and provide the strongest evidence as assessed by quality scores. The AHS is a large, prospective cohort study conducted in Iowa and North Carolina that enrolled over 8900 male and female participants between 1993 and 1997; it was designed to explore potential causes of disease among farmers and their families and among commercial pesticide applicators. Data were collected using either a self-administered questionnaire or a telephone interview. Asthma, as determined by self-reported physician diagnosis after the age of 20, was present in 2.7% of female and 2.2% of male farmers. The strength of the AHS data lies in the study's large sample size and analysis of specific pesticide groups. However, as the study population includes only individuals who are occupationally exposed, the degree of exposure may not be generalizable to the broader population. For farm women, exposure assessment included frequency of use, lifetime days of pesticide application, years on a farm, and total years of pesticide use. For male farmers/applicators, exposure assessment was based on lifetime pesticide use of 50 specific pesticides: ever use, frequency of use, number of years used and decade of first use, pesticide use practices, and use of personal protective equipment. This information was used to create two metrics of lifetime pesticide use: lifetime days of use and intensity-adjusted lifetime days of use. In addition to pesticide application information, there were also two measures indicative of ever having experienced elevated pesticide exposure: pesticide poisoning and high pesticide exposure events.

The results of the AHS showed that 12 of the 48 pesticides studied were associated with an increase in allergic asthma in male farmers, while 4 were associated with an increase in nonallergic asthma.[1184] Three insecticides had statistically significant ORs exceeding 2.0 for allergic asthma, that is, the OP insecticides coumaphos and parathion, and the organochlorine insecticide heptachlor. Two fumigants also add ORs in excess of 2.0, that is, 80/20 mixed carbon tetrachloride/carbon disulfide and EDB. Self-reported high pesticide exposure events were associated with both allergic and nonallergic asthma. Of the 12 pesticides associated with allergic asthma, 10 also showed significant exposure–response trends when evaluating high- and low-exposure categories based on the median number of intensity-adjusted lifetime days of use for each pesticide.

Considering only farm women ($n = 25{,}814$) in the AHS, 10 pesticides were found to be associated with allergic asthma and one with nonallergic asthma.[1061] Ten pesticides included: two herbicides, that is, 2,4-D and glyphosate; seven insecticides, that is, a carbamate (carbaryl), OPs (coumaphos, parathion, malathion, and phorate), an organochlorine (DDT), a pyrethroid (permethrin), and one fungicide (metalaxyl). Of these, the OP insecticides parathion and coumaphos again showed the strongest associations, as did the fungicide metalaxyl. The insecticide permethrin was the only exposure associated with nonatopic asthma in women.

Results from a Lebanese case–control study also found that asthmatic cases, as independently confirmed by a hospital pulmonologist reassessing the answers to a self-administered questionnaire, had higher odds of exposure to pesticides (OR = 2.32, 95% CI = 1.47–3.68).[1185] Exposure was also determined through a self-administered questionnaire that inquired as to domestic, occupational, and paraoccupational exposure as well as residential proximity to pesticide-treated fields, and included a pooled category for any exposure type; however, pesticide type was not specified. Importantly, this study showed a positive association between nonoccupational (including domestic and environmental) exposure and the odds of being asthmatic. However, the results could not be attributed to a specific pesticide, resulting in a relatively lower quality score than that of the AHS.

Two cross-sectional studies showed null and inverse associations between pesticide exposure and asthma. A European study used urinary ET as a biomarker of the carbamate fungicide ethylene bis-dithiocarbamate (EBDC) exposure[1186] to confirm increased exposure in 248 occupationally exposed farmers working in various industries, including grape, vegetable, potato, and flower bulb growing. In this study, diagnoses of asthma, wheeze, asthma attack, and chest tightness were reported more often by nonexposed controls, resulting in an inverse association. These EBDC fungicides do not have cholinergic activity, which may explain the negative association.

Similarly, a 2003 repeat cross-sectional study in Arkansas compared 135 pesticide aviators and 118 community-based controls and reached null conclusions, although spot monitoring of one aviation firm showed exposures that were undetectable or below the acceptable limit to pesticides including OPs and pyrethroids, which could also explain the null outcome suggestive of effective protection measures.[1187] Both of these studies had quality assessment scores below 13 points, with the Jones[1187] study scoring only 9 points. High loss to follow-up, poor exposure and confounder measurements, and selection bias from incentive recruiting methods contributed to the lower score.

Asthma in children: Seven studies assessed the association between pesticide exposure and a diagnosis of asthma in children; all reported a positive association with the exception of a Canadian farm study that reported no association. However, the studies differed markedly in both study population and exposure index. Four studies measured postnatal exposures in different age groups, while one study investigated prenatal exposure. Insecticides, herbicides, fungicides, and DDE were studied, and all were found to be associated with asthma and wheeze. Pre- and antenatal exposures were most strongly associated with asthmatic outcomes and maternal, but not paternal, exposures were correlated with increased risk of asthma and wheeze in children.

Two studies of a prospective Spanish cohort by Sunyer[1188,1189] were of relatively higher quality than others in this topic area, with quality scores of 18 out of 20 points. The remaining studies in this section scored between 12 and 14 points. Retrospective exposure assessment, lack of pesticide specificity, and questionnaire-based exposure measurements contributed to the lower scores.

Four population-based birth cohorts and one study using data from the Children's Health Study were consistent in reporting an association between exposure to pesticides in the first year of life and higher odds of asthma and wheeze.[155,1057,1188–1190] Specifically, Sunyer found that *in utero* exposure to the organochlorine insecticide metabolite DDE was associated with wheeze at age 4[1188] and asthma at age 6[1189] in a Spanish cohort. Notably, in the Spanish birth cohort, breast feeding showed a protective association with both wheeze and diagnosed asthma, despite bottle-fed children showing decreased DDE blood levels relative to breastfed children at age 4.[1188] Tagiyeva[1190] found that maternal exposure to both biocides (i.e., products that control unwanted organisms through chemical or biological means) and fungicides during pregnancy or 21 months postnatally was associated with childhood wheeze from birth to 81 months in a birth cohort study from the United Kingdom; however, only postnatal exposure was associated with asthma at 91 months. In contrast, from the Children's Health Study, Salam[1057] found that exposure to herbicides and pesticides occurring before, but not after, the first year of life was associated with an increased risk of asthma.

One cohort study used T-helper 1 (Th1) and T-helper 2 (Th2) cytokine measurements as biomarkers of allergic asthma and reported on the association between agricultural environments and asthma at age 2.[155] Maternal occupational exposure to agriculture pesticides, assumed to be predominantly OP and pyrethroid insecticides, as well as exposure to any agricultural field workers living in the household were significantly associated with both increased levels of Th2 cells and asthma and wheeze at 2 years of age ($p < 0.05$). Increased expression of Th2 cytokines has been previously shown to be associated with allergic asthma, contributing to its development through the recruitment of mast cells and eosinophils to the child's airways.[1191–1193]

A large ($n = 3291$ participants) questionnaire-based cross-sectional study reported that both occupational and nonoccupational exposure to pesticides in Lebanese schoolchildren aged 5–16 years resulted in an increase of asthma and chronic cough, chronic phlegm, and wheeze.[1065] Residential pesticide exposure was most strongly associated with recurrent wheeze, while occupational exposure of a household member was most strongly associated with asthma (OR = 4.61, 95% CI = 2.06–10.29). Interestingly, both this study and the Duramad[155] study described previously showed that adults exposed to pesticides at work "take home" exposures to their children, posing a greater risk of children developing asthma than either the use of pesticides within the home or exposure from residential community to spraying. The Lebanese study did not specify whether prenatal exposures were accounted for, while Duramad[155] did take into account *in utero* exposure.

A second large cohort study ($n = 3405$ children) used retrospective data from the Ontario Farm Family Health Study (OFFHS) to determine the association between *in utero* exposure to agricultural pesticides and the development of asthma and other health outcomes, including allergy and chronic bronchitis.[1194] A total of 173 cases were identified through self-report of a doctor's diagnosis of asthma, of which 114 had been exposed prenatally. No significant associations were reported between parental use of any pesticide and the development of asthma.

Chronic Obstructive Pulmonary Diseases

Three studies found significant positive associations between pesticide exposure and prevalent chronic bronchitis, while one Canadian study had results approaching significance only for female subjects (Weselak,[1194]). Of studies reporting a significant association, two were based on data from the AHS and received scores of 14 out of 20 points, and one was a case–control study of Lebanese adults scoring slightly lower. While all three studies demonstrated an effect of occupational exposures, the case–control study showed that nonoccupational exposures are also associated with the development of chronic bronchitis.

Hoppin[1195] studied farmers (20,400 male pesticide applicators and 508 female applicators) and found that 3% ($n = 654$) reported a history of physician-diagnosed chronic bronchitis diagnosed after age 20. Prevalent chronic bronchitis was significantly associated with 11 of the 49 pesticides studied in the adjusted model, with ORs ranging from 1.20 (herbicide chlorimuron-ethyl; 95% CI = 1.02–1.52) to 1.50 (organochlorine insecticide heptachlor; 95% CI = 1.19–1.89). Of the 18 pesticides significant in the unadjusted model, 14 were insecticides (i.e., 2 carbamates, 5 organochlorines, 5 OPs, and 2 pyrethroids) and 4 were herbicides. None showed a clear dose–response trend, although prevalence was increased for applicators with a history of high pesticide exposure events. The second AHS investigated 21,500 nonsmoking female spouses of HS-enrolled subjects. Valcin[1196] found an association of prevalent chronic bronchitis with the "ever" use of five pesticides. The herbicide paraquat had the highest OR (1.91; 95% CI = 1.02–3.55), followed by the herbicides cyanazine and MeBr, organochlorine insecticide DDT, and OP insecticide dichlorvos.

Any exposure to pesticides was also found to be positively associated with chronic bronchitis in a case–control study of Lebanese adults (OR = 2.46, 95% CI = 1.53–3.94).[1197] Regional exposure (i.e., living in a region heavily treated with pesticides), local exposure (i.e., living near a field treated with pesticides), and nonoccupational exposure (i.e., personal use) were all significantly associated with a diagnosis of chronic bronchitis. Occupational exposure resulted in the highest OR (15.92; 95% CI = 3.50–72.41). The lower score of this study resulted from its nonspecific exposure information.

Chronic bronchitis in children: A single study investigated exposure to pesticides during pregnancy and the development of chronic bronchitis and cough, as well as asthma, hay fever and allergies in children of Ontario farm families.[1194] No significant associations were reported between cough and bronchitis and prenatal exposure to agricultural pesticides. However, when stratified by sex, the risk of developing cough and bronchitis increased after exposure to insecticides, approaching significance for *female offspring* (OR = 2.29, 95% CI = 0.95–5.35). Similarly, the use of the herbicide *dicamba* (3,6-dichloro-2-methoxybenzoic acid) and the carbamate insecticide carbaryl increased the risk of developing cough and bronchitis when both sexes were analyzed together. Unfortunately, all data were collected retrospectively through the OFFHS, meaning that participants were asked to recall exposures that occurred in the past, and that information about the age of diagnosis of the children was not collected. These factors contributed to a relatively low quality score of 11 points out of 20.

Lung Function and Respiratory Symptoms

The review included 15 studies that investigated lung function, as measured by ventilator function tests and self-reported respiratory symptoms. All included studies focused on occupationally exposed adults in various settings, with the exception of one study of individuals residing in a pesticide spray zone. All studies were cross-sectional with the exception of the AHS and a study in Colorado, and included populations in Costa Rica, Spain, Croatia, Palestine, India, Sri Lanka, Philippines, Brazil, Ethiopia, and Lebanon.[1198]

Common measurements employed in the following studies included symptom questionnaires (to determine the presence or absence of chronic cough or phlegm, wheeze, diagnosis of asthma, chronic bronchitis, and dyspnea) and lung function measurements. Lung function measurements included: flow measurements, that is, maximum expiratory flow volume (MEFV), forced vital capacity (FVC), forced expiratory volume in the first second (FEV1), and the forced expiratory flow (FEF) at 75%, 50%, and the last 25% of the FVC (i.e., FEF25, FEF50, and FEF75); lung volume measurements, that is, total lung capacity (TLC), functional residual capacity (FRC), and residual volume (RV); and diffusing capacity, that is, diffusion capacity of the lung to absorb carbon monoxide (DLCO).

Twelve out of thirteen studies found significant positive associations between exposure to pesticides, primarily insecticides and herbicides, and the development of abnormal respiratory symptoms, as well as decreased performance on lung function tests. However, results were inconsistent across studies with respect to which lung tests were abnormal. In addition, many studies did not specify the pesticide(s) studies, making conclusions about the relative effect of different chemical groups difficult, and employed self-reported questionnaire-based exposure measurements.[1198]

Farm worker studies: Two Costa Rican studies investigated agricultural workers and respiratory outcomes. A high-quality cross-sectional study, score 17 out of 20 points, reported that for each unit increase in the total cumulative paraquat index (based on detailed work history), the odds of chronic cough increased by 1.8 (95% CI = 1.0–3.1), while the odds of shortness of breath with wheeze increased by 2.3 (95% CI = 1.2–5.1).[34] However, chronic bronchitis, persistent wheeze, and asthma were not associated with increased paraquat exposure and no difference in pulmonary function measures, interstitial thickening, or restrictive lung disease was seen between exposure groups. Fieten[1199] reported a significant association between exposure to chlorpyrifos and the development of wheeze and shortness of breath among exposed women. When the results were stratified by smoking status, nonsmoking women in this study had significantly increased odds of wheeze following exposure to chlorpyrifos (an OP insecticide), terbufos (an OP insecticide), and the herbicide paraquat (N,N'-dimethyl-4,4'-bipyridinium dichloride), with exposure to chlorpyrifos showing the strongest association (OR = 6.7, 95% CI = 1.6–28.0).

A cross-sectional study of 1379 Brazilian agricultural workers by Faria [1200] found that specific pesticide application activities were positively associated with symptoms of asthma and chronic respiratory disease, particularly among women, with associated ORs ranging from 1.82 (for washing clothes up to 2 days per month) to 2.54 (for cleaning equipment >2 days per month). Pesticide exposure included insecticides, fungicides, and herbicides, although no pesticide class was associated with symptoms. Peiris-John[152] compared Sri Lankan farmers with environmentally exposed freshwater fishermen and with marine fishermen living away from OP insecticide-sprayed areas. Farmers were found to have significantly lower FVC/FEV1 ratios than did both fishermen groups, with the FVC/FEV1 ratio decreasing during the spraying season compared with before the start of spraying. This study, which scored 16 out of 20 points, also reported that occupational, but not environmental, exposure led to decreased lung function results. A final cross-sectional study by Ejigu[1201] investigated health effects in Ethiopian farmers, and found that cough, phlegm, and wheeze were significantly more prevalent in farm workers than in controls ($p < 0.05$); however, the study received a very poor quality score and did not name specific pesticides.

A cross-sectional study in the Philippines of 102 cut-flower farmers[1202] exposed to 8 types of OPs reported symptoms of cough in 40% and abnormal peak flows in 88% of those examined. Red blood cell cholinesterase levels were depressed, but no baseline measurements were made. A cross-sectional study in Colorado of 761 farm residents and spouses[1203] with a history of pesticide poisoning examined respiratory symptoms, in addition to assessing lung function by spirometry in 196 individuals. In nonsmokers, pesticide poisoning remained a significant predictor of cough with an OR of 2.44 (95% CI $=$ 1.23–4.86).

Pesticide sprayer studies: A study of 89 pesticide sprayer and 25 farm worker controls in Granada, Spain, assessed respiratory function abnormalities following long-term exposure to pesticides; it used lung function tests in addition to investigating the contribution of paraoxonase (PON1) polymorphism on these outcomes.[159] The classes of pesticides most commonly used in the crop season studies were: insecticides (i.e., neonicotinoids, OPs, carbamates, and organochlorines), fungicides (e.g., dithiocarbamates), and herbicides (i.e., bipyridyls). Exposed subjects were more likely to experience irritative symptoms and tearing, while all other respiratory outcomes did not differ between groups. Paradoxically, sprayer status was associated with higher FEV1 and FEF 25%–75% and OP insecticide exposure was associated with higher FVC values, considered to be chance findings or a "healthy worker effect." Despite these results, exposure to endosulfan (an organochlorine insecticide) was associated with a significantly higher risk of respiratory symptoms (OR $=$ 3.68, 95% CI $=$ 1.16–11.68). In terms of restrictive lung changes, exposure to neonicotinoid insecticides was predictive of lower TLC ($p = 0.013$), RV ($p = 0.001$), and FRC ($p = 0.015$). Exposure to bipyridyls was associated with a fall in diffusing capacity, suggesting subtle changes in the alveolar–capillary membrane ($p = 0.041$).

This study[159] was the only one to analyze isoforms of PON1, a gene coding for an enzyme that hydrolyzes OP pesticides. It is hypothesized that the R isoform of PON1, which is related to polymorphism in PON1, is more highly active than other isoforms, and therefore will hydrolyze OP pesticides at a higher rate, resulting in a reduced effect of exposure. In the current study, subjects who carried the R isoform were found to have a three times lower risk of reporting symptoms related to occupational pesticide exposure, but did not differ in performance on lung function measures.

Two studies reported on the respiratory outcomes of male pesticide sprayers exposed to OP insecticides. Mekonnen and Agonafir[1204] report that in 109 Ethiopian farm sprayers, exposure to the OP insecticides chlorpyrifos, diazinon, and malathion resulted in reduced FVC and FEV1 in the youngest age group studies (15–24-year-olds), but did not show a significant positive association in the older age groups. This may indicate that the younger age group is more vulnerable to spraying. The prevalence of cough, breathlessness, wheeze, and phlegm did not differ significantly between exposed workers and the 69 farm area controls. Similarly, an Indian study of 376 agricultural pesticide sprayers expose to OP and carbamate insecticides found that pesticide sprayers had lower mean FVC, FEV1, FEV1/FVC ratio, and PEFR relative to 348 controls ($p < 0.001$).[1070] In addition, significantly more farmers were both diagnosed with COPD and showed an increased prevalence of respiratory symptoms, including wheeze, cough, loss of breath, and chronic bronchitis. However, the prevalence of asthma was not found to be increased in agricultural workers relative to controls.

A single study that investigated the lung function and respiratory symptoms of 250 male Palestinian farmers aged 22–77 years reported null associations.[167] This study had poor exposure attainment, using only two questions: one regarding how many hours subjects sprayed pesticides per year and the other inquiring as to current pesticide use. The use of personal protective equipment was also assessed. The authors suggest that the negative results may be attributable to an increased use of personal protective equipment in this population. However, the prevalence of chronic cough, wheeze, and breathlessness was found to be high.

Pesticide plant worker studies: Two studies with small sample size investigated the respiratory effects of occupational exposure to pesticides among pesticide plant workers and found associations with decreased lung function. In a Croatian study, female pesticide plant workers were at increased risk of chronic cough, dyspnea, and nasal catarrh.[1205] Male pesticide plant workers were more likely than unexposed controls to experience dyspnea and nasal catarrh. The authors did not specify the type of pesticide being processed by the plant. Both male and female pesticide workers showed significantly lower FVC, FEF50, and FEF25 relative to predicted values (control subjects were not tested), while the difference between observed and predicted values for FEV1 measurements was not significant. Similarly, workers exposed to pyrethroids and carbamate pesticides in Lebanon had increased odds of abnormal respiratory function, including FEV, FEV1/FVC ratio, and relative FEF 25%–75%, with the largest effect seen for relative FEF 25%–75% after adjusting for smoking status (OR = 16.5, 95% CI = 2.5–140.3).[151]

Agricultural health study: Hoppin[1206] analyzed data from the AHS to compare pesticide exposure and respiratory outcomes between farmers and commercial applicators. Farmers' reports of wheeze in the past year were positively associated with current use of: the herbicides alachlor, atrazine, EPTC, petroleum oil, and trifluralin; the OP insecticide malathion; and permethrin used on animals. Commercial applicators' reports of wheeze in the last year were positively associated with current use of the herbicide chlorimuron-ethyl and the OP insecticides dichlorvos and phorate. For both groups, significant dose–response trends were observed for both chlorimuron-ethyl and chlorpyrifos.

Nonoccupational: Petrie[1207] completed a before and after respiratory symptom survey of 292 residents of a New Zealand neighborhood sprayed with aerial *Bacillus thuringiensis* (Foray 48B0, an insecticide used to kill the larval stage of butterflies and moths). Resident health complaints increased after spraying; however, there was no significant increase in reports of cough or wheeze. The rate of resident reports of irritated throat did, however, double after spraying. This study received the second lowest score in this section, scoring only 9 out of 20 points, primarily due to using small area ecological exposure measurement as opposed to individual assessment.

Overview of Restrictive Lung Function Changes

Peiris-John,[152] as described above in the section "Lung Function and Respiratory Symptoms," found 25 Sri Lankan OP-exposed farmers to have significantly lower FVC, suggestive of restrictive lung function changes. The study pointed out that in this group, limited expansion of the thorax and/or reduced lung compliance were possibly due to thickening of the alveolar–capillary membrane.

As mentioned above by Schenker,[34] it is known that paraquat exposure in high doses causes oxidative damage to the lung, pulmonary fibrosis, and respiratory failure, raising concern that chronic, low-level exposures to paraquat may result in interstitial fibrosis. The study of 219 Cost a Rican paraquat sprayer, however, while finding increases in cough and in shortness of breath with wheeze, found no difference in pulmonary function measures indicative of interstitial thickening or restrictive lung disease between exposure groups.

An additional study, Hernandez[159] found that in 89 sprayers with exposure to bipyridilium herbicides, there was a fall in the diffusing capacity of the lungs, and that exposure to neonicotinoid insecticides was related to lower pulmonary volumes (i.e., TLC, RV, and FRC), suggestive of restrictive lung disease.

Respiratory Tract Infections

Three studies investigated the relationship between DDE and lower respiratory tract infections (LRTIs) in infants. All three were cohort studies scoring 15 points or above and assessed the association of both pre- and postnatal exposures with LRTIs. Two studies found an effect of *in utero* exposure, although one was positive only for upper respiratory tract infections (URTIs) but not for LRTIs, while the third paradoxically showed a protective effect of higher levels of postnatal DDE exposure.

A high-quality cohort study based in Catalonia, Spain, studied the association between maternal organochlorines and LRTIs in 521 infants.[1208] Only DDE was associated with LRTIs in infants during both the first 6 months of life (OR = 1.68, 95% CI = 1.06–2.66) and at age 14 months (OR = 1.52, 95% CI = 1.05–2.21). Results did not differ between infants who were breastfed and those who were not, suggesting that the effect occurred prenatally, a result that is consistent with other studies investigating pre- and postnatal pesticide exposure and respiratory outcomes. The authors suggest that this effect may be caused by immunologic suppression by DDE, which would suggest longer-lasting effects on both the immune and respiratory systems following exposure. This claim is corroborated by previous studies in both animals and humans linking increased DDE exposure to suppressed immune function.[1209–1211] Longer-lasting effects from LRTIs earlier in life may include the development of asthma.[1212]

A study in Nunavik, Canada, of Inuit infants and their mothers looked at both LRTI and URTI at 6 and 12 months of age.[1213] Adjusting for other confounders, they found that prenatal exposure to DDE in the 2nd quartile was associated with a 1.56 times higher risk of developing URTIs at age 6 months (95% CI = 1.05–2.33) and a 1.34 times higher risk at 12 months (95% CI = 1.00–1.78). No effect was seen in comparing the 3rd and 4th quartiles of exposure with the referent group. No significant association was shown between postnatal exposures and either type of respiratory infection. A third study by Glynn[1210] did not find a positive association in studying 190 pregnant women in Sweden and their infants at 3 months of age. Paradoxically, they found that higher levels of exposure to DDE were associated with a decreased risk of respiratory infections in infants (OR = 0.18, 95% CI = 0.06–0.60). It is important to note that the effects of other organochlorines such as CB congeners could not be differentiated from those of DDE in either of these studies.

Interstitial Lung Disease

Sarcoidosis: The association between environmental occupational exposures and sarcoidosis was investigated in a multicenter case–control study in the United States with 706 cases and matched controls.[1214] The diagnosis of sarcoidosis was found to be positively associated with exposure to insecticides at work, either agricultural or industrial (OR = 1.61, 95% CI = 1.13–2.28). Unfortunately, information about specific categories of insecticides was not collected and the exposure index was designed to capture environmental exposure broadly, resulting in the potential for misclassification of exposure causing a medium quality score.

Hypersensitivity pneumonitis: The most common type of hypersensitivity pneumonitis is farmer's lung, estimated by the Canadian Centre or Occupational Health and Safety to affect as many as 2%–10% of Canadian farm works.[1215] Hoppin[1206] studied farmer's lung among farmers in the AHS. "Ever" use of organochlorine or carbamate insecticides (e.g., DDT, lindane, and aldicarb) was associated with a diagnosis of farmer's lung (OR = 1.34, 95% CI = 1.04–1.74 and OR = 1.32, 95% CI = 1.03–1.68, respectively). High pesticide exposure events were also associated with increased odds of farmer's lung. High pesticide exposure events were defined as a positive answer to the question. "Have you ever had an incident or experience while using any type of pesticide which caused you unusually high personal exposure?" It was suggested that exposure to these pesticides may stimulate immune function and enhance the hypersensitivity effect of agents such as thermoactinomyces and other bacteria in moldy hay that cause farmer's lung. The study received a quality score of 14.5 out of 20 points and was the only study to look specifically at farmer's lung.

Limitations

Organic solvents present in many pesticide formulations may synergistically or independently contribute to outcomes. In addition, the generalizability of these studies to average environmental exposures is uncertain, as most studies were undertaken in the agricultural context. However, not only are pesticides frequently used indoors but also, as shown by Duramad,[155] indirect exposure through parental occupation or residential proximity are significant factors in the development of respiratory symptoms.

Overall, there is evidence that exposure to pesticides, and to OP or carbamate insecticides in particular, is associated with the development of respiratory symptoms and a spectrum of obstructive and restrictive lung diseases. Studies of asthma in children reported an association between maternal exposure to OP and organochlorine insecticides, as indicated by the presence of DDE, while respiratory tract infections in infants were linked to maternal exposure to organochlorine insecticide metabolites in two of three reviewed studies[1198] as suggested in Chapter 1.

Twelve studies investigated the effects of asthma, of which nine were of medium to high quality, found a positive association between OP and carbamate insecticides and atopic asthma, reporting a statistically significant OR above 2.0. This association was found for occupational, domestic, and environmental exposures, particularly after exposure to the OP insecticides parathion and coumaphos. While the possibility remains that these results could reflect the aggravation of pre existing asthma, asthma-related respiratory problems are nonetheless associated with pesticide exposure. In children, the evidence is consistent, all included studies finding a positive association between asthma and related respiratory problems and pesticide exposure, specifically maternal exposure to organochlorine insecticide (indicated by the presence of DDE), OP insecticide, biocide, and fungicide. Specifically, *in utero* and postnatal exposures in the first year of life were associated with asthma and wheeze up to 6 years of age. Breastfeeding was shown to have a protective effect, despite increased DDE levels in the infants.

The evidence linking chronic bronchitis to pesticide exposure in adults is not as prolific or as robust as that concerning asthma. While three studies did find a positive effect, the resulting ORs were below 2.0, with large CIs. In particular, two studies that used data from the AHS[1198] found an association between exposure to insecticides and the development of chronic bronchitis. Organochlorine, OP, carbamate, and pyrethroid insecticides all showed associations in farmers, while the herbicide paraquat showed the strongest relationship in their spouses through paraoccupational exposure. In addition, the only study to investigate chronic bronchitis in children found that only the association between insecticide exposure and the development of chronic cough and bronchitis approached significance.

Studies of occupational workers across many industries that use pesticides (e.g., farming, pesticide plant work, and pesticide spraying) showed a subtle yet persistent association between decreased lung function and exposure to a broad range of herbicides and insecticides. Exposure to the OP insecticide chlorpyrifos resulted in a particularly strong association with wheeze, chronic cough, and shortness of breath in many studies. Studying these occupationally exposed populations linked OP and carbamate insecticides in particular with decreased FEV1/FVC ratios, indicative of obstruction, as well as decreased FEF 25%–75%. These outcomes may reflect effects of chronic exposures and possibly direct toxic effects on the airways due to inhibition of acetylcholinesterase and resulting bronchoconstriction as well.

Exposure to neonicotinoid insecticides and organochlorine also showed associations with decreased lung function. The negative effects of pesticides on measures of lung function were more pronounced in younger study populations, and showed a dose–response relationship across exposure categories in studies able to assess this metric. Finally, sarcoidosis and farmer's lung (i.e., hypersensitivity pneumonitis) were both associated with occupational exposure to insecticides. The risk of developing farmer's lung was increased after exposure to organochlorine and carbamate insecticides in particular.

The relationship between respiratory tract infections in children and exposure to organochlorine insecticide (indicated by the presence of DDE) was assessed in three high-quality studies with varying results. Two studies showed a positive association between *in utero* exposure and respiratory tract infections, while a third paradoxically showed that higher levels during pregnancy were in fact protective.[1198] In addition, one study found that URTIs, but notLRTIs, in infants were associated with increased exposure to organochlorines.

The sum of the evidence would indicate that reducing or eliminating exposure to all pesticide types, and to OP and organochlorine insecticides in particular, would be prudent in both occupational and domestic settings with respect to preventing negative respiratory health consequences. While the study of agricultural occupational pesticide exposure and negative health outcomes remains challenging, the accumulation of studies showing significant associations between exposure and asthma, chronic obstructive lung diseases, and decreased lung function highlights the importance of reducing exposure when possible and utilizing proper personal protective equipment when exposure is unavoidable.

Discussion

January 2010 EDTA/DMPS challenge test was performed and it found to have elevated levels. The lead levels were 12 times the reference range. The patient began weekly chelation using 2000 mg IV EDTA immediately following intravenous glutathione. After several months, he experiences extreme fatigue and muscle soreness following the infusions. Chelation treatment was discontinued until January 2011. He experienced rhabdomyolysis with CPK at 1600, elevated myoglobin, cola-colored urine, and acute pain in both thigh and biceps muscle. Treatment was discontinued. He described that it was activated by EDTA, glutathione, and vitamins as well as hyperthermic conditions. The patient visited a neurologist who ruled out carnitine deficiency and suspected a glycogen storage disorder, biopsy suggested. A calcium deficiency was identified but it is still questionable as to whether or not the calcium deficiency may be contributing to the rhabdomyolysis, but hyperthermic conditions were still precipitating the symptoms.

The objective of this case presentation was to find the cause of the rhabdomyolysis in this particular patient. These triggers were found: EMF smart meter, Xanax, EDTA, serotonin syndrome, hypocalcemia, hyperthermia, heavy metals, autoimmune, hyperglycemic, hypothyroidism, and pesticides.

On February 28, 2014, 52,277 people reported to have side effects when taking Xanax. Among them, 308 people (0.59%) have rhabdomyolysis *in vitro*, alprazolam is bound (80%) to human serum protein. Serum albumin accounts for the majority of the binding. Drug products, along with their effect on increasing alprazolam AUC, are as follows: ketoconazole, 3.98-fold; itraconazole 2.70-fold; nefazodone 1.98-fold; fluvoxamine 1.96-fold (Contraindication: Xanax).

In addition to the relatively common (i.e., greater that 1%) untoward events enumerated in the table above, the following adverse events have been reported in association with the use of benzodiazepines: dystonia, irritability, concentration difficulties, anorexia, transient amnesia or memory impairment, loss of coordination, fatigue, seizures sedation, slurred speech, jaundice, musculoskeletal weakness, pruritus, diplopia, dysarthria, changes in libido, menstrual irregularities, incontinence, and urinary retention.

TREATMENT OF SENSITIVITY

Treatment for chemical sensitivity due to pesticide overload is not much different than treatment for other chemical sensitivities (Volume 5). It is clear that rigid avoidance of new exposures will aid in clearing. Heat depuration physical therapy appears to help remove these substances. Injection therapy is often necessary due to the allergic-like diathesis that occurs from inhalant, food, and chemical exposure to the insecticides. Also, nutrition[4] replacements to keep the detoxification systems fueled are extremely important. Immune modulation with a substance such as transfer factor, autogenous lymphocytic reaction,[4] and immune globulin[4] supplementations when indicated is often necessary in the severely damaged. In one series of patients who were treated in the ECU, we note that 26 of 33 patients decreased their organochlorine pesticide levels significantly ($p < 0.001$) with just avoidance alone. Oxygen therapy 2 hours per day at 4–8 L/minute can help[4]; so can autogenous lymphocytic factor if the T-cells are low, and gamma globulin supplementation if the subsets of gamma globulin are low.

Also, what was noted was that with time, even though they continued to improve, 18 patients developed new levels of toxics in their blood. Thus, new exposures were possible, but not probable, and since their symptoms continue to improve, we think that autotransfusion occurred from fat membrane stores. This autotransfusion factor has also been observed in patients undergoing heat depuration therapy and hospitalized ECU patients.

REFERENCES

1. Abdollahi, M., A. Ranjbar, S. Shadnia, S. Nikfar, A. Rezaie. 2004. Pesticides and oxidative stress: A review. *Med. Sci. Monit.* 10(6):141–147.
2. De Souza, A., R. Medeiros Ados, A. C. De Souza, M. Wink, I. R. Siqueira, M. B. Ferreira, L. Fernandes, M. P. Loayza Hidalgo, I. L. Torres. 2011. Evaluation of the impact of exposure to pesticides on the health of the rural population: Vale do Taquari, State of Rio Grande do Sul (Brazil). *Cien. Saude Colet.* 16(8):3519–3528.
3. Mostafalou, S., M. Abdollahi. 2012. Concerns of environmental persistence of pesticides and human chronic diseases. *Clin. Exp. Pharmacol.* 2(3):1000–1108.
4. Rea, W. J. 1994. *Chemical Sensitivity: Sources of Total Body Load, Vol.* 2, Boca Raton: Lewis Publishers.
5. Noncommunicable Diseases. World Health Organization. [Accessed February 29, 2016] http://www.who.int/topics/noncommunicable_diseases/en/
6. Randolph, T. G. 1962. *Human Ecology and Susceptibility to the Chemical Environment.* Springfield, IL: Charles C. Thomas Publisher.
7. Dickey, L. D. 1976. *Clinical Ecology.* Springfield, IL: Charles C. Thomas Publisher.
8. Rea, W. J. 1988. Inter-relationships between the environment and premenstrual syndrome. In *Functional Disorders of the Menstrual Cycle*, M. G. Brush and E. M. Goudsmit, eds. John Wiley & Sons Ltd.
9. Abou-Donia, M. B. 2003. Organophosphorus ester-induced chronic neurotoxicity. *Arch. Environ. Health: Int. J.* 58(8):484–497.
10. Hennies, K., H. P. Neitzke, H. Voigt. 2000. Mobile telecommunications and health.
11. National Coalition Against the Misuse of Pesticides (NCAMP). 1990. Chemical watch factsheet: Pyrethrins. *Pestic. You J.* 10(1):12.
12. Mueller-Beilschmidt, D. 1990. Toxicology and environmental fate of synthetic pyrethroids. *J. Pest. Reform.* 10(3):32–37.
13. National Coalition Against the Misuse of Pesticides (NCAMP). 1991. Chemical watch: Cyfluthrin. *Pestic. You J.* 11:5–6.
14. U.S. Environmental Protection Agency. 1982. *Recognition and Management of Pesticide Poisonings*, 3rd ed., p. 14. Washington, DC: U.S. Environmental Protection Agency. EPA-540/9-80-005.
15. O'Brien, R. D. 1960. *Toxic Phosphorus Esters: Chemistry, Metabolism, and Biological Effects.* New York: Academic Press.
16. Ecobichon, D. J. 1991. Toxic effects of pesticides. In *Casarett and Doull's Toxicology: The Basic Science of Poisons*, 4th ed., M. O. Amdur, J. Doull, C. D. Klaassen, eds., p. 576. New York: Pergamon Press.
17. Levine, W. G. 1983. Excretion mechanisms. In *Biological Basis of Detoxication*, J. Caldwell, W. B. Jakoby, eds., p. 260. New York: Academic Press.
18. Calabrese, E. J. 1980. *Nutrition and Environmental Health: The Influence of Nutritional Status on Pollutant Toxicity and Carcinogenicity, Vol. I, The Vitamins*, p. 61. New York: John Wiley & Sons.
19. Calabrese, E. J. 1980. *Nutrition and Environmental Health: The Influence of Nutritional Status on Pollutant Toxicity and Carcinogenicity, Vol. I, The Vitamins*, p. 62. New York: John Wiley & Sons.
20. Sipes, I. G., A. J. Gandolf. 1986. Biotransformation of toxicants. In *Casarett and Doull's Toxicology: The Basic Science of Poisons*, 3rd ed., C. D. Klaassen, M. O. Amdur, J. Doull, eds., p. 85. New York: Macmillan.
21. Calabrese, E. J. 1980. *Nutrition and Environmental Health: The Influence of Nutritional Status on Pollutant Toxicity and Carcinogenicity, Vol. I, The Vitamins*, p. 290. New York: John Wiley & Sons.
22. Feaster, J. P., C. H. Van Middleton, G. K. Davis. 1972. Zinc-DDT interrelationships in growth and reproduction in the rat. *J. Nutr.* 102:523–528.

23. Laseter, J. L., I. R. Deleon, W. J. Rea, J. R. Butler. 1983. Chlorinated hydrocarbon pesticides in environmentally sensitive patients. *Clin. Ecol.* 2:3–12.

24. Levine, M. J. 2007. *Pesticides: A Toxic Time Bomb in Our Midst.* Westport, CT: Praeger.

25. Torres-Sánchez, L., S. J. Rothenberg, L. Schnaas, M. E. Cebrián, E. Osorio, M. D. Hernández, R. M. García-Hernández, C. D. Rio-Garcia, M. S. Wolff, L. López-Carrillo. 2007. In utero p,p′-DDE exposure and infant neurodevelopment: A perinatal cohort in Mexico. *Environ. Health Perspect.* 115(3):435–439.

26. Torres-Sánchez, L., L. Schnaas, M. E. Cebrián, M. D. Hernández, E. O. Valencia, R. M. Hernández, L. López-Carrillo. 2009. Prenatal dichlorodiphenyldichloroethylene (DDE) exposure and neurodevelopment: A follow-up from 12 to 30 months of age. *Neurotoxicology* 30(6):1162–1165.

27. Eskenazi, B., A. R. Marks, A. Bradman, L. Fenster, C. Johnson, D. B. Barr, N. P. Jewell. 2006. In utero exposure to dichlorodiphenyltrichloroethane (DDT) and dichlorodiphenyldichloroethylene (DDE) and neurodevelopment among young Mexican American children. *Pediatrics* 118(1):233–241.

28. Ribas-Fitó, N., M. Torrent, D. Carrizo, J. Julvez, J. O. Grimalt, Sunyer J. 2007. Exposure to hexachlorobenzene during pregnancy and children's social behavior at 4 years of age. *Environ. Health Perspect.* 115(3):447–450.

29. Ribas-Fitó, N., M. Torrent, D. Carrizo, L. Munoz-Ortiz, J. Julvez, J. O. Grimalt, J. Sunyer. 2006. In utero exposure to background concentrations of DDT and cognitive functioning among preschoolers. *Am. J. Epidemiol.* 164(10):955–962.

30. Sagiv, S. K., J. K. Nugent, T. B. Brazelton, A. L. Choi, P. E. Tolbert, L. M. Altshul, S. A. Korrick. 2008. Prenatal organochlorine exposure and measures of behavior in infancy using the neonatal behavioral assessment scale (NBAS). *Environ. Health Perspect.* 116(5):666–673.

31. Sagiv, S. K., S. W. Thurston, D. C. Bellinger, P. E. Tolbert, L. M. Altshul, S. A. Korrick. 2010. Prenatal organochlorine exposure and behaviors associated with attention deficit hyperactivity disorder in school-aged children. *Am. J. Epidemiol.* 171(5):593–601.

32. Ribas-Fitó, N., E. Cardo, M. Sala, M. Eulalia de Muga, C. Mazon, A. Verdu, M. Kogevinas, J. O. Grimalt, J. Sunyer. 2003. Breastfeeding, exposure to organochlorine compounds, and neurodevelopment in infants. *Pediatrics* 111(5):580–585.

33. Saiyed, H. et al. 2003. Effect of endosulfan on male reproductive development. *Environ. Health Perspect.* 111(16):1958–1962.

34. Schenker, M. B., M. Stoecklin, K. Lee, R. Lupercio, R. Jorge Zeballos, P. Enright, T. Hennessy, L. A. Beckett. 2004. Pulmonary function and exercise-associated changes with chronic low-level paraquat exposure. *Am. J. Respir. Crit. Care. Med.* 170(7):773–779.

35. Bhatia, R., R. Shiau, M. Petreas, J. M. Weintraub, L. Farhang, B. Eskenazi. 2005. Organochlorine pesticides and male genital anomalies in the child health and development studies. *Environ. Health Perspect.* Feb; 113(2):220–224.

36. Villanueva, C. M. 2005. Atrazine in municipal drinking water and risk of low birth weight, preterm delivery, and small-for-gestational-age status. *Occup. Environ. Med.* 62(6):400–405.

37. Rauh, V. A., R. Garfinkel, F. P. Perera, H. F. Andrews, L. Hoepner, D. B. Barr, R. Whitehead, D. Tang, R. W. Whyatt. 2006. Impact of prenatal chlorpyrifos exposure on neurodevelopment in the first 3 years of life among inner-city children. *Pediatrics* 118(6).

38. Fenster, L., B. Eskenazi, M. Anderson, A. Bradman, A. Hubbard, D. B. Barr. 2007. In utero exposure to DDT and performance on the Brazelton neonatal behavioral assessment scale. *Neurotoxicology* 28(3):471–477.

39. Eggesbø, M., H. Stigum, M. P. Longnecker, A. Polder, M. Aldrin, O. Basso, C. Thomsen, J. Utne Skaare, G. Becher, P. Magnus. 2009. Levels of hexachlorobenzene (HCB) in breast milk in relation to birth weight in a Norwegian cohort. *Environ. Res.* 109(5):559–566.

40. Sunyer, J., M. Torrent, L. Munoz-Ortiz, N. Ribas-Fito, D. Carrizo, J. Grimalt, J. M. Anto, P. Cullinan. 2005. Prenatal dichlorodiphenyldichloroethylene (DDE) and asthma in children. *Environ. Health Perspect.* 113(12):1787–1790.

41. Sunyer, J., R. Garcia-Esteban, M. Alvarez, M. Guxens, F. Goñi, M. Basterrechea, M. Vrijheid, S. Guerra, J. M. Antó. 2010. DDE in mothers' blood during pregnancy and lower respiratory tract infections in their infants. *Epidemiology* 21(5):729–735.

42. Dallaire, F., E. Dewailly, G. Muckle, C. Vézina, S. W. Jacobson, J. L. Jacobson, P. Ayotte. 2004. Acute infections and environmental exposure to organochlorines in inuit infants from Nunavik. *Environ. Health Perspect.* 112:1359–1364.

43. Glynn, A., A. Thuvander, M. Aune, A. Johannisson, P. O. Darnerud, G. Ronquist, S. Cnattingius. 2008. Immune cell counts and risks of respiratory infections among infants exposed pre- and postnatally to organochlorine compounds: A prospective study. *Environ. Health.* 7:62.

44. Venners, S. A. 2005. Preconception serum DDT and pregnancy loss: A prospective study using a bio-marker of pregnancy. *Am. J. Epidemiol.* 162(8):709–16.

45. Carmichael, S. L., A. H. Herring, A. Sjödin, R. Jones, L. Needham, C. Ma, K. Ding, G. M. Shaw. 2010. Hypospadias and halogenated organic pollutant levels in maternal mid-pregnancy serum samples. *Chemosphere* 80(6):641–646.

46. Harley, K. G., A. R. Marks, A. Bradman, D. B. Barr, B. Eskenazi. 2008. DDT exposure, work in agriculture, and time to pregnancy among farmworkers in California. *J. Occup. Environ. Med.* 50(12):1335–1342.

47. Toft, G., A. M. Thulstrup, B. A. Jönsson, H. S. Pedersen, J. K. Ludwicki, V. Zvezday, J. P. Bonde. 2010. Fetal loss and maternal serum levels of 2,2′,4,4′,5,5′-hexachlorbiphenyl (CB-153) and 1,1-dichloro-2,2-bis(p-chlorophenyl)ethylene (p,p′-DDE) exposure: A cohort study in Greenland and two European populations. *Environ. Health* 9(1):22.

48. Axmon, A. 2006. Time to pregnancy as a function of male and female serum concentrations of 2,2′4,4′5,5′-hexachlorobiphenyl (CB-153) and 1,1-dichloro-2,2-bis (p-chlorophenyl)-ethylene (p,p′-DDE). *Human Reproduction* 21(3):657–665.

49. Brucker-Davis, F. et al. 2010. Exposure to selected endocrine disruptors and neonatal outcome of 86 healthy boys from Nice area (France). *Chemosphere* 81(2):169–176.

50. Salazar-García, F., E. Gallardo-Díaz, P. Cerón-Mireles, D. Loomis, V. H. Borja-Aburto. 2004. Reproductive effects of occupational DDT exposure among male malaria control workers. *Environ. Health Perspect.* 112(5):542–547.

51. Sugiura-Ogasawara, M., Y. Ozaki, S. Sonta, T. Makino, K. Suzumori. 2003. PCBs, hexachlorobenzene and DDE are not associated with recurrent miscarriage. *Am. J. Reprod. Immunol.* 50(6):485–489.

52. Waliszewski, S. M., R. M. Infanzon, S. G. Arroyo, R. V. Pietrini, O. Carvajal, P. Trujillo, P. M. Hopward-Jones. 2005. Persistent organochlorine pesticides levels in blood serum lipids in women bearing babies with undescended testis. *Bull. Environ. Contam. Toxicol.* 75(5):952–959.

53. Bianca, S., G. Li Volti, M. Caruso-Nicoletti, G. Ettore, P. Barone, L. Lupo, S. Li Volti. 2003. Elevated incidence of hypospadias in two Sicilian towns where exposure to industrial and agricultural pollutants is high. *Reprod. Toxicol.* 17(5):539–545.

54. Fernandez, M. F., B. Olmos, A. Granada, M. J. Lopez-Espinosa, J. M. Molina-Molina, J. M. Fernandez, M. Cruz, F. Olea-Serrano, N. Olea. 2007. Human exposure to endocrine-disrupting chemicals and prenatal risk factors for cryptorchidism and hypospadias: A nested case-control study. *Environ. Health Perspect.* 115(suppl. 1):8–14.

55. Sagiv, S. K., P. E. Tolbert, L. M. Altshul, S. A. Korrick. 2007. Organochlorine exposures during pregnancy and infant size at birth. *Epidemiology* 18(1):120–129.

56. Weiss, J. M., O. Bauer, A. Bluthgen, A. K. Ludwig, E. Vollersen, M. Kaisi, S. Al-Hasani, K. Diedrich, M. Ludwig. 2006. Distribution of persistent organochlorine contaminants in infertile patients from Tanzania and Germany. *J. Assist. Reprod. Genet.* 23(9–10):393–399.

57. Tadevosyan, N. S., A. E. Tadevosyan, M. S. Petrosyan. 2009. Pesticides application in agriculture of Armenia and their impact on reproductive function in humans. *NAMJ* 3(2):41–48.

58. Cocco, P., D. Fadda, A. Ibba, M. Melis, M. G. Tocco, S. Atzeri, G. Avataneo, M. Meloni, F. Monni, C. Flore. 2005. Reproductive outcomes in DDT applicators. *Environ. Res.* 98(1):120–126.

59. Cioroiu, M., D. Tarcau, R. Mocanu, S. Cucu-Man, B. Nechita, M. Luca. 2010. Organochlorine pesticides in colostrums in case of normal and preterm labor (IASI, Romania). *Sci. Total Environ.* 408(13):2639–2645.

60. Giordano, F. et al. 2010. Maternal exposures to endocrine disrupting chemicals and hypospadias in offspring. *Birth Defects Res. A Clin. Mol. Teratol.* 88(4):241–250.

61. Pathak, R., R. S. Ahmed, A. K. Tripathi, K. Guleria, C. S. Sharma, S. D. Makhijani, B. D. Banerjee. 2009. Maternal and cord blood levels of organochlorine pesticides: Association with preterm labor. *Clin. Biochem.* 42(7–8):746–749.

62. Siddiqui, M. K., S. Srivastava, S. P. Srivastava, P. K. Mehrotra, N. Mathur, I. Tandon. 2003. Persistent chlorinated pesticides and intra-uterine foetal growth retardation: A possible association. *Int. Arch. Occup. Environ. Health* 76(1):75–80.

63. Torres-Arreola, L., G. Berkowitz, L. Torres-Sanchez, M. Lopez-Cervantes, M. E. Cebrian, M. Uribe, L. Lopez-Carrillo. 2003. Preterm birth in relation to maternal organochlorine serum levels. *Ann. Epidemiol.* 13(3):158–162.

64. Wojtyniak, B. J. et al. and the INUENDO research group. 2010. Association of maternal serum concentrations of 2,2′,4,4′5,5′-hexachlorobiphenyl (CB-153) and 1,1-dichloro-2,2-bis (p-chlorophenyl)-ethylene (p,p′-DDE) levels with birth weight, gestational age and preterm births in Inuit and European populations. *Environ. Health* 9:56.

65. Gladen, B. C., Z. A. Shkiryak-Nyzhnyk, N. Chyslovska, T. D. Zadorozhnaja, R. E. Little. 2003. Persistent organochlorine compounds and birth weight. *Ann. Epidemiol.* 13(3):151–157.

66. Jusko, T. A., T. D. Koepsell, R. J. Baker, T. A. Greenfield, E. J. Willman, M. J. Charles, S. W. Teplin, H. Checkoway, I. Hertz-Picciotto. 2006. Maternal DDT exposures in relation to fetal and 5-year growth. *Epidemiology* 17(6):692–700.

67. Neta, G., L. R. Goldman, D. Barr, B. J. Apelberg, F. R. Witter, R. U. Halden. 2011. Fetal exposure to chlordane and permethrin mixtures in relation to inflammatory cytokines and birth outcomes. *Environ. Sci. Technol.* 45(4):1680–1687.

68. Pierik, F. H., M. A. Klebanoff, J. W. Brock, M. P. Longnecker. 2007. Maternal pregnancy serum level of heptachlor epoxide, hexachlorobenzene, and beta-hexachlorocyclohexane and risk of cryptorchidism in offspring. *Environ. Res.* 105(3):364–369.

69. Farhang, L., J. M. Weintraub, M. Petreas, B. Eskenazi, R. Bhatia. 2005. Association of DDT and DDE with birth weight and length of gestation in the child health and development studies, 1959–1967. *Am. J. Epidemiol.* 162(8):717–725.

70. Brucker-Davis, F., K. Wagner-Mahler, I. Delattre, B. Ducot, P. Ferrari, A. Bongain, J. Y. Kurzenne, J. C. Mas, P. Fénichel; Cryptorchidism Study Group from Nice Area. 2008. Cryptorchidism at birth in Nice area (France) is associated with higher prenatal exposure to PCBs and DDE, as assessed by colostrum concentrations. *Hum. Reprod.* 23(8):1708–1718.

71. Cole, D. C., B. Wainman, L. H. Sanin, J. P. Weber, H. Muggah, S. Ibrahim. 2006. Environmental contaminant levels and fecundability among non-smoking couples. *Reprod. Toxicol* 22(1):13–19.

72. Fenster, L., B. Eskenazi, M. Anderson, A. Bradman, K. Harley, H. Hernandez, A. Hubbard, D. B. Barr. 2006. Association of in utero organochlorine pesticide exposure and fetal growth and length of gestation in an agricultural population. *Environ. Health Perspect.* 114(4):597–602.

73. Gesink Law, D. C., M. A. Klebanoff, J. W. Brock, D. B. Dunson, M. P. Longnecker. 2005. Maternal serum levels of polychlorinated biphenyls and 1,1-dichloro-2,2-bis(p-chlorophenyl)ethylene (DDE) and time to pregnancy. *Am. J. Epidemiol.* 162(6):523–532.

74. Longnecker, M. P., B. C. Gladen, L. A. Cupul-Uicab, S. P. Romano-Riquer, J. P. Weber, R. E. Chapin, M. Herandez-Avila. 2007. In utero exposure to the antiandrogen 1,1-dichloro-2,2-bis(p-chlorophenyl) ethylene (DDE) in relation to anogenital distance in male newborns from Chiapas, Mexico. *Am. J. Epidemiol.* 165(9):1015–1022.

75. Damgaard, I. N., N. E. Skakkebaek, J. Toppari, H. E. Virtanen, H. Shen, K. W. Schramm, J. H. Petersen, T. K. Jensen, K. M. Main. 2006. Persistent pesticides in human breast milk and cryptorchidism. *Environ. Health Perspect.* 114(7):1133–1138.

76. Khanjani, N., M. R. Sim. 2006. Maternal contamination with dichlorodiphenyltrichloroethane and reproductive outcomes in an Australian population. *Environ. Res.* 101(3):373–379.

77. Khanjani, N., M. R. Sim. 2006. Reproductive outcomes of maternal contamination with cyclodiene insecticides, hexachlorobenzene and beta-benzene hexachloride. *Sci. Total Environ.* 368(2–3):557–564.

78. Levario-Carrillo, M., D. Amato, P. Ostrosky-Wegman, C. Gonzalez-Horta, Y. Corona, L. H. Sanin. 2004. Relation between pesticide exposure and intrauterine growth retardation. *Chemosphere* 55(10):1421–1427.

79. Ochoa-Acuna, H., J. Frankenberger, L. Hahn, C. Carbajo. 2009. Drinking-water herbicide exposure in Indiana and prevalence of small-for-gestational-age and preterm delivery. *Environ. Health Perspect.* 117(10):1619–1624.

80. Puertas, R. et al. 2010. Prenatal exposure to mirex impairs neurodevelopment at age of 4 years. *Neurotoxicology* 31(1):154–160.

81. Rea, W. J., H. C. Liang. 1991. Effects of pesticides on the immune system. *J. Nutr. Med.* 2:399–410.

82. Radomski, J. L., W. B. Deichmann, A. A. Rey, T. Merkin. 1971. Human pesticide blood levels as a measure of body burden and pesticide exposure. *Toxicol. Appl. Pharmacol.* 20:175–185.

83. Dale, W. E., A. Curley, C. Cueto Jr. 1966. Hexane extractable chlorinated insecticides in human blood. *Life Sci.* 5:47–54.

84. Hunter, C. G., J. Robinson, M. Roberts. 1969. Pharmacodynamics of dieldrin (HEOD). *Arch. Environ. Health* 18:12–21.

85. Brow, V. K. H., C. G. Hunter, A. Richardson. 1964. A blood test diagnostic of exposure to aldrin and dieldrin. *Br. J. Ind. Med.* 21:283–286.

86. Garrettson, L. K., A. Curley. 1969. Dieldrin: Studies in a poisoned child. *Arch. Environ. Health* 19:814–822.

87. Wislocki, P. G., G. T. Miwam, A. Y. H. Lu. 1980. Reactions catalyzed by the cytochrome P-450 system. In *Enzymatic Basis of Detoxication*, Vol. I, W. B. Jakoby, ed., p. 150. Orlando: Academic Press.

88. Hunter, C. G., J. Robinson, A. Richardson. 1963. Chlorinated insecticide content of human body fat in southern England. *Br. Med. J.* 1:221–224.

89. Hoffman, W. S., H. Adler, W. I. Fishbein, F. C. Bauer. 1967. Relation of pesticide concentrations in fat to pathological changes in tissues. *Arch. Environ. Health* 15:758–765.

90. Hayes, W. J., A. Curley. 1968. Storage and excretion of dieldrin and related compounds. *Arch. Environ. Health* 16:155–162.

91. Kazantzik, G., A. I. G. McLaughlin, P. F. Prior. 1964. Poisoning in industrial workers by the insecticide aldrin. *Br. J. Ind. Med.* 21:46–51.

92. Avar, P., G. Czegledi-Janko. 1970. Occupational exposure to aldrin: Clinical and laboratory findings. *Br. J. Ind. Med.* 27:279–282.

93. Dale, W. E., A. Curley, C. Cuero Jr. 1966. Hexane extractable chlorinated insecticides in human blood. *Life Sci.* 5:47–54.

94. Bell, A. 1960. Aldrin poisoning: A case report. *Med. J. Aust.* 2:698–700.

95. Baselt, R. C. 1982. *Disposition of Toxic Drugs and Chemicals in Man*, 2nd ed., pp. 21–22. Davis, CA: Biomedical Publications.

96. Baselt, R. C. 1982. *Disposition of Toxic Drugs and Chemicals in Man*, 2nd ed., pp. 293–294. Davis, CA: Biomedical Publications.

97. Davies, G. M., I. Lewis. 1956. Outbreak of food-poisoning from bread made of chemically contaminated flour. *Br. Med. J.* 2:393–398.

98. Weeks, D. E. 1967. Endrin-food-poisoning. *Bull. World Health Organ.* 37:499–512.

99. Rea, W. J. 1992. *Chemical Sensitivity*, Vol. 1, pp. 47, 155. Boca Raton, FL: Lewis Publishers.

100. Harrington, J. M., E. L. Baker Jr., D. S. Folland, J. W. Saucier, S. H. Sandifer. 1978. Chlordane contamination of municipal water system. *Environ. Res.* 15:155–159.

101. Collins, I. S., W. A. Crawford. 1976. Chlordane. *Med. J. Aust.* 1:762.

102. Furie, B., S. Trubowitz. 1976. Insecticides and blood dyscrasias. *J. Am. Med. Assoc.* 235:1720–1722.

103. Baxter, D. 1988. *Chlordane: A Pesticide Review, Health and Environmental Effects and Alternatives*, p. 4. Washington, DC: National Coalition Against the Misuse of Pesticides.

104. Feaster, J. P., C. H. Van Middelem, G. K. Davis. 1972. Zinc-DDT interrelationships in growth and reproduction in the rat. *J. Nutr.* 102:523–528.

105. Stehr-Green, P. A., J. C. Wohleb, W. Royce, S. L. Head. 1988. An evaluation of serum pesticide residue levels and liver function in persons exposed to dairy products contaminated with heptachlor. *JAMA* 259(3):372–377.

106. Schmid, R. 1960. Cutaneous porphyria in Turkey. *N. Engl. J. Med.* 263:397–398.

107. De Matteis, F., B. E. Prior, C. Rimington. 1961. Nervous and biochemical disturbances following hexachlorobenzene intoxication. *Nature* 191:363–366.

108. Richter, E., A. Schmid. 1976. Hexachlorbenolgehalt im Vollblut von Kindern. *Arch. Toxicol.* 35:141–147.

109. Siyali, D. S. 1972. Hexachlorobenzene and other organochloride pesticides in human blood. *Med. J. Aust.* 1:1063–1066.

110. Burns, J. E., F. M. Miller, E. D. Gomes, R. A. Albert. 1974. Hexachlorobenzene exposure from contaminated DCPA in vegetable spraymen. *Arch. Environ. Health* 29:192–194.

111. Burns, J. E., F. M. Miller. 1975. Hexachlorobenzene contamination: Its effects in a Louisiana population. *Arch. Environ. Health* 30:44–48.

112. Currier, M. F., C. D. McClimans, G. Barna-Lloyd. 1980. Hexachlorobenzene blood levels and the health status of men employed in the manufacture of chlorinated solvents. *J. Toxicol. Environ. Health* 6:367–377.

113. Schmid, R. 1960. Cutaneous porphyria in Turkey. *N. Engl. J. Med.* 263:397–398.

114. De Matteis, F., B. E. Prior, C. Rimington. 1961. Nervous and biochemical disturbances following hexachlorobenzene intoxication. *Nature* 191:363–366.

115. Cam, C., G. Nigogosyan. 1963. Acquired toxic cutanea tarda due to hexachlorobenzene. *JAMA* 183:90–93.

116. Peters, H. A. 1976. Hexachlorobenzene poisoning in Turkey. *Fed Proc.* 35(12):2400–2403.

117. Courtney, K. D. 1979. Hexachlorobenzene (HCB): A review. *Environ. Res.* 20:225–266.

118. Baselt, R. C. 1982. *Disposition of Toxic Drugs and Chemicals in Man*, 2nd ed., p. 370. Davis, CA: Biomedical Publications.

119. Milby, T. H., A. J. Samuels, F. Ottoboni. 1968. Human exposure to lindane: Blood lindane levels as a function of exposure. *J. Occup. Med.* 10:584–587.

120. Radomski, J. L., W. B. Deichmann, A. A. Rey, T. Merkin. 1971. Human pesticide blood levels as a measure of body burden and pesticide exposure. *Toxicol. Appl. Pharmacol.* 20:175–185.

121. Baumann, K., J. Angerer, R. Heinrich, G. Lehnert. 1980. Occupational exposure to hexachlorocyclohexane. I Body burden of HCH-isomers. *Int. Arch. Occup. Environ. Health* 47:119–127.

122. Ginsburg, C. M., W. Lowry, J. S. Reisch. 1977. Absorption of lindane (gamma benzene hexachloride) in infants and children. *J. Pediatr.* 91:998–1000.

123. Czegledi-Janko, C., P. Avar. 1970. Occupational exposure to lindane: Clinical laboratory findings. *Br. J. Ind. Med.* 27:283–286.

124. Loge, J. P. 1965. Aplastic anemia following exposure to benzene hexachloride (lindane). *JAMA.* 193:110–114.

125. West, I. 1967. Lindane and hematologic reactions. *Arch. Environ. Health* 15:97–101.

126. Morgan, D. P., E. M. Stockdale, R. J. Roberts, A. W. Walter. 1980. Anemia associated with exposure to lindane. *Arch. Environ. Health* 35:307–310.

127. Danopoulos, E., K. Mellissinos, G. Katsas. 1953. Serious poisoning by hexachlorocyclohexane. *Arch. Ind. Hyg. Occup. Med.* 8:582–587.

128. Murphy, S. D. 1986. Toxic effects of pesticides. In *Casarett and Doull's Toxicology: The Basic Science of Poisons*, 3rd ed., C. D. Klaasen, M. O. Amdur, J. Doull, eds., p. 549. New York: Macmillan.

129. Young, J. F., T. J. Haley. 1978. A pharmacokinetic study of pentachlorophenol poisoning and the effect of forced diuresis. *Clin. Toxicol.* 12:41–48.

130. Kuratsune, M. 1976. Epidemiologic studies on Yusho. In *PCB Poisoning and Pollution*, K. Higuchi, ed., p. 231. New York: Academic Press.

131. Proctor, N. H., J. P. Hughes. 1978. *Chemcial Hazards of the Workplace*, p. 404. Philadelphia: J. B. Lippincott.

132. Armstrong, R. W., E. R. Eichner, D. E. Klein, W. F. Barthel, J. V. Bennett, V. Jonsson, H. Bruce, L. E. Loveless. 1969. Pentachlorophenol poisoning in a nursery for newborn infants. II. Epidemiologic and toxicologic studies. *J. Pediatr.* 75:317–325.

133. U.S. Environmental Protection Agency. 1982. *Recognition and Management of Pesticide Poisonings*, 3rd ed., p. 19. Washington, DC: U.S. Environmental Protection Agency. EPA-540/9-80-005.

134. Gaines, T. B., R. D. Kimbrough. 1970. Oral toxicity of mirex in adult and suckling rats. *Arch. Environ. Health* 21:7–14.

135. Gaines, T. B. 1969. Acute toxicity of pesticides. *Toxicol. Appl. Pharmacol.* 14:515–534.

136. Innes, J. R. M. et al. 1969. Bioassay of pesticides and industrial chemicals for tumorigenicity in mice: A preliminary note. *J. Natl. Cancer Inst.* 42:1101–1114.

137. Waters, E. M., J. E. Huff, H. B. Gerstner. 1977. Mirex: An overview. *Environ. Res.* 14:212–222.

138. Menzer, R. E., J. O. Nelson. 1986. Water and soil pollutants. In *Casarett and Doull's Toxicology: The Basic Science of Poisons*, 3rd ed., C. D. Klaasen, M. O. Amdur, J. Doull, eds., p. 549. New York: Macmillan.

139. Anon. 1976. *Preliminary Report of Kepone Levels Found in Human Blood from the General Population of Hopewell, Virginia*. Research Triangle Park, NC: Health-Effects Research Laboratory, U.S. Environmental Protection Agency.

140. Adir, J., Y. H. Caplan, B. C. Thompson. 1978. Kepone serum half-life in humans. *Life Sci.* 22:699–702.

141. Dutheil, F., P. Beaune, C. Tzourio, M. Loriot, A. Elbaz. 2010. Interaction between ABCB1 and professional exposure to organochlorine insecticides in Parkinson disease. *Arch. Neurol.* 67(6).

142. Carson, R., L. Darling, L. Darling. 1962. *Silent Spring*. Boston: Houghton Mifflin.

143. Endosulfan to Be Banned, Poses 'unacceptable Risks' to Farm Workers and Wildlife, EPA Says—Environmental Health News. [Accessed March 02, 2016] http://www.environmentalhealthnews.org/ehs/news/endosulfan-ban

144. U.S. Environmental Protection Agency. 1982. *Recognition and Management of Pesticide Poisonings*, 3rd ed., p. 1. Washington, DC: U.S. Environmental Protection Agency. EPA-540/9-80-005.

145. U.S. Food and Drug Administration. 1987. *Food and Drug Administration Pesticide Program: Residues in foods*. Washington, DC: U.S. Food and Drug Administration.

146. Greenlee, A. R., T. E. Arbuckle, P. H. Chyou. 2003. Risk factors for female infertility in an agricultural region. *Epidemiology* 14(4):429–436.

147. Eskenazi, B., K. Harley, A. Bradman, E. Weltzien, N. P. Jewell, D. B. Barr, C. E. Furlong, N. T. Holland. 2004. Association of in utero organophosphate pesticide exposure and fetal growth and length of gestation in an agricultural population. *Environ. Health Perspect.* 112(10):1116–1124.

148. Mekonnen, Y. 2002. Pesticide sprayers' knowledge, attitude and practice of pesticide use on agricultural farms of ethiopia. *Occup. Med.* 52(6):311–15.

149. Ruckart, P. Z., K. Kakolewski, F. J. Bove, W. E. Kaye. 2003. Long-term neurobehavioral health effects of methyl parathion exposure in children in mississippi and ohio. *Environ. Health Perspect.* 112(1):46–51.

150. Whyatt, R. M. et al. 2004. Prenatal insecticide exposures and birth weight and length among an urban minority cohort. *Environ. Health Perspect.* 112(10):1125–1132.
151. Salameh, P., M. Waked, I. Baldi, P. Brochard. 2005. Spirometric changes following the use of pesticides. *East Mediterr. Health J.* 11(1–2):126–136.
152. Peiris-John, R. J., D. K. Ruberu, A. R. Wickremasinghe, W. van-der-Hoek. 2005. Low-level exposure to organophosphate pesticides leads to restrictive lung dysfunction. *Respir. Med.* 99(10):1319–1324.
153. Young, J. G., B. Eskenazi, E. A. Gladstone, A. Bradman, L. Pedersen, C. Johnson, D. B. Barr, C. E. Furlong, N. T. Holland. 2005. Association between in utero organophosphate pesticide exposure and abnormal reflexes in neonates. *Neurotoxicology* 26(2):199–209.
154. Grandjean, P., R. Harari, D. B. Barr, F. Debes. 2006. Pesticide exposure and stunting as independent predictors of neurobehavioral deficits in Ecuadorian school children. *Pediatrics* 117(3):e546–e556.
155. Duramad, P., K. Harley, M. Lipsett, A. Bradman, B. Eskenazi, N. T. Holland, I. B. Tager. 2006. Early environmental exposures and intracellular Th1/Th2 cytokine profiles in 24-month-old children living in an agricultural area. *Environ. Health Perspect.* 114(12):1916–1922.
156. Wolff, M. S., S. Engel, G. Berkowitz, S. Teitelbaum, J. Siskind, D. B. Barr, J. Wetmur. 2007. Prenatal pesticide and PCB exposures and birth outcomes. *Pediatr. Res.* 61(2):243–250.
157. Engel, S. M., G. S. Berkowitz, D. B. Barr, S. L. Teitelbaum, J. Siskind, S. J. Meisel, J. G. Wetmur, M. S. Wolff. 2007. Prenatal organophosphate metabolite and organochlorine levels and performance on the Brazelton Neonatal Behavioral Assessment Scale in a multiethnic pregnancy cohort. *Am. J. Epidemiol.* 165(12):1397–1404.
158. Eskenazi, B., A. R. Marks, A. Bradman, K. Harley, D. B. Barr, C. Johnson, N. Morga, N. P. Jewell. 2007. Organophosphate pesticide exposure and neurodevelopment in young Mexican-American children. *Environ. Health Perspect.* 115(5):792–798.
159. Hernandez, A. F., I. Casado, G. Pena, F. Gil, E. Villanueva, A. Pla. 2008. Low level of exposure to pesticides leads to lung dysfunction in occupationally exposed subjects. *Inhal. Toxicol.* 20(9):839–849.
160. Sanchez-Lizardi, P., M. K. O'Rourke, R. J. Morris. 2008. The effects of organophosphate pesticide exposure on Hispanic children's cognitive and behavioral functioning. *J. Pediatr. Psychol.* 33(1):91–101.
161. Handal, A. J., S. D. Harlow, J. Breilh, B. Lozoff. 2008. Occupational exposure to pesticides during pregnancy and neurobehavioral development of infants and toddlers. *Epidemiology* 19(6):851–859.
162. Boers, D. et al. 2008. Asthmatic symptoms after exposure to ethylenebisdithiocarbamates and other pesticides in the Europit field studies. *Hum. Exp. Toxicol.* 27(9):721–727.
163. Abdel Rasoul, G. M., M. E. Abou Salem, A. A. Mechael, O. M. Hendy, D. S. Rohlman, A. A. Ismail. 2008. Effects of occupational pesticide exposure on children applying pesticides. *Neurotoxicology* 29(5):833–838.
164. Lu, C., C. Essig, C. Root, D. S. Rohlman, T. McDonald, S. Sulzbacher. 2009. Assessing the association between pesticide exposure and cognitive development in rural Costa Rican children living in organic and conventional coffee farms. *Int. J. Adolesc. Med. Health* 21(4):609–621.
165. Barr, D. B., C. V. Ananth, X. Yan, S. Lashley, J. C. Smulian, T. A. Ledoux, P. Hore, M. G. Robson. 2010. Pesticide concentrations in maternal and umbilical cord sera and their relation to birth outcomes in a population of pregnant women and newborns in New Jersey. *Sci. Total Environ.* 408(4):790–795.
166. Eskenazi, B., K. Huen, A. Marks, K. G. Harley, A. Bradman, D. B. Barr, N. Holland. 2010. PON1 and neurodevelopment in children from the CHAMACOS study exposed to organophosphate pesticides in utero. *Environ. Health Perspect.* 118(12):1775–1781.
167. Abu Sham'a, F., M. Skogstad, K. Nijem, E. Bjertness, P. Kristensen. 2010. Lung function and respiratory symptoms in male Palestinian farmers. *Arch. Environ. Occup. Health* 65(4):191–200.
168. Marks, A. R., K. Harley, A. Bradman, K. Kogut, D. B. Barr, C. Johnson, N. Calderon, B. Eskenazi. 2010. Organophosphate pesticide exposure and attention in young Mexican-American children: The CHAMACOS study. *Environ. Health Perspect.* 118(12):1768–1774.
169. Bouchard, M. F., D. C. Bellinger, R. O. Wright, M. G. Weisskopf. 2010. Attention-deficit/hyperactivity disorder and urinary metabolites of organophosphate pesticides. *Pediatrics* 125(6):e1270–e1277.
170. Harari, R., J. Julvez, K. Murata, D. Barr, D. C. Bellinger, F. Debes, P. Grandjean. 2010. Neurobehavioral deficits and increased blood pressure in school-age children prenatally exposed to pesticides. *Environ. Health Perspect.* 118(6):890–896.
171. Xu, X., W. N. Nembhard, H. Kan, G. Kearney, Z. J. Zhang, E. O. Talbott. 2011. Urinary trichlorophenol levels and increased risk of attention deficit hyperactivity disorder among US school-aged children. *Occup. Environ. Med.* 68(8):557–561.
172. Horton, M. K., A. Rundle, D. E. Camann, D. B. Barr, V. A. Rauh, R. M. Whyatt. 2011. Impact of prenatal exposure to piperonyl butoxide and permethrin on 36-month neurodevelopment. *Pediatrics* 127(3):e699–e706.

173. Bouchard, M. F. et al. 2011. Prenatal exposure to organophosphate pesticides and IQ in 7-year old children. *Environ. Health Perspect.* 119(8):1189–1195.

174. Rauh, V., S. Arunajadai, M. Horton, F. Perera, L. Hoepner, D. B. Barr, R. Whyatt. 2011. 7-year neurodevelopmental scores and prenatal exposure to chlorpyrifos, a common agricultural pesticide. *Environ. Health Perspect.* 119(8):1196–1201.

175. Engel, S. M., J. Wetmur, J. Chen, C. Zhu, D. B. Barr, R. L. Canfield, M. S. Wolff. 2011. Prenatal exposure to organophosphates, paraoxonase 1, and cognitive development in childhood. *Environ. Health Perspect.* 119(8):1182–1188.

176. Handal, A. J., S. D. Harlow. 2009. Employment in the Ecuadorian cut-flower industry and the risk of spontaneous abortion. *BMC Int. Health Hum. Rights* 9:25.

177. Waller, S. A., K. Paul, S. E. Peterson, J. E. Hitti. 2010. Agricultural-related chemical exposures, season of conception, and risk of gastroschisis in Washington State. *Am. J. Obstet. Gynecol.* 202(3):241.e1–241.e6.

178. Chevrier, C., G. Limon, C. Monfort, F. Rouget, R. Garlantezec, C. Petit, G. Durand, S. Cordier. 2011. Urinary biomarkers of prenatal atrazine exposure and adverse birth outcomes in the PELAGIE birth cohort. *Environ. Health Perspect.* 119(7):1034–1041.

179. Koestner, A., S. Norton. 1991. Nervous system. In *Handbook of Toxicologic Pathology*, W. M. Haschek, C. G. Rousseaux, eds., p. 653. San Diego: Academic Press.

180. Murphy, S. D. 1986. Toxic effects of pesticides. In *Casarett and Doull's Toxicology: The Basic Science of Poisons*, 3rd ed., C. D. Klaassen, M. O. Amdur, J. Doull, eds., p. 528. New York: Macmillan.

181. Miyata, M., T. Namba, K. Horiuchi, S. Ishikawa. 1991. Participation of environmental factors in allergic conjunctivitis. *Neurophthalmol. Jpn.* 8:171–176.

182. Hayes, W. J. Jr., ed. 1982. *Pesticides Studied in Man*, pp. 284–425. Baltimore, MD: Williams & Wilkins.

183. Murphy, S. D. 1986. Toxic effects of pesticides. In *Casarett and Doull's Toxicology: The Basic Science of Poisons*, 3rd ed., C. D. Klaassen, M. O. Amdur, J. Doull, eds., p. 531. New York: Macmillan.

184. Johnson, M. K. 1982. The target of initiation of delayed neurotoxicity by organophosphorus esters: Biochemical studies and toxicological applications. *Rev. Biochem. Toxicol.* 4:141–212.

185. Ecobichon, D. J. 1982. Organophosphorus ester insecticides. In *Pesticides and Neurological Diseases*, D. J. Ecobichon, R. M. Joy, eds., p. 151. Boca Raton, FL: CRC Press.

186. Chabra, M. L., G. C. Sepaha, S. R. Jain, R. R. Bhagwat, J. D. Khandekar. 1970. ECG and necropsy changes in organophosphorus compound (malathion) poisoning. *Indian J. Med. Sci.* 24:424–429.

187. Khandekar, J. D. 1971. Organophosphate poisoning. *JAMA.* 217:1864.

188. Ludomirsky, A. et al. 1982. Q-T prolongation and polymorphous ("Torsade de Pointes") ventricular arrhythmias associated with organophysphorus insecticide. *Am. J. Cardiol.* 49:1154–1158.

189. Hayes, W. J. Jr. 1982. *Pesticides Studied in Man*, pp. 284–434. Baltimore, MD: Williams & Wilkins.

190. Xintaras, C., J. R. Burg, S. Tanaka, S. T. Lee, B. L. Johnson, C. A. Cotrrill, J. Bender. 1978. *NIOSH Health Survey of Velsicol Pesticide Workers: Occupational Exposure to Leptophos and Other Chemicals*. Washington, DC: U.S. Government Printing Office.

191. Namba, T., C. T. Notle, J. Jackrel, D. Grob. 1971. Poisoning due to organophosphate insecticides: Acute and chronic manifestations. *Am. J. Med.* 50:475–492.

192. Morgan, D. P. 1982. *Recognition and Management of Pesticide Poisoning*, 3rd ed., Washington, DC: U.S. Environmental Protection Agency.

193. Hayes, W. J. 1982. *Pesticides Studied in Man*. Baltimore: Williams & Wilkins.

194. Cherniack, M. G. 1986. Organophosphorus esters and polyneuropathy. *Ann. Intern. Med.* 104(2):264–266.

195. Johnson, M. K. 1980. The mechanism of delayed neuropathy caused by some organophosphorus esters: Using the understanding to improve safety. *J. Environ. Sci. Health, Part B* 15(6):823–41.

196. Soliman, S. A., J. Farmer, A. Curley. 1982. Is delayed neurotoxicity a property of all organophosphorus compounds? A study with a model compound: Parathion. *Toxicology* 23(4):267–79.

197. Wilson, B. W., M. Hooper, E. Chow, J. N. Seiber, J. B. Knaak. 1985. Assessment of farmworker risk from organophosphate-induced delayed neuropathy. *Discussion of Risk Assessment ACS Symposium Series Dermal Exposure Related to Pesticide Use*, pp. 479–491.

198. Xintaras, C., J. R. Burg, S. Tanaka, S. T. Lee, B. L. Johnson, C. A. Cotrrill, J. Bender. 1978. *NIOSH Health Survey of Velsicol Pesticide Workers: Occupational Exposure to Leptophos and Other Chemicals*. Washington, DC: U.S. Government Printing Office.

199. Lotti, M., A. Moretto, R. Zoppellari, R. Dainese, N. Rizzuto, G. Barusco. 1986. Inhibition of lymphocytic neuropathy target esterase predicts the development of organophosphate-induced delayed polyneuropathy. *Arch. Toxicol.* 59(3):176–79.

200. Rowntree, D. W., S. Nevin, A. Wilson. 1950. The effects of diisopropylfluorophosphonate in schizophrenia and manic depressive psychosis. *J. Neurol. Neurosurg. Psychiatry* 13(1):47–62.

201. Howkrs, M.B., E. Goodman, M. Van Sim. 1964. Some behavioral changes in man following anticholinksterase administration. *J. Nerv. Ment. Dis.* 138(4):383–89.

202. Brown, H. W. 1971. Electroencephalographic changes and disturbance of brain function following human organophosphate exposure. *Northwestern Med.* 70:845–846.

203. Dille, J. R., P. W. Smith. 1964. Central nervous system effects of chronic exposure to organophosphate insecticides. *Aerospace Med.* 35:475–478.

204. Duffy, F. H., J. L. Burchfiel, P. H. Bartels, M. Gaon, V. M. Sim. 1979. Long-term effects of an organophosphate upon the human electroencephalogram. *Toxicol. Appl. Pharmacol.* 47(1):161–76.

205. Levin, H. S., R. L. Rodnitzky. 1976. Behavioral effects of organophosphate pesticides in man. *Clin. Toxicol.* 9(3):391–405.

206. Rodnitzky, R. L., H. S. Levin, D. L. Mick. 1975. Occupational exposure to organophosphate pesticides, a neurobehavioral study. *Arch. Environ. Health* 7:441–471.

207. Sharp, D. S., B. Eskenazi, R. Harrison, P. Callas, A. H. Smith. 1986. Delayed health hazards of pesticide exposure. *Ann. Rev. Public Health* 7:441–471.

208. Tabershaw, I. R., W. C. Cooper. 1966. Sequelae of acute organophosphate poisoning. *J. Occup. Med.* 8:5–20.

209. Savage, E. P., T. J. Keefe, L. M. Mounce, R. K. Heaton, J. A. Lewis, P. J. Burcar. 1988. Chronic neurological sequelae of acute organophosphate pesticide poisoning. *Arch. Environ. Health Int. J.* 43(1):38–45.

210. Ishikawa, S., H. Hikita, M. Hayashi, T. Tamai. 1974. *Environmental Pollutants in Blood of Behcet's Disease—Organochlorine Pesticide and PCB: Study on Etiology, Treatment, and Prevention of Behcet's Disease,* pp. 156–160. Behcet's Disease Research Committee of Japan, Ministry of Welfare.

211. Wallace, L. A. 1987. The total exposure assessment methodology (TEAM) study, summary and analysis, Vol. 1, pp. 90–115. Washington, DC: U.S. Environmental Protection Agency. EPA-600-6-87-002A.

212. Abou-Donia, M. B. 1994. Organophosphorus pesticides. In *Handbook of Neurotoxicology,* L. W. Chang, R. S. Dyer eds., pp. 419–447. New York: Marcel Dekker.

213. Koelle, G. B. 1946. Protection of cholinesterase against inevitable inactivation by diisopropyl fluorophosphate in vitro. *J. Pharmacol. Exp. Ther.* 88:232–37.

214. Abou-Donia, M. B. 1992. *Neurotoxicology.* pp. 3–24. Boca Raton, FL: CRC Press.

215. Sussman, J. L., M. Harel, F. Frolow. 1992. Atomic structure of acetylcholinesterase from Torpedo californica. A prototypic acetylcholine-binding protein. *Science* 253:872–78.

216. Whittaker, M. 1994. The pseudocholinesterase variants: Esterase levels and increased resistance to fluoride. *Acta Genet. Basel.* 14:281–85.

217. Lockridge, O. 1990. Genetic variants of human serum cholinesterase influence metabolism of the muscle relaxant succinylcholine. *Pharmacol. Ther.* 47:35–60.

218. Mackness, B., M. I. Mackness, S. Arrol, W. Turkie, P. N. Durrington. 1997. Effect of the molecular polymorphisms of human paraoxonase (PONI) on the rate of hydrolysis of paraoxon. *Br. J. Pharmacol.* 122:265–68.

219. Davies, H. G., R. J. Richter, M. Keifer, C. A. Broomfield, J. Sowalla, C. E. Furlong. 1996. The effect of the human serum paraoxonase polymorphism is reversed with diazoxon, soman, and sarin. *Nat. Genet.* 14:334–36.

220. Morita, H., N. Yanagisawa, T. Nakajima, M. Shimizu, H. Hirabayashi, H. Okudera, M. Nohara, Y. Midorikawa, S. Mimura. 1995. Sarin poisoning in Matsumoto, Japan. *Lancet* 346:290–93.

221. Okumura, T., N. Takasu, S. Ishimatsu, S. Miyanoki, A. Mitsuhashi, K. Kumada, K. Tanaka, S. Hinohara. 1995. Report on 640 victims of the Tokyo subway sarin attack. *Ann. Emerg. Med.* 28:129–35.

222. Yokoyama, K., S. Araki, K. Murata, M. Nishikitani, T. Okumura, S. Ishimatsu, N. Takasu, R. F. White. 1998. Chronic neurobehavioral effects of Tokyo subway sarin poisoning in relation to posttraumatic stress disorder. *Arch. Environ. Health.* 53:249–56.

223. Masuda, N., M. Takatsu, H. Morinari. 1995. Sarin poisoning in Tokyo subway. *Lancet* 345:1446–47.

224. Smith, M. I., E. Elvove, W. H. Frazier. 1930. The pharmacological action of certain phenol esters with special reference to the etiology of so-called ginger paralysis. *Public Health Rep.* 45:2509–24.

225. Johnson, M. K. 1975. The delayed neuropathology caused by some organophosphorous esters: Mechanism and challenge. *Crit. Rev. Toxicol.* 2:289–316.

226. Abou-Donia, M. B. 1981. Organophosphorous ester-induced delayed neurotoxicity. *Annu. Rev. Pharmacol. Toxicol.* 21:511–548.

227. Abou-Donia, M. B., L. M. Lapadula. 1990. Mechanisms of organophosphorus ester-induced delayed neurotoxicity: Type I and type II. *Annu. Rev. Pharmacol. Toxicol.* 30:405–440.

228. Cavanagh, J. B., G. N. Patangia. 1995. Changes in the central nervous system in the cat as the result of tri-o-cresylphosphate poisoning. *Brain* 88:165–180.

229. Himuro, K., S. Murayama, K. Nishiyama, T. Shinoe, H. Iwase, M. Nagao, T. Takatori, I. Kanazawa. 1998. Distal sensory axonopathy after sarin intoxification. *Neurology* 51:1195–1197.

230. Davies, O. R., P. R. Holland. 1972. Effect of oximes and atropine upon the development of delayed neurotoxic signs in chickens following poisoning by DFP and sarin. *Biochem. Pharmacol.* 21:3145–3151.

231. Abou-Donia, M. B. et al. 1996. Triphenylphosphine (TPP): A type III organophosphorous compound-induced delayed neurotoxic agent (OPIDN). *Toxicologist* 30:311.

232. Abdel-Rahman, A. A. et al. 1997. Daily treatment of triphenylphosphine (TPP) produces organophosphorous-induced delayed neurotoxicity (OPIDN). *Toxicologist* 36:19.

233. Abou-Donia, M. B. 1992. Triphenyl phosphite: A type II organophosphorus compound-induced delayed neurotoxic agent. In *Organophosphates: Chemistry, Fates, and Effects. Part IV: Toxic Effects—Organismal*, J. E. Chambers, P. E. Levi, eds., pp. 327–351. San Diego, CA: Academic Press.

234. Bloch, H., A. Hottinger. 1943. Uber die spezifitat der cholinesterase-hemmung durch tri-o-kresyl phosphat. *Int. Z. Vitaminforsch* 13:90.

235. Earl, C. J., R. H. S. Thompson. 1952. The inhibitory action of triortho-cresyl phosphate and cholinesterases. *Br. J. Pharmacol.* 7:261–269.

236. Aldridge, W. N., J. M. Barnes. 1966. Further observations on the neurotoxicity of organophosphorus compounds. *Biochem. Pharmacol.* 15:541–547.

237. Johnson, M. K. 1969. The delayed neurotoxic effect of some organophosphorus compounds. *Br. Med. Bull.* 114:711–717.

238. Lotti, M. 1992. The pathogenesis of organophosphate delayed neuropathy. *Crit. Rev. Toxicol.* 21:465–487.

239. Curtes, J. P., P. Develay, J. P. Hubert. 1981. Late peripheral neuropathy due to acute voluntary intoxication by organophosphorous compounds. *Clin. Toxicol.* 18:1453.

240. de Jager, A. E., T. W. van Weerden, H. J. Houthoff, J. G. de Monchy. 1981. Polyneuropathy after massive exposure to parathion. *Neurology* 31:603–605.

241. Stamboulis, E., A. Psimaras, D. Vassilopoulos. 1991. Neuropathy following acute intoxication, with mercarbam (Opester). *Acta Neurol. Scand.* 83:198.

242. Winrow, C. J., M. L. Hemming, D. M. Allen, G. B. Quistad, J. E. Casida, C. Barlow. 2003. Loss of neuropathy target esterase in mice links organophosphate exposure to hyperactivity. *Nat. Genet.* 33:477–485.

243. Bus, J., J. Maurissen, B. Marable, J. Mattsson. 2003. Association between organophosphate exposure and hyperactivity? *Nat. Genet.* 34(3):235.

244. Abou-Donia, M. B. 1995. Involvement of cytoskeletal proteins in the mechanisms of organophosphorous ester delayed neurotoxicity. *Clin. Exp. Pharmacol. Physiol.* 22:358–359.

245. Schulman, H. 1988. *Advances in Second Messenger and Phosphorylation Research.* pp. 39–111. New York: Raven Press.

246. Patton, S. E., D. M. Lapadula, M. B. Abou-Donia. 1986. Relationship of tri-o-cresyl phosphate-induced delayed neurotoxicity to enhancement of in vitro phosphorylation of hen brain and spinal cord. *J. Pharmacol. Exp. Ther.* 239:597–605.

247. Suwita, E., D. M. Lapadula, M. B. Abou-Donia. 1986. Calcium and calmodulin-enhanced in vitro phosphorylation of hen brain cold-stable microtubules and spinal cord neurofilament triplet proteins after a single oral dose of tri-ocresyl phosphate. *Proc. Natl. Acad. Sci. USA* 83:6174–6178.

248. Abou-Donia, M. B., M. E. Viana, R. P. Gupta, J. K. Anderson. 1993. Enhanced calmodulin binding concurrent with increased kinase dependent phosphorylation of cytoskeletal proteins following a single subcutaneous injection of diisopropyl phosphorofluoridate in hens. *Neurochem. Res.* 22:165–173.

249. Gupta, R. P., M. B. Abou-Donia. 1998. Tau proteins-enhanced Ca2+/calmodulin (CaM)-dependent phosphorylation by the brain supernatant of diisopropyl phosphorofluoridate (DFP)-treated hen: Tau mutants indicate phosphorylation of more amino acids in tau by CaM kinase II. *Brain Res.* 813:32–43.

250. Gupta, R. P., M. B. Abou-Donia. 1994. In vivo and in vitro effects of diisopropyl phosphorofluoridate (DFP) on the rate of hen brain tubulin polymerization. *Neurochem. Res.* 19:435–444.

251. Gupta, R. P., M. B. Abou-Donia. 1995. Neurofilament phosphorylation and [125I] calmodulin binding by Ca2+/calmodulin-dependent protein kinase in the brain subcellular fractions of diisopropyl phosphorofluoridate (DFP)-treated hen. *Neurochem. Res.* 20(9):1095–1105.

252. Gupta, R. P., M. B. Abou-Donia. 1995. Diisopropyl phosphorofluoridate (DFP) treatment alters calcium-activated proteinase activity and cytoskeletal proteins of the hen sciatic nerve. *Brain. Res.* 677:162–166.

253. Gupta, R. P., G. Bing, J. S. Hong, M. B. Abou-Donia. 1998. cDNA cloning and sequencing of Ca2+/calmodulin-dependent protein kinase II alpha subunit and its mRNA expression in diisopropyl phosphorofluoridate (DFP)-treated hen central nervous system. *Mol. Cell Biochem.* 181:29–39.

254. Gupta, R. P., M. B. Abou-Donia. 1999. Tau phosphorylation by diisopropyl phosphorofluoridate (DFP)-treated hen brain supernatant inhibits its binding with microtubules: Role of Ca2+/calmodulin-dependent protein kinase II in tau phosphorylation. *Biochem. Pharmacol.* 53:1799–1806.

255. Gupta, R. P., T. V. Damodaran, M. B. Abou-Donia. 2000. C-fos mRNA induction in the central and peripheral nervous systems of diisopropyl phosphorofluoridate (DFP)-treated hens. *Neurochem. Res.* 25(3):327–334.

256. Gupta, R. P., A. A. Abdel-Rahman, K. F. Jensen, M. B. Abou-Donia. 2000. Altered expression of neurofilament subunits in diisopropyl phosphorofluoridate (DFP)-treated hen spinal cord and their presence in axonal aggregates. *Brain Research* 878(1–2):32–47. DOI: 10.1016/S0006-8993(00)02642-1.

257. Damodaran, T. V., M. B. Abou-Donia. 2000. Alterations in levels of mRNAs coding for glial fibrillary acidic protein (GFAP) and vimentin genes in the central nervous system of hens treats with diisopropyl phosphorofluoridate (DFP). *Neurochem. Res.* 25:809–816.

258. Jensen, K. F., D. M. Lapadula, J. K. Anderson, N. Haykal-Coates, M. B. Abou-Donia. 1992. Anomalous phosphorylated neurofilament aggregations in central and peripheral axons of hens treated with trior-tho-cresyl phosphate (TOCP). *J. Neurosci. Res.* 33:455–460.

259. Abou-Donia, M. B. et al. 2003. Organophosphorus ester-induced chronic neurotoxicity. 58(8):487, 490.

260. Jamal, G. 1997. Neurological syndromes of organophosphorus compounds. *Adverse Drug React. Toxicol. Rev.* 16:133–70.

261. Gershon, S., F. B. Shaw. 1961. Psychiatric sequelae of chronic exposure to organophosphorous insecticides. *Lancet* 1:1371–1374.

262. Dille, J. R., P. W. Smith. 1964. Central nervous system effects of chronic exposure to organophosphate insecticides. *Aerosp. Med.* 35:475–478.

263. Metcalf, D. R., J. H. Holmes. 1969. EEG, psychological and neurological alterations in humans with organophosphorous exposure. *Ann. N. Y. Acad. Sci.* 160:357–365.

264. Duffy, F. H., J. L. Burchfield, P. H. Bartels, M. Gaon, V. M. Sim. 1979. Long-term effects of an organophosphate upon the human electroencephalogram. *Toxicol. Appl. Pharmacol.* 47:161–176.

265. Pilkington, A., D. Buchanan, G. A. Jamal, R. Gillham, S. Hansen, M. Kidd, J. F. Hurley, C. A. Soutar. 2001. An epidemiological study of the relations between exposure to organophosphate pesticides and indices of chronic peripheral neuropathy and neuropsychological abnormalities in sheep farmers and dippers. *Occup. Environ. Med.* 58(11):702–710.

266. Russell, R., J. Macri. 1979. Central cholinergic involvement hyper-reactivity. *Pharmocol. Biochem. Behav.* 10:43–48.

267. Joubert, J., P. H. Joubert. 1988. Chorea and psychiatric changes in organophosphate poisoning. A report of 2 further studies. *S. Afr. Med. J.* 74:32–34.

268. Rosenstock, L., M. Keifer, W. E. Daniell, R. McConnell, K. Claypoole. 1991. Chronic central nervous system effects of acute organophosphate pesticide intoxication. *Lancet* 338:223–227.

269. Steenland, K., B. Jenkins, R. G. Ames, M. O'Malley, D. Chrislip, J. Russo. 1994. Chronic neurological sequelae to organophosphate pesticide poisoning. *Am. J Public. Health* 84:731–736.

270. Callender, T. J., L. Morrow, K. Subramanian. 1994. Evaluation of chronic neurological sequelae after acute pesticide exposure using SPECT brain scans. *J. Toxicol. Environ. Health* 41:275–84.

271. Stephens, R., A. Spurgeon, I. A. Calvert, J. Beach, L. S. Levy, H. Berry, J. M. Harrington. 1995. Neuropsychological effects of long-term exposure to organophosphates in sheep dip. *Lancet* 345:1135–1139.

272. Colosio, C., M. Tiramani, M. Maroni. 2003. Neurobehavioral effects of pesticides: State of the art. *Neurotoxicology* 24:577–591.

273. Scremin, O., T. M. Shih, L. Huynh, M. Roch, R. Booth, D. J. Jenden. 2003. Delayed neurologic and behavioral effects of subtoxic doses of cholinesterase inhibitors. *J. Pharmacol. Exp. Ther.* 304: 1111–1119.

274. Echbichon, D. J., R. M. Joy. 1995. *Pesticides and Neurological Diseases*, 2nd ed., Boston and London: CRC Press.

275. Savage, E. P., T. F. Keefe, L. M. Mounce, R. K. Heaton, J. A. Lewis, P. J. Burcar. 1988. Chronic neurological sequelae of acute organophosphates pesticide poisoning. *Arch. Environ. Health* 43:38–45.

276. Maroni, M., J. Jarvisalo, L. La Ferla. 1986. The WHO-UNDP epidemiological study on the health effects of exposure to organophosphorous pesticides. *Toxicol. Lett.* 33:115–123.

277. McConell, R., M. Keifer, L. Rosenstock. 1994. Elevated quantitative vibrotactile threshold among workers previously poisoned with methamidophos and other organophosphate pesticides. *Am. J. Ind. Med.* 25:325–334.

278. Yokoyama, K., K. Araki, K. Murata, M. Nishikitani, T. Okumura, S. Ishimatsu, N. Takasu. 1998. A preliminary study on delayed vestibulo-cerebellar effects of Tokyo Subway sarin poisoning in relation to gender difference: Frequency analysis of postural sway. *J. Occup. Environ. Med.* 40(1):17–21.

279. Rodnitzky, R. L., H. S. Levin, D. L. Mick. 1975. Occupational exposure to organophosphate pesticides. *Arch. Environ. Health* 30:98–103.

280. Maizlish, N., M. Schenker, C. Weisskopf, J. Seiber, S. Samuels. 1987. A behavioral evaluation of pest control workers with short-term, low-level exposure to the organophosphate diazinon. *Am. J. Indust. Med.* 12:153–172.

281. Daniell, W., S. Barnhart, P. Demers, L. G. Costa, D. L. Eaton, M. Miller, L. Rosenstock. 1992. Neuropsychological performance among agricultural pesticide applicators. *Environ. Res.* 59(1):217–228.

282. Beach, J. R., A. Spurgeon, R. Stephens, T. Heafield, I. A. Calvert, L. S. Levy, J. M. Harrington. 1996. Abnormalities on neurological examination among sheep farmers exposed to organophosphate pesticides. *Occup. Environ. Med.* 53(8):520–525.

283. London, L., J. E. Myers, V. Neil, T. Taylor, M. L. Thompson. 1997. An investigation into neurological and neurobehavioral effects of long-term agrochemical use among deciduous fruit farm workers in the Western Cape, South Africa. *Environ. Res.* 73(1–2):132–145.

284. Bazylewicz-Walckzak, B., W. Majzakova, M. Szymczak. 1999. Behavioral effects of occupational exposure to organophosphorous pesticides in female greenhouse plantin workers. *Neurotoxicology* 20(5):819–826.

285. Steenland, M. 1996. Chronic neurological effects of organophosphate pesticides. *Br. Med. J.* 312:1311–1312.

286. Levin, H. S., R. L. Rodnitzky, D. L. Mick. 1976. Anxiety associated with exposure to organophosphorous compounds. *Arch. Gen. Psychiatry* 33:225–228.

287. Kaplan, J. G., J. Kessler, N. Rosenberg, D. Pack, H. H. Schaumburg. 1993. Sensory neuropathy associated with Dursban (chlorpyrifos) exposure. *Neurology.* 43:2193–2196.

288. Stokes, L., A. Stark, E. Marshall, A. Narang. 1995. Neurotoxicity among pesticide applicators exposed to organophosphates. *Occup. Environ. Health* 52:648–653.

289. Fielder, N., R. G. Feldman, J. Jacobson, A. Rahill, A. Wetherell. 1996. The assessment of neurobehavioral toxicity: SOGOMSEC joint report. *Environ. Health Perspect.* 104(suppl. 2):179–191.

290. Srivastava, A. K., B. N. Gupta, V. Bihari, N. Mathur, L. P. Srivastava, B. S. Pangtey, R. S. Bharti, P. Kumar. 2000. Clinical, biochemical and neurobehavioral studies on workers engaged in the manufacture of quinalphos. *Food Chem. Toxicol.* 38(1):65–69.

291. Nishiwaki, Y., K. Maekawa, Y. Ogawa, N. Asukai, M. Minami, K. Omae; Sarin Health Effects Study Group. 2001. Effects of sarin on the nervous system in rescue team staff members and police officers 3 years after the Tokyo subway sarin attack. *Environ. Health Perspect.* 109:1169–1173.

292. Durham, W. F., H. R. Wolfe, G. E. Quinby. 1965. Organophosphorus insecticides and mental alertness. *Arch. Environ. Health* 10:55–66.

293. Tabershaw, I. R., W. C. Cooper. 1966. Sequelae of acute organic phosphate poisoning. *J. Occup. Med.* 8:5–20.

294. Petras, J. M. 1981. Soman neurotoxicity. *Fundam. Appl. Toxicol.* 1:242–249.

295. Faro, M. D., W. F. Windle. 1969. Transneuronal degeneration in brains of monkeys asphyxiated at birth. *Exp. Neurol.* 24:38–53.

296. McDonough, J. H., L. W. Dochterman, C. D. Smith, T. M. Shih. 1995. Protection against nerve agent-induced neuropathology, but not cardiac pathology, is associated with the anticonvulsant action of drug treatment. *Neurotoxicology* 15:123–132.

297. Kadar, T., G. Cohen, R. Sahar, D. Alkalai, S. Shapira. 1992. Long-term study of brain lesions following soman, in comparison to DFP and metrazol poisoning. *Hum. Exp. Toxicol.* 11:517–523.

298. Kadar, T., S. Shapira, G. Cohen, R. Sahar, D. Alkalay, L. Raveh. 1995. Sarin-induced neuropathology in rats. *Hum. Exp. Toxicol.* 14(3):252–259.

299. Veronesi, B., K. Jones, C. Pope. 1990. The neurotoxicity of subchronic acetylcholinesterase (AChE) inhibition in rat hippocampus. *Toxicol. Appl. Pharmacol.* 104:440–456.

300. Abdel-Rahman, A., A. K. Shetty, M. B. Abou-Donia. 2002. Acute exposure to sarin increases blood brain barrier permeability and induces neuropathological changes in the rat brain: Dose-response relationships. *Neuroscience* 113(3):721–741.

301. McDonald, B. E., L. G. Costa, S. D. Murphy. 1988. Spatial memory impairment and central muscarinic receptor loss following prolonged treatment with organophosphates. *Toxicol. Lett.* 40:47–56.

302. Rafaelle, K., D. Olton, Z. Annau. 1990. Repeated exposure to diisopropylfluorophosphate (DFP) produces increased sensitivity to cholinergic antagonists in discrimination retention and reversal. *Psychopharmacology (Berl.)* 100:267–274.

303. Bushnell, P. J., S. S. Padilla, T. Ward, C. N. Pope, V. B. Olszyk. 1991. Behavioral and neurochemical changes in rats dosed repeatedly with diisopropyl fluorophosphate. *J. Pharmacol. Exp. Ther.* 256:741–750.

304. Kassa, J., M. Koupilova, J. Vachek. 2001. The influence of low-level sarin inhalation exposure on spatial memory in rats. *Pharmacol. Biochem. Behav.* 70:175–179.

305. Prendergast, M. A., A. V. Terry Jr., J. J. Buccafusco. 1997. Chronic, low-level exposure to diisopropyl fluorophosphate causes protracted impairment of spatial navigation learning. *Psychopharmacology (Berl.).* 130:276–284.

306. Prendergast, M. A., A. V. Terry Jr., J. J. Buccafusco. 1998. Effects of chronic low-level organophosphate exposure on delayed recall, discrimination and spatial learning in monkeys and rats. *Neurotoxicol. Teratol.* 20:115–122.

307. Shih, T. M., S. M. Duniho, J. H. McDonough. 2003. Control of nerve agent-induced seizures is critical for neuroprotection and survival. *Toxicol. Appl. Pharmacol.* 188:69–80.

308. Lemercier, G., P. Carpentier, H. Setenac-Roumanou, P. Morelis. 1983. Histological and histochemical changes in the central nervous system of the rat poisoned by an irreversible anticholinesterase organophosphorous compound. *Acta Neuropathol.* 61:123–129.

309. Petras, J. M. 1994. Neurology and neuropathology of Soman-induced brain injury: An overview. *J. Exp. Anal. Behav.* 61:319–329.

310. Carpentier, P., I. S. Delamanche, M. Le Bert, G. Blanchet, C. Bouchaud. 1990. Seizurerelated opening of the blood brain barrier induced by soman: Possible correlation with the acute neuropathology observed in poisoned rats. *Neurotoxicology* 11:493–508.

311. Clement, J. G., B. Broxup. 1993. Efficacy of diazepam and avizafone against soman-induced neuropathology in brain of rats. *Neurotoxicology* 14:485–504.

312. Shih, T. M., T. A. Koviak, B. R. Capacio. 1991. Anticonvulsants for poisoning by the organophosphorous compound Soman: Pharmacological mechanisms. *Neurosci. Biobehav. Rev.* 15:349.

313. Pazdernik, T. L., M. R. Emerson, R. Cross, S. R. Nelson, F. E. Samson. 2001. Soman-induced seizures: Limbic activity, oxidative stress, and neuroprotective proteins. *J. Appl. Toxicol.* 21:S87–S94.

314. deGroot, D. M. G., E. P. B. Bierman, P. L. B. Bruijnzeel, P. Carpentier, B. M. Kulig, G. Lallement, B. P. Melchers, I. H. Philippens, A. H. van Huygevoort. 2001. Beneficial effects of TCP on soman intoxication in guinea pigs: Seizures, brain damage, and learning behavior. *J. Appl. Toxicol.* 21:S57–S65.

315. Taysee, L., J. H. Calvet, J. Buee, D. Christin, S. Delamanche, P. Breton. 2003. Comparative efficacy of diazepam and avizafone against sarin-induced neuropathology and respiratory failure in guinea pigs: Influence of atropine dose. *Toxicology* 188:197–209.

316. Abou-Donia, M. B. et al. 2003. Organophosphorus ester-induced chronic neurotoxicity. 58(8):487, 490.

317. Kim, Y. B., G. H. Hur, S. Shin, D. E. Sok, J. K. Kang, Y. S. Lee. 1999. Organophosphate-induced brain injuries: Delayed apoptosis mediated by nitric oxide. *Environ. Toxicol. Pharmacol.* 7:147–152.

318. Abdel-Rahman, A. A., A. M. Dechkovskaia, L. B. Goldstein, S. H. Bullman, W. Khan, E. M. El-Masry, M. B. Abou-Donia. 2004. Neurological deficits induced by malathion, DEET and permethrin, alone or in combination in adult rats. *J. Toxicol. Environ. Health A* 67:331–356.

319. McLeod, C. G., A. W. Singer, D. G. Harrington. 1984. Acute neuropathology in soman-poisoned rats. *Neurotoxicology* 5:53–58.

320. Churchill, L., T. L. Pazdernik, J. L. Jackson. 1985. Soman-induced brain lesions demonstrated by muscarinic receptor autoradiography. *Neurotoxicology* 6:81–90.

321. Baille, V., F. Dorandeu, P. Carpentier, J. C. Bizot, P. Filliat, E. Four, J. Denis, G. Lallement. 2001. Acute exposure to a low or mild dose of soman: Biochemical, behavioral and histopathological effects. *Pharmacol. Biochem. Behav.* 69:561–569.

322. Sidell, F. R. 1974. Soman and sarin: Clinical manifestations and treatment of accidental poisoning by organophosphates. *Clin. Toxicol.* 7(1):1–17.

323. West, I. 1968. Sequelae of poisoning from phosphate ester pesticides. *Ind. Med. Surg.* 37(11):832.

324. Namba, T., C. T. Nolte, J. Jackrel, D. Grob. 1971. Poisoning due to organophosphate insecticides. *Am. J. Med.* 50:475.

325. Kilburn, K. H. 1999. Evidence for chronic neurobehavioral impairment from chlorpyrifosa, and organophosphate insecticide (Dursban) used indoors. *Environ. Epidemiol. Toxicol.* 1:153–162.

326. Blondell, J., V. A. Dobozy. 1997. *Review of Chlorpyrifos Poisoning Data.* Washington, DC: U.S. Environmental Protection Agency.

327. Abou-Donia, M. B., A. A. Abdel-Rahman, L. B. Goldstein, A. M. Dechkovskaia, D. U. Shah, S. L. Bullman, W. A. Khan. 2003. Sensorimotor deficits and increased brain nicotinic acetylcholine receptors following exposure to chlorpyrifos and/or nicotine in rats. *Arch. Toxicol.* 77:452–458.

328. Abdel-Rahman, A. A., A. M. Dechkovskaia, H. Mehta-Simmons, X. Guan, W. Khan, M. Abou-Donia. 2003. Increased expression of glial fibrillary acidic protein in cerebellum and hippocampus: Differential effects on neonatal brain regional acetylcholinesterase following maternal exposure to combined chlorpyrifos and nicotine. *J. Toxicol. Environ. Health A* 66:2047–2066.

329. Eng, L. F., R. S. Ghirnikar. 1994. GFAP and astrogliosis. *Brain Pathol.* 4:229–237.

330. Olney, J. W., T. de Gubareff, J. Labruyere. 1983. Seizure-related brain damage induced by cholinergic agents. *Nature* 301:520–522.

331. Dawson, V. L., T. M. Dawson, E. D. Lonedon, D. S. Bredt, S. H. Snyder. 1991. Nitric oxide mediates glutamate neurotoxicity in primary cortical cultures. *Proc. Natl. Acad. Sci. USA* 88:6368–6371.

332. Solberg, Y., M. Belkin. 1997. The role of excitotoxicity in organophosphorus nerve agents central poisoning. *Trends Pharmacol. Sci.* 8:183–185.

333. Raveh, L., S. Chapman, G. Cohen, D. Alkalay, E. Gilat, I. Rabinovitz, B. A. Weissman. 1999. The involvement of the NMDA receptor complex in the protective effect of anticholinergic drugs against soman poisoning. *Neurotoxicology* 20:551–560.

334. Dawson, T. M., V. L. Dawson, S. H. Snyder. 1992. A novel neuronal messenger molecule in brain: The free radical, nitric oxide. *Ann. Neurol.* 32:297–311.

335. Montague, P. R., C. D. Gancayco, M. J. Winn, R. B. Marchase, M. J. Friedlander. 1994. Role of NO production in NMDA receptor-mediated neurotransmitter release in cerebral cortex. *Science* 263(5149):973–977.

336. Bagetta, G., R. Massoud, P. Rodino, G. Federici, G. Nisticò. 1993. Systematic administration of lithium chloride and tacrine increases nitric oxide synthase activity in the hippocampus of rats. *Eur. J. Pharmacol.* 237:61–64.

337. Kim, Y. B. et al. 1997. A role of nitric acid oxide in organophosphate-induced convulsions. *Environ. Toxicol. Pharmacol.* 1(3):53–56.

338. Thompson, C. B. 1995. Apoptosis in the pathogenesis and treatment of disease. *Science* 267:1456–1462.

339. Tsujimoto, Y. 1997. Apoptosis and necrosis: Intracellular ATP level as a determinant for cell death modes. *Cell Death Differ.* 4:429–434.

340. Murphy, A. N., G. Fiskum, M. F. Beal. 1999. Mitochondria in neurodegeneration: Cell life and death. *J. Cereb. Blood Flow Metab.* 19:231–245.

341. Floyd, R. A. 1999. Antioxidants, oxidative stress, and degenerative neurological disorders. *Proc. Soc. Exp. Biol. Med.* 222:236–245.

342. Gupta, R. P., D. Milatovic, W. D. Dettbarn. 2001. Depletion of energy metabolites following acetylcholinesterase inhibitor-induced status epilepticus: Protection by antioxidants. *Neurotoxicology*; 22:271–82.

343. Lieberman, A. D., M. R. Craven, H. A. Lewis, J. H. Nemenzo. 1998. Genotoxicity from domestic use of organophosphate pesticides. *J. Occup. Environ. Med.* 40(11):954–957.

344. Abou-Donia, M. B. et al. 2003. Organophosphorus ester-induced chronic neurotoxicity. 58(8):487, 490.

345. Sberna, G., J. Saez-Valero, Q. X. Li, C. Czech, K. Beyreuther, C. L. Masters, C. A. McLean, D. H. Small. 1998. Acetylcholinesterase is increased in the brains of transgenic mice expressing the C-terminal fragment (CT100) of the beta-amyloid protein precursor of Alzheimer's disease. *J. Neurochem.* 71:723–731.

346. Calderon, F. H., R. von Bernhardi, G. De Ferrari, S. Luza, R. Aldunate, N. C. Inestrosa. 1998. Toxic effects of acetylcholinesterase on neuronal and glial-like cells in vitro. *Mol. Psychiatry* 3:247–255.

347. Damodaran, T. V., K. H. Jones, A. G. Patel, M. B. Abou-Donia. 2003. Sarin (nerve agent GB)-induced differential expression of mRNA coding for the acetylcholinesterase gene in the rat central nervous system. *Biochem. Pharmacol.* 65:2041–2047.

348. Yang, L., H. Heng-Yi, X. J. Zhang. 2002. Increased expression of intranuclear AChE involved in apoptosis of SK-N-SH cells. *Neurosci. Res.* 42:261–268.

349. Andres, C., S. Seidman, R. Beeri, R. Timberg, H. Soreg. 1998. Transgenic acetylcholinesterase induces enlargement of murine neuromuscular junctions but leaves spinal cord synapses intact. *Neurochem. Int.* 32:449–456.

350. Abou-Donia, M. B., K. R. Wilmarth, K. F. Jensen. 1996. Neurotoxicity resulting from coexposure to pyridostigmine bromide, DEET, and permethrin: Implications of Gulf War chemical exposures. *J. Toxicol. Environ. Health* 48:35–56.

351. Kurt, T. L. 1998. Epidemiological association in U.S. veterans between Gulf War illness and exposure to anticholinesterases. *Toxicol. Lett.* 11:1–5.

352. Anger, W. K., D. Storzbach, L. M. Binder. 1999. Neurobehavioral deficits in Persian Gulf veterans: Evidence from a population-based study. *J. Int. Neuropsychol. Soc.* 5:203–212.

353. McCauley, L. A., G. Rischitelli, W. E. Lambert. 2001. Symptoms of Gulf War veterans possibly exposed to organophosphate chemical warfare agents at Khamisiyah, Iraq. *Int. J. Occup. Environ. Health* 7:3170–3175.

354. Storzbach, D., K. A. Campbell, L. M. Binder. 2000. Psychological differences between veterans with and without Gulf War unexplained symptoms. *Psychosom. Med.* 62:726–735.

355. White, R. F., S. P. Proctor, T. Heeren. 2001. Neuropsychological functions in Gulf War veterans: Relationship to self-reported toxicant exposures. *Am. J. Ind. Med.* 40:42–44.

356. Institute of Medicine of the National Academies. 1995. *Health Consequences of Service during the Persian Gulf War: Initial Findings and Recommendation for Immediate Action.* Washington, DC: National Academies Press.

357. Augerson, W. S. 2000. *A Review of the Scientific Literature as It Pertains to Gulf War Illnesses. Chemical and Biological Warfare Agents,* Vol. 5, Santa Monica, CA: RAND Corporation.

358. Hyams, K. C., F. S. Wignall, R. Roswell. 1995. War syndromes and their evaluation: From the U.S. Civil War to the Persian Gulf War. *Ann. Intern. Med.* 125:398–405.

359. Baker, D. G., C. L. Mendenhall, L. A. Simbart. 1997. Relationship between posttraumatic stress disorder and self-reported physical symptoms in Persian Gulf War veterans. *Arch. Intern. Med.* 157:2076–2078.

360. Horner, R. D. et al. 2003. Occurrence of amyotrophic lateral sclerosis among Gulf War veterans. *Neurology* 61:742–749.

361. Haley, R. W. 2003. Excess incidence of ALS in young Gulf War veterans. *Neurology* 61:750–756.

362. Freudenthal, R. L., L. Rausch, J. K. Gerhart, M. L. Barth, C. R. Mackerer, E. C. Bisinger. 1993. Subchronic neurotoxicity of oil formulations containing either tricresyl phosphate or tri-orthocresyl phosphate. *J. Am. Coll. Toxicol.* 12:409–416.

363. Daughtrey, W., R. Biles, B. Jortner. 1996. Subchronic delayed neurotoxicity evaluation of jet engine lubricants containing phosphorus additives. *Fundam. Appl. Toxicol.* 32:244–249.

364. National Coalition Against the Misuse of Pesticides. 2005. Lawn pesticide facts and figures. 25(2): 1–17.

365. Frawley, J. P., H. N. Fuyat, E. C. Hagen, J. R. Blake, O. G. Fitzhigh. 1957. Marked potentiation mammalian toxicity from simultaneous administration of two anticholinesterase compounds. *J. Pharmacol. Exp. Ther.* 121:96–106.

366. Lotti, M., A. Moretto. 2005. Organophosphate-induced delayed polyneuropathy. *Toxicol. Rev.* 24(1):37–49.

367. Kamel, F., J. A. Hoppin. 2004. Association of pesticide exposure with neurologic dysfunction and disease. *Environ. Health Perspect.* 112:950–958.

368. Steenland, K., R. B. Dick, R. J. Howell, D. W. Chrislip, C. J. Hines, T. M. Reid, E. Lehman, P. Laber, E. F. Krieg Jr., C. Knott. 2000. Neurologic function among termiticide applicators exposed to chlorpyrifos. *Environ. Health Perspect.* 108:293–300.

369. Lotti, M. 2002. Low-level exposures to organophosphorus esters and peripheral nerve function. *Muscle Nerve* 25(4):492–504.

370. Starks, S. E., J. A. Hoppin, F. Kamel, C. F. Lynch, M. P. Jones, M. C. Alavanja, D. P. Sandler, F. Gerr. 2012. Peripheral nervous system function and organophosphate pesticide use among licensed pesticide applicators in the agricultural health study. *Environ. Health Perspect.* 120(4):515–520.

371. Cole, D. C., F. Carpio, J. Julian, N. Leon. 1998. Assessment of peripheral nerve function in an Ecuadorian rural population exposed to pesticides. *J. Toxicol. Environ. Health A* 55(2):77–91.

372. Pilkington, A., D. Buchanan, G. A. Jamal, R. Gillham, S. Hansen, M. Kidd, J. F. Hurley, C. A. Soutar. 2001. An epidemiological study of the relations between exposure to organophosphate pesticides and indices of chronic peripheral neuropathy and neuropsychological abnormalities in sheep farmers and dippers. *Occup. Environ. Med.* 58(11):702–710.

373. Stokes, L., A. Stark, E. Marshall, A. Narang. 1995. Neurotoxicity among pesticide applicators exposed to organophosphates. *Occupat. Environ. Med.* 52(10):648–653.

374. Dow AgroSciences' New GM Corn: The Return of Agent Orange? Mercola.com. [Accessed March 07, 2016] http://articles.mercola.com/sites/articles/archive/2012/02/12/dow-agrosciences-developed-new-genetically-modified-crops.aspx

375. Stubbs, H. A., J. Harris, R. C. Spear. 1984. A proportionate mortality analysis of California agricultural workers, 1978–1979. *Am. J. Ind. Med.* 6:305–320.

376. Burmeister, L. E. 1981. Cancer mortality in Iowa farmers, 1971–1978. *J. Natl. Cancer Inst.* 66(3):461–464.

377. Burmeister, L. E., G. D. Everett, S. F. Lier, P. Isacson. 1983. Selected cancer mortality and farm practices in Iowa. *Am. J. Epidemiol.* 118(1):72–77.

378. Cantor, K., G. Everett, A. Blair, G. L. Schuman, P. Isacson. 1985. Farming and non-Hodgkin's lymphoma (abstract). *Am. J. Epidemiol.* 122(3):535.

379. Schumacher, M. C. 1985. Farming occupations and mortality from non-Hodgkin's lymphoma in Utah, a case-control study. *J. Occup. Med.* 27(8):580–584.

380. Saftlas, A. E., A. Blair, K. P. Cantor, L. Hanrahan, H. A. Anderson. 1987. Cancer and other causes of death among Wisconsin farmers. *Am. J. Ind. Med.* 11:119–129.

381. Pearce, N. E., A. H. Smith, D. O. Fisher. 1985. Malignant lymphoma and multiple myeloma linked with agricultural occupations in a New Zealand cancer registry-based study. *Am. J. Epidemiol.* 121(2):225–237.

382. Alavanja, M. C. R., G. A. Rush, P. Stewart, A. Blair. 1987. Proportionate mortality study of workers in the grain industry. *J. Natl. Cancer Inst.* 78(2):247–252.

383. Burmeister, L. E., S. E. Van Lier, P. Isacson. 1982. Leukemia and farm practices in Iowa. *Am. J. Epidemiol.* 115(5):720–728.

384. Blair, A., G. Everett, K. Cantor, R. Gibson, L. Schuman, P. Isacson, W. Blattner, S. Van Lier. 1985. Leukemia and farm practices (abstract). *Am. J. Epidemiol.* 122(3):535.

385. Blair, A., T. L. Thomas. 1979. Leukemia among Nebraska farmers: A death certificate study. *Am. J. Epidemiol.* 110(3):264–273.

386. Blair, A., D. W. White. 1985. Leukemia cell types and agricultural practices in Nebraska. *J. Occup. Med.* 40(4):211–214.

387. Delzell, W., S. Grufferman. 1985. Mortality among white and nonwhite farmers in North Carolina, 1976–1978. *Am. J. Epidemiol.* 12(3):391–402.

388. Milham, S. Jr. 1971. Leukemia and multiple myeloma in farmers. *Am. J. Epidemiol.* 91(1):307–310.

389. Gallagher, R. P., W. J. Thrlefall, J. J. Spinelli, P. R. Band. 1984. Occupational mortality patterns among British Columbia farm workers. *J. Occup. Med.* 26(12):906–908.

390. Everett, G., A. Blair, K. Cantor, R. Gibson, S. Van Lier. 1985. Environmental chemical exposures as risk factors for leukemia and non-Hodgkin's lymphoma (abstract). *Am. J. Epidemiol.* 122(3):535–536.

391. Cantor, K. P., A. Blair. 1984. Farming and mortality from multiple myeloma: A case-control study with the use of death certificates. *J. Natl. Cancer Inst.* 72(2):251–255.

392. Nandakumar, A., B. K. Armstrong, N. H. deKlerk. 1986. Multiple myeloma in western Australia: A case-control study in relation to occupation, father's occupation, socioeconomic status, and country of birth. *Int. J. Cancer* 37:223–226.

393. Wiklund, K. 1986. Trends in cancer risks among Swedish agricultural workers. *J. Natl. Cancer Inst.* 77(3):657–664.

394. Riihimaki, V., S. Asp, S. Hernberg. 1982. Mortality of 2,4-dichlorophenoxy acetic acid and 2,4,5-trichlorophenoxyacetic acid herbicide applicators in Finland. First report of an ongoing prospective study. *Scand. J. Work Environ. Health* 8:37–42.

395. Morris, P. D., T. D. Koepsell, J. R. Daling, J. W. Taylor, J. L. Lyon, G. M. Swanson, M. Child, N. S. Weiss. 1986. Toxic substance exposure and multiple myeloma: A case-control study. *J. Natl. Cancer Inst.* 76(6):987–994.

396. McDowall, M., R. Balarajan. 1984. Testicular cancer and employment in agriculture. *Lancet* 1:510–511.

397. Miles, P. K., G. R. Newell, D. E. Johnson. 1984. Testicular cancer associated with employment in agriculture and oil and natural gas extraction. *Lancet* 1:207–209.

398. Wiklund, K. 1986. Testicular cancer among agricultural workers and licensed pesticide applicators in Sweden. *Scand. J. Work Environ. Health* 12:630–631.

399. Wong, O., W. Borkcer, H. V. Davis, G. S. Nagle. 1984. Mortality of workers potentially exposed to organic and inorganic brominated chemicals, DBCP, TRIS, PBB, and DDT. *Br. J. Ind. Med.* 41:15–25.

400. Prabhakar, J. M. 1978. Possible relationship of insecticide exposure to embryonal cell carcinoma (letter). *J. Am. Med. Assoc.* 240:288.

401. Stemhagen, A., J. Slade, R. Altman, J. Bill. Occupational risk factors and liver cancer. *Am. J. Epidemiol.* 117(4):443–454.

402. Stubbs, H. A., J. Harris, R. C. Spear. 1984. A proportionate mortality analysis of California agricultural workers, 1978–1979. *Am. J. Ind. Med.* 6:305–320.

403. Austin, H., E. Delzell, S. Gufferman, R. Levine, A. S. Morrison, P. Stolley, P. Cole. 1988. Case-control study of hepato-cellular carcinoma, occupation and chemical exposures. *J. Occup. Med.* 29:665–669.

404. Gallagher, R. P., W. J. Threlfall, E. Jeffries, P. R. Band, J. Spinelli, A. J. Coldman. 1984. Cancer and aplastic anemia in British Columbia farmers. *J. Natl. Cancer Inst.* 72(6):1311–1315.

405. Mabuchi, K., A. M. Lilienfeld, L. M. Snell. 1980. Cancer and occupational exposure to arsenic: A study of pesticide workers. *Prev. Med.* 9:51–77.

406. Alavanja, M. C. R., H. Malker, R. B. Haves. 1987. Occupational cancer risk associated with the storage and bulk handling of agricultural foodstuff. *J. Toxicol. Environ. Health* 22(3):247–254.

407. Barthel, E. 1981. Increased risk of lung cancer in pesticide-exposed male agricultural workers. *J. Toxicol. Environ. Health* 8:1027–1040.

408. Blair, A., D. J. Grauman, J. H. Lubin. 1983. Lung cancer and other causes of death among licensed pesticide applicators. *J. Natl. Cancer Inst.* 71(1):31–37.

409. Wang, H. H., B. MacMahon. 1979. Mortality of pesticide applicators. *J. Occup. Med.* 21(11):741–744.

410. Coggon, D., B. Pannet, P. D. Winter, E. D. Acheson, J. Bonsall. 1986. Mortality of workers exposed to 2 methyl-4-chlotophenoxyacetic acid. *Scan. J. Work Environ. Health* 12:448–454.

411. Musicco, M., G. Filippini, B. M. Bordo, A. Melotto, G. Morello, F. Berrino. 1982. Gliomas and occupational exposure to carcinogens: Case-control study. *Am. J. Epidemiol.* 116(5):782–790.

412. Paganelli, A., V. Gnazzo, H. Acosta, S. L. López, A. E. Carrasco. 2010. Glyphosate-based herbicides produce teratogenic effects on vertebrates by impairing retinoic acid signaling. *Chem. Res. Toxicol.* 23(10):1586–1595. DOI: 10.1021/tx1001749.

413. Benbrook, C. B. 2012. Impacts of genetically engineered crops on pesticide use in the U.S.—The first sixteen years. *Environ. Sci. Eur.* 24:2190–4715.

414. Paganelli, A., Gnazzo, V., Acosta, H., López, S.L., Carrasco, A.E. 2010. Glyphosate-based herbicides produce terato-genic effects on vertebrates by impairing retinoic acid signaling. *Chem. Res. Toxicol.* 23(10):1586–1595. DOI: 10.1021/tx1001749.

415. Swanson, N., A. Leu, J. Abrahamson, B. Wallet. 2014. Genetically engineered crops, glyphosate and the deterioration of health in the United States of America. *J. Org. Syst.* 9:6–37.

416. Hoy, J. A., P. G. Hallock, T. Haas, R. D. Hoy. 2011. Observations of Brachygnathia superior (underbite) in wild ruminates in Western Montana, USA. *Wildl. Biol. Pract.* 7(2):15–29.

417. Huber, Col D. M. 2011. Genetic engineering. Roundup or roundup-ready crops may be causing animal miscarriages and infertility. *Global Research.* [Accessed March 8, 2016] http://www.globalresearch.ca/genetic-engineering-roundup-or-roundup-ready-crops-may-be-causing-animal-miscarriages-and-infertility/23335

418. Graves, L. 2016. Roundup: Birth Defects Caused by World's Top-Selling Weedkiller, Scientists Say. *The Huffington Post.* [Accessed March 08] http://www.huffingtonpost.com/2011/06/24/roundup-scientists-birth-defects_n_883578.html

419. Samsel, A., S. Seneff. 2013. Glyphosate's suppression of cytochrome P450 enzymes and amino acid biosynthesis by the gut microbiome: Pathways to modern diseases. *Entropy* 15(4):1416–1463.

420. The Horrific Truth about Monsanto's Roundup Herbicide. Mercola.com. [Accessed March 08, 2016] http://articles.mercola.com/sites/articles/archive/2013/06/09/monsanto-roundup-herbicide.aspx

421. USDA: NASS. 2013. *Agricultural Chemical Usage—Field Crops and Potatoes. USDA Economics, Statistics and Market Information System.* Albert R. Mann Library. Cornell University.

422. Hoy, J. A., R. D. Hoy, D. Seba, T. H. Kerstetter. 2002. Genital abnormalities in white-tailed deer (*Odocoileus virginianus*) in west-central Montana: Pesticide exposure as a possible cause. *J. Environ. Biol.* 23:189–197.

423. Swanson, N., A. Leu, J. Abrahamson, B. Wallet. 2014. Genetically engineered crops, glyphosate and the deterioration of health in the United States of America. *J. Org. Syst.* 9:6–37.

424. Xu, X. C., N. Brinker, A. Leu, J. Abrahamson, B. W. Wallet, J. A. Graham. 2006. Pesticide compositions containing oxalic acid. U.S. Patent No. 6992045 B2.

425. Hoy, J. A., G. T. Haas, R. D. Hoy, P. Hallock. 2011. Observations of brachygnathia superior in wild ruminants in Western Montana, USA. *Wildl. Biol. Pract.* 7:15–29.

426. Hoy, J., N. Swanson. 2015. The high cost of pesticides: Human and animal diseases. *Poult. Fish. Wildl. Sci.* 03(01):132.

427. Schroeder, K. 2005. The effect of hypothyroidism on hearing loss susceptibility. *Hearing J.* 58:10–12.

428. Kumar, J., R. Gordillo, F. J. Kaskel, C. M. Druschel, R. P. Woroniecki. 2009. Increased prevalence of renal and urinary tract anomalies in children with congenital hypothyroidism. *J. Pediatr.* 154:263–266.

429. El-Seraga, H. B. 2004. Hepatocellular carcinoma: Recent trends in the United States. *Gastroenterology* 127:527–534.

430. Chen, J. G., S. W. Zhang. 2011. Liver cancer epidemic in China: Past, present and future. *Semin. Cancer Biol.* 21:59–69.

431. Lyons, G. 2008. *Effects of Pollutants on the Reproductive Health of Male Vertebrate Wildlife—Males under Threat.* CHEM Trust. www.printguy.co.uk

432. Huang, Y., H. Gauvreau, J. Harding. 2012. Diagnostic investigation of porcine periweaning failure-to-thrive syndrome: Lack of compelling evidence linking to common porcine pathogens. *J. Vet. Diagn. Invest.* 24:96–106.

433. Chernyak, S. M., C. P. Rice, L. L. McConnell. 1996. Evidence of currently used pesticides in air, ice, fog, seawater and surface microlayer in the Bering and Chukchi seas. *Mar. Pollut. Bull.* 32:410–419.

434. Seba, D. B., J. M. Prospero. 1971. Pesticides in the lower atmosphere of the Northern Equatorial Atlantic Ocean. *Atmos. Environ.* 5:1043–1050.

435. Román, G. C. 2007. Autism: Transient in utero hypothyroxinemia related to maternal flavonoid ingestion during pregnancy and to other environmental antithyroid agents. *J. Neurol. Sci.* 262:15–26.

436. Howe, C. M., M. Berrill, B. D. Pauli, C. C. Helbing, K. Werry, N. Veldhoen. 2004. Toxicity of glyphosate-based pesticides to four North American frog species. *Environ. Toxicol. Chem.* 23:1928–1938.

437. Huber, D. M. 2010. What's new in agricultural chemical and crop interactions. *Fluid J.* 18:1–3.

438. Rolland, R. R. 2000. A review of chemically-induced alterations in thyroid and vitamin A status from field studies of wildlife and fish. *J. Wildl. Dis.* 36(4):615–635.

439. Hamlin, H. J., L. J. Guillette, Jr. 2010. Birth defects in wildlife: The role of environmental contaminants as inducers of reproductive and developmental dysfunction. *Syst. Biol. Reprod. Med.* 56:113–121.

440. Steinrücken, H. C., N. Amrhein. 1980. The herbicide glyphosate is a potent inhibitor of 5-enolpyruvyl-shikimic acid-3-phosphate synthase. *Biochem. Biophys. Res. Commun.* 94:1207–1212.

441. Samsel, A., S. Seneff. 2013. Glyphosates suppression of cytochrome P450 enzymes and amino acid biosynthesis by the gut microbiome: Pathways to modern diseases. *Entropy* 15:1416–1463.

442. Johal, G. S., D. M. Huber. 2009. Glyphosate effects on diseases of plants. *Eur. J. Agron.* 31:144–152.

443. Samsel, A., S. Seneff. 2015. Glyphosate, pathways to modern diseases III: Manganese neurological diseases, and associated pathologies. *Surg. Neurol. Int.* 6:45.

444. Schroeder, J. P., S. Raverty, E. Zabek, C. E. Cameron, A. Eshghi, D. Bain, R. Wood, Capt. L. Rhodes, B. Hanson. 2009. Investigation into the microbial culture and molecular screening of exhaled breaths of endangered southern resident killer whales (SRKW) and pathogen screening of the sea surface microlayer (SML) in Puget Sound. *Proceedings of the Puget Sound Georgia Basin Ecosystem*, pp. 1–8. Washington State Convention and Trade Center, Seattle, WA. February 1–8, 2009.

445. Perrone, S., S. Negro, M. L. Tataranno, G. Buonocore. 2010. Oxidative stress and antioxidant strategies in newborns. *J. Matern. Fetal Neonatal Med.* 23:63–65.

446. Friel, J. K., R. W. Friesen, S. V. Harding, L. J. Roberts. 2004. Evidence of oxidative stress in full-term healthy infants. *Pediatr. Res.* 56:878–882.

447. Gitto, E., S. Pellegrino, P. Gitto, I. Barberi, R. J. Reiter. 2009. Oxidative stress of the newborn in the pre- and postnatal period and the clinical utility of melatonin. *J. Pineal Res.* 46:128–139.

448. Ogihara, T. et al. 1996. New evidence for the involvement of oxygen radicals in triggering neonatal chronic lung disease. *Pediatr. Res.* 39:117–119.

449. Cole, D. J. 1985. Mode of action of glyphosate—A literature analysis. In *The Herbicide Glyphosate*, E. Grossbard, D. Atkinson, eds., pp. 48–74. London: LexisNexis Butterworths.

450. Kearney, P. C., D. D. Kaufman, eds. 1988. *Herbicides Chemistry: Degradation and Mode of Action*. USA: CRC Press.

451. Zaidi, A., M. S. Khan, P. Q. Rizvi. 2005. Effect of herbicides on growth, nodulation and nitrogen content of green gram. *Agron. Sustain. Dev.* 25:497–504.

452. DeLorenzo, M. E., L. Serrano. 2003. Individual and mixture toxicity of three pesticides; atrazine, chlorpyrifos, and chlorothalonil to the marine phytoplankton species *Dunaliella tertiolecta*. *J. Environ. Sci. Health B* 38:529–538.

453. Pettis, J. S., E. M. Lichtenberg, M. Andree, J. Stitzinger, R. Rose, D. van Engelsdorp. 2013. Crop pollination exposes honey bees to pesticides which alters their susceptibility to the gut pathogen *Nosema ceranae*. *PLoS One* 8:e70182.

454. Colborn, T., F. S. vom Saal, A. M. Soto. 1993. Developmental effects of endocrine-disrupting chemicals in wildlife and humans. *Environ. Health Perspect.* 101:378–384.

455. Vandenberg, L. N. et al. 2012. Hormones and endocrine-disrupting chemicals: Low-dose effects and nonmonotonic dose responses. *Endocr. Rev.* 33:378–455.

456. Thongprakaisang, S., A. Thiantanawat, N. Rangkadilok, T. Suriyo, J. Satayavivad. 2013. Glyphosate induces human breast cancer cells growth via estrogen receptors. *Food Chem. Toxicol.* 59:129–136.

457. Guillette, L. J. Jr., D. A. Crain, A. A. Rooney, D. B. Pickford. 1995. Organization versus activation: The role of endocrine-disrupting contaminants (EDCs) during embryonic development in wildlife. *Environ. Health Perspect.* 103:157–164.

458. Oakes, D. J., J. K. Pollak. 1999. Effects of a herbicide formulation, Tordon 75D®, and its individual components on the oxidative functions of mitochondria. *Toxicology* 136:41–52.

459. Li, C., H. M. Zhou. 2011. The role of manganese superoxide dismutase in inflammation defense. *Enzyme Res.* 2011: 6 p. Article ID 387176.

460. Swanson, N. S., M. W. Ho. 2014. Scandal of glyphosate reassessment in Europe. *Inst. Sci. Soc.* 63:8–9.

461. Mesnage, R., B. Bernay, G. E. Séralini. 2013. Ethoxylated adjuvants of glyphosate-based herbicides are active principles of human cell toxicity. *Toxicology* 313:122–128.

462. Mesnage, R., N. Defarge, J. Spiroux de Vendômois, G. E. Séralini. 2014. Major pesticides are more toxic to human cells than their declared active principles. *Biomed. Res. Int.* 2014:8 p. Article ID 179691. PMC3955666.

463. Peixoto, F. 2005. Comparative effects of the Roundup and glyphosate on mitochondrial oxidative phosphorylation. *Chemosphere* 61:1115–1122.

464. Lee, H. L., H. R. Guo. 2011. The hemodynamic effects of the formulation of glyphosate-surfactant herbicides. In *Herbicides, Theory and Applications*, S. Soloneski, M. L. Larramendy, eds., InTech. ISBN: 978-953-307-975-2. Available from: http://www.intechopen.com/books/herbicides-theory-and-applications/thehemodynamic-effects-of-the-formulation-of-glyphosate-surfactant-herbicides

465. Suzuki, T., H. Nojiri, H. Isono, T. Ochi. 2004. Oxidative damages in isolated rat hepatocytes treated with the organochlorine fungicides captan, dichlofluanid and chlorothalonil. *Toxicology* 204:97–107.

466. Lee, C. H., C. P. Shih, K. H. Hsu, D. Z. Hung, C. C. Lin. 2008. The early prognostic factors of glyphosate-surfactant intoxication. *Am. J. Emerg. Med.* 26(3):275–281.

467. Lee, H. L., C. D. Kan, C. L. Tsai, M. J. Liou, H. R. Guo. 2009. Comparative effects of the formulation of glyphosate-surfactant herbicides on hemodynamics in swine. *Clin. Toxicol. (Phila)* 47:651–658.

468. Markussen, M. D. K., M. Kristensen. 2010. Cytochrome P450 monooxygenase-mediated neonicotinoid resistance in the house fly *Musca domestica* L. *Pestic. Biochem. Physiol.* 98:50–58.

469. Rapporteur member state, Germany. 1998. Monograph on Glyphosate. Annex B5: Toxicology and metabolism. In *Glyphosate DAR*, released by German government agency BVL on CD 3:45.

470. Wertz, P. W., D. T. Downing. 1984. Cholesteryl sulfate: The major polar lipid of horse hoof. *J. Lipid Res.* 45:1320–1323.

471. Rossignol, D. A., S. J. Genuis, R. E. Frye. 2014. Environmental toxicants and autism spectrum disorders: A systematic review. *Transl. Psychiatry* 4:e360.

472. CDC Reports 1 in 50 American Children Diagnosed with Autism—NVIC Newsletter. National Vaccine Information Center (NVIC). [Accessed March 09, 2016] http://www.nvic.org/NVIC-Vaccine-News/April-2013/CDC-Reports-1-in-50-American-Children-Diagnosed-wi.aspx

473. National Health Statistics Reports. Centers for Disease Control and Prevention. 2016. [Accessed March 09, 2016] http://www.cdc.gov/nchs/products/nhsr.htm

474. Dr. Swanson: GMOs Cause Increase in Chronic Diseases, Infertility and Birth Defects—Sustainable Pulse. Sustainable Pulse. 2013. [Accessed March 09, 2016] http://sustainablepulse.com/2013/04/27/drswanson-gmos-and-roundup-increase-chronic-diseases-infertility-and-birth-defects/#.VuBEuX0rIsZ

475. Seneff, S., R. Davidson, J. Liu. 2012. Is cholesterol sulfate deficiency a common factor in preeclampsia, autism, and pernicious anemia? *Entropy* 14(11):2265–2290.

476. Seneff, S., R. Davidson, J. Liu. 2012. Empirical data confirm autism symptoms related to aluminum and acetaminophen exposure. *Entropy* 14(11):2227–2253.

477. Fantle, W. 2013. State of Fever. *The Cultivator: News from the Cornucopia Institute*. [Accessed March 9, 2016] http://www.cornucopia.org/wp-content/uploads/2013/06/Summer-Cultivator-for-website.pdf

478. Pesticides Tied to Lower IQ in Children. *Science News*. [Accessed March 09, 2016] https://www.sciencenews.org/article/pesticides-tied-lower-iq-children?mode=magazine

479. Koc, F., D. Yelden, Z. Kekec. 2007. Myeloneuritis due to acute organophosphate (DDVP) intoxication. *Toxicol. Lett.* 172:1538–1547.

480. Johnson, F. O., W. D. Atchison. 2009. The role of environmental mercury, lead and pesticide exposure in development of amyotrophic lateral sclerosis. *Neurotoxicology* 30(5):761–765.

481. Rinat, Z. 2016. Panel Says Pesticides Are Harming People, Killing Birds. Haaretz.com. [Accessed March 09].

482. Petrelli, G., I. Figa-Talamanca, L. Lauria, A. Mantovani. 2003. Spontaneous abortion in spouses of greenhouse workers exposed to pesticides. *Environ. Health Prev. Med.* 8(3):77–81.

483. Hanke, W., P. Romitti, L. Fuortes, W. Sobala, M. Mikulski. 2003. The use of pesticides in a Polish rural population and its effect on birth weight. *Int. Arch. Occup. Environ. Health* 76(8):614–620.

484. Dabrowski, S., W. Hanke, K. Polanska, T. Makowiec-Dabrowska, W. Sobala. 2003. Pesticide exposure and birthweight: An epidemiological study in Central Poland. *Int. J. Occup. Med. Environ. Health* 16(1):31–39.

485. Sallmen, M., J. Liesivuori, H. Taskinen, M. L. Lindbohm, A. Anttila, L. Aalto, K. Hemminki. 2003. Time to pregnancy among the wives of Finnish greenhouse workers. *Scand. J. Work Environ. Health* 29(2):85–93.

486. Pierik, F. H., A. Burdorf, J. A. Deddens, R. E. Juttmann, R. F. A. Weber. 2004. Maternal and paternal risk factors for cryptorchidism and hypospadias: A case-control study in newborn boys. *Environ. Health Perspect.* 112(15):1570–1576.

487. Berkowitz, G. S., J. G. Wetmur, E. Birman-Deych, J. Obel, R. H. Lapinski, J. H. Godbold, I. R. Holzman, M. S. Wolff. 2004. In utero pesticides exposure, maternal paraoxonase activity, and head circumference. *Environ. Health Perspect.* 112(3):388–391.

488. Salam, M. T., Y. F. Li, B. Langholz, F. D. Gilliland; Children's Health Study. 2004. Early-life environmental risk factors for asthma: Findings from the Children's Health Study. *Environ. Health Perspect.* 112(6):760–765.

489. Newman, L. S. et al.; ACCESS Research Group. 2004. A case control etiologic study of sarcoidosis: Environmental and occupational risk factors. *Am. J. Respir. Crit. Care Med.* 170(12):1324–1330.

490. Idrovo, A. J., L. H. Sanin, D. Cole, J. Chavarro, H. Caceres, J. Narvaez, M. Restrepo. 2005. Time to first pregnancy among women working in agricultural production. *Int. Arch. Occup. Environ. Health* 78(6):493–500.

491. Ronda, E., E. Regidor, A. M. Garcia, V. Dominguez. 2005. Association between congenital anomalies and paternal exposure to agricultural pesticides depending on mother's employment status. *J. Occup. Environ. Med.* 47(8):826–828.

492. Lacasana, M., H. Vazquez-Grameix, V. H. Borja-Aburto, J. Blanco-Munoz, I. Romieu, C. AguilarGarduno, A. M. Garcia. 2006. Maternal and paternal occupational exposure to agricultural work and the risk of anencephaly. *Occup. Environ. Med.* 63(10):649–656.

493. Meyer, K. J., J. S. Reif, D. N. Veeramachaneni, T. J. Luben, B. S. Mosley, J. R. Nuckols. 2006. Agricultural pesticide use and hypospadias in eastern Arkansas. *Environ. Health Perspect.* 114(10):1589–1595.

494. Zhu, J. L., N. H. Hjollund, A. N. Andersen, J. Olsen. 2006. Occupational exposure to pesticides and pregnancy outcomes in gardeners and farmers: A study within the Danish national birth cohort. *J. Occup. Environ. Med.* 48(4):347–352.

495. Brouwers, M. M., W. F. J. Feitz, L. A. J. Roelofs, L. A. L. M. Kiemeney, R. P. E. De Gier, N. Roeleveld. 2007. Risk factors for hypospadias. *Eur. J. Pediatr.* 166(7):671–678.

496. Handal, A. J., S. D. Harlow. 2009. Employment in the Ecuadorian cut-flower industry and the risk of spontaneous abortion. *BMC Int. Health Hum. Rights* 9:25.

497. Eckerman, D. A., L. S. Gimenes, R. C. de Souza, P. R. L. Galvao, P. N. Sarcinelli, J. R. Chrisman. 2007. Age related effects of pesticide exposure on neurobehavioral performance of adolescent farm workers in Brazil. *Neurotoxicol. Teratol.* 29(1):164–175.

498. Roberts, E. M., P. B. English, J. K. Grether, G. C. Windham, L. Somberg, C. Wolff. 2007. Maternal residence near agricultural pesticide applications and autism spectrum disorders among children in the California Central Valley. *Environ. Health Perspect.* 115(10):1482–1489.

499. Weselak, M., T. E. Arbuckle, D. T. Wigle, D. Krewski. 2007. In utero pesticide exposure and childhood morbidity. *Environ. Res.* 103(1):79–86.

500. Zuskin, E., J. Mustajbegovic, E. N. Schachter, J. Kern, V. Deckovic-Vukres, I. Trosic, A. Chiarelli. 2008. Respiratory function in pesticide workers. *J. Occup. Environ. Med.* 50(11):1299–1305.

501. Settimi, L. et al. 2008. Spontaneous abortion and maternal work in greenhouses. *Am. J. Ind. Med.* 51(4):290–295.

502. Hoppin, J. A., D. M. Umbach, S. J. London, C. F. Lynch, M. C. Alavanja, D. P. Sandler. 2006. Pesticides and adult respiratory outcomes in the agricultural health study. *Ann. N Y Acad. Sci.* 1076:343–354.

503. Hoppin, J. A., D. M. Umbach, G. J. Kullman, P. K. Henneberger, S. J. London, M. C. Alavanja, D. P. Sandler. 2007. Pesticides and other agricultural factors associated with self-reported farmer's lung among farm residents in the agricultural health study. *Occup. Environ. Med.* 64(5):334–341.

504. Carbone, P., F. Giordano, F. Nori, A. Mantovani, D. Taruscio, L. Lauria, I. 2006. Figà-Talamanca. Cryptorchidism and hypospadias in the Sicilian district of Ragusa and the use of pesticides. *Reprod. Toxicol.* 22(1):8–12.

505. Fear, N. T., K. Hey, T. Vincent, M. Murphy. 2007. Paternal occupation and neural tube defects: A case-control study based on the Oxford Record Linkage Study register. *Paediatr. Perinat. Epidemiol.* 21(2):163–168.

506. Bretveld, R. W., M. Hooiveld, G. A. Zielhuis, A. Pellegrino, I. A. van Rooij, N. Roeleveld. 2008. Reproductive disorders among male and female greenhouse workers. *Reprod. Toxicol.* 25(1):107–114.

507. Felix, J. F., M. F. Van Dooren, M. Klaassens, W. C. J. Hop, C. P. Torfs, D. Tibboel. 2008. Environmental factors in the etiology of esophageal atresia and congenital diaphragmatic hernia: Results of a case-control study. *Birth Defects Res. A Clin. Mol. Teratol.* 82(2):98–105.

508. Hoppin, J. A., D. M. Umbach, S. J. London, P. K. Henneberger, G. J. Kullman, M. C. Alavanja, D. P. Sandler. 2008. Pesticides and atopic and nonatopic asthma among farm women in the Agricultural Health Study. *Am. J. Respir. Crit. Care Med.* 177(1):11–18.

509. Hoppin, J. A., D. M. Umbach, S. J. London, P. K. Henneberger, G. J. Kullman, J. Coble, M. C. Alavanja, L. E. Beane Freeman, D. P. Sandler. 2009. Pesticide use and adult-onset asthma among male farmers in the Agricultural Health Study. *Eur. Respir. J.* 34(6):1296–1303.

510. Hougaard, K. S., H. Hannerz, H. Feveile, J. P. Bonde, H. Burr. 2009. Infertility among women working in horticulture: A follow-up study in the Danish Occupational Hospitalization Register. *Fertil. Steril.* 91(suppl. 4):1385–1387.

511. Dugas, J., M. J. Nieuwenhuijsen, D. Martinez, N. Iszatt, P. Nelson, P. Elliott. 2010. Use of biocides and insect repellents and risk of hypospadias. *Occup. Environ. Med.* 67(3):196–200.

512. Burdorf, A., T. Brand, V. W. Jaddoe, A. Hofman, J. P. Mackenbach, E. A. Steegers. 2011. The effects of work-related maternal risk factors on time to pregnancy, preterm birth and birth weight: The Generation R Study. *Occup. Environ. Med.* 68(3):197–204.

513. Sathyanarayana, S., O. Basso, C. J. Karr, P. Lozano, M. Alavanja, D. P. Sandler, J. A. Hoppin. 2010. Maternal pesticide use and birth weight in the agricultural health study. *J. Agromed.* 15(2):127–136.

514. Brender, J. D., M. Felkner, L. Suarez, M. A. Canfield, J. P. Henry. 2010. Maternal pesticide exposure and neural tube defects in Mexican Americans. *Ann. Epidemiol.* 20(1):16–22.

515. Petit, C., C. Chevrier, G. Durand, C. Monfort, F. Rouget, R. Garlantezec, S. Cordier. 2010. Impact on fetal growth of prenatal exposure to pesticides due to agricultural activities: A prospective cohort study in Brittany, France. *Environ. Health* 9:71.

516. Cosgrove, M. 2016. French Study Finds Pesticides and Herbicides in Pregnant Women. French Study Finds Pesticides and Herbicides in Pregnant Women. 2009. [Accessed March 09, 2016] http://www.digitaljournal.com/article/274327

517. Marks, A. R., K. Harley, A. Bradman, K. Kogut, D. B. Barr, C. Johnson, N. Calderon, B. Eskenazi. 2010. Organophosphate pesticide exposure and attention in young Mexican-American children: The CHAMACOS study. *Environ. Health Perspect.* 118(12):1768–1774.

518. Rauh, V. A., R. Garfinkel, F. P. Perera, H. F. Andrews, L. Hoepner, D. B. Barr, R. Whitehead, D. Tang, R. W. Whyatt. 2006. Impact of prenatal chlorpyrifos exposure on neurodevelopment in the first 3 years of life among inner-city children. *Pediatrics* 118(6):e1845–e1859.

519. Sagiv, S. K., S. W. Thurston, D. C. Bellinger, P. E. Tolbert, L. M. Altshul, S. A. Korrick. 2010. Prenatal organochlorine exposure and behaviors associated with attention deficit hyperactivity disorder in school-aged children. *Am. J. Epidemiol.* 171(5):593–601.

520. Xu, X., W. N. Nembhard, H. Kan, G. Kearney, Z. J. Zhang, E. O. Talbott. 2011. Urinary trichlorophenol levels and increased risk of attention deficit hyperactivity disorder among US school-aged children. *Occup. Environ. Med.* 68(8):557–561.

521. Ribas-Fitó, N., M. Torrent, D. Carrizo, J. Julvez, J. O. Grimalt, J. Sunyer. 2007. Exposure to hexachlorobenzene during pregnancy and children's social behavior at 4 years of age. *Environ. Health Perspect.* 115(3):447–450.

522. Rauh, V., S. Arunajadai, M. Horton, F. Perera, L. Hoepner, D. B. Barr, R. Whyatt. 2011. Seven-year neurodevelopmental scores and prenatal exposure to chlorpyrifos, a common agricultural pesticide. *Environ. Health Perspect.* 119(8):1196–1201.

523. Puertas, R. et al. 2010. Prenatal exposure to mirex impairs neurodevelopment at age of 4 years. *Neurotoxicology* 31(1):154–160.

524. Engel, S. M., J. Wetmur, J. Chen, C. Zhu, D. B. Barr, R. L. Canfield, M. S. Wolff. 2011. Prenatal exposure to organophosphates, paraoxonase 1, and cognitive development in childhood. *Environ. Health Perspect.* 119(8):1182–1188.

525. Hirabayashi, Y., T. Inoue. 2011. The low-dose issue and stochastic responses to endocrine disruptors. *J. Appl. Toxicol.* 31(1):84–88.

526. Myers, J. P., R. T. Zoeller, F. S. vom Saal. 2009. A clash of old and new scientific concepts in toxicity, with important implications for public health. *Environ. Health Perspect.* 117(11):1652–1655.

527. Vandenberg, L. N. et al. 2012. Hormones and endocrine-disrupting chemicals: Low-dose effects and nonmonotonic dose responses. *Endocr. Rev.* 33(3):378–455. Available online at http://edrv.endojournals.org/content/early/2012/03/14/er.2011-1050.full.pdf+html

528. Knapp, M., D. King, A. Healey, C. Thomas. 2011. Economic outcomes in adulthood and their associations with antisocial conduct, attention deficit and anxiety problems in childhood. *J. Ment. Health Policy Econ.* 14(3):137–147.

529. Fletcher, J., B. Wolfe. 2009. Long-term consequences of childhood ADHD on criminal activities. *J. Ment. Health Policy Econ.* 12(3):119–138.

530. von Stumm, S., I. J. Deary, M. Kivimäki, M. Jokela, H. Clark, G. D. Batty. 2011. Childhood behavior problems and health at midlife: 35-year follow-up of a Scottish birth cohort. *J. Child Psychol. Psychiatry* 52(9):992–1001.

531. Muir, T., M. Zegarac. 2001. Societal costs of exposure to toxic substances: Economic and health costs of four case studies that are candidates for environmental causation. *Environ. Health Perspect.* 109(suppl. 6):885–903.

532. Handal, A. J., B. Lozoff, J. Breilh, S. D. Harlow. 2007. Neurobehavioral development in children with potential exposure to pesticides. *Epidemiology* 18(3):312–320.

533. Proctor, N. H., J. P. Hughes. 1978. *Chemical Hazards of the Workplace*, p. 432. Philadelphia: J. B. Lippincott.

534. National Coalition Against the Misuse of Pesticides. 1989. Chemical watch factsheet. *Permethrin. Pestic. You J.* 9(4):32.

535. National Coalition Against the Misuse of Pesticides. 1988. Chemical watch factsheet. *Permethrin. Pestic. You J.* 8(2):25.

536. Corbel, V., M. Stankiewicz, C. Pennetier, D. Fournier, J. Stojan, E. Girard, M. Dimitrov, J. Molgó, J. M. Hougard, B. Lapied. 2009. Evidence for inhibition of cholinesterases in insect and mammalian nervous systems by the insect repellent deet. *BMC Biol.* 7(1):47.

537. Levinsky, W. J., R. V. Smalley, P. N. Hillyer, R. L. Shindler. 1970. Arsine hemolysis. *Arch. Environ. Health* 20:436.

538. Henry, M., M. Beguin, F. Requier, O. Rollin, J. F. Odoux, P. Aupinel, J. Aptel, S. Tchamitchian, A. Decourtye. 2012. A common pesticide decreases foraging success and survival in honey bees. *Science* 336(6079):348–350.

539. Goulson, D., S. O'connor, F. L. Wackers, P. R. Whitehorn. 2012. Neonicotinoid pesticide reduces bumble bee colony growth and queen production. *Science* 336(6079):351–52.

540. Huff, E. A. 2011. Leaked Document: EPA Knowingly Approved Bee-killing Pesticide. *NaturalNews*. January 05. [Accessed March 10, 2016] http://www.naturalnews.com/030921_EPA_pesticides.html

541. Pettis, J. S., D. vanEngelsdorp, J. Johnson, G. Dively. Pesticide exposure in honey bees results in increased levels of the gut pathogen Nosema. *Naturwissenschaften*. 99(2):153–158. doi: 10.1007/s00114-011-0881-1.

542. Mussen, E. 1990. California crop pollination. *Glean. Bee Cult.* 118:646–647.

543. Pimentel, D., H. Lehman. 1993. *The Pesticide Question: Environment, Economics, and Ethics*. New York: Chapman & Hall.

544. Pimentel, D., H. Acquay, M. Biltonen, P. Rice, M. Silva, J. Nelson, V. Lipner, S. Giordano, A. Horowitz, M. D'Amore. 1993. Assessment of environmental and economic impacts of pesticide use. *Pestic. Ques.* 47–84.

545. ICAITI. 1977. *An Environmental and Economic Study of the Consequence of Pesticide Use in Central American Cotton Production. Guatemala City, Guatemala*. Final Report, Central American Research Institute for Industry, United Nations Environmental Program.

546. Reddy, V. R., D. N. Baker, F. D. Whisler, R. E. Fye. 1987. Application of GOSSYM to yield decline in cotton. Systems analysis of effects of herbicides on growth, development and yield. *Argon. J.* 79:42–47.

547. Oka, I. N., D. Pimentel. 1976. Herbicide (2, 4-D) increases insect and pathogen pests on corn. *Science* 193:239–240.

548. Pimentel, D. 1994. Insect population responses to environmental stress and pollutants. *Environ. Rev.* 2(1):1–15.

549. Barnes, C. J., T. L. Lavy, J. D. Mattice. 1987. Exposure of non-applicator personnel and adjacent areas to aerially applied propanil. *Bull. Environ. Contam. Toxicol.* 39:126–133.

550. Akesson, N. B., W. E. Yates. 1984. Physical parameters affecting aircraft spray application. In *Chemical and Biological Controls in Forestry*, W. Y. Garner, J. Harvery, eds., pp. 95–111. Washington, DC: Am. Chem. Soc. (Ser. 238).

551. Mazariegos, F. 1985. *The Use of Pesticides in the Cultivation of Cotton in Central America*. Guatemala: United Nations Environment Program, Industry and Environment, July/August/September.

552. Hall, F. R. 1991. Pesticide application technology and integrated pest management (IPM). In *Handbook of Pest Management in Agriculture*, Vol. II, D. Pimentel, ed., pp. 135–170. Boca Raton, FL: CRC Press.

553. Hanner, D. 1984. Herbicide drift prompts state inquiry. *Dallas Morning News*.

554. NAS. 1989. *Alternative Agriculture*. Washington, DC: National Academy of Sciences.

555. Cornell. 2003. *Common Pesticides in Groundwater*. [Accessed March 10, 2016] http://pmep.cce.cornell. Edu/facts-slides-self/slide/set/gwater09.html

556. Holmes, T., E. Neilsen, L. Lee. 1988. *Managing Groundwater Contamination in Rural Areas. Rural Development Perspectives*. Washington, DC: US Department of Agriculture (Economic Research Series).

557. USGS. 1996. *Pesticides Found in Ground Water below Orchards in the Quincy and Pasco Basin*. [Accessed March 11, 2016] http://wa.water.usgs.gov/ccpt/pubs/fs-171-96.html

558. EPA. 1990. *Natural Pesticide Survey—Summary*. Washington, DC: U.S.A. Environmental Protection Agency.

559. USGS. 1995. *Pesticides in Public Supply Wells of Washington State*. [Accessed March 11, 2016] http://wa.water.usgs.gov/ccpt/pubs/fs-122-96.html

560. Well Owner. 2003. *The Use of Ground Water*. [Accessed March 11, 2016] http://www.wellowner.org/useof.html

561. CEQ. 1980. *The Global 2000 Report to the President of the US Entering the 21st Century.* New York: Pergamon Press.

562. Unnevehr, L. J. et al. 2003. *Frontiers in Agricultural Research: Food, Health, Environment, and Communities.* Washington, DC: National Academies of Science.

563. Barometer. 1991. *Too Much Beer Kills Thousands.* Oregon State University Barometer, May 14.

564. Mineua, P. et al. 1999. Poisoning of raptors with organophosphorus and carbamate pesticides with emphasis on Canada, US and UK. *J. Raptor Res.* 33(1):1–37.

565. Balcomb, R. 1986. Songbird carcasses disappear rapidly from agricultural fields. *Auk* 103:817–821.

566. White, D. H., C. A. Mitchell, L. D. Wynn, E. L. Flickinger, E. J. Kolbe. 1982. Organophosphate insecticide poisoning of Canada geese in the Texas Panhandle. *J. Field Ornithol.* 53:22–27.

567. Flickinger, E. L., K. A. King, W. F. Stout, M. M. Mohn. 1980. Wildlife hazards from Furadan 3G applications to the rice in Texas. *J. Wildl. Manage.* 44:190–197.

568. Flickinger, E. L., G. Juenger, T. J. Roffe, M. R. Smith, R. J. Irwin. 1991. Poisoning Canada geese in Texas by parathion sprayed for control of Russian wheat aphid. *J. Wildl. Dis.* 27:265–268.

569. EPA. 1989. *Carbofuran: A Special Review Technical Support Document.* Washington, DC: US Environmental Protection Agency, Office of Pesticides and Toxic Substances.

570. Stone, W. B., P. B. Gradoni. 1985. Wildlife mortality related to the use of the pesticide diazinon. *Northeastern Environ. Sci.* 4:30–38.

571. ABCBirds. 2003. Pesticides and Birds Campaign. [Accessed March 10, 2016] http://abcbirds.org/pesticides/pesticideindex.htm

572. CWS. 2003. *Pesticides and Wild Birds.* Canadian Wildlife Service. [Accessed March 10, 2016] http://www.cws-scf.ec.gc.ca/hww-fap/hww-fap.cfm?ID_species-90&lang=e

573. Potts, G. R. 1986. *The Partridge: Pesticides, Predation and Conservation.* London: Collins.

574. Mineau, P. 1988. Avian mortality in agroecosystems. The case against granule insecticides in Canada. In *Field Methods for the Environment Effects of Pesticides British Crop Protection Council (BPCP), Monograph 40*, M. P. Greaves, B. D. Smith, eds., British Crop Protection Council (BPCP), pp. 3–12. Thornton Heath, London: Gordon and Breach Science Publishers.

575. Elliot, J. E., R. J. Norstrom, J. A. Keith. 1988. Organochlorines and eggshell thinning in northern gannets *(Sula bassanus)* from Eastern Canada 1968–1984. *Environ. Poll.* 52:81–102.

576. Asia Times. 2001. *India/Pakistan.* [Accessed March 10, 2016] http://www.atimes.com/ind-pak/CF14Df01.html

577. D'Anieri, P., D. M. Leslie, M. L. McCormack. 1987. Small mammals in glyphosate-treated clearcuts in Northern Maine. *Can. Field Naturalist* 101:547–550.

578. USFWS. 1988. *1985 Survey of Fishing,* Hunting and Wildlife Associated Recreation, Washington, DC: US Fish and Wildlife Service, US Department of the Interior.

579. Dobbins, J. 1986. *Resources Damage Assessment of the T/V Puerto Rican Oil Spill Incident.* James Dobbins Report to NOAA. Washington, DC: Sanctuary Program Division.

580. Boutin, C., K. E. Freemark, D. E. Kirdk. 1999. Spatial and temporal patterns of bird use of farmland in Southern Ontario. *Can. Filed Naturalist* 113(3):430–460.

581. Millar, J. G. 1995. Fish and Wildlife Service's proposal to reclassify the bald eagle in most of the lower 48 states. *J. Raptor. Res.* 29(1):71.

582. Pimentel, D., U. Stachow, D. A. Takacs, H. W. Brubaker, A. R. Dumas, J. J. Meaney, J. A. S. O'Neil, D. E. Onsi, D. B. Corzilius. 1992. Conserving biological diversity in agricultural/forestry systems. *Bioscience* 42:354–362.

583. Atlas, R. M., R. Bartha. 1987. *Microbiol Biology: Fundamental and Application,* 2nd ed., Menlo Park, CA: Benjamin Cummings Co.

584. Pimentel, D. 1997. Pest management in agriculture. In *Techniques for Reducing Pesticide Use: Environmental and Economic Benefits*, D. Pimentel, ed., pp. 1–11. Chichester, UK: John Wiley & Sons.

585. Edwards, C. A., J. R. Lofty. 1982. Nitrogenous fertilizers and earthworm populations in agricultural soils. *Soil Biol. Biochem.* 14:515–521.

586. Stringer, A., C. Lyons. 1974. The effect of benomyl and thiophanate-methyl on earthworm populations in apple orchards. *J. Pestic. Sci.* 5:189–196.

587. Potter, D. A., S. K. Braman. 1991. Ecology and management of turfgrass insects. *Ann. Rev. Entomol.* 36:383–406.

588. PCC. 2002. News Bites. [Accessesd March 11, 2016] http://pccnaturalmarkets.com/sc/0205/newsbites.html

589. Rea, W. J. 1996. Pesticides. *J. Nutr. Environ. Med.* 6(1):55–124.

590. Bhopal Trial: Eight Convicted over India Gas Disaster. BBC News. 2010. [Accessed March 11, 2016] http://news.bbc.co.uk/2/hi/south_asia/8725140.stm

591. Varma, R., D. R. Varma. 2005. The Bhopal Disaster of 1984. *Bull. Sci. Technol. Soc.*

592. Madhya Pradesh Government: Bhopal Gas Tragedy Relief and Rehabilitation Department, Bhopal. Mp.gov.in. [Accessed March 11, 2016].

593. WebCite Query Result. WebCite Query Result. [Accessed March 11, 2016] http://www.webcitation.org/5qmWBEWcb

594. Eckerman, I. 2005. *The Bhopal Saga—Causes and Consequences of the World's Largest Industrial Disaster.* India: Universities Press Private Ltd.

595. Company Defends Chief in Bhopal Disaster. DealBook Company Defends Chief in Bhopal Disaster Comments. [Accessed March 11, 2016] http://dealbook.nytimes.com//2009/08/03/company-defends-chief-in-bhopal-disaster/

596. U.S. Exec Arrest Sought in Bhopal Disaster. CBSNews. [Accessed March 11, 2016] http://www.cbsnews.com/news/us-exec-arrest-sought-in-bhopal-disaster/

597. Eckmann, I. 1976. *Methyl Isocyanate.* New York: Union Carbide Corporation. F-41443A-7/76.

598. Eckmann, I. 1978. *Carbon Monoxide, Phosgene and Methyl Isocyanate. Unit Safety Procedures Manual.* Bhopal: Union Carbide India Limited, Agricultural Products Division.

599. O'Brien, R. D. 1960. Toxic phosphorus esters. In *Chemistry, Metabolism and Biological Effects.* p. 28. New York: Academic Press.

600. Lowengart, R. A., J. M. Peters, C. Cicionic, J. Buckley, L. Bernstein, S. Preston-Martin, E. Rappaport. 1987. Childhood leukemia and parents' occupational and home exposures. *J. Natl. Cancer Inst.* 79(1):39–46.

601. Epstein, S. S. 1983. Problems of causality, burdens of proof and restitution: Agent orange diseases. *TRIAL* 91:138.

602. Schmidt, K. F. 1992. *Puzzling over a poison: On closer inspection, the ubiquitous pollutant dioxin appears more dangerous than ever.* U.S. News and World Report, April 6, p. 61.

603. Murphy, S. D. 1986. Toxic effects of pesticides. In *Casarett and Doull's Toxicology: The Basic Science of Poisons,* 3rd ed., C. D. Klaasen, M. O. Amdur, J. Doull, eds., p. 555. New York: Macmillan.

604. Young, A. L., J. A. Calcagin, C. H. Thalken, J. W. Tromblay. 1978. *The Toxicology, Environmental Fate and Human Risk of Herbicide Orange and Its Dioxin.* USAF OEHL. Technical Report, 78–92. National Technical Information Service (AD-Ao62-143). Springefield, VA: U. S. Department of Commerce.

605. Jennings, A. M., G. Wild, J. D. Ward, A. Milfordward. 1988. Immunological abnormalities 17 years after accidental exposure to 2, 3, 7 8-tetrachlorodibenzo-p-dioxin. *Br. J. Ind. Med.* 45:701–704.

606. Anon. 1989. Dioxin via skin: A hazard at low doses? *Sc. News* 135(9):141.

607. Brewster, D. W., Y. B. Banks, A. M. Clark, L. S. Birnbaum. 1989. Comparative dermal absorption of 2, 3, 7, 8-tetrachlorodibenzo-p-dioxin and three polychlorinated dibenzofurans. *Toxicol. Appl. Pharmacol.* 97:156–166.

608. Baselt, R. C., ed. 1982. *Disposition of Toxic Drugs and Chemicals in Man,* 2nd ed., p. 242. Davis, CA: Biomedical Publications.

609. Hanify, J. A., P. Metcalf, C. L. Nobbs, K. J. Worsley. 1981. Aerial spraying of 2,4,5-T and human birth malformations: An epidemiological investigation. *Science* 212:349–351.

610. Industry Wary of Dioxin Guidelines. WSJ. [Accessed March 11, 2016] http://www.wsj.com/articles/SB10001424052970203899504577131094244269500

611. U.S. Environmental Protection Agency. 1982. *Recognition and Management of Pesticide Poisonings,* 3rd ed., p. 24. Washington, DC: U.S. Environmental Protection Agency. EPA-540/9-80-005.

612. Rea, W. J. 1992. *Chemical Sensitivity,* p. 221. Boca Raton, FL: Lewis Publishers.

613. Rea, W. J. 1992. *Chemical Sensitivity,* p. 883. Boca Raton, FL: Lewis Publishers.

614. Matthew, H., A. Logan, M. F. A. Woodruff, B. Heard. 1968. Paraquat poisoning—Lung transplantation. *Br. Med. J.* 3:759–763.

615. Spangenberg, T., H. Grahn, H. Schalk, K. H. Kuck. 2012. Paraquatintoxikation. *Med Klin Intensivmed Notfmed Medizinische Klinik—Intensivmedizin Und Notfallmedizin.* 107(4):270–274.

616. Rea, W. J. 1992. *Chemical Sensitivity,* p. 886. Boca Raton, FL: Lewis Publishers.

617. Pan, Y., W. J. Rea, A. R. Johnson, E. J. Fenyves. 1989. Formaldehyde sensitivity. *Clin. Ecol.* 6(3):79–84.

618. Hayes, W. J. Jr. 1982. *Pesticides Studied in Man,* pp. 14–25. Baltimore, MD: Williams & Wilkins.

619. Rea, W. J., A. R. Johnson, S. Youdim, E. J. Fenyves, N. Samadi. 1986. T & B lymphocyte parameters measured in chemically sensitive patients and controls. *Clin. Ecol.* 4(1):11–14.

620. Perelygin, V. M., M. B. Shpirt, O. A. Aripov, V. I. Ershova. 1971. Effect of some pesticides on immunological response reactivity. *Gigiena I Sanitariya* 12:29–33.

621. Latimer, J. W., H. S. Siegel. 1974. Immune response in broilers fed technical grade DDT (Antibodies). *Poult. Sci.* 53(3):1078–1083.

622. Atakaev, S. T., I. B. Boiko, V. A. Ilina. 1978. Effect of pesticides on the immunological state of the body. *Gigiena I Sanitariya* 8:7–10.

623. Klotz, V. I., R. A. Bahayantz, V. G. Brysin, A. Safarova. 1978. Effect of pesticides on the immunological reactivity of the body of animals and man. *Gigiena I Sanitariya* 9:35–36.

624. Wiltrout, R. W., C. D. Ercegovich, W. S. Ceglowski. 1978. Humoral immunity in mice following oral administration of selected pesticides. *Bull. Environ. Contam. Toxicol.* 20(3):423–443.

625. Koller, L. D., N. Issacson-Keskvliet, J. H. Exon, J. A. Brauner, N. M. Patton. 1979. Synergism of methylmercury and selenium producing enhanced antibody formation in mice. *Arch. Environ. Health* 34(4):248–252.

626. Loose, L. D., K. A. Pittman, K. F. Benitz, J. B. Silkworth. 1977. Polychlorinated biphenyl and hexachlorobenzene induced humoral immunosuppression. *J. Reticuloendothel. Soc.* 22(3):253–271.

627. Loose, L. D., J. B. Silkworth, K. A. Pittman, K. F. Benitz, W. S. Mueller. 1978. Impaired host resistance to endotoxin and malaria in polychlorinated biphenyl and hexachlorobenzene-treated mice. *Infect. Immun.* 20(1):30–35.

628. Silkworth, J. B., L. D. Loose. 1980. Environmental chemical induced modification of cell-mediated immune responses. *Adv. Exp. Med. Biol.* 121/A:499–522.

629. Evdokimov, E. S. 1974. Effect of organochlorine pesticides on animals. *Veterinarua* 12:94–95.

630. Street, J. C., R. P. Sharma. 1975. Alteration of induced cellular and humoral immune responses by pesticides and chemicals of environmental concern: Quantitivative studies of immunosuppression by DDT, arochlor 1254, carbaryl, carbofuran, methylparathion. *Toxicol. Appl. Pharmacol.* 32(3):587–602.

631. Friedman, G. I. 1967. Effect of sevin, chlorophos, and DDT on some specific and nonspecific indexes of the immunobiological and general reactivity of an organism (problems of toxic action of low intensity). Vop. GIG U.S.S.R.:Tr. Nauch Sess Akad. Med. Nauk U.S.S.R.

632. Gahliks, J., E. M. Adkari, N. Yolen. 1973. DDT and immunological responses. I. Serum antibodies and anaphylactic shock in guinea pigs. *Arch. Environ. Health* 26(6):305–308.

633. Gahliks, J., T. A. Zuhaidy, E. Askari. 1975. DDT and immunological responses. 3 reduced anaphylaxic and mast cell population in rats fed DDT. *Arch. Environ. Health.* 30(2):81–84.

634. Askari, E. M., J. Gahliks. 1976. DDT and immunological responses. I. Altered histamine levels and anaphylactic shock in guinea pigs. *Arch. Environ. Health* 26(6):309–331.

635. Rea, W. J. 1979. The environmental aspects of ear, nose, and throat disease. Part I. *J.C.E.O.R.L. Allergy* 41(7):41–56.

636. Jakoby, W. B., ed. 1980. *Enzymatic Basis of Detoxification*, Vol. 2. New York: Academic Press.

637. Reeves, W. G., J. S. Cameron, S. G. O. Johansson, C. S. Ogg, D. K. Peters, R. O. Weller. 1975. Seasonal nephritic syndrome. *Clin. Allergy* 5:121–137.

638. Giurgen, R., C. Witterberger, G. Frecus, S. Maniciolea, M. Borsa, D. Coprea, S. Ilyes. 1978. Effects of some organochlorine pesticides on the immunological reactivity of white rats. *Arch. Exp. Veterinarmed* 32(5):769–774.

639. Desi, I., L. Varga, I. Farkas. 1978. Studies on the immunosuppressive effect of organochlorine and organophosphoric pesticides in subacute experiments. *J. Hyg. Epidemiol. Microbiol. Immunol.* 22(1):115–122.

640. Glick, B. 1974. Antibody-mediated immunity in the presence of Mirex and DDT. *Poul. Sci.* 53(4):1476–1485.

641. Aripdzhanov, T. M. 1973. Effect of the pesticides Anthio and Milbex on the immunological reactivity and certain autoimmunological reactivity and certain autoimmune processes of the body. *Gigiena I Sanitariya* 7:39–42.

642. Koller, L. D., J. H. Exon, J. G. Roan. 1976. Immunological surveillance and toxicity in mice exposed to the organophosphate pesticide, leptophos. *Environ. Res.* 12(3):238–242.

643. Olefir, A. I. 1974. *Effect of chemical substances on the formation of acquired immunity.* U.S. NTIS Report AD-A008261, p. 9.

644. Olefir, A. I., O. P. Minister, R. E. Sova. 1977. Interrelation of indexes of natural body resistance during chronic poisoning with chlorophos, polychloropinene, and sevin. *Gigiena I Sanitariya* 4:25–28.

645. Olefir, A. I. 1978. Immunological reactivity of the pregnancy of animals affected by pesticides. *Gigiena I Sanitariya* 2:103–104.

646. Shubik, V. M., M. A. Nevstrueva, S. A. Kalnitskii, R. E. Levshits, G. N. Merkushev, E. M. Pilschik, T. V. Ponomareva. 1976. Effect of chronic entera administration of radioactive and chemical substances on the immune response. *G Ig. Otsenka Faktorov Radiats Neradiats Prir Ikh Komb* 87–91.

647. National Coalition Against the Misuse of Pesticides. 1989. Chemical watch factsheet. *Chlorpyrifes. Pestic. You J.* 9:41.

648. Street, J. C., R. P. Sharma. 1974. Quantitative aspects of immunosuppression by selected pesticides. *Toxicol. Appl. Pharmacol.* 29(1):135–136.

649. Dawkliker, W. B., A. N. Hicks, S. A. Levinson, K. Stewart, R. J. Brawn. 1979. Effects of pesticides on the immune response. (U. S. NTIS Report PB 80-1309834). *Environ. Sci. Technol.* 14(2):204–210.

650. Doull, J., M. C. Bruce. 1986. Origin and scope of toxicology. In *Casarett and Doull's Toxicology: The Basic Science of Poisons*, C. D. Klaassen, M. O. Amdur, J. Doull, eds., pp. 3–10. New York: Macmillan.

651. Street, J. C. 1981. Pesticides and the immune system. In *Immunologic Considerations in Toxicology*, Vol. I, R. P. Sharma, ed., pp. 45–66. Boca Raton, FL: CRC Press.

652. Moore, J. A., J. G. Zinkl, J. G. Vos. 1973. Effect on TCDD on immune system of lab animals. *Environ. Health Perspect.* 5:149–165.

653. Thigen, J. E., R. E. Faith, E. E. McConnell, J. A. Moore. 1975. Increased susceptibility to bacterial infection as a sequela to exposure to 2,3,7,8-tetrachlorodibenzo-p-dioxin. *Infect. Immun.* 12(6):1319–1324.

654. Allen, J. R., J. P. van Miller. 1977. Health implications of 2,3,7,8-tetrachlorodibenzo-p-dioxin (TCDD) exposure in primates. In *Pentachlorophenol*, K. R. Rao, ed., pp. 371–379. New York: Plenum Press.

655. Faith, R. E., J. A. Moore. 1977. Impairment of thymus-dependent immune functions by exposure of the developing immune system to 2,3,7,8-tetrachlorodibenzo-p-dioxin (TCDD). *J. Toxicol. Environ. Health* 3(3):451–464.

656. Thomas, R. T., R. D. Hinsdill. 1979. The effect of perinatal exposure to tetrachlorodibenzo-p-dioxin on the immune response of young mice. *Drug Chem. Toxicol.* 2(1–2):77–78.

657. Luster, M. I., R. E. Faith, L. D. Lawson. 1979. Effects of 2,3,7,8-tetrachlorodibenzofuran (TCDF) on the immune system in guinea pigs. *Drug Chem. Toxicol.* 2(1–2):49–60.

658. Williams, G. M., J. H. Weisberger. 1986. Chemical carcinogens. In *Casarett and Doull's Toxicology: The Basic Science of Poisons*, C. D. Klaassen, M. O. Amdur, J. Doull, eds., pp. 99–173. New York: Macmillan.

659. Bertschler, J., J. R. Butler, G. F. Lawlis, W. J. Rea, A. R. Johnson. 1985–1986. Psychological components of environmental illness: Factor analysis of changes during treatment. *Clin. Ecol.* 3(2):85–94.

660. Mauck, B., J. B. Lucot, S. Paton, R. D. Grubbs. 2010. Cholinesterase inhibitors and stress: Effects on brain muscarinic receptor density in mice. *Neurotoxicology* 31(5):461–467.

661. Hayden, K. M., M. C. Norton, D. Darcey, T. Ostbye, P. P. Zandi, J. C. S. Breitner, K. A. Welsh-Bohmer. 2010. Occupational exposure to pesticides increases the risk of incident AD: The cache county study. *Neurology* 74(19):1524–1530.

662. Weisskopf, M. G., M. F. Bouchard, D. C. Bellinger, R. O. Wright. 2010. Attention-deficit/hyperactivity disorder and urinary metabolites of organophosphate pesticides. *Pediatrics 125(6)*.

663. Wang, N. N., H. Dai, L. Yuan, Z. K. Han, J. Sun, Z. Zhang, M. Zhao. 2010. Study of paraoxonase-1 function on tissue damage of dichlorvos. *Toxicol. Lett.* 196(2):125–132.

664. Alter, G., D. Organiziak, W. J. Rea. Low level chemical toxicity: Relevance to chemical agent defense. *PsycEXTRA Dataset*.

665. Yilmazlar, A., G. Özyurt. 1977. Brain involvement in organophosphate poisoning. *Environ. Res.* 74(2):104–109.

666. Sorodoc, L., C. Lionte, E. Largu, O. Petris. 2011. Benefits of butyrylcholinesterase reactivability testing in organophosphate poisoning. *Hum. Exp. Toxicol.* 30(11):1769–1776.

667. Mostafalou, S., M. Abdollahi. 2013. Pesticides and human chronic diseases: Evidences, mechanisms, and perspectives. *Toxicol. Appl. Pharmacol.* 268(2):157–177.

668. Abdul-Ghani, M. A., R. A. DeFronzo. 2008. Mitochondrial dysfunction, insulin resistance, and type 2 diabetes mellitus. *Curr. Diab. Rep.* 8(3):173–178.

669. Kim, J. A., Y. Wei, J. R. Sowers. 2008. Role of mitochondrial dysfunction in insulin resistance. *Circ. Res.* 102(4):401–414.

670. Lowell, B. B., G. I. Shulman. 2005. Mitochondrial dysfunction and type 2 diabetes. *Science* 307(5708):384–387.

671. Ma, Z. A., Z. Zhao, J. Turk. 2012. Mitochondrial dysfunction and β-cell failure in type 2 diabetes mellitus. *Exp. Diabetes Res.* 2012:703538.

672. Johri, A., M. F. Beal. 2012. Mitochondrial dysfunction in neurodegenerative diseases. *J. Pharmacol. Exp. Ther.* 342(3):619–630.

673. Martin, L. J. 2012. Biology of mitochondria in neurodegenerative diseases. *Prog. Mol. Biol. Transl. Sci.* 107:355–415.

674. Lin, M. T., M. F. Beal. 2006. Mitochondrial dysfunction and oxidative stress in neurodegenerative diseases. *Nature* 443(7113):787–795.

675. Langston, J. W. 1996. The etiology of Parkinson's disease with emphasis on the MPTP story. *Neurology* 47(6 suppl. 3):S153–S160.

676. Caboni, P., T. B. Sherer, N. Zhang, G. Taylor, H. M. Na, J. T. Greenamyre, J. E. Casida. 2004. Rotenone, deguelin, their metabolites, and the rat model of Parkinson's disease. *Chem. Res. Toxicol.* 17(11):1540–1548.

677. Gomez, C., M. J. Bandez, A. Navarro. 2007. Pesticides and impairment of mitochondrial function in relation with the parkinsonian syndrome. *Front. Biosci.* 12:1079–1093.

678. Ilivicky, J., J. E. Casida. 1969. Uncoupling action of 2,4-dinitrophenols, 2-trifluoromethylbenzimid-azoles and certain other pesticide chemicals upon mitochondria from different sources and its relation to toxicity. *Biochem. Pharmacol.* 18(6):1389–1401.

679. Ranjbar, A., M. H. Ghahremani, M. Sharifzadeh, A. Golestani, M. Ghazi-Khansari, M. Baeeri, M. Abdollahi. 2010. Protection by pentoxifylline of malathion-induced toxic stress and mitochondrial damage in rat brain. *Hum. Exp. Toxicol.* 29(10):851–864.

680. Jamshidi, H. R., M. H. Ghahremani, S. N. Ostad, M. Sharifzadeh, A. R. Dehpour, M. Abdollahi. 2009. Effects of diazinon on the activity and gene expression of mitochondrial glutamate dehydrogenase from rat pancreatic Langerhans islets. *Pest. Biochem. Physiol.* 93(1):23–27.

681. Pournourmohammadi, S., S. N. Ostad, E. Azizi, M. H. Ghahremani, B. Farzami, B. Minaie, B. Larijani, M. Abdollahi. 2007. Induction of insulin resistance by malathion: Evidence for disrupted islets cells metabolism and mitochondrial dysfunction. *Pest. Biochem. Physiol.* 88:346–352.

682. Lee, H. K. 2011. Mitochondrial dysfunction and insulin resistance: The contribution of dioxin-like substances. *Diabetes Metab. J.* 35(3):207–215.

683. Lim, S., S. Y. Ahn, I. C. Song, M. H. Chung, H. C. Jang, K. S. Park, K. U. Lee, Y. K. Pak, H. K. Lee. 2009. Chronic exposure to the herbicide, atrazine, causes mitochondrial dysfunction and insulin resistance. *PLoS One* 4(4):e5186.

684. Ahmad, R., T. A. Teripathi, P. Tripathi, R. Singh, S. Singh, R. K. Singh. 2010. Studies on lipid peroxidation and non-enzymatic antioxidant status as indices of oxidative stress in patients with chronic myeloid leukaemia. *Singapore Med. J.* 51(2):110–115.

685. Ciobica, A., M. Padurariu, I. Dobrin, C. Stefanescu, R. Dobrin. 2011. Oxidative stress in schizophrenia—focusing on the main markers. *Psychiatr. Danub.* 23(3):237–245.

686. Fendri, C., A. Mechri, G. Khiari, A. Othman, A. Kerkeni, L. Gaha. 2006. Oxidative stress involvement in schizophrenia pathophysiology: A review. *Encéphale* 32(2 Pt 1):244–252.

687. Lushchak, V. I., D. V. Gospodaryov. 2012. *Oxidative Stress and Diseases*. InTechOpen: InTech.

688. Nathan, F. M., V. A. Singh, A. Dhanoa, U. D. Palanisamy. 2011. Oxidative stress and antioxidant status in primary bone and soft tissue sarcoma. *BMC Cancer* 11:382.

689. Grosicka-Maciag, E. 2011. Biological consequences of oxidative stress induced by pesticides. *Postepy Hig. Med. Dosw.* 65:357–366.

690. Olgun, S., H. P. Misra. 2006. Pesticides induced oxidative stress in thymocytes. *Mol. Cell. Biochem.* 290(1–2):137–144.

691. Slaninova, A., M. Smutna, H. Modra, Z. Svobodova. 2009. A review: Oxidative stress in fish induced by pesticides. *Neuro Endocrinol. Lett.* 30(suppl. 1):2–12.

692. Soltaninejad, K., M. Abdollahi. 2009. Current opinion on the science of organophosphate pesticides and toxic stress: A systematic review. *Med. Sci. Monit.* 15(3):RA75–90.

693. Abdollahi, M., S. Mostafalou, S. Pournourmohammadi, S. Shadnia. 2004. Oxidative stress and cholinesterase inhibition in saliva and plasma of rats following subchronic exposure to malathion. *Comp. Biochem. Physiol. C. Toxicol. Pharmacol.* 137(1):29–34.

694. Abdollahi, M., A. Ranjbar, S. Shadnia, S. Nikfar, A. Rezaie. 2004. Pesticides and oxidative stress: A review. *Med. Sci. Monit.* 10(6):141–147.

695. Braconi, D. B. G., M. Fiorani, C. Azzolini, B. Marzocchi, F. Proietti, G. Collodel, A. Santucci. 2010. Oxidative damage induced by herbicides is mediated by thiol oxidation and hydroperoxides production. *Free Radic. Res.* 44(8):891–906.

696. Mostafalou, S., M. Abdollahi. 2012. Concerns of environmental persistence of pesticides and human chronic diseases. *Clin. Exp. Pharmacol.* S5:e002.

697. Singh, C., I. Ahmad, A. Kumar. 2007. Pesticides and metals induced Parkinson's disease: Involvement of free radicals and oxidative stress. *Cell. Mol. Biol. (Noisyle-Grand)* 53(5):19–28.

698. Kanthasamy, A., K. M. S. Kaul, S. V. Anantharam, A. G. Kanthasamy. 2002. A novel oxidative stress dependent apoptotic pathway in pesticide-induced dopaminergic degeneration in PD models. *J. Neurochem.* 81(s1):76.

699. Sharma, H., P. Zhang, D. S. Barber, B. Liu. 2010. Organochlorine pesticides dieldrin and lindane induce cooperative toxicity in dopaminergic neurons: Role of oxidative stress. *Neurotoxicology* 31(2):215–222.

700. Mostafalou, S., M. A. Eghbal, A. Nili-Ahmadabadi, M. Baeeri, M. Abdollahi. 2012. Biochemical evidence on the potential role of organophosphates in hepatic glucose metabolism toward insulin resistance through inflammatory signaling and free radical pathways. *Toxicol. Ind. Health* 28(9):840–851.

701. Teimouri, F., N. Amirkabirian, H. Esmaily, A. Mohammadirad, A. Aliahmadi, M. Abdollahi. 2006. Alteration of hepatic cells glucose metabolism as a non-cholinergic detoxication mechanism in counteracting diazinon-induced oxidative stress. *Hum. Exp. Toxicol.* 25(12):697–703.

702. Begum, K., P. S. Rajini. 2011. Augmentation of hepatic and renal oxidative stress and disrupted glucose homeostasis by monocrotophos in streptozotocin-induced diabetic rats. *Chem. Biol. Interact.* 193(3):240–245.

703. Poovala, V. S., V. K. Kanji, H. Tachikawa, A. K. Salahudeen. 1998. Role of oxidant stress and antioxidant protection in acephate-induced renal tubular cytotoxicity. *Toxicol. Sci.* 46(2):403–409.

704. Shah, M. D., M. Iqbal. 2010. Diazinon-induced oxidative stress and renal dysfunction in rats. *Food Chem. Toxicol.* 48(12):3345–3353.

705. Tomita, M., T. Okuyama, H. Katsuyama, T. Ishikawa. 2006. Paraquat-induced gene expression in rat kidney. *Arch. Toxicol.* 80(10):687–693.

706. Xu, C., B. Bailly-Maitre, J. C. Reed. 2005. Endoplasmic reticulum stress: Cell life and death decisions. *J. Clin. Invest.* 115(10):2656–2664.

707. Back, S. H., S. W. Kang, J. Han, H. T. Chung. 2012. Endoplasmic reticulum stress in the beta-cell pathogenesis of type 2 diabetes. *Exp. Diabetes Res.* 2012:618396.

708. Kim, M. K., H. S. Kim, I. K. Lee, K. G. Park. 2012. Endoplasmic reticulum stress and insulin biosynthesis: A review. *Exp. Diabetes Res.* 2012:509437.

709. Scheuner, D., R. J. Kaufman. 2008. The unfolded protein response: A pathway that links insulin demand with beta-cell failure and diabetes. *Endocr. Rev.* 29(3):317–333.

710. Doyle, K. M., D. Kennedy, A. M. Gorman, S. Gupta, S. J. Healy, A. Samali. 2011. Unfolded proteins and endoplasmic reticulum stress in neurodegenerative disorders. *J. Cell. Mol. Med.* 15(10):2025–2039.

711. Lindholm, D., H. Wootz, L. Korhonen. 2006. ER stress and neurodegenerative diseases. *Cell Death Differ.* 13(3):385–392.

712. Koumenis, C. 2006. ER stress, hypoxia tolerance and tumor progression. *Curr. Mol. Med.* 6(1):55–69.

713. Lee, A. S., L. M. Hendershot. 2006. ER stress and cancer. *Cancer Biol. Ther.* 5(7):721–722.

714. Dickhout, J. G., R. E. Carlisle, R. C. Austin. 2011. Interrelationship between cardiac hypertrophy, heart failure, and chronic kidney disease: Endoplasmic reticulum stress as a mediator of pathogenesis. *Circ. Res.* 108(5):629–642.

715. Tabas, I. 2010. The role of endoplasmic reticulum stress in the progression of atherosclerosis. *Circ. Res.* 107(7):839–850.

716. Chinta, S. J., A. Rane, K. S. Poksay, D. E. Bredesen, J. K. Andersen, R. V. Rao. 2008. Coupling endoplasmic reticulum stress to the cell death program in dopaminergic cells: Effect of paraquat. *Neuromol. Med.* 10(4):333–342.

717. Yang, W., E. Tiffany-Castiglioni, H. C. Koh, I. H. Son. 2009. Paraquat activates the IRE1/ASK1/JNK cascade associated with apoptosis in human neuroblastoma SH-SY5Y cells. *Toxicol. Lett.* 191(2–3):203–210.

718. Chen, Y. Y., G. Chen, Z. Fan, J. Luo, Z. J. Ke. 2008. GSK3 beta and endoplasmic reticulum stress mediate rotenone-induced death of SK-N-MC neuroblastoma cells. *Biochem. Pharmacol.* 76(1):128–138.

719. Hossain, M. M., J. R. Richardson. 2011. Mechanism of pyrethroid pesticide-induced apoptosis: Role of calpain and the ER stress pathway. *Toxicol. Sci.* 122(2):512–525.

720. Chen, Y. W. et al. 2010. Pyrrolidine dithiocarbamate (PDTC)/Cu complex induces lung epithelial cell apoptosis through mitochondria and ER-stress pathways. *Toxicol. Lett.* 199(3):333–340.

721. Pesonen, M., M. Pasanen, J. Loikkanen, A. Naukkarinen, M. Hemmila, H. Seulanto, T. Kuitunen, K. Vahakangas. 2012. Chloropicrin induces endoplasmic reticulum stress in human retinal pigment epithelial cells. *Toxicol. Lett.* 211(3):239–245.

722. Skandrani, D., Y. Gaubin, B. Beau, J. C. Murat, C. Vincent, F. Croute. 2006. Effect of selected insecticides on growth rate and stress protein expression in cultured human A549 and SH-SY5Y cells. *Toxicol. In Vitro* 20(8):1378–1386.

723. Skandrani, D., Y. Gaubin, C. Vincent, B. Beau, J. Claude Murat, J. P. Soleilhavoup, F. Croute. 2006. Relationship between toxicity of selected insecticides and expression of stress proteins (HSP, GRP) in cultured human cells: Effects of commercial formulations versus pure active molecules. *Biochim. Biophys. Acta* 1760(1):95–103.

724. Gies, E., I. Wilde, J. M. Winget, M. Brack, B. Rotblat, C. A. Novoa, A. D. Balgi, P. H. Sorensen, M. Roberge, T. Mayor. 2010. Niclosamide prevents the formation of large ubiquitin-containing aggregates caused by proteasome inhibition. *PLoS One* 5(12):e14410.

725. Paul, S. 2008. Dysfunction of the ubiquitin–proteasome system in multiple disease conditions: Therapeutic approaches. *Bioessays* 30(11–12):1172–1184.

726. Sun, F., V. Anantharam, C. Latchoumycandane, A. Kanthasamy, A. G. Kanthasamy. 2005. Dieldrin induces ubiquitin–proteasome dysfunction in alpha-synuclein overexpressing dopaminergic neuronal cells and enhances susceptibility to apoptotic cell death. *J. Pharmacol. Exp. Ther.* 315(1):69–79.

727. Chou, A. P., N. Maidment, R. Klintenberg, J. E. Casida, S. Li, A. G. Fitzmaurice, P. O. Fernagut, F. Mortazavi, M. F. Chesselet, J. M. Bronstein. 2008. Ziram causes dopaminergic cell damage by inhibiting E1 ligase of the proteasome. *J. Biol. Chem.* 283(50):34696–34703.

728. Wang, X. F., S. Li, A. P. Chou, J. M. Bronstein. 2006. Inhibitory effects of pesticides on proteasome activity: Implication in Parkinson's disease. *Neurobiol. Dis.* 23(1):198–205.

729. Yang, W., E. Tiffany-Castiglioni. 2007. The bipyridyl herbicide paraquat induces proteasome dysfunction in human neuroblastoma SH-SY5Y cells. *J. Toxicol. Environ. Health A* 70(21):1849–1857.

730. Yang, W., L. Chen, Y. Ding, X. Zhuang, U. J. Kang. 2007. Paraquat induces dopaminergic dysfunction and proteasome impairment in DJ-1-deficient mice. *Hum. Mol. Genet.* 16(23):2900–2910.

731. Chou, A. P., S. Li, A. G. Fitzmaurice, J. M. Bronstein. 2010. Mechanisms of rotenone induced proteasome inhibition. *Neurotoxicology* 31(4):367–372.

732. Gonzalez, C. D., M. S. Lee, P. Marchetti, M. Pietropaolo, R. Towns, M. I. Vaccaro, H. Watada, J. W. Wiley. 2011. The emerging role of autophagy in the pathophysiology of diabetes mellitus. *Autophagy* 7(1):2–11.

733. Levine, B., G. Kroemer. 2008. Autophagy in the pathogenesis of disease. *Cell* 132(1):27–42.

734. Gonzalez-Polo, R. A., M. Niso-Santano, M. A. Ortiz-Ortiz, A. Gomez-Martin, J. M. Moran, L. Garcia-Rubio, J. Francisco-Morcillo, J. Zaragoza, G. Soler, J. M. Fuentes. 2007. Inhibition of paraquat-induced autophagy accelerates the apoptotic cell death in neuroblastoma SH-SY5Y cells. *Toxicol. Sci.* 97(2):448–458.

735. Niso-Santano, M., J. M. Bravo-San Pedro, R. Gomez-Sanchez, V. Climent, G. Soler, J. M. Fuentes, R. A. Gonzalez-Polo. 2011. ASK1 overexpression accelerates paraquat-induced autophagy via endoplasmic reticulum stress. *Toxicol. Sci.* 119(1):156–168.

736. Zucchini-Pascal, N., G. de Sousa, R. Rahmani. 2009. Lindane and cell death: At the crossroads between apoptosis, necrosis and autophagy. *Toxicology* 256(1–2):32–41.

737. Jungmann, G. 1966. Arsenic cancer in vintagers. *Landarzt* 42(28):1244–1247.

738. Roth, F. 1958. Uber den Bronchialkrebs Arsengeschadigter Winzer. *Virchows Arch.* 331(119–137).

739. Thiers, H., D. Colomb, G. Moulin, L. Colin. 1967. Arsenical skin cancer in vineyards in the Beaulolais (Fr.). *Ann. Dermatol.* 94:133–158.

740. Penel, N., D. Vansteene. 2007. Cancers and pesticides: Current data. *Bull. Cancer* 94(1):15–22.

741. Baldi, I., P. Lebailly. 2007. Cancers and pesticides. *Rev. Prat.* 57(suppl. 11):40–44.

742. Alavanja, M. C., M. R. Bonner. 2012. Occupational pesticide exposures and cancer risk: A review. *J. Toxicol. Environ. Health B Crit. Rev.* 15(4):238–263.

743. Jaga, K., C. Dharmani. 2005. The epidemiology of pesticide exposure and cancer: A review. *Rev. Environ. Health* 20(1):15–38.

744. Weichenthal, S., C. Moase, P. Chan. 2010. A review of pesticide exposure and cancer incidence in the Agricultural Health Study cohort. *Environ. Health Perspect.* 118(8):1117–1125.

745. Van Maele-Fabry, G., V. Libotte, J. Willems, D. Lison. 2006. Review and meta-analysis of risk estimates for prostate cancer in pesticide manufacturing workers. *Cancer Causes Control* 17(4):353–373.

746. Van Maele-Fabry, G., S. Duhayon, D. Lison. 2007. A systematic review of myeloid leukemias and occupational pesticide exposure. *Cancer Causes Control* 18(5):457–478.

747. Van Maele-Fabry, G., S. Duhayon, C. Mertens, D. Lison. 2008. Risk of leukaemia among pesticide manufacturing workers: A review and meta-analysis of cohort studies. *Environ. Res.* 106(1):121–137.

748. Lee, W. J., A. Blair, J. A. Hoppin, J. H. Lubin, J. A. Rusiecki, D. P. Sandler, M. Dosemeci, M. C. Alavanja. 2004. Cancer incidence among pesticide applicators exposed to chlorpyrifos in the Agricultural Health Study. *J. Natl. Cancer Inst.* 96(23):1781–1789.

749. Lee, W. J., J. A. Hoppin, A. Blair, J. H. Lubin, M. Dosemeci, D. P. Sandler, M. C. Alavanja. 2004. Cancer incidence among pesticide applicators exposed to alachlor in the Agricultural Health Study. *Am. J. Epidemiol.* 159(4):373–380.

750. Lee, W. J., D. P. Sandler, A. Blair, C. Samanic, A. J. Cross, M. C. Alavanja. 2007. Pesticide use and colorectal cancer risk in the Agricultural Health Study. *Int. J. Cancer* 121(2):339–346.

751. George, J., Y. Shukla. 2011. Pesticides and cancer: Insights into toxicoproteomic-based findings. *J. Proteomics* 74(12):2713–2722.

752. Rakitsky, V. N., V. A. Koblyakov, V. S. Turusov. 2000. Nongenotoxic (epigenetic) carcinogens: Pesticides as an example. A critical review. *Teratog. Carcinog. Mutagen.* 20(4):229–240.

753. Purdue, M. P., J. A. Hoppin, A. Blair, M. Dosemeci, M. C. Alavanja. 2007. Occupational exposure to organochlorine insecticides and cancer incidence in the Agricultural Health Study. *Int. J. Cancer* 120(3):642–649.

754. Beane Freeman, L. E., M. R. Bonner, A. Blair, J. A. Hoppin, D. P. Sandler, J. H. Lubin, M. Dosemeci, C. F. Lynch, C. Knott, M. C. Alavanja. 2005. Cancer incidence among male pesticide applicators in the Agricultural Health Study cohort exposed to diazinon. *Am. J. Epidemiol.* 162(11):1070–1079.

755. van Bemmel, D. M., K. Visvanathan, L. E. Beane Freeman, J. Coble, J. A. Hoppin, M. C. Alavanja. 2008. S-ethyl-N,N-dipropylthiocarbamate exposure and cancer incidence among male pesticide applicators in the agricultural health study: A prospective cohort. *Environ. Health Perspect.* 116(11):1541–1546.

756. Mahajan, R., A. Blair, C. F. Lynch, P. Schroeder, J. A. Hoppin, D. P. Sandler, M. C. Alavanja. 2006. Fonofos exposure and cancer incidence in the agricultural health study. *Environ. Health Perspect.* 114(12):1838–1842.

757. Spinelli, J. J., C. H. Ng, J. P. Weber, J. M. Connors, R. D. Gascoyne, A. S. Lai, A. R. Brooks-Wilson, N. D. Le, B. R. Berry, R. P. Gallagher. 2007. Organochlorines and risk of non-Hodgkin lymphoma. *Int. J. Cancer* 121(12):2767–2775.

758. Alavanja, M. C. et al. 2003. Use of agricultural pesticides and prostate cancer risk in the Agricultural Health Study cohort. *Am. J. Epidemiol.* 157(9):800–814.

759. Lynch, S. M., R. Mahajan, L. E. Beane Freeman, J. A. Hoppin, M. C. Alavanja. 2009. Cancer incidence among pesticide applicators exposed to butylate in the Agricultural Health Study (AHS). *Environ. Res.* 109(7):860–868.

760. Multigner, L., J. R. Ndong, A. Giusti, M. Romana, H. Delacroix-Maillard, S. Cordier, B. Jegou, J. P. Thome, P. Blanchet. 2010. Chlordecone exposure and risk of prostate cancer. *J. Clin. Oncol.* 28(21):3457–3462.

761. Band, P. R., Z. Abanto, J. Bert, B. Lang, R. Fang, R. P. Gallagher, N. D. Le. 2011. Prostate cancer risk and exposure to pesticides in British Columbia farmers. *Prostate* 71(2):168–183.

762. Samanic, C., J. Rusiecki, M. Dosemeci, L. Hou, J. A. Hoppin, D. P. Sandler, J. Lubin, A. Blair, M. C. Alavanja. 2006. Cancer incidence among pesticide applicators exposed to dicamba in the agricultural health study. *Environ. Health Perspect.* 114(10):1521–1526.

763. Koutros, S. et al. 2009. Heterocyclic aromatic amine pesticide use and human cancer risk: Results from the U.S. Agricultural Health Study. *Int. J. Cancer* 124(5):1206–1212.

764. Kang, D. et al. 2008. Cancer incidence among pesticide applicators exposed to trifluralin in the Agricultural Health Study. *Environ. Res.* 107(2):271–276.

765. Hou, L. et al. 2006. Pendimethalin exposure and cancer incidence among pesticide applicators. *Epidemiology* 17(3):302–307.

766. Andreotti, G., L. E. Freeman, L. Hou, J. Coble, J. Rusiecki, J. A. Hoppin, D. T. Silverman, M. C. Alavanja. 2009. Agricultural pesticide use and pancreatic cancer risk in the Agricultural Health Study Cohort. *Int. J. Cancer* 124(10):2495–2500.

767. Garabrant, D. H., J. Held, B. Langholz, J. M. Peters, T. M. Mack. 1992. DDT and related compounds and risk of pancreatic cancer. *J. Natl. Cancer Inst.* 84(10):764–771.

768. Alavanja, M. C. et al. 2004. Pesticides and lung cancer risk in the agricultural health study cohort. *Am. J. Epidemiol.* 160(9):876–885.

769. Dennis, L. K., C. F. Lynch, D. P. Sandler, M. C. Alavanja. 2010. Pesticide use and cutaneous melanoma in pesticide applicators in the agricultural heath study. *Environ. Health Perspect.* 118(6):812–817.

770. Pimentel, D., K. Hart. 2001. Pesticide use: Ethical, environmental, and public health implications. In *New Dimensions in Bioethics: Science, Ethics and the Formulation of Public Policy*, W. Galston, E. Shurr, eds., Boston, MA: Kluwer Academic Publishers.

771. Colborn, T., J. P. Myers, D. Dumanoski. 1996. *Our Stolen Future: How We Are Threatening Our Fertility, Intelligence, and Survival: A Scientific Detective Story.* New York: Dutton.

772. NAS. 1987. *Regulating Pesticides in Food.* Washington, DC: National Academy of Sciences.

773. Law, S., K. Basu, S. Banerjee, B. Begum, S. Chaudhuri. 2006. Cord blood-derived plasma factor (CBPF) potentiates the low cytokinetic and immunokinetic profile of bone marrow cells in pesticide victims suffering from acquired aplastic anaemia (AAA): An in Vitro Correlate. *Immunol. Investigations* 35(2):209–25.

774. Roberts, J. H. 1963. Aplastic anaemia due to pentachlorophenol and tetrachlorophenol. *South. Med. J.* 56:632.

775. Aksoy, M., K. Dincol, T. Akgun, S. Erdem, G. Dincol. 1971. Haematological effects of chronic benzene poisoning in 217 workers. *Br. J. Indust. Med.* 2:296–301.

776. Yardley-Jones, A., D. Anderson, D. V. Parke. 1991. The toxicity of benzene and its metabolism and molecular pathology in human risk assessment. *Br. J. Indust. Med.* 48:437–442.

777. Howard, P. H. 1991. Pesticides. In *Handbook of Environmental Fate and Exposure Data for Organic Chemicals*, Vol. 3, Chelsea, MI: Lewis.

778. Camitta, B. M., E. D. Thomas, D. G. Nathan, R. P. Gale, K. J. Kopecky, J. M. Rappeport, G. Santos, E. C. Gordon-Smith, R. Strob. 1979. A prospective study of androgens and bone marrow transplantation for treatment of severe aplastic anaemia. *Blood* 53:504–514.

779. Kansu, E., A. J. Erslev. 1976. Aplastic anaemia with "hot pockets." Scand. *J. Haematol.* 17:326–334.

780. Yang, C. W. Z., L. Li. 1962. Studies of bone marrow of aplastic anaemia: Preliminary classification study. *J. Chin. Intern. Med.* 12:757.

781. Shadduck, R. K. 2001. *Williams Haematology*, pp. 375–390. New York: McGraw-Hill Company.

782. Morstyn, G., W. Sheridan. 1996. *Cell Therapy*. Cambridge, UK: Cambridge University Press.

783. Storb, R., R. L. Prentice, E. D. Thomas. 1977. Marrow transplantation for treatment of aplastic anaemia. An analysis of factors associated with graft rejection. *N. Eng. J. Med.* 296:61–66.

784. Tooze, J. A., J. C. Marsh, G. E. C. Smith. 1999. Clonal evolution of aplastic anaemia to myelodysplasia/ acute myeloid leukaemia and paroxymal nocturnal haemoglobinuria. *Leuk. Lymphoma* 33:231–241.

785. Socie, G., S. Rosenfeld, N. Frickhofen, E. Gluckman, A. Tichelli. 2000. Late clonal diseases of treated aplastic anaemia. *Semin. Haematol.* 37:91–101.

786. Dexter, T. M., T. C. Allen, L. G. Lajtha. 1977. Conditions controlling the proliferation of hemopoietic stem cells in vitro. *J. Cell Physiol.* 91:335–342.

787. Verfaille, C. M. 1993. Soluble factors produced by Human Bone Marrow stroma increase cytokine-induced-proliferation and maturation of primitive hematopoietic progenitors while preventing their terminal differentiation. *Blood* 82:2045–2052.

788. Owen, M. E. 2002. In *Marrow Stromal Cell Culture*, J. N. Beresford, M. E. Owen, eds., pp. 1–9. Cambridge: Cambridge University Press.

789. Sanchez-Medal, L., J. P. Castanedo, F. Garcia-Rojas. 1963. Insecticides and aplastic anaemia. *N. Eng. J. Med.* 269:1365–1371.

790. Rugman, F. P., R. Cosstick. 1990. Aplastic anaemia associated with organochlorine pesticide: Case reports and review of evidence. *J. Clin. Pathol.* 43:98–110.

791. Fleming, L. E., M. A. Timeny. 1993. Aplastic anaemia and pesticides. *JOM* 35:1106–1112.

792. Knospe, W. H., W. H. Crosby. 1971. Aplastic anaemia: A disorder of the bone marrow sinusoidal microcirculation rather than stem-cell failure? *Lancet* 1:20–26.

793. Thomas, E. D., R. Storb, E. R. Giblett, B. Longpre, P. L. Weiden, A. Fefer, R. Witherspoon, R. A. Clift, C. D. Buckner. 1976. Recovery from aplastic anaemia following attempted marrow transplantation. *Exp. Haematol.* 4:97–102.

794. Ershler, W. B., J. Ross, J. L. Finlay, N. T. Shahidi. 1980. Bone marrow microenvironment defect in congenital hypoplastic anaemia. *N. Eng. J. Med.* 302:1321–1327.

795. Schrezenmeier, H., M. Gerok, H. Heimpel. 1992. Assessment of frequency of haematopoietic stem cells in aplastic anaemia by limiting dilution type long term marrow culture. *Expl. Haematol.* 20:806.

796. Brodsky, R. A. 1998. Biology and management of acquired severe aplastic anaemia. *Curr. Op. Oncol.* 10:95–99.

797. Gluckman, E., R. Rokicka-Milewska, I. Hann, E. Nikiforakis, F. Tavakoli, S. Cohen-Scali, A. Bacigalupo. 2002. Results and follow-up of a phase III randomized study of recombinant human granulocyte stimulating factor as support for immunosuppressive therapy in patients with severe aplastic anaemia. *Brit. J. Haematol.* 119:1075–1082.

798. Powell, K. 2005. It's the ecology, stupid. *Nature* 435:268–270.

799. Basu, K. 2003. *Structure-Function Correlationship of the Pluripotent Cells of Bone Marrow in Health and Disease: An Immunological Approach Towards the Haematopoietic Microenvironment versus Biological Response Modifiers.* Ph.D. thesis. Jadavpur University, Kolkata, India.

800. Forraz, N., R. Pettengell, C. P. Mc Guckin. 2002. Haematopoietic and neuroglial progenitor are promoted during cord blood ex-vivo expansion. *Brit. J. Haematol.* 119(4):888.

801. Law, S., D. Maiti, A. Palit, D. Majumder, K. Basu, S. Chaudhuri, S. Chaudhuri. 2001. Facilitation of functional compartmentalization of Bone marrow cells in leukemic mice by biological response modifiers: An immunotherapeutic approach. *Immun. Lett.* 76:145–152.

802. Law, S., B. Begum, S. Chaudhuri. 2003. Pluripotent bone marrow cells in leukemic mice elicit enhanced immune reactivity following sheep erythrocyte administration in vivo: A possible S-LFA3 interactive immunotherapy. *J. Exp. Clin. Cancer Res.* 22(2):421–429.

803. Law, S., D. Maiti, A. Palit, S. Chaudhuri. 2003. Role of Biomodulators and involvement of protein tyrosine kinase on stem cell migration in normal and leukaemic mice. *Immunol. Lett.* 86(3):287–290.

804. Law, S., S. Chaudhuri. 2004. Stem cells: Biomedical kinetics and application. *USTA* 6:5–17.

805. Saito, H. K., A. M. Hatakc, K. M. Dvorak, A. D. Leiferman, N. Donenberg, K. Arai, J. Ishizaka. 1988. Selective differentiation and proliferation of hematopoietic cells induced by recombinant human interleukins. *Proc. Natl. Acad. Sci.* 85:2288.

806. Gratkowski, H. 1974. *Herbicidal drift control: Aerial spray equipment, formulations, and supervision.* U.S.D.A. Forest Service General Technical Report PNW-14. Portland, OR: Pacific Northwest Forest and Range Experiment Station.

807. von Rumker, R. 1975. *A Study of the Efficiency of the Use of Pesticides in Agriculture.* Washington, DC: U.S. Environmental Protection Agency, Office of Pesticide Programs. EPA-540/9-75-025.

808. Heifetz, R. M., S. S. Taylor. 1989. Mother's milk or mother's poison? Pesticides in breastmilk. *J. Pest. Reform* 9(3):15–17.

809. U.S. House of Representatives. 1990. Statement of Jay Feldman, national coordinator: National Coalition Against the Misuse of Pesticides, before the Select Committee on Children, Youth and Families, September 13, 1990, Washington, DC.

810. National Coalition Against the Misuse of Pesticides. 1992. Lawn pesticide facts and figures. *Pesticide Regulation Hanbook A Guide for Users.* CRC Press.

811. Bazell, R. 1989. Cancer warp. *N. Republic* 201(25):12.

812. Calabrese, E. J. 1986. *Age and Susceptibility to Toxic Substances.* New York: John Wiley & Sons.

813. Spyker, J. M., D. L. Avery. 1977. Neurobehavioral effects of prenatal exposure to the organophosphate diazinon in mice. *J. Toxicol. Environ. Health* 3:989–1002.

814. Paigen, B. 1986. Children and toxic chemicals. *J. Pest. Reform* 6:2–3.

815. Lowengart, R. A., J. M. Peters, C. Cicionic, J. Buckley, L. Bernstein, S. Preston-Martin, E. Rappaport. 1987. Childhood leukemia and parents' occupational and home exposures. *J. Natl. Cancer Inst.* 79(1):39–46.

816. Behan, P. O., B. A. G. Haniffah. 1994. Chronic fatigue syndrome: A possible delayed hazard of pesticide exposure. *Clin. Infect. Dis.* 18(suppl. 1):S54.

817. Cooper, G. S., C. G. Parks, E. L. Treadwell, E. W. St Clair, G. S. Gilkeson, M. A. Dooley. 2004. Occupational risk factors for the development of systemic lupus erythematosus. *J. Rheumatol.* 31(10):1928–1933.

818. Gold, L. S., M. H. Ward, M. Dosemeci, A. J. De Roos. 2007. Systemic autoimmune disease mortality and occupational exposures. *Arthritis Rheum.* 56(10):3189–3201.

819. Parks, C. G., B. T. Walitt, M. Pettinger, J. C. Chen, A. J. de Roos, J. Hunt, G. Sarto, B. V. Howard. 2011. Insecticide use and risk of rheumatoid arthritis and systemic lupus erythematosus in the Women's Health Initiative Observational Study. *Arthritis Care Res. (Hoboken)* 63(2):184–194.

820. Walsh, N. 2016. Pesticides Linked to RA, Lupus Risk. [Accessed March 15, 2016] http://www.medpagetoday.com/Rheumatology/Arthritis/24625

821. Stroud, R. M., L. J. W. Miercke, J. O'Connell, S. Khademi, J. K. Lee, J. Remis, W. Harries, Y. Robles, D. Akhavan. 2003. Glycerol facilitator GlpF and the associated aquaporin family of channels. *Curr. Opin Struct. Biol.* 13(4):424–31.

822. Alderton, L. E., L. G. Spector, C. K. Blair, M. Roesler, A. F. Olshan, L. L. Robison, J. A. Ross. 2006. Child and maternal household chemical exposure and the risk of acute leukemia in children with Down's syndrome: A report from the Children's Oncology Group. *Am. J. Epidemiol.* 164(3):212–221.

823. Carozza, S. E., B. Li, K. Elgethun, R. Whitworth. 2008. Risk of childhood cancers associated with residence in agriculturally intense areas in the United States. *Environ. Health Perspect.* 116(4): 559–565.

824. Turner, M. C., D. T. Wigle, D. Krewski. 2010. Residential pesticides and childhood leukemia: A systematic review and meta-analysis. *Environ. Health Perspect.* 118(1):33–41.

825. Alexander, F. E. et al. 2001. Transplacental chemical exposure and risk of infant leukemia with MLL gene fusion. *Cancer Res.* 61(6):2542–2546.

826. Buckley, J. D. et al. 1989. Occupational exposures of parents of children with acute nonlymphocytic leukemia: A report from the Childrens Cancer Study Group. *Cancer Res.* 49(14):4030–4037.

827. Buckley, J. D., C. M. Buckley, K. Ruccione, H. N. Sather, M. J. Waskerwitz, W. G. Woods, L. L. Robison. 1994. Epidemiological characteristics of childhood acute lymphocytic leukemia. Analysis by immunophenotype. The Childrens Cancer Group. *Leukemia* 8(5):856–864.

828. Infante-Rivard, C., D. Labuda, M. Krajinovic, D. Sinnett. 1999. Risk of childhood leukemia associated with exposure to pesticides and with gene polymorphisms. *Epidemiology* 10(5):481–487.

829. Lafiura, K. M., D. M. Bielawski, N. C. Posecion Jr., E. M. Ostrea Jr., L. H. Matherly, J. W. Taub, Y. Ge. 2007. Association between prenatal pesticide exposures and the generation of leukemia-associated T(8;21). *Pediatr. Blood Cancer* 49(5):624–628.

830. Laval, G., A. J. Tuyns. 1988. Environmental factors in childhood leukaemia. *Br. J. Ind. Med.* 45(12):843–844.

831. Leiss, J. K., D. A. Savitz. 1995. Home pesticide use and childhood cancer: A case-control study. *Am. J. Public Health* 85(2):249–252.

832. Ma, X., P. A. Buffler, R. B. Gunier, G. Dahl, M. T. Smith, K. Reinier, P. Reynolds. 2002. Critical windows of exposure to household pesticides and risk of childhood leukemia. *Environ. Health Perspect.* 110(9):955–960.

833. Magnani, C., G. Pastore, L. Luzzatto, B. Terracini. 1990. Parental occupation and other environmental factors in the etiology of leukemias and non-Hodgkin's lymphomas in childhood: A case-control study. *Tumori* 76(5):413–419.

834. Meinert, R., P. Kaatsch, U. Kaletsch, F. Krummenauer, A. Miesner, J. Michaelis. 1996. Childhood leukaemia and exposure to pesticides: Results of a case-control study in northern Germany. *Eur. J. Cancer* 32A(11):1943–1948.

835. Menegaux, F., A. Baruchel, Y. Bertrand, B. Lescoeur, G. Leverger, B. Nelken, D. Sommelet, D. Hemon, J. Clavel. 2006. Household exposure to pesticides and risk of childhood acute leukaemia. *Occup. Environ. Med.* 63(2):131–134.

836. Monge, P., C. Wesseling, J. Guardado, I. Lundberg, A. Ahlbom, K. P. Cantor, E. Weiderpass, T. Partanen. 2007. Parental occupational exposure to pesticides and the risk of childhood leukemia in Costa Rica. *Scand. J. Work Environ. Health* 33(4):293–303.

837. Mulder, Y. M., M. Drijver, I. A. Kreis. 1994. Case-control study on the association between a cluster of childhood haematopoietic malignancies and local environmental factors in Aalsmeer, The Netherlands. *J. Epidemiol. Community Health* 48(2):161–165.

838. Rau, A. T., A. Coutinho, K. S. Avabratha, A. R. Rau, R. P. Warrier. 2012. Pesticide (endosulfan) levels in the bone marrow of children with hematological malignancies. *Indian Pediatr.* 49(2):113–117.

839. Reynolds, P., J. Von Behren, R. B. Gunier, D. E. Goldberg, M. Harnly, A. Hertz. 2005. Agricultural pesticide use and childhood cancer in California. *Epidemiology* 16(1):93–100.

840. Rudant, J. et al. 2007. Household exposure to pesticides and risk of childhood hematopoietic malignancies: The ESCALE study (SFCE). *Environ. Health Perspect.* 115(12):1787–1793.

841. Rull, R. P., R. Gunier, J. Von Behren, A. Hertz, V. Crouse, P. A. Buffler, P. Reynolds. 2009. Residential proximity to agricultural pesticide applications and childhood acute lymphoblastic leukemia. *Environ. Res.* 109(7):891–899.

842. Shu, X. O., Y. T. Gao, L. A. Brinton, M. S. Linet, J. T. Tu, W. Zheng, J. F. Fraumeni Jr. 1988. A population-based case-control study of childhood leukemia in Shanghai. *Cancer* 62(3):635–644.

843. Soldin, O. P., H. Nsouli-Maktabi, J. M. Genkinger, C. A. Loffredo, J. A. Ortega-Garcia, D. Colantino, D. B. Barr, N. L. Luban, A. T. Shad, D. Nelson. 2009. Pediatric acute lymphoblastic leukemia and exposure to pesticides. *Ther. Drug Monit.* 31(4):495–501.

844. Alavanja, M. C., A. Blair, M. N. Masters. 1990. Cancer mortality in the U.S. flour industry. *J. Natl. Cancer Inst.* 82(10):840–848.

845. de Chrisman, J. R., S. Koifman, P. de Novaes Sarcinelli, J. C. Moreira, R. J. Koifman, A. Meyer. 2009. Pesticide sales and adult male cancer mortality in Brazil. *Int. J. Hyg. Environ. Health* 212(3):310–321.

846. Cuneo, A., F. Fagioli, I. Pazzi, A. Tallarico, R. Previati, N. Piva, M. G. Carli, M. Balboni, G. Castoldi. 1992. Morphologic, immunologic and cytogenetic studies in acute myeloid leukemia following occupational exposure to pesticides and organic solvents. *Leuk. Res.* 16(8):789–796.

847. Brown, L. M., A. Blair, R. Gibson, G. D. Everett, K. P. Cantor, L. M. Schuman, L. F. Burmeister, S. F. Van Lier, F. Dick. 1990. Pesticide exposures and other agricultural risk factors for leukemia among men in Iowa and Minnesota. *Cancer Res.* 50(20):6585–6591.

848. Beard, J., T. Sladden, G. Morgan, G. Berry, L. Brooks, A. McMichael. 2003. Health impacts of pesticide exposure in a cohort of outdoor workers. *Environ. Health Perspect.* 111(5):724–730.

849. Delzell, E., S. Grufferman. 1985. Mortality among white and nonwhite farmers in North Carolina, 1976–1978. *Am. J. Epidemiol.* 121(3):391–402.

850. Merhi, M., H. Raynal, E. Cahuzac, F. Vinson, J. P. Cravedi, L. Gamet-Payrastre. 2007. Occupational exposure to pesticides and risk of hematopoietic cancers: Meta-analysis of case-control studies. *Cancer Causes Control* 18(10):1209–1226.

851. Ciccone, G., D. Mirabelli, A. Levis, G. Gavarotti, G. Rege-Cambrin, L. Davico, P. Vineis. 1993. Myeloid leukemias and myelodysplastic syndromes: Chemical exposure, histologic subtype and cytogenetics in a case-control study. *Cancer Genet. Cytogenet.* 68(2):135–139.

852. Van Maele-Fabry, G., S. Duhayon, C. Mertens, D. Lison. 2008. Risk of leukaemia among pesticide manufacturing workers: A review and meta-analysis of cohort studies. *Environ. Res.* 106(1):121–137.

853. Clavel, J., D. Hemon, L. Mandereau, B. Delemotte, F. Severin, G. Flandrin. 1996. Farming, pesticide use and hairy-cell leukemia. *Scand. J. Work Environ. Health* 22(4):285–293.

854. Bonner, M. R., B. A. Williams, J. A. Rusiecki, A. Blair, L. E. Beane Freeman, J. A. Hoppin, M. Dosemeci, J. Lubin, D. P. Sandler, M. C. Alavanja. 2010. Occupational exposure to terbufos and the incidence of cancer in the Agricultural Health Study. *Cancer Causes Control* 21(6):871–877.

855. Mills, P. K. 1998. Correlation analysis of pesticide use data and cancer incidence rates in California counties. *Arch. Environ. Health* 53(6):410–413.

856. Miligi, L., A. S. Costantini, A. Veraldi, A. Benvenuti, P. Vineis. 2006. Cancer and pesticides: An overview and some results of the Italian multicenter case-control study on hematolymphopoietic malignancies. *Ann. N. Y. Acad. Sci.* 1076:366–377.

857. Cantor, K. P., W. Silberman. 1999. Mortality among aerial pesticide applicators and flight instructors: Follow-up from 1965–1988. *Am. J. Ind. Med.* 36(2):239–247.

858. Orsi, L. et al. 2007. Occupation and lymphoid malignancies: Results from a French case-control study. *J. Occup. Environ. Med.* 49(12):1339–1350.

859. Flower, K. B., J. A. Hoppin, C. F. Lynch, A. Blair, C. Knott, D. L. Shore, D. P. Sandler. 2004. Cancer risk and parental pesticide application in children of Agricultural Health Study participants. *Environ. Health Perspect.* 112(5):631–635.

860. Persson, B., M. Fredriksson, K. Olsen, B. Boeryd, O. Axelson. 1993. Some occupational exposures as risk factors for malignant lymphomas. *Cancer* 72(5):1773–1778.

861. Cerhan, J. R., K. P. Cantor, K. Williamson, C. F. Lynch, J. C. Torner, L. F. Burmeister. 1998. Cancer mortality among Iowa farmers: Recent results, time trends, and lifestyle factors (United States). *Cancer Causes Control* 9(3):311–319.

862. van Balen, E., R. Font, N. Cavalle, L. Font, M. Garcia-Villanueva, Y. Benavente, P. Brennan, S. de Sanjose. 2006. Exposure to non-arsenic pesticides is associated with lymphoma among farmers in Spain. *Occup. Environ. Med.* 63(10):663–668.

863. Khuder, S. A., E. A. Schaub, J. E. Keller-Byrne. 1998. Meta-analyses of non-Hodgkin's lymphoma and farming. *Scand. J. Work Environ. Health* 24(4):255–261.

864. Buckley, J. D., A. T. Meadows, M. E. Kadin, M. M. Le Beau, S. Siegel, L. L. Robison. 2000. Pesticide exposures in children with non-Hodgkin lymphoma. *Cancer* 89(11):2315–2321.

865. Kristensen, P., A. Andersen, L. M. Irgens, P. Laake, A. S. Bye. 1996. Incidence and risk factors of cancer among men and women in Norwegian agriculture. *Scand. J. Work Environ. Health* 22(1):14–26.

866. Cantor, K. P. 1982. Farming and mortality from non-Hodgkin's lymphoma: A case-control study. *Int. J. Cancer* 29(3):239–247.

867. Kross, B. C., L. F. Burmeister, L. K. Ogilvie, L. J. Fuortes, C. M. Fu. 1996. Proportionate mortality study of golf course superintendents. *Am. J. Ind. Med.* 29(5):501–506.

868. Cantor, K. P., A. Blair, G. Everett, R. Gibson, L. F. Burmeister, L. M. Brown, L. Schuman, F. R. Dick. 1992. Pesticides and other agricultural risk factors for non-Hodgkin's lymphoma among men in Iowa and Minnesota. *Cancer Res.* 52(9):2447–2455.

869. Morrison, H. I., R. M. Semenciw, K. Wilkins, Y. Mao, D. T. Wigle. 1994. Non-Hodgkin's lymphoma and agricultural practices in the prairie provinces of Canada. *Scand. J. Work Environ. Health* 20(1):42–47.

870. Chiu, B. C., B. J. Dave, A. Blair, S. M. Gapstur, S. H. Zahm, D. D. Weisenburger. 2006. Agricultural pesticide use and risk of t(14;18)-defined subtypes of non-Hodgkin lymphoma. *Blood* 108(4):1363–1369.

871. Purdue, M. P., J. A. Hoppin, A. Blair, M. Dosemeci, M. C. Alavanja. 2007. Occupational exposure to organochlorine insecticides and cancer incidence in the Agricultural Health Study. *Int. J. Cancer* 120(3):642–649.

872. De Roos, A. J., S. H. Zahm, K. P. Cantor, D. D. Weisenburger, F. F. Holmes, L. F. Burmeister, A. Blair. 2003. Integrative assessment of multiple pesticides as risk factors for nonHodgkin's lymphoma among men. *Occup. Environ. Med.* 60(9):E11.

873. Ritter, L., D. T. Wigle, R. M. Semenciw, K. Wilkins, D. Riedel, Y. Mao. 1990. Mortality study of Canadian male farm operators: Cancer mortality and agricultural practices in Saskatchewan. *Med. Lav.* 81(6):499–505.

874. Eriksson, M., L. Hardell, M. Carlberg, M. Akerman. 2008. Pesticide exposure as risk factor for non-Hodgkin lymphoma including histopathological subgroup analysis. *Int. J. Cancer* 123(7):1657–1663.

875. Zhong, Y., V. Rafnsson. 1996. Cancer incidence among Icelandic pesticide users. *Int. J. Epidemiol.* 25(6):1117–1124.

876. Hardell, L., M. Eriksson. 1999. A case-control study of non-Hodgkin lymphoma and exposure to pesticides. *Cancer* 85(6):1353–1360.

877. Hardell, L., M. Eriksson, M. Nordstrom. 2002. Exposure to pesticides as risk factor for non-Hodgkin's lymphoma and hairy cell leukemia: Pooled analysis of two Swedish case-control studies. *Leuk. Lymphoma* 43(5):1043–1049.

878. Hoar, S. K., A. Blair, F. F. Holmes, C. D. Boysen, R. J. Robel, R. Hoover, J. F. Fraumeni Jr. 1986. Agricultural herbicide use and risk of lymphoma and soft-tissue sarcoma. *JAMA* 256(9):1141–1147.

879. McDuffie, H. H., P. Pahwa, J. R. McLaughlin, J. J. Spinelli, S. Fincham, J. A. Dosman, D. Robson, L. F. Skinnider, N. W. Choi. 2001. Non-Hodgkin's lymphoma and specific pesticide exposures in men: Cross-Canada study of pesticides and health. *Cancer Epidemiol. Biomarkers Prev.* 10(11):1155–1163.

880. Meinert, R., J. Schuz, U. Kaletsch, P. Kaatsch, J. Michaelis. 2000. Leukemia and nonHodgkin's lymphoma in childhood and exposure to pesticides: Results of a registerbased case-control study in Germany. *Am. J. Epidemiol.* 151(7):639–646 (discussion 647–650).

881. Miligi, L., A. S. Costantini, A. Veraldi, A. Benvenuti, P. Vineis. 2006. Cancer and pesticides: An overview and some results of the Italian multicenter case-control study on hematolymphopoietic malignancies. *Ann. N. Y. Acad. Sci.* 1076:366–377.

882. Nordstrom, M., L. Hardell, A. Magnuson, H. Hagberg, A. Rask-Andersen. 1998. Occupational exposures, animal exposure and smoking as risk factors for hairy cell leukaemia evaluated in a case-control study. *Br. J. Cancer* 77(11):2048–2052.

883. Pearce, N. E., A. H. Smith, D. O. Fisher. 1985. Malignant lymphoma and multiple myeloma linked with agricultural occupations in a New Zealand Cancer Registry-based study. *Am. J. Epidemiol.* 121(2):225–237.

884. Schroeder, J. C. et al. 2001. Agricultural risk factors for t(14;18) subtypes of non-Hodgkin's lymphoma. *Epidemiology* 12(6):701–709.

885. t Mannetje, A. et al. 2008. High risk occupations for non-Hodgkin's lymphoma in New Zealand: Case-control study. *Occup. Environ. Med.* 65(5):354–363.

886. Vajdic, C. M. et al. 2007. Atopy, exposure to pesticides and risk of non-Hodgkin lymphoma. *Int. J. Cancer* 120(10):2271–2274.

887. Woods, J. S., L. Polissar, R. K. Severson, L. S. Heuser, B. G. Kulander. 1987. Soft tissue sarcoma and non-Hodgkin's lymphoma in relation to phenoxyherbicide and chlorinated phenol exposure in western Washington. *J. Natl. Cancer Inst.* 78(5):899–910.

888. Zahm, S. H., D. D. Weisenburger, P. A. Babbitt, R. C. Saal, J. B. Vaught, K. P. Cantor, A. Blair. 1990. A case-control study of non-Hodgkin's lymphoma and the herbicide 2,4-dichlorophenoxyacetic acid(2,4-D) in eastern Nebraska. *Epidemiology* 1(5):349–356.

889. Zahm, S. H., D. D. Weisenburger, R. C. Saal, J. B. Vaught, P. A. Babbitt, A. Blair. 1993. The role of agricultural pesticide use in the development of non-Hodgkin's lymphoma in women. *Arch. Environ. Health* 48(5):353–358.

890. Burmeister, L. F., G. D. Everett, S. F. Van Lier, P. Isacson. 1983. Selected cancer mortality and farm practices in Iowa. *Am. J. Epidemiol.* 118(1):72–77.

891. Cerhan, J. R., K. P. Cantor, K. Williamson, C. F. Lynch, J. C. Torner, L. F. Burmeister. 1998. Cancer mortality among Iowa farmers: Recent results, time trends, and lifestyle factors (United States). *Cancer Causes Control* 9(3):311–319.

892. Landgren, O., R. A. Kyle, J. A. Hoppin, B. L. E. Freeman, J. R. Cerhan, J. A. Katzmann, S. V. Rajkumar, M. C. Alavanja. 2009. Pesticide exposure and risk of monoclonal gammopathy of undetermined significance in the Agricultural Health Study. *Blood* 113(25):6386–6391.

893. Lope, V., B. Perez-Gomez, N. Aragones, G. Lopez-Abente, P. Gustavsson, N. Plato, J. P. Zock, M. Pollan. 2008. Occupation, exposure to chemicals, sensitizing agents, and risk of multiple myeloma in Sweden. *Cancer Epidemiol. Biomarkers Prev.* 17(11):3123–3127.

894. Daniels, J. L. et al. 2001. Residential pesticide exposure and neuroblastoma. *Epidemiology* 12(1):20–27.

895. Feychting, M., N. Plato, G. Nise, A. Ahlbom. 2001. Paternal occupational exposures and childhood cancer. *Environ. Health Perspect.* 109(2):193–196.

896. Walker, K. M., S. Carozza, S. Cooper, K. Elgethun. 2007. Childhood cancer in Texas counties with moderate to intense agricultural activity. *J. Agric. Saf. Health* 13(1):9–24.

897. Giordano, F., V. Dell'Orco, F. Giannandrea, L. Lauria, P. Valente, I. Figa-Talamanca. 2006. Mortality in a cohort of pesticide applicators in an urban setting: Sixty years of follow-up. *Int. J. Immunopathol. Pharmacol.* 19(suppl. 4):61–65.

898. Littorin, M., R. Attewell, S. Skerfving, V. Horstmann, T. Moller. 1993. Mortality and tumour morbidity among Swedish market gardeners and orchardists. *Int. Arch. Occup. Environ. Health* 65(3):163–169.

899. Kogevinas, M. et al. 1995. Soft tissue sarcoma and non-Hodgkin's lymphoma in workers exposed to phenoxy herbicides, chlorophenols, and dioxins: Two nested case-control studies. *Epidemiology* 6(4):396–402.

900. Magnani, C., G. Pastore, L. Luzzatto, M. Carli, P. Lubrano, B. Terracini. 1989. Risk factors for soft tissue sarcomas in childhood: A case-control study. *Tumori* 75(4):396–400.

901. Bunin, G. R., J. D. Buckley, C. P. Boesel, L. B. Rorke, A. T. Meadows. 1994. Risk factors for astrocytic glioma and primitive neuroectodermal tumor of the brain in young children: A report from the Children's Cancer Group. *Cancer Epidemiol. Biomarkers Prev.* 3(3):197–204.

902. Cordier, S., M. J. Iglesias, C. Le Goaster, M. M. Guyot, L. Mandereau, D. Hemon. 1994. Incidence and risk factors for childhood brain tumors in the Ile de France. *Int. J. Cancer* 59(6):776–782.

903. Davis, J. R., R. C. Brownson, R. Garcia, B. J. Bentz, A. Turner. 1993. Family pesticide use and childhood brain cancer. *Arch. Environ. Contam. Toxicol.* 24(1):87–92.

904. Efird, J. T. et al. 2003. Farm-related exposures and childhood brain tumours in seven countries: Results from the SEARCH International Brain Tumour Study. *Paediatr. Perinat. Epidemiol.* 17(2):201–211.

905. Gold, E., L. Gordis, J. Tonascia, M. Szklo. 1979. Risk factors for brain tumors in children. *Am. J. Epidemiol.* 109(3):309–319.

906. Holly, E. A., P. M. Bracci, B. A. Mueller, S. Preston-Martin. 1998. Farm and animal exposures and pediatric brain tumors: Results from the United States West Coast Childhood Brain Tumor Study. *Cancer Epidemiol. Biomarkers Prev.* 7(9):797–802.

907. Pogoda, J. M., S. Preston-Martin. 1997. Household pesticides and risk of pediatric brain tumors. *Environ. Health Perspect.* 105(11):1214–1220.

908. Rosso, A. L., M. E. Hovinga, L. B. Rorke-Adams, L. G. Spector, G. R. Bunin. 2008. A case-control study of childhood brain tumors and fathers' hobbies: A Children's Oncology Group study. *Cancer Causes Control* 19(10):1201–1207.

909. Ruder, A. M. et al. 2006. The Upper Midwest Health Study: A case-control study of primary intracranial gliomas in farm and rural residents. *J. Agric. Saf. Health* 12(4):255–274.

910. Searles Nielsen, S., R. McKean-Cowdin, F. M. Farin, E. A. Holly, S. Preston-Martin, B. A. Mueller. 2010. Childhood brain tumors, residential insecticide exposure, and pesticide metabolism genes. *Environ. Health Perspect.* 118(1):144–149.

911. Blair, A., D. J. Grauman, J. H. Lubin, J. F. Fraumeni Jr. 1983. Lung cancer and other causes of death among licensed pesticide applicators. *J. Natl. Cancer Inst.* 71(1):31–37.

912. Wilkins III, J. R., T. Sinks. 1990. Parental occupation and intracranial neoplasms of childhood: Results of a case-control interview study. *Am. J. Epidemiol.* 132(2):275–292.

913. Smith-Rooker, J. L., A. Garrett, L. C. Hodges, V. Shue. 1992. Prevalence of glioblastoma multiforme subjects with prior herbicide exposure. *J. Neurosci. Nurs.* 24(5):260–264.

914. Musicco, M., M. Sant, S. Molinari, G. Filippini, G. Gatta, F. Berrino. 1988. A case-control study of brain gliomas and occupational exposure to chemical carcinogens: The risk to farmers. *Am. J. Epidemiol.* 128(4):778–785.

915. Figa-Talamanca, I., I. Mearelli, P. Valente, S. Bascherini. 1993. Cancer mortality in a cohort of rural licensed pesticide users in the province of Rome. *Int. J. Epidemiol.* 22(4):579–583.

916. Provost, D., A. Cantagrel, P. Lebailly, A. Jaffre, V. Loyant, H. Loiseau, A. Vital, P. Brochard, I. Baldi. 2007. Brain tumours and exposure to pesticides: A case-control study in southwestern France. *Occup. Environ. Med.* 64(8):509–514.

917. Rodvall, Y., A. Ahlbom, B. Spannare, G. Nise. 1996. Glioma and occupational exposure in Sweden, a case-control study. *Occup. Environ. Med.* 53(8):526–532.

918. Viel, J. F., B. Challier, A. Pitard, D. Pobel. 1998. Brain cancer mortality among French farmers: The vineyard pesticide hypothesis. *Arch. Environ. Health* 53(1):65–70.

919. Wesseling, C., D. Antich, C. Hogstedt, A. C. Rodriguez, A. Ahlbom. 1999. Geographical differences of cancer incidence in Costa Rica in relation to environmental and occupational pesticide exposure. *Int. J. Epidemiol.* 28(3):365–374.

920. Samanic, C. M., A. J. De Roos, P. A. Stewart, P. Rajaraman, M. A. Waters, P. D. Inskip. 2008. Occupational exposure to pesticides and risk of adult brain tumors. *Am. J. Epidemiol.* 167(8):976–985.

921. Zheng, T., K. P. Cantor, Y. Zhang, S. Keim, C. F. Lynch. 2001. Occupational risk factors for brain cancer: A population-based case-control study in Iowa. *J. Occup. Environ. Med.* 43(4):317–324.

922. Merletti, F. et al. 2006. Occupational factors and risk of adult bone sarcomas: A multicentric case-control study in Europe. *Int. J. Cancer* 118(3):721–727.

923. Holly, E. A., D. A. Aston, D. K. Ahn, J. J. Kristiansen. 1992. Ewing's bone sarcoma, paternal occupational exposure, and other factors. *Am. J. Epidemiol.* 135(2):122–129.

924. Moore, L. E., L. Gold, P. A. Stewart, G. Gridley, J. R. Prince, S. H. Zahm. 2005. Parental occupational exposures and Ewing's sarcoma. *Int. J. Cancer* 114(3):472–478.

925. Keller-Byrne, J. E., S. A. Khuder, E. A. Schaub. 1997. Meta-analyses of prostate cancer and farming. *Am. J. Ind. Med.* 31(5):580–586.

926. Dosemeci, M., R. N. Hoover, A. Blair, L. W. Figgs, S. Devesa, D. Grauman, J. F. Fraumeni Jr. 1994. Farming and prostate cancer among African-Americans in the southeastern United States. *J. Natl. Cancer Inst.* 86(22):1718–1719.

927. Chamie, K., R. W. DeVere White, D. Lee, J. H. Ok, L. M. Ellison. 2008. Agent Orange exposure, Vietnam War veterans, and the risk of prostate cancer. *Cancer* 113(9):2464–2470.

928. Sharma-Wagner, S., A. P. Chokkalingam, H. S. Malker, B. J. Stone, J. K. McLaughlin, A. W. Hsing. 2000. Occupation and prostate cancer risk in Sweden. *J. Occup. Environ. Med.* 42(5):517–525.

929. Forastiere, F., A. Quercia, M. Miceli, L. Settimi, B. Terenzoni, E. Rapiti, A. Faustini, P. Borgia, F. Cavariani, C. A. Perucci. 1993. Cancer among farmers in central Italy. *Scand. J. Work Environ. Health* 19(6):382–389.

930. Dich, J., K. Wiklund. 1998. Prostate cancer in pesticide applicators in Swedish agriculture. *Prostate* 34(2):100–112.

931. Meyer, T. E., A. L. Coker, M. Sanderson, E. Symanski. 2007. A case-control study of farming and prostate cancer in African-American and Caucasian men. *Occup. Environ. Med.* 64(3):155–160.

932. Fleming, L. E., J. A. Bean, M. Rudolph, K. Hamilton. 1999. Cancer incidence in a cohort of licensed pesticide applicators in Florida. *J. Occup. Environ. Med.* 41(4):279–288.

933. Mills, P. K., R. Yang. 2003. Prostate cancer risk in California farm workers. *J. Occup. Environ. Med.* 45(3):249–258.

934. Settimi, L., A. Masina, A. Andrion, O. Axelson. 2003. Prostate cancer and exposure to pesticides in agricultural settings. *Int. J. Cancer* 104(4):458–461.

935. MacLennan, P. A., E. Delzell, N. Sathiakumar, S. L. Myers, H. Cheng, W. Grizzle, V. W. Chen, X. C. Wu. 2002. Cancer incidence among triazine herbicide manufacturing workers. *J. Occup. Environ. Med.* 44(11):1048–1058.

936. Morrison, H., D. Savitz, R. Semenciw, B. Hulka, Y. Mao, D. Morison, D. Wigle. 1993. Farming and prostate cancer mortality. *Am. J. Epidemiol.* 137(3):270–280.

937. Band, P. R., N. D. Le, R. Fang, M. Deschamps, R. P. Gallagher, P. Yang. 2000. Identification of occupational cancer risks in British Columbia. A population-based case-control study of 995 incident breast cancer cases by menopausal status, controlling for confounding factors. *J. Occup. Environ. Med.* 42(3):284–310.

938. Dolapsakis, G., I. G. Vlachonikolis, C. Varveris, A. M. Tsatsakis. 2001. Mammographic findings and occupational exposure to pesticides currently in use on Crete. *Eur. J. Cancer* 37(12):1531–1536.

939. Brophy, J. T., M. M. Keith, K. M. Gorey, E. Laukkanen, D. Hellyer, A. Watterson, A. Reinhartz, M. Gilberston. 2002. Occupational histories of cancer patients in a Canadian cancer treatment center and the generated hypothesis regarding breast cancer and farming. *Int. J. Occup. Environ. Health* 8(4):346–353.

940. Duell, E. J., R. C. Millikan, D. A. Savitz, B. Newman, J. C. Smith, M. J. Schell, D. P. Sandler. 2000. A population-based case-control study of farming and breast cancer in North Carolina. *Epidemiology* 11(5):523–531.

941. Mills, P. K., R. Yang. 2005. Breast cancer risk in Hispanic agricultural workers in California. *Int. J. Occup. Environ. Health* 11(2):123–131.

942. Teitelbaum, S. L., M. D. Gammon, J. A. Britton, A. I. Neugut, B. Levin, S. D. Stellman. 2007. Reported residential pesticide use and breast cancer risk on Long Island, New York. *Am. J. Epidemiol.* 165(6):643–651.

943. Forastiere, F., A. Quercia, M. Miceli, L. Settimi, B. Terenzoni, E. Rapiti, A. Faustini, P. Borgia, F. Cavariani, C. A. Perucci. 1993. Cancer among farmers in central Italy. *Scand. J. Work Environ. Health* 19(6):382–389.

944. Lo, A. C., A. S. Soliman, H. M. Khaled, A. Aboelyazid, J. K. Greenson. 2010. Lifestyle, occupational, and reproductive factors and risk of colorectal cancer. *Dis. Colon Rectum* 53(5):830–837.

945. Alguacil, J. et al. 2000. Risk of pancreatic cancer and occupational exposures in Spain. PANKRAS II Study Group. *Ann. Occup. Hyg.* 44(5):391–403.

946. Ji, B. T. et al. 2001. Occupational exposure to pesticides and pancreatic cancer. *Am. J. Ind. Med.* 39(1):92–99.

947. Kauppinen, T., T. Partanen, R. Degerth, A. Ojajarvi. 1995. Pancreatic cancer and occupational exposures. *Epidemiology* 6(5):498–502.

948. Lo, A. C., A. S. Soliman, N. El-Ghawalby, M. Abdel-Wahab, O. Fathy, H. M. Khaled, S. Omar, S. R. Hamilton, J. K. Greenson, J. L. Abbruzzese. 2007. Lifestyle, occupational, and reproductive factors in relation to pancreatic cancer risk. *Pancreas* 35(2):120–129.

949. Partanen, T., T. Kauppinen, R. Degerth, G. Moneta, I. Mearelli, A. Ojajarvi, S. Hernberg, H. Koskinen, E. Pukkala. 1994. Pancreatic cancer in industrial branches and occupations in Finland. *Am. J. Ind. Med.* 25(6):851–866.

950. Buzio, L., M. Tondel, G. De Palma, C. Buzio, I. Franchini, A. Mutti, O. Axelson. 2002. Occupational risk factors for renal cell cancer. An Italian case-control study. *Med. Lav.* 93(4):303–309.

951. Fear, N. T., E. Roman, G. Reeves, B. Pannett. 1998. Childhood cancer and paternal employment in agriculture: The role of pesticides. *Br. J. Cancer* 77(5):825–829.

952. Hu, J Y Mao, K. White. 2002. Renal cell carcinoma and occupational exposure to chemicals in Canada. *Occup. Med. (Lond.)* 52(3):157–164.

953. Karami, S. et al. 2008. Renal cell carcinoma, occupational pesticide exposure and modification by glutathione S-transferase polymorphisms. *Carcinogenesis* 29(8):1567–1571.

954. Mellemgaard, A., G. Engholm, J. K. McLaughlin, J. H. Olsen. 1994. Occupational risk factors for renal-cell carcinoma in Denmark. *Scand. J. Work Environ. Health* 20(3):160–165.

955. Olshan, A. F., N. E. Breslow, J. M. Falletta, S. Grufferman, T. Pendergrass, L. L. Robison, M. Waskerwitz, W. G. Woods, T. J. Vietti, G. D. Hammond. 1993. Risk factors for Wilms tumor. Report from the National Wilms Tumor Study. *Cancer* 72(3):938–944.

956. Tsai, J., W. E. Kaye, F. J. Bove. 2006. Wilms' tumor and exposures to residential and occupational hazardous chemicals. *Int. J. Hyg. Environ. Health* 209(1):57–64.

957. Brownson, R. C., M. C. Alavanja, J. C. Chang. 1993. Occupational risk factors for lung cancer among nonsmoking women: A case-control study in Missouri (United States). *Cancer Causes Control* 4(5):449–454.

958. Bumroongkit, K., B. Rannala, P. Traisathit, M. Srikummool, Y. Wongchai, D. Kangwanpong. 2008. TP53 gene mutations of lung cancer patients in upper northern Thailand and environmental risk factors. *Cancer Genet. Cytogenet.* 185(1):20–27.

959. Pesatori, A. C., J. M. Sontag, J. H. Lubin, D. Consonni, A. Blair. 1994. Cohort mortality and nested case-control study of lung cancer among structural pest control workers in Florida (United States). *Cancer Causes Control* 5(4):310–318.

960. Rusiecki, J. A. et al. 2006. Cancer incidence among pesticide applicators exposed to metolachlor in the Agricultural Health Study. *Int. J. Cancer* 118(12):3118–3123.

961. Van Leeuwen, J. A., D. Waltner-Toews, T. Abernathy, B. Smit, M. Shoukri. 1999. Associations between stomach cancer incidence and drinking water contamination with atrazine and nitrate in Ontario (Canada) agroecosystems, 1987–1991. *Int. J. Epidemiol.* 28(5):836–840.

962. Mills, P. K., R. C. Yang. 2007. Agricultural exposures and gastric cancer risk in Hispanic farm workers in California. *Environ. Res.* 104(2):282–289.

963. Jansson, C., N. Plato, A. L. Johansson, O. Nyren, J. Lagergren. 2006. Airborne occupational exposures and risk of oesophageal and cardia adenocarcinoma. *Occup. Environ. Med.* 63(2):107–112.

964. Mills, P. K., G. R. Newell, D. E. Johnson. 1984. Testicular cancer associated with employment in agriculture and oil and natural gas extraction. *Lancet* 1(8370):207–210.

965. Ward, M. H., B. A. Kilfoy, P. J. Weyer, K. E. Anderson, A. R. Folsom, J. R. Cerhan. 2010. Nitrate intake and the risk of thyroid cancer and thyroid disease. *Epidemiology* 21(3):389–395.

966. Fortes, C., S. Mastroeni, F. Melchi, M. A. Pilla, M. Alotto, G. Antonelli, D. Camaione, S. Bolli, E. Luchetti, P. Pasquini. 2007. The association between residential pesticide use and cutaneous melanoma. *Eur. J. Cancer* 43(6):1066–1075.

967. Mahajan, R., A. Blair, J. Coble, C. F. Lynch, J. A. Hoppin, D. P. Sandler, M. C. Alavanja. 2007. Carbaryl exposure and incident cancer in the Agricultural Health Study. *Int. J. Cancer* 121(8):1799–1805.

968. Wiklund, K. 1983. Swedish agricultural workers. A group with a decreased risk of cancer. *Cancer* 51(3):566–568.

969. Tarvainen, L., P. Kyyronen, T. Kauppinen, E. Pukkala. 2008. Cancer of the mouth and pharynx, occupation and exposure to chemical agents in Finland [in 1971–95]. *Int. J. Cancer* 123(3):653–659.

970. Tisch, M., P. Schmezer, M. Faulde, A. Groh, H. Maier. 2002. Genotoxicity studies on permethrin, DEET and diazinon in primary human nasal mucosal cells. *Eur. Arch. Otorhinolaryngol.* 259(3):150–153.

971. Donna, A., P. Crosignani, F. Robutti, P. G. Betta, R. Bocca, N. Mariani, F. Ferrario, R. Fissi, F. Berrino. 1989. Triazine herbicides and ovarian epithelial neoplasms. *Scand. J. Work Environ. Health* 15(1):47–53.

972. Brender, J. D., M. Felkner, L. Suarez, M. A. Canfield, J. P. Henry. 2010. Maternal pesticide exposure and neural tube defects in Mexican Americans. *Ann. Epidemiol.* 20(1):16–22.

973. de Siqueira, M. T., C. Braga, J. E. Cabral-Filho, L. G. Augusto, J. N. Figueiroa, A. I. Souza. 2010. Correlation between pesticide use in agriculture and adverse birth outcomes in Brazil: An ecological study. *Bull. Environ. Contam. Toxicol.* 84(6):647–651.

974. Benachour, N., G. E. Seralini. 2009. Glyphosate formulations induce apoptosis and necrosis in human umbilical, embryonic, and placental cells. *Chem. Res. Toxicol.* 22(1):97–105.

975. Brucker-Davis, F., K. Wagner-Mahler, I. Delattre, B. Ducot, P. Ferrari, A. Bongain, J. Y. Kurzenne, J. C. Mas, P. Fenichel. 2008. Cryptorchidism at birth in Nice area (France) is associated with higher prenatal exposure to PCBs and DDE, as assessed by colostrum concentrations. *Hum. Reprod.* 23(8):1708–1718.

976. Perera, F. P. et al. 2003. Effects of transplacental exposure to environmental pollutants on birth outcomes in a multiethnic population. *Environ. Health Perspect.* 111(2):201–205.

977. Garry, V. F., D. Schreinemachers, M. E. Harkins, J. Griffith. 1996. Pesticide appliers, biocides, and birth defects in rural Minnesota. *Environ. Health Perspect.* 104(4):394–399.

978. Dugas, J., M. J. Nieuwenhuijsen, D. Martinez, N. Iszatt, P. Nelson, P. Elliott. 2010. Use of biocides and insect repellents and risk of hypospadias. *Occup. Environ. Med.* 67(3):196–200.

979. Petit, C., C. Chevrier, G. Durand, C. Monfort, F. Rouget, R. Garlantezec, S. Cordier. 2010. Impact on fetal growth of prenatal exposure to pesticides due to agricultural activities: A prospective cohort study in Brittany, France. *Environ. Health* 9:71.

980. Schreinemachers, D. M. 2003. Birth malformations and other adverse perinatal outcomes in four U.S. Wheat-producing states. *Environ. Health Perspect.* 111(9):1259–1264.

981. Enoch, R. R., J. P. Stanko, S. N. Greiner, G. L. Youngblood, J. L. Rayner, S. E. Fenton. 2007. Mammary gland development as a sensitive end point after acute prenatal exposure to an atrazine metabolite mixture in female Long–Evans rats. *Environ. Health Perspect.* 115(4):541–547.

982. Nassar, N., P. Abeywardana, A. Barker, C. Bower. 2010. Parental occupational exposure to potential endocrine disrupting chemicals and risk of hypospadias in infants. *Occup. Environ. Med.* 67(9):585–589.

983. Winchester, P. D., J. Huskins, J. Ying. 2009. Agrichemicals in surface water and birth defects in the United States. *Acta Paediatr.* 98(4):664–669.

984. Greenlee, A. R., T. M. Ellis, R. L. Berg. 2004. Low-dose agrochemicals and lawn-care pesticides induce developmental toxicity in murine preimplantation embryos. *Environ. Health Perspect.* 112(6):703–709.

985. Qiao, D., F. J. Seidler, T. A. Slotkin. 2001. Developmental neurotoxicity of chlorpyrifos modeled in vitro: Comparative effects of metabolites and other cholinesterase inhibitors on DNA synthesis in PC12 and C6 cells. *Environ. Health Perspect.* 109(9):909–913.

986. Rauch, S. A., J. M. Braun, D. B. Barr, A. M. Calafat, J. Khoury, A. M. Montesano, K. Yolton, B. P. Lanphear. 2012. Associations of prenatal exposure to organophosphate pesticide metabolites with gestational age and birth weight. *Environ. Health Perspect.* 120(7):1055–1060.

987. Richard, S., S. Moslemi, H. Sipahutar, N. Benachour, G. E. Seralini. 2005. Differential effects of glyphosate and roundup on human placental cells and aromatase. *Environ. Health Perspect.* 113(6):716–720.

988. Rocheleau, C. M., P. A. Romitti, L. K. Dennis. 2009. Pesticides and hypospadias: A metaanalysis. *J. Pediatr. Urol.* 5(1):17–24.

989. Swan, S. H., C. Brazil, E. Z. Drobnis, F. Liu, R. L. Kruse, M. Hatch, J. B. Redmon, C. Wang, J. W. Overstreet. 2003. Geographic differences in semen quality of fertile U.S. males. *Environ. Health Perspect.* 111(4):414–420.

990. Anway, M. D., A. S. Cupp, M. Uzumcu, M. K. Skinner. 2005. Epigenetic transgenerational actions of endocrine disruptors and male fertility. *Science* 308(5727):1466–1469.

991. Swan, S. H., R. L. Kruse, F. Liu, D. B. Barr, E. Z. Drobnis, J. B. Redmon, C. Wang, C. Brazil, J. W. Overstreet. 2003. Semen quality in relation to biomarkers of pesticide exposure. *Environ. Health Perspect.* 111(12):1478–1484.

992. Snijder, C. A., M. M. Brouwers, V. W. Jaddoe, A. Hofman, N. Roeleveld, A. Burdorf. 2011. Occupational exposure to endocrine disruptors and time to pregnancy among couples in a large birth cohort study: The Generation R Study. *Fertil. Steril.* 95(6):2067–2072.

993. Cavieres, M. F., J. Jaeger, W. Porter. 2002. Developmental toxicity of a commercial herbicide mixture in mice: I. Effects on embryo implantation and litter size. *Environ. Health Perspect.* 110(11):1081–1085.

994. Tiido, T., A. Rignell-Hydbom, B. Jonsson, Y. L. Giwercman, L. Rylander, L. Hagmar, A. Giwercman. 2005. Exposure to persistent organochlorine pollutants associates with human sperm Y:X chromosome ratio. *Hum. Reprod.* 20(7):1903–1909.

995. Fei, X., H. Chung, H. S. Taylor. 2005. Methoxychlor disrupts uterine Hoxa10 gene expression. *Endocrinology* 146(8):3445–3451.

996. Tiido, T. et al. 2006. Impact of PCB and p, p′-DDE contaminants on human sperm Y:X chromosome ratio: Studies in three European populations and the Inuit population in Greenland. *Environ. Health Perspect.* 114(5):718–724.

997. Gray Jr., L. E., J. Ostby, E. Monosson, W. R. Kelce. 1999. Environmental antiandrogens: Low doses of the fungicide vinclozolin alter sexual differentiation of the male rat. *Toxicol. Ind. Health* 15(1–2):48–64.

998. Joshi, C., B. Bansal, N. D. Jasuja. 2011. Evaluation of reproductive and developmental toxicity of cypermethrin in male albino rats. *Toxicol. Environ. Chem.* 93(3):593–602.

999. Meeker, J. D., L. Ryan, D. B. Barr, R. Hauser. 2006. Exposure to nonpersistent insecticides and male reproductive hormones. *Epidemiology* 17(1):61–68.

1000. Oliva, A., A. Spira, L. Multigner. 2001. Contribution of environmental factors to the risk of male infertility. *Hum. Reprod.* 16(8):1768–1776.

1001. Orton, F., E. Rosivatz, M. Scholze, A. Kortenkamp. 2011. Widely used pesticides with previously unknown endocrine activity revealed as in vitro antiandrogens. *Environ. Health Perspect.* 119(6):794–800.

1002. Stanko, J. P., R. R. Enoch, J. L. Rayner, C. C. Davis, D. C. Wolf, D. E. Malarkey, S. E. Fenton. 2010. Effects of prenatal exposure to a low dose atrazine metabolite mixture on pubertal timing and prostate development of male Long–Evans rats. *Reprod. Toxicol.* 30(4):540–549.

1003. Wang, H. et al. 2011. Maternal cypermethrin exposure during lactation impairs testicular development and spermatogenesis in male mouse offspring. *Environ. Toxicol.* 26(4):382–394.

1004. Baldi, I., A. Cantagrel, P. Lebailly, F. Tison, B. Dubroca, V. Chrysostome, J. F. Dartigues, P. Brochard. 2003. Association between Parkinson's disease and exposure to pesticides in southwestern France. *Neuroepidemiology* 22(5):305–310.

1005. Ascherio, A., H. Chen, M. G. Weisskopf, E. O'Reilly, M. L. McCullough, E. E. Calle, M. A. Schwarzschild, M. J. Thun. 2006. Pesticide exposure and risk for Parkinson's disease. *Ann. Neurol.* 60(2):197–203.

1006. Barbeau, A., M. Roy, G. Bernier, G. Campanella, S. Paris. 1987. Ecogenetics of Parkinson's disease: Prevalence and environmental aspects in rural areas. *Can. J. Neurol. Sci.* 14(1):36–41.

1007. Barlow, B. K., E. K. Richfield, D. A. Cory-Slechta, M. Thiruchelvam. 2004. A fetal risk factor for Parkinson's disease. *Dev. Neurosci.* 26(1):11–23.

1008. Butterfield, P. G., B. G. Valanis, P. S. Spencer, C. A. Lindeman, J. G. Nutt. 1993. Environmental antecedents of young-onset Parkinson's disease. *Neurology* 43(6):1150–1158.

1009. Baldi, I., P. Lebailly, B. Mohammed-Brahim, L. Letenneur, J. F. Dartigues, P. Brochard. 2003. Neurodegenerative diseases and exposure to pesticides in the elderly. *Am. J. Epidemiol.* 157(5):409–414.

1010. Ritz, B., Yu. 2000. Parkinson's disease mortality and pesticide exposure in California 1984–1994. *Int. J. Epidemiol.* 29(2):323–329.

1011. Barlow, B. K., D. W. Lee, D. A. Cory-Slechta, L. A. Opanashuk. 2005. Modulation of antioxidant defense systems by the environmental pesticide maneb in dopaminergic cells. *Neurotoxicology* 26(1):63–75.

1012. Chan, D. K. et al. 1998. Genetic and environmental risk factors for Parkinson's disease in a Chinese population. *J. Neurol. Neurosurg. Psychiatry* 65(5):781–784.

1013. Schulte, P. A., C. A. Burnett, M. F. Boeniger, J. Johnson. 1996. Neurodegenerative diseases: Occupational occurrence and potential risk factors, 1982 through 1991. *Am. J. Public Health* 86(9):1281–1288.

1014. Caudle, W. M., J. R. Richardson, M. Wang, G. W. Miller. 2005. Perinatal heptachlor exposure increases expression of presynaptic dopaminergic markers in mouse striatum. *Neurotoxicology* 26(4):721–728.

1015. Costello, S., M. Cockburn, J. Bronstein, X. Zhang, B. Ritz. 2009. Parkinson's disease and residential exposure to maneb and paraquat from agricultural applications in the central valley of California. *Am. J. Epidemiol.* 169(8):919–926.

1016. Dick, F. D. et al. 2007. Environmental risk factors for Parkinson's disease and parkinsonism: The Geoparkinson study. *Occup. Environ. Med.* 64(10):666–672.

1017. Jia, Z., H. P. Misra. 2007. Developmental exposure to pesticides zineb and/or endosulfan renders the nigrostriatal dopamine system more susceptible to these environmental chemicals later in life. *Neurotoxicology* 28(4):727–735.

1018. Priyadarshi, A., S. A. Khuder, E. A. Schaub, S. Shrivastava. 2000. A meta-analysis of Parkinson's disease and exposure to pesticides. *Neurotoxicology* 21(4):435–440.

1019. Elbaz, A., J. Clavel, P. J. Rathouz, F. Moisan, J. P. Galanaud, B. Delemotte, A. Alperovitch, C. Tzourio. 2009. Professional exposure to pesticides and Parkinson disease. *Ann. Neurol.* 66(4):494–504.

1020. Priyadarshi, A., S. A. Khuder, E. A. Schaub, S. S. Priyadarshi. 2001. Environmental risk factors and Parkinson's disease: A metaanalysis. *Environ. Res.* 86(2):122–127.

1021. Fall, P. A., M. Fredrikson, O. Axelson, A. K. Granerus. 1999. Nutritional and occupational factors influencing the risk of Parkinson's disease: A case-control study in southeastern Sweden. *Mov. Disord.* 14(1):28–37.

1022. Purisai, M. G., A. L. McCormack, S. Cumine, J. Li, M. Z. Isla, D. A. Di Monte. 2007. Microglial activation as a priming event leading to paraquat-induced dopaminergic cell degeneration. *Neurobiol. Dis.* 25(2):392–400.

1023. Firestone, J. A., T. Smith-Weller, G. Franklin, P. Swanson, W. T. Longstreth, Jr., H. Checkoway. 2005. Pesticides and risk of Parkinson disease: A population-based case-control study. *Arch. Neurol.* 62(1):91–95.

1024. Richardson, J. R., W. M. Caudle, M. Wang, E. D. Dean, K. D. Pennell, G. W. Miller. 2006. Developmental exposure to the pesticide dieldrin alters the dopamine system and increases neurotoxicity in an animal model of Parkinson's disease. *FASEB J.* 20(10):1695–1697.

1025. Fong, C. S., R. M. Wu, J. C. Shieh, Y. T. Chao, Y. P. Fu, C. L. Kuao, C. W. Cheng. 2007. Pesticide exposure on southwestern Taiwanese with MnSOD and NQO1 polymorphisms is associated with increased risk of Parkinson's disease. *Clin. Chim. Acta* 378(1–2):136–141.

1026. Frigerio, R., K. R. Sanft, B. R. Grossardt, B. J. Peterson, A. Elbaz, J. H. Bower, J. E. Ahlskog, M. de Andrade, D. M. Maraganore, W. A. Rocca. 2006. Chemical exposures and Parkinson's disease: A population-based case-control study. *Mov. Disord.* 21(10):1688–1692.

1027. Gatto, N. M., M. Cockburn, J. Bronstein, A. D. Manthripragada, B. Ritz. 2009. Well-water consumption and Parkinson's disease in rural California. *Environ. Health Perspect.* 117(12):1912–1918.

1028. Gorell, J. M., C. C. Johnson, B. A. Rybicki, E. L. Peterson, R. J. Richardson. 1998. The risk of Parkinson's disease with exposure to pesticides, farming, well water, and rural living. *Neurology* 50(5):1346–1350.

1029. Hancock, D. B., E. R. Martin, G. M. Mayhew, J. M. Stajich, R. Jewett, M. A. Stacy, B. L. Scott, J. M. Vance, W. K. Scott. 2008. Pesticide exposure and risk of Parkinson's disease: A family-based case-control study. *BMC Neurol.* 8:6.

1030. Hertzman, C., M. Wiens, B. Snow, S. Kelly, D. Calne. 1994. A case-control study of Parkinson's disease in a horticultural region of British Columbia. *Mov. Disord.* 9(1):69–75.

1031. Hubble, J. P., J. H. Kurth, S. L. Glatt, M. C. Kurth, G. D. Schellenberg, R. E. Hassanein, A. Lieberman, W. C. Koller. 1998. Gene-toxin interaction as a putative risk factor for Parkinson's disease with dementia. *Neuroepidemiology* 17(2):96–104.

1032. Koller, W., B. Vetere-Overfield, C. Gray, C. Alexander, T. Chin, J. Dolezal, R. Hassanein, C. Tanner. 1990. Environmental risk factors in Parkinson's disease. *Neurology* 40(8):1218–1221.

1033. Manthripragada, A. D., S. Costello, M. G. Cockburn, J. M. Bronstein, B. Ritz. 2010. Paraoxonase 1, agricultural organophosphate exposure, and Parkinson disease. *Epidemiology* 21(1):87–94.

1034. Menegon, A., P. G. Board, A. C. Blackburn, G. D. Mellick, D. G. Le Couteur. 1998. Parkinson's disease, pesticides, and glutathione transferase polymorphisms. *Lancet* 352(9137):1344–1346.

1035. Ritz, B. R., A. D. Manthripragada, S. Costello, S. J. Lincoln, M. J. Farrer, M. Cockburn, J. Bronstein. 2009. Dopamine transporter genetic variants and pesticides in Parkinson's disease. *Environ. Health Perspect.* 117(6):964–969.

1036. Seidler, A., W. Hellenbrand, B. P. Robra, P. Vieregge, P. Nischan, J. Joerg, W. H. Oertel, G. Ulm, E. Schneider. 1996. Possible environmental, occupational, and other etiologic factors for Parkinson's disease: A case-control study in Germany. *Neurology* 46(5):1275–1284.

1037. Semchuk, K. M., E. J. Love, R. G. Lee. 1992. Parkinson's disease and exposure to agricultural work and pesticide chemicals. *Neurology* 42(7):1328–1335.

1038. Tanner, C. M. et al. 2009. Occupation and risk of parkinsonism: A multicenter case-control study. *Arch. Neurol.* 66(9):1106–1113.

1039. Tanner, C. M. et al. 2011. Rotenone, paraquat, and Parkinson's disease. *Environ. Health Perspect.* 119(6):866–872.

1040. Wang, A., S. Costello, M. Cockburn, X. Zhang, J. Bronstein, B. Ritz. 2011. Parkinson's disease risk from ambient exposure to pesticides. *Eur. J. Epidemiol.* 26(7):547–555.

1041. Zorzon, M., L. Capus, A. Pellegrino, G. Cazzato, R. Zivadinov. 2002. Familial and environmental risk factors in Parkinson's disease: A case-control study in north-east Italy. *Acta Neurol. Scand.* 105(2):77–82.

1042. Parron, T., M. Requena, A. F. Hernandez, R. Alarcon. 2011. Association between environmental exposure to pesticides and neurodegenerative diseases. *Toxicol. Appl. Pharmacol.* 256(3):379–385.

1043. Tyas, S. L., J. Manfreda, L. A. Strain, P. R. Montgomery. 2001. Risk factors for Alzheimer's disease: A population-based, longitudinal study in Manitoba, Canada. *Int. J. Epidemiol.* 30(3):590–597.

1044. Bonvicini, F., N. Marcello, J. Mandrioli, V. Pietrini, M. Vinceti. 2010. Exposure to pesticides and risk of amyotrophic lateral sclerosis: A population-based case-control study. *Ann. Ist. Super. Sanita* 46(3):284–287.

1045. Burns, C. J., K. K. Beard, J. B. Cartmill. 2001. Mortality in chemical workers potentially exposed to 2,4-dichlorophenoxyacetic acid (2,4-D) 1945–94: An update. *Occup. Environ. Med.* 58(1):24–30.

1046. Choy, S., J. W. Kim. 2011. A case of amyotrophic lateral sclerosis in a worker treating pesticide wastes. *Korean J. Occup. Environ. Med.* 23(4):480–487.

1047. Das, K., C. Nag, M. Ghosh. 2012. Familial, environmental, and occupational risk factors in development of amyotrophic lateral sclerosis. *N. Am. J. Med. Sci.* 4(8):350–355.

1048. Doi, H., H. Kikuchi, H. Murai, Y. Kawano, H. Shigeto, Y. Ohyagi, J. Kira. 2006. Motor neuron disorder simulating ALS induced by chronic inhalation of pyrethroid insecticides. *Neurology* 67(10):1894–1895.

1049. McGuire, V., W. T. Longstreth, Jr., L. M. Nelson, T. D. Koepsell, H. Checkoway, M. S. Morgan, G. van Belle. 1997. Occupational exposures and amyotrophic lateral sclerosis. A population-based case-control study. *Am. J. Epidemiol.* 145(12):1076–1088.

1050. Kanavouras, K., M. N. Tzatzarakis, V. Mastorodemos, A. Plaitakis, A. M. Tsatsakis. 2011. A case report of motor neuron disease in a patient showing significant level of DDTs, HCHs and organophosphate metabolites in hair as well as levels of hexane and toluene in blood. *Toxicol. Appl. Pharmacol.* 256(3):399–404.

1051. Morahan, J. M., R. Pamphlett. 2006. Amyotrophic lateral sclerosis and exposure to environmental toxins: An Australian case-control study. *Neuroepidemiology* 27(3):130–135.

1052. Pamphlett, R. 2012. Exposure to environmental toxins and the risk of sporadic motor neuron disease: An expanded Australian case-control study. *Eur. J. Neurol.* 19(10):1343–1348.

1053. Qureshi, M. M., D. Hayden, L. Urbinelli, K. Ferrante, K. Newhall, D. Myers, S. Hilgenberg, R. Smart, R. H. Brown, M. E. Cudkowicz. 2006. Analysis of factors that modify susceptibility and rate of progression in amyotrophic lateral sclerosis (ALS). *Amyotroph. Lateral Scler.* 7(3):173–182.

1054. Morton, W. E., E. D. Crawford, R. A. Maricle, D. D. Douglas, V. H. Freed. 1975. Hypertension in Oregon pesticide-formulating workers. *J. Occup. Med.* 17(3):182–185.

1055. Antov, G., A. Aianova. 1980. Effect of the pesticide, fundazol, on the myocardium of rats with experimental atherosclerosis. *Probl. Khig.* 5:58–67.

1056. Zamzila, A. N., I. Aminu, S. Niza, M. R. Razman, M. A. Hadi. 2011. *Chronic Organophosphate Pesticide Exposure and Coronary Artery Disease: Finding a Bridge.* IIUM Research, Invention and Innovation Exhibition (IRIIE). p. 141. ISBN 978-983-3142-14-9.

1057. Salam, M. T., Y. F. Li, B. Langholz, F. D. Gilliland. 2004. Early-life environmental risk factors for asthma: Findings from the Children's Health Study. *Environ. Health Perspect.* 112(6):760–765.

1058. Draper, A., P. Cullinan, C. Campbell, M. Jones, A. Newman Taylor. 2003. Occupational asthma from fungicides fluazinam and chlorothalonil. *Occup. Environ. Med.* 60(1):76–77.

1059. Hoppin, J. A., D. M. Umbach, S. J. London, M. C. Alavanja, D. P. Sandler. 2002. Chemical predictors of wheeze among farmer pesticide applicators in the Agricultural Health Study. *Am. J. Respir. Crit. Care Med.* 165(5):683–689.

1060. Kolmodin-Hedman, B., A. Swensson, M. Akerblom. 1982. Occupational exposure to some synthetic pyrethroids (permethrin and fenvalerate). *Arch. Toxicol.* 50(1):27–33.

1061. Hoppin, J. A., D. M. Umbach, S. J. London, P. K. Henneberger, G. J. Kullman, M. C. Alavanja, D. P. Sandler. 2008. Pesticides and atopic and nonatopic asthma among farm women in the Agricultural Health Study. *Am. J. Respir. Crit. Care Med.* 177(1):11–18.

1062. Lessenger, J. E. 1992. Five office workers inadvertently exposed to cypermethrin. *J. Toxicol. Environ. Health* 35(4):261–267.

1063. Slager, R. E., J. A. Poole, T. D. LeVan, D. P. Sandler, M. C. Alavanja, J. A. Hoppin. 2009. Rhinitis associated with pesticide exposure among commercial pesticide applicators in the Agricultural Health Study. *Occup. Environ. Med.* 66(11):718–724.

1064. Moretto, A. 1991. Indoor spraying with the pyrethroid insecticide lambda-cyhalothrin: Effects on spraymen and inhabitants of sprayed houses. *Bull. World Health Organ.* 69(5):591–594.

1065. Salameh, P. R., I. Baldi, P. Brochard, C. Raherison, B. Abi Saleh, R. Salamon. 2003. Respiratory symptoms in children and exposure to pesticides. *Eur. Respir. J.* 22(3):507–512.

1066. Vandenplas, O., J. P. Delwiche, J. Auverdin, U. M. Caroyer, F. B. Cangh. 2000. Asthma to tetramethrin. *Allergy* 55(4):417–418.

1067. Wagner, S. L. 2000. Fatal asthma in a child after use of an animal shampoo containing pyrethrin. *West. J. Med.* 173(2):86–87.

1068. Weiner, B. P., R. M. Worth. 1969. Insecticides: Household use and respiratory impairment. *Hawaii Med. J.* 28(4):283–285.

1069. Arifkhanova, S. I., K. M. Ubaidullaeva, I. V. Liverko. 2007. Mucociliary transport in patients with chronic obstructive lung disease from the cotton-growing areas of Uzbekistan. *Probl. Tuberk. Bolezn. Legk.* (2):29–31.

1070. Chakraborty, S., S. Mukherjee, S. Roychoudhury, S. Siddique, T. Lahiri, M. R. Ray. 2009. Chronic exposures to cholinesterase-inhibiting pesticides adversely affect respiratory health of agricultural workers in India. *J. Occup. Health* 51(6):488–497.

1071. Barczyk, A., E. Sozanska, W. Pierzchala. 2006. The influence of occupational exposure to pesticides on the frequency of chronic obstructive pulmonary diseases. *Wiad. Lek.* 59(9–10):596–600.

1072. Ubaidullaeva, K. M. 2006. The clinical and functional features of chronic obstructive lung disease in patients with organic chlorine pesticides in blood. *Probl. Tuberk. Bolezn. Legk.* (9):21–23.

1073. Hoppin, J. A., M. Valcin, P. K. Henneberger, G. J. Kullman, D. M. Umbach, S. J. London, M. C. Alavanja, D. P. Sandler. 2007. Pesticide use and chronic bronchitis among farmers in the Agricultural Health Study. *Am. J. Ind. Med.* 50(12):969–979.

1074. Faria, N. M., L. A. Facchini, A. G. Fassa, E. Tomasi. 2005. Pesticides and respiratory symptoms among farmers. *Rev. Saude Publica* 39(6):973–981.

1075. LeVan, T. D., W. P. Koh, H. P. Lee, D. Koh, M. C. Yu, S. J. London. 2006. Vapor, dust, and smoke exposure in relation to adult-onset asthma and chronic respiratory symptoms: The Singapore Chinese Health Study. *Am. J. Epidemiol.* 163(12):1118–1128.

1076. Valcin, M., P. K. Henneberger, G. J. Kullman, D. M. Umbach, S. J. London, M. C. Alavanja, D. P. Sandler, J. A. Hoppin. 2007. Chronic bronchitis among nonsmoking farm women in the agricultural health study. *J. Occup. Environ. Med.* 49(5):574–583.

1077. Lee, D. H., M. W. Steffes, A. Sjodin, R. S. Jones, L. L. Needham, D. R. Jacobs, Jr. 2010. Low dose of some persistent organic pollutants predicts type 2 diabetes: A nested case-control study. *Environ. Health Perspect.* 118(9):1235–1242.

1078. Montgomery, M. P., F. Kamel, T. M. Saldana, M. C. Alavanja, D. P. Sandler. 2008. Incident diabetes and pesticide exposure among licensed pesticide applicators: Agricultural Health Study, 1993–2003. *Am. J. Epidemiol.* 167(10):1235–1246.

1079. Kouznetsova, M., X. Huang, Ma, L. Lessner, D. O. Carpenter. 2007. Increased rate of hospitalization for diabetes and residential proximity of hazardous waste sites. *Environ. Health Perspect.* 115(1):75–79.

1080. Everett, C. J., E. M. Matheson. 2010. Biomarkers of pesticide exposure and diabetes in the 1999–2004 national health and nutrition examination survey. *Environ. Int.* 36(4):398–401.

1081. Saldana, T. M., O. Basso, J. A. Hoppin, D. D. Baird, C. Knott, A. Blair, M. C. Alavanja, D. P. Sandler. 2007. Pesticide exposure and self-reported gestational diabetes mellitus in the Agricultural Health Study. *Diabetes Care* 30(3):529–534.

1082. Patel, C. J., J. Bhattacharya, A. J. Butte. 2010. An Environment-Wide Association Study (EWAS) on type 2 diabetes mellitus. *PLoS One* 5(5):e10746.

1083. Peiris-John, R. J., J. K. Wanigasuriya, A. R. Wickremasinghe, W. P. Dissanayake, A. Hittarage. 2006. Exposure to acetylcholinesterase-inhibiting pesticides and chronic renal failure. *Ceylon Med. J.* 51(1):42–43.

1084. Wanigasuriya, K. P., R. J. Peiris-John, R. Wickremasinghe, A. Hittarage. 2007. Chronic renal failure in North Central Province of Sri Lanka: An environmentally induced disease. *Trans. R. Soc. Trop. Med. Hyg.* 101(10):1013–1017.

1085. Siddharth, M., S. K. Datta, S. Bansal, M. Mustafa, B. D. Banerjee, O. P. Kalra, A. K. Tripathi. 2012. Study on organochlorine pesticide levels in chronic kidney disease patients: Association with estimated glomerular filtration rate and oxidative stress. *J. Biochem. Mol. Toxicol.* 26(6):241–247.

1086. Chevrier, C., G. Limon, C. Monfort, F. Rouget, R. Garlantezec, C. Petit, G. Durand, S. Cordier. 2011. Urinary biomarkers of prenatal atrazine exposure and adverse birth outcomes in the PELAGIE birth cohort. *Environ. Health Perspect.* 119(7):1034–1041.

1087. Bolognesi, C. 2003. Genotoxicity of pesticides: A review of human biomonitoring studies. *Mutat. Res.* 543:251–272.

1088. Bull, S., K. Fletcher, A. R. Boobis, J. M. Battershill. 2006. Evidence for genotoxicity of pesticides in pesticide applicators: A review. *Mutagenesis* 21(2):93–103.

1089. Guy, R. C. 2005. Toxicity testing, mutagenicity. In *Encyclopedia of Toxicology*, P. Wexler, B. D. Anderson, A. D. Peyster et al. eds., Elsevier Inc.

1090. Costa, C., S. Silva, J. Neves, P. Coelho, S. Costa, B. Laffon, J. Snawder, J. P. Teixeira. 2011. Micronucleus frequencies in lymphocytes and reticulocytes in a pesticide exposed population in Portugal. *J. Toxicol. Environ. Health A* 74(15–16):960–970.

1091. Ergene, S., A. Celik, T. Cavas, F. Kaya. 2007. Genotoxic biomonitoring study of population residing in pesticide contaminated regions in Goksu Delta: Micronucleus, chromosomal aberrations and sister chromatid exchanges. *Environ. Int.* 33(7):877–885.

1092. Garaj-Vrhovac, V., D. Zeljezic. 2002. Assessment of genome damage in a population of Croatian workers employed in pesticide production by chromosomal aberration analysis, micronucleus assay and Comet assay. *J. Appl. Toxicol.* 22(4):249–255.

1093. Carbonell, E., M. Puig, N. Xamena, A. Creus, R. Marcos. 1990. Sister chromatid exchange in lymphocytes of agricultural workers exposed to pesticides. *Mutagenesis* 5(4):403–405.

1094. Rupa, D. S., P. P. Reddy, K. Sreemannarayana, O. S. Reddi. 1991. Frequency of sister chromatid exchange in peripheral lymphocytes of male pesticide applicators. *Environ. Mol. Mutagen.* 18(2):136–138.

1095. Dhawan, A., M. Bajpayee, D. Parmar. 2009. Comet assay: A reliable tool for the assessment of DNA damage in different models. *Cell Biol. Toxicol.* 25(1):5–32.

1096. Grover, P., K. Danadevi, M. Mahboob, R. Rozati, B. S. Banu, M. F. Rahman. 2003. Evaluation of genetic damage in workers employed in pesticide production utilizing the Comet assay. *Mutagenesis* 18(2):201–205.
1097. Mostafalou, S., M. Abdollahi. 2012. Current concerns on genotoxicity of pesticides. *Int. J. Pharmacol.* 8(6):473–474.
1098. Shadnia, S., E. Azizi, R. Hosseini, S. Khoie, S. Fouladdel, A. Pajoumand, N. Jalali, M. Abdollahi. 2005. Evaluation of oxidative stress and genotoxicity in organophosphorous insecticides formulators. *Hum. Exp. Toxicol.* 24:439–445.
1099. Zeljezic, D., V. Garaj-Vrhovac. 2001. Chromosomal aberration and single cell gel electrophoresis (Comet) assay in the longitudinal risk assessment of occupational exposure to pesticides. *Mutagenesis* 16(4):359–363.
1100. Lebailly, P., C. Vigreux, C. Lechevrel, D. Ledemeney, T. Godard, F. Sichel, J. Y. LeTalaer, M. Henry-Amar, P. Gauduchon. 1998. DNA damage in mononuclear leukocytes of farmers measured using the alkaline comet assay: Modifications of DNA damage levels after a one-day field spraying period with selected pesticides. *Cancer Epidemiol. Biomarkers Prev.* 7(10):929–940.
1101. Peluso, M., F. Merlo, A. Munnia, C. Bolognesi, R. Puntoni, S. Parodi. 1996. (32)P-postlabeling detection of DNA adducts in peripheral white blood cells of greenhouse floriculturists from western Liguria, Italy. *Cancer Epidemiol. Biomarkers Prev.* 5(5):361–369.
1102. Carbonell, E., N. Xamena, A. Creus, R. Marcos. 1993. Cytogenetic biomonitoring in a Spanish group of agricultural workers exposed to pesticides. *Mutagenesis* 8(6):511–517.
1103. De Ferrari, M., M. Artuso, S. Bonassi, S. Bonatti, Z. Cavalieri, D. Pescatore, E. Marchini, V. Pisano, A. Abbondandolo. 1991. Cytogenetic biomonitoring of an Italian population exposed to pesticides: Chromosome aberration and sister-chromatid exchange analysis in peripheral blood lymphocytes. *Mutat. Res.* 260(1):105–113.
1104. Dulout, F. N., M. C. Pastori, O. A. Olivero, M. Gonzalez Cid, D. Loria, E. Matos, N. Sobel, E. C. de Bujan, N. Albiano. 1985. Sister-chromatid exchanges and chromosomal aberrations in a population exposed to pesticides. *Mutat. Res.* 143(4):237–244.
1105. Garry, V. F., R. E. Tarone, I. R. Kirsch, J. M. Abdallah, D. P. Lombardi, L. K. Long, B. L. Burroughs, D. B. Barr, J. S. Kesner. 2001. Biomarker correlations of urinary 2,4-D levels in foresters: Genomic instability and endocrine disruption. *Environ. Health Perspect.* 109(5):495–500.
1106. Lander, B. F., L. E. Knudsen, M. O. Gamborg, H. Jarventaus, H. Norppa. 2000. Chromosome aberrations in pesticide-exposed greenhouse workers. *Scand. J. Work Environ. Health* 26(5):436–442.
1107. Bolognesi, C., M. Parrini, F. Merlo, S. Bonassi. 1993. Frequency of micronuclei in lymphocytes from a group of floriculturists exposed to pesticides. *J. Toxicol. Environ. Health* 40(2–3):405–411.
1108. Gomez-Arroyo, S., Y. Diaz-Sanchez, M. A. Meneses-Perez, R. Villalobos-Pietrini, J. De Leon-Rodriguez. 2000. Cytogenetic biomonitoring in a Mexican floriculture worker group exposed to pesticides. *Mutat. Res.* 466(1):117–124.
1109. Pasquini, R., G. Scassellati-Sforzolini, G. Angeli, C. Fatigoni, S. Monarca, L. Beneventi, A. M. DiGiulio, F. A. Bauleo. 1996. Cytogenetic biomonitoring of pesticide-exposed farmers in central Italy. *J. Environ. Pathol. Toxicol. Oncol.* 15(1):29–39.
1110. Laurent, C., P. Jadot, C. Chabut. 1996. Unexpected decrease in cytogenetic biomarkers frequencies observed after increased exposure to organophosphorous pesticides in a production plant. *Int. Arch. Occup. Environ. Health* 68(6):399–404.
1111. Jablonicka, A., H. Polakova, J. Karelova, M. Vargova. 1989. Analysis of chromosome aberrations and sister-chromatid exchanges in peripheral blood lymphocytes of workers with occupational exposure to the mancozeb-containing fungicide Novozir Mn80. *Mutat. Res.* 224(2):143–146.
1112. Zeljezic, D., V. Garaj-Vrhovac. 2002. Sister chromatid exchange and proliferative rate index in the longitudinal risk assessment of occupational exposure to pesticides. *Chemosphere* 46(2):295–303.
1113. Rupa, D. S., P. P. Reddy, K. Sreemannarayana, O. S. Reddi. 1991. Frequency of sister chromatid exchange in peripheral lymphocytes of male pesticide applicators. *Environ. Mol. Mutagen.* 18(2):136–138.
1114. Rupa, D. S., P. Rita, P. P. Reddy, O. S. Reddi. 1988. Screening of chromosomal aberrations and sister chromatid exchanges in peripheral lymphocytes of vegetable garden workers. *Hum. Toxicol.* 7(4):333–336.
1115. Weinhold, B. 2006. Epigenetics: The science of change. *Environ. Health Perspect.* 114(3):A160–A167.
1116. Anway, M. D., M. K. Skinner. 2006. Epigenetic transgenerational actions of endocrine disruptors. *Endocrinology* 147(suppl. 6):S43–S49.
1117. Guerrero-Bosagna, C., M. Settles, B. Lucker, M. K. Skinner. 2010. Epigenetic transgenerational actions of vinclozolin on promoter regions of the sperm epigenome. *PLoS One* 5(9).
1118. Zama, A. M., M. Uzumcu. 2009. Fetal and neonatal exposure to the endocrine disruptor methoxychlor causes epigenetic alterations in adult ovarian genes. *Endocrinology* 150(10):4681–4691.

1119. Tao, L., S. Yang, M. Xie, P. M. Kramer, M. A. Pereira. 2000. Effect of trichloroethylene and its metabolites, dichloroacetic acid and trichloroacetic acid, on the methylation and expression of c-Jun and c-Myc protooncogenes in mouse liver: Prevention by methionine. *Toxicol. Sci.* 54(2):399–407.

1120. Tao, L., S. Yang, M. Xie, P. M. Kramer, M. A. Pereira. 2000. Hypomethylation and overexpression of c-jun and c-myc protooncogenes and increased DNA methyltransferase activity in dichloroacetic and trichloroacetic acid-promoted mouse liver tumors. *Cancer Lett.* 158(2):185–193.

1121. Kim, K. Y., D. S. Kim, S. K. Lee, I. K. Lee, J. H. Kang, Y. S. Chang, D. R. Jacobs, M. Steffes, D. H. Lee. 2010. Association of low-dose exposure to persistent organic pollutants with global DNA hypomethylation in healthy Koreans. *Environ. Health Perspect.* 118(3):370–374.

1122. Rusiecki, J. A., A. Baccarelli, V. Bollati, L. Tarantini, L. E. Moore, E. C. Bonefeld-Jorgensen. 2008. Global DNA hypomethylation is associated with high serum-persistent organic pollutants in Greenlandic Inuit. *Environ. Health Perspect.* 116(11):1547–1552.

1123. Song, C., A. Kanthasamy, V. Anantharam, F. Sun, A. G. Kanthasamy. 2010. Environmental neurotoxic pesticide increases histone acetylation to promote apoptosis in dopaminergic neuronal cells: Relevance to epigenetic mechanisms of neurodegeneration. *Mol. Pharmacol.* 77(4):621–632.

1124. Jones, P. A., S. B. Baylin. 2002. The fundamental role of epigenetic events in cancer. *Nat. Rev. Genet.* 3(6):415–428.

1125. Ziech, D., R. Franco, A. Pappa, V. Malamou-Mitsi, S. Georgakila, A. G. Georgakilas, M. I. Panayiotidis. 2010. The role of epigenetics in environmental and occupational carcinogenesis. *Chem. Biol. Interact.* 188(2):340–349.

1126. Maslansky, C. J., G. M. Williams. 1981. Evidence for an epigenetic mode of action in organochlorine pesticide hepatocarcinogenicity: A lack of genotoxicity in rat, mouse, and hamster hepatocytes. *J. Toxicol. Environ. Health* 8(1–2):121–130.

1127. Skinner, M. K., M. D. Anway. 2007. Epigenetic transgenerational actions of vinclozolin on the development of disease and cancer. *Crit. Rev. Oncog.* 13(1):75–82.

1128. Habibi, E., A. Masoudi-Nejad, H. M. Abdolmaleky, S. J. Haggarty. 2011. Emerging roles of epigenetic mechanisms in Parkinson's disease. *Funct. Integr. Genomics* 11(4):523–537.

1129. Kwok, J. B. 2010. Role of epigenetics in Alzheimer's and Parkinson's disease. *Epigenomics* 2(5):671–682.

1130. Oates, N., R. Pamphlett. 2007. An epigenetic analysis of SOD1 and VEGF in ALS. *Amyotroph. Lateral Scler.* 8(2):83–86.

1131. Burrell, A. M., A. E. Handel, S. V. Ramagopalan, G. C. Ebers, J. M. Morahan. 2011. Epigenetic mechanisms in multiple sclerosis and the major histocompatibility complex (MHC). *Discov. Med.* 11(58):187–196.

1132. Simmons, R. A. 2007. Developmental origins of diabetes: The role of epigenetic mechanisms. *Curr. Opin. Endocrinol. Diabetes Obes.* 14(1):13–16.

1133. Gravina, S., J. Vijg. 2010. Epigenetic factors in aging and longevity. *Pflugers Arch.* 459(2):247–258.

1134. Dwivedi, R. S., J. G. Herman, T. A. McCaffrey, D. S. Raj. 2011. Beyond genetics: Epigenetic code in chronic kidney disease. *Kidney Int.* 79(1):23–32.

1135. Lund, G., S. Zaina. 2011. Atherosclerosis: An epigenetic balancing act that goes wrong. *Curr. Atheroscler. Rep.* 13(3):208–214.

1136. Pournourmohammadi, S., M. Abdollahi. 2011. Toxicity and biomonitoring; gene expression. In *Anticholinesterase Pesticides: Metabolism, Neurotoxicity, and Epidemiology*, T. Satoh, R. Gupta, eds., Hoboken, NJ: Wiley.

1137. Rahimi, R., M. Abdollahi. 2007. A review on the mechanisms involved in hyperglycemia induced by organophosphorous pesticides. *Pest. Biochem. Physiol.* 88:115–121.

1138. Abdollahi, M., M. Donyavi, S. Pournourmohammadi, M. Saadat. 2004. Hyperglycemia associated with increased hepatic glycogen phosphorylase and phosphoenolpyruvate carboxykinase in rats following subchronic exposure to malathion. *Comp. Biochem. Physiol. C Toxicol. Pharmacol.* 137:343–347.

1139. Karami-Mohajeri, S., M. Abdollahi. 2011. Toxic influence of organophosphate, carbamate, and organochlorine pesticides on cellular metabolism of lipids, proteins, and carbohydrates: A systematic review. *Hum. Exp. Toxicol.* 30:1119–1140.

1140. Everett, C. J., E. M. Matheson. 2010. Biomarkers of pesticide exposure and diabetes in the 1999–2004 national health and nutrition examination survey. *Environ. Int.* 36(4):398–401.

1141. Montgomery, M. P., F. Kamel, T. M. Saldana, M. C. Alavanja, D. P. Sandler. 2008. Incident diabetes and pesticide exposure among licensed pesticide applicators: Agricultural Health Study, 1993–2003. *Am. J. Epidemiol.* 167(10):1235–1246.

1142. Saldana, T. M., O. Basso, J. A. Hoppin, D. D. Baird, C. Knott, A. Blair, M. C. Alavanja, D. P. Sandler. 2007. Pesticide exposure and self-reported gestational diabetes mellitus in the Agricultural Health Study. *Diabetes Care* 30(3):529–534.

1143. Thayer, K. A., J. J. Heindel, J. R. Bucher, M. A. Gallo. 2012. Role of environmental chemicals in diabetes and obesity: A national toxicology program workshop report. *Environ. Health Perspect.* 120(6):779–789.

1144. Crisp, T. M. et al. 1998. Environmental endocrine disruption: An effects assessment and analysis. *Environ. Health Perspect.* 106(suppl. 1):11–56.

1145. PAN. 2009. *List of Lists: A Catalogue of Lists of Pesticides Identifying Those Associated with Particularly Harmful Health or Environmental Impacts.* P. A. Network.

1146. McKinlay, R., J. A. Plant, J. N. Bell, N. Voulvoulis. 2008. Endocrine disrupting pesticides: Implications for risk assessment. *Environ. Int.* 34(2):168–183.

1147. Kojima, H., S. Takeuchi, T. Nagai. 2010. Endocrine disrupting potential of pesticides via nuclear receptors and aryl hydrocarbon receptor. *J. Health Sci.* 56(4):374–386.

1148. Lemaire, G., P. Balaguer, S. Michel, R. Rahmani. 2005. Activation of retinoic acid receptor-dependent transcription by organochlorine pesticides. *Toxicol. Appl. Pharmacol.* 202(1):38–49.

1149. Rochman, B. 2016. Pregnant women awash in chemicals. Is that bad for the baby? [Accessed date March 21, 2016] http://healthland.time.com/2011/01/14/pregnant-women-awash-in-chemicals-is-that-bad-for-baby/

1150. Jarrell, J., S. Chan, R. Hauser, H. Hu. 2005. Longitudinal assessment of PCBs and chlorinated pesticides in pregnant women from Western Canada. *Environ. Health* 4:10.

1151. Butler Walker, J., L. Seddon, E. McMullen, J. Houseman, K. Tofflemire, A. Corriveau, J. P. Weber, C. Mills, S. Smith, J. Van Oostdam. 2003. Organochlorine levels in maternal and umbilical cord blood plasma in Arctic Canada. *Sci. Total Environ.* 302(1–3):27–52.

1152. Common Menu Bar Links. 2012. Canada Health Act Annual Report 2010–2011 (Health Canada, 2011). [Accessed March 22, 2016] http://www.hc-sc.gc.ca/hcs-sss/pubs/cha-lcs/2011-cha-lcs-ar-ra/index-eng.php

1153. Environment Canada Water Science and Technology Directorate

1154. Fokina, K. V., V. P. Bezuglyi. 1978. Role of chlora and organophosphate pesticide complexes in the etiology of cerebral atherosclerosis. *Vrach. Delo* (4):19–23.

1155. Anand, S., S. Singh, U. N. Saikia, A. Bhalla, Y. P. Sharma, D. Singh. 2009. Cardiac abnormalities in acute organophosphate poisoning. *Clin. Toxicol.* 47:230–235.

1156. Kiss, Z., T. Fazekas. 1979. Arrhythmias in organophosphate poisonings. *Acta Cardiol.* 34:323–30.

1157. Lee, E., C. A. Burnett, N. Lalich, L. L. Cameron, J. P. Sestito. 2002. Proportionate mortality of crop and livestock farmers in the United States, 1984–1993. *Am. J. Ind. Med.* 42:410–20.

1158. Fleming, L. E., O. Gomez-Marin, D. Zheng, F. Ma, D. Lee. 2003. National Health Interview Survey mortality among US farmers and pesticide applicators. *Am. J. Ind. Med.* 43:227–33.

1159. Blair, A. et al. 2005. Mortality among participants in the agricultural health study. *Ann. Epidemiol.* 15:279–85.

1160. Mills, P. K., J. J. Beaumont, K. Nasseri. 2006. Proportionate mortality among current and former members of the United Farm Workers of America, AFL-CIO, in California 1973–2000. *J. Agromed.* 11:39–48.

1161. Blair, A., M. Dosemeci, E. F. Heineman. 1993. Cancer and other causes of death among male and female farmers from twenty-three states. *Am. J. Ind. Med.* 23:729–42.

1162. Schreinemachers, D. M. 2006. Mortality from ischemic heart disease and diabetes mellitus (type 2) in four U.S. wheat-producing states: A hypothesis–generating study. *Environ. Health Perspect.* 114:186–93.

1163. Mills, K. T., A. Blair, L. E. Freeman, D. P. Sandler, J. A. 2009. Hoppin. Pesticides and myocardial infarction incidence and mortality among male pesticide applicators in the Agricultural Health Study. *Am. J. Epidemiol.* 170:892–900.

1164. McDuffie, H. H. 1994. Women at work: Agriculture and pesticides. *J. Occup. Med.* 36:1240–1246.

1165. Dayton, S. B., D. P. Sandler, A. Blair, M. Alavanja, L. E. Beane Freeman, J. A. Hoppin. 2010. Pesticide use and myocardial infarction incidence among farm women in the agricultural health study. *J. Occup. Environ. Med.* 52(7):693–97.

1166. Hoppin, J. A., F. Yucel, M. Dosemeci, D. P. Sandler. 2002. Accuracy of self-reported pesticide use duration information from licensed pesticide applicators in the Agricultural Health Study. *J. Expo. Anal. Environ. Epidemiol.* 12:313–318.

1167. United States Environmental Protection Agency. 2006. *Organophosphorus Cumulative Risk Assessment–2006 Update.* US EPA.

1168. Meisinger, C., A. Schuler, H. Lowel. 2004. Postal questionnaires identified hospitalizations for self-reported acute myocardial infarction. *J. Clin. Epidemiol.* 57:989–992.

1169. Rosamond, W. D., J. M. Sprafka, P. G. McGovern, M. Nelson, R. V. Luepker. 1995. Validation of self-reported history of acute myocardial infarction: Experience of the Minnesota Heart Survey Registry. *Epidemiology* 6:67–69.

1170. Ninomiya, J. K., G. L'Italien, M. H. Criqui, J. L. Whyte, A. Gamst, R. S. Chen. 2004. Association of the metabolic syndrome with history of myocardial infarction and stroke in the Third National Health and Nutrition Examination Survey. *Circulation* 109:42–46.

1171. Cooper, G. S., S. A. Ephross, C. R. Weinberg, D. D. Baird, E. A. Whelan, D. P. Sandler. 1999. Menstrual and reproductive risk factors for ischemic heart disease. *Epidemiology* 10:255–259.

1172. Wang, Y., S. A. Hwang, E. L. Lewis-Michl, E. F. Fitzgerald, A. D. Stark. 2003. Mortality among a cohort of female farm residents in New York State. *Arch. Environ. Health* 58:642–648.

1173. Rosamond, W. D., L. E. Chambless, A. R. Cooper, L. S. Folsom, D. E. Conwill, L. Clegg, C. H. Wang, G. Heiss. 1998. Trends in the incidence of myocardial infarction and in mortality due to coronary heart disease, 1987 to 1994. *N. Engl. J. Med.* 339:861–7.

1174. Triant, V. A., H. Lee, C. Hadigan, S. K. Grinspoon. 2007. Increased acute myocardial infarction rates and cardiovascular risk factors among patients with human immunodeficiency virus disease. *J. Clin. Endocrinol. Metab.* 92:2506–12.

1175. Szema, A. M., S. A. Hamidi, S. David Smith, H. Benveniste. 2013. VIP gene deletion in mice causes cardiomyopathy associated with upregulation of heart failure genes. *PLoS ONE* 8(5).

1176. Wanigasuriya, K. P., R. J. Peiris-John, R. Wickremasinghe, A. Hittarage. 2007. Chronic renal failure in North Central Province of Sri Lanka: An environmentally induced disease. *Trans. R. Soc. Trop. Med. Hyg.* 101(10):1013–1017.

1177. Peiris-John, R. J., J. K. Wanigasuriya, A. R. Wickremasinghe, W. P. Dissanayake, A. Hittarage. 2006. Exposure to acetylcholinesterase-inhibiting pesticides and chronic renal failure. *Ceylon Med. J.* 51(1):42–43.

1178. Siddharth, M., S. K. Datta, S. Bansal, M. Mustafa, B. D. Banerjee, O. P. Kalra, A. K. Tripathi. 2012. Study on organochlorine pesticide levels in chronic kidney disease patients: Association with estimated glomerular filtration rate and oxidative stress. *J. Biochem. Mol. Toxicol.* 26(6):241–247.

1179. Hernandez, A. F., T. Parron, R. Alarcon. 2011. Pesticides and asthma. *Curr. Opin. Allergy Clin. Immunol.* 11(2):90–96.

1180. Henneberger, P. K. et al. 2003. Work-related reactive airways dysfunction syndrome cases from surveillance in selected US states. *J. Occup. Environ. Med.* 45(4):360–368.

1181. Selgrade, M. K. et al. 2006. Induction of asthma and the environment: What we know and need to know. *Environ. Health Perspect.* 114(4):615–619.

1182. Proskocil, B. J., D. A. Bruun, J. K. Lorton, K. C. Blensly, D. B. Jacoby, P. J. Lein, A. D. Fryer. 2008. Antigen sensitization influences organoposphorus pesticide-induced airway hyperreactivity. *Environ. Health Perspect.* 116(3):381–388.

1183. Senthilselvan, A., H. H. McDuffie, J. A. Dosman. 1992. Association of asthma with use of pesticides: Results of a cross-sectional survey of farmers. *Am. J. Respir. Dis.* 146(4):884–887.

1184. Hoppin, J. A., D. M. Umbach, S. J. London, P. K. Henneberger, G. J. Kullman, J. Coble, M. C. Alavanja, L. E. Beane Freeman, D. P. Sandler. 2009. Pesticide use and adult-onset asthma among male farmers in the Agricultural Health Study. *Eur. Respir. J.* 34(6):1296–1303.

1185. Salameh, P., M. Waked, I. Baldi, P. Brochard, B. A. Saleh. 2006. Respiratory diseases and pesticide exposure: A case-control study in Lebanon. *J. Epidemiol. Community Health* 60(3):256–261.

1186. Boers, D. et al. 2008. Asthmatic symptoms after exposure to ethylenebisdithiocarbamates and other pesticides in the Europit field studies. *Hum. Exp. Toxicol.* 27(9):721–727.

1187. Jones, S. M., A. W. Burks, H. J. Spencer, S. Lensing, P. K. Roberson, J. Gandy, R. M. Helm. 2003. Occupational asthma symptoms and respiratory function among aerial pesticide applicators. *Am. J. Ind. Med.* 43(4):407–417.

1188. Sunyer, J., M. Torrent, L. Munoz-Ortiz, N. Ribas-Fito, D. Carrizo, J. Grimalt, J. M. Antó, P. Cullinan. 2005. Prenatal dichlorodiphenyldichloroethylene (DDE) and asthma in children. *Environ. Health. Perspect.* 113(12):1787–1790.

1189. Sunyer, J., M. Torrent, R. Garcia-Esteban, N. Ribas-Fito, D. Carrizo, I. Romieu, J. M. Antó, J. O. Grimalt. 2006. Early exposure to dichlorodiphenyldichloroethylene, breastfeeding and asthma at age six. *Clin. Exp. Allergy* 36(10):1236–1241.

1190. Tagiyeva, N., G. Devereux, S. Semple, A. Sherriff, J. Henderson, P. Elias, J. G. Ayres. 2010. Parental occupation is a risk factor for childhood wheeze and asthma. *Eur. Respir. J.* 35(5):987–993.

1191. Izuhara, K., H. Saito. 2006. Microarray-based identification of novel biomarkers in asthma. *Allergol. Int.* 55(4):361–367.

1192. Umetsu, D. T., J. J. McIntire, O. Akbari, C. Macaubas, R. H. DeKruyff. 2002. Asthma: An epidemic of dysregulated immunity. *Nat. Immunol.* 3(8):715–720.

1193. Wills-Karp, M. 2001. Asthma genetics: Not for the TIMid? *Nat. Immunol.* 2(12):1095–1096.

1194. Weselak, M., T. E. Arbuckle, D. T. Wigle, D. Krewski. 2007. In utero pesticide exposure and childhood morbidity. *Environ. Res.* 103(1):79–86.
1195. Hoppin, J. A., M. Valcin, P. K. Henneberger, G. J. Kullman, D. M. Umbach, S. J. London, M. C. Alavanja, D. P. Sandler. 2007. Pesticide use and chronic bronchitis among farmers in the Agricultural Health Study. *Am. J. Ind. Med.* 50(12):969–979.
1196. Valcin, M., P. K. Henneberger, G. J. Kullman, D. M. Umbach, S. J. London, M. C. Alavanja, D. P. Sandler, J. A. Hoppin. 2007. Chronic bronchitis among nonsmoking farm women in the Agricultural Health Study. *J. Occup. Environ. Med.* 49(5):574–583.
1197. Salameh, P. R., M. Waked, I. Baldi, P. Brochard, B. A. Saleh. 2006. Chronic bronchitis and pesticide exposure: A case-control study in Lebanon. *Eur. J. Epidemiol.* 21(9):681–688.
1198. Sanborn, M. 2012. *Systematic Review of Pesticide Health Effects.* Ontario College of Family Physicians.
1199. Fieten, K. B., H. Kromhout, D. Heederik, B. van Wendel de Joode. 2009. Pesticide exposure and respiratory health of indigenous women in Costa Rica. *Am. J. Epidemiol.* 169(12):1500–1506.
1200. Faria, N. M. X., L. A. Facchini, A. G. Fassa, E. Tomasi. 2005. Pesticides and respiratory symptoms among farmers. *Rev. Saude Publica* 39(6):973–981.
1201. Ejigu, D., Y. Mekonnen. 2005. Pesticide use on agricultural fields and health problems in various activities. *East Afr. Med. J.* 82(8):427–432.
1202. Del Prado-Lu, J. L. 2007. Pesticide exposure, risk factors and health problems among cutflower farmers: A cross sectional study. *J. Occup. Med. Toxicol.* 2:9.
1203. Beseler, C., L. Stallones. 2009. Pesticide poisoning and respiratory disorders in Colorado farm residents. *J. Agric. Saf. Health* 15(4):327–334.
1204. Mekonnen, Y., T. Agonafir. 2004. Lung function and respiratory symptoms of pesticide sprayers in state farms of Ethiopia. *Ethiop. Med. J.* 42(4):261–266.
1205. Zuskin, E., J. Mustajbegovic, E. N. Schachter, J. Kern, V. Deckovic-Vukres, I. Trosic, A. Chirelli. 2008. Respiratory function in pesticide workers. *J. Occup. Environ. Med.* 50(11):1299–1305.
1206. Hoppin, J. A., D. M. Umbach, S. J. London, C. F. Lynch, M. C. Alavanja, D. P. Sandler. 2006. Pesticides and adult respiratory outcomes in the Agricultural Health Study. *Ann. N. Y. Acad. Sci.* 1076:343–354.
1207. Petrie, K. J., M. Thomas, E. Broadbent. 2003. Symptom complaints following aerial spraying with biological insecticide Foray 48B. *N. Z. Med. J.* 116(1170):U354.
1208. Sunyer, J., R. Garcia-Esteban, M. Alvarez, M. Guxens, F. Goni, M. Basterrechea, M. Vrijheid, S. Guerra, J. M. Antó. 2010. DDE in mothers' blood during pregnancy and lower respiratory tract infections in their infants. *Epidemiology* 21(5):729–735.
1209. Daniel, V., W. Huber, K. Bauer, C. Suesal, C. Conradt, G. Opelz. 2002. Associations of DDT and DDE blood levels with plasma Il-4. *Arch. Environ. Health.* 57(6):541–547.
1210. Glynn, A., A. Thuvander, M. Aune, A. Johannisson, P. O. Darnerud, G. Ronquist, S. Cnattingius. 2008. Immune cell counts and risks of respiratory infections among infants exposed pre- and postnatally to organochlorine compounds: A prospective study. *Environ. Health* 7:62.
1211. Vine, M. F., L. Stein, K. Weigle, J. Schroeder, D. Degnan, C. K. Tse, L. Backer. 2001. Plasma 1,1-dichloro-2,2-bis(p-chlorophenyl)ethylene (DDE) levels and immune response. *Am. J. Epidemiol.* 153(1):53–63.
1212. Sigurs, N., L. Bjarmason, F. Sigurbergsson, B. Kjellman. 2000. Respiratory syncytial virus bronchiolitis in infancy is an important risk factor of asthma and allergy at age 7. *Am. J. Respir. Crit. Care Med.* 161(5):1501–1507.
1213. Dallaire, F., E. Dewailly, G. Muckle, C. Vezina, S. W. Jacobson, J. L. Jacobson, P. Avotte. 2004. Acute infections and environmental exposure to organochlorines in Inuit infants from Nunavik. *Environ. Health Perspect.* 112(14):1359–1365.
1214. Newman, L. S. et al.; ACCESS Research Group. 2004. A case control etiologic study of sarcoidosis: Environmental and occupational risk factors. *Am. J. Respir. Crit. Care Med.* 170(12):1324–1330.
1215. Canadian Centre for Occupational Health and Safety (CCOHS). 2008. Farmer's lung. Available online at http://www.ccohs.ca/oshanswers/diseases/farmers_lung.html
1216. Cohn, W. J., J. J. Boylan, R. V. Blanke, M. W. Fariss, J. R. Howell, P. C. Guzelian. 1978. Treatment of chlordecone (kepone) toxicity with cholestyramine. *N. Engl. J. Med.* 298:243–248.
1217. O'Callahan, J. P. 2003. Neurotoxic esterase: Not so toxic? *Nat. Genet.* 33:1–2.
1218. Shintani, T., D. J. Klionsky. 2004. Autophagy in health and disease: A double-edged sword. *Science* 306(5698):990–995.
1219. van Wijngaarden, E., P. A. Stewart, A. F. Olshan, D. A. Savitz, G. R. Bunin. 2003. Parental occupational exposure to pesticides and childhood brain cancer. *Am. J. Epidemiol.* 157(11):989–997.
1220. Wilkins III, J. R., R. A. Koutras. 1988. Paternal occupation and brain cancer in offspring: A mortality-based case-control study. *Am. J. Ind. Med.* 14(3):299–318.

1221. Ortega Jacome, G. P., R. J. Koifman, R. G. T. Monteiro, S. Koifman. 2010. Environmental exposure and breast cancer among young women in Rio de Janeiro, Brazil. *J. Toxicol. Environ. Health A* 73(13–14):858–865.

1222. Ren, A., X. Qiu, L. Jin, J. Ma, Z. Li, L. Zhang, H. Zhu, R. H. Finnell, T. Zhu. 2011. Association of selected persistent organic pollutants in the placenta with the risk of neural tube defects. *Proc. Natl. Acad. Sci. U. S. A.* 108(31):12770–12775.

1223. Stephenson, J. 2000. Exposure to home pesticides linked to Parkinson disease. *JAMA* 283(23):3055–3056.

1224. Sherman, J. D. 1996. Chlorpyrifos (Dursban)-associated birth defects: Report of four cases. *Arch. Environ. Health* 51(1):5–8.

1225. O'Donnell, C. J., R. J. Glynn, T. S. Field, R. Averback. 1999. Misclassification and under-reporting of acute myocardial infarction by elderly persons: Implications for community-based observational studies and clinical trials. *J. Clin. Epidemiol.* 52:745–51.

1226. Rea, W. J. et al. 1984. Pesticides and brain function changes. *Clinical Ecology* II(3):145–150.

1227. Pimentel, D. 2005. Environmental and economic costs of the application of pesticides primarily in the United States. *Environment, Development and Sustainability* 7(2):229–252.

1228. Liang, H.-C., W. J. Rea. *Chemical Sensitivity.* Vol. 2, p. 916. CRC Press, Inc.

1229. Shile, B. D., D. P. Sandler, A. Blair et al. 2010. *Pesticide Use and Myocardial Infarction Incidence Among Farm Women in the Agricultural Health Study*, Wolters Kluwer Health, Inc.

8 Terpenes and Terpenoids

INTRODUCTION

Terpenes (isoprenes) are the natural odors and colors of many plants and building materials to which the individual with chemical sensitivity may be constantly exposed and which may cause an ongoing exacerbation of symptoms. Terpenes rival the output of methane from the Earth. In quantity, they are very important for the survival and optimum functioning of the natural environment. Because terpene sensitivity is quite common among the individuals with chemical sensitivity and because it is a major aggravating factor for their illness and a deterrent to their recovery, we dedicate a separate chapter to this subject.

The most common terpene in the body is the isoprene unit, 2-methyl 1,3-butadiene, which builds cholesterol. It is an analog of isopentyl phosphate. It also emanates from refineries as one of the largest chemicals. Breath analysis in over 500 chemically sensitive patients show 1,3-butadiene as the number one entity that is respired.

Even though terpenes rival methane as an outdoor pollutant, they are also found indoors. They can be a major deterrent to health, as we have seen many times. Many patients with chemical sensitivity and chronic degenerative disease are made ill by pine, cedar, and other terpene odors in the home. Many are ingredients of cleaning solutions. Table 8.1 shows the indoor terpenes that are common and can be measured.

FORMULATION

The terpenes are a class of natural products or hydrocarbons having structural relationship with isoprene or some of its multiple.[1] Isoprene and porphin are building blocks of natural substances. Porphins are building blocks of natural substances such as heme, cytochrome, corroles, etc. Isoprene consists of five carbon atoms attached to eight hydrogen atoms (C_5H_8).[2] It is 2-methyl-1,3-butadiene $(CH_2C(CH_3)CH=CH_2)$; terpenoids $(HC=CH)$ are oxygenated derivatives of hydrocarbons or new compounds structurally related to isoprene. They are isolated from sources other than plants and are often included in the class of terpenes.[1,2] More than 5000 structurally determined terpenes are known.[1] Many of these have also been synthesized in the laboratory.[1] Indoor air analysis of a house showed terpenes and acetic acid made by the chemical reaction of terpenes.

ISOPRENE: ISOTERPENE

Isoprene (short for isoterpene) or 2-methyl-1,3 butadiene is a common organic compound with the formula $CH_2=C(CH_3)CH=CH_2$. Under standard conditions, isoprene is a colorless liquid. However, this compound is highly volatile because of its low boiling point, and it will produce the noxious but pleasant odor of wood pollutants that can disturb many patients with chemical sensitivity. Terpenes can trigger many reactions in the body, including all of the major systems. Not only is it present in natural substances but it is also released into the air by oil refineries.

Isoprene (C_5H_8) is the monomer of natural rubber and also a common structure motif to an immense variety of other naturally occurring compounds, collectively termed as the isoprenoids. Molecular formulas of isoprenoids are multiples of isoprene in the form of $(C_5H_8)_n$, and this is termed the isoprene rule. The functional isoprene units in biological systems are dimethylallyl diphosphate (DMADP) and its isomer isopentenyldisphosphate/diphosphate (IDP).

TABLE 8.1

Measured Indoor Terpenes

d-Limonene

α-Pinene

β-Pinene

Eucalyptol

β-Phellandrene

Campene

2-Turpentine

Source: Environmental Health Center-Dallas, 2013.

The singular terms *isoprene* and *terpene* are synonymous, whereas the plurals *isoprenes* and *terpenes* refer to *terpenoids* (isoprenoids).

NATURAL SOURCES OF TERPENES

Isoprene is produced and emitted into the atmosphere by many species of trees. Major producers are oak, poplar, eucalyptus, coniferous (pine, cedar, etc.), and some legumes. As stated in the introduction, the isoprene components are the most significant in making cholesterol. The yearly emission of isoprene emissions by vegetation is around 600 Tg with half of that coming from tropical broadleaf trees and the remainder coming from shrubs.[3] The emission of terpenes is almost equivalent to the emission of methane into the atmosphere and accounts for one-third of all hydrocarbons released into the atmosphere. After its release, isoprene is converted by free radicals (like the hydroxyl [OH] radical) and to a lesser extent by ozone[4] into various species, such as aldehydes (Table 8.2), hydroperoxides, organic nitrates, and epoxides, which then mix into water droplets and help create aerosols and haze.[5,6]

These substances are very disturbing to individuals with chemical sensitivity and chronic degenerative disease who are also sensitive to odors. While most in the field acknowledge that isoprene emission affects aerosol formation, whether isoprene increases or decreases aerosol formation is debatable.

A second major effect of isoprene on the atmosphere is that in the presence of nitric oxides (NO_x) it contributes to the formation of tropospheric ozone, which is one of the leading air pollutants in many countries. It has been shown to bother individuals with chemical sensitivity. Isoprene itself is normally not regarded as a pollutant, as it is a natural product available from plants. However, it can cause sensitivity and sickness in the patient with chemical sensitivity and chronic degenerative disease. The formation of tropospheric ozone is only possible in the presence of high levels of NO_x, which comes almost exclusively from industrial activities. In fact, isoprene can have an opposite effect and quench ozone formation under low levels of NO_x.

ISOPRENE PRODUCTION FROM PLANTS

Isoprene is made through the methylerythritol 4-phosphate pathway (MEP pathway, also called the nonmevalonate pathway) in the chloroplasts of plants. One of the two end products of the MEP pathway, DMADP, is catalyzed by the inside isoprene synthase to form isoprene. Therefore, an inhibitor that blocks the MEP pathway, such as fosmidomycin, also block isoprene formation. Isoprene emission increases dramatically with temperature and maximizes at around 40°C (Figure 8.1).

This presence has led to the hypothesis that isoprene may protect plants against heat stress (thermotolerance) hypothesis. Emission of isoprene is also observed in some bacteria, and this is thought to come from nonenzymatic degradation from DMADP.

TABLE 8.2

Volatile Organic Compounds and Aldehydes: Indoor Air Analysis—Terpenes and Terpenoids

VOCs and Aldehydes	CAS#	Test Results (µg/m³)	Reference Levels (µg/m³)	Agency	Comparison to Reference Levels
L-Camphor-acetic acid and pinene	76-22-2	14	2	1/	700.0%
Acetic acid	64-19-7	15	25	1/	60.0%
Formaldehyde	50-00-0	9	20	2/	45.0%
Furfural	98-01-1	3	8	1/	37.5%
Acetaldehyde	74-07-0	16	45	1/	35.6%
Benzene	174-43-2	1	4.5	1/	22.2%
Benzaldehyde	100-52-7	2	9	1/	22.2%
Tolualdehyde	529-20-4	1	9	1/	11.1%
Isopropyl alcohol	67-63-1	40	492	1/	8.1%
Butyraldehyde	123-72-8	1	14	1/	7.1%
Hexaldehyde	66-25-1	5	80	1/	6.3%
1-Dodecanol	112-53-8	3	100	1/	3.0%
Heptanal	111-71-7	1	40	1/	2.5%
Myrcene	123-35-3	2	100	1/	2.0%
Valeraldehyde	110-62-3	2	100	1/	2.0%
Nonyl aldehyde	124-19-6	2	150	1/	1.3%
α-Terpinolene	586-62-9	1	100	1/	1.0%
α-Pinene	80-56-8	2	350	1/	0.6%
1-Methyl-4-(1-methylethyl) benzene	99-87-6	1	275	1/	0.4%
Ethyl alcohol	64-17-5	6	1880	1/	0.3%
β-Pinene	117-91-3	1	350	1/	0.3%
Tetradecane	629-59-4	1	350	1/	0.3%
Acetic acid, ethyl ester	141-78-6	4	1440	1/	0.3%
Toluene	108-88-3	3	1200	1/	0.3%
1,1,1-Trichlorothane	71-55-6	1	1080	1/	0.1%
1,8-Cineole	470-82-6	2	n/l	n/l	n/l
4-Terpineol	562-74-3	1	n/l	n/l	n/l
Acetic acid, butyl ester	123-86-4	2	n/l	n/l	n/l
Hexamethylcyclotrisiloxane	541-54-8	27	n/l	n/l	n/l
Dimethylsilane	1111-74-6	27	n/l	n/l	n/l
6-Methyl-t-hepten-5-one	110-93-0	1	n/l	n/l	n/l
Ethyl octanoate	106-32-1	1	n/l	n/l	n/l
Total other VOCs as toluene		32			
Total VOCs and aldehydes		231	<200		115.5%

Note: Terpenes can be converted to acetic acid and aldehydes.

Isoprene emission in plants is controlled both by the availability of substrate (DMADP) and by enzyme (isoprene synthase) activity. In particular, light, CO_2, and O_2 dependencies of isoprene emission are controlled by substrate availability, whereas temperature dependency of isoprene emission is regulated both by substrate level and enzyme activity.

Isoprene emission appears to be a mechanism that trees use to combat abiotic stresses.[5] In particular, isoprene has been shown to protect against moderate heat stresses ($\sim$40°C). It was proposed that isoprene emission was specifically used by plants to protect against large fluctuations in leaf temperature. This accounts for the output in the summer, which is greater than the output in the winter. In Texas, in summer, temperatures range from 100°F to 110°F for the months of June, July, and August, when the terpene haze can be seen in both the city and the country.

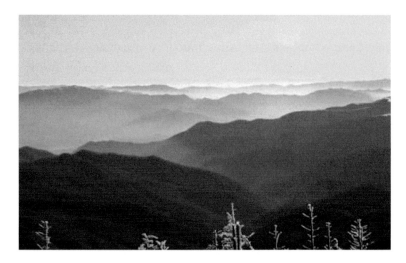

FIGURE 8.1 **(See color insert.)** Picture of terpene haze. (From https://earthdata.nasa.gov/user-resources/sensing-our-planet/volatile-trees.)

Isoprene is incorporated into and helps stabilize cell membranes in response to heat stress, conferring some tolerance to heat spikes. Isoprene may also confer some resistance to reactive oxygen species.[7] The amount of isoprene released from isoprene-emitting vegetation depends on leaf mass, leaf area, light (particularly photosynthetic photon flux density, or PPFD), and leaf temperature. Thus, during the night, little isoprene is emitted from tree leaves, whereas daytime isoprene emissions are expected to be substantial during hot and sunny days. Up to 20 μg/g dry leaf weight occurs in many oak species.[8]

In general, the most common hydrocarbon found in the human body are terpenes.[9,10] The estimated production rate of isoprene in the human body is 0.15 μmol/(kg/hour), equivalent to ~17 mg/day for a person weighing 70 kg. Isoprene is also common in low concentrations in many foods. Isoprene is used for the formulation of cholesterol. Isoprenes have properties used in the stabilization of patients with chemical sensitivity and chronic degenerative disease. We have successfully used the intradermal neutralization technique for many terpenes in patients with chemical sensitivity in order to stabilize their chemically triggered problem. These terpenes include cedar, pine, juniper, hogwort, and many others. Individuals with chemical sensitivity function poorly when triggered by excess terpenes. By using the intradermal neutralization technique, physicians can aid patients in relieving their symptoms.

In the industrial process, isoprene was first isolated by thermal decomposition of natural rubber.[11] It is most readily available industrially as a by-product of the thermal cracking of naphtha or oil and as a side product in the production of ethylene. Refineries emanate much 1,3-butadiene 2-methyl; about 800,000 tons of butadiene is produced annually. About 95% of the isoprene production is used to produce *cis*-1,4-polyisoprene—a synthetic version of natural rubber. Many patients with chemical sensitivity are sensitive to the synthetic rubber.

Natural rubber is a polymer of isoprene—most often *cis*-1,4-polyisoprene—with a molecular weight of 100,000–1,000,000. Typically, a few percent of other materials, such as proteins, fatty acids, resins, and inorganic materials, are found in high-quality natural rubber. Some natural rubber sources such as gutta-percha are composed of *trans*-1,4-polyisoprene, a structural isomer that has similar, but not identical properties.[10]

Gutta-percha has been used for years in dental fillings (as root canals) when coupled with silver and mercury amalgams. Many patients with chemical sensitivity are sensitive to gutta-percha.

Isoprene is a common structural motif in biological systems. The isoprenoids (e.g., the carotenes are tetraterpenes) are derived from isoprene. Also derived from isoprene are phytol, retinol (vitamin A), tocopherol (vitamin E), dolichols, and squalene. Heme A has an isoprenoid tail, and lanosterol, a sterol precursor in animals, is derived from squalene and hence from isoprene. The functional isoprene units in biological systems DMADP and its isomer IDP are used in the biosynthesis of naturally occurring isoprenoids such as carotenoids, quinones, lanosterol derivatives (e.g., steroids), and the parental chains of certain compounds (e.g., phytol chain or chlorophyll). We frequently have to use interdermal neutralization for some of these substances, such as vitamins A and E.

CARCINOGENICITY

Significantly, isoprene is reasonably anticipated to be a human carcinogen based on sufficient evidence of carcinogenicity from studies in experimental animals. This observation of toxicity may be used in the patient with chemical sensitivity who is already sensitive to isoprene.

CASE STUDIES IN EXPERIMENTAL ANIMALS

Exposure to isoprene by inhalation caused tumors at several different tissue sites in mice and rats.[12] In mice of both sexes, isoprene caused blood vessel cancer (hemangiosarcoma) and benign or malignant tumors of the Harderian gland (adenoma or carcinoma) and the lung (alveolar/bronchial adenoma or carcinoma).[13] In male mice, it also caused cancer of the hematopoietic system (histiocytic sarcoma) and benign or malignant tumors of the liver (hepatocellular adenoma or carcinoma) and for stomach (squamous cell papilloma or carcinoma). In rats of both sexes, isoprene caused benign or malignant tumors of the mammary gland (fibroadenoma or carcinoma) and kidney (renal cell adenoma or carcinoma). In male rats, it also caused benign tumors of the testes (adenoma).[12-14] Inhaled isoprene appeared to initiate or trigger chemical sensitivity and some chronic degenerative diseases.

Isoprene is the 2-methyl analog of 1,3-butadiene, an industrial chemical that has been identified as a carcinogen in humans and experimental animals.[15-17]

The isoprene analog isopentenyl pyrophosphate is a building block of cholesterol synthesis, and levels of exhaled isoprene correlate with cholesterol synthesis.[18,19] Isoprene and butadiene are metabolized to monoepoxide and diepoxide intermediates by liver microsomal cytochrome P450-dependent monooxygenases from several species, including humans.[15,16,18] These intermediates may be detoxified by hydrolysis (catalyzed by epoxide hydrolase) or conjugation with glutathione (catalyzed by glutathione S-transferase).

The diepoxide intermediates of isoprene and butadiene cause mutations in *Salmonella typhimurium*, whereas the monoepoxides of isoprene and parent compounds did not. In mammalian cells *in vitro*, isoprene did not cause sister chromatid exchange, chromosomal aberrations, or micronucleus formation,[12,16] but it did cause DNA damage in human peripheral blood mononuclear cells and human leukemia cells when incubated with microsomal enzymes.[20] In mice exposed *in vivo*, isoprene and 1,3-butadiene caused sister chromatid exchange in bone marrow cells and micronucleus formation in peripheral blood erythrocytes.[21,22] Sites at which both isoprene and butadiene caused tumors in rodents include liver, lung, Harderian gland, stomach, hematopoietic tissue, and circulatory system in mice and the mammary glands, kidney, and testes in rats.[16,17] Harderian gland tumors caused by isoprene in mice had a frequency of unique mutations of the K-*ras* proto-oncogene (A–T transversions at codon 61).[23]

There is no evidence to suggest that mechanisms by which isoprene causes tumors in experimental animals would not also operate in humans.

No epidemiological studies were identified that evaluated the relationship between human cancer and exposure specifically to isoprene.

The majority of isoprene produced commercially is used to make synthetic rubber (*cis*-polyisoprene), most of which is used to produce vehicle tires. The second and third largest uses are in the production of styrene–isoprene–styrene block polymers and butyl rubber (isobutane–isoprene copolymer).[18]

Isoprene is recovered as a by-product of thermal cracking of naphtha or gas and oil from C_5 streams in refineries.[16,18] The isoprene yield is about 2%–5% of the ethylene yield. Demand for isoprene in the United States grew 6.5% annually from 1985 to 1992.[16] In 1994, isoprene production in the United States was about 619,000,000 pounds, almost 29% more than in 1992. Estimated isoprene production capacity for eight facilities was 598 million pounds in 1996, based on estimates of isoprene content of product stream available from ethylene production via heavy liquids. In 2009, isoprene was produced by 22 manufacturers worldwide, including 12 U.S. producers.[24] It was available from 23 suppliers, including 12 U.S. suppliers.[25] The U.S. imports of isoprene (purity 95% by weight) increased from 0 in 1989 to a peak of 144 million pounds in 2003. Imports declined to 19.6 million pounds in 2004, the lowest level since 1992, but remained nearly 32 million pounds from 2005 through 2008. During this period, the U.S. exports of isoprene ranged from 7.9 million to 39.6 million pounds (in 2006).[26] Reports filed from 1986 until 2002 under the U.S. Environment Protection Agency's Toxic Substances Control Act Inventory Update Rule indicated that the U.S. production plus imports of isoprene totaled 100–500 million pounds.[27a]

Isoprene is formed endogenously in humans at a rate of 0.15 μmol/kg of body weight per hour, equivalent to ca. 2–4 mg/kg per day.[27b]

The major hydrocarbon in human breath, accounting for 70% of exhaled hydrocarbons, is 1,3-butadiene-2 methyl.[28] Table 8.3 shows the concentrations in human blood range from 1.0 to 4.8 μg/L[29]

Isoprene is produced at higher rates in males than females. The rate of isoprene production increases with age until the age of 29.[30] It is lower in young children than adults by a factor of about 2.4.[31] In

TABLE 8.3

Breath Analysis of a 55-Year-Old White Female Typical of Isoprene Being the Most Common Emanation but Coupled with Other Toxics—EHC-Dallas

Breath Abundance	Compounds	Sources
512.56	1,3-Butadiene 3-Methyl or (isoprene) 2-Methyl	1. Natural emanation from trees, legumes 2. Natural rubber 3. Synthetic rubber 4. Normal human generates isoprene at rate of 17 mg/day
109.96	Oxirane-methyl (ethylene) (isopropyl)	
47.5	Butanane-2-methyl	
47.5	Pentane	Natural gas
29.75	Ethylparaben	Food preservative
29.72	Benzoic acid, 4-ethoxy-, ethyl ester	
29.72	Ethoxybenzhydrazine	
17.42	4-Amino-1-butanol	
17.43	4-Penten-2one	
17.42	Isopropyl (alcohol)	
9.53	Hexane	
5.51	Hydrazine-methyl	
5.43	3-Heradecane	
5.37	1,3-Cycloheptatriene	
5.37	Cyclobutane, 2-propenylidene	
5.33	1,3-2H-Isobenzoforanone, 4,7-dimethyl	
5.33	3 (2H) Benzofuranone	
5.33	Benzene acetaldehyde, 2,5-trimethyl	
5.25	Penture 2-Bromo	
5.25	Penture 2-Methyl	

Source: Environmental Health Center - Dallas 2013.

a study of 30 adult volunteers, the mean isoprene concentration measured in alveolar breath was 118 ppb, with a range of 0–474 ppb.[32] After 20–30 minutes of exercise, isoprene concentration in exhaled air decreased to a range of 0–40 ppb.[33] Smoking one cigarette increased the concentration of isoprene in exhaled air by 70%.[34] Isoprene is also produced endogenously by other animals. Production rates reported for rats and mice were 1.9 and 0.4 μmol/kg of body weight per hour, respectively.[35]

Foods of plant origin would be expected to be a source of daily exposure to isoprene, since isoprene is emitted by agricultural crops and is the basic structural unit in countless natural products found in foods such as terpenes and vitamins A and K.[16] Isoprene has been reported to occur in the essential oil of oranges, hops, carrot roots, and roasted coffee.[16,36]

Isoprene is emitted from plants and trees and is generally present in the environment at low concentrations.[36] Isoprene emissions from many types of plants have been estimated under various climatic conditions in order to evaluate their importance in global climate change.[37–46] Annual global isoprene emissions, estimated at 175 billion to 503 billion kg (386 billion to 1109 billion pounds), account for an estimated 57% of the total global natural volatile organic compound emissions.[47] The average biogenic emission rate factor for isoprene in the U.S. woodlands is 3 mg/m^2 per hour (compared with 5.1 mg/ m^2) for the total volatile organic compounds.[48] Isoprene concentrations in biogenic emissions range from 8% to 91% of total volatile organic compounds, averaging 58%. Because isoprene biosynthesis is associated with photosynthesis, isoprene emissions are negligible during night.[50] Because isoprene is emitted primarily by deciduous trees, emissions are seasonal, being highest in the summer and lowest in the winter.[48,49] The south central and southeastern areas of the United States have the highest biogenic emissions.[48,50] The half-life of atmospheric isoprene has been estimated at 0.5 hour by reacting with nitric oxide, 4 hours by reaction with hydroxyl radicals, and 19 hours by reacting with ozone.[51]

Exposure to pollutants along with exposure to terpene emissions can explain why some patients with chemical sensitivity and chronic degenerative disease remain ill (due to exposure to terpenes).

Anthropogenic sources of isoprene in the atmosphere include ethylene production by naphtha cracking, wood pulping, oil fires, woodburning stoves and fireplaces, other biomass combustion, tobacco smoking (200–400 μg per cigarette), and gasoline and exhaust from turbines and automobiles.[51,52] Isoprene has been measured as one of the most volatile organic compounds in the ambient air in regions with industrial pollution and in urban residential and rural areas as an indicator of the potential for ozone formation. Thus, isoprene is a key indicator for regional air quality, as well as being a component of the global carbon cycle.[53–57]

The reported concentration of isoprene in ambient air in the United States ranges from 1 to 21 parts per billion carbon (ppbC). Isoprene accounts for <10% of nonmethane hydrocarbons in ambient air. Biogenic hydrocarbons may contribute more to total atmospheric hydrocarbons under stagnant atmospheric conditions.[58,59] The major sources of isoprene in ambient air appear to be biogenic emissions at rural sites and vehicular emissions in urban areas.[60,61] Where the source is primarily biogenic, the isoprene concentration slowly increases during the day, reaching a peak in the middle of the day, when photosynthesis is the highest. Where vehicular emissions are the primary source, the isoprene concentration peaks during the morning and evening rush hours and is low in the middle of the day.[62] One study concluded that in summer at least 80% of the isoprene at a rural site was due to biogenic emissions, but that in winter more than 90% of residential isoprene was from urban air-mass mixing.[53] Where industrial emissions are the primary source of isoprene, the concentration may peek at night, or there may be no peak at all.[63,64] A patient with chemical sensitivity usually experiences more problems at night.

The primary source of isoprene in indoor air is environmental tobacco smoke. Isoprene was found to be the major component of hydrocarbons in the air of a smoky café (10 patrons smoking, 10 not smoking) (16.7%) and in sidestream smoke (29.2%).[65] In November 1992, a monitoring survey in homes and workplaces in the greater Philadelphia area found mean isoprene concentrations in personal air samples of 4.65 μg/m^3 in 60 nonsmoking homes, 18.15 μg/m^3 in 29 homes with smokers, 5.29 μg/m^3 in 51 not nonsmoking workplaces, and 22.80 μg/m^3 in 28 workplaces that allowed smoking.[66] A survey in the lower Rio Grande Valley of Texas reported a median summertime isoprene concentration of 2.90 μg/m^3 in three indoor air samples, compared with 0.40 μg/m^3 for three indoor air samples with no smoking.[67] Natural terpenes in the homes of nonsmokers can arise from pine and cedar wood and in some cases, camphor. Other conifer woods can severely disturb the patient with chemical sensitivity. Often these woods and furniture made from conifers must be removed from the home of a person with chemical sensitivity in order for him or her to get well.

Air-monitoring data were collected at three U.S. facilities that produced isoprene monomers or polymers. Of the samples, 98.5% showed concentrations of <10 ppm, and 91.3% showed <1 ppm.[68,69] The National Occupational Hazard Survey conducted from 1972 to 1974 estimated that 58,000 workers in over three industries potentially were exposed to isoprene.[70] The National Occupational Exposure Survey conducted from 1981 to 1983 estimated in a more limited survey that 3700 workers, including 578 women, in four industries were potentially exposed to isoprene.[71]

In 1989, a sweet-tasting protein, *pentadin*, was discovered and isolated in the fruit of ouvi (*Pentadiplandra brazzeana* baillon), a climbing shrub growing in some tropical countries in Africa.[72] The fruit has been consumed by the apes and the natives for a long time. The berries of the plant are incredibly sweet. African locals call them "J'oublie" (French for "I forget") because their taste helps nursing infants forget their mother's milk.[73] Pentadin brazen[74] discovered in 1994, is also a sweet-tasting protein discovered in an African fruit. Pentadin's molecular weight is estimated to be 122 kDa. It is reported to be 500 times sweeter than sucrose on a weight basis. With its sweetness, there is a slow onset and decline of this substance, similar to monellin and thaumatin—however, pentadin's sweet profile is closer to monellin's than thaumatin's.[72]

Biological formation of terpenes occurs when two molecules of acetic acid give rise to *mevalonic acid* ($C_6H_{12}O_2$), which converts to isopentenyl pyrophosphate, which contains the five-carbon isoprene skeleton.

2 mol acetic acid → mevalonic acid ($C_6H_{12}O_2$) → isopentenyl pyrophosphate → isoprene.

Acetic acid comes from vinegar and is a descaling agent and photographic film inhibitor; it is used in electroplating, as a solvent for paints; it is used in the production of vinyl acetate, as a chemical reagent, it is used in production of polyethylene phosphate, and as a photolab anhydrate. Further transformations of the compound result in the true terpenes and terpenoids. The true terpenes are grouped according to the specific number of isoprene units (C_5H_8) in a molecule; for example, monoterpenes ($C_{10}H_{16}$) contain two units; sesquiterpenes ($C_{15}H_{24}$) contain three; diterpenes ($C_{20}H_{32}$),[75] triterpenes ($C_{30}H_{48}$),[76] and tetraterpenes ($C_{40}H_{64}$). Polyterpenes such as rubber and gutta-percha (used in root canals for teeth repairs contain 1000–5000 isoprene units joined in a long chain.

Exposure to terpenes may occur in various ways. Some of the more common include living in a home of pine or cedar wood, living in an area surrounded by pine trees, having Christmas trees in the house, using scented cleaners, using paints and paint cleaners containing turpentines, using pine resins for building materials, and/or building in areas where cedars, sage, creosote bushes, or camphorproducing trees proliferate. Often, the odors of many plants, such as hogwort, ragweed, and cut grass, are worse than the pollen and last longer than a year, severely exacerbating symptoms of individuals with chemical sensitivity, who come in contact with them. Because rubber floors and other synthetic rubbers output terpenes, they can also cause problems for individuals with chemical sensitivity.

The term *essential oils* comes from alchemists who hoped to find the essence of nature.[77] Instead, they discovered liquids with aromatic odors in the flowers, leaves, and roots of plants and trees, especially conifers and citrus trees. Many of these odors have been found to trigger sensitivity in those who are chemically sensitive.

After 1,3-butadiene 2-methyl and α-pinene, the most important terpene found is oil of turpentine. Other important terpenes are present in the oils of oranges, lemons, and verbena and are generally termed limonene, α-pinene, and d-limonene. These terpenes are frequently found in the breath analysis of patients with chemical sensitivity. The 1,3-butadiene 2-methyl (Table 8.4) is also often present in the patient with chemical sensitivity. It is usually number 1.

TABLE 8.4
Breath Test for Volatile Organic Compounds

Medication/supplements taken in the last 3 days: 48-year-old female

Chemical formula for librium, gabapentin

Librium: 7 chloro-2-(methylamino)-5-phenyl-3H-1,4-venzodiazepine 4-oxide hydrochloride ($H_{14}ClN_3OClH$)

Gabapentin: 1-(aminomethyl)cyclohexane acetic acid ($C_9H_{17}NO_2$)

Breath Abundance	Chemical	Origin/Formula	Properties/Major Uses
182.5	1,3-Butadiene(2-methyl-)	Natural/synthetic (C_5H_8)	Monomer of isoprene commonly used for building cholesterol. Isoprene is made through the nonmevalonate pathway (*MEP) in the chloroplast of plants; inhibitors like fosmidomycin that block the MEP pathway also block isoprene formation. Marker for disorder of cholesterol metabolism—hypercholesterolemia. Natural isoprene is not regarded as a pollutant. Turpentine produced and emitted by oaks, poplars, eucalyptus, and some legumes. Converted by free radicals and to a lesser extent by ozone into various species. Organic nitrates and epoxides help to create aerosol haze. Protects plant against heat stress. Carcinogen increases up to the age of 25. As a monomer in the production of synthetic rubber and plastics. Product of ethanol.
30.75	Ethylparaben	Synthetic $C_9H_{10}O_3$	Antifungal preservative, human endocrine disruptor—preservative in cosmetics and pharmaceuticals, food additive to inhibit fungal growth.
30.75	2-Ethoxybenzhydrazide	Synthetic $C_9H_{12}N_2O_2$	Food additive E number E214. Pharmaceutical intermediates. Many organic synthesis.
30.75	Benzoic acid, 4-ethoxy-, ethyl ester	Synthetic C_7HO_2	Motor fuel antiknock agent. Made by oxidation of toluene. Determine the heat capacity of a bomb calorimeter. Artificial flavors. Plasticizers, extraction of phenol. Food preservatives.
11.03	Cyclohexanol-5-methyl-2-(1-methylethyl)-1a,b,5a)	Natural/synthetic $C_{10}H_{20}O$	Additives to cosmetics, aftershaves, suntan lotions, and essential oils. Menthol from mint oils or made synthetically from coal tar. Opposite to capsaicin property to the skin, giving the skin cool sensation. Cough drops, local anesthetic for minor sore throat, minor muscle aches.
5.57	Benzene,2,4-dimethyl-1-methylpropyl)-	Synthetic C_8H_{10}	Manufacture of isophthalic acid (copolymer, alter the properties of polyethylene terephthalate making it suitable for making soft drink bottles).
5.57	Benzenecataldehyde, A,2,5-trimethyl	Synthetic	Component of tobacco smoke, pesticide methyl benzene acetaldehyde, fragrance products.
5.01	4,5,6,7-Tetramethylphthalide	Synthetic $C_8H_2ClO_2$	Fungicide, agriculture, forestry, fisheries. Partial ortho-xylene oxidation produces phthalide as a by-product. Part of volatile essential oil.
5.01	Benzene, 1,3-bis(1-formylethyl)-	Synthetic $C_{12}H_{14}O_2$	Pharmaceutical compound.
5.01	2,3,5,6-Tetramethylterephthalaldehyde	Synthetic $C_{12}H_{14}O_2$	Pharmaceutical research, cosmetic composition, sun screen.

(Continued)

TABLE 8.4 (*Continued*)
Breath Test for Volatile Organic Compounds

Breath Abundance	Chemical	Origin/Formula	Properties/Major Uses
4.75	Benzene, 1-methoxy-4(1-propenyl)-	Natural $C_{10}H_{12}O$	Found in anise, fennel, anise myrtle, liquorices, and star anise. Flavoring substance. Very sweet (13 times sweeter than sugar). Alcoholic drinks, seasoning, confectionery applications, oral hygiene products, natural berry flavors. Manufacture of drugs anisyldithiothione, anethold, dithione, anethole, trithione, insect repellent against mosquitoes.
4.75	5-Methoxyindane	Synthetic $C_{10}H_{12}O$	"Dual fingerprint reagents" are chemical formulations, which produce with latent fingerprints in a single-step intermediate in making anti-inflammatory agents. Intermediate chemical in making SSRI drugs.
4.75	Estragole	Natural $C_{10}H_{12}O$	Natural phenylpropene. Primary constituent of essential oil of tarragon (60%–75% of the oil). Found in essential oil of basil (23%–8%), pine oil, turpentine, fennel, anise *Syzygium anisatum*. Perfume, food additive for flavor (strong, sweet, and 2002 tarragon). Genotoxic carcinogenic.
4.06	Benzaldehyde, 2,4-dimethyl-	Synthetic $C_{10}H_{16}O$	Flavor and fragrance agents: smells like naphthyl, cherry, almond, spice, cherry, and vanilla.
6.06	Benzaldehyde, 3,5-dimethyl-	Natural/synthetic $C_9H_{10x}O$	Plastic additives. Pharmaceutical intermediate. Flavoring fragrance.
3.67	Eucalyptol	Natural $C_{10}H_{18}O$	Natural eucalyptus oil, camphor laurel, bay leaves, tea tree, mugwort, sweet basil, wormwood, rosemary, sage. Flavoring fragrance, mouthwash, cough suppressants, insecticide, insect repellent.
3.67	Cyclohexanemethanol, 4-hydroxy-a-a,4-trimethyl-	Natural $C_{10}HO_2$	Oil of turpentine, oregano, thyme, eucalyptus. Used for chronic bronchitis in United States. Currently used as expectorants in Guaifenesin.
3.67	Trifluoroacetyl-a-terpineol	Natural/synthetic $C_{12}H_{17}F_3O_2$	Found in pine tree; pine smoke used to dry tea. Also manufactured from 1-pinene. Lilac odor. Common ingredient in perfumes, cosmetics flavors, essential oil of *Rosmarinus officinalis*, oil used for rheumatic pain, kettle hop flavorants in beer, wines.
3.67	Pentane,2,2,3-trimethyl-	Petrochemical/synthetic C_8H_{18}	Isomer of octane. Important component of gasoline. Insoluble in water. Lighter than water. Antiknock agent along with iso-octane

Camphene is a solid terpene obtained from camphor. Some flowers, such as violet, produce oil odors for a whole day after picking.[78] These terpene odors will exacerbate symptoms in patients with chemical sensitivity who are sensitive to them. Table 8.4 shows a patient who is sensitive to terpenes and terpenoids.

The essential oils of plants contain an abundance of monoterpenes, sesquiterpenes, and diterpenes. The most common structural monoterpenes are derivatives of geraniol, the main constituent of geranium oil. Menthol is the chief component of peppermint oil. d-Limonene composes over 90% of lemon oil. α-Pinene is found in the oil of rosemary. Camphor is the main component of sage oil. Iridoids are interesting monoterpenes, which have been isolated from ants. Monoterpenes are used in flavor and perfume industries because of their attractive odors, high volatilities, and low molecular weights.[78] Most of these are synthesized and usually trigger symptoms in individuals with chemical sensitivity. Several monoterpenes are found in turpentine. The rosin acids are diterpenes. Vitamin A is the best-known open-chain diterpene. The triterpenes that are obtainable from shark liver oil may be converted to cholesterol and many other steroids. The carotenoid pigments are the best-known tetraterpenes. The function of terpenes in plants, which has been previously described as being a protectant for heat and other organisms, is not always so clear. Terpenes sometimes possess toxic properties that link to the protection of the species. Animals do not eat some types of terpenes. The same protective properties appear to trigger and exacerbate symptoms in individuals with chemical sensitivity.

Sesquiterpenes include zingiber (the constituent in ginger oil), cadinene (from oil cubebs), α-santonin (from plants of *Artemisia*), and alphacoranes, cedranes, and chamigranes (from various species of woods, such as Alaskan cedar). Others are caryophyllanes, illudanes, and humulenes, which occur in hops. The fastest-growing group is the perhydroazulenes (quaianes and guaiacum wood oil).[78] Quaianes and quaianolides constitute the largest group isolated from fungi, marine organisms, or plants.[78] The sesquiterpene lacones quaianolides have remarkable cytotoxic properties.[78] At present, the reaction of individuals with chemical sensitivity to sesquiterpenes is unknown; however, it should be evaluated in view of patients known reaction to other terpenes.

Diterpenes emanate from the resins of various coniferous species. Abietic acid derivatives are the principal product of rosin, a resin that comes mainly from pine and has a variety of industrial uses, most of which exacerbate sensitivity in the individual who is chemically sensitive. Labdanes and clerodanes are the "bitter" principle of bark, roots, and stems (from clerodane and horehound).[78]

Sesquiterpenes, a class of terpenes identified in 1965, are C_{25} compounds isolated from protective waxes and coatings of insects or from fungal sources. Examples are retigeranic acid and ophiobolin A. It is unknown whether these will exacerbate symptoms in individuals who are chemically sensitive.

Tetraterpenes do not possess the structural complexity and stereochemical structure of the lower terpenes (those under C_{40}). Most are carotenoid pigments exemplified by α-carotene. They are found in the chloroplast of all green plants and in some algae. An example may be regarded as degraded carotene and as such may explain why some patients with chemical sensitivity cannot tolerate it. However, most patients with chemical sensitivity generally are able to tolerate carotenes.

Polyterpenes usually consist of 500–5000 cis-linked isoprene units. They are natural rubbers from Heva and Guayule, which arise due to a generic error. The polymers are found in only about 1% of the plant kingdom. Some individuals with chemical sensitivity do not tolerate rubbers. Often, however, it is an additive, such as carbon disulfide, that is a triggering agent to which they react, thus confusing accurate definition of the triggering agent.

Terpenes have found to be toxic. Experimental studies using 20 different species of the Compositae plant family indicated that *Cnicus benedictus* (blessed thistle), *Chrysanthemum leucanthemum* (marguerite, oxide daisy), and *Helianthus debilis* (dwarf sunflower) are "strong sensitizers" and thus may exacerbate chemical sensitivity.[75] *Helenium amarum* (bitterweed), *Gaillardia amblyodon* (blanket flower), *Artemisia ludoviciana* (prairie sage), *Ambrosia trifida* (giant ragweed), and *Solidago virgaurea* (goldenrod) are medium sensitizers.[75] The odor of giant ragweed is particularly well known to exacerbate chemical sensitivity. Only a weak, or no, sensitizing capacity was found in 12 species, including cornflower, wormwood, mugwort, coltsfoot, and dandelion.[75]

TABLE 8.5

Typical Terpenes Found in Homes and Levels Found

Compound	4555-1 Bedroom		4555-2 Bedroom		4555-3 Living Room		Typical Sources
	µg/m³	ppbv	µg/m³	ppbv	µg/m³	ppbv	
d-Limonene	20.9	3.8	9.5	1.7	18.6	3.3	Cleaners,
α-Pinene	45.6	8.2	19.8	3.6	43.0	7.7	disinfectants,
β-Pinene	16.2	2.9	6.7	1.2	16.5	3.0	fragrances,
d-Carene	23.6	4.2	11.1	2.0	21.0	3.8	perfumes, and
Eucalyptol	14.5	2/3	4.8	0.8	11.1	1.8	wood products
β-Phellandrene	18.5	3.3	8.3	1.5	17.0	3.1	
Camphene	2.9	0.5	1.8	0.3	3.5	0.6	
Myrcene	7.4	1.3	3.0	0.5	7.7	1.4	
Linalool	4.3	0.9	0.1	<0.1	<0.1	<0.1	
L-Camphor	2.5	0.4	<0.1	<0.1	0.2	<0.1	Medicinal products
Menthol	0.8	,0.1	<0.1	<0.1	1.0	0.2	and air fresheners

However, we have seen patients with chemical sensitivity who were sensitive to these, especially mugwort. In a considerable number of species, cross-reactivities have been noted that were apparently dependent on the occurrence of sesquiterpene lactones, which have an x-methylene group exocyclic to the lactone in common.[75] The presence of an x-methylene y-lactone group appears to be virtually essential in bringing about a sensitivity to Compositae[79] (Table 8.5).

One hundred and eighty species of Compositae have been shown to cause allergic contact dermatitis in gardeners, nursery workers, amateur gardeners, florists, and breeders in Europe.[76 80] Farmers, roadmen, land workers, or others who work mainly outdoors have been adversely affected by widely distributed weeds that are members of the Compositae family. They often suffer from "airborne contact dermatitis."[81–86] These weeds will exacerbate the sensitivity of those with chemical sensitivity if they are exposed to even minute quantities.

Species of Compositae are used as drugs. These include yarrow, absinth, tansy, arnica, and camomile.[78] Dandelion and elecampane serve as animal fodder.[78] Folk and medicinal remedies have dictated the use of coltsfoot, yarrow, arnica, and common marigold for various ills.[78] When ingested, these may exacerbate chemical sensitivity or at times temporarily aid it.

Terpinolene is a constituent of some vegetable oils and of some pine species.[87] Terpinolene was found to induce eczematous lesions on the hands and forearms of a 49-year-old woman whose occupation involved the use of a special machine cleaner.[88] It might be considered a pheromone due to its presence in the cephalic secretions of the Australian termite.[89] This substance is used by veterinarians for its antiviral properties.[78] It is also used in foods as an artificial flavor, which may exacerbate chemical sensitivity.[78]

BIOLOGICAL RESPONSES

Anderson[90] has shown that ~30% of the air contaminants in new homes are terpenes or terpenoids areas. This high incidence has also been the experience at the EHC-Dallas and the EHC-Buffalo. Clearly, many patients react to these terpenes/terpenoids with symptoms of asthma, headache, rhinosinusitis, vasculitis, gastrointestinal upset, and genitourinary imbalance; others experience short-term memory loss, lack of concentration, confusion, etc.

The odors of some terpenes seem quite toxic; we have seen patients with chemical sensitivity become quite ill following relocation from areas of high man-made pollution to less chemically polluted rural, semiarid, and arid regions that are high in natural terpenes. These regions, though less mechanized, can pose severe problems for patients with chemical sensitivity because of the presence of terpenes of sage, juniper, mountain cedar, pine, creosote, and various other plants.

Occupational exposure to cedar and pine woods and pine resins (colophony) can cause asthma and chronic lung disease. Prior studies suggest that plicatic and abietic acids are responsible for the asthmatic reactions that occur in cedar wood and colophony workers. Studying rat and human lung cells by Ayars et al.[91] showed that both types of acids caused dose- and time-dependent lysis of the alveolar epithelial cells. If these acids were injected into the lungs of rats, bronchial epithelial sloughing occurred. These researchers presumed that repeated exposures promoted chronic lung disease, which was probably a type of chemical sensitivity, in these workers and also in electrical workers who were exposed to pure resin.

Exacerbation of chemical sensitivity has been observed in patients living in homes where large amounts of pine and cedar were used for construction, for example, in paneling, chairs, desks, cupboards, and furnishings. At the EHC-Dallas and the EHC-Buffalo, we have observed many patients with chemical sensitivity who could not tolerate their homes because of exposure to pine and cedar. They had to either move or do a thorough job of sealing areas in which emissions occurred so that no odor emanated into the air. Table 8.3 shows a 55-year-old female's breath analysis with a lot of isoprene (1,3-butadiene 2-methyl).

A case report in literature described a 40-year-old male known to react to zinc oxide plaster who presented with acute eczema of the face, hands, and arms. His problems began 2 days after he had planted 100 *Cupressus leylandii* shrubs. The adhesive in zinc oxide plaster is colophony, a pine tar distillate that contains abietic acid and other related terpenes, as does the essential oil from *Cupressus* leaf (++), *Cupressus* leaf extract in ether (+++) abietic acid 20% pet (+), and Spanish colophony 20% pet (+++).[92] The latex of *Euphorbia virgata* has been found to contain various skin-irritant esters of the diterpene ingenol.[93] In a carcinogenic assay, acetone extract of this latex produces squamous cell papilloma.[78] One of the initiator-promoters for skin carcinogenesis was identified as 3-O-2-methyl-decanoyl ingenol.[78] The patient improved after removal of the plaster around the windows and sinks. The colophony emanating from the plaster was likely the reason.

DIAGNOSIS OF TERPENE SENSITIVITY

Diagnosis of terpene sensitivity is usually performed by intradermal injection, inhalation, and oral challenge. At the EHC-Dallas, we tested patients with chemical sensitivity who were thought by history to be bothered by terpene odors. The results of our intradermal studies are presented in Tables 8.6 and 8.7. There were 368 intradermal challenges with 270 positives and 98 negatives. These sensitivities appeared to be a part of the overall chemical sensitivity, as evidenced by the patients who had proven sensitivities to both intradermal and double-blind inhaled challenge (Table 8.6). These patients had to avoid terpenes as much as possible and take neutralizing injections of terpene extract in order to improve their condition. Many terpenes have been identified through breath analysis. 1,3-Butadiene is the most frequently identified. Other common terpenes found in breath analysis include pine, tree, grass, ragweed, and Mt. Cedar (Table 8.3). Tables 8.8a and 8.8b show the inhaled and intradermal challenges of other toxics as well as some terpenes in chemically and terpene-sensitive patients.

TREATMENT OF TERPENE SENSITIVITY

At the EHC-Dallas and the EHC-Buffalo, our policy is to avoid terpenes and use the intradermal injection or sublingual method to neutralize patients with chemical sensitivity to various terpenes as part of their treatment regimen. This treatment appears to give them much more latitude of movement when injection contents are expanded to contain both indoor and outdoor terpene contaminants.

TABLE 8.6

Symptoms in 90 Terpene-Sensitive Patients with Chemical Sensitivity after Intradermal Inhaled Provocation

Symptoms	No. of Patients	No. of Positive	% Positive
Saline—control	96	0	0
Cephalgia	90	52	57.8
Ear, nose, throat	90	28	31.1
Toxic brain syndrome	90	48	53.3
Myalgia	90	18	20.0
Neurological	90	22	24.4
Asthma	90	28	31.1
Vasculitis	90	22	24.4
Dermatitis	90	4	4.4
Immune deregulation	90	16	17.8

Source: Environmental Health Center-Dallas, 2010—performed under environmentally controlled area.

TABLE 8.7

Intradermal Test Provoking Symptoms or Signs in 76 Patients with Chemical Sensitivity—EHC-Dallas, 2012

Terpenes	No. of Patients	No. of Positive	% Positive
Saline	76	0	0
Pine terp	76	46	60.5
Tree terp	72	28	38.9
Grass terp	74	6	8.1
Ragweed terp	72	20	27.8
Mt. Cedar terp	74	14	18.9

Source: Environmental Health Center-Dallas-2012.
Note: Dilutions—1/25–1/3000; +—performed under environmentally less polluted conditions.

TABLE 8.8a

Intradermal and Inhalant Challenge of Chemicals in 45 Terpene-Sensitive Patients with Chemical Sensitivity Intradermal Test Performed under Environmentally Less Polluted Conditions

Chemicals	No. Tested	No. Positive	%	Dosage (ppm)
Cigarette smoke	42	35	83.3	Ambient
Orris root	42	40	95.2	Ambient
Ethanol	41	35	85.4	<0.50
Formaldehyde	18	18	100.0	<0.20
Newsprint	39	28	71.8	Ambient
Perfume	39	26	66.7	Ambient
Phenol	17	9	52.9	<0.20
Chlorine	11	6	54.5	<0.33
Pesticides	–	–	–	<0.0034
Placebo	45	0	0	Normal saline

Source: Environmental Health Center-Dallas, 2013.

TABLE 8.8b

Inhalant Chemicals	No. Tested	No. Positive	%	Dosage
Cigarette smoke	42	35	83.3	Ambient < odor threshold
Orris root	45	30	66.0	Ambient < odor threshold
Ethanol	21	16	76.2	<0.50 ppb
Formaldehyde	18	15	83.3	<0.20 ppb
Newsprint	40	40	200.0	Ambient
Perfume	45	45	100.0	Ambient
Phenol	22	15	68.2	<0.20 ppb
Chlorine	23	12	52.2	<0.33 ppb
Pesticides	21	18	85.7	<0.0034 ppb
Placebo control	45	0	0.0	Normal saline

Note: Newsprint and perfume under dosage should be ambient < odor threshold.

Documented in Table 8.3 is the high degree of reactivity the patient with chemical sensitivity experiences with terpene challenge. We have also found a high degree of cross-reactivity of terpenes with other toxic chemicals in the sensitive patient; intradermal neutralization given on a regular schedule will often markedly decrease overall reactivity.

At the EHC-Dallas and the EHC-Buffalo, we have treated over 7000 patients with avoidance and injections with the neutralizing doses for terpenes without problems. The average duration of therapy is 1–1 1/2 years. Patients usually take the injections every 4 days. On greater exposure, they may take up to four injections per day, although the extract from the average exposure has been found to be extremely effective.

Neutralization for grass terpenes is particularly efficacious in patients who are ill due to cutting grass. Pine terpene extract will help individuals who are terpene sensitive and have many pine trees around their house or who are exposed to pine inside their home. These antigen injections for terpenes are only useful with a mild-to-moderate exposure; however, they will not allow the individual who is severely terpene sensitive to stay in a room with pine floor and panels for a long time because the total environment load is too high.

In conclusion, terpenes are a significant factor in the initiation, exacerbation, and propagation of some cases of chemical sensitivity. Awareness of whether the individual with chemical sensitivity comes in contact with these terpenes will help clinicians to treat more readily their patient's illness.

Some of the literature show the cases of unusual terpene problems.

CAMPHOR

Camphor is a waxy, flammable, white or transparent solid with a strong aromatic odor.[3] It is a terpenoid with the chemical formula $C_{10}H_{16}O$. It is found in the wood of camphor laurel (*Cinnamomum camphora*), a large evergreen tree found in Asia (particularly in Sumatra, Borneo, and Taiwan), and also of *Dryobalanops aromatic*, a giant of the Bornean forests. It also occurs in some other related trees in the laurel family, notably *Ocotea usambarensis*. Dried rosemary leaves (*Rosmarinus officinalis*), in the mint family, contain up to 23% camphor. It can also be synthetically produced from oil of turpentine. It is used for its scent, as an ingredient in cooking (mainly in India), as an embalming fluid, for medicinal purposes, and in religious ceremonies. A major source of camphor in Asia is camphor basil, also made from pine terpene. This also occurs in the United States. Norcamphor is a camphor derivative with the three methyl groups replaced by hydrogen.

The patient and family moved into a house built in the Cedar Hill area of Dallas in 1968. The patient immediately smelled a peculiar odor which was not pungent but just an odor. The family replaced carpet with ceramic floors, which generally improved the odor of the house. However, the odor still persisted. Air analysis showed the analysis of camphor, acetic acid, and α- and β- pinene. Numerous odors of aldehyde and acetic acid were also measured. It was thought that the odors from the pine terpenes combined with acetic acid caused the camphor. The patient underwent intradermal provocative skin tests which confirmed sensitivity to the pine terpenes. Apparently, the camphor odor was due to the combination of the pine terpenes and acetic acid that was also found in the air.

PRODUCTION

Camphor can be produced from α-pinene, which is abundant in the oils of coniferous trees and can be distilled from turpentine produced as a side product of chemical pulping. With acetic acid as the solvent and with catalysis by a strong acid, α-pinene readily rearranges into camphene, which in turn undergoes Wagner–Meerwein rearrangement into the isobornyl cation, which is captured by acetate to give isobornyl acetate. Hydrolysis into isoborneol followed by oxidation gives racemic camphor. By contrast, camphor occurs naturally as D-camphor, the (R)-enantiomer.

USES

Modern uses include camphor as a plasticizer for nitrocellulose (see Celluloid) as a moth repellent, as an antimicrobial substance, in embalming, and in fireworks. Solid camphor releases fumes that form a rust-preventative coating, and is therefore stored in tool chests to protect tools against rust.[94]

Some folk remedies state camphor deters snakes and other reptiles due to its strong odor. Similarly, camphor is believed to be toxic to insects and is thus sometimes used as a repellent.[95] Camphor crystals are sometimes used to prevent damage to insect collections by other small insects. They are also used as a cough suppressant.

Its effects on the body include tachycardia, vasodilation in skin (flushing), slower breathing, reduced appetite, increased secretions and excretions such as perspiration, and diuresis.[96]

Camphor is poisonous in large doses. It produces symptoms of irritably, disorientation, lethargy, muscle spasms, vomiting, abdominal cramps, convulsions, and seizures.[97–99] Lethal doses in adults are in the range of 50–500 mg/kg (orally). Generally, 2 g causes serious toxicity and 4 g is potentially lethal.[100]

In ancient and medieval Europe, camphor was used as an ingredient in sweets.

Currently, camphor is used as a flavoring, mostly for sweets, in Asia. It is widely used in cooking, mainly for desserts, in India where it is known as kachka karpooram or "pachha karpoora."

Camphor is readily absorbed through the skin and produces a feeling of cooling similar to that of menthol, and acts as mild local anesthetic and antimicrobial substance. There are anti-itch gels and cooling gels with camphor as the active ingredient. Camphor is an active ingredient (along with menthol) in vapor-steam products, such as Vicks VapoRub.

This case report of camphor ingestion in a 15-month-old child illustrates the potential toxicity of a common household product.

Oral ingestion of camphor is unusual, given that these products have both unpleasant taste and texture. This patient ingested 70 mL of an over-the-counter medicated ointment containing 4.73% camphor, 2.6% menthol, and 1.2% eucalyptus oil. While the concentration of camphor in this product is low, an estimated 280 mg/kg of camphor was consumed. With significant ingestion of camphor (>50 mg/kg), neurologic toxicity is common. In this patient, prolonged generalized tonic–clonic seizure activity was noted $\sim$2 hours post single acute ingestion of camphor. This delay in onset of seizure activity is atypical, as seizures have previously been noted to occur in the 90 minutes following ingestion.

Readily available medicated ointments containing camphor have the potential for serious or fatal consequences when ingested by children.

COMMON SUBSTANCES CONTAINING CAMPHOR

VicksVapoRub, Vicks Inhaler, and Dencorub, which are highly toxic, are readily absorbed from skin but most toxic exposure is from ingestion.

CASE REPORT

A 66-year-old female was brought to the University Clinic for Toxicology in Skopje, with status epilepticus, after several generalized tonic–clonic seizures. On arrival, the patient was somnolent, with heavy headache, hypotensive (14/9 kPa), with partial amnesia, relaxed muscles, small amount of blood in mouth, and specific odor. Five minutes later, during standard examination, the patient developed another generalized tonic–clonic seizure. A dose of 10 mL i.v. diazepam was administered to stabilize the patient, and a few minutes later, the patient woke up. Heteroanamnesis taken from her husband showed that she had another similar convulsion 10 days ago; EEG, CT, and MRI performed previously did not show any abnormalities. The specific smell, repeated seizures, and especially the dermal application of Kamfart crème confirmed the suspicion of poisoning with camphor. The toxicological examination showed a positive result. After excluding the camphor crème, the patient did not manifest any seizures.

CLUSTER OF CHILDREN WITH SEIZURES CAUSED BY CAMPHOR POISONING

In 2009, Khine et al.[101] described a number of cases of camphor-associated seizure activity resulting from the availability of imported camphor products in certain ethnic populations who use them as a natural remedy.

They present three cases of seizures associated with imported, illegally sold camphor in young children who presented to a large, urban children's hospital in Bronx, New York, during a 2-week period.

The children's ages ranged from 15 to 36 months. Two children ingested camphor, and one child was exposed to repetitive rubbing of camphor on her skin. All three patients required pharmacologic intervention to terminate the seizures. One patient required bag-valve-mask ventilation for transient respiratory depression. All three patients had leukocytosis, and two patients had hyperglycemia. Exposure occurred as a result of using camphor for spiritual purposes, cold remedy, or pest control. After identification of these cases, the New York City Department of Health released a public health warning to keep camphor products away from children. Similar warnings were issued later by other state health departments.

These cases highlight the toxicity associated with camphor usage in the community and that inappropriate use of illegally sold camphor products is an important public health issue.

Guilbert et al.[102] describes a case of a young child who lived in Hong Kong who presented with a severe status epilepticus after a return flight from Paris. Routine laboratory tests failed to establish a cause. The parents reported that the nanny had given an abdominal massage to the child with an unlabeled solution reported to have antiflatulence effects. Toxicological analysis of this solution revealed the presence of camphor. Although the highly toxic effects of camphor have long been established, the present case illustrates that camphor continues to be a source of pediatric exposure. This case highlights the importance of systematic questioning and recalls the extreme danger associated with camphor even when administered transcutaneously.

According to Gouin,[103] this case report of camphor ingestion by a 15-month-old child illustrates the potential toxicity of a common household product.

Readily available medicated ointments containing camphor have the potential for serious or fatal consequences when ingested by children.

According to Mendanha et al.,[104] terpenes are considered potent skin permeation enhancers with low toxicity. Electron paramagnetic resonance (EPR) spectroscopy of the spin label 5-doxyl stearic acid (5-DSA) was used to monitor the effect of sesquiterpene nerolidol and various monoterpenes on membrane fluidity in erythrocyte and fibroblast cells. In addition, the hemolytic levels and cytotoxic effects on cultured fibroblast cells were also measured to investigate possible relationships between the cellular irritation potentials of terpenes and the ability to modify membrane fluidity. All terpenes increased cell membrane fluidity with no significant differences between the monoterpenes, but the effect of sesquiterpene was significantly greater than that of the monoterpenes. The IC(50) values for the terpenes in the cytotoxicity assay indicated that 1,8-cineole showed lower cytotoxicity and α-terpineol and nerolidol showed higher cytotoxicity. The correlation between the hemolytic effect and the IC(50) values for fibroblast viability was low ($R = 0.61$); however, in both tests, nerolidol was among the most aggressive of terpenes and 1,8-cineole was among the least aggressive. Obtaining information concerning the toxicity and potency of terpenes could aid in the design of topical formulations optimized to facilitate drug absorption for the treatment of many skin diseases.

SENSITIVE METHOD FOR DETERMINATION OF ALLERGENIC FRAGRANCE TERPENE HYDROPEROXIDES USING LIQUID CHROMATOGRAPHY COUPLED WITH TANDEM MASS SPECTROMETRY HAS BEEN SHOWN

According to Rudback et al.,[105] different compositions of monoterpenes are utilized for their pleasant scent in cosmetics and perfumes. However, the most commonly used fragrance terpenes easily oxidize upon contact with air, forming strongly skin-sensitizing hydroperoxides. Due to their thermolability and low UV absorbance, detection methods for hydroperoxides are scarce. For the first time, a simple and sensitive method using LC/ESI-MS/MS was developed to quantitatively determine hydroperoxides from the common fragrance compounds—linalool, linalyl acetate, and limonene. The method was applied to autoxidized petitgrain oil and sweet orange oil. A separation was accomplished using a C3 column. The method LOD for the investigated hydroperoxides in the essential oils was below 0.3 μg/mL, corresponding to 0.3 ppm. For prevention purposes and according to EU regulations, concentrations in cosmetics exceeding 100 ppm in "rinse-off" and 10 ppm in "stay-on" products of linalool and limonene must be labeled. However, the products may still contain allergens, such as hydroperoxides, formed by oxidative degradation of their parent terpenes. The sensitivity and selectivity of the presented LC/MS/MS method enables detection of hydroperoxides from the fragrance terpenes linalool, linalyl acetate, and limonene. However, for routine measurements, the method requires further validation.

MONOTERPENE AND WOOD DUST EXPOSURES: WORK-RELATED SYMPTOMS AMONG FINNISH SAWMILL WORKERS

According to Rosenberg et al.,[106] monoterpenes and wood dust are released into the work environment during sawing of fresh wood. Symptoms related to exposure to monoterpenes and wood dust include irritation of the eyes, mucous membrane, and skin.

They studied 22 sawhouse workers, who processed pine and spruce in 1997–1999. Exposure to monoterpenes was assessed by determining monoterpenes in air and verbenols in urine by gas chromatography using flame ionization detection. Wood dust was determined gravimetrically.

Exposures to monoterpenes (geometric mean, GM) among sawhouse workers were 61–138 mg/m³ and 2.0–13 mg/m³ during processing of pine and spruce, respectively. Urinary verbenol correlated well with workers' exposure to the α-pinene fraction of monoterpenes. The inhalable dust concentration in the breathing zone was 0.5–2.2 mg/m³ during pine processing and 0.4–1.9 mg/m³ during spruce processing. The prevalence of symptoms, in the eyes or respiratory tract, was high during both seasons and in connection with either tree species.

The highest monoterpene concentration (GM), in the breathing zone, measured during processing of pine, was less than one-fourth of the Finnish occupational exposure limit (OEL, 570 mg/m³). Verbenol concentrations in postshift urine samples reflected accurately the exposure to monoterpenes. The concentrations of inhalable dust (GM) were less than one-half the Finnish OEL (5 mg/m³). No significant differences in dust exposure were observed among tree species processed. Work-related symptoms appeared to correlate with monoterpene exposure during processing of pine and with wood dust exposure during processing of spruce.

According to Pei et al.,[107] two new triterpenes, (1α,3β,8α,9β,10α,13α,14β)-9,10-dimethyl-25,26-dinorolean-5-en-1,3-diol (1) and (1α,3β,6β)-olean-12-en-1,3,6-triol (2) were isolated from the leaves of *Aleurites fordii*, together with five known triterpenes. The structures of isolates were established by one-dimensional (1D) and 2D NMR spectroscopy data along with MS analysis. Of the isolated compounds, 1, 2, and 4 (daturadiol) displayed moderate cytotoxicities against two or more human cancer cell lines in HepG2 (hepatocellular carcinoma), SK-OV-3 (ovarian carcinoma), A-549 (lung carcinoma), and SNU-1 (gastric carcinoma).

METABOLISM OF THE ABORTIFACIENT TERPENE, (*R*)-(+)-PULEGONE, TO A PROXIMATE TOXIN, MENTHOFURAN

According to Gordon et al.,[108] (*R*)-(+)-pulegone, the major monoterpene component of the abortifacient mint oil, pennyroyal oil, is metabolized by hepatic microsomal monooxygenases of the mouse to a hepatotoxin. The formation of a toxic metabolite is apparently mediated by cytochromes P-450 of the phenobarbital class inasmuch as phenobarbital pretreatment of mice increases, whereas β-naphthoflavone pretreatment decreases the extent of hepatic necrosis caused by pulegone. Furthermore, two inhibitors of cytochromes P-450, cobaltous chloride and piperonyl butoxide, block toxicity. An analog of (*R*)-(+)-pulegone that was labeled with deuterium in the allylic methyl groups was found to be significantly less hepatotoxic than the parent compound. The results indicate that oxidation of an allylic methyl group is required for generation of a hepatotoxic metabolite. Menthofuran was identified as a proximate toxic metabolite of (*R*)-(+)-pulegone, and investigations with (*R*)-(+)-pulegone-d6 and 18O₂ strongly indicate that menthofuran is formed by a sequence of reactions that involve: (1) oxidation of an allylic methyl group, (2) intramolecular cyclization to form a hemiketal, and (3) dehydration to form the furan.

OCCUPATIONAL HEALTH GUIDELINE FOR TURPENTINE

PERMISSIBLE EXPOSURE LIMIT

The current OSHA standard for turpentine is 100 parts of turpentine per million parts of air (ppm) averaged over an 8-hour work shift. This may also be expressed as 560 mg of turpentine per cubic meter of air (mg/m³).

EFFECTS OF OVEREXPOSURE

1. *Short-term exposure*: Overexposure to turpentine may cause irritation of the eyes, nose, throat, lungs, and skin. It may also cause headache, dizziness, and painful, urination or dark red urine. Greater exposure may cause unconsciousness and death.
2. *Long-term exposure*: Prolonged overexposure causes skin irritation. Skin sensitization can occur.

RECOMMENDED MEDICAL SURVEILLANCE

The following medical procedures should be made available to each employee who is exposed to turpentine at potentially hazardous levels:

1. *Initial medical screening*: Employees should be screened for the history of certain medical conditions (listed below) which might place the employee at increased risk from turpentine exposure.
   a. *Skin disease:* Turpentine is a skin defatting agent and sensitizer and can cause dermatitis on prolonged exposure. Persons with preexisting skin disorders may be more susceptible to the effects of this agent.
   b. *Liver disease:* Although turpentine is not known as a liver toxin in humans, the importance of this organ in the biotransformation and detoxification of foreign substances should be considered before exposing persons with impaired liver function.
   c. *Kidney disease:* Turpentine has been reported to cause albuminuria and hematuria in humans and special consideration should be given to those with a history of impaired renal function.
   d. *Chronic respiratory disease:* In persons with impaired pulmonary function, especially those with obstructive airway diseases, the breathing of turpentine might cause exacerbation of symptoms due to its irritant properties.
2. *Periodic medical examination*: Any employee developing the above-listed conditions should be referred for further medical examination.

SUMMARY OF TOXICOLOGY

Turpentine vapor is a mucous membrane irritant and, at higher concentrations, a convulsant. The LC50 for rats is 3590 ppm for 1 hour and 2150 ppm for 6 hours; hyperpnea, ataxia, tremors, and convulsions were noted. In cats, 1440 ppm produced disturbances in equilibrium and convulsions in 30–60 minutes; paralysis occurred in 150–180 minutes. In human subjects, 750–1000 ppm for several hours caused irritation of the eyes, headache, dizziness, nausea, and tachycardia; 1878 ppm for 1–4 hours was considered definitely toxic. Heavy overexposure is also reported to cause irritation of the nose and throat, cough, headache, vertigo, and irritation of the kidneys and bladder manifested by transient albuminuria and hematuria. However, there is little evidence that turpentine vapor at lower concentration of 75–200 ppm is said to be moderately irritating. The liquid is also a defatting agent and causes skin irritation. Some persons may develop skin hypersensitivity. Mild intoxication from skin absorption has been reported.

SANITATION

Skin that becomes contaminated with turpentine should be promptly washed or showered with soap or mild detergent and water to remove any turpentine.

Employees who handle liquid turpentine should wash their hands thoroughly with soap or mild detergent and water before eating, smoking, or using toilet facilities.

COMMON OPERATIONS AND CONTROLS

The following list includes some common operations in which exposure to turpentine may occur and control methods which may be effective in each case:

Operation	Controls
Used in the manufacture of synthetic pine oil and insecticides, and in β-pinene resins, flavors, and perfumes	Local exhaust Ventilation process enclosure, personal protective equipment
Used in the preparation of polishes; used in the manufacture of synthetic camphor, and used in paints	Local exhaust Ventilation process enclosure; personal protective equipment

Terpenes can be devastating to the chemically sensitive individuals and must be eliminated and/or neutralized for them in order to stay well.

REFERENCES

1. Anon. 1982. *McGraw-Hill Encyclopedia of Science and Technology*, Vol. 13, pp. 583–586. New York: McGraw-Hill.
2. Anon. 1985. *The New Encyclopedia Britannica*, Vol. 2, 15th ed., p. 647. Chicago, IL: Encyclopedia Britannica.
3. Guenther, A., T. Karl, P. Harley, C. Wiedinmyer, P. I. Palmer, C. Geron. 2006. Estimates of global terrestrial isoprene emissions using MEGAN (Model of Emissions of Gases and Aerosols from Nature). *Atmos. Chem. Phys.* 6(11):3181–3210.
4. IUPAC Subcommittee on Gas Kinetic Data Evaluation. 2007. Data Sheet OX_VOC7.
5. Science Daily. 7 August 2009. Organic Carbon Compounds Emitted by Trees Affect Air Quality.
6. Science News. 6 August 2009. A Source of Haze.
7. Sharkey, T. D., A. E. Wiberley, A. R. Donohue. 2007. Isoprene emission from plants: Why and how. *Ann. Bot.* 101(1):5–18.
8. Vickers, C. E., M. Possell, C. I. Cojocariu, V. B. Velikova, J. Laothawornkitkul, A., Ryan, P. M. Mullineaus, C. N. Hewitt. 2009. Isoprene synthesis protects transgenic tobacco plants from oxidative stress. *Plant Cell Environ.* 32(5): 520–531.
9. Benjamin, M. T., M. Sudol, L. Bloch, A. M. Winer. 1996. Low-emitting urban forests: A taxonomic methodology for assigning isoprene and monoterpene emission rates. *Atmos. Environ.* 30(9):1437–1452.
10. Gelmont, D., R. A. Stein, J. F. Mead. 1981. Isoprene—The main hydrocarbon in human breath. *Biochem. Biophys. Res. Commun.* 99(4):1456–1460.
11. King, J., H. Koc, K. Unterkofler, P. Mochalski, A. Kupferthaler, G. Teschl, S. Teschl, H. Hinterhuber, A. Amann. 2010. Physiological modeling of isoprene dynamics in exhaled breath. *J. Theoret. Biol.* 267(4):626–637.
12. NTP. 1995. *NTP Technical Report on the Toxicity Studies of Isoprene (CAS No. 78-79-5) Administered by Inhalation to Fe44/N Rats and B6C3F1 Mice*. NTP Technical Report Series No. 31. Research Triangle Park, NC: National Toxicology Program, pp. 1–G5.
13. Placke, M. E., L. Griffis, M. Bird, J. Bus, R. L. Persing, L. A. Cox, Jr. 1996. Chronic inhalation oncogenicity study of isoprene in B6C3F1 mice. *Toxicology* 113(1–3):253–262.
14. Melnick, R. L., R. C. Sills. 2001. Comparative carcinogenicity of 1,3-butadiene, isoprene, and chloroprene in rats and mice. *Chem. Biol. Interact.* 135–136:27–42.
15. Gervasi, P. G., L. Citti, M. Del Monte. 1985. Mutagenicity and chemical reactivity of epoxidic intermediates of the isoprene metabolism and other structurally related compounds. *Mutat. Res.* 156(1–2):77–82.
16. NTP. 1999. NTP Report on Carcinogens Background Document for Isoprene. National Toxicology Program. http://ntp.niehs.nih.gov/files/Isoprene.pdf
17. NTP. 1999. *NTP Toxicology and Carcinogenesis Studies of Isoprene (CAS No. 78-79-5) Administered by Inhalation to Ferr/N Rats and B6C3F1 Mice*. NTP Technical Report Series no. 31. Research Triangle Park, NC: National Toxicology Program, pp. 1–G5.

18. IARC. 1994. Isoprene. In *Some Industrial Chemicals*. IARC Monographs on the Evaluation of Carcinogenic Risk of Chemicals to Humans, Vol. 60, pp. 215–232. Lyon, France: International Agency for Research on Cancer.

19. Rieder, J., P. Lirk, C. Ebenbichler, G. Gruber, P. Prazeller, W. Lindinger, A. Amann. 2001. Analysis of volatile organic compounds: Possible applications in metabolic disorders and cancer screening. *Wien. Klin. Wochenschr.* 113(5–6):181–185.

20. Fabiani, R., P. Rosignoli, A. Bartolomeo, R. Fuccelli, G. Morozzi. 2007. DNA-damaging ability of isoprene and isoprene mono-epoxide (EPOX I) in human cells evaluated with the comet assay. *Mutat. Res.* 629(1):7–13.

21. Tice, R. R. 1988. The cytogenetic evaluation of in vivo genotoxic and cytotoxic activity using rodent somatic cells. *Cell Biol. Toxicol.* 4(4):475–486.

22. Tice, R. R., R. Boucher, C. A. Luke, D. E. Paquette, R. L. Melnick, M. D. Shelby. 1988. Chloroprene and isoprene: cytogenetic studies in mice. *Mutagenesis* 3(2):141–146.

23. Hong, H. L., T. R. Devereux, R. L. Melnick, S. R. Eldridge, A. Greenwell, J. Haseman, G. A. Boorman, R. C. Sills. 1997. Both K-*ras* and H-*ras* protooncogene mutations are associated with Harderian gland tumorigenesis in B6C3F$_1$ mice exposed to isoprene for 26 weeks. *Carcinogenesis* 18(4):783–789.

24. SRI. 2009. *Directory of Chemical Producers*. Menlo Park, CA: SRI Consulting. Database edition. Last accessed July 13, 2009.

25. Chem Sources. 2009. Chem Sources—Chemical Search. Chemical Sources International. http://www.chemsources.com/chemonline.html and search on isoprene. Last accessed July 7, 2009.

26. USITC. 2009. USITC Interactive Tariff and Trade DataWeb. United States International Trade Commission. http://dataweb.usitc.gov/scripts/user_set.asp and search on HTS no. 2901242000. Last accessed July 7, 2009.

27a. EPA. 2004. *Non-confidential IUR Production Volume Information*. US Environmental Protection Agency. http://www.epa.gov/oppt/iur/tools/data/2002-vol.html and search on CAS number.

27b. Taalman, R. 1996. Isoprene: Background and issues. *Toxicology* 113(1–3):242–246.

28. Gelmont, D., R. A. Stein, J. F. Mead. 1981. Isoprene—The main hydrocarbon in human breath. *Biochem. Biophys. Res. Commun.* 99(4):1456–1460.

29. Cailleux, A., M. Cogny, P. Allain. 1992. Blood isoprene concentrations in humans and in some animal species. *Biochem. Med. Metab. Biol.* 47(2):157–160.

30. Lechner, M., B. Moser, D. Niederseer, A. Karlseder, B. Holzknecht, M. Fuchs, S. Colvin, H. Tilg, J. Rieder. 2006. Gender and age specific differences in exhaled isoprene levels. *Respir. Physiol. Neurobiol.* 154(3):478–483.

31. Taucher, J., A. Hansel, A. Jordan, R. Fall, J. H. Futrell, W. Lindinger. 1997. Detection of isoprene in expired air from human subjects using proton-transfer-reaction mass spectrometry. *Rapid Commun. Mass Spectrom.* 11(11):1230–1234.

32. Turner, C., P. Spanel, D. Smith. 2006. A longitudinal study of breath isoprene in healthy volunteers using selected ion flow tube mass spectrometry (SIFT-MS). *Physiol. Meas.* 27(1):13–22.

33. Senthilmohan, S. T., D. B. Milligan, M. J. McEwan, C. G. Freeman, P. F. Wilson. 2000. Quantitative analysis of trace gases of breath during exercise using the new SIFT-MS technique. *Redox. Rep.* 5(2–3):151–153.

34. Senthilmohan, S. T., M. J. McEwan, P. F. Wilson, D. B. Milligan, C. G. Freeman. 2001. Real-time analysis of breath volatiles using SIFT-MS in cigarette smoking. *Redox. Rep.* 6(3):185–187.

35. Peter, H., H. J. Wiegand, H. M. Bolt. 1987. Pharmacokinetics of isoprene in mice and rats. *Toxicol. Lett.* 36(1):9–14.

36. Taalman, R. 1996. Isoprene: Background and issues. *Toxicology* 113(1–3):242–246.

37. Mayrhofer, S., U. Heizmann, E. Magel, M. Eiblmeier, A. Müller, H. Rennenberg, R. Hampp, J. P. Schnitzler, J. Kreuzwieser. 2004. Carbon balance in leaves of young poplar trees. *Plant Biol.* 6(6):730–739.

38. Parra, R., S. Gasso, J. M. Baldasono. 2004. Estimating the biogenic emissions of non-methane volatile organic compounds from the North Western Mediterranean vegetation of Catalonia Spain. *Sci. Total Environ.* 329(1–3):241–259.

39. Schnitzler, J. P., M. Graus, J. Kreuzwieser, U. Heizmann, H. Rennenberg, A. Wisthaler, A. Hansel. 2004. Contribution of different carbon sources to isoprene biosynthesis in poplar leaves. *Plant Physiol.* 135(1):152–160.

40. Schnitzler, J. P., I. Zimmer, A. Bachl, M. Arend, J. Fromm, R. J. Fischbach. 2005. Biochemical properties of isoprene synthase in poplar (Populus x canescens). *Planta* 222(5):777–786.

41. Pegoraro, E., A. Rey, G. Barron-Gafford, R. Monson, Y. Malhi, R. Murthy. 2005. The interacting effects of elevated atmospheric CO_2 concentration, drought and leaf-to-air vapour pressure deficit on ecosystem isoprene fluxes. *Oecologia* 146(1):120–129.

42. Sasaki, M., Y. Nakamura, K. Fujita, Y. Kinugawa, T. Lida, Y. Urahama. 2005. Relation between phase structure and peel adhesion of poly (styrene-isoprene-styrene) triblock copolymer/tackifier blend system. *J. Adhes. Sci. Tech.* 19(16):1445–1457.

43. Sharkey, T. D. 2005. Effects of moderate heat stress on photosynthesis: Importance of thylakoid reactions, rubisco deactivation, reactive oxygen species, and thermotolerance provided by isoprene. *Plant Cell. Environ.* 28(3):269–277.

44. Moukhtar, S., C. Couret, L. Rouil, V. Simon. 2006. Biogenic volatile organic compounds (BVOCs) emissions from *Abies alba* in a French forest. *Sci. Total Environ.* 354(2–3):232–245.

45. Simon, V., L. Dumergues, J. L. Ponche, L. Torres. 2006. The biogenic volatile organic compounds emission inventory in France: Application to plant ecosystems and the Berre-Marseilles area (France). *Sci. Total Environ.* 372(1):164–182.

46. Tambunan, P., S. Baba, A. Kuniyoshi, H. Iwasaki, T. Nakamura, H. Yamasaki, H. Oku. 2006. Isoprene emission from tropical trees in Okinawa Island, Japan. *Chemosphere* 65(11):2138–2144.

47. Guenther, A., C. N. Hewitt, D. Erickson, R. Fall, C. Geron, T. Graedel, P. Harleyh, L. Klinger, M. Lerdau, W.A. McKay, T. Pierce, B. Schdes, R. Steinbrecher, T. Tallamaya, J. Taylor, P. Zimmerman. 1995. A global model of natural volatile organic compound emissions. *J. Geophys. Res. Atmos.* 100(D5):8873–8892.

48. Guenther, A., P. Zimmerman, M. Wildermuth. 1994. Natural volatile organic compound emission rate estimates for US woodland landscapes. *Atmos. Environ.* 28(6):1197–1210.

49. Fuentes, J. D., D. Wang. 1999. On the seasonality of isoprene emissions from a mixed temperate forest. *Ecol. Appl.* 9(4):1118–1131.

50. Lamb, B., D. Gay, H. Westberg, T. Pierce. 1993. A biogenic hydrocarbon emission inventory for the USA using a simple forest canopy model. *Atmos. Environ. Part A Gen. Top.* 27(11):1673–1690.

51. HSDB. 2009. Hazardous Substances Data Bank. National Library of Medicine. http://toxnet.nlm.nih.gov/cgi-bin/sis/htmlgen?HSDB and search on CAS number. Last accessed: July 7, 2009.

52. Adam, T., S. Mitschke, T. Streibel, R. R. Baker, R. Zimmermann. 2006. Quantitative puff-by-puff-resolved characterization of selected toxic compounds in cigarette mainstream smoke. *Chem. Res. Toxicol.* 19(4):511–520.

53. Borbon, A., P. Coddeville, N. Locoge, J. C. Galloo. 2004. Characterising sources and sinks of rural VOC in eastern France. *Chemosphere* 57(8):931–942.

54. Guo, H., S. C. Lee, P. K. Louie, K. F. Ho. 2004. Characterization of hydrocarbons, halocarbons and carbonyls in the atmosphere of Hong Kong. *Chemosphere* 57(10):1363–1372.

55. Kuster, W. C., B. T. Jobson, T. Karl, D. Riemer, E. Apel, P. D. Goldan, F. C. Fehsenfeld. 2004. Intercomparison of volatile organic carbon measurement techniques and data at La Porte during the TexAQS2000 Air Quality Study. *Environ. Sci. Technol.* 38(1):221–228.

56. Warneke, C., S. Cato, J. A. De Gouw, P. T. Goldan, W. C. Kuster, M. Shao, E. R. Lovejoy, R. Fall, F. C. Fehsenfeld. 2005. Online volatile organic compound measurements using a newly developed proton-transfer ion-trap mass spectrometry instrument during New England Air Quality Study—Intercontinental Transport and Chemical Transformation 2004: Performance, intercomparison, and compound identification. *Environ. Sci. Technol.* 39(14):5390–5397.

57. Helen, H., H. Hakola, L. Pirjola, T. Laurila, K. H. Pystynen. 2006. Ambient air concentrations, source profiles and source apportionment of 71 different C_2-C_{10} volatile organic compounds in urban and residential areas of Finland. *Environ. Sci. Technol.* 40(1):103–108.

58. Altschuller, A. 1983. Natural volatile organic substances and their effect on air quality in the United States. *Atmos. Environ.* 17(11):2131–2165.

59. Hagerman, L. M., V. P. Aneja, W. A. Lonneman. 1997. Characterization of non-methane hydrocarbons in the rural southeast United States. *Atmos. Environ.* 31(23):4017–4038.

60. Borbon, A., H. Fontaine, M. Veillerot, N. Locoge, J. C. Galloo, R. Guillermo. 2001. An investigation into the traffic-related fraction of isoprene at an urban location. *Atmos. Environ.* 35(22):3749–3760.

61. So, K. L., T. Wang. 2004. C_3-C_{12} non-methane hydrocarbons in subtropical Hong Kong: spatial-temporal variations, source-receptor relationships and photochemical reactivity. *Sci. Total Environ.* 328(1–3):161–74. SRI. 2009. *Directory of Chemical Producers*. Menlo Park, CA: SRI Consulting. Database edition. Last accessed July 13, 2009.

62. Borbon, A., N. Locoge, M. Veillerot, J. C. Galloo, R. Guillermo. 2002. Characterisation of NMHCs in a French urban atmosphere: overview of the main sources. *Sci. Total Environ.* 292(3):177–191.

63. Zhao, W. X., P. K. Hopke, T. Karl. 2004. Source identification of volatile organic compounds in Houston, Texas. *Environ. Sci. Technol.* 38(5):1338–1347.

64. Chiang, H. L., J. H. Tsai, S. Y. Chen, K. H. Lin, S. Y. Ma. 2007. VOC concentration profiles in an ozone non-attainment area: A case study in an urban and industrial complex metroplex in southern Taiwan. *Atmos. Environ.* 41(9):1848–1860.

65. Barrefors, G., G. Petersson. 1993. Assessment of ambient volatile hydrocarbons from tobacco smoke and from vehicle emissions. *J. Chromatogr.* 643(1–2):71–76.

66. Heavner, D. L. 1996. Determination of volatile organic compounds and respirable suspended particulate matter in New Jersey and Pennsylvania homes and workplaces. *Environ. Int.* 22(2):159–183.

67. Mukerjee, S. 1997. An environmental scoping study in the lower Rio Grande Valley of Texas—III. Residential micro environmental monitoring of air, house dust, and soil. *Environ. Int.* 23(5):657–673.

68. Leber, A. P. 2001. Overview of isoprene monomer and polyisoprene production processes. *Chem. Biol. Interact.* 135–136:169–173.

69. Lynch, J. 2001. Occupational exposure to butadiene, isoprene and chloroprene. *Chem. Biol. Interact.* 135–136:207–214.

70. NIOSH. 1976. *National Occupational Hazard Survey (1972–74). DHEW (NIOSH) Publication No. 78-114.* Cincinnati, OH: National Institute for Occupational Safety and Health.

71. NIOSH. 1990. National Occupational Hazard Survey (1981–83). National Institute for Occupational Safety and Health. Last updated: July 1, 1990. http:// www.cdc.gov/noes/noes1/40940sic.html

72. Van der Wel, H., G. Larcon, C. M. Hladik, G. Hallekant, D. Glaser. 1989. Isolation and characterization of pentadin, the sweet principle of *Petadiplandra brazzeana* Baillon. *Chem. Senses* 14:75–79.

73. UW-Madison professor makes a sweet discovery. 10:57 p.m., November 4, 2002. Jason Stein for the *State Journal.*

74. Ming, D., G. Hellekant. 1994. Brazzein, a new high-potency thermostable sweet protein from *Pentadiplandra brazzeana* B. *FEBS Lett.* 355(1):106–108.

75. Zeller, W., M. de Gols, B. M. Hausen. 1985. The sensitizing capacity of Compositae plants. VI. Guinea pig sensitization experiments with ornamental plants and weeds using different methods. *Arch. Dermatol. Res.* 277:28–35.

76. Burry, J. N., R. Kuchel, J. G. Read, J. Kirk. 1973. Australian bush dermatitis: Compositae dermatitis in South Australia. *Med. J. Aust.* 1:110–116.

77. Anon. 1980. *Encyclopedia International*, Vol. 118, p. 6. New York: Lexicon publications.

78. Anon. 1982. *McGraw-Hill Encyclopedia of Science and Technology*, Vol. 13, pp. 583–586. New York: McGraw-Hill. (This is verbatim #1).

79. Mitchell, J. C., T. A. Geissman, G. Dupuis, G. H. N. Towers. 1971. Allergic contact dermatitis caused by Artemisia and Chrysanthemum species. The role of sesquiterpene lacones. *J. Invest. Dermatol.* 56:98–101.

80. Mitchell, J. C., G. Dupuis. 1971. Allergic contact dermatitis from sesquiterpenoids of the Compositae family of plants. *Br. J. Dermatol.* 84:139–150.

81. Brunsting, L. A., C. R. Anderson. 1931. Ragweed dermatitis. *JAMA* 103:1285–1290.

82. Grater, W. C. 1975. Hypersensitivity dermatitis from American weeds and other poison ivy. *Ann. Allergy* 35:159–164.

83. Pathak, M. A., F. Daniels, Jr., T. B. Fitzpatric. 1962. The presently known distribution of furocoumarins (psoralens) in plants. *J. Invest. Dermatol.* 39:225.

84. Howe, J. S. 1887. Dermatitis venenata caused by *Leucanthemum vulgare*. *Boston Med. Surg. J.* 116:227–229.

85. Shlmire, B. 1940. Contact dermatitis from vegetation; patch testing and treatment with plant oleoresius. *South. Med. J.* 33:337–346.

86. Slater, B. J., J. L. Noris, N. Francis. 1946. Ragweed dermatitis. *Occup. Med.* 2:298–300.

87. Fenaroli, T. 1975. *Handbook of Flavor Ingredients*, Vol. 2, 2nd ed., p. 523. Cleveland, OH: CRC Press.

88. Gastelain, P. Y., J. P. Camoin, J. Jouglard. 1980. Contact dermatitis to terpene derivatives in a machine cleaner. *Contact Dermat.* 6:358–360.

89. Moore, B. P. 1968. Studies on the chemical composition and function of the cephalic gland secretion in Australian termites. *J. Insect. Physiol.* 14:33.

90. Andersen, I. 1972. Technical notes—Relationships between outdoor and indoor air pollution. *Atmos. Environ.* 6:275–278.

91. Ayars, G. H., L. C. Altman, C. E. Frazier, E. Y. Chi. 1989. The toxicity of constituents of cedar and pine woods to pulmonary epithelium. *J. Allergy Clin. Immunol.* 83:610–618.

92. Hindson, C., F. Lawlor, A. Downey. 1982. Cross sensitivity between zinc oxide-plaster and *Cupressus Leylandii* shrubs. *Contact Dermat.* 7:335–360.

93. Upadhyay, R., R. Samiyeh, A. Tafazuli. 1981. Tumor promoting and skin irritant diterpene esters of *Euphorbia virgata* latex. *Neoplasma* 28(5):555–558.

94. Tips for Cabinet Making Shops, Campur USP Natural Powder. Universal Preserv-a-Chem Inc.

95. *The Housekeeper's Almanac, or, the Young Wife's Oracle! for 1840!. No. 134.* New York: Elton, 1840. Print.

96. Church, J. 1797. An inaugural Dissertation on Camphor: Submitted to the examination of the Rev. John Ewing, S.S.T.P. provost; the trustees & medical faculty of the University of Pennsylvania, on the 12th of May, 1797; for the degree of Doctor of Medicine. University of Philadelphia: Printed by John Thompson. Retrieved January 18, 2013.

97. Camphor overdose. Medline. NIH. Retrieved January 19, 2012.

98. Martin D., J. Valdez, J. Boren, M. Mayersohn. 2004. Dermal absorption of camphor, menthol, and methyl salicylate in humans. *J. Clin. Pharmacol.* 44(10):1151–1157. doi: 10.1177/0091270004268409. PMID 15342616.

99. Uc A., W. P. Bishop, K. D. Sanders. 2000. Camphor hepatotoxicity. *South. Med. J.* 93(6): 596–598. doi: 10.1097/00007611-200006000-00011.PMID 10881777.

100. Poisons Information Monograph: Camphor. International Programme on Chemical Safety.

101. Khine H., D. Weiss, N. Graber, R. S. Hoffman, N Esteban-Cruciani, J. R. Avner. 2009. A cluster of children with seizures caused by camphor poisoning. *Pediatrics* 123(5):1269–1272. doi: 10.1542/peds.2008-2097

102. Guilbert J., C. Flamant, F. Hallalel, D. Doummar, A. Frata, S. Renolleau. 2007. Anti-flatulence treatment and status epilepticus: A case of camphor intoxication. *Emerg. Med. J.* 24(12): 859–860. doi: 10.1136/emj.2007.052308

103. Gouin, S., H. Patel. 1996. Unusual cause of seizure. *Pediatr. Emerg. Care* 12(4):298–300.

104. Mendanha, S. A., S. S. Moura, J. L.V. Anjos, M. C. Valadares, A. Alonso. 2013. Toxicity of terpenes on fibroblast cells compared to their hemolytic potential and increase in erythrocyte membrane fluidity. *Toxicol. In Vitro.* 27(1):323–329.

105. Rudbäck J., N. Islam, U. Nilsson, A. T. Karlberg. 2013. A sensitive method for determination of allergenic fragrance terpene hydroperoxides using liquid chromatography coupled with tandem mass spectrometry. *J. Sep. Sci.* 36(8):1370–1378. doi: 10.1002/jssc.201200855. Epub 2013 Mar 22.

106. Rosenberg C., T. Liukkonen, T. Kallas-Tarpila, A. Ruonakangas, R. Ranta, M. Nurminen, I. Welling, P. Jäppinen. 2002. Monoterpene and wood dust exposures: Work-related symptoms among Finnish sawmill workers. *Am. J. Ind. Med.* 41(1):38–53.

107. Pei, Y. H., O. K. Kwon, J. S. Lee, H. J. Cha, K. S. Ahn, S. R. Oh, H. K. Lee, Y. W. Chin. 2013. Triterpenes with cytotoxicity from the leaves of *Vernicia fordii*. *Chem Pharm Bull. (Tokyo)* 61(6):674–677.

108. Gordon W. P., A. C. Huitric, C. L. Seth, R. H. McClanahan, S. D. Nelson. 1987. The metabolism of the abortifacient terpene, (R)-(+)-pulegone, to a proximate toxin, menthofuran. *Drug Metab Dispos.* 15(5):589–594.

9 Therapeutic Use of Stress to Provoke Recovery

The Perspective of a Holistic Psychiatrist/Psychoanalyst

Martha Stark, MD

INTRODUCTION

In the evocative words of Ernest Hemingway,[1] "The world breaks everyone, and afterward, many are strong at the broken places." This same sentiment is captured by[2] in his well-known aphorism, "That which does not kill us makes us stronger."

My goal has long been to create a holistic conceptual framework that captures the essence of what is involved in the process of healing, be it of mind or of body. To that end, I have coined the word MindBodyMatrix, a term that speaks to the complex interdependence of mind and body; it also reflects a keen appreciation for the intimate and precise relationship between the health and vitality of the mind and that of the body. Throughout this chapter, I will be using the terms such as system, living system, living matrix, and MindBodyMatrix interchangeably.

STRESSFUL STUFF HAPPENS

Stressful stuff happens. However, it will be how well we are ultimately able to manage its impact—psychologically, physiologically, and energetically—that will make all the difference. In other words, it will be how well we are ultimately able to cope with the impact of stress in our lives that will either impede our growth by compromising our functionality or trigger our growth by forcing us to evolve to a higher level of functionality.

As a psychoanalyst and holistic psychiatrist who has worked intensively with patients suffering from chronic health problems, I have had the opportunity to observe the emergence of various themes and patterns in the evolution of patients from compromised functionality to more robust capacity. I believe that I am therefore in a position to put forth some rough guidelines for treating the underlying disease process in patients suffering from chronic fixed-name illnesses—whether primarily mental (examples include mood disorders, anxiety disorders, and personality disorders, to name but a few) or primarily physical (examples include chemical sensitivity, chronic fatigue syndrome, electromagnetic hypersensitivity, fibromyalgia, and autoimmune disorders, to name but a few).

In this chapter, I will be offering a perspective that I hope can be used by integrative healthcare practitioners and interested laypersons as a conceptual framework for reversing underlying chronic dysfunction and restoring the resilience, adaptability, and regulatory capacity of the MindBodyMatrix.

CAPACITY TO COPE WITH STRESS

Recently, I have begun to formulate a conceptual framework that captures the essence of what I believe must happen if a patient with long-standing psychiatric and medical issues is ever to evolve from compromised functionality to more robust capacity or, as we shall soon see, from dysfunctional defense to more functional adaptation.

Over the years, I have come increasingly to appreciate the significance of something that is at once both completely obvious and quite profound, namely, that it will be input from the environment and the patient's capacity to process, integrate, and adapt to this input that will ultimately enable the patient to get better. More specifically, however, it will actually be stressful input from the environment and the patient's capacity to process, integrate, and adapt to the impact of this stressful input that will not only provoke recovery but also promote strengthening at the broken places.

ENVIRONMENTAL STRESSORS

Here, I am using the term "environment" to encompass the living and the nonliving; the external and the internal; and the psychological, the physiological, and the energetic. Environmental stressors may therefore take the form of such challenges as an anxiety-provoking but ultimately health-promoting interpretation; the accumulation of metabolic waste products in the body; an interpersonal disappointment; exposure to the aluminum found in antiperspirants or the mercury found in dental amalgams; psychological, physical, or sexual abuse; contact with a carcinogenic pesticide (like the insect-repellent DEET); the loss of a parent; or the ingestion of endocrine disruptors (like the phthalates found in plastic bottles).

In my own psychoanalytic writings on the impact of stress, I have found it clinically useful to conceive of psychological stressors (especially relevant in the early-on parent–child relationship) as involving both the presence of bad (parental errors of commission) and the absence of good (parental errors of omission); both too much that was bad between parent and child and not enough that was good; trauma and abuse on the one hand, deprivation and neglect on the other—environmental toxicities and environmental deficiencies that were internally recorded and structuralized as psychic scars in the developing mind of the young child.

In other words, both toxicities and deficiencies are environmental stressors, the cumulative impact of which will potentially compromise the health and vitality of the MindBodyMatrix or—and this is the central tenet of my chapter—potentially benefit the health and vitality of the MindBodyMatrix.

CORRECTING FOR TOXICITIES AND DEFICIENCIES

As I will later demonstrate, *lightening the system's load* (to correct for toxicities) and *replenishing the system's reserves* (to correct for deficiencies) will facilitate the flow of information and energy throughout the system's vast network of interconnected channels. The more seamless that flow, the better able will the system be to process, integrate, and adapt to the impact of the myriad environmental stressors to which it is being continuously exposed. The more effective the processing, integrating, and adapting, the more resilient will the system be and the better able not only to manage the impact of stress but also to benefit from that stress.

Psychiatric and medical interventions that lighten the load, replenish the reserves, and facilitate the flow of information and energy will therefore reinforce the system's adaptability and revitalize the system's capacity to transform dysfunctional defenses (mobilized in the face of environmental stressors that are simply too much to be managed) into more functional adaptations (when their impact is ultimately able to be managed).

TRANSFORMATION OF DEFENSE INTO ADAPTATION: FROM LESS EVOLVED TO MORE EVOLVED

Although defenses are less healthy and less evolved and adaptations more healthy and more evolved, both are self-protective mechanisms that speak to the lengths to which a system will go in order to preserve its homeostatic balance in the face of environmental challenge.

In other words, defense and adaptation are actually flip sides of the same coin; defenses always have an adaptive function, just as adaptations do also serve to defend. As such, defenses and adaptations have a yin–yang relationship, representing, as they do, not opposing but complementary forces. In fact, just as in quantum mechanics, where particles and waves are thought to be different manifestations of a single reality (depending upon the observer's perspective), so, too, defense and adaptation are conjugate pairs demonstrating this same duality (both–and, not either–or).

However, here, I am making a distinction between, on the one hand, *defensive reactions* that are mobilized in the immediate aftermath of challenge and are automatic, knee-jerk, stereotypic, and rigid and, on the other hand, *adaptive responses* that unfold in the aftermath of challenge only over time and are therefore more processed, integrated, flexible, and complex.

The system defends when the impact of a stressor is too much to be processed and integrated; the system adapts when that impact is ultimately able to be processed and integrated. Defenses are needed to survive, but adaptations enable us to thrive.

In fact, it could be said that being able to adapt is a story about having the capacity to make a virtue out of necessity (also known as to make a silk purse out of a sow's ear) because it involves managing with finesse—and ultimately to one's benefit—the variety of life stressors to which one will inevitably be exposed over the course of one's life.

The transformation of less healthy defensive reaction into more healthy adaptive response is eloquently captured by the concept of evolving from cursing the darkness to lighting a candle.

POSITIVE (AMPLIFYING) FEEDBACK LOOP

Indeed, if the integrative practitioner focuses on reinforcing the underlying integrity of the living system and thereby facilitating the ease with which information and energy can be transmitted throughout its expanse, then the system's ability to evolve from reacting defensively to responding adaptively will be revived.

In other words, if the orderedness and fluidity of the living system are being continuously reinforced, then the system's ability to process and integrate the potentially disruptive impact of environmental stressors will be revitalized, such that the net result of stressful input will be a honing of the system's capacity not only to cope with but also to benefit from, the impact of stressful environmental input—this benefits the result of ongoing provocation of the system, which serves to fine-tune its resilience and trigger its reconstitution at ever higher levels of functionality, coherence, and adaptive capacity.

I am speaking about the existence of a positive (amplifying) feedback loop, whereby a system that is beginning to function a little more effectively by virtue of its reinforced ability to process and integrate the impact of environmental stressors will give rise to an even more functional system that is able to handle even more effectively the impact of the multitude of environmental stressors to which it is being continuously exposed—all of which highlights how critically important it is that the integrative practitioner remain ever focused on reinforcing the structural integrity of the MindBodyMatrix and thereby restoring the ease of flow of information and energy throughout its entirety.

DISORDER AND DISEASE

In essence, the conceptual framework that I am proposing conceives of the healing process—with respect to both mind and body—as one that requires the holistic practitioner to be exquisitely attuned to the system's capacity to cope with stress, which in turn will be a story about the system's ability to process and integrate the impact of environmental impingement, which in turn will be a reflection of the underlying orderedness of the MindBodyMatrix and the resultant ease with which information and energy can be propagated throughout its expanse—lack of order manifesting as *disorder* and disrupted ease of flow manifesting as *disease*.

And so it is that we speak about psychiatric disorders/diseases and of medical disorders/diseases.

In turn, disarray of the crystalline matrix and the resultant disrupted flow[3] will interfere with the system's ability to process, integrate, and adapt to the impact of stressful environmental input, which will then further compromise the resilience of the system and its capacity to cope with the stress of life.[4]

The term "disorder" is a particularly auspicious one inasmuch as it speaks to the idea not only of randomness (the less than optimally ordered distribution of molecules in the living matrix) but also of ill health, both mental and physical. Indeed, psychiatric and medical disorders are fundamentally about the disordered distribution of molecules in the crystalline array that constitutes the living matrix and, because of this disorder, disruption to the ease of flow of information and energy throughout its vast network—disease.

But whether the primary involvement is of mind or body, disorder (i.e., disrupted orderedness within the MindBodyMatrix) and disease (i.e., disrupted ease of flow within the MindBodyMatrix) are implicated in the generation of chronic health problems—both psychiatric and medical.

From this it follows that the journey from disorder and disease to health and vitality requires that the system's infrastructure be ordered and fluid, thereby allowing for the near-instantaneous transmission of regulatory information and vibratory energy throughout the extensive network of communication channels constituting the MindBodyMatrix.

In essence, optimal health (both mental and physical) is a story about orderedness and ease of flow within the living matrix—both of which properties will enable the system to cope with the stress of life by mobilizing not low-level defenses that will further compromise the system's integrity but higher-level adaptations that will buttress its resilience and regulatory capacity.

SELF-ORGANIZING SYSTEMS RESIST PERTURBATION

In the language of complexity theory,[5–7] I here conceptualize the MindBodyMatrix as a complex adaptive, self-organizing chaotic system. The living matrix is *complex* (which speaks to the intricate interdependence of the system's constituent components), *adaptive* (which speaks to the system's capacity to benefit from experience), *self-organizing* (which speaks to the spontaneous emergence of system-wide patterns arising from the interplay of the system's components), and *chaotic* (which speaks to the system's underlying orderedness despite its apparent randomness—an orderedness that will emerge as the system evolves over time).

How do patients advance from an unhealthy state of *disorder* (be it psychiatric or medical) to a healthy state of orderedness? Krebs[8] reminds us that we must never lose sight of the fact that self-organizing (chaotic) systems resist perturbation. No matter how compromised their functionality, self-organizing systems—fueled as they are by their homeostatic tendency to remain constant over time—are inherently resistant to change; they have an inertia that must be overcome if the system is ever to evolve from dysfunctionality to more robust capacity.

CHALLENGE TO PROVIDE IMPETUS AND SUPPORT TO PROVIDE OPPORTUNITY

In this chapter, I will therefore be developing the idea that a holistic practitioner, in order to expedite advancement of the patient from impaired health to a state of well-being, must challenge the system (whenever possible) and support the system (whenever necessary), all with an eye to jumpstarting the system's innate ability to self-repair in the face of environmental threat.[9–11]

More specifically, my contention will be that in reaction/response to—stressful—therapeutic interventions, the patient will either react defensively (when challenged) or respond adaptively (when supported), the net result of which will be the therapeutic induction, over time, of healing cycles of defensive collapse and adaptive reconstitution at ever higher levels of resilience, vitality, and mastery.

Indeed, the patient's journey from illness to wellness will involve progression through these iterative cycles of disruption and repair as the patient evolves from chaos and dysfunction to coherence and functionality.

Resistance to Change

Let me illustrate this fundamental principle by speaking about the almost universal resistance to change manifested by psychiatric patients.

Consider a patient who is clinging tenaciously to dysfunctional defenses that had once served her but that have long since outlived their usefulness. As a self-organizing system, the patient must be sufficiently perturbed (i.e., impacted) by input from the outside (i.e., the therapist's interventions) that there will be impetus (i.e., force needed to bring about change) for the patient to relinquish her attachment to these deeply entrenched, maladaptive patterns of acting, reacting, and interacting—that have come to define her characteristic (defensive) stance in the world—in favor of more adaptive ways of acting, reacting, and interacting.

In essence, the therapist's interventions must have enough stressful impact that they will challenge the homeostatic balance (i.e., the status quo) of the patient's dysfunctional defenses. By the same token, the therapist's interventions must also provide enough support that this input, in combination with the patient's inborn striving toward health (i.e., her resilience), will prompt the patient to evolve to ever higher levels of adaptive capacity and wholesome balance. As a result, her dysfunctional actions, reactions, and interactions will become transformed into more functional ways of being and doing.

Complementarity of Challenge and Support

If the therapist offers only gratification and support, then there will be nothing that needs to be mastered and nor will there be much impetus for transformation and growth. However, therapeutic input that provides an optimal level of stress (in the form of anxiety-provoking but ultimately health-promoting interventions offering just the right balance of frustration and gratification, just the right combination of challenge and support) will ultimately provoke not only reversal of underlying dysfunction but also optimization of functionality by tapping into the patient's intrinsic striving toward health and inborn ability to self-correct in the face of environmental perturbation.

In truth, support and optimal challenge work in concert. Whereas optimal challenge will trigger recovery and revitalization by prompting the system to adapt, support will facilitate that adaptation by reinforcing the system's underlying resilience and restoring its reserves, thereby honing the system's ability to cope with—and, even, benefit from—stressful environmental input.

In sum, challenge is necessary for jumpstarting recovery but recovery also requires support; by the same token, support is necessary for transformation and growth but recovery also requires challenge.

In other words, challenge of the patient's underlying dysfunction will create the impetus for destabilization; but its support will create the opportunity for restabilization—at a higher level of functionality, resilience, and capacity.

GOLDILOCKS PRINCIPLE AND OPTIMAL STRESS

My contention is that the psychiatric patient will react/respond in any one of three ways to psychotherapeutic interventions that alternately challenge and then support, support and then challenge.

Too much challenge, too much anxiety, too much stress will overwhelm and prompt defense because it will be too much to be processed and integrated—in other words, it will be traumatic stress.[12]

Too little challenge, too little anxiety, too little stress will offer too little impetus for transformation and growth and will serve, instead, to reinforce the (dysfunctional) status quo.

But just the right amount of challenge, just the right amount of anxiety, just the right amount of stress—to which the father of stress, Hans Selye,[13] referred as eustress and to which I[9-11] and others[14] refer as optimal stress—will provide just the right amount of therapeutic leverage needed to promote, after initial disruption, reconstitution at a higher level of integration, functionality, and self-regulatory capacity.

In essence, the therapeutic induction of an optimal level of anxiety supports the adage that no pain, no gain.

SANDPILE MODEL AND THE PARADOXICAL IMPACT OF STRESS

Long intriguing to chaos theorists has been the sandpile model,[15] which is believed to offer a dramatic depiction of the cumulative impact, over time, of environmental impingement on open systems. Evolution of the sandpile is governed by some complex mathematical formulas and is well known in many scientific circles; but the sandpile model is rarely applied to living systems and has never been used to demonstrate either the adaptability and resilience of the living system or the paradoxical impact of stress on it.

Not Just "In Spite Of" But "By Way Of"

My contention, however, is that this simulation model provides an elegant visual metaphor for how we are continuously refashioning ourselves at ever higher levels of complexity and integration—not just in spite of stressful input from the outside but by way of that input.

Amazingly enough, the grains of sand being steadily added to a gradually evolving sandpile are the occasion for both its disruption and its repair. Not only do the grains of sand being added precipitate partial collapse of the sandpile but they also become the means by which the sandpile will be able to build itself back—each time at a new level of homeostasis (more specifically, each time at a new allostatic set point).[16] The system will therefore have been able not only to manage the impact of the stressful input but also to benefit from that impact.

And, as the sandpile evolves, an underlying pattern will begin to emerge, characterized by recursive cycles of disruption and repair, destabilization and restabilization, defensive collapse and adaptive reconstitution at ever higher levels of integration, balance, and harmony.

In essence, the grains of sand represent environmental challenges, the mastery of which will fuel the underlying system's evolution from chaos and disorder to coherence and orderedness.

DIFFERENCE BETWEEN A POISON AND A MEDICATION

The noted sixteenth-century Swiss physician Paracelsus[17] is credited with having written that the difference between a poison and a medication is the dosage thereof. And, I would add, the system's capacity—a function of its underlying resilience—to process, integrate, and ultimately adapt to the impact of that stressor.

Stressful input, therefore, is inherently neither bad (poison) nor good (medication), which is to say that the therapist's interventions are inherently neither toxic (poison) nor therapeutic (medication).

Rather, the dosage of the stressor, the underlying resilience and adaptability of the system (which, as we have seen, is a reflection of its underlying orderedness and fluidity), and the intimate edge[18] between stressor and system will determine whether the system, in reaction/response to the environmental stimulus, defends and devolves to ever greater disorganization (disorder and disease) or adapts and evolves, by way of a series of healing cycles, to ever more complex levels of organization and dynamic balance.

In other words, if the interface between stressor and system is such that the stressor is able to provoke recovery within the system, then what would have been poison becomes medication, what would have constituted toxic input becomes therapeutic input, what would have been deemed traumatic stress becomes optimal stress, and what would have overwhelmed becomes transformative.

I am, of course, speaking here about the therapeutic use of stress to provoke recovery by activating the body's innate ability to heal itself.[19,16,20–22]

A poem by Christopher Logue (2004)[49] that speaks directly to the system's ability to adapt to stressful input is entitled "Come to the Edge":

Come to the edge. We might fall. Come to the edge. It's too high!
COME TO THE EDGE! And they came and he pushed and they flew …

HORMETIC (BIPHASIC) DOSE–RESPONSE RELATIONSHIP

If the MindBodyMatrix cannot process, integrate, and adapt to stressful input, then, over time, the health of the system will become increasingly compromised. However, as has already been noted, if the MindBodyMatrix is able to process, integrate, and ultimately adapt to the potentially devastating impact of the myriad environmental stressors to which it is being continuously exposed, then over time the system will evolve, through iterative cycles of destabilization and restabilization, to ever higher levels of health not just in spite of the stressful input but by way of that input—this benefits the result of tapping into the wisdom of the body[19] and jumpstarting the system's innate ability to self-correct in the face of optimal challenge.

Ordinarily, a linear dose–response relationship is assumed to exist between the dose of a toxin and the clinical response. In other words, if something (like stress) is generally thought to be bad for you, then it will be bad for you at whatever the dose—no matter how small.

So how might we understand the seemingly paradoxical response of the MindBodyMatrix to stress? Why is it that high doses of stress might be toxic whereas lower doses of stress would be therapeutic?

Hormesis—which means, literally, to excite—is the term used to describe this biphasic relationship that exists between the dose of an agent and its clinical response.

Although long marginalized in the toxicological literature (which has historically embraced a linear no-threshold model whereby toxins are thought to be toxic at whatever their dose and to become ever more toxic at ever higher doses), the concept of hormesis is now slowly gaining acceptance in some academic circles, largely through the extraordinary research efforts of Edward Calabrese,[23,24] an avant-garde toxicologist who believes that the hormetic effect is an almost universal biological phenomenon. Calabrese's contention is that the biphasic dose response is a manifestation of the system's adaptive response to stress, a modest overcompensation, Calabrese suggests, in the face of threatened disruption to homeostatic balance.

In other words, because of the hormetic (biphasic) effect, there is not always a simple linear relationship between the dose of a stressor and the clinical response.

By the same token, because of the hormetic (biphasic) effect, optimally stressful therapeutic interventions will enable the patient to advance from suboptimal health and depleted vitality to optimal health and revitalized well-being. By initially prompting destabilization of the (dysfunctional) status quo of the patient's defensive structures, these optimally stressful interventions—as long as they provide just the right balance of challenge and support—will ultimately tap into the body's innate ability to heal itself in the face of threatened disruption to its homeostatic balance, thereby triggering repair and restabilization of the system at ever higher levels of integration, self-regulatory capacity, and functionality.[9–11]

HOMEOSTASIS AND THE STRESS RESPONSE: WALTER B. CANNON AND HANS SELYE

CANNON'S WISDOM OF THE BODY

Walter B. Cannon devoted decades of scientific study to the body's efforts to maintain the constancy of its internal environment in the face of stressful challenge. In 1932, Cannon, in his seminal volume entitled *The Wisdom of the Body*, introduced the concept of homeostasis to describe the various regulatory mechanisms utilized by the body to preserve or, if lost, to restore the constancy of its internal environment. Cannon's interest was in the ongoing compensatory micro adjustments that the body mobilizes in an effort to maintain this dynamic equilibrium in the face of environmental stressors.

SELYE'S STRESS OF LIFE

Hans Selye, author of the 1978 classic *The Stress of Life*, took up where Cannon had left off. Long intrigued by the body's nonspecific response to generic unpleasantness, Selye developed the idea of a general adaptation syndrome, a three-stage model that he conceived in order to address not just the impact on the body of the usual and customary stresses of everyday life with which Cannon had been primarily concerned but also the cumulative impact, over time, of unusual or extreme stress.

Selye's three-stage general adaptation syndrome speaks directly to the body's ongoing efforts to restore its homeostatic balance when challenged by not just acute but also chronic stress.

The first is the alarm stage of the acute stress response, characterized by heightened arousal and mobilization of the body's defenses in an effort to preserve its dynamic equilibrium.

If the stress persists, however, the body will transition into the second stage (the early chronic stage) of the stress response, namely, resistance and adaptation, characterized by intensification of the body's defensive efforts—all with an eye either to fending off (resisting) the stressor and/or to making whatever internal adjustments are necessary in order to live with (adapt to) the stressor.

Although the body's efforts to compensate by resisting and adapting enable the body to manage the impact of the stressors, the body cannot keep this up for the duration and, eventually, its reserves will become depleted.

Selye posited that if indeed stress continues indefinitely, then the body will transition into the third stage (the late chronic stage) of the general adaptation syndrome, namely, exhaustion. Now the body begins to break down. No longer able to resist or adapt, no longer able to maintain its internal constancy, no longer able to preserve its homeostatic balance, and no longer able to defy the inexorable forces of entropy, the exhausted body, overloaded from the cumulative impact of toxicities and depleted from the cumulative impact of deficiencies, will collapse, accompanied by progressive decline in structure and function. Loss of the body's adaptability, loss of the body's regulatory capacity, and loss of the body's resilience will characterize this final stage of maladaptation, decompensation, and dyshomeostasis.

Depletion of the body's adaptation reserves signals the onset of such disease processes as chemical sensitivity, chronic heart disease, chronic obstructive pulmonary disease, environmental illness, autoimmune disease, chronic skin conditions, chronic inflammatory bowel disease, type 2 diabetes, and chronic degenerative disease, to name a few. Once the overloaded and depleted system has devolved into this third and final stage of the stress response, the system will no longer be able to return to its erstwhile baseline of health and vitality. In the words of Thomas Wolfe,[25] "You can't go home again."

OPEN VERSUS CLOSED SYSTEM

Admittedly, a closed system, which (by definition) does not allow for the free exchange of information and energy between itself and its surroundings, will, over time, ultimately lose its battle to entropy (a thermodynamic term used to describe a closed system's progressive deterioration from orderedness to disorder).

But if a system is open (as is the living system) and therefore able to receive regulatory input from the outside, the system—despite its depleted state—will can be revitalized, at least to some extent. If its load can be lightened (to correct for toxicities), its reserves replenished (to correct for deficiencies), and its flow facilitated (to expedite the processing and integrating of environmental challenge), then the system will still have a fighting chance to recover its health—even if the set point (which becomes the new normal) is now lower.

And, as has been noted repeatedly throughout this chapter, it will then be optimal stress (i.e., just the right balance of challenge and support) that will be able, once again, to provoke the newly reconfigured system to continue its evolution (although its baseline will now be the new, albeit lower, set point) through iterative cycles of disruption and repair to ever more robust (even if still compromised) health.

PRECIPITATING DISRUPTION IN ORDER TO TRIGGER REPAIR

In essence, the therapeutic intent of the holistic practitioner is to precipitate disruption in order to trigger repair. Because, as noted earlier, self-organizing systems resist perturbation, the provocation of rupture in order to galvanize recovery must be instigated again and again if the system is to evolve from dysfunctional defense to more functional adaptation.

And so it is that the patient's dysfunctional defensive structures must be sufficiently impacted by the therapist's stressful input that their foundation will indeed become weakened. By the same token, however, progressive unsettling of the foundation will force the patient to tap into underlying resilience in order to restore homeostatic balance in the face of optimal challenge—the net result of which will be the eventual emergence of orderedness from chaos as low-level defenses that were growth-disrupting become transformed into higher-level adaptations that are more growth-promoting.

MINIMAL LOAD, OPTIMAL LOAD, AND OVERLOAD: FROM STABILITY THROUGH INCREASING COMPLEXITY TO CHAOS

Based upon study of the sandpile model, I postulate that—whatever the biological system, whatever the agent (poison or medication), whatever the endpoint (health-promoting or disease-promoting), and biochemical individuality notwithstanding[26]—three distinct stages will inevitably emerge along the dose–response curve (here intended to represent the response, over time, of a single system to ongoing environmental input):

1. *Minimal load*: The initial stage during which the system's homeostatic mechanisms will allow it to preserve both its status quo and its level of complexity.
2. *Optimal load*: A compensatory stage during which the system's underlying resilience will enable it to evolve to ever higher levels of complexity as it advances, over time, through iterative cycles of defensive collapse—a *minor avalanche* in chaos theory—and adaptive reconstitution.
3. *Overload*: The terminal stage of decompensation during which the overburdened system—the load having exceeded the system's adaptive capacity—will sustain catastrophic collapse—a *major avalanche* in chaos theory—and devolve to a much lower level of complexity.

In other words, recursive cycles of disruption and repair will continue indefinitely, until some indeterminate point in time when a critical threshold will have been reached, a tipping point,[27] a saturation point, a point of toxic accumulation[28–32] that will trigger a devastating, cataclysmic breakdown of the system—and the whole process will then begin anew, but this time from an entirely different baseline of complexity.

The nonlinear evolution of a chaotic system proceeds as follows: From stability and perpetuation of the status quo (when the system, in the face of minimal load, is maintaining itself, by way of ongoing homeostatic adjustments, at a baseline level of complexity) through increasing complexity (when the system, in the face of optimal load, is evolving to ever newer levels of homeostatic balance and ever higher levels of complexity) to chaos (when the system, in the face of overload and having exhausted its adaptation reserves, collapses entirely, devolving to a much lower level of complexity).

With respect to the dose–response curve, I am therefore proposing that we consider the x-axis (the dose) to reflect the element of time and the y-axis (the response) to reflect the level of complexity in the system—a lower level of complexity going hand in hand with defensive reactions and a higher level of complexity going hand in hand with adaptive responses.

My contention is that all living systems, in response to input from the outside, will evolve from minimal load through optimal load to overload; from minimal stress through optimal stress to traumatic stress[13,4]; from unadapted through adapted to maladapted; from uncompensated through modestly overcompensated to decompensated; and from a state of homeostasis (which speaks to a single set point) through states of allostasis (which speak to ever-changing set points as the system adapts to ever-changing environmental conditions, in the process ever increasing its allostatic load)[28-33] to a state of dyshomeostasis (which speaks to the system's inability to preserve any balance at all in the face of allostatic overload).

In other words, I believe that all living systems—by virtue of the fact that they are open, complex adaptive, self-organizing, and chaotic—will evolve, given enough time, from stability through increasing complexity to chaos. Why, one wonders, do living systems evolve in this manner? For the very same unfathomable reason that a sandpile, in response to ongoing input from the outside, advances through its cycles…

ALLOSTATIC LOAD

The concept of an allostatic (total body) load that is becoming ever more burdensome as the system evolves, over time, offers a framework for understanding the transitioning of a system from the early chronic stage of Selye's stress response (when the system, by way of ongoing defense and adaptation, is still struggling to preserve its dynamic equilibrium in the face of manageable challenge) to the late chronic stage of Selye's stress response (when the system, its energetic and nutrient reserves depleted, collapses from overload and exhaustion).

With respect to this ever-increasing allostatic load, the price paid for psychological adaptation is significantly less than the price paid (initially latent but, ultimately, more overt) for physiological adaptation. In fact, despite psychological bruises and scars sustained along the way and the resultant loss of innocence, emotional maturity can usually be achieved over time without exacting such a toll that the system crashes into the late chronic stage of the stress response. In contradistinction to this, the attainment of physiological maturity (a euphemism for aging) will often, sadly, be accompanied by the unfortunate transitioning from early chronic stress (Selye's second stage) to late chronic stress (Selye's third stage).

This transitioning to the final stage of the stress response occurs because the various physiological adaptations accompanying the aging process may take such a toll on the system and the allostatic load increase so much that stressors once constituting an optimal challenge (triggering defense and adaptation) will now constitute a traumatic challenge. In other words, physiological stressors that might once have been managed by way of defense and adaptation are no longer able to be handled because of the system's decreasing resilience and consequent inability to maintain a dynamic equilibrium. As a result, with the passage of time, the system may crash into the late chronic stage of dyshomeostasis, maladaptation, and fixed-name disease.

Along these same lines of an ever-increasing allostatic load accompanied by ever more compromise in functioning of the underlying system, more than 40 years ago, the author of this volume William J. Rea (in the tradition of Theron Randolph, the father of clinical ecology) introduced the model of a rain barrel becoming gradually filled with drops of rain—to the point of overflow—to represent visually the cumulative (albeit often subtle) impact, over time, of stress on the body. The capacity of the barrel speaks to the body's capacity to tolerate environmental stressors, overt clinical symptoms manifesting only once the barrel has become filled to the brim, signifying that the point of toxic accumulation has been reached—although, even prior to this critical point of overflow, as the total body load is steadily increasing, there will be subclinical dysfunction, imbalance, and disharmony.[28-31]

In essence, Rea's Rain Barrel Model, with its highlighting of the critically important tipping point reached once the barrel has become filled to overflowing (i.e., once the allostatic load has reached a critical mass), offers an elegant way to conceptualize the trigger for the transitioning of the system from Selye's second stage of the stress response (when the system, despite its ever-increasing underlying dysfunction, is still struggling—by way of defending and adapting—to preserve its dynamic balance) to the third stage of the stress response (when the depleted and exhausted system, having reached the limits of its adaptive capacity, collapses into chronic fixed-name disease).

Obviously, in order for the patient to remain in Selye's second stage (where defense and adaptation are still resources upon which the system can rely), it will be critically important that whatever adaptations (psychological or physiological) the system must make in order to preserve its internal constancy, the price they demand not be too great. The higher the cost, the heavier the allostatic load and the more depleted the adaptation reserves. And once the adaptive capacity of an overburdened and exhausted system has been exceeded, the system will crash, marking its transition into the third stage of Selye's stress response—and the onset of chronic disease.

In order to maintain, for as long as possible, the system's ability to cope with stress (through defense and adaptation), thereby forestalling the system's transitioning into the stage of late chronic disease, it is therefore critically important that therapeutic interventions target the system's allostatic load and adaptation reserves. In an ongoing manner, treatments must hone in on correcting for both the system's toxicities (by lightening the total body load, thereby easing its allostatic load) and the system's deficiencies (by replenishing the total body reserves, thereby reinforcing its adaptation reserves).

These carefully tailored interventions are specifically designed to prevent overflow of the rain barrel by restoring the resilience of a compromised matrix.

REA'S RAIN BARREL AND STARK'S SANDPILE

The sandpile model that I have presented here is intended to complement, not replace, the model of the rain barrel. However, instead of a rain barrel to which drops of rain are being added, it is a sandpile to which grains of sand are being added.

Both Rea's Rain Barrel and Stark's Sandpile offer a visual representation of the cumulative impact, over time, of stress on an open system, whereas the focus of the rain barrel model is on one critical moment in time, the focus of the sandpile model is on a series of such moments over the course of time. In other words, the rain barrel model speaks to what happens when one specific critical threshold is reached; the sandpile model, on the other hand, speaks to what happens over and over again, each time a critical threshold is reached, namely, partial collapse of the sandpile, then its partial recovery, partial collapse, then its partial recovery, periodic cycles of disruption and repair, disruption, and repair—until such time as a final critical threshold is reached and the sandpile collapses altogether.

So, too, as earlier discussed, Selye's stress response speaks to the cumulative impact, over time, of stress on an open system—whereas the focus of Selye's triphasic stress response is on linear progression from preadapted to adapted to maladapted as health and vitality become increasingly compromised and adaptation reserves increasingly depleted (Selye likens it to the progression from childhood to adulthood to senescence), the focus of the sandpile model is on nonlinear progression of a complex adaptive system through iterative cycles of collapse, recovery, collapse, recovery, the system each time reconstituting at ever higher levels of order and complexity, even as the system's underlying stability and balance are becoming increasingly compromised.

Then, at some indeterminate point in time, the periodicity of disruption and repair will give way to a devastating, cataclysmic collapse of the entire sandpile once the tipping point has been reached—a major avalanche, a sandpile-flattening event, total breakdown, irretrievable structural damage as irreparable disorder replaces the erstwhile order.

Unlike Selye's stress response, the focus of the sandpile model is on the reversibility of disorder and dysfunction and on the resilience of a system that is able continuously evolve, in the face of ongoing challenge and in defiance of the inexorable force of entropy, to ever newer heights by virtue of its intrinsic structure and its openness to regulatory input from the environment, even as the system is becoming ever more compromised in its underlying structure and ever more dangerously balanced at the edge of chaos (the point between orderedness and true chaos).

It is really quite extraordinary, and the clinical implications profound, that stress itself can provide the means by which a complex adaptive system open to regulatory input from the outside can reconstitute over and over again, something new emerging each time, a regrouping, a new orderedness, a realignment, even as the underlying structure is becoming ever less perfectly configured and ever less precisely ordered.

Adaptive reconstitution at ever newer homeostatic (or, more accurately, allostatic) set points will enable partial recovery of the sandpile's structural integrity and partial reversal of its underlying disorder and dysfunction. However, this structural reorganization will give only the appearance of a return to normal because, in truth, the reorganization will have been accomplished at the expense of the system's overall stability and balance. Nonetheless, iterative cycles of partial collapse, then partial recovery, partial defensive collapse, and then partial adaptive reconstitution at ever higher levels of orderedness and complexity will continue indefinitely, with the sandpile growing ever bigger, even as it is becoming ever more undermined in structure and function, ever less stable, and ever less balanced.

WEB OF LIFE

Whether described as the ground regulation system,[34,35] the biological terrain,[50] the connective tissue matrix,[3] the extracellular matrix,[28–32] the living matrix,[36–38,51] or the MindBodyMatrix,[9,10] the living system is an intricate web of interdependent living tissue that extends from the surface of the body to its innermost recesses, ultimately penetrating every cell in the body. This vast regulatory network of complex and interwoven pathways allows for the high-speed transmission of regulatory information and vibratory energy throughout the body's expanse and is therefore ultimately responsible for the body's innate ability to regulate and repair itself.

It is a ground regulation system that includes the connective tissue or extracellular matrix, the cytoskeleton or cellular matrix, the nuclear matrix, and the molecular structures linking these matrices.[32] More specifically, this web of life comprises a continuous meshwork of connective tissue fibers (glycoproteins that are either structural, like collagen and elastin, or cross-linking, like fibronectin and laminin) dispersed throughout an amorphous ground substance (a colloidal gel consisting primarily of large sugar–protein complexes). These sugar–protein complexes—proteoglycan/glycosaminoglycan (PG/GAG) macromolecules—contain a positively charged, core protein backbone (PG) to which negatively charged, highly polymerized glycan side chains (GAGs) are attached. These GAGs stand out from the PG backbone in a bristle-like fashion and are surrounded by, and tightly bound to, polarized water molecules.

In the language of solid-state physics, the branch of physics that studies highly ordered systems (like crystalline solids), we now understand this ground regulation system to be a liquid crystal with semiconducting properties.[3] In other words, because the living matrix is a highly ordered array of molecules (primarily glycoproteins, PG/GAGs, and water) closely packed and tightly organized in a crystal-like lattice structure, it has the semiconducting properties of a crystal and, as such, allows for the near-instantaneous flow of regulatory information and vibratory energy throughout the entire fabric of the body.

It is this crystallinity that enables the living matrix (with its protein backbone, its sugar–protein side chains, and its tightly bound layers of water) to conduct electrons and other subatomic energetic entities (i.e., units of information and energy) at about the speed of light, transmitting both information (in much the way that a phone line transmits information) and energy (in much the way that the wire to a toaster transmits energy). The living matrix is therefore the ideal vehicle for this astoundingly complex and extraordinarily effective global communication system responsible for preserving homeostatic balance within the body.

From this, it follows that the architecture of the connective tissue matrix accounts for not only its tensile strength and structural integrity but also its ability continuously to process and integrate, at lightning-fast speeds, the impact of environmental perturbations. It is not therefore too much of a stretch to hypothesize that it is this connective tissue meshwork of interconnected collagen fibers and the semifluid ground substance in which those fibers are immersed that account in large part for the resilience, adaptability, and capacity of the MindBodyMatrix to reconstitute itself in the face of environmental challenge.

Whether the units of information and energy are described as electrons, biophotons, or energy quanta; whether the flow is of discontinuous particles or continuous waves; whether the transport system involves collagen fibrils outside the cells, microtubules inside the cells, or sugar–protein macromolecules in the interstitial ground substance; whether propagation is by way of layers of electrically charged water, the perineural DC system,[39] acupuncture meridians, or energy channels[3,40]; and whether the speed of transmission is the speed of semiconductivity or the speed of light or simply instantaneous, many of the research scientists who devote themselves to the study of these esoteric concepts share a common dream, namely, to unravel the secret of life by studying the inner workings, on the most elemental level, of the living system.

When the concept of homeostasis was first introduced by Cannon,[19] his focus was on regulatory organ systems, most especially the autonomic nervous and endocrine systems. In a little known but brilliant volume published more than 20 years ago and entitled *Matrix and Matrix Regulation: Basis for a Holistic Theory in Medicine*, however, Alfred Pischinger[34] presents a fairly compelling case for the idea that maintenance of balance within the body is accomplished by way of the ground regulation system (also known as the connective tissue or extracellular matrix, or, simply, the living matrix). His contention is that nerve endings and capillary networks are embedded within this matrix; but nowhere do they have direct contact with functioning cells. And so it is not simply regulatory organ systems but the ground regulation system itself that makes possible the maintenance of balance within the body.

It is therefore crucial that this matrix operate as effectively as possible because the health and vitality of the body's cells are entirely dependent upon it.

FACILITATING THE FLOW

In order to optimize the flow of information and energy throughout the living system, it is essential that the body be kept as uncongested, nutrient-rich, well-oxygenated, alkaline, electron-rich, negatively charged, energetically unblocked, well-balanced, relaxed, well-rested, and structurally aligned as possible.

Of course, regular exercise will also be critical for maintaining the system's resilience and adaptability. Most effective is high-intensity interval training, an exercise strategy that alternates periods of short intense anaerobic exercise with less intense recovery periods. As with psychotherapeutic interventions that alternately challenge and support, here too, cycles of anaerobic activity alternating with aerobic activity appear to be associated with fine-tuning the matrix and optimizing functionality.

Furthermore, in order to regulate gene expression and protein function, it will be important that there be adequate methylation of the various components of the ground regulation system, easily enough obtained by way of nutrient supplementation with such methyl donors as folic acid, vitamin B12, trimethylglycine (TMG), dimethylglycine (DMG), *S*-adenosylmethionine (SAM-e), and dimethylaminoethanol (DMAE).

Particularly critical for maintenance of a healthy and vital living matrix will be water, the presence of which will allow the matrix to function as a liquid crystal, thereby making possible the high-speed, body-wide propagation of information and energy necessary to ensure the resilience of the matrix, its adaptability, and its capacity to reconstitute at ever higher levels of order, coherence, and integration.

LIGHTENING THE LOAD AND REPLENISHING THE RESERVES

Whatever the focus, more specific therapeutic interventions must ultimately aim to facilitate the flow of information and energy throughout the entire fabric of the body in order to allow the living system not only to manage the impact of environmental challenge but also to benefit from it.

Until the flow of information and energy has been reinstated, the system's resilience, adaptability, and capacity to tolerate the stress of life will remain compromised. However, once the orderedness and fluidity of the system's infrastructure have been restored with targeted treatments that correct for internal toxicities and deficiencies, the system's capacity to reverse the underlying disease processes will be revitalized—mental and physical well-being recovered.

There are many different customized therapies that will offer just the right balance of challenge and support needed to optimize overall MindBodyHealth. With respect to determining the appropriate dose, however, one must never forget that the difference between a poison and a medication is the dosage thereof (and the system's capacity to process, integrate, and adapt to its impact). This means, of course, that whatever treatments are administered, they must provide just the right mix of challenge and support because a lot of a good thing can be toxic and a little of a bad thing can be therapeutic.

With that said, treatment modalities must either eliminate bad (e.g., by way of heavy metal chelation to remove toxic metals like lead, aluminum, and arsenic that have bioaccumulated in the body's tissues) or supplement with good (e.g., by way of oxygen therapy to support oxidative phosphorylation in the mitochondria and the aerobic production of energy) or, as is true for many treatments, do both (e.g., by way of saunas and deep tissue massage, both of which not only relieve muscular tension, lymphatic congestion, and energy blockages but also facilitate the flow of nutrients into, and waste products out of, the cells).

With respect to lightening the total body load, first and foremost, of course, will be avoidance of those substances (whether ingested, inhaled, or absorbed) to which a patient might be reactive.

However, beyond avoidance, there are a number of targeted therapies (in addition to the aforementioned chelation, saunas, and deep tissue massage) that are specifically designed to lighten the total body load: antioxidants (to reduce oxidative stress caused by free radicals), detox foot pads, ionic foot baths, enemas, and colonics. Although some of these approaches are controversial, their therapeutic intent is the same, namely, to reduce toxicities that are interfering with the propagation of information and energy through the ground regulation system so that environmental stressors can be more easily processed and assimilated by a now more ordered and fluid MindBodyMatrix.

There are also a number of targeted therapies (in addition to the aforementioned oxygen therapy, saunas, and deep tissue massage) that are specifically designed to replenish the total body reserves: love, support, probiotics, prebiotics, organic food, digestive enzymes, essential fatty acids, amino acids, other nutritional supplementation, phytonutrients, alkaline water, restful sleep, a light box, earthing, and neodymium magnets.

And then some interventions both lighten the load and replenish the reserves, that is, they get both bad out and good in. In addition to saunas and deep tissue massage, these treatments include sensorimotor psychotherapy, eye movement desensitization and reprocessing (EMDR), psychomotor psychotherapy (PBSP), somatic experiencing, psychoanalysis, yoga, lymphatic drainage, the chi machine, craniosacral therapy, Reiki, shiatsu, frequency-specific microcurrent (FSM), ayurvedic medicine, traditional Chinese medicine (TCM), acupuncture, therapeutic touch, reflexology, and chiropractic—to name a few.

Lightening the body load and replenishing the body reserves will reinforce the system's resilience and capacity to tolerate the stress of life.

A more reinforced, coherent, and functional infrastructure—one that has now become both more ordered and more fluid—will enhance the system's capacity to process and integrate the impact of environmental impingement, which in turn will reinforce the system's resilience and adaptability and mark its transitioning from a dysfunctional state of disorder and disease to a more functional one of orderedness, ease of flow, resilience, adaptability, and regulatory capacity.

In essence, ongoing lightening of the load and replenishing of the reserves will provide the stressful input needed—optimal stress—to fuel recursive cycles of disruption and repair, defensive collapse, and adaptive reconstitution at ever higher levels of synergy, the rhythms of mind and body now synchronized and in harmonic resonance.

RESILIENCE: CONTINUOUS ADJUSTMENT TO INSTABILITY

How well the MindBodyMatrix is able to process and integrate environmental perturbations will be a reflection of the system's underlying health, more specifically, a reflection of its resilience, its regulatory capacity, and its ability to adapt.

Of note is the fact that implicit in the conceptualization of self-regulatory capacity as a story about the system's ability to restore its homeostatic balance in the face of challenge is the compelling idea that a living system will be able to preserve its stability only by way of continuous adjustment to instability. Indeed, in 1965, two obstetricians made an intriguing discovery about the paradoxical relationship between regularity of the fetal heart rate and fetal mortality. They observed that the more metronome-like the heartbeat, the less likely the fetus would be to survive. In other words, the regularity of the fetal heart rate was found to be highly correlated with fetal death. By the same token, the obstetricians observed that the greater the heart rate variability (i.e., the more variable the heart's beat-to-beat intervals), the more likely the fetus would be to survive.[41] This regulatory capacity, critically important for the maintenance of health, has been described as "the ability to survive change by changing."[42]

Charles Richet,[43] a French physiologist, was also addressing this seeming paradox when he made the following observation about the living system: "In a sense <the living being> is stable because it is modifiable. ... the slight instability is the necessary condition for the true stability of the organism."

In essence, health speaks to the capacity continuously to adjust to ongoing environmental perturbation and adaptively to reorganize at ever newer homeostatic (allostatic) set points.

THERAPEUTIC USE OF STRESS TO PROVOKE PHYSIOLOGICAL HEALING

Before I discuss in detail the therapeutic use of stress to provoke psychological healing by activating the system's innate capacity to heal itself, I would like to make a brief reference to a variety of treatment modalities that demonstrate the therapeutic use of stress to provoke physiological recovery.

HOMEOPATHY

In the late eighteenth century, a German physician, Samuel Hahnemann, developed the field of homeopathy, the basic principle of which is that like cures like (also known as the *Law of Similars*). By administering very small doses of substances known to cause the symptoms of a particular disease, homeopathic remedies induce a cure of these symptoms (and of the underlying disease process) by stimulating the body's innate ability to heal itself.[44]

The key to the effectiveness of a homeopathic remedy is the administration of minute doses of a potentized substance, which means that the substance has been serially diluted (each dilution increasing its effectiveness) and succussed (the solution then shaken vigorously) in order to release its full energetic potential. Advocates of homeopathy believe that although homeopathic solutions are so highly diluted that no detectable amounts of the substance remain, the solutions nonetheless contain a memory of the substance. The body is thought to recognize the energetic signature of the substance and then to react to its imprinted memory.

Well-known examples of homeopathic remedies are the treatment of a rattlesnake bite with a highly diluted solution of snake venom or the treatment of high fevers and throbbing headaches with a highly diluted solution of belladonna, the toxic substance extracted from the poisonous herb of that name (also known as the deadly nightshade).

HOMEOPATHY VERSUS ALLOPATHY

To highlight the distinction between allopathy and homeopathy: Allopathy is the conventional, mainstream method of treating diseases; it does so not by attending to the underlying disease process but by treating its symptoms (and signs) with substances that produce effects opposite to those produced by the disease—in other words, by offering symptomatic relief. Examples include the use of antipyretics to treat fevers, anti-inflammatories to reduce swelling and inflammation, antitussives to suppress coughs, antihypertensives to decrease blood pressure, antiemetics to ease nausea and prevent vomiting, and anticonvulsants to stop seizures.

Homeopathy, however, is more attuned to the underlying disease process and aims to treat diseases with substances that produce effects similar to those produced by the disease but with doses so small that the body's natural healing processes will be triggered.

In other words, whereas allopathy involves prescribing an antisymptom remedy to correct for the symptom, homeopathy involves creating, as the remedy, a diluted version of the symptom itself in order to jumpstart the body's inborn self-healing mechanisms, thereby correcting the underlying disease process itself.

IMMUNOTHERAPY

In any event, holistic practitioners contend that administering either a single small dose of allergen or a series of such low doses, over a period of time, will stimulate the body's immune system and promote the body's resistance to subsequent exposures to that allergen. The various forms of immunotherapy (which include vaccinations) prepare the body for future challenges by inducing tolerance (also known as acquired tolerance or adaptive immunity) and include such immune-strengthening techniques as provocation–neutralization, enzyme-potentiated desensitization (EPD), low-dose antigen (LDA) therapy, and Nambudripad's allergy elimination technique (NAET). The theory behind such treatments is that single or intermittent exposures to doses that do not overwhelm the body—and, instead, provide an optimal challenge—will prompt the body to adapt, thereby promoting resistance to subsequent exposures.

ACUPUNCTURE

Acupuncture is a procedure involving the stimulation, with very fine needles, of specific acupuncture points along the surface of the body in an effort to correct imbalances in the flow of information and energy along the meridians that form a continuous communication network throughout the expanse of the body. By simulating an injury without actually seriously damaging the tissue, the healing cascade is activated. In essence, the mild stimulus is thought to tune up the repair channels, thereby restoring the flow of energy, relieving pain, and curing any number of mental and physical conditions.

DEEP TISSUE MASSAGE

Deep tissue massage involves the application of intense and focused pressure to deep muscles and connective tissue (fascia) in order to relieve chronic muscle tension, reduce stress hormone levels, activate the parasympathetic nervous system, stimulate the release of serotonin and endorphins (endogenous morphine), increase the flow of lymph, and promote relaxation. After the body, in response to the stress of the pressure, first (defensively) guards, the body will then (adaptively) release. In essence, the optimal stress of a deep tissue massage will cause first a defensive reaction (in the form of a reflexive tightening) and then an adaptive response (in the form of a more relaxed going-with-the-flow).

EXERCISE

Well known to athletes is the fact that moderate exercise, in the form of, say, every-other-day workouts, provides an optimal challenge to the body; it creates microtears that the body is then able to repair on those alternate days when the body is at rest.

PROLOTHERAPY

Based upon the concept that cause irritation or injury will stimulate healing, prolotherapy (also known as proliferation therapy or regenerative injection therapy) is a highly effective treatment for chronic ligament and tendon weakness. It involves injecting a mildly irritating solution (e.g., dextrose, water, and a local anesthetic like lidocaine) into the affected ligament or tendon in order to induce a mild inflammatory reaction, which will then activate the body's healing process, resulting ultimately in overall strengthening of the damaged connective tissue and alleviation of the pain. Prolotherapy is believed by several holistic practitioners to be significantly more effective than cortisone injections because these latter injections, although providing immediate short-term pain relief, will, because of the catabolic effect of steroid hormones over the long term, cause destruction of tissue and exacerbation of pain.

In sum, just as with the sandpile model, treatment modalities that provide just the right combination of challenge and support will enable the body to progress from illness to wellness by jumpstarting the body's inborn ability to self-heal in the face of optimal stress.

THERAPEUTIC USE OF STRESS TO PROVOKE PSYCHOLOGICAL RECOVERY

As earlier suggested, with respect to the psychotherapeutic process, the catalyst for progressive transformation of less healthy defense into more healthy adaptation will be working through the cumulative impact of optimally stressful therapeutic interventions that afford just the right balance of challenge and support—challenge (such that the patient's defenses, no matter how seemingly intractable, will become temporarily destabilized) and support (such that the patient, after working through the disruption, will have the opportunity adaptively to restabilize at a higher level of integration, balance, and harmony).

Working through these recursive cycles of disruption and repair will enable the patient ultimately to evolve to a level of functionality, adaptive capacity, and resilience that will render unnecessary unhealthy defenses to which she had desperately clung in a self-sabotaging attempt to avoid confronting the myriad anxiety-provoking realities in her life—both past and present.

In order to bring about this undermining of the patient's dysfunctional defenses and the subsequent creation of impetus and opportunity for their replacement with more functional self-protective mechanisms, we will repeatedly present the patient with optimally stressful interventions that alternately challenge and then support, support and then challenge. If we want first to increase the patient's anxiety and then decrease it, we will first challenge and then support. However, if we want first to decrease the patient's anxiety and then increase it, we will first support and then challenge. Either way, our aim is to find that delicate balance between too much anxiety and too little anxiety; it will then be the therapeutic generation within the patient of this incentivizing anxiety that will optimize her potential for transformation and growth.

And so it comes to conclusion that the patient's dysfunctional defensive structures must be perturbed enough by the therapist's anxiety-provoking interventions that there will be both impetus and opportunity for adaptive reconstitution of these structures at a higher, more functional level.

PSYCHOTHERAPEUTIC INTERVENTIONS THAT ALTERNATELY CHALLENGE AND THEN SUPPORT

The therapist will be able to facilitate this working-through process by constructing psychotherapeutic interventions strategically designed either to challenge the patient by directing her attention to where she is not (but where the therapist would want the patient to be) or to support the patient by resonating with where she is (and where the patient would seem to need to be).

More specifically, with her finger ever on the pulse of the patient's level of anxiety and capacity to tolerate further challenge, the therapist will therefore alternately challenge (by reminding the patient of what she really does—albeit reluctantly—know) and support (in some situations, by resonating empathically with what the patient finds herself thinking, feeling, or doing in order not to have to know and, in other situations, by resonating empathically with the pain of the patient's grief as she begins to let herself know).

I have developed several prototypical psychotherapeutic statements (including a conflict statement and a disillusionment statement) that capitalize upon the idea that the therapeutic use of optimal stress can indeed expedite the psychotherapeutic endeavor by precipitating rupture in order to trigger repair.[45,9,10] These strategically constructed interventions will alternately increase the patient's anxiety (by confronting her with her knowledge of some uncomfortable reality) and then decrease the patient's anxiety (by resonating empathically with her experience of that uncomfortable reality)—again, all with an eye to generating an optimal level of destabilizing stress and incentivizing anxiety.

ANXIETY-PROVOKING BUT ULTIMATELY GROWTH-PROMOTING CONFLICT STATEMENTS

Interestingly, the first of these anxiety-provoking but ultimately growth-promoting interventions first names the patient's adaptive capacity to know an uncomfortable reality and then resonates empathically with the patient's defensive need to deny such knowledge. These conflict statements are specifically designed to call to the patient's attention the conflict that exists within her between, on the one hand, what she really does know and, on the other hand, what she finds herself resorting to in order not to have to know.

The format of these optimally stressful conflict statements is as follows: "You know ..., *but* you find yourself thinking, feeling, doing ... in order not to have to know." In other words, the patient knows; but, because the anxiety elicited by that knowledge is too much to manage she finds herself needing to mobilize a (dysfunctional) defense in order not to have to know.

ANXIETY-PROVOKING BUT ULTIMATELY GROWTH-PROMOTING DISILLUSIONMENT STATEMENTS

The second of these anxiety-provoking but ultimately growth-promoting interventions also first names the patient's adaptive capacity to know an uncomfortable reality but then resonates empathically with the patient's dawning ability to experience it. These disillusionment statements are specifically designed to facilitate the patient's grieving by highlighting, on the one hand, the disillusioning reality that the patient is beginning to confront and, on the other hand, the patient's new-found ability to let herself begin to feel the actual pain of her grief about it.

The format of these optimally stressful disillusionment (or grieving) statements is as follows: "You know ..., and it breaks your heart ..." In other words, the patient knows; but, because the anxiety elicited by that knowledge is—for whatever complex mix of reasons—more manageable, she has the adaptive capacity to let herself experience the pain of it.

Whether the therapist utilizes these conflict statements and disillusionment statements or constructs other psychotherapeutic interventions that alternately increase the patient's anxiety (by directing her to where she does not want to be) and then decrease the patient's anxiety (by validating where she is), the underlying principle will be the therapeutic use of stress to provoke recovery.

In whatever way the therapist alternately challenges and then supports the patient's deeply ingrained defensive patterns, all such interventional efforts—rendered with compassion and without judgment—will reflect a deep appreciation for the patient's ambivalent attachment to these defenses for which she admittedly pays a price but that also serve her.

HEALING CYCLES OF DISRUPTION AND REPAIR

In sum, the healing process—to be effective in bringing about deep and lasting change—must involve this therapeutic induction of healing cycles of disruption and repair in reaction/response to the therapist's optimally stressful interventions, such that the patient, after initial defensive collapse, will be able subsequently to reconstitute adaptively at ever higher levels of accountability, empowerment, and complex understanding.

COMPLEMENTARY MODES OF PSYCHOTHERAPEUTIC ACTION

My contention is that psychotherapy affords patients the opportunity for belated mastery of early-on psychological traumas that were simply too overwhelming to be managed at the time they were inflicted. Instead of being processed and gradually organized into healthy psychic structure and adaptive capacity, the unassimilated traumatizing experiences were split off and their chaotic memory traces stored internally, where they then wreaked havoc on the MindBodyMatrix in the form of any number of manifest psychological and physiological symptoms (the aforementioned chronic depression, despair, unremitting anxiety, generalized musculoskeletal pain, adrenal fatigue, brain fog, persistent insomnia, reflexive irritability, and uncontrollable impulsivity, to name but a few).

Elsewhere,[45] I have proposed that the therapeutic action of psychodynamic psychotherapy can be conceptualized as having been divided, historically, into roughly three different schools of thought regarding the healing process—schools of thought that are complementary, not conflicting.

Each of the three perspectives focuses on some aspect of the patient's defenses—be it the patient's resistance to acknowledging painful truths about the self (Model 1), the patient's refusal to confront—and grieve—painful truths about her objects (Model 2), or, under the sway of her repetition compulsion, the patient's reenactment of unmastered childhood dramas on the stage of her life and in the therapy (Model 3). By the same token, each of the three perspectives approaches the healing process somewhat differently—Model 1 is more *cognitive*, Model 2 is more *affective*, and Model 3 is more *relational*.

In any event, the patient's resistances (Model 1), her relentless pursuits (Model 2), and her compulsive and unwitting reenactments (Model 3) are the dysfunctional defenses to which she clings in order not to have to know, not to have to feel, and not to have to take ownership of what she plays out on the stage of her life. As such, they serve to block out the immediate pain of her grief about all the early-on privations, deprivations, and injuries that were simply too overwhelming for her to cope with at the time.

The three schools of psychodynamic thought therefore address different aspects of the therapeutic action; but all three perspectives address transformation of chaotic and less evolved defenses into coherent and more evolved adaptations to the stress of life.

Transformation of Resistance into Awareness

Model 1, enhancement of knowledge within, is the interpretive perspective of classical psychoanalysis, a drive–defense model that focuses on the patient's unmodulated drives and self-protective defenses, a model that offers the neurotically conflicted patient an opportunity to gain greater self-awareness and insight into her inner workings, so that she can make more informed decisions about her life, become more master of her destiny, and channel her now more modulated energies into actualized potential.

Transformation of Relentlessness into Acceptance

Model 2, provision of corrective experience for, is a more contemporary perspective, one that focuses on the patient's psychological deficiencies, these psychic scars the result of early-on absence of good in the form of parental deprivation and neglect. This deficiency-compensation perspective is one that offers the patient an opportunity in the here-and-now relationship with her therapist both to grieve the early-on parental failures and to experience symbolic restitution. As the patient makes her peace with the reality that the people in her world were not, and will never be, all that she would have wanted them to be, she will evolve to a place of greater acceptance and inner peace.

Transformation of Reenactment into Accountability

Model 3, engagement in relationship with, is another contemporary perspective, one that focuses on the patient's psychological toxicities, these psychic scars the result of early-on presence of bad in the form of parental trauma and abuse. The essence of the stance such a patient will come to assume in relation to her therapist is best captured by the late Warren Zevon[46] in a rock song entitled "If You Won't Leave Me I'll Find Someone Who Will." This third model of therapeutic action conceives of the therapy as offering the patient a stage upon which to play out, symbolically, her unresolved childhood dramas but ultimately, as a result of negotiating at the intimate edge of authentic engagement with her therapist, to encounter a different response this time. The outcome will indeed be a better one because the therapist will be able to facilitate resolution by bringing to bear her own, more evolved capacity to process and integrate on behalf of a patient who truly does not know how. As the patient is confronted with the sobering reality of what she has been unconsciously reenacting in her relationships, she will evolve to a place of greater accountability for her actions, reactions, and interactions.

Internal Dynamics versus Affective Experience versus Relational Dynamics

To summarize: Over the course of the treatment, the therapist must remain ever attuned to the dysfunctional defenses that the patient has mobilized as a reaction to life stressors that were simply too much to be processed and integrated at the time. So whether, in the moment, the therapist is focused on the patient's internal dynamics (Model 1), the patient's affective experience (Model 2), or the patient's relational dynamics (Model 3), the therapist will alternately challenge the patient's defensive structures (when possible) and support those structures (when necessary).

These optimally stressful psychotherapeutic interventions, which both challenge and support, will therefore be utilized to provide the impetus for temporary disorganization of the dysfunctional status quo and then compensatory reorganization at a higher level of therapeutic understanding and adaptive capacity. Again and again, these strategically formulated interventions (like the grains of sand in the sandpile model of chaos theory) will prompt destabilization in order to trigger restabilization at ever higher levels of orderedness and complexity.

CONCLUSION

The journey from disorder and disease to health and vitality—from illness to wellness—requires the system's infrastructure to be ordered and fluid. In fact, orderedness and fluidity within the MindBodyMatrix are a prerequisite for the achievement of optimal health. As noted earlier, the more ordered the crystalline matrix, the easier will be the flow of regulatory information and vibratory energy throughout its expanse; the more seamless the flow, the better able will the system be to process, integrate, and adapt to the impact of environmental stressors; and the better able the system is to adapt to the impact of environmental challenge, the more resilient will the system be and the more optimal its health. Whether the focus is on mind or body, the goal of any treatment must therefore be to restore the system's intrinsic orderedness and fluidity, that is, its resilience, so that stressful challenges can be mastered and the system evolve to ever higher levels of functionality and complexity.

Again, bad stuff happens. However, it will be how well an individual is able to deal with the impingement (i.e., process and integrate it) that will make of it either a growth-disrupting (sandpile-destabilizing) event or a growth-promoting (sandpile-restabilizing) opportunity.

Whether the primary target is mind or body and the clinical manifestation therefore psychiatric or medical, the critical issue will be the ability of the MindBodyMatrix to handle stress through adaptation. Again, too much stress will overwhelm and prompt defense; too little stress will offer too little opportunity for transformation and growth; but just the right amount of stress—optimal stress—will provide just the right amount of therapeutic leverage needed to induce, after initial disruption, adaptive reconstitution at ever higher levels of synergy, the rhythms of mind and body now synchronized and in harmonic resonance.

Without challenge, there will be no impetus for recovery from chronic illness; without support, there will be no such opportunity.

All of this prompts me to wonder: Is there not a certain beauty in brokenness, a beauty never achieved by things unbroken? If a bone is fractured and then heals, the area of the break will be stronger than the surrounding bone and will not again easily fracture. Are we, too, not stronger at our broken places? And is there not a certain beauty in brokenness, a quiet strength we acquire from having survived adversity and hardship and having mastered the experience of disappointment, heartbreak, and devastation? And, then, when we finally rise above it, don't we rise up in quiet triumph, even if only we notice...

REFERENCES

1. Hemingway, E. 1929. *A Farewell to Arms.* New York: Charles Scribner's Sons.
2. Nietzsche, F. 1899. *The Twilight of the Idols: Or How to Philosophise with a Hammer.* London, England: T. Fisher Unwin.
3. Oschman, J. 2000. *Energy Medicine: The Scientific Basis.* London, England: Churchill Livingstone.
4. Selye, H. 1978. *The Stress of Life.* New York: McGraw-Hill Book Co.
5. Strogatz, S. 1994. *Nonlinear Dynamics and Chaos: With Applications to Physics, Biology, Chemistry, and Engineering.* Cambridge, MA: Perseus Books.
6. Kauffman, S. 1995. *At Home in the Universe: The Search for the Laws of Self-Organization and Complexity.* New York: Oxford University.
7. Buchanan, M. 2000. *Ubiquity: Why Catastrophes Happen.* New York: Three Rivers Press.
8. Krebs, C. 1998. *A Revolutionary Way of Thinking.* Melbourne, Australia: Hill of Content Publishing Co. Pty. Ltd.
9. Stark, M. 2008. Hormesis, adaptation, and the sandpile model. *Crit. Rev. Toxicol.* 38(7):641–644.
10. Stark, M. 2012. The sandpile model: Optimal stress and hormesis. *Dose Response* 10(1):66–74.
11. Stark, M. 2014. Optimal stress, psychological resilience, and the sandpile model. In *Hormesis in Health and Disease*, S. Rattan, E. Le Bourg, eds., pp. 201–224. Boca Raton: CRC Press/Taylor & Francis.
12. van der Kolk, B. 2006. *Traumatic Stress: The Effects of Overwhelming Experience on Mind, Body, and Society.* New York: Guilford Press.
13. Selye, H. 1974. *Stress without Distress.* New York: Harper & Row.
14. Scott, C. 2009. *Optimal Stress.* Hoboken, NJ: Wiley.
15. Bak, P. 1999. *How Nature Works: The Science of Self-Organized Criticality.* Gottingen Germany: Copernicus Publications.
16. Sapolsky, R. M. 1994. *Why Zebras Don't Get Ulcers.* New York: W. H. Freeman and Co.
17. Paracelsus, T. 2004. *The Archidoxes of Magic.* Turner R. (trans). Temecula, CA: Ibis Publishing.
18. Ehrenberg, D. 1992. *The Intimate Edge: Extending the Reach of Psychoanalytic Interaction.* New York: W. W. Norton & Co.
19. Cannon, W. B. 1932. *The Wisdom of the Body.* New York: W. W. Norton & Co.
20. McEwen, B. S. 1998. Stress, adaptation, and disease: Allostasis and allostatic load. *Ann. NY Acad. Sci.* 840:33–44.
21. Bland, J. 1999. *Genetic Nutritioneering.* New York: McGraw-Hill Book Co.
22. McEwen, B. S. 2002. *The End of Stress as We Know It.* Washington, DC: Joseph Henry Press.
23. Calabrese, E. J., L. A. Baldwin. 2003. Hormesis: The dose-response revolution. *Annu. Rev. Pharmacol. Toxicol.* 43:175–197.
24. Mattson, M. P., E. J. Calabrese. 2009. *Hormesis: A Revolution in Biology, Toxicology and Medicine.* New York: Humana Press.
25. Wolfe, T. 2011. *You Can't Go Home Again.* New York: Scribner.
26. Williams, R. 1998. *Biochemical Individuality.* New York: McGraw-Hill Book Co.
27. Gladwell, M. 2002. *The Tipping Point: How Little Things Can Make a Big Difference.* Boston, MA: Back Bay Books.
28. Rea, W. J. 1992. *Chemical Sensitivity.* Vol. 1. Boca Raton, FL: CRC Press/Lewis Publishers.

29. Rea, W. J. 1994. *Chemical Sensitivity: Sources of Total Body Load.* Vol. 2. Boca Raton, FL: CRC Press/Lewis Publishers.

30. Rea, W. J. 1995. *Chemical Sensitivity: Clinical Manifestations of Pollutant Overload.* Vol. 3. Boca Raton, FL: CRC Press/Lewis Publishers.

31. Rea, W. J. 1996. *Chemical Sensitivity: Tools, Diagnosis and Method of Treatment.* Vol. 4. Boca Raton, FL: CRC Press/Lewis Publishers.

32. Rea, W. J., K. Patel. 2010. *Reversibility of Chronic Degenerative Disease and Hypersensitivity: Regulating Mechanisms of Chemical Sensitivity.* Vol. 1. Boca Raton, FL: CRC Press/Taylor & Francis.

33. Schulkin, J. 2012. *Allostasis, Homeostasis, and the Costs of Physiological Adaptation.* Cambridge, England: Cambridge University Press.

34. Pischinger, A. 1991. *Matrix and Matrix Regulation: Basis for a Holistic Theory in Medicine.* Madrid, Spain: Medicina Biologica.

35. Heine, H. 2000. *Homotoxicology and Ground Regulation System.* Baden-Baden, Germany: Aurelia-Verlag.

36. Lipton, B. 2007. *The Biology of Belief: Unleashing the Power of Consciousness, Matter & Miracles.* Carlsbad, CA: Hay House.

37. McTaggart, L. 2008. *The Field: The Quest for the Secret Force of the Universe.* New York: Harper Perennial.

38. Sheldrake, R. 2009. *Morphic Resonance: The Nature of Formative Causation.* South Paris, ME: Park Street Press.

39. Becker, R., G. Selden. 1998. *The Body Electric: Electromagnetism and the Foundation of Life.* New York: William Morrow and Company/HarperCollins.

40. Ho, M. W. 2008. *The Rainbow and the Worm: The Physics of Organisms.* Singapore, China: World Scientific Publishing Company.

41. Hon, E. H., S. T. Lee. 1965. Electronic evaluations of the fetal heart rate patterns preceding fetal death, further considerations. *Am. J. Obstet. Gynae.* 87:814–826.

42. Meadows, D. 2008. *Thinking in Systems: A Primer.* White River Junction, VT: Chelsea Green Publishing.

43. Richet, C. 1900. *Functions of Defense: Dictionnaire de Physiologie* 4, Paris, FR: F. Alcan.

44. Neumayer, P. 2014. *Hahnemann's Legacy.* Colorado Springs, CO: CreateSpace Independent Publishing Platform.

45. Stark, M. 1999. *Modes of Therapeutic Action: Enhancement of Knowledge, Provision of Experience, and Engagement in Relationship.* Northvale, NJ: Jason Aronson.

46. Zevon, W. 1996. *I'll Sleep When I'm Dead.* Burbank, CA: Elektra Records.

47. Stark, M. 1994. *Working with Resistance.* Northvale, NJ: Jason Aronson.

48. Stark, M. 1994. *A Primer on Working with Resistance.* Northvale, NJ: Jason Aronson.

49. Logue, C. 2004. Come to the Edge. *New Numbers.* London: Cape. pp. 65–66.

50. Bernard, C. 1957. *An Introduction to the Study of Experimental Medicine* (originally published in 1865); first English translation by Henry Copley Greene, published by Macmillan & Co., Ltd., 1927.

51. Braden, G. 2007. *The Divine Matrix: Bridging Time, Space, Miracles, and Belief.* California: Hay House.

Index

A